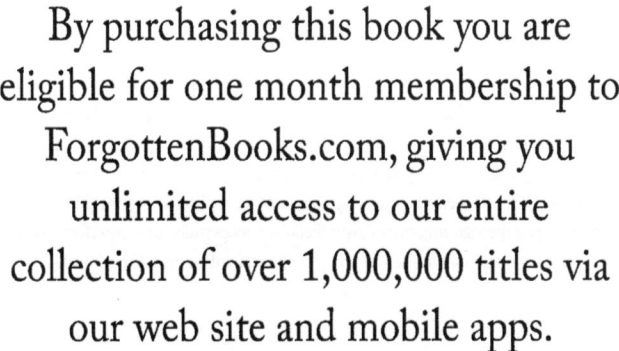

ISBN 978-0-265-53066-5
PIBN 10861500

CONDENSED

Materia Medica

BY

C. HERING,

REVISED, ENLARGED AND IMPROVED

BY

E. A. FARRINGTON, M. D.,

PROFESSOR OF MATERIA MEDICA.

FOURTH EDITION.

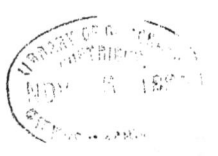
PHILADELPHIA:
BOERICKE & TAFEL.
1894.

T. B. & H. B. COCHRAN, PRINTERS.

LANCASTER, PA.

TO

DR. CHAS. G. RAUE,

HIS FORMER PUPIL AND ASSISTANT, FOR SEVEN YEARS HIS COLLEAGUE AS

PROFESSOR IN THE HAHNEMANN COLLEGE, OF PHILADELPHIA,

AND FOREVER HIS TRUE FRIEND, THIS BOOK

IS DEDICATED.

CONSTANTINE HERING.

PREFACE.

In placing this work before the profession, the author wishes it to be understood that it is not with any desire to have such condensed work supersede the study and use of the more complete Materia Medica; nor is it on account of any supposed incorrectness or unreliability of the original works of Hahnemann, for these, after nearly three-fourths of a century of daily searching scrutiny, must be accepted as bearing the imprint of being wrought by a master mind—almost intuitive perception having guided in the work.

The real object in preparing this work has been to give in a condensed form, to the student of Homœopathy, such absolutely necessary material as would enable him, in a comparatively short time, to gain knowledge of such important leading symptoms and conditions as are characteristic of each remedy—knowledge which is imperatively necessary for everyday practice. The large and more complete works present by their size, if by nought else, great obstacles to the rapid acquirement of a practical knowledge of the genius of each remedy. In order to overcome this, efforts have been made in the past to condense the material of the larger works. Clinical experience only can verify symptoms obtained through provings; this we are gaining daily, and profiting thereby. Year by year we have been enabled, through such experience, to separate wheat from tares. We have now garnered at least a fair percentage of good wheat—and the harvest season is not yet over.

The material for this work has been culled from the manuscript and other material collected for a much larger work on verified and important symptoms, viz., "Guiding Symptoms," now in process of publication, on which many years of careful research have been bestowed.

Not all of our remedies are herein given, inasmuch as this work is intended for a text-book, a manual, not a complete Materia Medica; and though it was desirable to condense, it was also necessary to give the really useful symptoms sufficiently complete to make up the picture of each remedy so as to be practically useful, thus making it impossible to give more remedies, without so increasing the bulk as to render the book unsuited to its purpose.

Regarding the arrangement of symptoms, it will be found to correspond to that used in the "Analytical Therapeutics;" for full explanation, see introduction to the same.

The symptoms of each remedy are divided into forty-eight chapters—thus, [1] Mind and disposition; this contains all mental states. [2] Sensorium, embracing over-sensitiveness and irritability of brain and senses; vertigo; dullness, etc. [3] Inner head, pains, etc. [4] Outer head, symptoms of bones, periosteum, skin, and hair; also motions and positions of head. [5] Sight and eyes. [6] Hearing and ears. [7] Smell and nose. [8] Face, including expression, etc. [9] Lower jaw, outer mouth, chin, and submaxillary glands. [10] Teeth and gums. [11] Taste, speech and tongue. [12] Inner mouth. [13] Palate and throat. [14] Desire for food and drink. [15] Effects ot eating and drinking. [16] Gastric symptoms. [17] Epigastric region. [18] Hypochondria. [19] Abdomen. [20] Rectum and anus, including emission of flatus, stools, hemorrhoids. [21] Urinary organs and urine. [22] Male functions and organs. [23] Female organs. [24] Pregnancy and parturition, including mammæ; also infants at the breast. [25] Voice and larynx. [26] Respiration. [27] Cough. [28] Inner chèst and lungs. [29] Heart and circulation. [30] Outer chest. [31] Neck and back. [32] Upper limbs. [33] Lower limbs. [34] All the limbs. [35] Rest, motion and position; modalities will be indexed so as to refer to chapter number. [36] Nerves; this chapter embraces symptoms pertaining more especially to the nervous system; trembling, spasms, weakness, lameness or paralysis. [37] Sleep and dreams. [38] Times of day, indexed. [39] Temperature and weather, indexed. [40] Chill, fever and sweat. [41] Attacks and periodicity, indexed. [42] Sides and relation to space, indexed. [43] Sensations; predominating feelings. [44] Tissues—in a work of this character but little need be said on this subject. In the "Guiding Symptoms" more prominence is given thereto. [45] Passive motion, contact, injuries, etc. [46] Skin. [47] Stages of life, constitution, diathesis, dyscrasia. [48] Relationship with other drugs. For convenience and to save space, some ot these headings have been shortened throughout the work.

The ❙ corresponding to the third degree of distinction in Bœnninghausen's Repertory, has here more significance than in the "Guiding Symptoms;" there it stands before symptoms verified by cures, here it marks in most instances characteristic symptoms.

The Greek letter θ (theta), is occasionally used (not as extensively as in the Guiding Symptoms) before the pathological or physiological state to which the symptom refers.

Every care has been bestowed that this might prove a reliable manual for the use of students, particularly the profession.

The thanks of the author are due to Dr. C. G. Raue, for his careful and systematic arrangement of the mind symptoms; to Drs. Korndœrfer and Farrington, for their assistance on the first edition, and to Drs. Knerr and Mohr, for assistance on the second; also to those friends who have kindly sent in corrections and additions.

CONSTANTINE HERING.

PREFACE TO THIRD EDITION.

IN the preparation of this, the third edition of HERING'S CONDENSED MATERIA MEDICA, **additions** have been made and a few typographical errors corrected, but in justice to the lamented author, no alterations have been made in the substance of the text as he left it.

More than twenty new remedies, arranged after the plan of the book, are given in full; and over forty partially proved drugs, with brief but distinctive indications, are added to the sections on "Relationship." These latter are arranged and classified in alphabetical order on page xviii.

Besides all this, about six hundred choice and well-attested symptoms have been incorporated in their proper places in the text. All the late works have been drawn upon for the new material, and even private sources have been unsparingly taxed; but still, great caution has been used in making selections. The plans and purposes of the book demand clinical as well as pathogenetic symptoms. But of the former sort only those have been employed which agree with the provings, and which show every evidence of genuineness. Such discrimination demands the exercise of one's best judgment, and the expenditure of much time. But it is believed the benefits to be derived far outweigh the trouble. The book is now offered to the profession and to students, not as a rival of other works, but as a rich treasury full of information common to Homœopathic literature, and also of gleanings from the vast collection which Dr. Hering made during a busy half-century of medical study and labor.

E. A. FARRINGTON.

Philadelphia, 1738 Green Street.
October 1st, 1884.

Publishers' Preface to Fourth Edition.

The third edition of HERING'S CONDENSED MATERIA MEDICA being exhausted the question of a fourth edition confronted the publishers. After due consideration it was determined to let the work of those masters in Homœopathy, Hering and Farrington, remain as they left it. Homœopathy is not a shifting changing science. This book is a true exponent of Homœopathy, and while it might be enlarged by the addition of new remedies it could not be improved upon in its sphere—A CONDENSED MATERIA MEDICA. So the old work is again brought out, unchanged. It is a book culled by Hering from the manuscript of his ten volume Guiding Symptoms, and it contains the cream of that large work. As Hering says: "Clinical experience only can verify symptoms obtained through provings;" and further: "We have now garnered at least a fair percentage of good wheat." That "good wheat" is to be found in this volume—a volume that, perhaps, contains fewer unverified symptoms than any other published; indeed it has been said that *every* symptom in this book has been verified at the bedside. Be that as it may, the HERING'S CONDENSED MATERIA MEDICA is undoubtedly one of the most helpful books to the physician ever published.

THE PUBLISHERS.

LIST OF REMEDIES.

(xiii)

LIST OF REMEDIES.

Name.	Abbreviation.
Calcarea ostrearum.	Calc. ostr.
Calcarea phosphorica.	Calc. phosph.
Camphora.	Camphor.
Cannabis Indica.	Cann. Ind.
Cannabis sativa.	Cann. sat.
Cantharis.	Canthar.
Capsicum.	Capsic.
Carbo animalis.	Carb. an.
Carbo vegetabilis.	Carb. veg.
Carduus marianus.	Card. mar.
Caulophyllum.	Cauloph.
Causticum.	Caustic.
Cepa.	Cepa.
Chamomilla.	Chamom.
Chelidonium.	Chelid.
Chininum sulfuricum.	Chin. sulf.
Cicuta virosa.	Cicut.
Cimicifuga (Actæa racemosa).	
Cimex lectularius.	Cimex.
Cina.	Cina.
Cinchona officinalis.	Cinch. off.
Cistus Canadensis.	Cist. Can.
Clematis erecta.	Clemat.
Cocculus.	Coccul.
Coffea.	Coffea.
Colchicum autumnale.	Colchic.
Collinsonia.	Collin.
Colocynthis.	Coloc.
Conium maculatum.	Conium.
Crocus sativus.	Crocus.
Crotalus.	Crotal.
Croton tiglium.	Crot. tigl.
Cuprum metallicum.	Cuprum.
Cyclamen Europæum.	Cyclam.
Digitalis purpurea.	Digit.
Dioscorea villosa.	Diosc. vill.
Dolichos.	Dolich.
Drosera rotundifolia	Droser.
Dulcamara.	Dulcam.
Elaterium.	Elat.
Erigeron.	Eriger.
Eupatorium perfoliatum.	Eupat. perf.
Eupatorium purpureum.	Eupat. purp.
Euphrasia.	Euphras.
Ferrum.	Ferrum.
Ferrum iodatum.	Ferr. iod.
Fluoricum acidum.	Fluor. ac.
Gambogia.	Gambog.
Gelsemium.	Gelsem.
Glonoinum.	Glonoin.
Gnaphalium.	Gnaphal.
Graphites.	Graphit.

LIST OF REMEDIES.

Name.	Abbreviation.
Nitric. acid.	Nitr. ac.
Nitrum.	Nitrum.
Nux moschata.	Nux mosch.
Nux vomica.	Nux vom.
Oleander.	Oleand.
Opium.	Opium.
Oxalicum acidum.	Ox. ac.
Pareira brava.	Pareir.
Paris quadrifolia.	Paris.
Petroleum.	Petrol.
Phosphorus.	Phosphor.
Phosphoricum acidum.	Phosph. ac.
Phytolacca decandra.	Phytol. dec.
Platina.	Platin.
Plumbum.	Plumbum.
Podophyllum peltatum.	Podoph.
Psorinum.	Psorin.
Ptelea trifoliata.	Ptel. trif.
Pulsatilla.	Pulsat.
Ranunculus bulbosus.	Ran. bulb.
Ranunculus sceleratus.	Ran. scel.
Rheum.	Rheum.
Rhododendron.	Rhodod.
Rhus toxicodendron.	Rhus tox.
Rumex crispus.	Rumex.
Rnta graveolens.	Ruta.
Sabadilla.	Sabad.
Sabina.	Sabin.
Sambucus nigra.	Sambuc.
Sanguinaria canadensis.	Sanguin.
Sarsaparilla.	Sarsap.
Secale cornutum.	Sec. corn.
Selenium.	Selen.
Senega.	Seneg.
Sepia.	Sepia.
Silicea.	Silic.
Spigelia.	Spigel.
Spongia tosta.	Spongia.
Squilla.	Squilla.
Stannum.	Stannum.
Staphisagria.	Staphis.
Sticta pulmonaria.	Sticta pulm.
Stramonium.	Stramon.
Sulphur.	Sulphur.
Sulphuricum acidum.	Sulph. ac.
Tabacum.	Tabac.
Taraxacum.	Tarax.
Tellurium.	Tellur.
Terebinthina.	Terebinth.
Theridion.	Therid.
Thuja.	Thuja.
Trillium pendulum.	Trill. pend.

ADDITIONS OF SINGLE SYMPTOMS.

Acalypha indica	to Relationship under			Phosphor.
Actæa spicata	"	"	"	Act. rac.
Allium sativum	"	"	"	Cepa.
Ant. sulph. aurat.	"		"	Ant. crud.
Arctium lappa	"	"	"	Bryon.
Argent. oxidat.	"	"	"	Arg. nitr.
Bellis perennis	"		"	Arnic.
Calc. hypophos.	"	"	"	Calc. phosph.
Calc. iod.			'	Apis.
Calendula			'	"
Cereus serp.			'	Cicut.
Chin. mur.	"		"	Cinchon.
Cinnabaris			"	Kali bich.
"	"	"	"	Thuja.
Cinnamomum	"	"	"	Secale.
Clem. vitalba	"		"	Clemat.
Coccus cacti			"	Thuja.
Condurango	"	"	'	Arum.
Cupr. ars.	"	"	"	Cuprum.
Gettysburg			'	Silic.
Guarea		"	"	Apis.
Helianthus			"	Chin. sulf.
Jaborandi		"	"	Agar.
Jatropha		"	"	Ver. alb.
Kali sulph.	"	"	"	Kali carb.
Lactic. acid.	"		"	Laches.
Merc. præc. rub.	"		"	Mercur.
Myosotis	'		"	Stannum.
Myrtus com.			"	Sulphur.
Nitr. spir. dulc.	"	"	"	Phosph. ac.
Physostigma	"	"	"	Agar.
Plantago major	"		"	Mercur.
Ricinus com.			"	Ver. alb.
Santonin.		"	"	Cina.
Senecio	"		"	Millef.
Silphium			"	Stannum.
Soda sulphite	"	"	"	Natr. carb.
Tarentula Cubensis	"		"	Cinch. off.
"	"	"	"	Laches.
Verbascum			"	Conium.
"		'	"	Platina.
Zincum picricum	"		:	Zinc.
" sulph.	"	"		"

(xviii)

CONDENSED

MATERIA MEDICA.

· ABIES CANADENSIS.

Hemlock Spruce. Gatchell. *Compositæ.*

² **Sensorium.** Tipsy feeling, swimming in the head, faint as if the top of the head were congested.

¹⁷ **Stomach.** ❙ Gnawing, hungry, faint feeling at the epigastrium; craves meat, pickles and other coarse foods.

ABIES NIGRA.

Black Spruce. Gatchell. *Compositæ.*

¹ **Mind.** ❙ Low-spirited.

⁶ **Ear.** Pain in the left external meatus.

¹³ **Throat.** Sensation of something sticking in the œsophagus towards its lower end.

¹⁴ **Appetite.** ❙ Lost mornings, but there is craving noon and night.

¹⁷ **Stomach.** ❙ Continual distressing sensation about the stomach as if everything was knotted up; worse whenever debilitated.

❙ Sensation as of an undigested hard-boiled egg in the stomach.

❙ Pain after a hearty meal.

²⁶ **Breathing.** Dyspnœa.

²⁹ **Heart.** Heavy, slow beating of the heart, sharp, cutting pains.

⁴⁸ **Relationship.** Compare *Nux vom.*, *Lactic acid* (latter feels as if all food lodges under upper end of sternum).

ABROTANUM.

Southern Wood. DEVENNTER. GATCHELL. CUSHING. *Compositæ.*

¹ **Mind.** Feeble, dull.
  Indolence, aversion to bodily motion.
  Good-humored or gloomy.
  ❙ Anxious, depressed. *θ* Gastralgia.
  ❙ Child cross, depressed, very peevish. *θ* Marasmus.
³ **Inner Head.** Left brain feels weaker.
  As if squeezed on the temporal regions.
⁴ **Outer Head.** Could not hold head up.
  Scalp sore; itching.
  Distended veins on forehead. See 29.
⁵ **Eyes.** ❙ Blue rings around the eyes; eyes looking dull.
  θ Chlorosis.
  Inflamed eyes.
⁶ **Ears.** Humming as of bees; wind rushes out of right ear.
⁷ **Nose.** Inner nose dry.
  ❙ Nosebleed with boys.
⁸ **Face.** ❙ Face wrinkled as if old. *θ* Marasmus.
  ❙ Comedones with emaciation.
  Face feels cold.
¹⁰ **Teeth.** Drawing, tearing in carious teeth.
¹¹ **Tongue, etc.** Acid taste.
  ❙ Slimy taste. *θ* Gastralgia.
¹² **Mouth.** Dry and sore; saliva increased.
¹⁴ **Desires. Aversions.** Gnawing hunger; ❙ ravenous appetite, all the while emaciating.
  Craves bread boiled in milk.
¹⁷ **Stomach.** Burning as from acidity.
  ❙ As if stomach were hanging or swimming in water, with
    coldness. *θ* Gastralgia.
  ❙ Pains cutting, gnawing, burning, < at night. *θ* Gastralgia.
¹⁹ **Abdomen.** Weak sinking in bowels.
  ❙ Distended abdomen. *θ* Hemorrhoidal colic. *θ* Chlorosis.
    θ Marasmus.
  ❙ Hard lumps in different parts of abdomen. *θ* Marasmus.
²⁰ **Stool, etc.** ❙ Food passes undigested. *θ* Marasmus.
  ❙ After suddenly checked diarrhœa. *θ* Marasmus.
  ❙ Alternate diarrhœa and constipation. *θ* Marasmus.
  ❙ Constipation. *θ* Gastralgia.
  ❙ Protruding piles, with burning, from touch or when
    passing.
  Piles worse when rheumatism abated.
  With inclination to stool, only blood passes.

²¹ **Urine.** Bladder full, urging; scanty urine.
²² **Male Sexual Organs.** ❙ Hydrocele of children.
²³ **Female Sexual Organs.** Darting in l. ovary; twitching
   in both ovaries.
   Dysmenorrhœa or suppressed menses.
²⁴ **Pregnancy.** ❙ Blood and moisture oozing from navel of the
   newborn.
²⁵ **Larynx.** Sudden hoarseness or weak voice.
²⁶ **Breathing.** Breathing impeded, difficult.
²⁷ **Cough.** Troublesome cough. *θ* Rheumatism.
²⁸ **Lungs.** Cold air causes raw feeling.
   ❙ Pressing sensation remains in affected side, impeding
   free breathing. *θ* Pleurisy.
²⁹ **Heart. Pulse.** ❙ Pain across chest, 'sharp and severe in
   region of heart. *θ* Rheumatism.
   ❙ Pulse weak and small. *θ* Chlorosis.
   ❙ Ebulitions with general heat, and distended veins on
   forehead and hands. *θ* Hemorrhoidal colic.
³⁰ **Outer Chest.** Drawing in muscles, worse from motion.
³¹ **Back.** Back weak with ovarian pains.
   ❙ Pains in sacrum. *θ* Hemorrhoidal colic.
   Sudden spinal inflammation; sudden aching pains in the
   back, better by motion, 36.
³² **Upper Limbs.** Aching from shoulder-joints to elbows.
   Aching in fingers, first r. then l. side.
   Pricking and coldness of finger tips. ˙
   Numb sensation in fingers.
   Distended veins, 29.
   ❙ Legs emaciated. *θ* Marasmus.
³³ **Lower Limbs.** Stitching, tearing, itching in old footsores.
   Drawing in ankle-joint.
   Dead cold feet.
³⁴ **Limbs in General.** ❙ Inability to move. *θ* Rheumatism.
   Back and limbs sore and lame, worse mornings awaking.
³⁵ **Position, etc.** Lies prone.
   Motion, see 28, 30, 31.
³⁶ **Nerves.** Weak, sickly feeling, when excited trembling.
   ❙ Lame and sore. *θ* Rheumatism.
   ❙ Weak and prostrated after influenza, see 4.
   Numbness, partial paralysis; spine affected.
³⁷ **Sleep.** ❙ Sleepless, restless. *θ* Hemorrhoidal colic.
   Frightful dreams and trembling on awaking.
³⁸ **Time.** Night, see 17. Morning, 31.
³⁹ **Temperature and Weather.** Cold air, see 28.
   ❙ Chilblains itch; frostbitten limbs.
⁴⁰ **Chill. Fever. Sweat.** Creeping chill in brain with prickling.
   ❙ High fever. *θ* Rheumatism.
   ❙ Hectic fever with chillness after influenza, very weaken-
   ing. *θ* Marasmus.

[41] **Attacks.** Sudden hoarseness, see 25.
[42] **Sides.** Left, see 3, 23.
  Right to left, 32.
[43] **Sensations.** Aching; coldness; deadness; pricking; sting-
  ing; itching; gnawing; drawing; darting; tearing;
  cutting; sticking; scraping; pressing; soreness; rawness;
  dryness; burning; hanging or swimming.
[44] **Tissues.** ▮ Gout in wrists and ankles.
  ▮ After suppressed gastralgia.
  Joints stiff with pricking—sore, lame, joints, < awaking.
  Contraction of limbs from cramps or colic.
  ▮ Inflammatory rheumatism before swelling.
  ▮ Chlorosis.
  ▮ Marasmus of children.
  Emaciations, see 8, 14.
[45] **Contact, Injuries, etc.** Worse from touch, 20.
[46] **Skin.** ▮ Skin flabby, hangs loose. *θ* Marasmus.
  ▮ Furunculus; after *Hepar sulph.*
[47] **Stages and States.** Children: emaciation.
  Boys: *θ* Nosebleed. *θ* Hydrocele.
  Newborn, 34.
[48] **Relationship.** After *Acon.* and *Bryon.*, pleurisy, see 28.
  After *Hepar*, see 46.
  Concordances: *Nux vom.*, *Agar.*

ABSINTHIUM.

Wormwood.   GATCHELL.   *Compositæ.*

[1] **Mind.** Forgets what happened before epileptic spasms; t.
  Brutal, insane; t.
  Terrifying hallucinations.
  Stupor alternating with dangerous violence.
[2] **Sensorium.** Drunken.
  Vertigo on rising; momentary unconsciousness. *θ* Epi-
  leptics.
  Insensible with the convulsions.
[3] **Inner Head.** Congestion of brain and spinal marrow.
[4] **Outer Head.** Wants to lie with head low.
  : Baldness and tinea.
[5] **Eyes.** Sight dim.
  Pain in balls.
  Eyes red, suffused with tears.
  Lids swollen, heavy, itch.
[6] **Ears.** ▮ Running from ears. *θ* After headache.

[8] **Face.** Foolish look.

Makes grimaces in epilepsy.

Rush of blood to face.

[9] **Lower Face.** Jaws firmly fixed.

Foams at the mouth in epilepsy.

[11] **Tongue, etc.** Bites his tongue in epilepsy; tongue thick, protruding, can scarcely talk.

Tongue trembling; seems paralyzed.

[13] **Throat.** Throat as if scalded; inflamed.

[15] **Eating.** Food lies heavy; as if not much would be assimilated.

[16] **Nausea and Vomiting.** Belching; nausea' and vomiting in the morning.

Nausea apparently in the region of gall-bladder.

[17] **Stomach.** Feels cold and oppressed.

[18] **Hypochondria.** Liver feels as if swollen, see 40.

Gall-bladder, see 16.

Pain in spleen, feels as if swollen.

[19] **Abdomen.** Bloated around waist and in abdomen.

Bloated with flatus.

[20] **Stool, etc.** Constipation and hemorrhoids.

Destroys worms.

[21] **Urine.** Constant desire to urinate.

Urine deep orange, of a strong smell, like horse's urine.

[22] **Male Sexual Organs.** Seminal emissions with relaxed parts.

[23] **Female Sexual Organs.** Darting pain in r. ovary.

Pains in uterus.

Promotes the menses.

ı Chlorosis.

[27] **Cough.** Cough with liver complaint.

[29] **Heart. Pulse.** Tremor of heart, felt toward the back.

Heart thumps, can be heard in scapular region.

[31] **Back.** Pain in sacrum.

[32] **Upper Limbs.** Pain in shoulders.

Trembling of limbs.

[33] **Lower Limbs.** ı Horses kick with hind legs towards the belly. θ Ascarides.

[34] **Limbs in General.** Limbs thrown about in epilepsy.

Pain in limbs; they swell.

[35] **Position, etc.** Rising, see 2.

Lying low, see 4.

Bends backwards in spasms.

[36] **Nerves.** Epilepsy; before the attack, trembling; during, loss of consciousness, he falls, see 8, 9, 11, 34; after, obtuse, dazed, weak, even general paralysis.

ı Epileptic attacks occurring in rapid succession.

Excited opisthotonos, grinding teeth. followed by stupor.

[37] **Sleep.** Night restless; disturbing dreams.

[38] **Time.** Morning, 16 ; night, 37.

[40] **Chill. Fever. Sweat.** Chill, heat, (with sleep) then sweat ; thirst in all stages.

Fevers in autumn, with swollen liver and spleen.

[41] **Attacks.** Attacks antepone.

[42] **Sides.** Right, 23.

[44] **Tissues.** Hyperæmia of brain, medulla, spine.

Ecchymosis in stomach, in endocardium and pericardium.

❙ Paralysis of inner organs.

[45] **Contact, Injuries, etc.** Bruises and inflammation following‚

[46] **Skin.** Jaundiced.

[47] **Stages and States.** Young people.

[48] **Relationship.** Collaterals: *Artem. vulg.*, *Abrot.*

Concordances: Alcohol; *Bellad.*, *Chamom.*, *Hyos.*, *Stramon.*

Lasting effects of its abuse much worse than those from spirituous liquors, opium or tobacco.

ACETICUM ACIDUM.

Vinegar.   C. HERING. $C_4 H_3 O_3.$

[1] **Mind.** Alternate stupor and delirium.

Violent delirium, with distention of belly and obstinate constipation.

Very dull and low spirited.

Anxiety ; grieves about his sickness and his children.

Extreme irritability of temper. θ With abdominal complaints.

[2] **Sensorium.** Vertigo, with feebleness and fainting.

Appears as if drunken, with heavy head.

[3] **Inner Head.** Headache from abuse of tobacco, opium, coffee or alcohol.

[4] **Outer Head.** Red patches on scalp, crusts between the hair.

Hair bristles.

[5] **Eyes.** Conjunctiva inflamed, accompanied by sour stomach.

False membrane, dense, yellow, white, tough, closely adherent; 48.

Flow of tears.

[7] **Nose.** Nosebleed.

Liable to freqnent catarrhal attacks.

[8] **Face.** Anxious, wild expression of countenance.

❙ Left cheek very red, with the fever. θ Croup.

Pale, waxen, emaciated.

[9] **Lower Face.** Lips become of a deep purple tint.

In upper part of joint of left jaw, aching ; increases on pressure and with motion.

¹⁰ **Teeth.** Teeth feel dull.
¹¹ **Tongue, etc.** Pain across root, impedes speech and moving jaw; scarcely able to walk.

Glands under tongue and on lower jaw swollen; sore to touch.
¹² **Inner Mouth.** Foul breath.
¹³ **Throat.** ❙ Children swallow with some difficulty, even a teaspoonful of water. θ Croup.

Difficult swallowing, has to eat very slowly.

Inflamed sore throat, ulcerated.

Indications of a white film, low down in fauces.
¹⁵ **Drinking.** ❙ No thirst, with fever. θ Croup.

❙ Great thirst. θ Dropsy, Diabetes, 21.
¹⁶ **Nausea and Vomiting.** Hot eructations, heat in stomach.

Nausea and sweat; retching or anxiety.

❙ Vomiting after every meal, with great thirst. θ Cancer.
¹⁷ **Stomach.** Contents of stomach feel as if in a ferment.

❙ Violent burning pain in stomach and in chest, followed by coldness of skin and cold sweat on forehead; burning worse lying on back.
¹⁹ **Abdomen.** Bellyache, with rumbling in bowels, diarrhœa and violent delirium; irritable. See 1.

❙ Ascites. See dropsy.
²⁰ **Stool, etc.** ❙ Diarrhœa liquid or undigested, with swelling of legs and feet. θ Phthisis.

❙ Diarrhœa in the later stages of abdominal typhus.

Costiveness with tympanitis and stupor.

Profuse hemorrhoidal bleeding.

Hemorrhage from bowels. θ After checked metrorrhagia.
²¹ **Urine.** ❙ Passes large quantities of pale urine. θ Diabetes mellitus, 21.
²² **Male Sexual Organs.** Very weakening, nightly emissions.
²⁴ **Pregnancy.** During pregnancy, sour belching and vomiting, with profuse water-brash and salivation, day and night.

After labor, hemorrhages (outward application of vinegar). Also when cold, pale, with difficult breathing. See 48.

Breasts greatly and painfully distended with milk. θ Mammary abscesses threatening.

Milk impoverished, bluish, transparent, of strong, sour taste and odor; deficient in caseine and butter.

Sucklings droop, lose flesh, get marasmus.
²⁵ **Larynx.** Hoarseness, with laryngeal irritation.

Lining membrane of larynx and windpipe covered with fibrinous exudation.

❙ Croup, especially when the face is bright red. (Diluted in water, ten drops in a tumbler of water with some sugar, a teaspoonful every hour or two.)

[26] **Breathing.** Difficult breathing, from laryngeal obstructions.

Hissing, rattling in throat.

Hurried and ·laborious.breathing.

[27] **Cough.** Croup-like sound; a hollow sound with each inhalation.

[29] **Heart and Pulse.** Pulse: 96 and full; full and irregular; accelerated and small, contracted; very weak and small.

[31] **Back.** Must lie on the abdomen to relieve pain in the spine. θ Myelitus.

[32] **Upper Limbs.** Sensation of lameness in wrists and hands.

[33] **Lower Limbs.** Weak and weary.

Lessened sensibility.

Œdematous swelling, with diarrhœa.

[35] **Position, etc.** Motion, 9, 11. Lying, 17, 31.

[37] **Sleep.** Sleeplessness, with other sufferings.

Sleep much broken, without any known cause.

[38] **Time.** Diarrhœa more in the morning.

Day and night: 24. Night: 22, 40.

[40] **Chill. Fever. Sweat.** Skin cold.

Flushes of heat more in outer parts, increasing the sweat.

Febrile heat, with a dry skin; in bilious, putrid and typhoid fevers. Typhus with delirium.

Profuse sweating; night-sweats.

Hectic fevers, with cough, dyspnœa, night-sweats, diarrhœa, œdema and emaciation.

[42] **Sides.** Left cheek red; maxilliary joint aches.

[43] **Sensations.** Burning on inner and outer parts.

Diminished sensibility on the whole surface of body.

[44] **Tissues.** Hemorrhages from nose, lungs, stomach, bowels, uterus.

Wasting away, great emaciation.

❙ General anasarca and dropsical affections of abdomen and legs, with great thirst.

[45] **Contact, Injuries, etc.** Touch: 11. Pressure: 9.

After bruising and spraining, if dry heat follows.

Burns and scalds.

Stings of wasps.

After the bite of a mad cat, lacerated wound, swollen upper and lower leg (externally and internally).

[46] **Skin.** Diseased cuticle separates in flakes.

❙ Skin pale and waxen. θ Dropsy.

Broad, flat, condylomata, dry or moist.

Nævi, warts, corns.

[48] **Relationship.** Antidotes to *Acet. ac.:* Large doses are best counteracted by *Magnesia* or *Calcar.;* fluid magnesia or lime-water, a teaspoonful in a cup of water taken in sips. Higher preparations: for the depressing, agoniz-

ing feeling : *Tabac.;* if insufficient : *Acon.;* for the gastric, pulmonary and febrile symptons : *Natr. mur.*, high ; may be followed by *Sepia.* It follows *China* in hemorrhage, 24. Compare with *Kali bich.* (but membrane on eye in latter more easily detached).

Acet. ac. is an antidote to all anæsthetic vapors; further to *Acon.*, *Asar.*, *Coffea*, *Euphorb.*, *Hepar*, *Ignat.*, *Opium*, *Stramon.*, *Tabac.* and *Alcohol.*

The sick have aversion to it in poisonings with *Agar. emet.*

Symptoms of *Bellad.*, *Mercur.* and *Laches.* are aggravated by it.

It follows well after *Cinchon.* in hemorrhages.

Disagrees when given after *Borax*, *Caustic.*, *Nux. vom.*, *Ran. bulb.*, *Sarsap.*

ACONITUM.

Monkshood.   HAHNEMANN.   *Ranunculaceæ.*

[1] **Mind.** Absent-mindedness; weakness of memory; cannot remember dates.

Clairvoyance, perception of distant things.

Ecstasy; fancies; delirium, especially at night.

Changing mood, now full of mirth, now disposed to tears.

❚ Afraid of a crowd or of crossing busy streets.

Fear of ghosts; of loss of reason; apprehensive of the future.

Fear of approaching death; predicts the day.

Anxiety inconsolable, piteous wailing; reproaches others for mere trifles; peevish, impatient; pusillanimity.

❚ Anxiety, restless, agonized tossing about.

Oversensitive; cannot bear light or noise; buzzing in the ears; will not be touched or uncovered.

Mood peevish, irritable, malicious; or sad, desponding.

After a fright, afraid in the dark. After fright with vexation or anger, heat, congestions, threatened abortion; ailments from fright following later.

Ailments from anger; from chagrin; child has spells of rage.

Imagines some part of the body is deformed, thinks from the stomach.

[2] **Sensorium.** Vertigo from congestion, as in the sun, after dry, cold winds; from anger, fright; from suddenly suppressed catamenia by emotions or cold.

Vertigo from a fall or contusion; face pale or red, but no stupor.

Vertigo on raising the head, especially after lying down in a warm room; nausea, vanishing of sight, loss of consciousness, nosebleed; or reeling as if drunk.

Fainting on rising from a recumbent position, with paleness of the face or congestion to the head.

³ **Inner Head.** Sunstroke, especially from sleeping in the rays of the sun.

Brain affections of children, with violent pain in head and oversensitiveness of eyes; or lying stupefied, with vomiting, bowels constipated.

Congestion, anxiety, with heat and redness of the face, or pale face; carotids pulsate strongly; pulse full, strong, or small and quick; worse toward evening. Ebullition, with anxiety.

Fulness and heaviness in the forehead, as if the whole brain would start out through the eyes.

Beating and shooting in the head.

Crampy sensation over the root of the nose, feels as if he would lose his senses; suppressed catarrh.

Headache, as if the brain were moved or raised; worse during motion, drinking, talking or sunlight.

Burning, as if the brain were moved by boiling water.

On going into a warm room, forehead feels as if compressed.

Pressure in forehead, temples and top of head.

Headache, with increased secretion of urine.

⁴ **Outer Head.** Sensation in the vertex as if pulled by the hair.

Sensation of crackling, as from bending tinsel, in temples, forehead and nose; worse toward evening, from motion; better from sitting.

Formication of the scalp, relieved by heat.

Cold sweat on the forehead.

⁵ **Eyes.** Aversion to light, particularly sunlight; light dazzles the eyes.

Optical illusions in dark colors or black.

Flickerings make him anxious, fears he might touch people passing by.

Eyes protuding, staring, distorted. θ Apoplexy. θ Asthma. θ Tetanus.

Pupils contracted, then dilated.

Eyes red, inflamed, vessels deep red, burning, pressive-shooting pains, especially on moving the balls; no discharge; conjunctivitis from exposure to cold, dry winds.

Violent pains, intense congestion; ophthalmia from suppressed gonorrhœa.

Upper half of the eyeball sore when moved.

Profuse lachrymation, with intense pain.

Conjunctivitis from cinders or other foreign bodies.

Lids hard, red, swollen, feel tense; hot, dry, burning and
sensitiveness to air; cold water relieves the dry heat.

⁶ **Ears.**   Extreme sensitiveness to noises; music unbearable,
goes through every limb; makes her sad.

Roaring in the ears.

Tearing in the left ear.

External ear hot, swollen, red, painfully sensitive.

⁷ **Nose.**   Smell acutely sensitive.

Nosebleed, bright red.

Coryza: violent sneezing, fever, thirst, restlessness; dry or
fluent; caused by dry, cold air or wind.

Coryza, with headache, roaring in the ears, fever, sleeplessness; especially if coryza has been suppressed by
exposure; better in the open air, worse from talking.

⁸ **Face.**   Anxious expression.

Face: red and pale alternately; one red, one pale cheek;
livid, lips blackish; bloated, unequally red; sensation
as if the face was growing larger.

General heat and redness of face, following coldness and
sunken look of the same.

On rising, the red face turns deadly pale.

Neuralgia of the trigeminus, left side; face red and hot;
restlessness, anguish; rolling about screaming.

Sensation as if the muscles were firmly but not spasmodically contracted, numbness, heavy feeling of the
whole face.

⁹ **Lower Face.**   Lips dry, black, peeling off; complaints on
the upper lip.

Burning, tingling, numbness of the lips.

Swelling of the lower jaw, with aching in the face.

Stitching thrusts in the lower jaw.

Mouth drawn to one side.   θ Convulsions.

¹⁰ **Teeth.**   Toothache from cold, from dry, cold winds, with
throbbing on one side, redness of the cheek, congestion
to head, great restlessness; left side.

Grinding the teeth.

Teeth sensitive to cold air; toothache in sound teeth.

¹¹ **Tongue, etc.**   Taste: bitter, except water; putrid; sweetish;
like rotten eggs; flat, nauseous, compels hawking of
tough mucus.

Trembling and temporary stammering.

Talking: 3, 7.

Tongue feels as if swollen, burning, prickling, tingling.

Numbness of mouth and tongue.

Tongue coated white or yellow-white.

¹² **Inner Mouth.**   Dryness of the mouth, tongue and lips.

Accumulation of water in the mouth.   θ Ascarides.

Orifices of the salivary ducts sore, as if corroded.

Saliva generally diminished.

¹³ **Throat.** Redness of soft palate and uvula.

Feeling of dryness, as if something had stuck in the throat.

Stinging in the throat; fauces dark red, burning.

Burning and numbness in the throat; throat almost insensible.

Pricking, burning in throat and along the eustachian tube, compelling swallowing.

Almost entire inability to swallow, with hoarseness.

When swallowing: stinging pains in throat; feels as if food remained in the region of the heart.

¹⁴ **Desires. Aversions.** Hunger and thirst excessive, but eats slowly.

Burning, unquenchable thirst.

Desire for: wine or brandy; beer; bitter drinks.

Loss of appetite or loathing of food, qualmishness.

¹⁵ **Eating and Drinking.** Better from cold drinks; anxiety relieved.

Drinking ice water causes cough; gastric catarrh, especially from drinking while overheated.

After eating, violent pain in the stomach, with warmth and tenderness; hiccough; nausea (after meat broths).

After wine, blood-spitting, congestions.

Smoking: aggravates palpitation; stupefies.

¹⁶ **Nausea and Vomiting.** Hiccough.

Nausea, with seat-worms; vomiting of lumbrici and of mucus.

Nausea in œsophagus or stomach, rarely in the throat.

Vomiting: of bile; of green masses; with bitter taste; of blood, of bloody mucus or of what has been drunk, followed by thirst.

Vomiting with anxiety, heat, thirst, profuse sweat and increased micturition.

¹⁷ **Stomach.** Pressure in the pit of the stomach, as from a weight; after repeated vomiting sensation of a cold stone there.

Burning from stomach up through the œsophagus to mouth.

Sudden excruciating pain, with gagging, retching, vomiting of blood, gasping; cold sweat on forehead; congestion of mucous lining of stomach. θ Stage of desquamation in scarlatina.

Region of stomach sensitive to touch.

¹⁸ **Hypochondria.** Anxious feeling in the præcordia.

Pressure or constriction in region of the liver, with oppression of breathing.

Tension and heaviness in the hypochondria.

Stitches in the region of the liver taking the breath.

Stitches and heat in the diaphragm.

[19] **Abdomen.** Colic forces him double, yet relieved in no position; inflammatory, after a cold.

Burning, cutting, darting in the bowels; worse from least pressure or lying on right side.

Abdomen hot to the touch, distended, sensitive; paroxysms of anguish.

Umbilical region hard, swollen. *θ* Seat-worms.

Meteorism, vomiting, inability to urinate.

Cutting extending in a circle, from spine to abdomen.

ı Incarcerated hernia, with bilious vomiting; hernia with excessive sensibility and inflammation, or with cold, clammy sweat.

[20] **Stool, etc.** Stool scanty, loose, frequent, with tenesmus; small, brown, painful, at last bloody. *θ* Dysentery.

White, with dark red urine.

Like chopped herbs. *θ* Summer complaint.

Bilious diarrhœa of infants, with colic.

Diarrhœa from getting wet; slimy, bloody stools, violent pains in the bowels; tenesmus, also between discharges.

Urging; slimy stools; intolerable nightly tingling, itching at the anus. *θ* Seat-worms.

Dysentery or inflammatory diarrhœa during hot days and cold nights.

Cutting, griping, followed by frequent urging to stool after anger or fright.

Alternate slimy stools and constipation. *θ* Icterus.

Constipation; clay-colored stools.

Bleeding piles, inflamed; stinging and pressure in anus.

[21] **Urine.** Sensitiveness of the renal region; shooting pains.

Micturition painful, difficult, drop by drop; frequent desire.

Urine scanty, fiery, scalding hot, dark red, turbid.

Brown, burning urine, with brick-colored sediment.

Enuresis, with thirst.

Diuresis, with headache or profuse sweat.

Retention or suppression of urine, with pressure in the bladder or stitches in the region of the kidneys; retention from cold especially in children, with much crying and restlessness.

Hæmaturia, with hemorrhoids of anus or bladder; burning distress in the urethra.

[22] **Male Sexual Organs.** Sexual desire increased; fits of lasciviousness.

Increased desire in the evening, with the heat and sweat.

Sexual desire decreased, with relaxed parts; tingling in parts.

Bruised pain in the testicles.

Testes feel swollen and hard.

Children reach with their hands to the genitals. θ Cystitis.

²³ **Female Sexual Organs.** Ovaritis, painful urging to urinate; high fever; also after the menstrual flow is suddenly checked.

Prolapsus uteri, occurring suddenly, with inflammation, bitter vomit, cold sweat, or dry, hot skin.

Metritis, sharp shooting pains, abdomen exceedingly tender.

Menses: generally too late, diminished, but too protracted; plethoric females who lead a sedentary life; tendency of blood to head and chest; profuse, with nosebleed; suppressed by fright, with vexation.

Leucorrhœa copious, tenacious, yellowish.

Labor-like pressing in the womb; has to bend double, but relieved in no position. θ Dysmenorrhœa.

Uterine hemorrhage active, much excitability, giddy, cannot sit up, fear of death.

²⁴ **Pregnancy.** During pregnancy, restless, fear of death, predicts the time to die.

Impending abortion from fright, with vexation; circulation excited, rapid breathing.

Labor-pains violent, follow in rapid succession; parts dry, tender, undilatable; contractions insufficient.

After-pains too painful, too long-lasting.

Milk fever, with delirium; mammæ hot.

Childbed fever, lochia suppressed, mammæ lax, empty; skin hot, dry; pulse hard, frequent or contracted; eyes wild, staring, glittering; tongue dry; abdomen inflated, sensitive.

Return of the lochia, when women commence going about after confinement.

Newborn children: asphyxia, apopletic symptoms, hot, purplish, breathless, pulseless; icterus; ophthalmia; retained urine.

²⁵ **Larynx.** Croaking voice.

Larynx sensitive to touch.

Laryngitis, with inflammatory fever; also with suffocative spasms (spasms of the glottis).

Laryngeal complaints after straining the voice.

Dryness in the windpipe causing a frequent little cough.

▮ Croup: awaking in first sleep; child in agony, impatient, tosses about; dry, short cough, but not much wheezing nor sawing breathing; cough and loud breathing during expiration; every expiration ending with a hoarse, hacking cough; after exposure to dry, cold winds.

²⁶ **Breathing.** Labored, anxious, or quick and superficial, short, when sleeping or raising one's self; deep, slow sighing.

Breath hot; hot feeling in lungs.

Asthma from active hyperæmia of lungs and brain, face red, eyes staring; after emotions; can talk but little at a time; loud, strong, noisy breathing, with open mouth.

Asthma after suppression of an acute rash; feeling of a band around the chest; muscles of the chest are rigid; occasionally vomiting, urine scanty, dark; after the paroxysm, the sputum is yellow or blood-streaked.

Agony, sits up straight, can hardly breathe; pulse like a thread, vomituritio; sweat, with anxiety; swelling under short ribs. *θ* After scarlatina.

Oppression of the chest when moving fast or ascending. *θ* Heart disease.

²⁷ **Cough.** Child grasps its throat every time it coughs.

Cough: dry and painful; short, dry, hacking, excited by tickling in the larynx; spasmodic, rough, croaking, with danger of suffocation; dry, hard, ringing.

Expectoration absent; or bloody; thick, white mucus.

Cough worse after taking cold; drinking cold water; from tobacco smoke; lying on either side; evening, night, more after midnight.

❙ Lying on the back partially relieves dry cough with nervous excitability.

²⁸ **Lungs.** Hæmoptysis: blood comes with up an easy hawking, hemming or slight cough; expression of anxiety; great fear of death; palpitation, quick pulse; stitches in the chest; caused by mental excitement; exposure to dry, cold air; after wine.

Stitches about the chest; cannot lie on the right side; only on the back; dry, hacking cough. *θ* Pleurisy.

Lancinating through the chest, with dry heat, difficult breathing, often violent chill.

Pressure, weight and burning under the sternum.

²⁹ **Heart. Pulse.** Oppression about the heart, burning flushes along the back.

Anxiety about the præcordia, heart beats quicker and stronger; fear of death.

Palpitation, with a feeling as if boiling water was poured in the chest.

Anxiety, difficulty of breathing, flying heat in face, sensation of something rushing into the head.

Feeling of fulness; pulse hard, strong, contracted; stitches at the heart; lies on the back, with raised shoulders; constriction of the chest.

Fainting with tingling.

During three beats, the apex strikes only one.

Pulse: full, hard, strong in fevers, inflammations; small, intermittent, irregular, in asthma; quicker than the beat of the heart; quick, hard, small in peritonitis; when slow, almost imperceptible, thread-like, with anxiety; full, hard and frequent, succeeding chill, during which it was small and weak.

31 Neck and Back. Tearing in nape of neck.

Painful stiff neck, worse moving the neck; pains down the neck to the right shoulder.

Bruised pain between the shoulders.

Drawing, tearing pain in the scapulæ.

❙ Pain in the back prevents his taking a deep inspiration.

Stiffness of the back.

Crawling in the spine, as from beetles; formication.

Numbness of small of back, extending into lower limbs.

Cutting pain in circles, from spine to abdomen.

Pain in the small of the back, especially at last lumbar vertebræ, as if beaten.

Spasms from inflammatory affections of the spine.

32 Upper Limbs. Tearing pain in the shoulder-joint.

Formication in arms, hands and fingers.

❙ Arms hang down powerless, as if paralized by blows.

❙ Numbness of the left arm; can scarcely move the hand; tingling of the fingers.

Shooting pains, tearing, erratic, in arms, forearms, wrists and finger-joints.

Paralysis of the wrists.

Creeping in the fingers while writing.

Red pimples on the back of the hands; stinging-itching.

Hands icy-cold; cold, sweaty palms.

33 Lower Limbs. Drawing-tearing, in left hip-joint on moving.

Shooting, tearing pains in legs, knees, ankle, toes, etc.

Limbs feel tired during repose.

Legs almost powerless; after sitting numbness.

Cramps in the calves.

Legs and feet feel numb; tingling, commencing in the feet and spreading upwards.

Sensation as if drops of cold water trickled down the front of the thighs.

Numbness in the gouty limb.

Hot pricking in the toes; toes "go to sleep" while walking.

Coldness of the feet and ankles; soles and toes cold and sweaty.

34 Limbs in General. Bruised, heavy feeling.

Numbness, icy-coldness and insensibility of hands and feet.

Hot hands and cold feet.

Rheumatic inflammation of the joints, worse evening and night; intense, bright red, shining swelling of the parts, sensitive to the least contact.

Lameness and numb feeling in affected parts; pain intolerable.

35 **Position, etc.** Rest: 33. Lying down: 2, 40; on right side: 19, 28; on either side: 27; on back, 27, 28, 29. Sitting: 4, 33, 46. Sits up straight: 26. Cannot sit up: 23. Rising: 2, 8. Must bend double: 19, 23. Motion: 3, 4, 5, 31, 33. Walking: 33. Moving fast: 26. Ascending: 26.

36 **Nerves.** Great irritation of the nervous system.

Convulsions of children, teething, heat, startings, twitches of single muscles; child gnaws its fists, frets, cries; costive or dark watery stools.

Trembling palpitation; muscles feel bruised.

Numbness, tingling; left side lame; paralysis of the limbs.

Jerks of left leg or arm; grinding teeth; comatose, restless, moaning.

Lassitude, bruised feeling and restlessness of the body.

37 **Sleep.** Sleepiness; spasmodic yawning.

Sleeplessness after midnight, with anxiety, restlessness, continual tossing about; eyes closed.

Sleeplessness caused by fear, fright, or anxiety, with fear of the future.

Dreams anxious, vivid.

38 **Time.** Evening: 3, 4, 22, 27, 34, 40. Night: 1, 25, 27, 34, 40, 43. After midnight: 27, 37.

39 **Temperature and Weather.** Sun: 3, 5, 46. Hot days and cool nights: 20. Warm room, 3. Open air: 7. Dry, cold wind: 2, 5, 7, 25, 28, 44. Cold water: 5. Getting wet: 20. Uncovering: 1, 40.

After cold land wind (W., N. W.) in coughs, croup, etc.

40 **Chill. Fever. Sweat.** Chill at the beginning violent, more in the evening after lying down, often with hot cheek and contracted pupils.

Chilly, if uncovered or touched.

With the chill: internal heat, anxiety, red cheeks; body chilly, hot forehead and ears, internal heat.

Shivering ascends from feet to chest.

Dry heat, with thirst, short breathing, quick, hard, full pulse.

Covered or affected parts sweat profusely; likes to be uncovered.

Profuse hot sweat during sleep (also in consumptives).

Bad effects from suppressed sweat.

42 **Sides.** Right: 31.

To be given in cases going from right to left; earache, faceache, toothache, arm numb.

Left to right: paralysis (the opposite with the sick).

43 **Sensations.** Burning, tingling and numbness.

Coldness and retarded venous circulation.

Oversensitive to pain; pains, especially at night, seem insufferable.

44 Tissues. Increased action of serous membranes, reddening their capiliary vessels.

Arterial system dominant; has but little effect on changed blood corpuscles; of no use in typhoid states.

Congestions with the mind symptoms.

Housemaid's knee, acute symptoms.

Glands painful, hot, swollen.

Burning through all the mucous membranes.

45 Contact, Injuries, etc. Touch: 1, 5, 17, 25, 34, 40. Pressure: 19. Contusion: 2. Fall: 2.

46 Skin. Red, shining, hot swellings; violent pains.

Dark, miliary rash.

Rash like measles, pains in the joints; dry, barking cough; cannot bear light; hot, dry skin.

Scarlet rash, with high fever.

Spots like flea-bites; itching unchanged by scratching.

Erysipelas, smooth skin; violent fever.

Erythema from the sun's rays; papular erythema.

Yellow skin. *θ*Jaundice.

Dryness and burning of the skin.

47 Stages and States. Children's diseases, with high fever.

Dark hair and eyes.

Persons leading a sedentary life.

Old age; sleeplessness.

Especially persons with tonicity (rigidity) of fibre.

Contraindicated in fevers which bring out eruptions or are otherwise salutary, unless there is agonizing tossing with dry skin.

48 Relationship. Antidotes to it: *Acet. ac., Paris, Vinum.*

Acon. is an antidote to *Bellad., Chamom., Coffea, Nux vom., Petrol., Sepia, Sulphur, Veratr.*

After *Acon.* follow well: *Arnic., Bellad., Bryon., Sepia* and *Sulphur ;* in gastric states, after pulmonary febrile affections: *Ipec.;* in colic: *Arsen.;* in cough: *Bryon., Spongia.*

Acon. may often be indicated after *Arnic., Coffea, Sulphur* and *Veratr.*

Mercur. follows well in dysentary.

Complementary to *Coffea,* in fever, sleeplessness, intolerance of pain; to *Arnic.* in bruises; and to *Sulphur,* high.

Ailments from *Acon.: Act. rac., Chamom., Coffea, Nux vom., Petrol., Sepia, Sulphur.*

Abuse of *Acon.* calls for *Sulphur.*

ACTÆA RACEMOSA.

Black Cohosh.   JEANES.   *Ranunculaceœ.*

[1] **Mind.**   Desire for solitude; to wander from place to place.
Answers questions hurriedly and evasively.
Would not answer at other times very loquacious.
Declares she will go crazy.
Weeping mood; dejection; anxiety; apprehensiveness.
❚ Melancholia from hyperæsthesia of nervous centres; hence with women, with inebriates, etc.
Fear of death—thinks she is going to die.
Mental depression, with suicidal tendency.
Suspicious, indifferent, taciturn, takes no interest in household matters.
Irritable, least thing that goes wrong makes her angry.
Mania following disappearance of neuralgia.
After fright, threatened abortion.
Aggravations from mental emotions.
Mind affected by business failure; by disappointed love.

[2] **Sensorium.**   Constant dull feeling in vertex.
Vertigo: head feels large and heavy; when stooping, head swims; on rising in morning; nausea when raising the head from the pillow.
Fainting fits.

[3] **Inner Head.**   Rush of blood to the head, brain feels too large for the cranium; after suppressed uterine discharges or suddenly ceasing pains.
Waving sensation in the brain.
Dull frontal headache relieved by pressure.
Great pain in head and eyeballs, increased by the slightest movement.
Severe pains in right side of head, back of orbit.
Aching and shooting pains in vertex, occiput, left temple, eye and ear; worse lying down; hysterical crying.
Top of head feels as if it would fly off.
❚ Head feels too large and throbs.   θ Intermittent fever.
Intense pain as if a bolt had been driven from neck to vertex, worse at every throb of the heart.

[5] **Eyes.**   Dark spots before the eyes, dilated pupils, double vision.
Intense pains in the eyeballs; worse from moving the head or eyes, and in the evening.
Severe pain in the centre of the eyeballs; worse in the morning, lasts all day; worse going up stairs.

[6] **Ears.**   Sensitive to least noise.

Singing in the left, later in both ears.

⁷ **Nose.** Coryza, dry in the evening, white mucus during the day; sneezing; aching pains in the head and eyes, sensitive to cold air, every inhalation seems to bring the cold air in contact with the brain.

⁸ **Face.** Wild, fearful expression.

Face pale; eyes large, sunken, surrounded by dark rings.

Forehead feels cold; deadly pale.

Neuralgia affecting the malar bone, pain goes off at night, reappears the next day.

Frequent flushes of heat, wants to be in the open air.

⁹ **Lower Face.** Under lip cracked, as if bitten.

Jaw sunken.

¹⁰ **Teeth.** Toothache in neuralgic and rheumatic patients.

¹¹ **Tongue, etc.** Taste: disagreeable; coppery.

Cannot speak a syllable, though she makes the effort.

Speaking: 27.

Tongue: clean, but pointed and trembling; swollen; coated light brown, more in the middle.

¹² **Inner Mouth.** Breath offensive.

Mouth and tongue feel hot and dry.

¹³ **Throat.** Dry spot in the throat, causing cough; dryness of the pharynx, with constant desire to swallow; fulness in the pharynx; uvula and palate swollen.

Hawks up a viscid, coppery tasting mucus.

¹⁴ **Desires. Aversions.** No thirst, slight feeling of hunger in stomach; rumbling in abdomen.

Appetite variable.

No appetite for dinner, wants to drink cold water; little at a time suffices.

¹⁶ **Nausea and Vomiting.** Eructations, with nausea, vomiting and headache.

Vomiting ot green substance; groans, raves, presses both hands to her head for relief.

¹⁷ **Stomach.** Acute, darting pains in the stomach.

Sinking or "goneness" in the epigastrium.

¹⁹ **Abdomen.** Periodical colicky pains, better bending double and after stool.

Flatulence, causing sensation of fulness.

Severe pains in bowels, small of back and down the limbs.

Excruciating pains in bowels, much rumbling and wind.

Sharp pain across the hypogastrium.

Abdominal muscles sore.

²⁰ **Stool, etc.** ▮ Frequent, thin, dark, offensive stools. θ Spotted fever.

Morning diarrhœa, of children.

Pains go from limbs to bowels, producing diarrhœa and partial retention of urine.

Alternate diarrhœa and constipation.

[21] **Urine.** Pressing in region of kidneys and small of back.
Irritable bladder.
Urine: profuse, pale, watery; bloody, frequent; scanty, feels hot.

[23] **Female Sexual Organs.** Spasms of the broad ligaments.
Ovarian pains shoot up to the side.
Severe pain in lower part of abdomen, worse by motion.
Bearing down in uterine region and small of back; limbs feel heavy, torpid.
Great tenderness on pressure over the uterine region.
Menses: profuse, early, dark, blood coagulated; scanty, slightly coagulated; sharp pains across abdomen, has to double up; labor-like pains; debility between periods, scanty flow between menses; suppressed by mental emotions, from cold, from fever.
Rheumatic dysmenorrhœa.
Epileptic or hysterical spasms at time of menses.
Leucorrhœa, with sensation of weight in the uterus.

[24] **Pregnancy.** Complaints in pregnancy; nausea; false labor-like pains; sharp pains across abdomen; sleeplessness; insanity.
Labor-pains severe, tedious or spasmodic, with fainting fits or cramps.
Cardiac neuralgia in parturition.
Convulsions in labor from nervous excitement.
"Shivers," first stage of labor.
After-pains, worse in the groins; oversensitiveness; nausea and vomiting.
Lochia: suppressed, by cold or emotions; watery, mixed with small clots.
Inframammary pains, worse left side.
Burning in the mammæ.

[25] **Larynx.** Hoarseness, worse in the evening; very sensitive to cold air.
Tickling in throat, with violent cough.

[26] **Breathing.** Frequent sighing.

[27] **Cough.** From a dry spot in the throat, spasmodic with pain in back of neck.
Cough at every attempt to speak, dry, short, constant at night.

[28] **Lungs.** Severe pain in the left chest, below fifth or sixth rib.
Pain in right side of chest, must lie quietly on back and press with the hand; breath short; slight cough.

[29] **Heart. Pulse.** Pains from the region of the heart, all over the chest and down the left arm; palpitation; unconsciousness; cerebral congestion; dyspnœa; face livid;

cold sweat on the hands; numbness of the body; the left arm numb and as if bound to the side.

Hearts action ceases suddenly; impending suffocation.

Pulse weak, irregular, eighty per minute; feeble in the morning, with trembling and weakness.

31 **Neck and Back.** Cramp in the muscles of the neck on moving the head.

I Violent, lightning-like pains in posterior spinal sclerosis.

Stiff neck from cold air, pain from moving even the hands.

I Sensitiveness of the spine, especially in the cervical and upper dorsal regions; pressure causes retching and nausea; soreness of all the muscles. θ Spotted fever.

I Heat in back of head extending down the back; during spasms, muscles of neck and shoulders sore afterwards.

Pain under left scapula.

I Head and neck retracted. θ Spotted fever.

Severe pain in the back, down the thighs and through the hips, with heavy pressing down.

Violent aching in small of back.

32 **Upper Limbs.** Pains in the muscles, worse from motion.

Left arm feels as if bound to the side.

Constant irregular motions of the left arm; arm useless.

Cold sweat on hands.

Hands tremble, especially when writing.

33 **Lower Limbs.** Joints swollen, heat in them.

Fearful pains through the lower limbs, like growing pains.

34 **Limbs in General.** Aching in the limbs.

Excessive muscular soreness.

Rheumatism affecting the belly of the muscles; cramping, stitching pains.

Uneasy feeling in limbs, causing restlessness.

35 **Position, etc.** Motion: 3, 23, 31; of head: 5; of eyes: 5; of handwriting: 32. Stooping: 2. Bending double: 19, 23. Raising head: 2. Rising: 2. Going up stairs: 5. Lying: 3; on back: 28.

33 **Nerves.** Trembling of the legs, twitching of the flexors.

Great debility between the menses.

Irregular motion of the limbs, worse left; legs unsteady.

Alternate tonic and clonic spasms.

Epilepsy, periodical convulsions, with uterine diseases.

Hysteric spasms.

37 **Sleep.** Comatose.

Sleeplessness: with excited brain; after nursing the sick.

Starts during sleep; restless.

Cannot sleep, because she feels numb all over.

Unrefreshing sleep.

38 **Time.** Day: 5, 7. Morning: 2, 5, 20, 29, 40. "11–12 M.:" 40. Evening: 5, 7, 25, 40. Night: 8, 27, 40.

[39] **Temperature and Weather.** Cold air: 7, 25, 31. Open air: 8.

[40] **Chill. Fever. Sweat.** Chilliness down the back, from 11 to 12 M.

Chilliness, then heat; languid, stretches her limbs, 10 A. M.

Feet and hands cold, then hot.

Chill, then heat, then sweat, alternating dry skin, 5 P. M.

Night-sweats. θ Diarrhœa.

Sweat smells offensive.

[41] **Attacks.** Periodical attacks of colic.

Pains come on suddenly.

Headache at intervals.

[42] **Sides.** Right: side of head, of chest, see 28.

Left: temple, see 3; inframammary pain, chest below 5th and 6th ribs, from heart down the arm, arm as if bound to side, motions in it, asleep, comp. 36, back below scapula.

Singing in ear: left then both.

[43] **Sensations.** Pricking all over.

Like electric shocks here and there.

Sharp, lancinating pains in various parts, associated with ovarian or uterine irritation.

General bruised feeling as if sore.

Whole body, especially the arms, feels numb.

[45] **Contact, Injuries, etc.** Pressure: 3, 16, 23, 28.

[46] **Skin.** Eruption of white pustules over the face and neck; sometimes large, red, papular.

Prickling, itching, heat of the whole surface.

[47] **Stages and States.** Climacteric years.

Nervousness from anxiety or overexertion.

Rheumatic persons.

Children, teething. θ Diarrhœa.

[48] **Relationship.** Collaterals: *Act. spic.*, and other Rannnculaceæ.

Acon. relieves the sleeplessness.

Act. spic., Byron. and *Pulsat.* similar in rheumatism. The first is preferable in rheumatism of small joints, tearing pains; joints ache after exercise.

Baptis. relieved headache and nausea.

Cauloph. similar in uterine and rheumatic affections.

Compare: *Pulsat., Sepia, Natr. mur., Lil. tig.* and *Ignat.*

AESCULUS HIPPOCASTANUM.

Horse Chestnut.   HELBIG.   *Sapindaceæ.*

[1] **Mind.** Depressed, low-spirited; irritable.

Unable to fix the attention.

[2] **Sensorium.** Confused feeling in the head, with giddiness.

[3] **Inner Head.** Dull pressure in forehead, slight nausea, followed at once by stitches in right hypochondrium.

Neuralgic darting from right to left across the forehead; followed by flying pains in the epigastrium.

Frequent flying pains through the temples.

Dull pain in the occiput, with flushes of heat over the occiput, neck and shoulders.

[4] **Outer Head.** Soreness of side of scalp rested on (right).

[5] **Eyes.** Flickering before the eyes.

Pupils dilated; contract slowly.

Eyes feel heavy and dull; balls feel sore and hot.

Burning and stinging deep in the left orbit, as if the pain surrounded the ball.

Painful aching over the left eye.

Twitching: of the lids; of the muscles under the left eye. Lachrymation.

[6] **Ears.** Burning in ears; pressure; ringing in the right.

[7] **Nose.** Dryness of the posterior nares and throat.   θ Coryza.

Fluent coryza, dull frontal headache, thin, watery discharge; burning, rawness; sensitiveness to inhaled air.

Stinging and burning in posterior nares and soft palate.

[8] **Face.** Pale, miserable appearance.

Flying heat and redness of the left side of the face.

Face swells after washing; rubbing causes red spots.

[11] **Tongue, etc.** Taste: sweet; bitter, afterward sweetish; metallic; oily or coppery with salivation.

Cannot control the tongue so as to form words rightly.

Tongue coated white or yellow; feels scalded.

Tip of the tongue sore, as if ulcerated.

[12] **Mouth.** Thick yellow phlegm in the mouth.

Salivation, oily taste; teeth as if covered with oil.

[13] **Throat.** Hawks up ropy mucus, of a sweetish taste.

Pricking in fauces; pressure as if something had lodged there.

Dryness, burning and constriction in fauces.

Tonsils dark, congested, swollen; worse the left; inclination to swallow, with dull aching pain, burning like fire.

Frequent neuralgic pains in the fauces.

[15] **Eating.** Stomach feels full, as if walls were thick, after eating.

[16] **Nausea and Vomiting.** Eructations: sour; greasy; bitter;
   taste of food; empty; thick mucus.
   Violent retching and vomiting; burning in stomach.
[17] **Stomach.** Pressure as from a stone in the pit of the stomach.
   Gnawing and emptiness in the stomach in the early morn-
   ing.
   Fluttering, faintness in stomach, burning, great distress.
   Periodical tightness in scrobiculus, with labored breathing.
[18] **Hypochondria.** Constant, severe aching, from the pit of
   the stomach to the right lower lobe of the liver.
   Tenderness in the right hypochondrium; stitches, follow-
   ing headache.
   Pinching pain in the right hypochondrium, with colic;
   pain through to the back on inspiring.
   Congestion of liver and portal system.
   Pain in the region of the spleen.
[19] **Abdomen.** Burning distress, soreness and aching at navel.
   Abdomen tender to touch; sense of fulness and throbbing
   in it.
   Rumbling in the bowels, with cutting about the navel.
   Cutting in the right inguinal region.
   Flatulent or flying pains in the bowels.
[20] **Stool, etc.** Passing fetid flatus.
   Soreness, burning, itching, fulness and urging at the anus.
   ❙ Dryness, heat and constriction of the rectum; rectum
   feels as if full of small sticks; knife-like pain in anus.
   Hemorrhoids purple; painful sensation of burning; seldom bleed; aching and lameness, or shooting in back.
   Prolapsus ani after stool; dull headache.
   Stool large, dry, hard and knotty; difficult, dark; mushy,
   light brown; first part hard, black, the last of about
   natural consistency, but white as milk.
[21] **Urine.** Frequent, scanty urination; pain in kidneys.
   Urine: dark, muddy, passed with much pain; scalding;
   hot; dark brown sediment; yellow, with thick white
   mucous sediment.
[23] **Female Sexual Organs.** Leucorrhœa dark yellow, thick
   and sticky; worse after menses; worse walking; cor-
   rodes the labia; aching in the sacrum and knees.
[24] **Pregnancy.** Sacro-iliac symphysis gives out while walking;
   must sit down; still better lying. θ Hemorrhoids.
[25] **Larynx.** Sensation of dryness and stiffness of the glottis
   and of the laryngo-pharyngeal mucous membrane.
   Hoarse voice.
[26] **Breathing.** Rapid, labored; with pain in r. lung. See 32.
[27] **Cough.** Dry, short, increased by swallowing and deep
   breathing; dry, hacking, caused by constriction of the
   fauces, with irritation of the epiglottis.

[28] **Lungs.** Raw feeling in the chest.

Lungs feel engorged, heavy.

Stitches through chest; stitches go from left to right side.

[29] **Heart. Pulse.** Darting in the region of heart, with fulness and palpitation.

Dull, aching, burning in the region of the heart.

Palpitation, heart's action full, heavy; can feel the pulsation all over the body.

Pulse: accelerated; soft, weak.

[31] **Neck and Back.** Lameness and weariness, in back of neck.

Aching between the shoulders.

Pains in right scapula and chest; worse inhaling.

Severe, dull, aching pain in lumbo-sacral region, affecting sacrum and hips; worse stooping forward and when walking.

[32] **Upper Limbs.** Left arm and hand much warmer, feel heavy and swollen.

Right arm feels paralyzed, cannot raise it.

Pricking, swollen feeling of hands after washing them.

Nails blue.

[33] **Lower Limbs.** Back and legs weak; can hardly walk, must lie down.

[34] **Limbs in General.** Joints stiff, aching and painful.

Limbs feel heavy.

[35] **Position, etc.** Lying: 24, 33. Motion: 44. Walking: 23, 24, 31, 33. Stooping: 31. Sitting: 24.

[36] **Nerves.** Flying, neuralgic pains.

Lameness and paralytic feelings: 31, 32, 33.

Feels faint, weak; weariness, faintness at the stomach.

[37] **Sleep.** Disposition to stretch and yawn.

Drowsy: falls asleep; on awaking, knows not where she is.

Awakened by burning pain in the stomach.

Mornings on awaking, sore and tired.

[38] **Time.** Morning: 17, 37, 44. Evening: 40.

[39] **Temperature and Weather.** Open air: 7. Washing: 32.

Heat of fire: 40.

[40] **Chill. Fever. Sweat.** Chilliness: creeping up and down the back, with burning in the anus; better from heat of fire.

Evening: fever, skin hot, dry; burning palms and soles.

Disposition to stretch and yawn; head aches, as if it would burst.

Flashes of heat over the occiput, face, neck and shoulders.

Sweat profuse, hot, with the fever.

[42] **Sides.** Right: hypochondria, see 18; groin, lung, see 26; inhaling, arm paralyzed. Left: pain in eyeball, red face, tonsil congested; heart, see 29; arm heavy.

Left to right: stitches through chest.

Tissues. Fulness as from too much blood: heart, head, skin.

Sore feeling of muscles, mornings on awaking and on motion.

Dryness of mucous membranes.

Mucous membranes swell.

⁴⁶ **Skin.** Formication: scalp, nose, fauces.

Itching of the body, especially about the waist.

⁴⁷ **Stages and States.** Hemorrhoidal tendency.

⁴⁸ **Relationship.** Collateral: *Æsc. glab.*

Concordances: *Aloes, Collin., Mercur., Nux vom., Podoph., Sulphur* (weak spine).

AETHUSA CYNAPIUM.

Fool's Parsley.   NENNING.   *Umbelliferæ.*

¹ **Mind.** Lies unconscious, dilated pupils, staring eyes (child).

Incapacity of mind to think, confused; idiocy.

Great sadness when alone; hallucinations and delirium.

Anxiety and restlessness, afterwards headache and colic.

Irritability, especially in the afternoon and in the open air.

² **Sensorium.** Vertigo: with sleepiness, can't lift the head up; giddiness ceases and head gets hot; with palpitation.

³ **Inner Head.** Violent pain, as if brain were dashed to pieces.

Pressing pain in the forehead, as if it would split, at its height vomiting and finally diarrhœa.

Headache ceases, with discharge of flatus downwards.

Stitches and pulsations in the head.

Distressing pain in the occiput, nape, and down the spine, better from bending stiffly backwards.

Sensation as if both sides of the head were in a vice.

⁵ **Eyes.** Objects seem much larger than natural.

Eyes brilliant, protruding; dilated pupils.

Chronic photophobia; scrofulous ophthalmia; swelling of the meibomian glands; edges of the lids inflamed, adhere at night, must be washed open in the morning.

⁶ **Ears.** Yellow discharge from right ear, with stitching pains.

⁷ **Nose.** Nose stopped up with thick mucus; frequent but ineffectual desire to sneeze.

⁸ **Face.** Expression of anxiety, with well-marked linea nasalis.

Face: puffed, spotted red; pale.

⁹ **Lower Face.** Chin and corners of the mouth feel cold.

¹⁰ **Teeth.** Stinging or tearing in the gums.

¹¹ **Tongue, etc.** Aphthæ in mouth and throat salivation.

Feeling as if the tongue were too long.

Taste: bitter; like cheese; like onions; sweetish in the morning.

Speech impeded, slow.

[13] **Throat.** Soft palate, red and swollen.

[14] **Desires. Aversions.** Burning thirst.

Desire for wine, or aggravation from its use.

[15] **Eating.** While eating: sudden heaviness in forehead.

After eating: pain below navel, lienteric stool, dry cough.

[16] **Nausea and Vomiting.** Violent sudden vomiting: of frothy white substance; of yellow fluid, followed by curdled milk and cheesy matter. Cannot bear milk in any form.

Vomiting of greenish phlegm, similar to the stools.

The milk is forcibly ejected soon after being taken; then weakness causes drowsiness. θ Nursing children.

Regurgitation of food an hour or so after eating.

[17] **Stomach.** Painful contractions of the stomach so severe as to prevent vomiting.

Tearing, rending pains in pit of stomach, extending to the œsophagus.

[18] **Hypochondria.** Lancinating in the right hypochondrium, in the afternoon.

Painful pressing, burning, stitching, left hypochondrium.

Shooting in left hypochondrium, often and long-continued.

Soreness and painfulness in both hypochondria.

[19] **Abdomen.** Coldness of abdomen and lower limbs, with aching of bowels, relieved by warm, wet applications.

Bluish-black swelling of the abdomen.

Colic, followed by vomiting, vertigo and weakness.

[20] **Stool, etc.** Diarrhœa: stools bright, yellowish, then green and slimy, later greenish-grey; green, thin, bilious or bloody mucus, stools undigested; greenish mucus, with bile, much pain and tenesmus.

[21] **Urine.** Pain in the kidneys, worse from sneezing, worse from deep inhalation and lying.

Cutting pains in bladder, with frequent calls to urinate.

Urine: red, sediment white; copious, clear as water; too frequent after exertion.

[22] **Male Sexual Organs.** Right testicle drawn up, with pain in kidneys.

[24] **Pregnancy.** Labor pains too weak, not regular.

[26] **Breathing.** Short breath, interrupted by hiccough.

[28] **Lungs.** Stitches in left side of chest.

[29] **Heart. Pulse.** Palpitation, with vertigo and headache.

Pulse: frequent, small, somewhat hard and unrythmical.

[31] **Back.** Sensation as if the small of the back were in a vice.

Painful furuncle in the sacral region.

[32] **Upper Limbs.** Numbness of the arms, aching about the scapulæ, extending to the arms.

Sensation as if the arms had become much shorter.

[33] **Lower Limbs.** Boring and shooting in lower limbs, with great weariness.

Lancinating and drawing from left hip into the thigh.

Laming ache in the middle of right thigh while sitting; better when moving.

Lancinating from right heel into the sole.

Crawling in the feet.

[35] **Position, etc.** Moving: 33. Walking: 46. Bending backwards: 3. Cannot stand: 36. Lying: 21.

[36] **Nerves.** Epileptiform spasms, with clenched thumbs, red face, eyes turned downwards, dilated, staring, immovable pupils, foam at the mouth, teeth set, pulse small, hard, accelerated.

Spasms, with stupor or delirium.

Restlessness, with excessive anguish.

Great weakness; children cannot stand; cannot hold up head.

[37] **Sleep.** Dozing of child after vomiting spells or after stool.

On falling asleep, rolling of eyes or slight convulsions.

[38] **Time.** Morning: 5. Afternoon: 1, 18. Night: 5.

[39] **Temperature and Weather.** Headache better walking in the open air.

Frequently indicated in summer.

Heat: 46. Moist warmth: 19. Room: 43. Open air: 1. Washing: 43.

[40] **Chill. Fever. Sweat.** Coldness, rigors, stiffness of the limbs.

[42] **Sides.** Right: 6, 18, 22, 33. Left: 18, 28, 33.

[43] **Sensations.** Sensation as if head, face and hands were swollen; worse after washing; better coming in room.

Sensation as of a band around the head and chest.

Sensation of parts as if in vice; head ; chest; small of back.

[44] **Tissues.** Ecchymosis, black and blue spots all over.

[46] **Skin.** Eruption itching when exposed to heat.

Liability to excoriation of the thighs when walking.

Red spots on the skin.

Little water blisters, itching in bed.

Tetters bleed easily.

Reddish-blue spots on trunk and left leg.

[47] **Stages and States.** Children, during dentition,

[48] **Relationship.** Collaterals: *Cicut., Conium., Œnanth, croc.*

Concordances: *Ant. crud* (vomiting of milk); *Arsen.; Asar.; Calc. ostr.* (vomiting of milk); *Cuprum ; Ipec.; Opium.*

It antidotes *Opium*, and is antidoted by vegetable acids.

AGARICUS MUSCARIUS, OR AMANITA.

Fly Fungus.   SCHRETER AND STAPF.   *Nat. order, Fungi.*

[1] **Mind.** Cannot find the proper word, uses wrong words; worse after exertion; sleepless nights.

Confusion of the head, heaviness, as after intoxication.

Ecstasy; fancies excited; makes verses.

Delirium, tries to get out of bed.

I Great exertion of power with delirium.

Great loquacity, convulsive motions of facial and cervical muscles, mostly right side, drawing head down to shoulder; merry, incoherent talk; followed by malaise.

Sings, talks, but does not answer questions.

Disinclined to answer questions.

Indisposed to perform any labor, especially mental.

She is indifferent, though naturally very solicitous.

Very much out of humor.

Protracted mental application or exciting debates bring on vertigo.

[2] **Sensorium.** Vertigo: when walking in the open air, reeling as if drunk; long-lasting, with great sensitiveness to cold air; momentary, from strong light of the sun.

Great weight in the head, it constantly falls backwards.

[3] **Inner Head.** Dull headache, especially in forehead; must move head to and fro and close the eyes as for sleep.

I Dull, drawing headache in morning, extending into root of nose, with nosebleed or thick mucous discharge.

Tearing and pressure in left half of the brain.

Pressing in right side, as if a nail were thrust in; worse sitting quietly; better moving slowly about.

Pain as though sharp ice touched the head or cold needles pierced it.

Violent oppressive pains, chiefly in forehead.

I Headaches of those who are subject to chorea, or who readily become delirious in fever or with pain; twitchings or grimaces.

[4] **Outer Head.** Sensation of coldness on right side of frontal bone, though warm to the touch.

Icy coldness in region of coronal suture after scratching.

Twitching of head and cervical muscles, worse on right side.

Drawing or stitching pains in head, shifting from side to side.

[5] **Eyes.** Feeling of weakness in eyes without having exerted them.

Indistinct sight; focal distance changes while reading; first grows shorter, then longer.

Dim sight; things look obscured, as from turbid water; muscæ volitantes; vibrating spectra, with vertigo.

Reads with difficulty, type seems to move. θ Diplopia.

Flickering before the eyes while writing.

Black spot before left eye.

Pupils dilated.

Viscid yellow humor gluing the lids; gum in canthi.

Burning in canthi; inner angles itch, burn and are red; worse from touch.

Frequent slight twitching in eyelids.

Twitching in the eyeballs; while reading, frequent twitching and pressing in left eyeball.

Spasms, with aching in left eyeball. θ Myopia.

Narrowing of space between eyelids.

Clonic spasms; lids open and close in quick succession.

Swelling of tear gland.

⁶ **Ears.** ❙ Redness, burning-itching of the ears, as if they had been frozen.

⁷ **Nose.** Smell sensitive; vinegar unbearable.

Frequent sneezing.

Nosebleed when blowing nose early in the morning.

Profuse fetid discharge from the nose.

Mucous membrane very sensitive.

Frequent dropping of clear water from nose, without coryza.

⁸ **Face.** Puffy, pale, blue under eyes, nose and lips blue.

Redness, with itching-burning, as from freezing.

Twitching of facial muscles.

Tearing in face and jaw-bones.

⁹ **Lower Face.** Trembling vibration in lips and muscles of lower jaw; convulsive shaking of lower jaw.

Pricking in the chin, as from needles.

¹⁰ **Teeth.** Tearing in lower molars, worse from cold air.

Swelling and bleeding of the gums.

Shooting from right lower teeth up to right side of head.

¹¹ **Tongue, etc.** Left side of tongue numb.

Tongue: dry; coated white, mornings; sore; smarting, burning tip, as from pepper.

Tremulous propulsion of the tongue; inarticulate speech. θ Chorea.

¹² **Inner Mouth.** Smell from mouth: offensive, like that after eating horse-radish.

¹³ **Throat.** Feeling of dryness of fauces and pharynx, causing contraction, as when drinking an astringent.

Great difficulty in swallowing, with ravenous appetite.

Throws up some flocculi or solid lumps of phlegm, almost without cough.

4

[14] **Desires. Aversions.** Much hunger, but no appetite early in the morning.

Burning thirst. θ Typhus.

[15] **Eating and Drinking.** Better for an hour after eating, while he is so exhausted; but great sleepiness remains.

After meat, heartburn.

[16] **Nausea and Vomiting.** Eructations: taste of rotten eggs or of apples; empty.

Nausea, vomiting.

[17] **Stomach.** Cardialgia lasting three hours after a meal; burning, changing into a dull pressure, like from a foreign body, with nausea.

Heavy sensation in the stomach.

[18] **Hypochondria.** Liver enlarged, congested.

Sharp stitches, as from needles, in the region of the liver; dull stitches during breathing.

Stitches under short ribs, left side.

Pulsation deep in the spleen.

[19] **Abdomen.** Loud rumbling in the bowels.

[20] **Stool, etc.** Grass green, bilious; thin, yellow, fecal, slimy; pappy, with cutting in the abdomen and much wind; bloody, dysenteric.

Diarrhœa mostly in the morning, after rising and eating, with much rumbling; crampy colic and passing of wind.

Passes much inodorous flatus.

[21] **Urine.** Urine: profuse, colorless; clear, lemon-colored.

Viscid, glutinous mucus from the urethra.

Weakness of sphincter vesicæ, with dribbling.

[22] **Male Sexual Organs.** Great desire for an embrace, the penis being relaxed.

Voluptuous itching of the genitals.

After coitus: great debility; profuse night-sweats; burning, itching of the skin; tension and pressure under ribs.

Spermatorrhœa, with pains and weakness in the thighs.

❚ Complaints after sexual debauches.

[23] **Female Sexual Organs.** Prolapsus uteri after cessation of menses.

❚ Bearing down pain almost intolerable.

Itching and irritation of the parts, with strong desire for an embrace.

Menses too profuse, with tearing, pressive pains in back and abdomen.

[24] **Pregnancy.** Nipples itch, burn, look red.

[25] **Larynx.** Scratching in throat when singing.

[26] **Breathing.** Oppression and constriction of the larynx; he fears suffocation.

Frequent deep inspiration.

Difficulty in breathing, as if the chest was too full; he

must breathe more deeply; also from muscular constriction.

²⁷ **Cough.** Violent coughs in isolated attacks, ending in repeated sneezing.

Convulsive, hacking cough, with oppressive sweat.

❙ Sudden convulsive coughs, worse forenoons.

Violent spasmodic cough at night.

Expectoration of small, transparent lumps, almost without cough, relieving the lungs.

²⁸ **Lungs.** Jerking stitches through right lung.

Oppression of the chest, in the region of the diaphragm, with drawing pains.

Tension in the lower part of the chest during motion and when sitting, taking away his breath.

²⁹ **Heart. Pulse.** Burning, shooting pains in region of heart, extending to left shoulder-blade; caused by deep inspiration and much worse from coughing, sneezing, hiccough.

Anxious sensation of pressure in heart, oppression on bending body.

Palpitation violent, strongly felt, worse evenings, with redness of face; on sitting down, some irregular strong beats; anxious oppression.

Constant feeling of a lump in the epigastrium, with pain under the sternum; drawing in region of diaphragm, sharp pains in left side.

Pulse: feeble, scarcely perceptible; becomes slower; small, irregular.

³¹ **Neck and Back.** Twitching of the cervical muscles.

Stiffness in the nape of the neck.

Peculiar sensation of weakness and stiffness between shoulders; extends to the neck.

Pain in the back, as after continued stooping.

Muscles feel bruised; on bending forward, feel short.

Spasmodic, pressive, drawing pain starts from back, extends to middle of chest and into œsophagus.

Violent shooting, burning pains, deep in the spine.

Aching along spine and limbs.

❙ Pain in lumbar region and sacrum; a sort of crick in the back; extends along to the nape of the neck.

Sensation of ants creeping along spine.

Spine sensitive to touch; worse mornings.

Every motion, every turn of body, causes pain in spine.

Sudden stitch in sacral region while walking in open air.

³² **Upper Limbs.** Violent laming pain in left hand and arm after palpitation commences.

Drawing pain from left upper arm to forearm; drawing in muscles of left forearm and down over the elbow.

Burning, itching pimples on the arms.

❙ Burning, itching on both hands, as if frozen; parts hot, swollen, red.

❙ Trembling of the hands.

Right hand unsteady while writing; arm feels paralyzed from much writing.

❙ Stiffness in fingers from gout.

³³ **Lower Limbs.** Twitching of the gluteal muscles.

Heaviness of the legs; languor.

Pains in legs, especially in region of right hip-joint, like from fatigue.

Violent pains in limbs, especially left hip under gluteal muscles.

Drawing, pressive pains in legs; especially in ankles.

Pains in legs most marked, standing or sitting; better when walking or from motion.

Dull pain along the tibia; drawing pains.

Toes itch and burn; are red and swollen, as if frost-bitten.

Cramp in the soles at night.

³⁴ **Limbs in General.** Frequent jumping of muscles.

Feels as if her limbs did not belong to her.

After repeated and severe epistaxis, great soreness and bruised feeling of joints of limbs.

Limbs cold, blue.

³⁵ **Position, etc.** Rest: symptoms generally worse. Motion: 3, 28, 31, 44. Walking: 2, 28, 31, 33, 44. Exertion: 1, 40. Sitting: 3, 28, 29. Bending; 29, 31.

³⁶ **Nerves.** Debility after coitus.

Tremor of whole body.

Paralysis of lower limbs, with slight spasms of arms.

Spasmodic motions, from simple involuntary motions and jerks of single muscles, to a dancing of the whole body.

Twitching of eyelids and eyeballs; trembling of legs and hands, debility; soreness of spine; worse at approach of thunder-storm.

❙ Involuntary movements while awake; ceasing during sleep.

Coma following the febrile excitement of dentition; eyes half open, showing the white; breathing not hurried, but often a deep inspiration, followed by a sigh and slight convulsive twitching of extremities.

Cramps in the hands and feet; body convulsed, as if a galvanic battery were applied to the spine.

³⁷ **Sleep.** Frequent yawning; before spasms, or paroxysms of headache.

Unusual sleepiness.

Uneasy, restless sleep; from violent itching and burning of the skin.

On falling asleep; starts, twitches; sudden complete
awaking.

Awakes often at night, is wide awake.

[38] **Time.** Morning: 3, 11, 14, 20 31, 44. Forenoon: 27, 44.
Evening: 29. Night: 27, 33, 40.

[39] **Temperature and Weather.** Very sensitive to cold air.
꜀ Chilblains, frost-bite.

Approach of thunder-storm: 36. Cold air: 10. Open
air: 2, 31, 40. In warm bed: 44.

[40] **Chill. Fever. Sweat.** Great chilliness in the open air,
strikes through the whole body.

Chilly on slight movement, or from raising the bedclothes.

Shiverings over the body, running from above downwards.

Heat slight, chiefly on upper part of body.

Sweat: greasy, but not offensive, all night, during sleep;
from slight exertion; often only on front of body; at
night, especially about legs; cold, on face, neck, chest.

[42] **Sides.** Symptoms often appear diagonally (right arm, left
leg, etc.).

Right: 3, 4, 10, 28, 33. Left: 3, 5, 11, 18, 29, 32, 33, 44.

[43] **Sensations.** Burning-itching and redness of various parts:
ears, nose, face, upper and lower limbs, like chilblains.

Pricking as from pins, burning.

Sensation in various parts, as if ice touched or as if ice-
cold needles were piercing the skin.

Corrosive biting now and then on the skin.

Formication, crawling.

Cramp-like pain in muscles, erratic, when sitting.

[44] **Tissues.** Makes the blood thin.

Veins swollen, with cool skin.

Muscles feel bruised from touch; better from walking.

Pains in long bones, as if bruised, after motion.

Pains in bones morning and forenoon, especially left tibia,
condyle of left elbow (like syphilitic pains, but better
rather than worse in warmth of bed).

Joints feel as if dislocated.

Obesity.

[45] **Contact, Injuries, etc.** Body sensitive to touch or pressure; burning in canthi; pain in spine, between vertebræ, muscles feel bruised; pricking in left thumb.

Worse from touch: 5, 31. After scratching: 4.

Slight blows cause ecchymoses.

[46] **Skin.** Burning-itching, redness and swelling, as from frost-
bites.

Miliary eruptions close and white, with intolerable burning, itching.

Itching stitches in various parts.

Violent itching between thumb and forefinger, left hand.

[47] **Stages and States.** Light hair; skin and muscles lax.
Old people with indolent circulation.
Venous erythism.

[48] **Relationship.** Similar to: *Act. rac.* (delirium of alcoholism);
chorea; spinal irritation; *Bellad.* (cerebral excitement,
but more in chorea); *Calc. ostr.* (alcoholism; icy-cold feeling on head); *Cannab. Ind.* (alcoholism; extravagant
fancies); *Cicut.* (spasms of eyes); *Codein.* (eyelids twitching, etc.); *Coffea* (ecstasy); *Hyosc.* (typhoid of drunkards;
loquacity, dancing, muscular twitchings, and with all
tremor, tendency to stupor and feeble pulse); *Ignat.* (hysterical or emotional chorea; sighing; convulsive cough;
twitches; laughing and crying); *Laches.* (loquacious delirium ; alcoholism ; typhoid of low type, tremulous protrusion of tongue; tremor, feeble pulse, livid extremities); *Mygale* (chorea); *Nux vom.* (chorea; alcoholism;
spinal irritation; convulsions; tremor; paraplegic symptoms; enlarged liver); *Opium* (alcoholism; chorea, with
spasmodic, angular jerks of flexors; hands tremble, slow
pulse); *Pulsat.* (spinal irritation ; chorea ; chilblains,
etc.); *Sepia* (icy-cold feeling on head ; jerks of head and
tongue, etc.); *Sticta* (chorea with jumping and dancing);
Stramon. (delirium tremens; singing, laughing, dancing;
extravagant recitals; loquacity; chorea, with gyratory
motions, etc.); *Tarant.* (chorea, one arm and leg constantly in motion); *Thea* (verbose; spinal irritation);
Ver. alb. (icy-cold feeling on head); *Zincum* (chorea).
Vinegar and Eau de Cologne induce fainting. *Sal Ammoniæ* also aggravates ; t.
Mushrooms will not grow in ground containing either iron
or coal.
Antidoted by: charcoal; coffee; wine; brandy; camphor;
fat or oil (relieves stomach); *Calc. ostr.* (relieves icy-coldness); *Pulsat.; Rhus tox.* (nightly backache).
Atropine is said to be antagonistic to *Muscarine*, but they
both, when topically used, dilate the pupil.
Muscarine is very similar to *Pilocarpine* (jaborandi), since
both cause arrest of heart's action; profuse sweat; salivation, lachrymation; contracted pupils, etc. *Muscarine*
acts more on the lachrymal glands, less on sweat and
salivary glands; *Pilocarpine* causes more urging to urinate. *Muscarine*, given internally, contracts the pupil
more than *Pilocarpine;* used topically, only the former
dilates the pupil. *Gelsem.* is here similar to *Muscarine*.
Follow well: *Bellad., Calc. ostr., Mercur., Opium, Pulsat.,
Rhus tox.* and *Silicea.*
Acted well after *Dulcam., Phosph. ac., Pulsat.* and *Cuprum*
had failed. θ Chronic diarrhœa.

Cured where *Bellad.*, *Stramon.* and *Hyosc.* failed.   θ Clonic spasms of eyes.

Compare in irritable weakness of accommodative apparatus of eye: *Physostigma* (pain after using eyes, muscæ volitantes, flashes of light, twitching of lids and around eyes; myopia); *Jaborandi* (spasm of accommodation, vision continually changing; eyes tire easily, are irritable).

AGNUS CASTUS.

Vitex Agnus Castus.   HAHNEMANN.   *Verbenaceæ.*

¹ **Mind.**   ∎ Absent-minded, reduced power of insight.
Low-spirited, fears of approaching death.
Despairing sadness; peevishness.
Anxious, fear and weakness.

² **Sensorium.**   After dulness in the head, a pressing, long-lasting headache, followed by vomiting and spasmodic trembling.
Heaviness of head and pressure in the neck, as if the head would fall forward.

³ **Inner Head.**   Tearing, with pressure in the temple and forehead, worse during motion.
Contractive headache above the temples from reading.
Pain in upper head, as from staying in a close room; looking to one point relieves it.

⁴ **Outer Head.**   Biting-itching on the scalp, worse evenings and when falling asleep.
Tension and chilliness in scalp, which is warm to touch.

⁵ **Eyes.**   Dilated pupils; photophobia.
Eyes burn when reading in the evening.
Corrosive itching over and on eyebrows and lids, and below eyes.

⁶ **Ears.**   Ringing or roaring in the ears.
Hardness of hearing.

⁷ **Nose.**   Illusion of smell; as of herring; musk.
Hard aching on dorsum of nose, relieved by pressure.

⁸ **Face.**   Corrosive itching on the cheeks.
Erysipelas on left cheek, spreading from nose over face and head.

⁹ **Lower Face.**   Rending-tearing under alveoli of r. lower jaw.

¹⁰ **Teeth.**   Teeth painful when touched by warm food or drink.
Throbbing, tearing toothache in left eye-tooth, small boil near the tooth, very painful to touch; in attacks.

¹¹ **Tongue, etc.**   Taste: metallic, coppery; bitter.
Tongue coated white.

[13] **Throat.** Corrosive itching in pit of throat.
[14] **Desires. Aversions.** Lessened appetite; thirstlessness.
[15] **Eating.** Abdomen distended after meals.
[16] **Nausea and Vomiting.** Hiccough; inclined to get angry; peevish.

Nausea in pit of stomach when standing; later, qualmishness in the abdomen, with pressing down, wants to support it.

Nausea as from eating fat food. θ Checked catamenia.
[17] **Scrobiculum.** Pinching in scrobiculum when sitting bent over.
[18] **Hypochondria.** Soreness in region of spleen.

Swelling and induration of the spleen. θ Intermittent.

Aching in region of liver, worse from touch.
[19] **Abdomen.** Rumbling in the abdomen during sleep.

Abdomen sensitive to pressure.

Incarcerated flatus.

Feels as if the entrails were sinking down, constantly inclined to support the bowels with the hands.

Violent contracting bellyache, coming suddenly in the morning, with bearing down. θ Suppressed menses.
[20] **Stool, etc.** Diarrhœa of children; chronic diarrhœa of adults.

Feels as if diarrhœa would set in, when standing; anguish, great weakness.

Great accumulation of wind; flatus smells like urine remaining long on the clothes.

Hard stools; constipation; difficult expulsion of soft stool.

When pressing at stool, discharge of prostatic fluid.

A sore feeling under the skin near the anus when walking.

Corrosive itching of the perineum; pruritus podicis.

Deep rhagades or fissures of the anus.

Ascarides.
[21] **Urine.** Pains in bladder.

Passes more urine.

When urinating, sometimes pain in lower abdomen, sometimes in the kidneys.

Red, turbid urine, with burning and pressure in urethra.

Emissions of prostatic fluid. See 20, 22.
[22] **Male Sexual Organs.** ∎ Sexual desire lessened, almost lost; impotence with spermatorrhœa.

Feeble erections, no sexual desire.

∎ Penis so relaxed that voluptuous fancies excite no erections.

∎ Testes cold, swollen, hard; penis small, flaccid.

∎ Impotence, with gleet, especially with those who have frequently had gonorrhœa.

∎ Yellow urethral discharge.

Itching of genitals.

I Gleet, with want of sexual desire or erections.

²³ **Female Sexual Organs.** Suppressed menses, with drawing
pain in the abdomen.

I A transparent leucorrhœal discharge passes imperceptibly
from the very relaxed parts.

Leucorrhœa, not copious, but spotting her linen yellow.

Hysteria, with maniacal lasciviousness.

²⁴ **Pregnancy.** Retained placenta.

I Milk scanty, or disappears.

Sterility.

²⁵ **Larynx.** Voice as if passing through wool.

²⁶ **Breathing.** Oppression on going up stairs.

Dyspnœa; worse in the evening.

²⁷ **Cough.** Cough: in the evening, in bed, before falling
asleep; with raising of blood, followed by copious
mucus; in paroxysms, with palpitation and nosebleed,
mostly in the morning; when inhaling cold air.

²⁸ **Lungs.** Feeling of dryness in the chest.

²⁹ **Pulse.** Slow and weak pulse, often imperceptible.

³⁰ **Outer Chest.** Pressure in region of sternum, worse when
breathing deeply.

³¹ **Back.** Sharp, deep stitches on and near the coccyx, to the
left, near sacrum and coccyx.

³² **Upper Limbs.** Hard pressure in right axilla and upper
arm, worse from touch or motion.

Swelling of finger-joints, tearing pains, arthritic nodes.

³³ **Lower Limbs.** Heaviness of right foot, as from a weight.

Lancinating pain in the right hip-joint, worse during motion, somewhat better in rest.

Legs much fatigued and swollen towards evening.

Cold knees.

Ankles swollen after a sprain.

Tearing, rending in feet and toes, worse on walking.

Feet easily turn under when walking on stone pavement.

³⁴ **Limbs in General.** Pain as if luxated.

³⁵ **Position, etc.** Motion: 3, 32, 23. Walking: 20, 33. Going up stairs: 26. Standing: 16, 20.

³⁶ **Nerves.** Spasmodic complaints of hypochondriacal men.

Great weakness: as from violent anguish; with depression of spirits; with agalactia.

Feels bruised all over.

³⁷ **Sleep.** Sleeplessness.

Awaking often, as if alarmed, startings.

Anxious dreams.

³⁸ **Time.** Morning: 19. Evening: 4, 5, 26, 27, 33, 40, 46.

³⁹ **Temperature and Weather.** Bad effects from getting feet
wet.

Warm things: 10.

⁴⁰ **Chill. Fever. Sweat.** Chilliness, internal with trembling, skin warm.

Slight chilliness towards evening, followed by heat, with headache, no thirst, slight delirium, tormenting, profuse sweat.

Chill and heat alternate.

Chilly all over, but only hands feel cold to touch.

Flushes of burning heat, mostly in face, with cold knees; evening in bed.

Sweat on the hands when walking in the open air.

Sweats easily.

⁴² **Sides.** Right: 4, 9, 32, 23. Left: 8, 31, 33.

⁴³ **Sensations.** Bruised feeling all over.

⁴⁴ **Tissues.** Inflammatory, rheumatic swelling of the joints. Gouty nodosities.

⁴⁵ **Contact. Injuries.** May be indicated in bruises or wounds. Sprains and luxations of joints; strains from overlifting. Prevents excoriation in walking.

Touch: 10, 16, 32. Pressure: 7.

⁴⁶ **Skin.** Gnawing or itching on different parts of the body, relieved temporarily by scratching.

Itching around the ulcers, in the evening.

· Yellow tint of skin.

⁴⁷ **Stages and States.** Lymphatic constitution.

"Old sinners," with impotence and gleet.

⁴⁸ **Relationship.** After *Agn. cast.* are useful: *Arsen., Bryon., Ignat., Lycop., Pulsat., Selen.* (impotence), *Sulphur.*

Antidotes to *Agn. cast.: Camphor., Natr. mur.* (the headache); strong solution of table salt.

AILANTHUS GLANDULOSA.

Tree of Heaven.   P. P. WELLS.   *Simarubeæ.*

¹ **Mind.** Torpor, stupor; stoic indifference.

Loss of memory.

Inability to concentrate mental effort; must read a subject several times, or add a column of figures over and over before correct.

Depression of spirits; frequent sighing.

Great anxiety; restlessness.

Constant muttering delirium.

² **Sensorium.** Vertigo: more when stooping; with nausea and cold sweat.

❙ Dizzy, face hot, cannot sit up; drowsy, yet very restless
and anxious; later insensible, with muttering delirium;
recognizes no one.   θ Scarlatina.

Feeling as if an electric current were passing through the
left side of head, or down to the extremities.

Apoplectic fulness of head.

³ **Inner Head.**   Headache, with nausea and giddiness.

Dull, heavy sensation in the forehead, with disinclination
to think or act.

Thick, heavy feeling in the base and right side of the
head.

Darting through temples and back of head, with confusion
of ideas; severe pain through temples on waking.

Dull headache, burning in eyes, oppression of chest.

Pain in the occiput.

⁴ **Outer Head.**   Beating in the occipital arteries.

Tender bruised sensation over the fronto-parietal suture.

⁵ **Eyes.**   Intolerance of light; tears from bright light, and
from the open air.

❙ Eyes suffused and congested, startled look when roused;
pupils dilated and sluggish; photophobia.

Burning, smarting and aching in the eyes.

Rough feeling in the left eye, as from dust.

Conjunctiva inflamed, towards the outer canthus.

Pus-like discharge, agglutinating the lids in the morning.

Dark blue circles around the eyes.

⁶ **Ears.**   Pain in the ear when swollowing.

Itching around the left ear at night; gets red when
scratched.

Parotid gland tender and enlarged.   θ Scarlatina.

⁷ **Nose.**   Loss of smell.

Coryza, with a rawness inside about the nostrils; the
whole nose and upper lip became covered with very
thick gray-brown scabs.

Fluent nasal catarrh, with sneezing.

❙ Copious, thin, ichorous, bloody discharge, without fetor.

Chronic catarrh, difficult breathing through the nose.

Dryness of the nose, secretion suppressed.

Itching and uneasy feeling around the nose.

⁸ **Face.**   Heat and redness of the face; mahogany color.

Chronic, speckled, spotted face; a kind of acne.

Irregular red spots of capillary congestion, like with
drunkards.

Swelling of the left side of face; puffed erysipelatous face.

Countenance indicating distress; great prostration.

⁹ **Lower Face.**   Small but deep, ragged ulcer near the angle
of the mouth; lips cracked.

Inflamed vesicles on the lower lip, chin bright red.

¹⁰ **Teeth.** ı Covered with a brown slime or sordes.

Tearing in left upper or lower teeth, face and head; worse on lying down, must walk about; better from pressure and towards morning.

¹¹ **Tongue, etc.** Tongue: thickly covered with a whitish coat; brown in the middle; moist, coated white, tip and edges livid; ı dry, parched and cracked.

Taste: insipid, flat; feverish. _θ_ Bronchial catarrh.

Water tastes brackish and flat.

¹³ **Throat.** Fauces and tonsils inflamed, with spots of incipient ulceration.

Throat tender, sore on swallowing, or on admitting air.

Hawking of mucus, constant effort to raise hard lumps of whitish matter.

ı Throat livid, swollen; tonsils studded with many deep, angry-looking ulcers, with scanty, fetid discharge; neck tender and swollen. _θ_ Scarlatina.

Throat swollen, dark red, almost purple. _θ_ Scarlatina.

Thyroid gland tender, enlarged.

¹⁴ **Desires. Aversions.** Appetite: capricious; poor, yet eats as usual.

Hunger and sense of emptiness during the chill.

Thirst for cold drinks.

¹⁵ **Eating and Drinking.** Food taken was speedily vomited.

¹⁶ **Nausea and Vomiting.** Sudden, violent vomiting when sitting up.

Vomiting, with stupor.

Nausea, vomiting, diarrhœa, spasmodic abdominal pains.

¹⁷ **Stomach.** Peculiar feeling of emptiness in stomach; pain.

¹⁸ **Hypochondria.** Oppression, like a stricture, below hypochondria; a very debilitating sensation with nausea.

Tenderness over the hepatic region.

¹⁹ **Abdomen.** Weak, burning, uneasy feeling in the bowels, as of approaching diarrhœa.

Tvmpanitis; slight rumbling in the bowels.

²⁰ **Stool, etc.** Dysentery, frequent painful stools, little fecal matter, much bloody mucus; very little fever.

Frequent watery stools expelled with great force.

ı Stools thin, watery, offensive, passing involuntarily with the urine.

ı Tapeworm.

²¹ **Urine.** Scanty or suppressed; passed unconsciously; acid.

²² **Male Sexual Organs.** Chancre-like sore on the prepuce.

²⁵ **Larynx.** Voice hoarse, failing.

Awoke in the morning, with almost entire loss of voice.

Croupy choking.

Oppression of bronchia, with dull headache.

²⁶ **Breathing.** Hurried, irregular, heavy. _θ_ Scarlatina.

Equable oppression, as though the chest were strapped; as if air-cells stuck together.

Asthmatic oppression in large bronchi; wheezing.

Shortness of breath, with dyspnœa.

²⁷ **Cough.** Dry, hacking constant; with oppression, burning, and pains in the chest; tight and wheezing, with scanty expectoration; pains through left lung; continual deep bronchial, without pain, worse from exercise.

Violent fits of coughing before retiring and on rising.

Coughs continually until she raises freely, then better.

Cough, with breathing somewhat oppressed; muco-purulent expectoration; free in the morning, sticky and scanty during the day.

Expectoration: at times mixed with blood, at times of blood alone; bitter, yellow, more mornings.

²⁸ **Lungs.** Excessive soreness and tenderness of lungs; feeling as if the air-cells were stuck together; tired feeling in the lungs.

Stitching and aching in the chest, under clavicle.

Burning in the right, aching in the left lung.

Sensation of fulness and smothering before expectoration.

²⁹ **Heart. Pulse.** Dull pain and contracted feeling in region of base of heart and through centre of left lung.

Pulse rapid and small; weak, sometimes scarcely perceptible, very frequent and irregular. θ Scarlatina.

³¹ **Neck and Back.** Itching around her neck.

Thickened, swollen feeling of the muscles of neck.

❙ Neck tender and very much swollen.

Constant aching between the shoulders.

Glands of the neck sore, with pain under the left scapula.

Constant sharp pain through the small of back and hips.

³² **Upper Limbs.** Large water blister on the end of the thumb, with smaller ones at the side of the finger nails.

Tingling in fingers and left arm on awaking.

³³ **Lower Limbs.** Numbness of left leg, with tingling, pricking pain in the foot and toes.

Severe pain in left foot, a tension while walking.

³⁴ **Limbs in General.** Feeling of uneasiness and aching restlessness.

Heaviness of the limbs.

Limbs feel as though they were asleep.

³⁵ **Position, etc.** Exertion: 27. Walking: 10, 33. Stooping: 2. Rising: 27. Sitting up: 16. Lying: 10.

³⁶ **Nerves.** Great debility, easily exhausted.

Electric thrill, starting from the brain, to the extremities.

Jerking cramps of the limbs during sleep.

Low, adynamic forms of disease, sudden and extreme prostration, torpor, vomiting, pulse small and rapid, purplish skin.

[37] **Sleep.** Very drowsy, restless, soon passes into insensibility.

Sleep disturbed, unrefreshing. Heavy sleep through the night.

Restless at night, talking and moaning in sleep, night-sweat, frequent waking.

Sleeps best on the right side. *θ* Bronchial affections.

[38] **Time.** During the day: 27. Morning: 5, 25, 27, 40. Evening: 27. Night: 6, 20, 37, 46. Toward morning: 10.

[39] **Temperature and Weather.** Open air: 5.

[40] **Chill. Fever. Sweat.** Chill, with hunger and sense of general emptiness.

Miliary eruption before the chill.

Chills, followed by flushes of heat, with severe pain in the head and soreness of the lungs.

Skin either very hot or cool to the touch.

Dry, hot skin, most in the morning, until noon.

Cold sweat stood out upon the skin. *θ* Verified in cholera.

[42] **Sides.** Right: 3, 18, 28, 37. Left: 2, 5, 6, 8, 10, 27, 28, 29, 31, 32, 33, 46.

[43] **Sensations.** Feeling of fulness everywhere.

Soreness, irritability and prickling or tingling.

Electric current from head into limbs.

[45] **Contact, Injuries, etc.** Pressure: 10.

Pressure of clothes feels uncomfortable.

[46] **Skin.** ❙ Eruption of miliary rash, in patches, with efflorescence between the points of rash of a dark, almost livid color; most on forehead and face.

Skin cold and dry, of livid color; after pressing with the finger the color returns very slowly.

Itching around left ear, back, face and neck at night; felt as if she would go crazy.

Large maculæ and bullæ, filled with a claret-colored serum. Petechiæ.

❙ Malignant scarlatina.

[47] **Stages and States.** The odor of the flowers affects the asthmatic; also women and children more than men; old people least of all.

Nervous, sensitive persons.

Bilious temperament, stout and robust.

[48] **Relationship.** Collaterals: *Ptelea* and the *Xanthoxyleæ*.

Antidotes to *Ailanth.*: *Aloe²ᵉ*, for the dull headache; *Rhus tox.* for the headache and erysipelatous face; *Nux vom.* for the general effects.

Concordances: *Amm. carb.; Arnic.* (sore lungs); *Arum triph.; Aloe; Baptis.; Bryon.; Gelsem.; Hyosc.; Laches.; Nitr. acid; Nux vom.; Phytol.; Prussic acid; Rhus tox.; Stramon.*

ALOE SOCOTRINA.

Socotrine Aloes.   HELBIG.   *Liliaceæ.*

[1] **Mind.** Lassitude, alternating with great mental activity.
> Great disinclination to mental labor; it fatigues him; general languor.
> Anxiety.
> Ill-humored; hypochondriacal, worse in cloudy weather.
> Hates people, repels everyone.
> Restlessness, with ebullitions of blood.
> After a nocturnal emission, fright at slight noises.

[2] **Sensorium.** Vertigo: as if everything whirled with her, worse on going up stairs or turning quickly; with anxiety when moving; everything seems insecure; better after nasal catarrh sets in.

[3] **Inner Head.** Congestion to head, compelling one to sit up.
> ❙ Headache across forehead, with heaviness of eyes and nausea; must make the eyes small.
> Obtuse frontal headache, incapacity for all mental work.
> Weight on the vertex; pressure in the forehead and occiput.
> Dull, pressive pain: in supraorbital region; in sinciput.
> Pressing outwards to the temples, with periodic heat of the face and flickering before the eyes.
> Stitches in the temples aggravated by every footstep.
> Headache after insufficient stool; with abdominal pains.
> Headaches with gastro-intestinal irritation and with coldness of lower limbs from afflux of blood to the cerebral centres; headaches better from cold applications.

[4] **Outer Head.** Sensitiveness of the scalp in spots.
> Dryness of the hair.
> Alopecia with chronic headaches.

[5] **Eyes.** Eyes glittering, somewhat red, prominent; unsteady, anxious look.
> ❙ Flickering before the eyes, with heat of face; scotoma.
> Yellow rings move before the eyes. (See 48.)
> Dimness before the eyes while writing.
> Pain deep in orbits, as if in muscles, worse on right side.

[6] **Ears.** Cracking in the ears when moving the jaw.
> Sticking pain in the left ear, later in the right.

[7] **Nose.** Nosebleed in bed after awaking.
> Coryza, with burning and pain in the nose; on sneezing, stitches in the umbilical region.

[8] **Face.** Heat of the face with the headache or when excited.
> Face: pale during cloudy weather; sickly, sunken.

[9] **Lower Face.** Lips: redder than usual; dry, cracked; moist, soreness of the borders; white, scaly.

[10] **Teeth.** Sensitiveness in a hollow molar; worse when eating; later a pustule appears on the gum near the diseased tooth.

[11] **Tongue, etc.** Taste: bitter, sour, like ink or iron; metallic. Tongue: coated yellowish-white; stiff; dry, red.

Severe fine stitches, from behind forward, in the under part of the tongue when moving it.

Yellow ulcers on tongue.

[12] **Inner Mouth.** Inflamed sore spots in the mouth, on the tongue, inside of cheeks.

Sickening smell from the mouth.

Increase of saliva.

[13] **Palate and Throat.** Fauces raw, hot, as if burned.

Palate swollen; arches of the velum palati pain on chewing hard food, or on yawning, worse in the evening, and in the morning on awaking; worse on empty swallowing.

Hawking of thick, jelly-like mucus, in lumps, from fauces and posterior nares; rawness and swollen feeling in pharynx.

[14] **Desires. Aversions.** Aversion to meat.

Longing for juicy articles; fruits, especially apples.

Thirst: with dryness of mouth; awakens at night.

[15] **Eating and Drinking.** Hungry during the diarrhœa; hungry after the morning stool.

Sour food does not agree.

Beer relieves pains in anus; drinking vinegar the colic.

Water causes pains in the stomach.

❚ Has to hurry to the closet immediately after eating or drinking.

[16] **Nausea and Vomiting.** Eructations: bitter; acrid; or sour.

Rising of flatulence toward the throat, with sensation as if vomiting were coming on.

Nausea: with frontal headache; with empty feeling in the stomach; with pain at the umbilicus.

Vomiting of blood.

[17] **Scrobiculum and Stomach.** Pain in the scrobiculum on making a false step.

Fullness in stomach, followed by distension of epigastrium.

[18] **Hypochondria.** Painfulness in the hypochondria, with chilliness and diarrhœa; painful weakness of the legs.

Stitches from spleen into chest, or drawing into the loins.

Hepatic region: burning; uneasiness, heat, pressure and tension; dull pain, worse on standing, bends forward.

Stitches from the liver into chest, obstructing respiration.

[19] **Abdomen.** Pulsation in the region of the navel.

Distension of the abdomen, especially the epigastrium.

with flatus moving about; worse after meals; during menstruation; on motion.

Gurgling of flatus in descending colon; worse after eating.

Abdomen painful, especially about the naval; twisting, griping about the navel, must sit bent forward; urging to stool, with passage only of offensive flatus.

The abdominal muscles pain when rising from a recumbent posture, or when touched, when standing erect, or when pressing to stool.

❙Heaviness: in the hypogastrium; in the rectum; dragging down in the abdomen.

²⁰ **Stool, etc.**   Heat, soreness and heaviness in the rectum.

Urging wakens at night, drives out of bed at 6 A. M.

Urging to stool, with passage of urine.

❙Urgency as with diarrhœa, only hot flatus passes, with great relief; it soon returns, with sensation of a plug wedged between the symphysis pubis and os coccygis.

❙Feces escape almost without being noticed.

Stools: small, brownish, slimy, half fluid; yellow pappy; bloody, jelly-like mucus, and feces with much sputtering flatus; stool and urine escape together.

❙Lumpy, watery stool.

Diarrhœa: in hot, damp weather; evening, night and morning; from vinegar; from cold, damp room; when walking or standing; when passing urine.

❙Hemorrhoids protrude like grapes, with constant bearing down in rectum.

❙Itching and burning in the anus; preventing sleep.

❙Weakness or loss of power of sphincter ani.

²¹ **Urine.**   Burning when urinating.

Frequent urging to urinate; worse at night; or in afternoon: urging so quick he can scarcely retain urine.

Urine: copious, pale, especially after stool; saffron-yellow, becoming cloudy; or scanty, hot; or bloody.

Sediment yellowish, like bran, or slimy.

²² **Male Sexual Organs.**   Sexual desire increased.

Seminal emissions; strong desire afterward.

Testicles cold; penis small; scrotum relaxed; epididymis sensitive, especially to touch or while walking.

Itching of the prepuce.

²³ **Female Sexual Organs.**   Fulness, heaviness in uterine region, with labor-like pains in loins and groin; worse standing.

Menses too early and too profuse.

Leucorrhœa of bloody mucus.

²⁴ **Pregnancy.**   Lameness, which seems to arise from a sense of weight and pressure into the pelvis; during pregnancy.

²⁵ **Larynx.**   Scraping in the larynx.

Voice husky; hawking.

26 Breathing. Whistling in the throat, as if something had fallen into the trachea.

Difficult respiration.

Respiration impeded by stitches through left side of chest.

27 Cough. With stitches in the right side of the larynx; sputa of yellow, tenacious mucus; cough with scratching in the throat.

28 Lungs. Congestion to chest; dry cough; bloody expectoration; even in incipient tuberculosis in the young.

Front of chest feels sore on deep inspiration.

Weakness of the chest.

29 Heart. Pulse. Strong beat of the heart occasionally; pain through to the left scapula.

Pulse: accelerated; weak, suppressed after vomiting; slow in the afternoon.

31 Neck and Back. Lumbago, alternating with headache; also with piles.

Stitches through the sacrum to the loins.

Pressure and heaviness in the sacral region while sitting; better from motion.

32 Upper Limbs. Heaviness of right arm; weakness of wrist-joints.

33 Lower Limbs. Weariness of the calves.

Weakness of the ankle-joint.

Soles of the feet pain when walking on the pavement.

Great toe feels as if sprained.

34 Limbs in General. Lameness, weariness in limbs; weakness in joints; often with the abdominal disturbances.

Pains, of short duration, as if bruised or dislocated (left forearm, right scapula, left ribs).

Pricking, dull twitching, drawing pains in the joints (fingers, knees, elbows).

35 Position, etc. Lying: 6. Sitting: 31. Standing: 18, 19, 20, 23. Must sit up: 3. Bending forwards: 18, 19. Rising: 19. Walking: 20, 22, 23. Every step: 3. False step: 17. Ascending stairs: 2. Turning quickly: 2. Motion: 2, 6, 11, 19, 28, 31.

36 Nerves. Paralytic drawing in the muscles.

General weakness, weariness, extreme prostration.

37 Sleep. Drowsy, dozing in the morning.

Awakened: by thirst; urgency to urinate; pollutions and sexual desire; pains in the back; chill.

Cannot sleep, heat and a crowd of thoughts busy him.

Oppressive dreams of danger, could not cry out; dreams of soiling himself.

38 Time. Morning: 13, 15, 20, 22, 37. Afternoon: 21, 29. Evening: 13, 20. Night: 15, 20, 21, 37, 40.

[39] **Temperature and Weather.** Cloudy weather: 1, 8. Damp weather: 20. Cold damp room: 20. Cold: 3, 23, 40. Warmth: 3. Open air: 19, 40.

[40] **Chill. Fever. Sweat.** Chilly: with coryza, in the cold open air; at stool, shivering.

Cold hands and feet in bed, preventing sleep.

Cold hands, warm feet.

Heat in spots, on the scalp or in the face.

Ebullitions, with anxiety and restlessness.

Sweat: smells strong; offensive on the genitals; at night, after drinking.

[41] **Attacks.** Sudden, quickly passing, urging to stool.

Pains of short duration.

[42] **Sides.** Right: 5, 6, 27, 32, 34. Left: 6, 9, 26, 29, 34. Left to right: 6.

[44] **Tissues.** Congestion to head and chest, especially to portal system.

Mucous membranes; especially causes the production of mucus in jelly-like lumps or "cakes."

Acts mainly on the rectal mucous lining.

[45] **Contact, Injuries, etc.** Touch: 14, 19, 22. Pressure: 33.

[46] **Skin.** Itching, especially of the legs.

Pimples on the abdomen.

Spots which, when scratched, pain and become sensitive.

[47] **Stages and States.** ❙ Old people. θ Colic and diarrhœa.

Phlegmatic, indolent persons.

[48] **Relationship.** *Aloe* has many symptoms like *Sulphur*, and is equally important in chronic diseases, with abdominal plethora, etc.

Similar to *Ailanth.* (dull, fronal headache); *Gum gutt.* (diarrhœa); *Amm. mur.* (abdominal and diarrhœic symptoms); *Nux vom.* (gastric, abdominal and uterine troubles; bad effects of sedentary habits); *Canthar.* (bladder).

Antidotes to *Aloe: Sulphur*, Mustard.

Camphor relieves for awhile.

Nux vom. and *Lycop.* relieve the earache.

Bellad. suits in congestion of eyes of local origin; *Aloe* of reflex; the characteristic for the latter is: redness of eyes with yellow vision.

ALUMINA, OR ARGILLÁ.

Pure Clay.　　　　HAHNEMANN.　　　　$Al_2\,O_3$.

[1] **Mind.** Mistakes in speaking, using words not intended.

Must be changed into some one else before he can see or speak.

Consciousness of his personal identity confused.

Time passes too slowly.

Seeing blood on a knife, she has horrid ideas of killing herself, though she abhors the idea.

Crying, against his will.

Low-spirited, trifling things appeared insurmountable.

Apprehensive of losing his reason.

Dread of death, without thought of suicide.

Variable mood, at one time confident, at another timid.

Peevish and whining, with heat of the ear lobes.

Sufferings follow anger.

Mental symptoms worse in the morning on awaking.

[2] **Sensorium.** Vertigo: everything turns with him in a circle with nausea, worse before breakfast; on opening the eyes, on stooping, better after breakfast, and from wiping the eyes.

Great dullness, with dread of falling forward.

Heaviness of the head, with pale, languid face.

Inability to walk, except with eyes open, and in daytime.

Cloudiness and drunken feeling, alternating with pain in the kidneys.

[3] **Inner Head.** Throbbing, frontal pains, worse going up stairs, or stepping.

Burning, pressive pain, with heat in the forehead, while standing or sitting, better in the open air.

Severe stitches in the brain, with nausea.

Headache, with constipation.

Headache relieved by lying quiet in bed.

[4] **Outer Head.** Itching of scalp, with dry, white scales.

Humid scurf, worse about the temples, bleeding when scratched, worse in the evening, or at new and full moon.

Scalp feels numb.

Pressure on forehead, as from a tight hat.

Pain as if the hair were pulled, with nausea.

Falling off and excessive dryness of the hair, scalp sore when the hair is touched.

[5] **Eyes.** White stars before the eyes, with vertigo.

Dim-sightedness, like looking through a fog.

Objects appear yellow.

Burning and pressure in the eyes.

❙ Eyes inflamed, itching at inner canthus, agglutination at night, and lachrymation by day, yellow halo around candle; hot or acrid tears.

Spasmodic closure of the lids at night, and burning in the eyes in the morning and evening.

❙ Eyelids thickened, dry, burning, smarting.

Nictitation from large papillæ of conjunctiva.

Inclination to stare.

Strabismus of either eye; loss of power of internal recti.

Sensation of coldness in the eyes, in the open air.

⁶ **Ears.** Humming; roaring; whistling; sound as of large bells.

Redness and heat of one ear, evenings.

Sensation as if something lay before the ear: on blowing the nose it is felt, on swallowing it is removed; snapping in the ears when chewing or swallowing; dull hearing; eustachian tubes plugged.

Stitches in the ears, evening or night.

⁷ **Nose.** Sense of smell weak.

Disposition to colds in head.

Fluent coryza, with frequent sneezing, free from one nostril, the other obstructed; lachrymation.

Chronic nasal catarrh, with scurfy, sore nostrils, and discharge of thick, yellow mucus.

Discharge of dry, hard, yellow-green mucus from nose; nose swollen, red and sore to touch, worse in the evening. ·

Violent pain in root of nose.

Copious, yellow, sour-smelling mucus, with sore nostrils.

Septum narium swollen, red and painful to touch.

· ❙ Redness of the nose.

❙ Point of nose cracked.

⁸ **Face.** Gloomy, pale, or alternately red and pale.

Itching of various parts of the face.

Tension of the skin of the face, as though white of egg had dried on it.

Bloated places, like bulbous excrescences.

Blood-boils on face and nose.

⁹ **Lower Face.** Tensive pain in articulation of jaw, when chewing or opening the mouth.

❙ Involuntary spasmodic twitching of lower jaw. θ Hemorrhage of bowels.

Upper lip covered with little blisters.

¹⁰ **Teeth.** Toothache, teeth feel loose and elongated, worse from chewing; in open air; evening.

Drawing toothache, extending to other parts, as down the larynx, neck, or shoulders.

Teeth covered with sordes.

· Swelling of gums, they bleed and ulcerate.
[11] **Tongue, etc.** Taste: sweetish, or fatty; almost lost. .
Tingling, itching on the tongue, must scratch it.
[12] **Mouth.** Musty, bad odor from mouth.
Small ulcers in mouth.
Saliva increased, although mouth may feel dry.
Sensation of soreness in mouth.
[13] **Throat.** Pressure in throat as from a plug, with soreness
and dryness.
Sensation of swelling in the sides of the throat.
Tightness from pharynx down to stomach, as if food
could not pass.
Pharynx looks dry, glazed and red.
Great dryness of throat, especially on awaking, voice
husky; sneezing, hawking, and sensation of lump in
throat.
Feeling of splinter in throat.
Copious, thick, tenacious mucus in throat, evening and
morning.
Thick mucus, dropping from posterior nares. See 25.
Ulcers in fauces, spongy; secreting a yellowish-brown,
badly-smelling pus; with boring pains from fauces to
right temple and head.
[14] **Desires. Aversions.** Longing for fruit and vegetables,
potatoes disagree.
Aversion to meat; to beer.
Thirst all day.
Appetite for starch, chalk; clean, white rags; charcoal,
cloves, acids, coffee or tea-grounds, dry rice, and other
indigestible things.
[15] **Eating and Drinking.** ❙ Worse from eating potatoes. See 16.
Worse from tobacco smoke.
All irritating things, like salt, wine, vinegar, pepper, etc.,
immediately start cough.
Throat sore after using onions in food.
Easily drunken from the weakest spirituous drinks.
Mucus in throat, tasting sweet, after dinner.
[16] **Nausea and Vomiting.** Eructations: sour; bitter, after
potatoes; worse evenings.
Heartburn.
Nausea, with chilliness, pale face, desire to lie down, faint-
ness; better after breakfast.
Mucous vomit.
[17] **Stomach.** Constriction and twisting in the stomach, extend-
ing up the œsophagus to the throat.
Stitches in pit of stomach, extending upwards to chest.
Drawing or oppressive pain going upward to chest and
throat.

[18] **Hypochondria.** Liver pains as if bruised, when stooping; stitches when rising again.

Tearing from the liver to hip.

Shooting pain in the region of the spleen.

[19] **Abdomen.** Abdomen seems to hang down heavily, like a load, when walking afternoons.

Reaching too high strains the abdominal muscles.

Pains worse sitting bent.

Pressing in both groins, toward sexual organs, evenings.

Stitching, pressing pain in region of abdominal ring, like from hernia.

Flatulent colic; **ı** painter's colic.

Colic in the morning.

[20] **Stool, etc.** **ı** Inactivity of the rectum; even the soft stool requires great straining.

ı No desire for and no ability to pass stool, until there is a large accumulation.

ı Stools: hard, dry and knotty; like sheep's dung, with cutting in anus, followed by blood.

Constipation of sucklings.

Diarrhœa; with urging in rectum; **ı** when she urinates.

Clots of blood pass from the anus.

Hemorrhoids worse in evening, better after night's rest.

Itching and burning at the anus; fistula ani.

Perineum: pressure when blowing the nose; sweats and is tender to touch.

[21] **Urine.** Pains in the kidneys, in alternation with a cloudiness, as if drunken.

Tenesmus vesicæ.

ı Urine voided while straining at stool, or cannot pass urine without such straining.

Urine: scanty with red sediment, in arthritic affections; copious and pale, in nervous diseases; with thick, white sediment; more frequent, copious and dark.

Feeling of weakness in bladder and genitals in the evening, with fear that he will wet the bed.

[22] **Male Sexual Organs.** Excessive sexual desire.

Involuntary emissions, followed by all his old symptoms.

Left testicle hard and very painful.

Tickling on the genitals and thighs.

[23] **Female Sexual Organs.** Menses: too early, short, scanty and of pale blood; too early, preceded by headache; delay, finally appear, being pale and scanty.

Leucorrhœa: acrid, corrosive; acrid, profuse, relieved by cold washing; transparent, profuse, during the day.

Painful throbbing in left side of vagina.

Stitches in left side of vulva, extending up to chest.

[24] **Pregnancy.** Gastric and abdominal symptoms during pregnancy.

[25] **Larynx.** Sensation of tightly adhering phlegm in the larynx, not removed by hawking or cough; wheezing on inspiration.

Tickling in larynx, with irritation to cough.

Rawness in larynx on awaking.

Sudden complete aphonia.

Hoarseness evening and night, especially toward morning.

Voice: has a nasal twang; husky and thick.   See 13.

[26] **Breathing.** Rattling, asthmatic breathing, worse coughing.

Oppression worse when sitting stooped; better straightening up or walking in open air.

Talking or singing makes him cough.

Breathing arrested by copious, thick, tenacious, saltish mucus.

[27] **Cough.**   Cough: dry, hacking, with frequent sneezing; from sensation as of loose skin hanging in throat; from elongated uvula; from talking or singing; short; causes pains in right temple and top of head, sometimes also difficult breathing; soon after waking in the morning; every morning a long attack of dry cough, ending in difficult raising of a little white mucus; with tearing pain and involuntary emission of urine, in old or withered looking people.

[28] **Lungs.**   Violent, oppressive pain in chest, worse at night.

Chest feels constricted, worse from sitting bent or stooping, better on straightening up or on walking.

Congestion of blood to chest and head, with redness of face and one ear, caused by suppressed hemorrhoidal flux.

Shooting stitches right to left in the afternoon, worse on going down stairs.

Talking increases soreness of chest; lifting aggravates or produces soreness in left chest.

Riding in a carriage gives pain in chest.

[29] **Heart.   Pulse.**   Awakes with palpitation.

Palpitation irregular, large and small beats intermix.

Pulse either unchanged or full and accelerated.

[31] **Neck.   Back.**   Shooting in right side of neck, posterior portion.

Pain in the back and small of back as if beaten.

Pain in back as if a hot iron were thrust through lower vertebræ.

Violent stitch in the middle of the back.

Gnawing pain in the back.

[32] **Upper Limbs.**   Pain, as from a sprain, in shoulder-joint, especially on raising the arm.

Sense of tightness in the arm, like from cold.

Burning on the arms and fingers, and in the left elbow, like from a glowing iron.

Arms feel heavy, as if paralyzed; go to sleep.

Rhagades worse in winter and from washing.

Nails brittle or thick.

Panaritium, with brittle nails, lancinating pains and tendeney to ulceration of the finger tips.

³³ **Lower Limbs.**   Nates go to sleep when sitting.

Great heaviness in the lower limbs, can scarcely drag them; when walking he staggers, and must sit down; evenings.

Burning and smarting-itching on the thighs, better from scratching.

Tearing in the knees and patellæ, or from knee to toes.

Numbness of the heel when stepping.

Pain in the sole of the foot on stepping, as though it were too soft and swollen.

Itching and redness of the toes.

³⁴ **Limbs in General.**   Arms and legs feel heavy.

Frequent stretching of limbs when sitting.

Trembling of the limbs.

Jerking and twitching of the limbs.

³⁵ **Position, etc.**   Better from moderate exercise in the open air.

Feels moderately well at night, but cannot lie on right side, on account of cough.

Motion of jaw: 9, 10.   Raising arm: 32.   Reaching: 19. Stepping: 3, 33.   Walking: 19, 26, 28, 33.   Going up stairs: 3.   Going down stairs: 28.   Sitting: 3, 19, 21, 34. Must sit down: 36. Sitting stooped: 26, 28. Standing: 3.   Stooping: 2, 28.   Straightening body up: 28.

³⁶ **Nerves.**   Much fatigued by talking.

❙ Faint and tired, must sit or lie down.

Involuntary movements of single parts.   ❙ Impaired co-ordination.

Spasms, with attacks of laughing and weeping; ❙ sudden jerks, starts from sleep; paralytic weakness; obstinate spastic anæmia.

Paralysis from spinal disease.

Rheumatic and traumatic paralysis in gouty persons.

³⁷ **Sleep.**   Sleepiness, with inclination to lie down.

Restless sleep, turns frequently, feels too warm, lies uncovered in unrefreshing slumber, with many dreams and frequent awaking.

Restless sleep, always awaking with palpitation of heart.

Dreams: anxious; of boat foundering; of ghosts; of thieves; confused.

³⁸ **Time.**   Morning: 1, 5, 13, 16, 19, 20, 27.   Afternoon: 19, 28. Evening: 4, 5, 6, 7, 10, 13, 16, 19, 20, 21, 25, 33, 40. Night: 5, 6, 24, 25, 28, 40.   Toward morning: 25. Day: 5, 23, 40.

[39] **Temperature and Weather.** Generally better in warmth, worse in cold air, out-doors.

Worse in-doors, while sitting.

Better walking, out doors, in mild weather.

Warmth in bed: 46. Open air: 3, 5, 10, 26. Winter: 32, 41. Cold washing: 23, 32.

[40] **Chill. Fever. Sweat.** Chill, with great thirst.

Internal chill and shivering, with desire for warmth of stove, with stretching and bending of limbs, worse after warm drink.

Chill during the day, heat at night.

Heat at night, with anxiety and sweat.

Heat in the evening, commencing in and spreading from the face, sometimes of only the right side.

Sweat at night, toward morning most profuse in face, frequently only on right side of face.

Entire inability to sweat.

[41] **Attacks.** At intervals sudden sharp pains, like a stab.

Worse new and full moon, skin symptoms.

Worse in winter, skin symptoms.

[42] **Sides.** Right: 18, 27, 31, 40. Left: 18, 22, 23, 28, 32. Right to left: 28. Below—upward: 13, 17, 23.

Upper left and lower right side most affected.

[43] **Sensations.** Sensation of constriction of internal organs.

Some parts of body feel larger.

Some parts—lower jaw and arms—feel shorter.

[44] **Tissues.** Emaciation; spare habit, and old people.

[45] **Contact, Injuries, etc.** Touch: 7, 20. Pressure of foot on ground: 33. Scratching: 11, 33. Riding in carriage: 28.

[46] **Skin.** Intolerable itching of whole body, especially when getting warm and in bed: scratches until the skin bleeds, which is then painful; itching and formication with flatulence, dry stools or diarrhœa.

Eruptions humid, scabby, sore, gnawing.

Ulcerated surface secretes yellow-brown, badly smelling pus.

Blood-boils: 8. Rhagades: 32. Bulbous excrescences: 8.

[47] **Stages and States.** Infancy: constipation, especially when artificial food is used.

Cholera infantum, stools green, acidity of primæ viæ.

❙ Constipation of sucklings.

Strasbismus.

Puberty: chlorosis, with longing for indigestible substances.

Dark complexion, excitable.

Mild disposition.

Lack of animal heat.

Spare habit.

Old people, hypochondriacal.

[48] **Relationship.** Similar to: *Bar. carb.* (hypochondriasis of aged; constipation); *Bryon.* (peevish, irritable; gastric and abdominal symptoms; constipation; throbbing headache; dry cough with vomiting; stitches in chest; dryness of mucous surfaces; fever, etc.); *Calc. ostr.; Chamom.* (useful as an intermediate remedy); *Conium* (old people; loss of power of internal recti of eyes); *Ferrum* (chlorosis; relaxed abdomen; disgust for meat, etc.); *Ferr. jod.* (profuse, transparent leucorrhœa); *Graphit.* (chlorosis; skin rough, chapped, itching; nails, blepharitis, etc.); *Ipec.; Laches.* (sad on waking; climaxis); *Pulsat.* (tearful, peevish; head, etc.; better in open air; ozæna; taste lost; averse to meat; chlorosis; scanty menses; complaints at puberty; lack of animal heat; soles of feet sore, worse walking; toes red, itching, etc.); *Plumbum* (colic; constipation, etc.); *Ruta* (loss of power of internal recti of eyes); *Sepia* (irritable, tearful; ozæna; scanty menses; puberty; prolapsus uteri; inactive rectum; weakness in urinary organs, etc.); *Silic.; Sulphur; Zincum* (inner canthus; granular lids).

Compare with the following in clergyman's sore throat: *Arg. nitr., Kali bich., Lycop.,* etc.

Alum. follows *Bryon., Laches., Sulphur;* and is followed by *Bryon.*

Alum. and *Bryon.* are complementary.

Chamom. is useful as an intermediate remedy.

Antidotes to *Alum.: Bryon:, Camphor, Chamom., Ipec.*

Alum. antidotes: lead poisoning, as in painter's colic; ailments from lead.

AMBRA.

Ambergris.   *Introduced by Hahnemann.*

[1] **Mind.** Memory impaired.

Comprehension slow, has to read everything three or four times, and then does not understand it.

Is not able to reflect upon anything properly, feels stupid.

Confusion of the head.

Difficult thinking in the morning.   θ Old people.

Distorted images, grimaces, diabolical faces crowd upon his fancy.

She is excited, loquacious; talking fatigues her; was unable to sleep at night.

Melancholy; great sadness; despair; melancholy following excessive mental excitation.

Fears of becoming crazy.

Anguish and sweat all over, at night.

[2] **Sensorium.** Had to lie down on account of vertigo and feeling of weakness in the stomach.

Music causes the blood to rush to the head.

[3] **Inner Head.** Pressure in forehead, with fear of becoming crazy.

Tearing: in forehead; in left temple up to the vertex; in right frontal eminence and behind the left ear.

Extremely painful tearing on top of head and apparently in whole upper half of brain, with paleness of face and coldness of left hand.

Pressive-drawing ascending from nape of neck, and extending through head towards forehead, considerable oppression remaining in lower part of occiput.

Dulness in the occiput.

Tearing pains predominate in the head.

[4] **Outer Head.** Falling off of the hair.

On the right side of the head, a spot, where the hair when touched pains, as if sore.

[5] **Eyes.** Dulness of vision, like looking through a mist.

Pressure and smarting in eyes, as from dust; lachrymation.

Pressure on eyes, which are difficult to open, and pain in them as if they had been closed too firmly, particularly in the morning.

Itching on the eyelid as if a stye were forming.

[6] **Ears.** Roaring and whistling in the ears, in the afternoon.

Crackling in left ear (like the sound made when winding a watch).

Hearing decreases; with cold sensation of abdomen.

Violent tearing pain in and behind right auricle.

Tearing in the right ear.

Crawling; itching and tickling in the ears.

Music aggravates cough.

Listening to music brings on congestion to head.

[7] **Nose.** Nosebleed, particularly in the morning.

Dried blood collects in the nose.

Nose stuffed up, paining as if sore, internally.

Long-continued dryness of nose, frequent irritation, as from sneezing.

[8] **Face.** Flushes of heat in the face.

Tearing in upper part of face, particularly near right ala nasi.

Pimples, and itching in the whiskers.

Painful swelling of cheek on upper jaw, with throbbing in gums.

Jaundiced color of face.

⁹ **Lower Face.** Lips hot.

Lips numb and dry in the morning on awaking.

¹⁰ **Teeth.** Drawing pain now in one and again in another tooth; increased by warmth, momentarily removed by cold; not aggravated by chewing and passes off after a meal; at the same time the inner portion of the gums was swollen.

Bleeding of the gums.

¹¹ **Tongue, etc.** Bitter taste in mouth in morning on awaking.

Sour taste after drinking milk.

Folds pain as if sore under the tongue, like small growths.

ı Ranula.

¹² **Mouth.** Fetor of the mouth, worse mornings. θ Pertussis.

Blisters in the mouth, pain as if burnt.

Smarting and cracked painful condition of the mouth.

¹³ **Throat.** Tearing pain in palate, extending into left ear.

Dryness of the throat in the morning.

Sore feeling in the throat during empty deglutition, and from outward pressure, not when swallowing food, with tension of the glands of the throat as if swollen.

Sore throat after exposure to a draught of air; stitching from the throat into the right ear, and pains particularly from motion of the tongue.

¹⁴ **Desires. Aversions.** Thirstlessness.

¹⁵ **Eating and Drinking.** Aggravation from warm drinks, especially from warm milk. Better after eating : 40.

¹⁶ **Nausea and Vomiting.** Eructations either empty, sour or bitter.

Heartburn: with abortive eructations; when walking in the open air; from drinking milk.

Every evening, sensation as of spoiled stomach and acrid risings up to the larynx.

Nausea after breakfast.

¹⁷ **Stomach.** Pressure and burning under the scrobiculum; belching removes it.

Pressure in the stomach and hypochondria.

Tension and pressure, or stitches and pressure in the stomach.

¹⁸ **Hypochondria.** Pressing pain in a small spot in the upper right side of the abdomen, though not felt to touch.

Tearing pain in the region of the spleen.

¹⁹ **Abdomen.** Distended abdomen; accumulation of much flatus, which subsides without being passed.

ı Sensation of coldness in the abdomen.

Coldness of one side of the abdomen.

Colic, sometimes followed by diarrhœa.

²⁰ **Stool, etc.** First copious, soft, light brown stools, after a few days, constipation.

Stool not hard, though large.

Frequent ineffectual desire for stool, this makes her very anxious, ❙ at this time the presence of other persons becomes unbearable.

Large flow of blood with the stool.

Itching in the anus; stitches.

²¹ **Urine.** Frequent micturition at night.

Urine when emitted is clouded, yellowish-brown, and deposits a brownish sediment, after which urine looks clear and yellow.

Sour-smelling urine. *θ* Whooping cough.

Urinates three times as much as the drink taken, especially in morning; followed by a dull pain in region of kidneys.

Sensation as if a few drops passed through the urethra.

²² **Male Sexual Organs.** Internal, strong, voluptuous sensation in the genital organs; nocturnal pollutions.

Itching pimple over the male genitals.

²³ **Female Sexual Organs.** Stitches in ovarian region, when drawing in the abdomen or pressing upon it.

❙ Discharge of blood between periods, at every little accident, as after every hard stool or after a walk a little longer than usual.

During the menses, the left leg becomes quite blue from distended varices, with pressive pain in the leg.

Thick, mucous leucorrhœa, increased from day to day, or leucorrhœa, at night, of bluish-white mucus; preceding each discharge, a stitch in the vagina.

Lying down aggravates the uterine symptoms.

Severe itching on the pudenda, must rub the parts.

Soreness and itching, with swelling of the labia.

²⁵ **Larynx.** Tickling in the throat, exciting cough.

Hoarseness and roughness of the voice, with accumulation of thick, tough mucus, easily thrown off by coughing.

Itching, scraping and soreness in the larynx and trachea.

Reading aloud or talking aggravates the cough.

²⁶ **Breathing.** Tightness of the chest, cannot take a deep breath or yawn fully.

Oppression felt in the chest and between the scapulæ.

Feeling of pressure in chest, worse during exhalation.

Asthma of old people and of children.

²⁷ **Cough.** Paroxysms of cough coming from deep in the chest, excited by violent tickling in the throat, evening without, morning with expectoration, generally of greyish-white, seldom of yellow mucus, of salty or sour taste, and often in large quantities.

❙ Violent spasmodic cough, with frequent eructations and hoarseness.

- Lifting a heavy weight aggravates the cough.
28 **Lungs.** Sensation of pressure deep in right chest; also in left chest or in upper part of chest.
Sensation of rawness in the chest.
Itching in the chest and thyroid gland.
29 **Heart. Pulse.** Anxiety at the heart, causing oppression of breathing, with flushes of heat.
Palpitation when walking in open air, with paleness of face.
Violent palpitation, with pressure in chest, as if a lump laid there, or as if chest was stuffed up.
Pulse accelerated, with ebullitions.
30 **Outer Chest.** Burning on the chest.
31 **Neck. Back.** Pressive, drawing pain in nape of neck.
Tearing in the left, or in both shoulders.
Rheumatic pains in the right side of the back.
Painful tension in the lumbar muscles.
32 **Upper Limbs.** Tearing in the left shoulder-joint.
Drawing, and as if sprained and lame in the shoulder.
Arms "go to sleep" during day, when at rest, as well as during night; numbness of left arm; tingling in thumb.
Tearing pains in the shoulder, elbow, forearm and hand.
Weakness of the fingers at night.
Long-lasting icy-coldness of the hands.
Stinging in the hands and fingers, like from insects.
Drawing in the fingers and thumb.
Itching in the palms of hands.
Cramp in hands sometimes when taking hold of anything.
Tips of the fingers are shrivelled.
Tearing, lancinating or itching, in tips of fingers and thumb.
33 **Lower Limbs.** Tearing pain, first in left, then in right hip-joint.
Sensation of contraction in (right) thigh, the limb seems to be shortened.
Tearing in nates, hip, knee, leg, ankle and foot.
Heaviness of the legs.
Sensation as if "gone to sleep" in both legs; has no firm step.
Cramp in the legs and in the calves nearly every night.
Cold feet.
Gouty pain in ball of great toes.
Itching on inner border of sole of the right foot, not relieved by scratching.
34 **Limbs in General.** Tearing or rheumatic pains, in parts of all the limbs.
Uncommon twitching in all the limbs and coldness of the body, at night.

Uneasiness, like a crawling, with anxiety, only by day.

Weariness, with painful soreness of all the limbs.

[35] **Position, etc.** Lying: 23. Must lie down: 2, 36. In bed, early in morning, weakness. Exercise: 40. Walking: 23; in open air: 16, 29. Motion of tongue: 13. Desire to bend and stretch limbs. Lifting heavy weights, 27.

[36] **Nerves.** ▮ Spasms and twitches in the muscular parts; ofte in nervous affections.

Arms and limbs "go to sleep" easily.

Great lassitude.

Hemiplegia, left side.

Weakness: of the whole body; of the knees, as if they would give way; of the feet, with loss of sensation; in the stomach, so that she must lie down.

[37] **Sleep.** Cannot sleep at night, yet knows not why.

Restless sleep, with anxious dreams.

Vexatious, anxious dreams and talking in sleep.

[38] **Time.** Morning: 5, 7, 9, 11, 12, 13, 21, 27, 34. Forenoon: 40. Afternoon: 6. Evening: 27, 40. Night: 1, 21, 23, 32, 33, 34, 37, 40. After midnight: 40. Day, 34. Day and night: 32. Every quarter hour: 40.

[39] **Temperature and Weather.** Warmth: 10. Cold: 10. Open air: 16. Draught of air: 13. Worse during the spring.

[40] **Chill. Fever. Sweat.** Chill in the forenoon, with lassitude and sleepiness, relieved by eating.

Chill of single parts of the body, with heat of the face.

Anxious flushes of heat returning every quarter hour, most violent towards evening.

Profuse sweat at night, worse after midnight and most on the affected side.

Profuse sweat, particularly on the abdomen and thighs, during exercise.

[41] **Attacks.** ▮ Cough in spasmodic paroxysms.

[42] **Sides.** Right: 3, 4, 6, 8, 13, 18, 28, 31, 33. Left: 3, 6, 13, 18, 23, 28, 31, 32. Left to right: 33. Behind forwards: 3.

[44] **Tissues.** Tearing in muscles and joints, often on one side.

Softening of the brain.

Emaciation.

[45] **Contact, Injuries, etc.** Soreness of parts after rubbing. Touch: 4. Chewing: 10. Scratching: 33. Pressure: 13, 23.

[46] **Skin.** Burning in the skin.

The tips of fingers become wrinkled.

Soreness of a wart on the finger.

Itch eruption is reproduced by it (*Ambra*).

Numbness of the skin.

Burning herpes.

[47] **Stages and States.** ❙ In old age.   θ Asthma.   θ Colds.
The so-called bilious or nervous-bilious temperament.

[48] **Relationship.**   Similar to *Arsen.* (cardiac asthma); *Act. rac.*
(night cough); *Castor.; Asaf.* (women who are nervous
and fail to react); *Coca* (embarrassed, bashful); *Coffea;*
Cinchon.; Ignat.

Kali brom. (increase of reflex action); *Moschus* (hysteric
asthma); *Nux vom.* (both suit nervous, thin, bilious persons); *Opium; Phosphor.* (asthma; nervous excitability;
"irritable weakness;" slender build, etc.); *Phosph. ac.;*
Pulsat.; Sepia; Staphis.; Sulphur; Sulph. ac. (cough and
belching); *Valer.* (nervousness, hysteria; lack of reaction
in nervous weakness); *Laches.* and *Sepia* (worse from
overlifting); *Laches., Ver. alb.* (cough with belching;
coldness, etc.).

Antidotes to *Ambra: Camphor, Coffea, Nux vom., Pulsat.,*
Staphis.

Ambra antidotes: *Staphis.* (especially the voluptuous itching of scrotum); *Nux vom.*

AMMONIUM CARBONICUM.

Smelling Salts.   HAHNEMANN. $2NH_4O, 3CO_2$.

[1] **Mind.** Forgetful, makes mistakes in writing and speaking.
Absent-minded.
Confusion and dulness of the head.
Aversion to work, not disposed for anything.
Gloomy, depressed, with feeling of impending trouble,
with sensation of coldness.
Anxious concern about one's sickness.
Anxiety, with inclination to weep.
Hearing others talk, or talking himself, affects him.

[2] **Sensorium.**   Frequent giddiness, as if the surroundings
were turning with him in a circle, in the morning after
rising, lasting the whole day, worse in evening; also at
night, when moving the head.
Congestion of blood to the head at night and when awaking, heat of the face.

[3] **Inner Head.**   Headache: in the morning in bed, with nausea and risings in throat, as if to vomit; in the morning,
but worse in the afternoon.
Boring, stitching headache at night.
Headache, thrusts in the forehead, as if it would burst.
Pulsating, beating and pressing in forehead, as if it would
6

burst; worse after eating; while walking in open air; better from pressure; in warm room.

Stitches in various parts of the head.

Tearing: in whole head; in temples; back of left ear, ascending to vertex.

Sensation of looseness of the brain; as if brain fell to the side toward which he leaned.

⁴ **Outer Head.** Drawing pain in periosteum of forehead, wakens from sleep in morning, passes off after rising.

Severe itching of the scalp, especially on the occiput.

Sensation as if hair would stand on end, with crawling and cold feeling on head, after coming into room from open air.

Scalp, even the hair, painful to touch.

⁵ **Eyes.** Double vision.

Aversion to light, with burning in eyes.

Optical illusions, particularly in white or bright colors.

Large black spot floats before eyes after sewing.

Cataract of the right eye.

Pressure on eyelids, that he cannot open them, even though internally awake.

Pressure, cutting and stitching in the eyes.

Smarting in the eyes and itching on the margin of lids.

Stye on the right upper eyelid, with tension.

Inflammation of the eyes; vision obscured.

Eyes bloodshot, with lachrymation.

⁶ **Ears.** Hard hearing; ear itches and discharges pus.

Humming before the ears.

Itching above the ears, spreads over the whole body.

Hard swelling of the right parotid gland.

Painful sensitiveness of the dull ear to loud noise.

⁷ **Nose.** When stooping, blood rushes to tip of nose.

❙ Nosebleed: when washing face in morning; after dinner.

Bloody mucus blown from nose frequently.

Burning water runs from the nose.

❙ Stoppage, mostly at night, must breathe through the mouth, with long-lasting coryza.

⁸ **Face.** Heat in face: with red cheeks; during mental exertion; during and after dinner.

Redness of left cheek.

Pale face, bloated.

Hard swelling of cheek, also of the parotid and cervical glands.

Pustulous eruption on forehead, cheeks, chin.

Small boils and indurations, emitting water and blood, on the cheek, at the corner of the mouth, and on the chin.

Freckles.

⁹ **Lower Face.** Herpetic eruption around the mouth.

Itching eruption on the lips.

Upper lip pains, as if cracked.

Lower lip cracked in the middle, bleeding and burning.

Painful burning blister on inside of the lower lip.

Blueness of the lips.

10 **Teeth.** Feel too long, too dull.

Violent toothache, evenings, immediately on going to bed.

Stitching pain in molars when biting, can use incisors only.

Drawing toothache during catamenia, better from eating; worse from warm fluids.

Sensation as of an ulcer at the root of a tooth.

Teeth fall out.

Gums very sensitive; bleed easily.

11 **Tongue, etc.** Taste: sweetish; of blood; offensive; bitter; of food, sourish or metallic.

Painful vesicles on the tongue.

Talking difficult at times, like from weakness of the parts, also from pain.

12 **Mouth.** Redness and inflammation of inner mouth and gullet; pain as if raw.

Sensation as if the mouth were swollen.

Great dryness of mouth and throat.

Much saliva must be ejected.

13 **Throat.** Pain in throat, as if the right tonsil were swollen when swallowing.

Enlarged tonsils, bluish, much offensive mucus there.

Sensation as if something had lodged in throat, impeding deglutition.

Burning pain in throat.

Putrid sore throat.

Tendency to gangrenous ulceration of tonsils.

14 **Desires. Aversions.** Continual thirst, no appetite.

Appetite: only for bread and cold food; for sweets.

Great hunger and appetite, yet a small quantity satiates.

15 **Eating and Drinking.** Cannot eat (noon) without drinking.

Worse during eating; heat in face, headache, nausea and prostration.

Worse after eating; nausea, pressure in stomach and forehead; speech becomes difficult.

16 **Nausea and Vomiting.** Hiccough, morning after the chill.

Eructations: empty; imperfect; taste of the food; sour.

Heartburn.

Nausea and vomiting of all that has been eaten; afterwards sour taste in mouth.

17 **Stomach.** Feels full, trembling.

Empty feeling in stomach.

Pressure in stomach after eating, or at night the clothes feel oppressive.

Heat in stomach, spreading through the bowels.

Pain in stomach, with tendency to water-brash.

18 **Hypochondria.** Pressure or sore feeling in right hypochondrium.

Stitches in left hypochondrium.

Splenic affections.

19 **Abdomen.** Pressure above the navel, like from a button.

Pressive pain in the left side of abdomen.

Sudden painful contraction of the bowels, extending to the epigastrium; better from pressure; on lying down it ceases.

Cutting pain, with retraction of abdominal walls.

Colic and pain between the scapulæ.

Stitches through the abdomen.

Elastic swelling (size of a fist) in the left groin, evenings; bruised pain therein; cannot lie on left side; on awaking, both swelling and pain gone.

20 **Stool, etc.** Painful diarrhœa.

Stool of feces and mucus.

Stools at first retarded, later soft.

Costiveness on account of hardness of feces.

Discharge of blood before and after stool.

Discharge of prostatic fluid after stool.

Protrusion of hemorrhoids after stool, with long-lasting pains, cannot walk; protrude also independent of the stool.

Burning at anus, prevents sleep at night; must rise from bed on account of this and tenesmus.

Itching at anus.

21 **Urine.** Pressure of urine on the bladder, with cutting pain.

Frequent urination at night; involuntary, in sleep towards morning.

Pale urine, with sandy sediment; whitish sediment.

22 **Male Sexual Organs.** Forcing (würgend) pain in the testicles and seminal cords; sensitiveness of testicles to touch, aggravated by erections.

Testicles and scrotum relaxed, necessitating a supporter.

Erections without sexual desire, mornings.

Violent sexual desire, almost without erections.

Seminal emissions almost every night.

Itching of the genitals.

23 **Female Sexual Organs.** Menses: premature, abundant, preceded by griping, colic, and want of appetite; too late, scanty and short; blackish, in clots, and passing off with pain in abdomen; acrid, makes the thighs sore; very slightly colored; copious at night, and when sitting and driving.

ı Cholera-like symptoms at the beginning of catamenia.

Leucorrhœa: watery, burning, from the uterus; acrid, profuse from the vagina.

Violent tearing in abdomen and vagina.

Swelling, itching and burning of the pudendum; with leucorrhœa.

25 **Larynx.** Hoarseness, cannot speak a loud word; aggravation from speaking; great dryness.

Larynx as if drawn shut from both sides of the throat.

26 **Breathing.** Great difficulty of breathing in going up even a few steps; less in the open air.

Dares not come into a warm room, in which he becomes deathly pale, and can do nothing but sit quiet.

Difficult breathing; causing short cough.

ı Asphyxia imminent in the course of a disease.

Shortness of breath and palpitation after every exertion.

ı Emphysema.

27 **Cough.** Cough: at night, about midnight, violent, about 3 or 4 A. M.; dry, particularly at night, like from "feather down" in throat; short, asthmatic, from irritation in larynx, with painful sensation of spasmodic contraction of chest.

Cough: with asthma, evening in bed; each time with stitch in scrobiculum.

28 **Lungs.** Burning in the chest.

Stitches in right chest: when stooping; when walking; when raising up in bed.

Stitches in left chest, prevent lying on left side.

Lower part of chest most affected.

29 **Heart. Pulse.** Frequent palpitation, with contraction of epigastrium and weak feeling in the pit of stomach.

Audible palpitation, with attacks of great anxiety, as if dying; cold sweat; involuntary flow of tears; unable to speak; loud, difficult breathing and trembling of hands. *θ* Angina pectoris.

Pulse hard, tense, frequent.

30 **Outer Chest.** Right mamma painful to touch.

Small pimple on the sternum; when touched feels as if a splinter was therein.

Red rash on chest.

31 **Neck. Back.** Lymphatic glands swollen.

Violent pain in small of back, with great coldness.

Pressive, drawing pain in small of back and loins, only when at rest, during the day; passing off when walking.

Stitches at the coccyx, where before there was itching.

32 **Upper Limbs.** Axillary glands painful and swollen.

Tearing, also bruised pains in the shoulder.

Weight and lameness in right arm; has no power in it, must let it hang; hand swollen.

Cramp in right arm, drawing it backward.
Cracking of elbow-joint when moved.
Boring pain in the olecranon depression.
Itching eruption on inside of the right forearm.
Pain in wrist; in back of hands; in fingers and thumbs.
Trembling of hands.
Cracking of skin of hands; peeling of skin from palms.
Hands look blue and veins distended, after washing in
    cold water.
  ▮ Inflammation of finger ends, whitlow.

³³ **Lower Limbs.** Restlessness in the legs.
Great weakness and languor of lower limbs.
Soreness between the limbs of children.
Violent pain in the hip-joint when walking.
Blue spot, with great burning, above the knee.
Boring and drawing pains in the knees.
Leg frequently "goes to sleep" when sitting or standing,
    also when lying on it at night.
Cramp in the leg.
Severe pain in the heels when awaking in the morning,
    as if ulcerated to the bone.
Heel hurts when standing or walking much, as if fester-
    ing; sometimes suppuration.
Tearing in ankle and bones of feet, ceases when warm in
    bed.
Cold feet, particularly when going to bed.
Trembling of the feet.
Ball of the great toe painful.
The great toe becomes red, swollen and painful, particu-
    larly in bed, evenings.

³⁴ **Limbs in General.** Pain in all the limbs at night, with
    gnawing pain in small of back.
Inclination to stretch the limbs.

³⁵ **Position, etc.** Dislikes to move.
Rest: 31. Lying: 19, 33. Must sit quiet: 26. Sitting:
    33. Standing: 33. Moving: 2, 32. Stooping: 7, 28.
    Raising up: 28. Rising: 4. Walking: 3 (in open air),
    28, 31, 33. Ascending: 26. Exertion: 26.

³⁶ **Nerves.** Debility: must lie down; and soreness of the
    whole body.

³⁷ **Sleep.** Must sleep in the afternoon, or the eyes pain.
Restless, unrefreshing sleep; tosses about.
Frequent, violent starting out of sleep, with great fear
    afterward.
Nightmare every night, sometimes in a sweat when awak-
    ing. θ Heart disease.
Somnolence, with blood over-carbonized.
Dreams: vivid; romantic; lewd; anxious; of danger and

want; of ghosts; of dying; of dead persons; offensive; of lice; of scolding.

Talks during sleep.

⁸⁸ Time.   Morning: 2, 3, 4, 7, 16, 21, 22, 33, 40. Afternoon: 37. Evening: 2, 10, 27, 33, 40. Day: 31, 40. Night: 2, 7, 17, 20, 21, 22, 27, 33, 34, 37, 40.   After midnight: 27.

³⁹ Temperature and Weather.   In wet, stormy weather, ill-humor, etc.

Very sensitive to cold air, out-doors.

Open air: 26, 40.   Warm room: 3, 26, 40.   Warm in bed: 33, 43.   Coming in room from open air: 4.   Washing: 7, 32.

Children dislike washing.   Worse from wet poultices.

⁴⁰ Chill.   Fever.   Sweat.   Chill evening; frequently alternating with heat, till toward midnight.

Chill increased in open air, lessened in warm room.

Heat, evening, particularly of the face; with cold feet.

Hectic fever.   θ Scurvy.

Sweat in the morning, mostly at the joints.

Sweat on lower part of body.

Continuous day or night-sweat.

⁴¹ Attacks.   Worse during new moon.

⁴² Sides.   Right: 5, 6, 13, 18, 28, 30, 32.   Left: 3, 8, 18, 19, 28.

⁴³ Sensations.   Drawing tension, as from shortening of the muscles.

Pain as if joints were sprained.

Tearing in joints, better in warmth of bed.

Pain as from festering under the skin.

⁴⁴ Tissues.   Hemorrhage from nose, gums and bowels.

Muscles soft and flabby, emaciation.   θ Scurvy.

Tendency to gangrenous degeneration of the parts.   θ Inflammation of vulva.

⁴⁵ Contact, Injuries, etc.   Touch: 4, 30.   Pressure: 3, 10, 19. Scratching: 46.

⁴⁶ Skin.   Violent itching; after scratching, burning blisters appear.

Itching lessened by scratching.

Upper half of body as red as scarlet.

❙ Malignant scarlatina, with somnolence, starting from sleep; dark red or putrid sore throat; sticky salivation; parotitis; external throat swollen; stertorous breathing; involuntary stools with excessive vomiting; body red, with miliary rash, or faintly developed eruption; threatened paralysis of brain.

Erysipelas of old people when cerebral symptoms are developed; while the eruption is still out, debility and soreness of the whole body; tendency to gangrenous destruction.

Sometimes relieves the nightly pains of felons.

Desquamation; receding scarlatina.

[47] **Stages and States.** Scrofulous children.

Stout women, who led a sedentary life, have various troubles in consequence, and readily catch cold in winter.

Erysipelas of old people.

[48] **Relationship.** Similar to its relatives, *Amm. mur.*, *Amm. phosph.*, etc., and to: *Ant. tart.* (emphysema, etc.; blood poisoned with carbonic acid); *Arnic.; Arsen.* (inflammations); *Aurum* (heart); *Apis* (scarlatina, miliaria; burning-stinging); *Bellad.; Coccul.* (muscular asthenopia); *Calc. ostr.* (parotitis in scarlatina; pale, flabby, etc.); *Hepar; Kali bichr.; Kali carb.; Laches.* (erysipelas); *Lauroc.; Natr. mur.* (muscular asthenopia); *Phosphor.; Pulsat.; Rhus tox.* (rash, scarlatina with parotitis, etc.); *Ruta* (muscular asthenopia); *Staphis.; Sulphur; Veratr.* (cholera-like symptoms during menses).

The presence of miliary rash may distinguish it from the sometimes similar *Bellad.* in scarlatina.

Inimical to *Laches.*

Antidote to: poisoning with *Rhus tox.;* stings of insects.

Antidoted by: *Arnic., Camphor., Hepar;* vegetable acids, fixed oils, as castor, linseed, almond and olive oils.

AMMONIUM MURIATICUM.

Sal Ammoniæ. NENNING. *Ammonium chloride, N H 4 Cl.*

[1] **Mind.** Desire to cry, and at times crying.

Disinclination to speak.

Involuntary aversion to certain persons.

Great earnestness.

Apprehensive and gloomy, like from internal grief.

Irritability or bad humor, mostly mornings.

[2] **Sensorium.** Vertigo and fulness of head; at times as if she would fall sideways.

[3] **Inner Head.** Heaviness in forehead, frequently during the day (internal sensation of heat and some sweat).

Pressure in forehead, toward root of nose, with sensation as if brain was torn.

Contractive pain in occiput.

Tearing mostly in right temple, thence through right side of face.

Stitches in left temple and side of head, and when stooping, in the vertex, with sensation as if head would split.

[4] **Outer Head.**   Itching of the scalp.

Itching pimples on right side of occiput.

[5] **Eyes.**   Mist before eyes, worse in bright light out-doors; better in room.

Sensation in left eye as if a body arose, which impeded sight.

Yellow spots before the eyes.

Flying spots and points before the eyes.

Burning of the eyes and lachrymation, at night.

Eyes gum together in morning, with burning in canthi after washing.

[6] **Ears.**   Humming and roaring in right ear.

Hard hearing, with discharge.

Itching in both ears, not relieved by scratching, with discharge of fluid ear-wax.

Stitches in the ears, also with boring or burning, mostly when walking in open air.

Digging and tearing in right ear; also at night, when lying thereon, a rooting and rolling, as if something would come out.

[7] **Nose.**   Loss of smell, with coryza.

Sore internally and at the edge of the nostrils.

Ulcerative pain in left nostril, with sensitiveness to touch.

External swelling of left nostril, with discharge of bloody crusts.

Bleeding from left nostril, preceded by itching.

Constant itching in nose, with irritation to blow it, and sensation as of a large, rough body up in the nose, with obstruction.

Coryza, with stoppage of nose, hoarseness and burning in larynx.

I Watery, acrid coryza, corroding the lip.

Frequent sneezing.

[8] **Face.**   Very pale face.

Burning heat of face, passes off in the open air.

Tearing in bones of face, especially in malar and lower maxilla.

Swelling of the cheek, with swelling of a gland under the angle of lower jaw, with beating, stitching pain.

[9] **Lower Face.**   Lips burn like fire.

Corners of mouth ulcerated.

Dry, shrivelled, cracked lips, must moisten them with the tongue, continually.

Pimples, blisters, on upper lip.

[10] **Teeth.**   Pain in a decayed root, ceases when pressed upon with the finger.

Stitching pain in upper incisors.

Swelling of gums of lower left side, with stitches up to left temple.

[11] **Tongue, etc.** Blister on tip of tongue, with burning pain.

[13] **Throat.** Stitches in throat, during and between deglutition, also when yawning.

External and internal swelling of throat, with pressing pain when swallowing, with drawing, stitching pain in the swollen submaxillary glands.

Sore throat, with viscid phlegm, so tough that it cannot be hawked up.

Dryness in throat.

[15] **Eating and Drinking.** No appetite.

Much thirst, especially evenings.

After eating: beating in breast near œsophagus, with heat of face and restless mood; sore spot behind soft palate relieved.

[16] **Nausea and Vomiting.** Hiccough, with stitches in chest.

Eructations: empty; bitter or tasting of food.

Nausea, with water-brash, after eating, with shudderings.

Regurgitation: of food; of bitter, sour water.

[17] **Stomach.** Empty or hungry feeling in stomach.

Sensation as from fasting, yet fulness in stomach, worse after breakfast.

Rooting and rolling in stomach, in morning, passes off after breakfast.

Gnawing in stomach, as if worms were in it.

Burning and stitching in scrobiculum, from thence drawing to the right axilla, and in the upper arm.

[18] **Hypochondria.** Intermittent pains in both hypochondria.

Stitching and burning in right hypochondrium, afternoons, when walking.

Splenic stitches, while sitting.

[19] **Abdomen.** Bellyache, griping pains about the navel.

Heaviness in lower abdomen, like from a load, with anxiety as if the abdomen would burst, ceases after sleep.

Distention of the abdomen.

Stitches in the abdomen, above the left hip.

Pain from right side of pubes, to hip and small of back.

Cutting and stitches from both ossa pubis to small of back, with urging to urinate, evenings.

[20] **Stool, etc.** Stitching or tearing pain in perineum, when walking.

❙ Burning in the rectum during, and for hours after, stool.

Green, slimy, diarrhœic stools, in the morning.

Diarrhœa, with soreness of anus, sore pustules near it.

Diarrhœa after eating, with pain in abdomen, back, small of back and limbs; much flatus.

Hard, crumbling stools, require great effort to expel.

Hemorrhoids, sore and smarting.

Hemorrhoids after suppressed leucorrhœa.

[21] **Urine.**   Frequent urging, with frequent urination.

Urging, yet only a few drops pass, until next stool, when it flows freely.

Profuse and frequent discharge during the night.

Deep yellow urine, with light, cloudy sediment.

Sediment like clay.

[22] **Male Sexual Organs.**   Stitches and beating in left spermatic cord.

Frequent erections.

[23] **Female Sexual Organs.**   ı Menses too early, with pain in abdomen and small of back, continuing at night; flow more profuse at night.   θ Prolapsus uteri.

Leucorrhœa: with tension of abdomen, without collection of wind; like white of eggs, preceded by griping about the navel; brown, slimy, unpainful, after every urination.

[25] **Larynx.**   Hoarseness, with burning in larynx, afternoon.

Frequent hawking, with expectoration of small lumps of mucus, with sensation of rawness in throat, back of uvula.

[26] **Breathing.**   Shortness of breath.

Heaviness of chest, when walking in the open air.

[27] **Cough.**   Dry, from tickling in the throat, night or day; dry in morning, with stitches in chest, or left hypochondrium, becomes loose in afternoon; loose at night, with stitches in left hypochondrium, lying on back, worse when turning on side; worse before eating or drinking cold things.

Expectoration of blood, following an itching in throat.

[28] **Lungs.**   Pressure and stitches in the chest, as if a morsel of food had lodged there.

Painful tension below the right breast.

Bruised pain in lower right chest.

Burning at small spots of the chest.

Beating, like a pulse, at a small spot in the left chest, only when standing, mornings.

[29] **Heart. Pulse.**   Tearing in region of heart, going from there into left forearm.

Pulse accelerated.

[30] **Outer Chest.**   Burning, itching, red spots on left chest, pale under pressure.

[31] **Neck. Back.**   Stiff neck, with pain from nape to between shoulders, when turning.

Tearing pains in side of neck, alternating with tearing in the cheek.

Pain in small of back, as if bruised or crushed, during rest or motion, also at night, in bed, could neither lie on back nor on side.

Bruised and sprained pain between the scapulæ.

Stitches in the left scapula.

Pinching in muscles of the right scapula.

Coldness in back and between the shoulders, not relieved by feather or wool covering, followed by itching.

❘ Severe pains in lumbo-sacral region.

32 Upper Limbs. Swelling of the axillary glands.

Rheumatic pain, first in right, then in left shoulder-joint.

Tearing in left arm, like in the tendons, to the fingers; ceases from strong motion.

Drawing and tearing, from right elbow to fingers.

Itching on inside of forearm, with eruption in bend of elbow.

Right forearm heavy and as if "asleep."

Tearing in left wrist, with swelling of back of hand.

Stitches and painful beating under nail of left thumb.

Skin peels off between thumb and forefinger of both hands.

33 Lower Limbs. Languor and weakness in lower limbs.

Pain in left hip, as if the tendons were too short, must limp when walking; when sitting, gnawing pain in the bone.

Tearing in thighs when sitting.

Stitches in knee-joint, evening, when sitting.

Hamstrings painful when walking, as if too short.

Cramp-like contraction in lower part of left leg.

Violent tearing (and stitches), with ulcerative pain in heels; at times relieved by rubbing; occurs also at night in bed.

Feet feel as if "asleep."

Cold feet, evening, in bed.

Itching in sole of right foot, evening.

Stitching in toes, coming slowly and going slowly.

34 Limbs in General. Tearing and painful jerks, now here, and again there, through all the limbs.

35 Position, etc. Pains in limbs better from motion.

Must walk bent, with uterine displacement.

Rest: 31. Lying: 6, 27. Sitting: 33. Standing, 28. Stooping: 3. Motion: 31, 32. Turning on side: 27. Turning head: 31. Walking: 18, 20, 33, 36.

36 Nerves. Ebullitions with anxiety, weakness, as if paralyzed.

Sudden prostration after dinner when walking in open air.

Great weakness, mornings.

37 Sleep. Constant yawning without sleepiness, mornings.

Sleepiness early in evening, eyelids fall shut; better after candle-light.

Cannot fall asleep before midnight, on account of cold feet.

Heat in head prevents sleep before midnight.

Restless sleep and waking after midnight.

Anxious, fearful dreams, starts out of sleep.

Dreams: of falling into water; of sickness; lascivious.

Wakes at 2 A. M. from violent cutting in abdomen.

Wakes at night: from sneezing, with tickling in throat causing cough; pain in small of back.

38 Time. Morning: 1, 5, 17, 27, 28, 36, 37, 40, 43. Afternoon:

18, 25, 27. Evening: 15, 19, 33, 37, 40, 46. Night: 5, 6, 21, 23, 31, 33, 37, 40. Day: 2. Day and night: 40. Night or day: 27.

[39] **Temperature and Weather.** Usually better in open air.
Open air: 5, 6, 8, 26, 36. Warm room: 40. Room: 5. Washing: 5.

[40] **Chill. Fever. Sweat.** Chill, with external coldness in the evening and from uncovering at night.
Chill running up the back.
Chill alternating every half hour with heat.
Heat, with red puffed up face, particularly in warm room and after bodily exertion.
Flushes of heat in frequent attacks, ending each time with sweat, which is most profuse in face, palms of hands and soles of feet.
Sweat day and night, following heat.
Profuse night-sweat over the whole body, most copious after midnight, and early in morning, in bed.

[41] **Attacks.** Stitching pain in toes, slowly coming and slowly going.
Flushes of heat in attacks: 40.

[42] **Sides.** Right: 3, 4, 6, 18, 19, 28, 31, 32, 33. Left: 3, 5, 7, 10, 19, 22, 27, 28, 31, 32, 33.
Scrobiculum to right arm: 17. Heart to left forearm: 29.
Shoulder-joints—right, then left: 32. Pubes to hip: 19.
Pubes to back: 19.

[43] **Sensations.** Blood seems in constant ebullition.
Bruised pain in whole body, in the morning after arising.

[45] **Contact, Injuries, etc.** Touch: 7. Pressure: 10. Scratching: 6.

[46] **Skin.** Itching on various parts of body, generally evenings, before going to bed, better afterward.
Fine rash over the whole body.
Rash-like measles.
Small-pox more on trunk and upper limbs.

[47] **Stages and States.** Suitable to those who are fat and sluggish; body fat, but legs thin.

[48] **Relationship.** Similar to its relatives and to: *Ant. crud.* (mucous membranes); *Aloe* (abdominal symptoms); *Arsen.* (catarrhs); *Arg. nitr.* (mucus in throat); *Calc. ostr.* (fat people; coldness between scapulæ; profuse menses); *Conium* (night cough); *Caustic.* (stiff joints, contractions of muscles; burning hoarseness); *Carb. veg.* (hoarseness; burning on chest, etc.); *Coloc.* (in colic); *Hepar; Iodine; Kali bichr.* (stringy mucus, etc); *Kali chlor.* (catarrh); *Kali hydr.* (pimples on the back, etc.); *Mercur.; Merc. corr.; Magn. mur.* (especially bloody sputum; crumbling stool; atonic bladder); *Natr. Mur.* (catarrh); *Nux. Vom.;*

Phosphor.; Rhus tox. (sprains; joints worse sitting, etc.);
Seneg. (fat people; mucous secretions; stitches in scapula
with lung affections, etc.); *Sepia* (blisters about joints;
atonic bladder, etc.); *Silic.; Sulphur.*
Aggravations from *Amm. mur.* are relieved by a hot bath.
Antidoted by: bitter almonds; *Coffea; Nux. vom.*

ANACARDIUM ORIENTALE.

Marking Nut.   STAPF.   *Anacardiaceæ.*

[1] **Mind.** ｜Great weakness and loss of memory.

Memory quite useless, particularly single names, mornings.
｜Difficult recollection.

From 9 to 10 P. M. first extreme excitement of fancy and
projective ideas; later, by degrees, becomes dull and
does not think at all.

Imagines he hears voice of mother or sister who are far away.

Feels as though he had two wills, one commanding to do
what the other forbids.

Extreme merriness; laughs when he should be earnest.

Every motion extremely awkward and sluggish.

Unsociability.

Aversion to work.

Sadness; looks on the anxious side of everything.
｜Hypochondriasis. θ Hemorrhoids and constipation.

Hypochondriac mood in forenoon, dejected and desponding, with foolish, clumsy actions.

He feels separated from the whole world and has so little
confidence in himself that he despairs of being able to
do that which is required of him.

Anxiety and feeling of impending misfortune.

Very indifferent and insensible to pleasant or unpleasant
circumstances.

Extremely irritable; passionate and contradictory.
｜Irresistible desire to curse and swear.

Exertion of mind brings on tearing, pressing headache in
forehead, temples and occiput.

[2] **Sensorium.** Vertigo: getting black before the eyes; when
walking; when stooping; as if surroundings, or self
were tottering; rising from stooping, feels as if turning
to the left.
｜Weakness of all the senses.

[3] **Inner Head.** Pressure: in the forehead, mornings when
awaking, and in the evening; in the right side of occiput.

Violent pressure in the right or left temple.

Dull pressure, like from a plug, on the left side of vertex.

Constrictive headache in the forehead, with very irritable mood, pains increase hourly; momentarily relieved by strong pressure; finally whole head affected.

Headache worse during mental work, with sensation of heat in the head; better during a meal, worse after.

Tearing pain in the occiput.

Stitches: over the right eye; in the left side of the head.

Throbbing headache.

Heat in the head.

Headache, worse during motion and work.

  ❙ Gastric and nervous headache.

⁴ **Outer Head.** Violent itching of the scalp; also on forehead.

Many lentil-sized boils on the scalp, with sore pain when touched or scratched.

⁵ **Eyes.** Great sensitiveness to light.

The light seems to have a halo around it.

Optical illusions in dark colors; flickering before eyes.

Short-sightedness.

Pupils first contracted, later dilated.

❙ Vision indistinct.

Pressure, like from a plug, on the upper margin of orbit.

Pressure on eyeball from before backwards.

⁶ **Ears.** Humming in the ears; roaring before the ears.

Hearing at times very weak, at others very acute.

Tearing or stitching pains in left ear; worse swallowing.

⁷ **Nose.** Illusory smell as of burning tinder, morning, rising.

Constant smell before nose like pigeon or chicken dung, especially when smelling his clothes or his body.

Smell seems quite lost, though the nose is not obstructed.

Red pustule in right nostril on the septum, with sore pain when touched.

Sneezing, followed by fluent coryza and lachrymation.

⁸ **Face.** Pale, wan looking; blue rings around the eyes.

White, scaly herpes on right cheek, near the upper lip.

⁹ **Lower Face.** Rough, scaly skin around the mouth, with crawling-itching.

Burning dryness of outer border of lips, almost like from pepper.

¹⁰ **Teeth.** Toothache on taking something warm in the mouth.

Toothache in one lower incisor, worse by contact with tongue and the open air; tearing in the teeth.

Teeth of lower jaw seem most affected.

Swelling of gums; bleeding of gums upon slight rubbing.

¹¹ **Tongue, etc.** Bitter taste in mouth after smoking tobacco.

Everything tastes like herring-brine.

❙ Flat, offensive taste in the mouth and of food.

Heaviness of tongue and sensation as if swollen; impedes speech; speech firmer and surer in afternoon than forenoon.

Tongue is white, and rough like a grater.

[12] **Mouth.** Fetid odor from mouth, without his perceiving it.
Painful vesicles in the mouth.

[13] **Throat.** Roughness in throat; sensation as of scraping in throat.

Sensation of rawness in throat during cough, after eating.

Firm, tough mucus comes in pharynx and lodges over posterior nares.

[14] **Desires. Aversions.** Constant thirst; yet drinking takes the breath, must stop frequently during a draught.

Thirst during the heat.

At times violent hunger, at others no appetite.

[15] **Eating and Drinking.** ▮ Symptoms disappear during dinner; begin anew after two hours.

Worse after eating; head, stomach and bowel symptoms.

[16] **Nausea and Vomiting.** Hiccough.

Eructations: empty, frequent fluid, causing choking; with spasmodic pain in stomach.

Heartburn after eating soup; burning, rising from stomach to throat.

Nausea in morning, with empty feeling in stomach.

Nausea, with retching, returning soon after drinking cold water, with vomiting of the water, accompanied by pain, as if the œsophagus were distended by a large ball.

Vomiting of ingesta, which gives relief, after the cough.

[17] **Stomach.** First, sensation of fasting in pit of stomach, then pressure in stomach.

Stitch in pit of stomach during inspiration.

Rumbling and fermentatinon in pit of stomach.

Weak digestion, with fulness and distention of abdomen.

[18] **Hypochondria.** Stitches in hypochondria.

[19] **Abdomen.** Pain around the navel, as if a dull plug were pressed into the intestines.

Continual rumbling in abdomen, especially in umbilical region.

Pinching and griping in the abdomen.

[20] **Stool, etc.** Moisture from the rectum.

▮ Great and urgent desire for stool, but with the effort the desire passes away, without an evacuation; the rectum seems powerless, with sensation as if plugged up.

Inactivity of rectum, even soft stool passed with difficulty.

Stools of very pale color.

Frequent profuse hemorrhage when at stool.

Itching at the anus.

[21] **Urine.** Constant desire to urinate.

Frequent urging with but small discharge.

Urine: clear as water; turbid when passed, deposits a dirty sediment; when shaken looks clay-colored.

22 **Male Sexual Organs.** Violent sexual desire.

Erections during the day.

Seminal emissions at night, without amorous dreams.

Cutting pain along the penis.

Voluptuous itching of scrotum, exciting sexual desire.

23 **Female Sexual Organs.** Leucorrhœa, with soreness, also causing itching.

24 **Pregnancy.** Nausea during pregnancy, worse before and after, better while eating.

25 **Larynx.** Voice hoarse and deep.

Talking excites cough.

26 **Breathing.** Shortness of breath, oppression in region of the sternum.

Anxiety in region of sternum, without pain, feels as if he must go into the open air and be busy.

27 **Cough.** Excited by: talking; tickling in trachea. Cough after eating, with vomiting of food; with pain in occiput.

Cough excited by fits of vexation; dyspnœa during and after spells; in children who have an uncontrollable temper.

Expectoration: of sweetish, flat tasting mucus; tenacious, greyish-yellow; purulent.

28 **Lungs.** Dull pressure, as from a plug in right side of chest.

Sharp stitches in the precordial region, extending thence to small of back.

29 **Heart. Pulse.** Stitch in the region of the heart; during inspiration, at night.

Stitches piercing through and through at the heart; each time two quickly succeeding each other.

Pulse general accelerated.

Beating in the blood-vessels.

30 **Outer Chest.** Itching on the chest.

31 **Neck. Back.** Stiffness of nape of neck.

Dull, intermittent pressure, like from a heavy load on right side of neck and on left acromion.

Painful tearing between the scapulæ.

32 **Upper Limbs.** Dull stitches in left scapula, return slowly and radiate on all sides.

Left arm "goes to sleep," also the fingers.

Sensation of weakness in the arms, with trembling.

Very painful strokes, like from a heavy body at the middle of the left upper arm.

Short, painful inward pressure here and there on forearms.

Cramp-like pain at metacarpo-phalangeal articulations.

Great feeling of dryness of the hands.

Hands, even the palms, covered with warts.

Numbness of the fingers.

33 **Lower Limbs.** Dull pressure, like from a plug, in the left glutei muscles.

Painful, dull, pointed pressure in the thigh, at times in rythmical intermission.

Painful uneasiness about the knees, with sensation of stiffness, as if bandaged or made tense, when sitting.

Wave-like stitches, here and there, in the legs.

Knees feel paralyzed, with stiffness and great lassitude, is scarcely able to walk.

Painful drawing in the tibia.

▮ Cramp in the calves when walking, or rising from a seat; better lying down.

Cramp-like pressure in the calves, externally.

Cramp-like, intermittent drawing, from heel up into calves.

Pain in ankle, as if sprained, when stepping on left foot.

Stitches in dorsum of foot.

Cramp-like, drawing and tearing pains, from toes to dorsum of foot.

Burning in soles of feet while sitting.

Coldness of feet in the morning.

34 **Limbs in General.** Tired feeling in the limbs.

Repeated tearings in paroxysms, through upper and lower limbs at the same time.

35 **Position, etc.** Restlessness of body, cannot keep still.

Must lie on the back.

Very faint on going up stairs.

Circulation excited while sitting.

Motion: 1, 3, 43. Walking: 2, 33, 43. Lying or sitting: 43. Stooping: 2.

Beginning walking is toilsome, by continuing to walk he feels better.

36 **Nerves.** Paralysis of single parts.

Trembling: from every motion; from going up stairs.

37 **Sleep.** Sleeplessness from restlessness.

Could not sleep well on account of itching.

Sound sleep until 9 A. M.

Vivid dreams at night, which recurred to him during the day, as if the things dreamed of had really happened.

Dreams: of fire; of dead bodies.

38 **Time.** Most prominent times of aggravation, morning, and evening until midnight.

Remission after midnight and during the day.

Morning: 1, 3, 7, 16, 33. Forenoon: 1, 11. Afternoon: 11. Evening: 1, 3, 40. Night: 22, 29, 37, 40. Day: 22, 37.

39 **Temperature and Weather.** Sensitive to draught; liable to take cold.

Open air: 10, 26, 46.   Warm room: 40.
Prefers sunny places, feels cold.

⁴⁰ **Chill. Fever. Sweat.** Shivering over the back, as if
   cold water were poured over it, with heat of the face.
   Internal chill, even in warm room.
   Heat of upper body, with cold feet, internal shiverings
   and hot breath.
   Heat from 4 P. M. till evening, daily; passing off after supper.
   Heat of left side.
   Evening, sweat on head, abdomen and back, even when
   sitting quiet.
   Night-sweat on abdomen and back.
   Clammy sweat in palms, particularly the left.
   Cool sweat with internal heat.
   Sweat lessened while eating.

⁴¹ **Attacks.** The attacks cease for one or two days and then
   continue again for a couple of days.
   Tertian and quartan intermittents.

⁴² **Sides.** Left side, or ❙ first left, then right.
   Right: 3, 7, 8, 28, 31.   Left: 3, 6, 31, 32, 33, 40.
   Pains pressing from without inwards.
   Before backwards: 5, 28.   Below upwards: 33.

⁴³ **Sensations.** Heaviness and fulness of whole body from
   playing the piano.
   Wants to lie or sit continually; can scarcely move a hand.
   Drawing and pains in every part of body.
   Pressing or penetrating pain as from plug, in different parts.
   ❙ Sensation as of a hoop or band around the part.

⁴⁴ **Tissues.** Cramp-like pains in muscles.
   Contraction of joints.
   Complaints of external parts.
   Emaciation.

⁴⁵ **Contact, Injuries, etc.** Touch: 4, 7, 10.   Pressure: 3.
   Itching generally aggravated, but sometimes improved or
   changed in location by scratching.
   Rubbing: 11.

⁴⁶ **Skin.** White herpetic spots.
   Burning and stinging herpes.
   Excessively itching eruptions.
   Blisters discharging a yellowish transparent liquid, hard-
   ening to a crust in the open air.
   Warts even on palms of hands.

⁴⁷ **Stages and States.** Frequently indicated in nervous and
   hysterical females.
   Old people.
   Women during pregnancy, gastric and nervous disorders.

⁴⁸ **Relationship.** Similar to: *Ant. tart.* (cough in high-tem-
   pered children; gaping, drowsy after cough); *Apis*

(skin); *Coriaria ruscifolia* (loss of memory, etc.); *Ferrum* (occiput pains in cough); *Iodium; Juglans; Lycop.; Nitr. ac.* (cursing); *Nux vom.; Phos. ac.* (brain); *Platin.; Pulsat.; Urt. ur.* (skin); *Zincum* (brain); *Pulsat.; Natr. mur.* (dry coryza); *Caustic.* (in writer's spasm).

Relatives: *Anac. occid., Comoc., Rhus glab., Rhus rad., Rhus tox., Rhus ven.*

Antidotes: *Coffea* and *Juglans.*

Anac. antidotes: *Rhus tox.*, especially if there are gastric symptoms, or the symptoms go from right to left.

It follows well after *Lycop., Pulsat.* and *Platin.*

After *Anac.: Platin.* follows well.

Belongs to the same family as the *Rhoes*, and there is a similarity with the *Terebinthineæ.*

Neither *Camphor* nor *Spir. nitr. dulc.* antidotes its effects, but for the anger and violence of mind, the smelling of raw coffee is a very effectual antidote.

ANTIMONIUM CRUDUM.

Native Sulphide of Antimony.   CASPARI SbS_3.

[1] **Mind.** Insensible; bed-sores formed, yet he complained of no pain.

Child delirious, drowsy, with nausea, hot and red face; pulse irregular; feverish heat; cries when washed in cold water; better washed in warm water.

❙ Loathing of life.

Inclined to suicide by shooting himself.

Great sadness and woeful mood.

Anxious reflection in relation to his present and future.

❙ Sentimental mood in moonlight, particularly ecstatic love.

❙ Child is fretful and peevish, does not wish to be touched or looked at.

Sulky, does not wish to speak with any one.

[2] **Sensorium.** Vertigo, nausea, nosebleed.

Weakness of the head.

Heaviness in forehead.

Rush of blood to the head.

[3] **Inner Head.** Slight, dull headache and vertigo, increased by ascending stairs.

Stupefying, dull headache in the forehead so violent that sweat broke out from anxiety; when walking in the open air.

In left temporal region: pressure inwards; drawing; slow pulsation with fine pricking.

❙Headache: after bathing in the river, with weakness of the limbs and aversion to food; from deranging stomach; drinking alcoholic drinks; after a chill; after suppressed eruption; from taking cold.

⁴ **Outer Head.** Small spot on left parietal bone, painful to touch.

Lentil-sized, flat tubercles here and there on the scalp, painful to pressure, crawling sensation around them.

Formicating itching on the scalp; losing the hair.

Disposition to take cold about the head after getting wet or bathing in cold water; worse in the evening and on getting warm; better in the open air and when at rest.

⁵ **Eyes.** Looking into the fire increases cough.

Eyes red, inflamed, with itching and nightly agglutination.

Eyes worse from glare of the snow.

Redness of the left eye, with aversion to light.

Pustules on the cornea, with profuse mucus; pustules on margins of lids and on face.

❙Soreness of outer canthi.

Gum in the canthi, forenoon.

Small, moist spot at the outer canthus, very painful when sweat comes in contact with it.

❙Lids red and inflamed.

❙Chronic blephar-ophthalmia of children.

⁶ **Ears.** Ringing before the ears, roaring in the ears.

A kind of deafness of right ear, as if a leaflet was lying before the tympanum; boring with the finger does not relieve it.

Drawing pain through the right ear and into the eustachian tube, after dinner.

Redness, burning and swelling of the left ear.

Otorrhœa.

⁷ **Nose.** Stoppage in nose.

Nosebleed: evenings; after headache, with giddiness; with rush of blood to head.

Coryza: fluent or dry.

Nose painful when breathing, as from inhalation of cold air or of acrid vapors.

❙Sore, cracked or crusty nostrils.

⁸ **Face.** Sad expression.

Face red. See 1.

Twitches in facial muscles.

Heat and itching on cheeks.

Pimples, pustules and boils on the face.

Eruption like nettle-rash.

Yellow crusted eruption on the left cheek, painful to touch and easily detached.

Suppurating and long-lasting eruption on cheeks.

⁹ **Lower Face.** Lips dry.

Cracks in the corners of the mouth.

Burning, stinging on the chin, as from a hot spark.

Small, honey-colored granules on chin, with sore feeling when touched.

¹⁰ **Teeth.** ❙ Toothache in hollow teeth, pain sometimes penetrates into the head; worse at night; after eating, and from cold water; touching the tooth with the tongue, causes pain as if nerve was torn; better walking in open air.

Stitches in the tooth when drawing air into mouth.

Jerking or gnawing pain in hollow teeth.

Gums detach from teeth and bleed easily.

¹¹ **Tongue, etc.** Taste: bitter or lessened.

Tongue coated: thick and white; milky white; yellow.

Much saltish saliva in the mouth.

Sore feeling and redness on border of tongue.

¹² **Mouth.** Dryness of the mouth.

Ptyalism, saltish-tasting saliva.

¹³ **Throat.** Rawness of palate, with expectoration of much mucus when clearing throat.

Must draw quantities of thick, yellowish mucus from posterior nares into throat, and expectorate it.

¹⁴ **Desires. Aversions.** Desire for acids and pickles.

Long-lasting loss of appetite, with disgust for all food.

Hunger early on waking, without appetite; eating does not relieve it; at the same time sense of emptiness in pit of stomach, and want of animal heat.

Intense thirst, with dryness of lips; more at night; or thirstlessness.

¹⁵ **Eating and Drinking.** ❙ Bread and pastry particularly occasion nausea and cutting colic.

Laziness with desire to lie down, after eating.

Fulness and tension, after eating, alternating with lightness, cheerfulness and activity of mind and body.

❙ After bad, sour wine, vomiting. θ Gastric catarrh.

After nursing, diarrhœa.

Nursing children throw up a little sour milk, as soon as they take the breast or bottle.

Worse from pork; from acids. θ Diarrhœa, whooping-cough.

¹⁶ **Nausea and Vomiting.** Hiccough after smoking tobacco.

❙ Belching with taste of what has been eaten.

Burning at pit of stomach like heartburn, with good appetite.

Nausea: after drinking a glass of wine; from overloading the stomach.

❙ Vomiting: of mucus and bile; slimy; of drink only; renewed by food or drink; persistent, tongue white, no thirst. θ Marasmus of children, gastric catarrh, etc.

Violent vomiting and diarrhœa.

¹⁷ **Stomach.** ❙ Stomach weak, easily disturbed digestion.

Painful sense of fulness of stomach, which is sore to pressure.

Pain at stomach as after too much eating, with distended but not hard abdomen.

Cramp-like pains at the stomach.

Burning, spasmodic pain at pit of stomach, driving to despair; is resolved to drown himself.

❙ Gastric catarrh; white tongue, nausea and vomiting;' cough; bowels loose or stools in lumps. Caused by: overeating, sour wine, hot weather, bathing; during measles; metastasis of gout or rheumatism.

¹⁸ **Hypochondria.** Slight tension in the hypochondria.

¹⁹ **Abdomen.** Abdomen very much distended.

Incarcerated flatus; costive.

Rumbling in the abdomen.

Pinching and sensation as if diarrhœa would come on.

Sensation of emptiness in intestines, going off after meal.

Colic, with loss of appetite, hard stool, red urine.

Violent cutting in abdomen, feeling of oppression coming from stomach, indisposition to work, dull mood and pain at stomach with eructations.

Hard gland in left groin, painful to pressure.

Cutting in the bowels with watery diarrhœa.

²⁰ **Stool, etc.** Acrid diarrhœa.

Stools: watery, with vomiting; watery; profuse; ❙ watery, with little, hard lumps, or containing undigested food; mucous mornings.

❙ Diarrhœa, worse from vinegar and other acids; sour wine; overheating; after cold bath; night and early morning.

❙ Alternate diarrhœa and constipation, with old people.

❙ Diarrhœa of old people.

❙ Difficult, hard stool, feces too large, costive, with incarcerated flatus. .

Stools white, dry, irregular. Hard lumps of curd.

Sensation of copious stool, but only flatus escapes, with finally very hard stool.

Pain in rectum during stool; feeling of soreness as if an ulcer had been torn open.

❙ Copious hemorrhage from bowels, with solid feces; hemorrhoidal.

❙ Mucous piles, pricking, burning; continuous mucous discharge, staining yellow; sometimes ichor oozes out.

²¹ **Urine.** Tenesmus of the bladder rouses him from sleep at night.

Frequent urination, with much mucus, intense burning in urethra and backache during emission.

Cutting in urethra while urinating.

Urine: gold-yellow, with scarcely perceptible cloud; brown-red; with small red corpuscles after standing twenty-four hours.

Involuntary urination.

22 **Male Sexual Organs.** Excited sexual desire, with uneasiness of whole body, which prevents him sitting long.

Nightly pollutions, with or without voluptuous dreams.

Itching: of penis; of tip of glans.

Biting, itching, as from salt on left side of scrotum.

23 **Female Sexual Organs.** Tenderness over the ovarian region; after catamenia has been checked by taking bath.

Pressure in the womb, as if something would come out.

Menses commence at an early period, are profuse, then cease; subsequently chlorosis.

Before menses, toothache, with boring into the temples.

Discharge of acrid water from the vagina, which caused a smarting down the thighs.

Leucorrhœa watery and containing lumps.

24 **Pregnancy.** During pregnancy: gastro-intestinal and hemorrhoidal affections.

25 **Larynx.** Feebleness of voice.

Loss of voice; from getting overheated; better after rest.

Violent spasms in the larynx and pharynx, as if the throat were filled with a plug, which becomes alternately thicker and thinner, accompanied by a feeling of soreness.

26 **Breathing.** Short, heavy breathing; dyspnœa.

Deep, sighing breathing, as from fulness of the chest, afternoon and after eating.

Oppression coming from stomach.

Constriction almost to suffocation.

When exhaling, sharp stitches in left cheek.

27 **Cough.** Frequent dry cough.

Cough shaking the whole body, with involuntary escape of copious urine.

Cough after rising in the morning, in attacks; as if arising from the abdomen; ▮ the first attack is always most severe, the subsequent ones weaker and weaker, until the last resemble only a hacking. θ Whooping-cough. θ Stomach cough.

Cough: in the hot sun; on coming into warm room from cold air; whooping-cough after measles.

Looking into the fire increases cough.

28 **Lungs.** Oppression and pressive pains in chest, more right.

Stitches in the chest.

▮ Pain in the chest with heat.

Burning and sticking in the chest.

29 **Heart. Pulse.** Violent palpitation of the heart.

Pulse extremely irregular; now accelerated and again
  slow, changing every few beats.

³⁰ **Outer Chest.** Severe continual itching upon the chest the
  whole day.

³¹ **Neck. Back.** Swelling of the cervical glands.

Spasmodic drawing pain in muscles of nape of neck, reaching to scapulæ, evening after lying down and in morning; aggravated by stooping, exerting arms and turning head to left.

Itching of neck and back.

Spasmodic stitches in right scapula when sitting.

Violent pain in small of back when rising from sitting;
  disappeared when walking.

³² **Upper Limbs.** Cracking in elbow-joint when moving it.

Drawing pain: in arms; in fingers and their joints.

ı Arthritic pains in fingers.

Finger nails do not grow as rapidly as formerly, and skin
  beneath the nail painfully sensitive.

ı Crushed finger nails grow in splits, and like warts, and
  with horny spots.

³³ **Lower Limbs.** Legs fall asleep while sitting quietly.

Painful drawing in hip joints.

Painful stiffness of the knee.

Pain just below the knee, as if it had been tied too tightly.

Drawing pain: in knees; in lower part of left tibia; in left
  heel; and tearing through right great toe. *θ* Gout.

Violent pain in lower limbs.

ı Large horny places on the soles, close to the toes.

Corns on soles and toes.

ı Great sensitiveness of soles when walking.

³⁴ **Limbs in General.** Convulsions and trembling of limbs.

Lassitude, tremulous fatigue and heaviness of all the limbs,
  as if coming out of the abdomen; with trembling of
  hands when writing and subsequent discharge of much
  stinking flatus; abdomen distended after dinner.

Rheumatic or gouty pains.

³⁵ **Position, etc.** Rest: 4, 25. Sitting: 31, 33. Stooping: 31.
  Lying: 15, 31. Rising: 31. Ascending: 3. Walking:
  10, 31, 33. Moving arm: 32. Writing: 34. Exertion
  of arms: 31. Turning head: 31.

³⁶ **Nerves.** Disposition to start, even at slight noises.

Twitching of muscles; of many parts of the body.

Great lassitude.

Convulsions with the vomiting.

³⁷ **Sleep.** ı Great sleepiness during the day; mostly in forenoon.

At 7 P. M. feels overwhelmed with sleep.

Coma. Deep, unfreshing sleep.

Slight raving during sleep.

Wakefulness, with shivering over the left side, on which
he does not lie; or with sexual desire and erections
when getting warm.

Frequent waking, as from fright.

Dreams: of quarreling; voluptuous; anxious, as if he
were to be hurt; horrible, about mutilation of men.

³⁸ **Time.** Morning: 14, 20, 27, 31, 40. Forenoon: 5, 37.
Noon: 40. Afternoon: 6, 20. Evening: 4, 7, 31, 37.
Night: 5, 10, 14, 20, 21, 22, 37, 40. Day: 40.

³⁹ **Temperature and Weather.** Getting warm: 4, 25, 37.
Warm room: 27, 40. Heat of sun: 27. Warm water: 1.
Bathing: 23; in river: 3, 4. Cold water: 1, 10, 20.
Open air: 3, 4, 10.

Worse in warm weather; ❙ exhaustion with night-sweats,
sleepiness, nausea, vomiting.

❙ Cannot bear the heat of the sun.

⁴⁰ **Chill. Fever. Sweat.** Chill predominating during the
. day, even in warm room.

Violent, shaking chill toward noon, with thirst (for beer).

Shivering over the back; feet cold as ice, with sweat on
rest of body.

Heat at night.

Sweat in the morning when awaking, which causes a
shriveling of the tips of the fingers.

Sweat, which returns at precisely the same hour, usually
every other (third) morning.

❙ After the sweat is over, heat and thirst return.

⁴¹ **Attacks.** Symptoms repeat every five, six or twelve weeks.
Returning periodically; coma, earache.

Sweat at same hour every other day.

⁴² **Sides.** Right: 6, 28, 31, 33. Left: 4, 5, 6, 8, 19, 22, 26, 33, 37.
Gout commencing right side going to the left.

⁴⁴ **Tissues.** Hemorrhages dark.

Dropsical swellings of the whole body.

❙ Mucous membranes generally affected.

Swelling pain and redness of the glands.

External parts turn black; dry gangrene.

Obesity of the young.

⁴⁵ **Contact, Injuries, etc.** Touch: 1, 4, 8, 9, 10. Pressure: 4,
17, 19. Boring in the ear: 6. Scratching: 46.

⁴⁶ **Skin.** Eruption like boils and blisters.

Pustules like varicella.

Itching of skin, feels sore when scratched.

Pimples and vesicles as from stings of insects, especially
on face and joints of extremities.

❙ Measle-like eruption; smooth warts; ❙ horny excrescences.

Boils on the perineum; burning around them.

Deep, spongy ulcers.

Eruption with thick, hard scabs; often honey-yellow.
Bed-sores: 2.
[47] **Stages and States.** Children.
Young people grow fat.
❙ Old people: alternate diarrhœa and constipation.
[48] **Relationship.** Similar to: *Apis* (skin); *Arsen.* (gastric catarrh, burning eruption, dropsy); *Amm. mur.* (mucous
flux); *Bryon.* (rheumatism, gastric symptoms, effects of
heat, etc.); *Chamom.; Hepar; Ipec.* (gastric ailments);
Mercur.; Nux vom.; Pulsat. (gastric symptoms, relief
in open air, mind, chills and fever, etc.); *Ran. bulb.*
(horny exanthemata); *Rhus tox.; Sulphur; Scilla.*
Related to: *Ipec.*, still more to *Lycop.* (Teste).
Similar in gastric vertigo to *Pulsat.;* gastric headache from
sour things, to *Pulsat.* or *Arsen.;* inflamed eyes to *Acon.*,
Euphras.; in toothache in hollow teeth, to *Pulsat.;* in
lessened appetite from summer heat, to *Bryon., Carb.
veg.;* cramp in stomach, to *Pulsat.* or *Ipec.;* watery di-
arrhœa, to *Ferrum;* after getting overheated, gastric
symptoms, to *Bryon.; Antim. sulph. aurat.*, preferable
for ashma from muco-pus in bronchi.
Useful after *Ipec.* or *Pulsat.* in intermittent.
❙ Polypi with *Pulsat.* and *Mercur.*
After *Ant. crud.* follow well: *Pulsat., Mercur., Sulphur..*
Antidotes to *Ant. crud.: Calcar., Hepar, Mercur.*
Ant. crud. antidotes: stings of insects.
Complementary: *Squilla.*

ANTIMONIUM TARTARICUM.

Tartar Emetic.   Stapf. $2[K(Sb\ O)C_4H_4O_6]H_2O.$

[1] **Mind.** Confusion of the head; with feeling as if he ought
to sleep.
The child will not allow itself to be touched without
whining and crying.
❙ Bad humor.   θ Bronchial catarrh.
Wild gaiety toward evening.
Apprehensive and restless.
Dreads being left alone, lest he should be very nervous.
Mental excitement.
Frightened at every trifle.
[2] **Sensorium.** Vertigo: on closing the eyes; on walking;
with flickering before the eyes; when lifting the head,
must lie down.

Heaviness of head.

3 Inner Head. Headache, as from a band compressing the forehead.

Pressive pains in the forehead, stitching extending downwards into the left eye.

Throbbing in right side of forehead.

Painful drawing in the right temple, extends down to the zygoma and upper jaw.

Tearing pains in the head.

Stitches in left parietal bone on stooping, extending forwards.

Trembling of the head, particularly when coughing.

4 Outer Head. Scalp very sensitive, with heaviness, of head.

5 Eyes. Flickering before the eyes.

Sees only as through a thick veil. Vanishing of sight.

ı Dim, swimming eyes. θ Diarrhœa.

Inflammation of conjunctiva, with much lachrymation.

Eyeballs pain, as if bruised,

Eyes feel tired, as if the lids would close.

Inclination to press the lids tightly together.

ı Ophthalmia rheumatica or arthritica.

6 Ears. Roaring in the ears.

Fluttering before the left ear, as from a large bird; at same time warmth of ear.

Twitching, tearing in right concha, evening on lying down; disappears in bed.

7 Nose. Sneezing, fluent coryza and chilliness, with loss of taste and smell.

Stoppage of nose, alternating with fluent coryza.

Nosebleed, followed by fluent coryza with sneezing.

Stupefying tension over root of nose, as from a band.

8 Face. Face: ı pale, sunken; pale, puffed, with coma; ı bluish.

ı Tearing pain in whole side of face, even head and neck of that side. θ Rheumatic toothache.

Burning heat of face.

Cold sweat on face.

Warm sweat on forehead and head from efforts to vomit.

Convulsive twitches in almost every muscle of the face.

9 Lower Face. Lips dry, scurfy.

Itching vesicles on lips.

Burning, as from hot coal, on right side of chin.

10 Teeth. Violent toothache in the morning.

Rheumatic toothache of intermittent type.

Gums bleed.

During dentition catarrhal hyperæmia.

11 Tongue, etc. Taste: flat; salty; sour; bitter; as from rotten eggs.

Food seems tasteless. Tobacco has no taste

ı Tongue: red, in streaks; very red, and dry in centre; covered with thick, white, pasty coat; coated very thinly white, with reddened papillæ, red edges.

Difficult, even painful, to move the tongue.

12 **Mouth.** Mouth so sore, can scarcely swallow, morning after rising.

Small circular patches like small-pox pustules, in and upon the mouth and tongue.

13 **Throat.** Sensation of soreness on posterior part of palate when not swallowing.

ı Much mucus in throat with short breathing.

Roughness in throat, with sensation as if a small leaf obstructed the windpipe on hawking.

Swallowing painful or impossible.

14 **Desires. Aversions.** Extraordinary appetite for apples, and thirst for cold water.

Desire for acids.

Much thirst, drinks little and often, or, absence of thirst.

Appetite diminished.

No desire for his tobacco.

15 **Eating and Drinking.** Food relieves, somewhat, the pressure in the abdomen.

16 **Nausea and Vomiting.** Violent hiccough.

Eructations: empty; acid; bitter; salty, nauseous fluid; taste of the food taken.

Qualmishness in stomach after dinner.

Nausea: ı causing anxiety; with slight pressure in pit of stomach, followed by headache in forehead; and incessant vomiting whole night, with diarrhœa; then yawning with profuse lachyrmation, followed by vomiting.

Vomiting: in any position, except lying on right side: with headache, trembling of hands; with great effort.

Vomit: green; tough, watery mucus, then pasty food, then fluid, mixed with bile.

ı Vomiting is followed with great languor, drowsiness, loathing, desire for cooling things. θ Diarrhœa.

Retching, then vomiting, followed by great prostration.

17 **Stomach.** Sensation as if stomach had been "overloaded;" eructations frequent, like foul eggs; sleep restless.

Violent pains at the epigastrium, which was tense.

Cramps in the stomach.

Pressure in pit of stomach.

Beating and throbbing, particularly in pit of stomach or abdomen, with great concern about the future.

18 **Hypochondria.** Region of liver sensitive to touch.

Icterus with pneumonia, especially of the right lung.

19 **Abdomen.** Abdomen feels as if stuffed full of stones, though he has eaten nothing, and it does not feel hard.

Pressure and aching in hypogastrium, with cold shivers.

Violent colic, as if the bowels would be cut to pieces.

Violent cutting and labor-like tearing, from above downwards across groins, through thighs down to knees.

Colic around the umbilicus.

Violent burning soreness in right groin.

Shifting of flatulence, with rumbling in bowels, diarrhœa.

²⁰ **Stool, etc.** Stitches in the rectum.

Copious alvine evacuation.

Stools; yellowish-brown; thin, bilious, mucous; liquid greenish, with heat at the anus; slimy, appear like yeast; of cadaverous smell.

Desire for stool ineffectual, though the bowels seem full and pressing.

²¹ **Urine.** Urine: dark brownish-red, turbid, of strong odor; becomes cloudy and deposits a violet-colored earthy sediment; scanty, last drops bloody, violent pains in the bladder; albuminous.

Burning in the urethra during, also after urinating.

²³ **Female Sexual Organs.** Menses too early, weak, and only for two days.

Before menses: pain in the groins and cold creepings.

Leucorrhœa of watery blood, worse when sitting; comes in paroxysms.

Pustules on external genitals.

²⁴ **Pregnancy.** Gastric derangements—vomiting of mucus; belching; disgust for food; salivation.

❙Child at birth pale, breathless, gasping, although the cord still pulsates. θ Asphyxia neonatorum.

²⁵ **Larynx.** Voice weak and changed in the evening.

Hoarseness in the morning, worse on talking.

❙Rattling of mucus when coughing or breathing.

❙Much rattling of mucus in trachea; cannot get it up.

❙Rattling, originating in upper bronchia, can be heard at a great distance. θ Bronchial catarrh.

❙Catarrhal croup, croup of adults.

❙Bronchioectasis and senile catarrh.

²⁶ **Breathing.** Rapid; short; heavy and anxious.

❙Dyspnœa; must be supported in a sitting posture.

❙Suffocated and oppressed about 3 A. M., must sit up to get air; after cough and expectoration she became better.

❙Child breathless and pale when born.

Great difficulty in expiration.

❙Respiration with great rattling of mucus.

²⁷ **Cough.** ❙Coughing and gaping consecutively.

❙Cough, if children get angry, also after eating; child vomits food and mucus.

❙Short cough with a shrill sound. θ Bronchial catarrh.

❚ Cough compels the patient to sit up, is moist and rattling, but no expectoration.

Catarrh provokes cough, though she had no power to cough.

Gasping for air, before every attack of cough.

Cough: with copious frothy expectoration or without expectoration.

❚ Cough grows less frequent, patient shows signs of " carbonized blood."

Scraping cough, with pus-like expectoration.

Bloody, slimy expectoration after hæmoptysis.

²⁸ **Lungs.** ❚ Chest seems full of phlegm, without ability to expectorate it.

Anxious, with oppression of the′ chest and rising of warmth from the heart.

So warm about the heart that she must let the arms sink down with general weakness.

Full feeling of the chest. Constriction of chest.

❚ Œdema of the lungs. ❚ Broncho-pneumonia.

²⁹ **Heart. Pulse.** Palpitation of the heart.

❚ Great precordial anxiety, with vomiting of mucus and bile.

Pulse: hard and quick, in old people; rapid, weak and trembling; small, contracted.

³⁰ **Outer Chest.** Crawling as of insects above the left mamma.

³¹ **Neck. Back.** Does not like anything to touch him; inclination to unbutton the collar of his shirt.

Cramp in the muscles of the neck.

Pain in the back as from fatigue, especially after eating and while sitting.

Sharp stitches in the region of kidneys on moving arms.

❚ Violent pain in sacro-lumbar region; the slightest effort to move causes retching and cold, clammy sweat.

³² **Upper Limbs.** Tearing and stitching pains.

Pain as from dislocation, in the right shoulder.

❚ Trembling·of the hands.

Hands cold and moist.

Finger tips appear dead, dry and hard; without sensation.

³³ **Lower Limbs.** Numbness and coldness in the legs.

Tension in the hamstrings on walking.

Rheumatic pains about the hips, thighs and calves.

Feet go "to sleep" immediately after sitting down.

Weariness in the feet. Cold feet.

³⁴ **Limbs in General.** Weakness; insensibility and coldness; heaviness.

Constant inclination to stretch.

Rheumatic and bruised sensation in limbs, on and shortly before rising.

³⁵ **Position, etc.** On lying down: 6. Sitting: 23, 26, 31, 33.

Lifting the head: 2. Rising: 34. Stooping: 3. Motion: 31, 36, 40. Moving the arms: 31. Inclined to stretch: 34. Walking: 2, 33.

[36] **Nerves.** Trembling: of whole body; internal; of head and paralytic trembling of hands on every motion.

Great restlessness. θ Bronchial catarrh.

Great weakness and lassitude.

Great prostration and sluggishness of the body.

Faintness.

Alternation of unsteadiness and syncope.

[37] **Sleep.** I Yawning; great sleepiness; irresistible inclination to sleep.

Had scarcely fallen asleep when he was seized with shocks and jerks, all of which came from the abdomen.

[38] **Time.** 3 A. M.: 26. Morning: 10, 12, 25. Evening: 1, 6, 25. Night: 16, 40. During the day: 40.

[39] **Temperature and Weather.** Open air: 2.

[40] **Chill. Fever. Sweat.** Chill; with external coldness, coming on at all times of the day, with somnolency; mostly with trembling and shaking; frequently as if cold water was poured over one.

Chill and heat alternating during the day.

Violent but not long-lasting heat succeeding a long chill, aggravated by every motion.

Long-lasting heat, after a short chill, with somnolency and sweat on the forehead.

Profuse sweat all over, also at night.

Sweat is frequently cold and clammy.

The affected parts sweat most profusely.

Sticky sweat.

[41] **Attacks.** Wave-like increase and decrease of pain in forehead.

[42] **Sides.** Rheumatic pains first in right hand then through both legs from above downwards, especially in knees.

Right: 4, 9, 16, 19, 32. Left: 3, 6, 30. Above downwards: 3, 19. Behind forwards: 3.

[44] **Tissues.** I Mucous membranes; catarrhal inflammation; conjunctivitis; gastritis, enteritis; laryngitis, tracheitis, bronchitis, extending even into the air-cells; cystitis.

I Pustular eruption: on the conjunctiva; face; mouth and fauces; œsophagus, stomach, jejunum; genitals. See 46.

[45] **Contact, Injuries, etc.** I The child wants to be carried, cries if any one touches it; will not let you feel the pulse.

[46] **Skin.** Red itching rash over the body.

Vesicular eruption over the body.

I Pustular eruption leaves bluish-red marks on face, also similar eruption on genitals and thighs, painful.

I Thick eruption like pocks, often pustular, as large as a pea.

Itching pustules; which soon dry up.

Itching in the skin.

❙ Eruption fails to appear and convulsions set in; varicella.

⁴⁸ **Relationship.** Similar to: *Acon.* (croup, spasm of larynx); *Arsen.* (asthma; heart symptoms; gastric catarrh, etc.); *Baryt. carb.; Bromine* (croup); *Camphor; Hepar; Iodium; Kali hydr.* (œdema pul., pneumonia); *Laches.* (dyspnœa on awakening, sensitive larynx, asthma, asphyxia, etc.); *Lycop.* (catarrh on the chest, but the spasmodic motion of alæ is replaced by dilated nostrils in *Ant. tart.*); *Veratr.* (both have diarrhœa, colic, vomiting, coldness, and craving for acids); *Ant. tart.* has more jerks, drowsiness and urging to urinate; *Veratr.* more cold sweat and fainting.

Similar to *Ipec.* (but has more drowsiness from defective respiration. It must supplant *Ipec.* when lungs seem to fail, patient becomes sleepy and the cough ceases or becomes less frequent).

Effects of vaccination when *Thuja* fails and *Silic.* is not indicated.

With *Phosphor.*, hydrocephaloid in wornout constitutions; also similar in laryngitis, pneumonia, etc.

Follow with *Silic.* for dyspnœa from foreign substances in the windpipe; *Pulsat.* in gonorrhœal suppression; *Tereb.* in symptoms from damp cellars.

Conium cures pustules on the genitals caused by *Ant. tart.*

Camphor., Ipec., Pulsat., Sepia, Sulphur follow *Ant. tart.* well.

Ant. tart. follows well after *Baryt. carb., Pulsat., Camphor.* and *Caustic.*

Antidotes to *Ant. tart.*: *Asaf., Cinchon., Coccul., Ipec., Lauroc., Opinm, Pulsat.* and *Sepia.*

Ant. tart. antidotes: *Sepia.*

APIS MELLIFICA.

Poison of the Honey Bee.   BRAUNS, 1835.   *Apium virus.*

¹ **Mind.** Loss of consciousness.

❙ Sopor interrupted by piercing shrieks.

Impaired memory. ❙ Absent-mindedness.

Awkwardness, lets everything fall from his hands.

Dulness of head; ❙ indifference.

Could not bring his thoughts to bear on anything.

Muttering delirium.

❙ Sudden shrill screams.   θ Hydrocephalus, etc.

Busy, restless, changing kind of work.

8

Delusive idea that he must run or hop, that he cannot
walk.

❙ Great tearfulness, cannot help crying.

Dread of death.

Apathy, hardness of hearing; happy expression.

Mood: iritable; hard to please; nervous.

Violence, amounting to frenzy.

❙ Jealousy (in women).

Manias, especially proceeding from sexual cause in women.

² **Sensorium.** Confused vertigo, worse sitting than when
walking, extreme when lying and on closing the eyes;
nausea and headache.

³ **Inner Head.** Brain feels tired; as if "gone to sleep," tingling.

Dull, heavy, tensive headache over the eyes, with pain
through the orbits.

Chronic headache, violent pain in forehead and temples,
at times involving the eyes, attended by vertigo, nausea,
and vomiting, must hold the head and eyes down.

Burning and throbbing in the head, worse by motion and
stooping, temporarily better by pressing the head firmly
with the hands; occasional sweat.

Aching in the occiput.

Violent drawing from the back of neck, extending behind
the left ear, spreading over left half in head.

Neuralgic pain, like a bee sting, in and about left temple.

Congestion to the head and face; fulness in the head.

❙ Child lies in torpor; delirium, sudden shrieking cries,
squinting, grinding teeth, boring head in pillow; one
side twitching, the other paralyzed; head wet from
sweating; urine scanty, milky; big toe turns up; nausea
while lying; breath offensive; tongue sore. θ Acute
hydrocephalus. θ After erysipelatous eruptions.

❙ Pain in occiput, with occasional sharp shrieks. θ Hydrocephalus.

❙ Chronic meningitis, with considerable cephalic disturbance and symptoms indicating threatening if not actual
effusion of serum into the cavity of the arachnoid.

❙ Hydrocephaloid; stupor; eyes red, head hot, shrill
shrieks; tongue dry, skin dry, hands cold and blue;
urine suppressed, abdomen tender; diarrhœa mucous,
offensive, involuntary, containing flakes of pus. See 20.

Hydrocephalic enlargement of the head.

⁴ **Outer Head.** ❙ Head feels swollen; integuments feel swollen
and stiff.

Hair falls out in spots.

Puffiness of scalp, forehead and around the eyes. θ Erysipelatous inflammation of scalp and face.

❙ Boring (backward) the head in the pillow.

I Fontanelle sunken.   *θ* Cholera infantum.

Copious sweat of the head, of musk-like order.

⁵ **Eyes.   I** Squinting; trembling of eyeball, worse at night.

Rolling the eyes.

Severe, darting, lancinating pains in the eyes.

I Burning, stinging, shooting pains.

I Conjunctiva injected, full of dark vessels; chemosis.

I Cornea: thick, having dark, smoky spots; greyish, smoky, opaque.

Ulcers on cornea; cicatrices; **I** staphyloma corneæ. See 48.

Conjunctivitis, photophobia, but cannot bear eyes covered.

I Scalding tears, profuse; great sensitiveness to light.

Lids: dark red, everted, swollen, excoriation of edges; granulated; swollen and very sensitive; **I** œdematous, with bag-like swelling under the eye; non-inflammatory œdema (like *Arsen.*); feel stiff.

⁶ **Ears.**   Hardness of hearing.

I Redness and swelling of both ears.

Raises the hand to the back of the ears with each scream.

⁷ **Nose.**   Thick, white, fetid, mucous discharge, mixed with blood.

I Nose swollen, red and œdematous.

I Boils in nostrils, better from cold.

⁸ **Face.**   Expression: happy, pleasant; of terror; apathetic; features distorted, face dark and much swollen; sunken, pale, sickly.

Face: pale; sallow; dark red; swollen, red and hot, with burning and piercing, more right side; œdematous, **I** waxy, pale.

Burning cheeks, with cold feet.

I Erysipelas of the face.

Stinging pain in left malar bone.

⁹ **Lower Face.**   Lips œdematous.

Raging, violent pains in the lips, extending to gums and head, finally to the whole body.

Roughness and tension in lips, especially upper.

Upper lip swollen, hot and red.

Lower lip chapped.

Burning: in the lips; on the chin.

I Bluish lips from asphyxia; constriction of the throat.

¹⁰ **Teeth.**   Jumping pain in left upper molars.

Sudden involuntary biting the teeth together.

Gums bleed easily.

Violent pain in gums.

Swelling and redness of gums and cheek, with sore pain and stinging in the teeth.

Dentition: **I** gums sacculated, look watery, child awakens with screams; red spots here and there on the skin.

¹¹ **Tongue, etc.** Bitter taste.

Inability to talk, or put the tongue out.

Dryness of tongue; fiery redness of buccal cavity, with painful tenderness.

Rawness, burning and painful stinging blisters along the edge of the tongue.

Tongue: red at the tip; swollen, looks dry, glossy; cracked, sore, ulcerated, or covered with vesicles; coated white; glossitis.

¹² **Mouth.** Dryness of mouth and fauces.

Scalding in the mouth and throat.

Fetid breath.

Viscid, tough, frothy saliva.

¹³ **Throat.** ı Tonsils swollen, bright red, stinging when swallowing.

Deep ulcers on tonsils or palate; erysipelatous and œdematous appearance around ulcers.

Œdema of the glottis.

Mucous membrane covered with dirty, greyish deposit.

Tenacious mucus in the throat.

Throat swollen, inside and outside; hoarse; breathing and swallowing difficult.

Small blisters filled with clear lymph, in clusters, on back part of throat.

¹⁴ **Desires. Aversions.** No appetite, nor desire for food.

Insatiable thirst; drinks often, but little at a time. θ In catarrh of chest, diarrhœa, diphtheria and some dropsies.

Thirstless. θ In cerebro-spinal meningitis, ovarian dropsy, ascites and pregnancy.

No thirst with the heat; mouth dry.

Craves milk, which relieves.

Appetite for sour things.

Child nurses by day, refuses at night. θ After vaccination.

¹⁵ **Eating and Drinking.** Continued swallowing relieves soreness and cough.

Vomits the food as soon as taken, followed by retching.

After eating: heaviness at stomach; diarrhœic discharge renewed.

¹⁶ **Nausea and Vomiting.** Bitter or acrid belching; heartburn up into throat; water-brash.

Nausea, with inclination to vomit.

Vomiting: of bile; of mucus, with red specks; of ingesta and slime; and diarrhœa.

¹⁷ **Stomach.** Burning heat in stomach.

Pit of stomach sensitive; burning as from acidity; irritability of stomach; fulness; pressure aggravates the pains.

Great soreness in the pit of stomach when touched.

¹⁸ **Hypochondria.** Violent burning pain under short ribs on both sides.

Sensation of soreness under the ribs.

Obliged to bend forward from a painful contractive feeling in the hypochondria.

ı Pain in hypochondriac regions, extending upwards.

[19] **Abdomen.**   Fulness and enlargement of abdomen.

Rumbling in abdomen.

Sickly feeling in abdomen, inclines him to sit quiet.

Violent cutting pains in the abdomen.

Soreness of the bowels and abdominal walls felt when pressing upon them, or sneezing.

ı Feeling as if intestines were bruised.   θ Dysentery. θ Ascites.

Aching, pressive pain in the hypogastrium, with bearing down in the uterus.

Burning, stinging in the bowels.

ı Peritonitis, with exudation; often with metritis; urine scanty, dark.

ı Walls of abdomen tense; sensitiveness of ileo-cœcal region.   θ Typhus.

[20] **Stool, etc.**   Throbbing in the rectum, with sensation in the anus as if stuffed full; tenesmus.

Diarrhœa: ı watery; yellow, with griping; watery and foul-smelling; watery, copious, black; greenish-yellow mucus, worse morning; slimy mucus and blood; frequent, bloody, painless; olive-green, slimy, profuse, full of bright red lumps; thin, yellow, with extreme weakness, stool with every motion of body, as if anus were constantly open.   .

Costive, with large, hard, difficult stools; stinging pains, and sensation in abdomen as from something tight, which would break if much effort were used.

ı Hemorrhage from bowels, with burning pains, excoriation of anus, constant tenesmus.   θ Prolapsus ani.

[21] **Urine.**   Renal pains, soreness on pressure or when stooping.

Frequent sudden attacks of pain along the ureters.

ı Great irritation of neck at bladder, with frequent and burning urination.

Frequent desire, with passage of only a few drops.

Strangury, stricture, retained urine or inflamed bladder after abuse of cantharides.

Difficult urination, with children.

Incontinence, with great irritation of the parts.

Urine: scanty, high colored; red, bloody, hot and scanty; scanty, fetid; scanty, reddish-brown; after standing, turbid; scanty, milky, albuminous; dark, with sediment like coffee grounds; containing uriniferous tubules and epithelium.

[22] **Male Sexual Organs.**   Frequent and long-lasting erections.

Swelling of testicles, more the right; violent itching and redness of scrotum, sore to touch.

▮ Dropsy of the scrotum; hydrocele.

²³ **Female Sexual Organs.** Sharp, cutting, lancinating pains in ovarian region, extending down thigh; worse right side; numbness in side and limb. θ Ovaritis. θ Ovarian tumor.

Feeling of weight, heaviness in ovarian region.

Right ovary enlarged, pain in left pectoral region, cough.

▮ Dropsy of the ovaries (right), or of the uterus.

Great tenderness over the uterine region, with bearing down pain; leucorrhœa and painful urination.

Heat and fulness of uterine region.

▮ Burning or stinging pains in region of uterus or ovaries.

Menorrhagia, with heaviness in the abdomen, faintness, uneasiness, restlessness, yawning; may have red spots on body, stinging like bee-stings.

Suppressed menses, with congested or inflamed ovaries. Amenorrhœa.

Dvsmenorrhœa, with scanty discharge of slimy blood.

Œdema of the labia.

Ovarian tumors.

Leucorrhœa: profuse, acrid, green.

²⁴ **Pregnancy.** ▮ Abortion during the early months.

Mammæ: burning, stinging, swelling, hardness and suppuration.

▮ Erysipelas of mammæ.

▮ Stinging, burning in scirrhus tumors of the mammæ, or in open cancer.

Menorrhagia accompanying pelvic peritonitis.

Ulceration of the navel in the newborn.

²⁵ **Larynx.** Hoarseness mornings, dryness, burning of larynx.

Speaking is painful; feels as if it wearied the pharynx, in which there is drawing pain.

Weak feeling in larynx.

▮ Œdema glottidis.

²⁶ **Breathing.** Breathing: hurried and difficult, with fever and headache; short, quick; difficult, worse bending forwards or backwards; worse lying on left side.

Great feeling of suffocation; cannot bear anything about the throat.

Oppression, worse ascending; worse in a warm room.

²⁷ **Cough.** Irritation to cough in the suprasternal fossa.

Severe cough, especially after lying and sleeping.

Cough: croupy; with ringing sound; dry, with gagging; with soreness of upper part of chest; with painful concussion of head.

Expectoration: seldom; sweetish or tasteless.

²⁸ **Lungs.** Sensation of soreness, as if bruised or beaten.

Dull, aching pain in left side of chest, near the middle of sternum, with sensation of fulness in the chest and short breath.

ı Hydrothorax. *θ* After pleurisy.

Stitches in left side of chest.

ı Burning, stinging pains throughout entire front of chest.

²⁹ **Heart. Pulse.** Sudden attack of acute pain just below the heart, soon extending diagonally toward the right chest.

Blowing sound with the diastole.

Pulse: accelerated, full and strong; feeble, scarcely perceptible at wrist; at times intermittent and imperceptible; wiry and frequent; ı hard, small and quick.

³⁰ **Outer Chest.** ı Chest feels as if beaten or bruised.

³¹ **Neck. Back.** Stiffness in the back of neck.

Rheumatic stitches in right side of neck.

Tensive pain from left shoulder to back of neck.

Burning and heat, like "prickly heat," on the back.

Lower posterior dorsal region, especially left, feels as if bruised.

Burning, pressing in coccygeal region, worse from any attempt to sit down; evening.

³² **Upper Limbs.** Violent rheumatism in right, later in left shoulder.

Lame feeling in the scapulæ.

Pressure under the scapulæ, painful when moving.

Drawing pains in the arms.

ı Œdema of the hands.

Sensation of numbness in fingers, especially the tips about the roots of the nails.

ı Panaritium, with burning, stinging and throbbing; very sensitive to touch; especially in "runrounds," after abuse of *Sulphur*.

³³ **Lower Limbs.** Sore pain about left hip-joint; later, weakness, unsteadiness, trembling in the joint.

Violent pain in left knee, more outside and to the front.

Sensation in the toes and whole feet as if too large, swollen and stiff; also at night on removing the boots.

Burning in the toes, with redness; feet cold.

ı Legs and feet waxy, pale, swollen, œdematous.

³⁴ **Limbs in General.** Trembling of hands and feet.

Limbs: numb; cold.

³⁵ **Position, etc.** Inclined to sit quiet: 19. Lying: 2; on left side: 26, 27. Sitting: 2, 31. Rising: 36. Motion: 3, 20, 32, 40. Walking: 2. Holds head and eyes down: 3. Stooping: 3, 21. Bending forwards or backwards: 26.

Better by changing position of painful parts, which were worse by lying down.

Pains are better while moving or walking.

36 Nerves. Trembling; nervous restlessness.

Tired, as if bruised in every limb and especially in the back, like after exertion; worse on rising after sitting.

Great prostration.

Left side motionless; now and then moves the right arm; convulsions, trembling and jerking of the limbs.

37 Sleep. Yawning.

❙ Great inclination to sleep, but cannot, from nervous restlessness.

Continuous deep sleep.

Restless sleep and incessant dreaming.

❙ Screams during sleep; also sudden starting.

Dreams: of journeying; of flying; of assembled people; unpleasant.

38 Time. Morning: 20, 25. 3 P. M.: 40. 4. P. M.: 1. Evening: 31, 40. Night: 5, 14, 33. Day: 14.

39 Temperature and Weather. Closed rooms, especially if overheated, are insupportable.

Inclination for open air.

Cold weather aggravates weakness and chest troubles.

Worse getting wet through, but better from washing or moistening the part in cold water.

40 Chill. Fever. Sweat. Chill about 3 P. M., worse in warmth; runs down the back, with great prostration.

Chilliness from the slightest motion, with heat of face and hands; toward evening.

Sensation of coldness without coldness of the skin; ague.

Skin burning hot all over, or gradually grows cool in some places, hot in others.

Heat, with inclination to uncover.

Dry, hot skin, or alternate dry and moist skin.

Sweat after trembling and fainting, then nettle-rash.

❙ During hot stage more or less violent headache, generally a continuous deep sleep. θ Intermittent.

❙ Sweating stage either absent or of a very light grade. θ Intermittent.

❙ Continuous low fever; no thirst; worse 3 P. M., is then very drowsy.

❙ Typhoid forms of fever, especially enteric, cerebral, exanthematic forms; febris nervosa putrida.

Thirst wanting during sweat; may or may not be present during heat, always thirst during the chill.

Apyrexia: pain under short ribs, left side; feet swollen; urine scanty; limbs and joints sore; restless; urticaria.

41 Attacks. Pains return periodically in diphtheria.

Sudden sharp paroxysms of pain.

Pains suddenly migrating from one part to another.

⁴² **Sides.** Right: 8, 22, 23, 31, 36.   Left: 3, 8, 10, 18, 23, 29,
      31, 33, 36, 40.   Left to right: 29, 31.   Right to left: 32.
      Below upwards: 18.   Above downwards: 23.

⁴³ **Sensations.** Burning, stinging like bee-stings, and soreness,
      seem to be the predominating painful sensations—while
      itching, tension and throbbing may or may not be
      painful.
      Numbness of external parts.

⁴⁴ **Tissues.** Affections of circulatory apparatus and fluid, drop-
      sies, phlebitis, varicose veins, ecchymosed spots, gan-
      grene, unhealthy suppuration.
      Periosteum inflamed.
      ı Serous membranes: inflamed; effusions; synovitis.
      Mucous membranes inflamed and catarrhal.
      Glands enlarged, inflamed.
      Muscles stiff, tender on pressure, somewhat swollen; rigid;
      rheumatic inflammation.
      Indurations: scirrhus, or open cancer.

⁴⁵ **Contact, Injuries, etc.** Touch: 17, 19, 22, 26, 32, 46.
      Pressure: 3, 17, 19, 21.   Cannot bear covering: 5.

⁴⁶ **Skin.** Stinging, burning, prickling, smarting, or itching of
      the skin; sensitiveness to the slightest touch.
      Skin very hot and red.
      Red spots on abdomen and other parts; burning, stinging.
      Intensely deep red rash.
      ı Scarlatina.
      Measle-like eruption.
      Small pustules, with burning, smarting, stinging; forming
      dry, scaly, laminated, brownish scabs.
      Body covered with large, white wheals, deep scarlet inter-
      spaces.
      ı Erysipelas, with bruised, sore pain and much swelling.
      White miliary eruption on chest and abdomen.
      Nettle-rash in warm weather, when one cannot sweat.
      Skin: pale, waxy, almost transparent; dark blue, almost
      black.
      Carbuncles, with burning, stinging pains.

⁴⁷ **Stages and States.** Strumous diathesis.
      Bilious, nervous temperament; women and children; es-
      pecially widows; girls, who though generally careful,
      become awkward, and let things fall while handling them.
      Old people, asthma.
      Those predisposed to miscarry should not receive *Apis*
      except in high potencies.

⁴⁸ **Relationship.** Antidotes to massive doses and in poison-
      ings: *Natr. mur.*, the substance, the solution, the poten-
      cies; sweet oil, as it contains table salt; onions; bleed-
      ing is decidedly a bad palliative, and is in most cases
      injurious.

Antidotes to potencies: after overdosing, *Ipec.*, low, relieved much; to drink coffee, seems indifferent; some have given *Apis*, high, *Laches.* and *Lact. ac.*

(Has been given in ailments from stings, and from anthrax infection.)

It is an antidote to *Canthar.* (ischuria, inflammation of bladder, acute Bright's disease); abuse of *Iodium, Cinchon., Digit.*

It follows well after vaccination (erysipelas, painless diarrhœa); after *Sulphur*, in panaritium.

After it follows well: *Graphit.* (tetter on ear-lobe); *Arsen.* (hydrothorax); *Phosphor.* (absorption of the false membrane in diphtheria); *Stramon.* after *Apis* has removed the jealousy in mania; *Lycop.* (in staphyloma); *Sulphur* (in hydrothorax, pleuritic effusion, hydrocephalus); *Iodium* (in puffy, swollen knee).

Complementary: *Natr. mur.*

Has been given in alternation in cases when the change of symptoms indicated it with: *Iodium* in swelling of knee; *Sulphur* in swollen eyes; *Hepar* in urticaria; *Mercur.* in ascites with peritonitis; *Lycop.* in staphyloma.

It often disagrees after *Rhus tox.* in eruptive diseases; and *Rhus tox.* given after *Apis* has often disagreed.

Collateral relation (belonging to the same family); *Bombus, Crabro, Vespa.*

It has cured where *Bellad.* failed in cough of horses; where *Bryon., Canthar., Digit., Helleb.*, etc., had failed in albuminuria after scarlatina; cases in which *Pulsat.*, seemingly indicated, failed, especially in uterine complaints; when *Thuja, Phosphor., Canthar.*, etc., had failed in affections of the prostate gland.

Concordances: *Acet. ac.* (dropsy); *Acon.; Anac.* (urticaria); *Apocyn. cannab.* (dropsy); *Arnic.* (bruised sore); *Arsen.* (typhoid forms; gangrene; dropsies; scarlatina; urticaria; chills); *Bellad.* (meningitis, especially of cerebral meninges; faucitis; erysipelas; scarlatina; glandular organs, etc.); *Bromin.* (swelling of ovary during menses); *Bryon.; Cantharides* (erysipelas, urinary symptoms); *Cinchon.; Colchic.* (rheumatism, etc.); *Crot. tig.* (urticaria); *Euphras.* (conjunctiva); *Ferrum; Graphit.; Hepar; Iodium* (swollen knee); *Laches.* (typhoid states; gangrene); *Lycop.; Mercur.; Natr. ars.; Natr. mur.* (chills; urticaria; tension in ovarian region, etc.); *Pulsat.; Rhus tox.* (eyes, but *Apis* has less suppuration; vesicular erysipelas, but darker than in *Apis*, and spreading left to right; typhoid states; restlessness, but in *Apis* more fidgitiness, etc.); *Rum. crisp.* (painless, greenish-yellow diarrhœa); *Sabin.* (ovarian and uterine symptoms); *Sepia; Silic.* (ovary and inverted nipple); *Sulphur* (tubercular meningitis; checked eruptions, especially urticaria; asthma; hydrothorax); *Tereb.* (urinary symptoms); *Therid.* (vertigo); *Thuja* (sycosis, evils of vaccination); *Urt. ur.; Zincum; Calc. iod.* (which has relieved conical cornea and staphyloma); *Guarea* (has cured conjunctivitis with marked chemosis).

APOCYNUM CANNABINUM.

Indian Hemp.   ALLENTOWN SCHOOL.   *Apocynaceæ.*

¹ **Mind.** Bewildered.
 Low-spirited and nervous. θ Ascites and chronic diarrhœa.
³ **Inner Head.** Heaviness of the head evenings; aching in the small of the back and limbs.
 Hydrocephalus; stupor, sight of one eye totally lost, the other eye slightly sensible; constant involuntary motion of one arm and leg; forehead projecting; sutures open. Stage of exudation.
⁵ **Eyes.** Heat, redness of the left eye, feeling as of sand in the eye; early in the morning.
⁷ **Nose.** Nostrils and throat filled with thick, yellow mucus, on waking in the morning.
⁸ **Face.** Bloated after lying down; passes off after sitting up.
¹¹ **Tongue, etc.** Taste: bitter, sub-acrid, in the fauces.
¹² **Mouth.** Dryness of the mouth on awaking; thirst.
 Constant spitting; increased secretion of mucus and saliva in mouth and fauces.
¹³ **Throat.** Thick, yellow mucus in the throat in the morning; unpleasant degree of heat.
¹⁴ **Desires. Aversions.** ❙ Great thirst, but water disagrees, causing pain, or is immediately thrown off. θ Dropsy.
¹⁵ **Eating and Drinking.** Distention about the stomach and hypochondria after a moderate meal.
¹⁶ **Nausea and Vomiting.** Nausea after sleep.
 Violent vomiting, prostration and drowsiness, cold skin. Distressing vomiting at intervals. θ Menorrhagia.
¹⁷ **Stomach.** Sinking at the stomach on awaking.
 ❙ Stomach so irritable not even a draught of water can be retained. θ Dropsy.
¹⁹ **Abdomen.** ❙ Ascites.
²⁰ **Stool, etc.** Bilious stool; loose, but not very copious.
 Bowels sluggish, but feces not hard or costive.

²¹ **Urine.** Scanty; no uneasiness.

Retention of urine, with paralysis of lower extremities.

Urine light, or sherry-yellow in color, no sediment on cooling.

²³ **Female Sexual Organs.** Amenorrhœa in young girls;. abdomen and legs bloated.

Metrorrhagia continuous or paroxysmal; fluid or clotted;. nausea, vomiting, palpitation; pulse quick, feeble, when moved; fainting, when raising the head from pillow.

²⁶ **Breathing.** Oppression of the chest on awaking.

Oppression about the epigastrium and chest, difficulty in getting breath enough to speak; after a light meal.

❙ Hydrothorax.

Irresistible disposition to sigh.

²⁷ **Cough.** Loose rattling, with oppression of the chest; short, dry; evening or night.

Scanty expectoration of white mucus.

²⁹ **Heart. Pulse.** Pulse 45 between attacks of vomiting;. feeble. θ Metrorrhagia.

³¹ **Neck. Back.** Slight soreness in region of kidneys when bringing muscles into action.

³³ **Lower Limbs.** Hard aching in both knees.

Œdema of the feet and ankles.

³⁴ **Limbs in General.** Itching in the limbs; weakness.

³⁵ **Position, etc.** Using muscles: 31. Raising the head, fainting: 23. Lying, face bloated, better sitting up: 8.

³⁶ **Nerves.** General restlessness with debility.

Involuntary motions one arm and leg. θ Hydrocephalus.

³⁷ **Sleep.** On going to bed desire for sleep, inability to sleep.

Drowsiness; vomiting; weakness.

Stupor.

Restlessness, little sleep.

³⁸ **Time.** Morning: 5, 7, 12, 13, 15, 16, 17. Evening: 3, 27, 37, 46. Night: 27.

⁴⁰ **Chill. Fever. Sweat.** Heat of the skin on going to bed.

Sweat: when the skin moistens, the dropsy improves.

⁴² **Sides.** Left: 5.

⁴⁴ **Tissues.** ❙ Excretions diminished, especially urine; sweat.

❙ Acute inflammatory dropsy.

❙ Dropsy: with great thirst, but water causes pain or is vomited, after typhus, scarlatina, cirrhosis; but mostly uncomplicated with organic disease.

Profuse (uterine) hemorrhages.

⁴⁶ **Skin.** Skin cold, with vomiting. See 16.

Skin hot, evening going to bed.

⁴⁸ **Relationship.** Concordances: *Acet. ac.;* ❙ *Apis* (which has no thirst in dropsies); *Arsen.; Bellad.; Bryon.; Cin-*

chon.; Colchic.; Digit. (dropsy; slow pulse); *Elat.;* ❚ *Helleb.* (hydrocephalus, ascites, etc.); *Kali carb.; Lycop.; Mercur.; Merc. sulph.; Scilla; Sulphur; Veratr.alb.*
❚ Dropsy after abuse of quinine.

ARALIA RACEMOSA.

Spikenard.   S. A. JONES.   *Araleaceæ.*

[7] **Nose.** Smarting soreness of posterior nares caused by passage of acrid mucus; with peculiar soreness of the alæ nasi, as if fissured.

[26] **Breathing.** Dry, wheezing respiration, sense of impending suffocation; whistling worse during inspiration, must sit up. θ Hay-asthma.

[27] **Cough.** ❚ Awakes and coughs, cannot again sleep because of it.

Sputum at acme of asthma scanty, then increased warm and saltish.

[28] **Lungs.** Raw, burning, sore feeling behind the whole length of the sternum and in each lung.

ARGENTUM METALLICUM.

Pure Metallic Silver.   *Introduced by Hahnemann.*

[1] **Mind.** Fear of apoplexy, particularly with palpitation of heart.

Ill-humor, with disinclination to talk.

Out of humor in forenoon; in afternoon copious nosebleed.

Restlessness, anxiety, which drives him from place to place.

[2] **Sensorium.** Dizziness on entering a room after a walk.

While slumbering in bed, before midnight, it seemed as if the head was falling out of bed; followed by a violent convulsive starting of body.

Felt suddenly giddy, and as if a mist were before the eyes.

Attacks of vertigo; he cannot think rightly.

When looking at running water, giddy.

❚ A crawling and whirling in the head, as if drunken.

[3] **Inner Head.** Congestion to the head, followed by redness of cheeks.

Cutting stitches from left ear into brain.

Pressing pain, with dulness in forehead, and drawing pressure in occiput.

Pressive, tearing pain, at temporal bones, worse by touch.

Painful sensation of emptiness in head, feeling as if it were hollow, with aching of the whole brain.

Left-sided headache, as if in the brain substance; at first only slight drawing, gradually becoming more violent; at its culmination raging as though a nerve was being torn, ceasing suddenly.

⁴ **Outer Head.** Tenderness on top of head, painful to touch.

Pressing, tearing pain in skull, principally in the temporal bones, renewed every day at noon, worse by pressure and touch, better in open air.

Aching of external parts of head.

⁵ **Eyes.** Sight vanishes.

Amaurosis of left eye, contracted pupil, insensible to light.

Violent itching of lids and in the corners of the eyes. θ Blepharitis.

Lids greatly swollen.

Pustules along edges of lids.

Any effort to separate lids causes edges to be drawn in.

Lids raw, sore, red, smarting.

Abundant purulent discharge.

⁶ **Ears.** Corrosive itching; scratching until bleeding ensues.

⁷ **Nose.** Tickling, crawling sensation in the nose, followed by nosebleed.

When blowing the nose, violent bleeding.

▮ Violent fluent coryza, with frequent sneezing, mornings.

⁸ **Face.** Pressing and tearing of the facial bones; drawing, tearing in the right zygoma.

Face straw-colored, including lips. θ Scirrhus of os uteri.

⁹ **Lower Face.** Swelling of upper lip, close under the nose.

¹⁰ **Teeth.** Severe aching in the decayed last molar, left side.

Teeth adhere together like from glue.

¹¹ **Tongue, etc.** Sore, burning blisters on tongue; tongue dry.

Speech impeded by much viscid saliva in the mouth.

¹² **Mouth.** Dryness in the mouth.

▮ Fetid breath. θ Scirrhus uteri.

¹³ **Throat.** Region of submaxillary glands swollen; the neck stiff; swallowing difficult, as from internal swelling; has to force every mouthful down the œsophagus.

Scratching sensation in the soft palate, as from something rough sticking there; felt most during empty swallowing, forcing him to swallow saliva.

Painful tension in fauces as from swelling, when yawning.

▮ Throat feels raw and sore during expiration, or when swallowing or coughing.

▮ Viscid, grey, jelly-like mucus in pharynx, easily hawked up; early morning.

▮ Anæsthesia of the fauces. *θ* Diphtheria.

▮ Tension in fauces on right side, felt only when gaping. *θ* Aphonia.

¹⁴ **Desires. Aversions.** Appetite increased; hungry after eating a full meal.

Desire for wine.

At times loss of appetite, with aversion to smoking.

Aversion to all food, even when thinking of it.

Want of thirst, even during the hot stage of the fever.

¹⁵ **Eating and Drinking.** During and after meals, sweating.

After dinner, nosebleed.

¹⁶ **Nausea and Vomiting.** Squeamish nausea in region of sternum, with vertigo and burning in scrobiculum.

Nauseous sensations with hunger; nausea in his dreams.

Vomiting, with the stool in the afternoon.

Bitter, acrid fluid rises up into the throat; heartburn.

¹⁷ **Stomach.** Burning in the stomach, ascending to the chest.

Anxiety and pressure in pit of stomach.

¹⁸ **Hypochondria.** Cutting stitch under the last left ribs.

¹⁹ **Abdomen.** Tympanitic puffing of right side of abdomen.

Sore to hard pressure; slowly lessened after wind passes.

Expansion and sensation of fulness in epigastrium, with hunger.

Loud croaking in the abdomen, with hunger.

Wind colic.

Distention of hypogastrium, which was exceedingly sensitive to contact.

Contraction and tension of the abdominal muscles; has to walk bent forward.

Bruised pain over left hip, and on whole left side of pelvis.

Tension in the groins.

Painful soreness in the whole abdomen, worse when riding in a carriage.

²⁰ **Stool, etc.** Frequent urging in lower part of rectum, with discharge of small quantities of soft stool.

Dry stool, like sand, after dinner.

Alvine evacuation irregular, often lienteric diarrhœa.

Diarrhœa with constant pain in left side of stomach.

Sore between the nates, around anus, and in groin, on moderate walking.

²¹ **Urine.** Turbid, sweetish, profuse at night. *θ* Diabetes.

Urine profuse at night; pale, fetid.

²² **Male Sexual Organs.** Seminal emissions almost every night, without erection, with atrophy of penis; after onanism.

Yellowish-greenish gonorrhœa, of an indolent character from beginning.

Very profuse gonorrhœa, with contusive pain in testicle.

Greyish ulcers, with shaggy borders, at the prepuce; at the same time in the throat.

Crushed pain in the testicles; clothing increases the pain on walking; also evenings in bed.

Scrotum and feet œdematous. *θ* Diabetes mellitus.

:23 **Female Sexual Organs.** ι Pains in the left ovary and loins.

Purulent, ichorous, sometimes bloody matter flows from uterine ulcers, filling room with an unbearable stench.

Neck of uterus looks spongy, deeply corroded.

Metrorrhagia, large lumps with violent pains, increased with every motion.

Hemorrhages at the approach of the climacteric period.

ι Prolapsus uteri; pain in left ovary; pain in small of back extending to the front and downwards.

:25 **Larynx.** ι Rawness and soreness in upper part of larynx, when coughing, not when swallowing.

ι Hoarseness; especially of professional singers, speakers, etc.

Cannot speak a loud word; constant tickling in the throat, provoking cough.

Laughing produces mucus in larynx and excites cough.

When stooping, or ascending stairs, mucus rises into the throat, easily brought up by a single cough.

A grey, gelatinous phlegm is easily raised from trachea.

ι Over the bifurcation of the trachea, a raw spot; hoarseness; worse when using the voice.

:26 **Breathing.** When reading aloud in the evening, he has to hem and hawk.

Stitches between the sixth and seventh ribs, worse when inhaling.

With a deep inhalation, pressing out pain below the second and third rib.

With every deep breath cutting on both sides on last ribs.

Violent stitches in chest impede inhalation and exhalation.

Want of breath, also in diabetes.

:27 **Cough.** Dry, caused by irritation in the bronchia, with a sore pain; drawing stitches on lowest rib, near spine; in attacks, rattling by day and in room, not at night, nor in open air; with easy expectoration, white, thickish, looking like boiled starch; ι from laughing; from dull cutting, which becomes a stitch, in the air-passages from below upwards, with mucus in chest.

Expectoration almost constant, day and evening.

28 **Lungs.** Stitches in right chest from within outwards, he can neither inhale nor exhale without feeling it.

ι Great weakness of the chest, worse left side.

29 **Heart. Pulse.** Beats sometimes omit.

Palpitation increased by sudden muscular exertion.

Full feeling in region of heart.

Frequent spasmodic, but painless twitchings of whole cardiac muscle, especially on lying on back; fears apoplexy.

Pulse: often unchanged; more frequently in evening, in
bed; slow in the morning.

³⁰ **Outer Chest.**   Cutting, left side, in cartilages of false ribs.

Chest feels sore to touch.

❙ Boil near last rib.

³¹ **Neck.   Back.**   The sterno-cleido-mastoid muscles hurt
when stretched by turning of head.

Itching between the shoulder-blades.

On right of pelvis, near sacrum, skin feels cold as if
touched with ice; returns after eating.

³² **Upper Limbs.**   Upper arms feel powerless, as after severe
labor.

Tearing in bones of arms, especially of hands and fingers.

A short paralytic drawing on the outside of upper arm;
on pressure it pains as if beaten; same in wrist-joint.

³³ **Lower Limbs.**   Stitches in the hip when walking.

From time to time crampy pains in the thighs.

Weariness about the hip-joints, worse walking; feel bruised
on hard pressure after rising.

Stiffness in the hips in the morning.

Knee pains as if bruised, while sitting.

Knees knock together when walking.

Calves feel as if too short on going down stairs.

When stepping, feet feel sore, as if ulcerated.

Feet œdematous, swollen.

Tearing in the feet, at times in the soles, dorsa, heels or
toes, in tarsal or metatarsal bones.

³⁴ **Limbs in General.**   Numbness in limbs, as if asleep.

All the limbs feel stiff.

Loss of power; after walking, unusual fatigue.   Heaviness.

Joints of hands and feet feel sore; drawing in the joints.

³⁵ **Position, etc.**   Motion: 13, 23, 36.   Exertion: 29.   Must
go from place to place: 1.   Walking: 20, 22, 23, 34.
Ascending: 25.   Descending: 33, 44.   Sitting; 33.
Bending forwards: 19. Stooping: 25.   Turning head:
31.   After rising: 33.   Lying: 29, 36.

³⁶ **Nerves.**   Painless twitching: around right shoulder and
right thigh; of right thumb, abducting it while writing.

Spasmodic, painful twitching of muscles on temple, forehead, and throat, near thyroid cartilage.

Convulsive shocks of whole body; after previous vertigo;
mostly when dropping off to sleep, preventing sleep.

Epileptic attacks, followed by delirious rage, jumping
about, striking those near.

Weary, forced to lie down and sleep.

Paralytic weakness on motion; bruised feeling.

Lame, weakness with all pains.

³⁷ **Sleep.** Gaping, drowsy; depressed in mind.

Like electric shocks on going to sleep.

Restless sleep; anxious, frightful dreams, on awaking believes them true.

Nausea in dreams.

On awaking: fatigue; upper arm weak, legs powerless.

³⁸ **Time.** Day: 27. Morning: 7, 13, 29, 33. Forenoon: 1, 40. Noon: 4. Afternoon: 1, 16, 40. Evening: 22, 26, 27, 29, 40. Night: 21, 27. Before midnight: 2, 40. After midnight: 40.

³⁹ **Temperature and Weather.** Better in open air: 4, 27. Entering warm room: 2. Uncovering: 40.

⁴⁰ **Chill. Fever. Sweat.** Coldness on small spots.

Chill: in the afternoon and evening, until asleep; before midnight, every time the bed clothes are raised.

Chilly, stupid; chill spreads from the back.

Heat in the forenoon without thirst, heat all over, but less on the head.

❚ Hectic, 11 A. M. to 12 M., or 1 P. M.

Sweats easily; during and after eating; upper part of body, or only front of body.

Sweat after midnight.

Sweat on abdomen, chest.

⁴¹ **Attacks.** Pains increase gradually, disappear suddenly.

Sudden momentary pains; belly, back, right shoulder, etc.

Cough in attacks.

⁴² **Sides.** Right: 3, 8, 28, 31, 36. Left: 3, 5, 10, 18, 19, 23, 28, 30, 32, 46. Below upwards: 3, 17, 27. Above downwards: 23. Within outwards: 28.

⁴³ **Sensations.** Soreness and rawness in internal organs.

Articular rheumatism, without swelling, with burning, lancinating pains, like from the sting of a wasp, severe at the knee, still more at the elbow.

Pains: as if sprained; as if beaten.

⁴⁴ **Tissues.** Drawing pains in maxillary and parotid glands.

❚ Acts on cartilages and joints.

Joints feel weak, sore; especially in lower limbs when descending.

Arthritic bruised pains in joints; boring.

Emaciation.

❚ Tenderness, pressure or tearing in the bones; gnawing, especially in the long bones, and in those of the face.

⁴⁵ **Contact, Injuries, etc.** Touch: 3, 4, 19, 30, 46. Pressure: 4, 19, 32, 33. Scratching: 6, 46. Riding in carriage: 19.

⁴⁶ **Skin.** Itching, unchanged by scratching.

Sore exanthemata, cannot bear to have them touched, even the motion of the skin is almost unbearable.

A pimple on left temple sore to the touch.

Stinging as from fleas here and there.

⁴⁷ **Stages and States.** Tall, thin people of irritable temperament.

Affections from onanism.

⁴⁸ **Relationship.** Cured gonorrhœa, after *Cannab.*, *Copaiva* and *Mercur.* failed.

Cured scirrhus of os tincæ, after *Conium*, *Cicuta*, *Sepia* and *Lycop.* failed.

Uterine and ovarian symptoms, similar to *Pallad.*, the latter on the right side; *Argent. met.* on the left.

❙ Ailments from abuse of mercury.

Antidotes to *Argent. met.*: *Mercur.*, *Pulsat.*

After *Argent. met.* follow well: *Calc. ostr.*, *Pulsat.*, *Sepia.*

Argent. met. follows well after *Alum.* and *Platin.*

A return of trembling palpitation four months after delivery, after being cured in the third month of pregnancy by *Argent. met.*, was relieved by *Rhus tox.*

Compare•*Stannum* in cough excited by laughing.

ARGENTUM NITRICUM.

Nitrate of Silver.   J. O. Mueller. $AgO, NO5$.

¹ **Mind.** Loss of consciousness; faint feeling.

❙ Loses his memory; frequently cannot find the right word, hence falters in speech; lies with closed eyes, shunning light and conversation.

Imbecility.

Time seems to pass very slowly.

Dulness of the head, mental confusion; dizziness; tendency to fall sideways.

Thinks about killing himself.

❙ Impulsive, must walk fast; frequent attacks of anxiety.

Indifference to occupation, loses all inclination for work; melancholic, believes he is despised by his family; believes that all his undertakings will fail.

Reserved; sad; taciturn, with dulness of the head and beating in the whole body.

❙ Feeling as if a cloud hung over him, with great depression; usually with sighing respiration, worse in a close room.

Easily frightened; fears the disease may result seriously; weeping mood.

Easily angered; from it cough and stitches in the chest.

Thinking intently increases headache and causes dimness of vision.

Noticing beating of heart increases it. See 36.

❚ Apprehension when ready to go to church or opera, bringing on diarrhœa.

² **Sensorium.** Vertigo: when walking with eyes closed, which alarms him ; staggers when walking in the dark, has to seize hold of things ; ❚ buzzing in ears ; general debility of the limbs and trembling ; vertigo and complete but transient blindness ; epilepsy.

Drowsy, dilated pupils ; green stools. θ Hydrocephaloid.

³ **Inner Head.** Congestion of blood to head and face.

Rush of blood, throbbing carotids, head seems too large ; relieved by tight bandage.

Boring in left frontal eminence, worse at night in warm bed.

Pressing pains sometimes on vertex, sometimes left frontal bone, relieved by pressure or by tight bandaging ; worse from any exhaustive mental labor ; letters would then run together.

Violent pressure in the forehead commencing over the eyes, spreading upwards to coronal suture ; in m$_{orning}$.

Hemicrania ; pressive, screwing, throbbing pain in one frontal protuberance, temple or into the bones of the face. At its height, trembling of the whole body, intense nausea, which ends in watery, bilious vomit ; lies senseless, eyes closed, shuns light and conversation.

Digging pains in the right hemisphere of the brain.

Digging, cutting motion through left hemisphere, from occiput to frontal protuberance, recurs frequently, increases and decreases rapidly.

⁴ **Outer Head.** Almost constant boring, cutting in bones of forehead, vertex, temples and face.

❚ Head feels much enlarged.

Itching, creeping, crawling, as from vermin ; roots of hair feel as if pulled upwards ; she had to scratch all the time.

Herpetic eruption on the occiput.

Burning in the scalp, which feels as if drawn tight ; cold feeling in eyes.

⁵ **Eyes.** Far-sighted.

Grey spots and serpent-like bodies moved before him.

Letters become blurred ; run together. See 3.

Photophobia, eyes filled with mucus.

Photophobia and weak sight, preventing his writing.

Vanishing of sight, he must constantly wipe away mucus.

Paralysis of accommodation from errors of refraction, glasses failing.

Eyes red, shuns light, after straining them while sewing ; worse in the warm room, better in the open air.

Conjunctiva towards inner canthus, is red and swollen,
· like pterygium.

Canthi as red as blood, the caruncula swollen, standing out
like a lump of red-flesh; clusters of intensely red vessels,
extend from inner canthus to the cornea.

❙Cornea opaque; ulceration of the cornea in newborn
infants; profuse purulent discharge from the lids.

Conjunctiva of ball and lids intensely congested; ❙bright
red granulations on lids; lids swollen, thick pus discharges.

Œdema of the lids and sensation of fulness, dryness and
heat, especially on moving the ball, which is sensitive
to touch; chemosis; non-excoriating lachrymation.

Lids crusty, swollen, thick; with pannus.

❙Ciliary blepharitis from being over a fire; better from
cold air and cold applications.   θ Ectropion.

⁶ **Ears.**   Dull hearing; complete deafness in typhus.

Ringing in the ears; whizzing and feeling of obstruction,
with hard hearing in left ear.

Stitches from right into left ear, with congestion to head.

Fulness and ringing in the ears.   θ Meningitis.

Tearing in the ears.

⁷ **Nose.**   Sense of smell blunted.

Smell as of pus before the nose; small ulcers in the nares.

Discharge of whitish pus, with clots of blood.

Coryza, with stupefying headache over the eyes, has to lie
down; sneezing chilliness, lachrymation, sickly look.

Violent itching of the nose.

⁸ **Face.**   Face sunken, pale, bluish; leaden colored; ❙old looking, ashen; ❙yellow, dirty looking.

Circumscribed red cheeks.

Left side swollen, with great heat and burning; lips much
swollen.

During attack of prosopalgia, sour taste.

Infraorbital neuralgia, left side.

⁹ **Lower Face.**   Hard, pale blotches on the vermillion border
of the upper lip, sore to the touch.

Lips: trembled when he spoke; lips and finger nails blue.

¹⁰ **Teeth.**   Teeth: sensitive to cold water; black.

Gums tender, bleed easily; neither painful nor swollen.

¹¹ **Tongue, etc.**   Taste: sweetish-bitter; sour; metallic, astringent; inky; lost.

Cannot talk; spasms of the muscles of tongue and throat.

Tongue coated white.

❙Tip of the tongue red, painful (see 17); papillæ erect,
prominent.

Tongue dry, hard as a chip, and black like the teeth.

Red streak down middle of tongue.

¹² **Mouth.**   Fetor from the mouth; morning.

Ptyalism.

Inner mouth covered with a whitish-grey coat.

[13] **Throat.** ❙ Uvula and fauces dark red.

❙ Thick tenacious mucus in the throat, obliging him to hawk; causing slight hoarseness.

Rawness, soreness; scraping in the throat.

❙ Sensation as if a splinter were lodged in the throat, when swallowing, breathing or moving the neck.

Wart-like excrescences feel like pointed bodies when swallowing.

Swallowing difficult.

Burning and dryness in fauces and pharynx.

Paroxysms of cramp in the œsophagus.

[14] **Desires. Aversions.** ❙ Irresistible desire for sugar.

❙ Loss of appetite; much thirst, or no thirst.

Desire for strong cheese.

[15] **Eating and Drinking.** Eating, or a swallow of wine, relieves the head; coffee aggravates.

Sour things lessen nausea.

Warm fluids relieve, cold aggravate the pains in stomach.

After drinking, dyspnœa.

Nausea after each meal, mostly after dinner, or after supper.

Fluids go "right through him." See 20.

[16] **Nausea and Vomiting.** ❙ Belching after every meal; stomach as if it would burst with wind; belching difficult, finally air rushes out with great violence.

Tasteless, or sour eructations.

Deathly nausea with headache, not abating after vomiting.

The vomited substances tinge the bedding black. θ Yellow fever.

Awakens at midnight, with oppression at stomach as from a heavy lump inducing vomiting; in the morning throws up a glairy mucus which can be drawn into strings; during the afternoon desire to vomit, tremulous weakness.

[17] **Stomach.** Small spot between the xyphoid and navel, sensitive to the slightest pressure; pain radiates in all directions; increases and decreases gradually. θ Gastrodynia.

Regularly towards midnight, attacks of pain preceded by vomiting of slimy and bilious fluid.

Constant drawing and gnawing, increasing daily to violent attacks, ending in vomiting of clear, saltish water.

❙ After ice cream, gastralgia, pain radiating in all directions, worse after food.

Stitches in the stomach, and short breathing.

Trembling; weakness at pit of stomach.

Fulness of the stomach; painful swelling at the pit, with great anxiety- θ Flatulent dyspepsia.

Stinging, ulcerative pain in the left side of stomach, worse from touch and deep inspiration.

Gastric catarrh after a long "spree;" tip of tongue red. See 11.

Ulceration of stomach, worse from cold food; mucous stools.

[18] **Hypochondria.** Region of the liver sensitive to pressure; periodical attacks of pain about liver and navel, with nausea, retching and vomiting of tough phlegm.

Tension as from a band around the hypochondria.

Spasms of the diaphragm.

[19] **Abdomen.** Fulness and heaviness of the abdomen, with anxiety, impeding respiration; after supper.

Rumbling, gurgling; wind cannot pass.

Tension of abdomen, cannot bear to be touched. See 17.

Constriction in the bowels, as if tightly tied with a band.

Stitches dart through the abdomen like electric shocks, especially when suddenly changing from rest to motion.

Bearing down in the hypogastrium.

Hemorrhoidal colic mornings, during cold, misty weather.

[20] **Stool, etc.** Stools: of green, fetid mucus, with noisy flatus at night; green, brown, bloody, fetid mucus, worse after midnight; slimy, watery, greenish, bloody, with tenesmus; green, watery, with sour taste in mouth; green flakes like spinach; bright yellow, thin, fetid, after weaning; before stool, fermentation.

❙ Green stool; sopor, large pupils.

Croupous inflammation of the rectum; thin, unshapely strips pass in masses, with burning, constriction and sore pain in left side of abdomen.

❙ Masses of epithelium connected by muco-lymph, looking red or green and shreddy, with severe bearing down in hypogastrium; advanced dysentery, with suspected ulceration.

Looseness after exalted imagination; chronic diarrhœa after mental shock.

Stool and urine passed involuntarily.

❙ Diarrhœa as soon as he drinks.

❙ Child is very fond of sugar, but diarrhœa results from eating it.

Constipation aggravates every complaint; alternates with diarrhœa; stools very dry. θ Epilepsy.

Tænia or thread-worms; the latter, especially with much itching at the anus.

[21] **Urine.** Acute pain about the kidneys, extending down the ureters to bladder; worse from the slightest touch or motion, even deep inspiration.

Ulcerative pain in middle of urethra, as from a splinter.

Urine dark red; no albumen; deposits red crystals of uric acid.

Urine passed unconsciously and uninterruptedly.

| Incontinence of urine at night; also by day.

| Urging to urinate; urine passes less easily and freely.

Urine burns while passing, urethra feels as if swollen, with feeling as if the last drops remained behind; profuse purulent urethral discharge.

Stream of urine spreads asunder.

Bleeding of urethra; painful erections.

²² **Male Sexual Organs.**   Impotence; erections, but they fail when coition is attempted.

Want of desire, organs shriveled.

Coition painful; urethra as if put on the stretch, or sensitive at its orifice.

Ulcers on the prepuce small, covered with pus; later spreading, bowl-shaped, with a tallow-like coating.

Contusive pain, with enlargement and hardening of right testicle.

²³ **Female Sexual Organs.**   Bleeding ulcers, the hemorrhages being of short duration.

Dreams of sexual gratification.

| Coition painful, followed by bleeding from the vagina.

| Prolapsus with ulceration of os or cervix uteri.

Menses: too early, profuse, long-lasting; with headache, cutting in small of back and groin; at night tormenting pressure in præcordia; internal trembling in epigastrium; irregular, too soon or too late, too copious or too scanty, but always with thick, coagulated blood.

| Metrorrhagia, with nervous erethism at change of life; also in young widows and those who have borne no children; returns in attacks; region of ovaries painful, with pains radiating to sacrum and thighs.

Leucorrhœa copious, yellow, corroding.

²⁴ **Pregnancy.**   Disposed to abortion.

| During pregnancy, stomach as if it would burst with wind; head feels expanded.

Nipples sore from nursing.

Puerperal convulsions; spasms preceded by a sensation of general expansion, mostly of face and head.

Sometimes just after an attack she lies quiet, but before another she becomes very restless.

Suckling infants die early; have marasmus.

²⁵ **Larynx.**   Internal soreness of the larynx and pit of the throat; worse in the morning.

Hoarse voice.

Phlegm in the larynx causing rattling, whistling breathing until removed in small lumps by cough.

Rawness, soreness high up in trachea, when coughing.

| Chronic laryngitis of singers, raising voice causes cough.

²⁶ **Breathing.**   Many people in room seem to take away his breath.

Motion, going up stairs or bodily exertion, causes asthmatic attacks, face congested, palpitation.

Short breathed, with deep sighs; much oppression; violent attacks of dry, spasmodic asthma, forcing him to rise and walk about.

Inclined to take a deep breath, but the effort causes asthma.

Upper abdominal walls are drawn in during inspiration; expand during expiration; the effort to breathe deeply takes away the breath at once. θ Paralysis of diaphragm.

Spasms of the respiratory muscles in cholera; great constriction and stitches in the epigastrium; cannot talk; drinking suffocates; even a handkerchief before the nose impedes breathing; agony, thinks of killing himself.

[27] **Cough.** Cough evenings; tobacco smoke becomes intolerable.

Irritating cough, tormenting evening and night.

Suffocative cough at noon.

Paroxysms of cough are brought on by: phlegm in larynx; irritation under the sternum; by a fit of passion; laughing; stooping; smoking; ascending stairs.

Expectoration purulent, mixed with light blood.

Catarrh at first dry, later loose, with rattling cough, profuse sweat, sickly look, hollow eyes, restless sleep; expectoration yellow.

Belching or straining to vomit, during the attack of cough.

[28] **Inner Chest.** Stitching pain in region of fifth rib, left side, with frequent blood spitting.

Bursting pain after going up stairs; has to press with both hands.

Aching, tensive pain in the chest in various places of the size of a half dollar.

[29] **Heart. Pulse.** Palpitation of the heart: with nausea; with asthma; violent, from the slightest mental emotion or sudden muscular exertion.

Heart's action irregular, intermittent, with an unpleasant sensation of fulness; exertion causes strong beating, worse when noticing it.

Constant anxious feeling in region of heart; burning feeling.

Pains about the heart, can hardly breathe; choking.

[30] **Outer Chest.** Violent pain in the muscles of the chest.

[31] **Neck. Back.** I Indurated glands on the neck, with suspicion of former syphilis.

Acute pains in the dorsal region after a fall.

Pain in the small of the back, relieved when standing or walking; but severe when rising from a seat.

Pain in back and lower ribs during pregnancy.

Weakness in sacro-iliac symphisis as if bones were loose.

Sense of weight in lower part of sacrum and os coccygis, better standing; worse sitting and with stool.

[32] **Upper Limbs.** Paralytic drawing pain in right arm.
Heaviness of the left arm.
Pimple on hand near wrist, feels as if a splinter was in it.
Spasmodic contraction of the abductors of the fingers, can
hardly separate them; fingers half clenched.
Hands tremble, cannot write.
Nails blue.
Numbness of finger-tips; left ring and little fingers in-
sensible.

[33] **Lower Limbs.** Lassitude of lower limbs, with dizziness as
from intoxication.
Debility and weakness of lower limbs the whole afternoon;
with sick feeling and dread of work.
Numbness of the lower extremities, with coldness.
Limbs, especially his knees, start up at night, awakening
him.
Calves weary, as after a long journey.
Pains in calves torment him all night.
Œdema of the feet.

[34] **Limbs in General.** ❙ Lassitude, weariness of forearms, legs,
Trembling. θ Paralysis.
Rheumatic tendency in right arm and thigh. θ Asthma.
During day, tormented with formication of arms and legs.
Chorea-like convulsive motion of limbs; legs drawn up;
arms jerked outward and upward.

[35] **Position, etc.** Motion: 19, 21, 26. Moving neck: 13. Walking: 2, 26, 31, 36. Walks fast: 1. Going up stairs: 26, 27,
28. Exertion: 26, 29. Lying: 1, 7, 24, 36. Sitting: 31.
Stooping: 27. Rising: 31. Standing: 31, 36. Changing
from rest to motion: 19.

[36] **Nerves.** Epilepsy from fright, during menstruation; at
night; pupils always dilated for a day or two before;
also vertiginous epilepsy, loss of vision.
Hysteria, with complete but transient blindness.
❙ Convulsions preceded by great restlessness.
Chorea, with tearing in legs.
Locomotor ataxia, lightning-like pains; vertigo (see 2),
gastric symptoms (q. v.).
Creeping, jerking in various parts, more in paralyzed parts.
❙ Periodical trembling of the body.
❙ Voluntary motion impossible; left side indescribably weak.
❙ Paraplegia from debilitating causes.
Traumatic paraplegia, also when from compression as in
Pott's disease.
So weak, must lie down; then becomes apathetic, with
yawning; cold shuddering.
Walks and stands unsteadily, after hard mental labor;
especially when he thinks himself unobserved.

[37] **Sleep.** Yawning and chilliness; soporous condition.

Is prevented from falling asleep by fancies and images hovering before his imagination.

After long, wearisome, fatiguing night watching.

Much excited at night; murmured constantly; nothing but shaking would arouse him; scarcely are his eyes open before he again closes them.

Sees departed friends, the dead, ghosts at night; dreams of putrid water, of serpents, which fill him with horror.

In the morning, dreams he is hungry; this awakens him, and he finds he has a violent spasm of the stomach, with hunger, nausea, flatulence.

[38] **Time.** Day: 34. Morning: 3, 12, 16, 19, 25, 37, 40. Noon: 27. Afternoon: 16, 33. Evening: 19, 27. Night: 3, 21, 23, 27, 33, 36, 37, 41, 46. Midnight: 16, 17. After midnight: 20.

[39] **Temperature and Weather.** Coming in room from open air: 40. Warmth: 3, 5, 15, 40, 46. Working over the fire: 5. Open air: 5. Cold: 5, 15. Cold, damp weather: 19.

[40] **Chill. Fever. Sweat.** Chilliness, with nausea; chilly, with many complaints.

Chilly, with cold hands and feet.

Constant chilliness up the back and over shoulders; worse after meals; worse coming into room from the open air.

Skin dry, but not very hot.

Temperature sunken.

Intermittent fever, with pulmonary hemorrhage; generally no thirst.

Profuse sweat; it stands out on the face in beads; stitches in the side, cough during the attack.

Morning sweat.

Sweat and chilliness, as soon as he gets warm in bed.

[41] **Attacks.** Increasing quickly and decreasing quickly, or gradually increasing and decreasing.

Pains in skull sometimes remit, and are followed by more violent hemicrania.

Asthmatic attacks at night, with rapid pulse.

Moral and nervous disturbances come on in quite regular paroxysms.

[42] **Sides.** Right: 3, 18, 22, 32, 34, 46. Left: 3, 6, 8, 17, 19, 20, 28, 32, 36, 46. Behind upwards: 3. Right to left: 6. Above downwards: 21. Pains radiate: 17, 23.

[43] **Sensations.** Sensation of expansion, head, face, etc.

Want of feeling; numbness in external parts.

Dreadful soreness in the flesh and limbs.

Like a splinter in various parts.

[44] **Tissues.** Emaciation, most marked in legs; withered look.

❙ Œdema of legs; ascites; affection of the liver.

Muscles rigid.

Sallowness rather than pallor; shortness of breath; gastric ulcer; chlorosis.

❙ Bone affection; especially caries of little bones.

Defective oxidation, destruction of red corpuscles, lessened temperature.

❙ Septic forms of scarlet fever.

⁴⁵ **Contact, Injuries, etc.** Touch: 5, 9, 17, 19, 21. Pressure: 3, 17, 18, 28. Tight bandage: 3. Must wipe the eyes: 5. Scratching: 4. After a fall: 31.

⁴⁶ **Skin.** Skin from a blue-grey, violet or bronze color, to real black; skin brown, tense, hard.

Itching, smarting, mostly of thighs and axillæ, when warm at night.

❙ Bluish-black eruption. _θ_ Scarlet fever.

❙ Erysipelatous bed-sores, left shoulder, sacrum, or both hips; centre covered with dry, bloody incrustations; black, hard on sacrum. _θ_ Typhus.

Pustulous ecthyma.

Wart-shaped excrescences on the skin.

⁴⁷ **Stages and States.** Melancholy; congestions to head and chest; nosebleed. Change of life; itching skin; flushes.

⁴⁸ **Relationship.** Antidotes to _Arg. nitr._: ❙ _Natr. mur._ (chemical and dynamic), _Arsen._ and milk.

Arg. nitr. antidotes _Amm. caust._

Boys' complaints, after tobacco.

According to Bœnninghausen, as antidotes to _Arg. nitr._ and also to _Nitr. ac._, are prominent, _Pulsat._, _Calcar._, _Sepia_, and next to these three, _Lycop._, _Mercur._, _Silic._, _Rhus tox._, _Phosphor._ and _Sulphur._

❙ _Coffea cruda_ increases nervous headache.

After _Arg. nitr._ had failed in flatulent indigestion, _Lycop._ cured.

It has been given with success: after _Bryon._ and _Spigel._, in dyspepsia; after _Spongia_ was given for a goitre, and myopia followed; after _Veratr._ for wind passing upwards in great quantities, inducing faintness.

Similar to: _Aurum; Cuprum; Kali bichr.; Laches.; Mercur.; Merc. corr.; Merc. iod.; Natr. mur.; Nitr. ac._

The main difference between the metal and the nitrite, is, that the latter acts more on mucous membranes, the skin, and especially on the bones and periosteum, and must be beneficial to herpetic patients, and the former acts especially on the cartilages.

Complaints from pressure of clothes; also in _Calcar._, _Bryon._, _Caustic_, _Lycop._, _Sarsap._ and _Stannum._

Argentum oxidum may be substituted when in chlorosis there are menorrhagia and tendency to diarrhœa. It is also applicable for metrorrhagia with uterine fibroid.

ARNICA MONTANA (RADIX).

Leopard's bane.   HAHNEMANN.   *Compositæ.*

[1] **Mind.** Unconscious; when spoken to answers correctly, but unconsciousness and delirium at once return.

❙ Stupefaction, loss of sight and hearing.   θ Concussion of brain.

❙ Stupor, with involuntary discharge of feces.   θ Typhus.

❙ Forgetful; what he reads quickly escapes his memory, even the word he is about speaking.   θ Typhus.

Absent-minded, thoughts wander from their object and dwell on images and fancies.

Confusion of head, changing to pressive right-sided headache.

Delirium, low murmuring.

❙ Delirium tremens.

❙ Sheds tears and makes exclamations.   θ After rage.

Picks the bedclothes.

She does not speak a word; declines answering questions, dislikes sympathy.

Indisposed to think; after a walk in the open air.

❙ Fears being touched or struck by persons coming toward him.   θ Gout.

❙ Fear of public places; agorophobia.

Hypochondriacal anxiety.

❙ Hopelessness; indifference.   θ After concussion.

Oversensitive mood, peevish, quarrelsome.

Frightened; unexpected trifles cause him to start.

Ailments from fright or anger.

❙ Violent attacks of anguish.   θ Angina pectoris.

[2] **Sensorium.** Vertigo; when moving the head she feels as if everything turned with her or was falling on her; from a too copious meal, nausea, with obscuration of sight; when shutting eyes; ears feel stopped up when speaking, etc.

Vertigo a stomaco lasse, with nausea, vomiting and diarrhœa.

[3] **Inner Head.** Pressive pain in forehead when walking, ascending stairs, reflecting or reading.

Pressive headache over the eyes and toward the temples, with sensation as if the tissues of the forehead were spasmodically contracted.

Pressive headache as if the head were being distended.

Pains over one eye, with compression in forehead and greenish vomiting.

Stitching, tearing pains in the left temple.

❚ Headache as from a nail thrust into the temple, with general sweat about 12 P. M., followed by faintness.

Pain as if a knife was drawn through the head transversely from the left side, followed by internal coldness of head.

Feels like a heavy weight, pressing-shooting in temples.

Burning in the brain, with natural heat of the body, night and morning; worse from motion, better at rest.

Heaviness in the middle of the brain.

❚ Apoplexy, loss of consciousness, with involuntary evacuations from bowels and bladder, paralysis (left-sided); pulse full, strong; stertor; sighing, muttering.

Exudations in brain and spine.

❚ Meningitis after mechanical or traumatic injuries.

❚ Bad effects from falls or blows on the head.

⁴ **Outer Head.**   Sensation as if integuments of forehead were spasmodically contracted.

Cold sensation at a small spot on the forehead.

Unbearable feeling as from ice on top of the head; after breakfast.

Burning or hot spots on top of the head.

⁵ **Eyes.**   Flickering before eyes, worse when reading or writing.

Dilated pupils; sensitiveness to light.

Diplopia after injuring the eye.

Loss of sight after a violent blow.

❚ Traumatic ulceration, with much hemorrhage into the anterior chamber.

❚ Retinal hemorrhage expedites absorption of clots.

Margin of upper lids painful when lids are moved, as if they were dry and slightly sore.

Œdema of dry, hot, inflamed lids, with much subconjunctival suggillation.

Congestion to the eyes; balls bloodshot.

❚ Inflammation of eyes, with suggillations after mechanical injuries.

Severe ciliary neuralgia; head hot, body cool.

⁶ **Ears.**   Noises in the ear caused by rush of blood to the head; with great sensitiveness to sound.

❚ Hard hearing.   θ From concussions.

Bruised pain in ears, stitches in and behind ears; with great sensitiveness to loud sounds; ears very dry.

Discharge of blood from the ear.

⁷ **Nose.**   Bruised pain in the nose.

❚ Nosebleed: preceded by tingling; copious after every exertion; from mechanical causes; after washing the face.

End of nose cold.

Swelling of nose.

❚ Violent sneezing, after overlifting the day before.

[8] **Face.**   Pale, sunken; sallow; red, swollen.

Red swelling of right cheek, with throbbing and pinching pain; swollen lips and great heat in head, with cold body.

Redness and burning in one cheek.

Dry heat in face toward evening, without thirst; nose cold.

[9] **Lower Face.**   Lips: burn; swollen and cracked.

Lower lip trembles.

Bruised pain in (right) articulation of jaw, from motion, early in morning.

Lower jaw hanging down.

[10] **Teeth.**   ı Toothache after operation, plugging, etc.

Excruciating pains, cutting, tearing in all teeth of right upper jaw, radiating to ear; worse from external warmth or from inhaling fresh air.

Tooth feels as if forced out of socket; throbbing toothache.

ı Gums sore, swollen.   θ Teething children.

ı Beating and tingling in the gums.   θ Toothache.

[11] **Tongue, etc.**   Taste: putrid; of rotten eggs; bitter.

Biting sensation on the tongue, with soreness, burning and stinging in the back part of the throat.

Tongue: coated white; dry, with a brown streak down the middle; dry or coated yellow.   θ Typhus.

[12] **Mouth.**   Dry, with much thirst.

ı Putrid smell from mouth.   θ Typhus.

[13] **Throat.**   Stinging in back of throat between acts of deglutition.

Chronic pains in fauces and larynx, worse for a long time after an animated talk.

[14] **Desires.   Aversions.**   Longing for vinegar or sour things; for alcoholic drinks.

Appetite lessened.

Repugnance to food.

Aversion: to meat; broth; milk; smoking tobacco.

Thirst for cold water, without fever.

[15] **Eating and Drinking.**   After eating distress in epigastrium (after a blow).

[16] **Nausea and Vomiting.**   ı Eructations: bitter and like rotten eggs, in the morning; empty.

Belches after coughing.

Hiccough.   θ Meningitis.

Nausea: empty vomiturition; burning-scratching in the throat; general relaxation during forenoon.

ı Vomiting of dark red coagula, mouth bitter; general soreness.

Vomits the least food; retching at night.

[17] **Stomach.**   Pinching, spasmodic griping in stomach, also with pulmonary and cardiac constriction, and with dysenteric stools.

Pressive, cutting pains in epigastrium; nausea and retching.

Stomach feels full with nausea and satiety.

Stomach distended with wind; pressure on præcordia, oppression of chest.

❙ Hæmatemesis from injuries; sore all over.

Heaviness in the stomach.

[18] **Hypochondria.** Stitches in region of liver; painful when turning in bed.

Pressure in region of liver; below the heart, day and night.

Stitches in the splenic region, with soreness on pressure.

[19] **Abdomen.** Hard swelling of the right side of abdomen, with severe pain when touched.

Sharp pains from side to side through abdomen.

Colic with strangury.

Pains around the naval when moving.

[20] **Stool, etc.** Undigested food; bloody; purulent; bloody, slimy mucus, with urging and violent bellyache; dark, bloody mucus, with sore, bruised feeling in abdomen; brown, fermented (like yeast); averse to food; fetid breath; very offensive, papescent, at times involuntary; involuntary during sleep; frequent, small, mucous.

❙ Dysentery with ischuria, or tenesmus of neck of bladder, with fruitless urging.

❙ Flatus smelling like rotten eggs.

Obstinate constipation after a blow on epigastrium.

[21] **Urine.** Agonizing pains in back and hips.

Piercing pains, as from knives plunged into the kidneys; chilly, inclined to vomit.

Chill followed by nephritic pains, nausea and vomiting, without relief.

❙ Bladder affections after mechanical injuries.

❙ Tenesmus from spasms of neck of bladder.

Bladder feels overfilled, ineffectual urging.

❙ Has to wait a long time for urine to pass.

❙ Involuntary urination at night during sleep.

❙ Constant urging while urine passes involuntary in drops.

Urine in small quantity, staining napkin yellow-brown.

Scanty, red urine, very offensive.

Frequent discharge of pale urine.

❙ Retention of urine from exertion.

❙ Ischuria with dysentery.

Urine dark brown, scanty; brick-dust sediment; red, in liver complaint; acid, increased specific gravity.

❙ Bloody urine; hæmaturia from mechanical causes.

Infants scream from pain in bladder.

[22] **Male Sexual Organs.** ❙ Penis and testicles swollen, purple-red; after injuries.

Spermatic cords painfully swollen, stitches in abdomen.

Phimosis from friction; parts bruised and much swollen.

Erysipelas of scrotum extending to the anus.

❙ Hydrocele caused by a bruise.

²³ **Female Sexual Organs.**   Metrorrhagia after coition.
Menses generally too soon; nausea in epigastrium.
Ulcers of uterus with a tendency to bleed.
Labia painfully swollen.
❙ Prolapsus, caused by concussion.

²⁴ **Pregnancy.**   ❙ Threatened abortion from falls, shocks, etc.;
nervous, excited; feels bruised.
Labor-pains: violent, yet they do but little good; weak, or
ceasing, wants to change position often; feels bruised.
❙ Soreness of parts after labor.
After-pains violent; return while suckling.
Constant dribbling of urine after labor.
Hemorrhages bright red or mixed with clots; head hot,
body cool.
❙ Sore nipples.
❙ Mastitis from bruises; erysipelatous inflammation.
❙ Asphyxia neonatorum.

²⁵ **Larynx.**   Voice deep; or low, muttering.
Hoarseness from over-using voice; also early in morning.
Raw, scraped sensation along trachea and bronchia.

²⁶ **Breathing.**   Breath fetid, short, panting.
Children when angry lose their breath altogether.
Dysynœa, head hot, face red, body cool.
❙ Asthma, with inclination to move about; sleepless, before
midnight; looks as if dying; with fatty heart.

²⁷ **Cough.**   Constant insupportable tickling in larynx and
trachea, causing cough day and night.   θ Pneumonia.
Dry slight cough from tickling low down in the trachea,
every morning after rising.
Paroxysms of cough at night during sleep, not awaking.
Tickling in lower part of trachea, and dry, hacking cough,
most at night; scanty, difficult expectoration of transparent, glairy slime, mixed with black dots, or bloody.
Expectoration: offensive, green, purulent, blood-streaked;
when loosened must be swallowed; day and evening.
❙ Whooping-cough; child cries before the paroxysm.
❙ Cough causes bloodshot eyes, nosebleed; expectoration
of foaming blood, or clots of blood; sometimes in evening of putrid tasting mucus, which must be swallowed.

²⁸ **Lungs.**   ❙ Hemorrhage after mechanical injuries; slight
spitting of black, thick, viscid blood, or bright red,
frothy blood, mixed with mucus and coagula.
Burning or rawness in the chest.
Chest sore when coughing, sputum blood-streaked; cannot
raise the loosened mucus.
Pressive pain in (right) chest, at a small spot, not increased
by motion, touch or inspiration.

10

Stitches in chest (left side), worse from a dry cough; worse from motion; from external pressure.

❙ Pleurisy after mechanical injuries; must continually change position, bed feels so hard.

❙ Pneumothorax from external injuries.

²⁹ **Heart. Pulse.** Stitches in cardiac region.

Region of base of heart feels as if bruised.

❙ "Strain of the heart" from violent running.

Palpitation after almost any exertion; goes off by rest.

Pain from liver through left chest and down left arm; veins on hand swollen, purplish; sudden pain, as if heart were squeezed, or, as if it got a shock.

❙ Pressure under the sternum, anguish, collapse; small, irregular pulse, dyspnœa; angina pectoris.

❙ Fatty degeneration of heart.

Pulse: accelerated, full, hard; sometimes quicker than beat of heart; intermittent, feeble, hurried, irregular; feeble fluttering.

³⁰ **Outer Chest.** ❙ Articulations and cartilaginous connections of chest feel as if beaten, when moving, breathing, or coughing.

Violent stitches in middle of left chest.

³¹ **Neck. Back.** Weakness of cervical muscles; they do not support the head steadily.

Great sensibility of cervical vertebræ to pressure.

Violent spinal pain, as from sudden rising after long stooping.

Right scapula and small of the back painful, as if beaten.

Bruised pain at inner portion of right scapula.

Sacrum pains, as if beaten.

³² **Upper Limbs.** Violent twitching pain from the left shoulder-joint to the middle finger.

Tingling in the arms.

Arms feel weary, as if bruised.

Sensation as if joints of the arms and wrists were sprained.

Tearing in tips of the left ring and little finger.

Cramps in fingers of left hand.

Acute bruised pain in the balls of the thumbs.

³³ **Lower Limbs.** Drawing, pressive pains in left hip-joint, thigh being extended, when sitting.

Hips pain as if sprained.

Formication; lame feeling; must often change position, bed or chair seems so hard; after exertion, long marches, etc.

Pain in thighs when walking, as from a blow.

Stitch, like from a needle, when touching the knee.

Knee-joints suddenly bending when standing, feet numb, insensible.

❙Hygroma patellæ.

Pain in the calf of the right leg, as from a blow, with lassitude of the legs.

Tarsal joint pains as if sprained.

Want of power in ankles and feeling of a heavy weight in each instep.

Hot erysipelatous inflammation and painfulness of foot.

Feet feel tired or inflamed after a walk.

Arthritic pains in foot, worse toward evening; fear passers may strike it; big toe-joint red, feels sprained.

³⁴ **Limbs in General.** Heaviness.

Paralytic pain in all joints during motion, as if bruised.

Limbs as if bruised at rest or in motion; painful concussion from jolting of carriage or stepping firmly.

❙Limbs ache as if beaten.

Tearing, with soreness, numbness, swelling, or tingling.

³⁵ **Position, etc.** Rest: 3, 29, 34. Motion: 3, 9, 19, 26, 28, 33, 34, 40, 43. Walking: 3, 33. Walking in open air: 1. Ascending: 3. Must change position: 24, 28, 33, 37. Exertion: 7, 29, 33. Moving head: 2. Turning in bed: 18. Attempting to sit up: 40. Sitting: 33. Standing: 33. Lying with head low: 37. Must lie down: 36.

³⁶ **Nerves.** Twitching of the muscles.

Whole body, especially skin and joints, excessively painful and sensitive.

Tired feeling, as after hard work or as if beaten.

Weary, bruised, sore. great weakness, must lie down, yet bed feels too hard.

❙Great sinking of strength.

Lassitude and sluggishness of the whole body; scarcely able to stand.

Paralysis: generally painful; left-sided (after apoplexy); partial, from concussion of the spine.

³⁷ **Sleep.** Sleepiness; too sleepy early in the evening.

Languor, drowsiness.

❙While answering, falls into a deep sleep before finishing.

Unrefreshing sleep, loud, blowing breathing.

Is often kept awake until 2 to 3 A. M. from heat, restlessness and constant desire to change position; or from prickling, stinging, biting, now here, now there, on the body.

On falling asleep: starts as in fright; is aroused by heat.

Lies preferably with head low, or horizontally.

Worse after a long sleep, or on awaking.

Dreams: vivid; frightful, of graves, black dogs, struck by lightning, etc.; unrefreshing, anxious.

³⁸ **Time.** Morning: 3, 9, 16, 25, 40. Forenoon: 40. Evening:

27, 33, 37, 40. Night: 3, 16, 21, 27, 37. Midnight: 3. Before midnight: 26. Day and night: 18, 27.

[39] **Temperature and Weather.** Inclination for open air; better in open air.

Sudden cooling after overheating, followed by a cough, like consumption.

Open air: 10. Warmth: 10. Washing: 7.

[40] **Chill. Fever. Sweat.** Chill felt worse in pit of stomach.

Chill most in evening, with much thirst already before chill.

Chill after every sleep.

Chilly internally, with external heat.

▮Chilly, with heat and redness of one cheek.

Chilly morning or forenoon; before chill, yawning, thirst for large quantities of water; drawing in periosteum.

▮Head alone, or face alone hot, body cold.

Dry, general heat after waking; early morning, violent thirst; uncovering makes him chilly; chilly even when moving in bed.

Heat, with indifference, stupor, drinks less.

Continuous heat, with such weakness, that when attempting to sit up he faints.

Flushes of heat; with thirst.

Great internal heat; hands and feet being cold.

Sweat: sour or offensive; sometimes cold; nightly sour.

Several transitory sweats all over at night, with anguish.

Hectic fever, emaciation; after a blow on stomach.

During apyrexia in intermittent fever, headache, yellow face, bitter taste, aversion to meat.

▮Fevers: intermittent; typhoid; traumatic.

[41] **Attacks.** Worse during the increase of the moon.

Periodical attacks of megrim.

Spasms of cough.

▮Heat in oft repeated short attacks.

[42] **Sides.** Right: 1, 8, 9, 10, 18, 19, 28, 31, 33. Left: 3, 18, 28, 29, 30, 32, 33, 46.

[43] **Sensations.** Pains insufferable, drive him crazy; increased by every motion or noise; change quickly from part to part; scratches at the wall or bed, apparently for relief.

Feels as if beaten or bruised.

Parts feel as if sprained, especially joints.

Tearing, drawing in outer parts.

Tingling in outer parts.

Bruised parts tingle, feel numb, or as if dead.

Torpidity from mechanical injuries or failure of vital powers.

[44] **Tissues.** ▮Concussions and contusions.

Bleeding of internal and external parts.

▮Inflammation of skin, cellular tissue; tender on pressure.

❙ Prevents suppuration.

❙ Burrowing pus, not painful.

Muscles rigid.

❙ Myalgia; particularly after overexertion.

Emaciation.

❙ Septic states; tendency to typhoid forms.

Hyperinosis is rather a contra-indication for *Arnic.*

❙ Gout and rheumatism.

Dropsy of internal parts.

Bones (periosteum) ache.   ❙ Osteo-myelitis (in beginning).

⁴⁵ **Contact, Injuries, etc.**   Touch: 1, 19, 28.   Pressure: 18, 28, 31, 44.

❙ Mechanical injuries : concussion of brain while there are unconsciousness, pallor, or drowsiness, weak, intermitting pulse, cold surface, and other indications of depressed vitality from shock.

⟡   Worse after riding; sick stomach from car riding.

❙ Everything on which he lies seems too hard.

❙ Sprains with much swelling, bluish redness, intense soreness.

❙ Contusions without laceration.

❙ Stings of bees or wasps; splinters.

❙ Compound fractures, and their profuse suppuration.

⁴⁶ **Skin.**   Hot, red, œdematous.

Hot, hard, shining swelling, from insect sting.

Petechiæ, ecchymoses.

❙ Many small, painful boils, one after another; extremely sore.

Red spots first on limb, then upon the trunk.

Bed-sores; especially sacral region and hips.

Erysipelatous inflammation, left hand dark blue.

Phlegmonous erysipelas.

Erythema nodosum.

Varicose ulcers: torpid; dirty, bluish bottom; no pus, but watery, fetid secretion, half transparent crusts, like thick glue, fetid.

Painful ulcers.

Corns (pare them and apply externally).

⁴⁷ **Stages and States.**   Dark hair, rigid muscles.

Plethoric; very red face.

Hydrogenoid constitution of Grauvogl.

❙ Compound fractures, and their profuse suppuration.

Light complexion, sandy hair, sanguine.   θ Whooping-cough.

Nervous, cannot stand pain.

Especially suitable to those who remain long impressed by even slight mechanical injuries.

⁴⁸ **Relationship.**   Antidotes to massive doses: *Camphor, Ipec.*

Antidotes to potencies: *Acon., Arsen., Chinchon., Ignat., Ipec.*

Arnic. antidotes: *Amm. carb., Cinchon., Cicut., Ferrum, Ignat., Ipec., Seneg.*

It follows well after: **ı** *Acon., Ipec., Veratr.;* after *Apis,* in hydrocephalus.

After it follow well: *Acon., Arsen., Bryon., Ipec., Rhus tox., Sulph. ac.*

Arnic. is indicated in ailments from spirituous liquors or from charcoal vapors.

ı Complementary to *Acon.*

Alternated successfully in cases where the change of symptoms indicate it, with *Acon.* and *Rhus tox.*

Injurious after the bite of a dog or any rabid or angry animal.

Wine increases the unpleasant effects of *Arnic.*

Hyper. is preferable in spinal concussions; and *Calend.* in wounds with loss of substance or with suppuration.

Cognates: *Acon.; Amm. carb.; Croton* (swashing in abdomen); *Arsen.; Baptis.; Bellad.; Bryon.· Chamom.; China; Euphras.* (injuries to eye); *Calend.; Ferrum; Hepar.; Hyper.; Hamam.; Ipec.; Mercur.; Pulsat.; Ran. scel.* (pains in intercostal muscles); *Rhus tox.; Ruta; Staphis.; Silic.; Symphyt.; Sulphur* (traumatic pleurisy); *Sulph. ac.; Veratr.; Bellis peren.* (wounds, boils, etc.; erysipelatous tendency).

ARSENICUM ALBUM.

Arsenious oxide.   HAHNEMANN. $As_2 O_3$.

ı Mind. Weakness of memory.

Confusion of the head.

Averse to meeting acquaintances, because he imagines having formerly offended them, though he knows not how.

Sad, tearful, anxious mood.

Fears to be left alone, lest he do himself bodily harm.

ı Determined to commit suicide, he suffers so.

Fears he will have to murder some one.

Sees vermin; throws away bugs by the handful.

Tears his body, injures his own person; insanity.

ı Dread of death when alone, or on going to bed.

Anxious and depressed fears, permanent loss of health.

ı Intense anxiety and with restlessness, worse after midnight; driving out of bed.

ı Great anxiety, with constriction of chest and dyspnœa.

❙ Great fear, restlessness, trembling, cold sweat, prostration. Self-willed and tearful.

❙ Vexation, with anxiety, restlessness and chilliness. Child captious, wants to be carried.

❙ Cannot find rest anywhere, changes place continually, wants to go from one bed to another.

² **Sensorium.**   Sensation as if the brain moved and beat against skull, during motion.

Vertigo, as if he would fall.   Vertigo of malarial origin, with hyperæsthesia of hearing, or during pregnancy; lips and face bluish; jugular veins undulate.

Vertigo, with loss of consciousness during coughing fits, in asthmatics.

Heaviness in the head, with humming in the ears; goes off in open air, but returns on entering the room.

³ **Inner Head.**   Intense frontal headache, with vertigo.

Drawing, pressive pain in right side of forehead.

Pain as if bruised or sore, over the nose and in the forehead, rubbing relieves temporarily.

Throbbing frontal headache over root of nose.   θ Ozæna.

Headache: beating; or pressure as from a load on brain; rising up in bed and motion aggravates; cold washing relieves temporarily, walking in open air permanently.

The pain in head and face is especially severe on left side; cannot lean or rest on that side.

⁴ **Outer Head.**   Erysipelatous burning and swelling of the head, with great weakness and coldness; worse at night.

❙ Can scarcely bear hair to be touched, scalp so sensitive.

Falling out of the hair.

Great sensitiveness of head to open air; wraps up head warmly.

❙ Chronic eruptions, with pustules and vesicles filled with pus.

⁵ **Eyes.**   ❙ Sensitive to light; photophobia.

Snow dazzles, with lachrymation.

Flickering before the eyes.

❙ Everything appears green; sees as through a white gauze.

Weakness of sight; dim sight.

Pupils contracted or dilated.

❙ Eyes sunken or protruding.

Yellowness of the sclerotica.

Pain in right eyeball, particularly during motion.

Pulsative throbbing in eyes, at every pulsation a stitch.

Feeling of sand in eyes.

❙ Violent burning in eyes.

Chronic trachoma, inner surface of lids rubs eyeballs; burning, etc.

Croupous conjunctivitis from ophthalmia neonatorum.

▮ Conjunctiva looks like a piece of raw beef.

Trembling of upper eyelid, with lachrymation.

▮ Eyelids œdematous and spasmodically closed; also for non-inflammatory œdema (like *Apis*).

Agglutination of lids.

▮ Edges of lids painful during motion, as if dry and rubbing on the ball.

Extreme redness of inner surface of lids, with uneasy sensation rather than pain.

▮ Burning in margins of eyelids.

▮ Ophthalmia of children, skin rough, dry and dirty looking; photophobia and profuse, acrid lachrymation; relieved by hot applications.

⁶ **Ears.** Unusual sensitiveness to sound.

Ringing in the ears.

Roaring in the ears, with each paroxysm of pain.

Hardness of hearing, cannot hear the human voice. (Compare *Phosphor.*)

Stitching, tearing from left meatus auditorius outwards, more in the evening.

Yellow discharge from the right ear, with dryness of the nose; the hearing is not weakened.

Discharges of cadaverous odor, profuse, ichorous.

⁷ **Nose.** Offensive smell before the nose.

Smells of pitch and sulphur alternately, before the nose.

▮ Cannot bear the smell or sight of food.

Dryness of the nasal cavity.

Discharge of burning mucus from the right nostril.

Fluent coryza, with frequent sneezing; with hoarseness and sleeplessness; with swollen nose; alternating with stoppage.

▮ Watery discharge causes burning and smarting at nostrils as if sore.

Distressing stoppage at the bridge of the nose.

Nosebleed after a fit of passion or vomiting.

▮ Knotty swelling of the nose.

⁸ **Face.** . Expression anxious, but not wild; distressed; of suffering; mental agony; surly; wild; hippocratic; sunken.

Appearance very pale; yellow, waxy; grey; earthy; livid, bluish; flushed; red and swollen.

▮ Œdematous swelling of face.

Twitching of facial muscles.

Tearing in left half of face.

▮ Burning, stinging pains, as from red hot needles.

Pimples and vesicles, with acrid discharge; itching, burning; worse at night, in cold air, better from warmth.

▮ Cancerous ulcers on the face; scabbing; burning pain

⁹ **Lower Face.** Severe pains along right inferior maxillary nerve.

Bites the tumbler when drinking.

| Sore lips and ulcers in the mouth.

| Eruptions on the lips.

Contractive quivering or jerking on one side of upper lip, especially when falling asleep.

[10] **Teeth.** Grinding of the teeth while asleep.

Teeth seem longer, become loose, and are sensitive to pressure and to cold water.

Pain in some of the teeth, as if loose and would fall out, pain not increased by chewing.

Jerking toothache, extending to the temple, relieved or removed by sitting up in bed and by external warmth.

| Toothache relieved by heat of stove.

| Swollen, bleeding gums, painful to touch.

[11] **Tongue, etc.** Taste: woody, dry; unpleasant; sweetish in throat; sour; metallic; bitter; putrid.

Food tastes: too salty; not salty enough; insipid; sour.

Beer tastes flat.

Loss of power of speech.

| Violent burning on the tongue.

| Swelling about root of tongue, externally and internally.

Coating: sides furred, with red streak down the middle and redness of tip; thickly furred, edges red; whitish; yellowish-white; as if painted white; brown.

| Tongue: dry, and morbidly red, with papillæ considerably raised at the tip; lead colored.

| Pale, doughy, takes print of teeth; neuralgia.

| Edge of tongue red, takes imprint of teeth.

| Gangrene of tongue; spots on tongue, burning like fire.

[12] **Mouth.** | Dryness of mouth with violent thirst.

Burning in mouth, pharynx and œsophagus.

Much saliva; must spit often.

Saliva decreased.

| Aphthæ in mouth; they become livid or bluish.

Painful blisters in mouth and on tongue.

[13] **Throat.** Dryness, soreness, scraping and burning in fauces and throat.

Sensation of constriction of throat.

Swallowing very difficult and painful.

Paralytic condition of pharynx and œsophagus.

Burning when swallowing; food goes down to region of larynx, when it is ejected again.

Diphtheritic membrane is dry looking and wrinkled.

[14] **Desires. Aversions.** Appetite increased.

Desire for: sour things; brandy; coffee; milk; lard.

Loss of appetite with increased thirst.

Aversion: to food; to butter.

Thirst and dryness of mouth, with peculiar thick white saliva.

Excessive thirst, drinking does not refresh.

❘ Drinks often, but a little at a time ; or may drink much and often. ❘ Frequent unquenchable thirst.

❘ Great thirst but water molests the stomach. *θ* Dropsy.

Burning thirst, without especial desire to drink.

¹⁵ **Eating and Drinking.** Gastro-intestinal symptoms worse: after ice; ❘ ice cream; ice water; vinegar; sour beer; tobacco (chewing); alcoholic drinks; bad sausages; cheese; fruits.

❘ Bad effects from inordinate use of spirituous liquors. *θ* Delirium tremens ; vomiting; diarrhœa; hemorrhages.

¹⁶ **Nausea and Vomiting.** ❘ Hiccough frequent ; also when fever ought to have come.

Abortive eructations; fruitless retching; irregular, convulsive action of stomach, instead of ordinary peristalsis.

Qualmishness 11 A. M. and 3 P. M.

❘ Nausea and complete loss of appetite.

Long-lasting nausea, with faintness, tremor; heat all over and shuddering.

❘ Violent vomiting of food and gastric fluids; vomit usually scanty.

Vomit: bitter ; green-yellow liquid ; ingesta ; brown, turbid matter; streaked with blood; blood; black; first water, then thick, glairy, or grass-green mucus, lastly blood.

❘ Also immediately after food or drink.

❘ Frequent vomiting with apprehension of death.

¹⁷ **Stomach.** ❘ Pressure in the region of the stomach ; weight, as of a stone.

Stomach tender to pressure.

❘ Intense heat and burning in stomach and pit of stomach.

Violent, tearing, boring pain and cramp, in the stomach and intestines.

Pain in the stomach relieved by sweet milk.

❘ Great anxiety about the epigastric region.

Epigastrium distended and hard ; and umbilicus sensitive to touch.

Pain in the pit of the stomach arresting breathing.

¹⁸ **Hypochondria.** Painful bloatedness in the right hypochondrium, with burning pain.

Pain in region of liver increased on pressure.

Stitches in right hypochondrium, extending to region of stomach, ending as violent pressure over whole abdomen.

Drawing, stitching pain under the left hypochondrium.

Tensive, pressive pain in spleen.

❘ Induration and enlargement of spleen and liver.

¹⁹ **Abdomen.** Abdomen distended and painful.

Rumbling in bowels.

Cutting pains in abdomen.

❙ Violent pains in abdomen, with great anguish, has no rest anywhere, rolls about on floor and despairs of life.

Pains about navel, aggravated by lying on back.

Pain in right side of abdomen, near lumbar region, spreading through abdomen to right groin and same side of scrotum.

Groins: contractive pain in left; as if sprained in right, when stooping; digging, burning like a boil; stitches.

❙ Swelling of inguinal gland.

²⁰ **Stool, etc.** Involuntary stools and urine.

❙ Diarrhœa after chilling stomach by taking cold substances.

Diarrhœa: slimy, green mucus; of pieces of mucus, with tenesmus and cutting pain in anus; stools small, with tenesmus, first dark green feces, afterwards dark green mucus; black mucus, with persistent vomiting; black, acrid and putrid; yellow, with tenesmus and burning pain; like dirty water; of blood and water.

Purging, with extreme coldness of the extremities.

❙ Diarrhœa worse after midnight, also in morning after rising.

Anus red and sore. ❙ Burning in anus.

Constipation with pain in the bowels.

Hemorrhoids: with stitching pain when walking or sitting, not when at stool; with burning pain, relieved by heat.

❙ Hemorrhages from bowels, dark, offensive.   θ Typhus.

²¹ **Urine.** Frequent urging, with profuse discharge.

Involuntary micturition.

Urine scanty, passed with difficulty, burning during discharge.

Retention of urine, as if the bladder were paralyzed.

Urine: dark brown; dark yellow; turbid; sediment of red sand; mixed with pus and blood.

Hæmaturia. ❙ Albuminuria.

❙ Uræmia, anguish with thoughts of murder, especially in drunkards.

²² **Male Sexual Organs.** Glans blue-red, swollen and cracked.

Excessively painful inflammation and swelling of the genitals, increasing almost to gangrene.

Herpes preputialis chronic (after failure of *Rhus*).

❙ Scrotum œdematous.

Emissions during diarrhœic stool.

²³ **Female Sexual Organs.** Increased sexual desire, with involuntary discharge of mucus.

Menses: too early; too profuse; exhausting menorrhagia.

Hemorrhage, with lancinating, burning pains; sudden of profuse dark blood.

During menses, sharp sticking in rectum, thence to anus and pubes.

Painful menses.

Amenorrhœa. Scanty pale menses.

Thin, whitish, offensive discharge instead of the menses.

❙ Leucorrhœa: profuse, yellowish, thick and corroding.

Stitches from the abdomen down into the vagina.

❙ Burning or tensive pain in the ovary.

❙ Pressive, stitching pains in region of right ovary.

❙ Drawing, stitching pain from region of ovary into the thigh, which feels numb and lame; worse from motion, bending, or sitting bent.

Burning, throbbing, lancinating pain in uterine region.

²⁴ **Pregnancy.** Burning pains in mammæ; relief from motion.

²⁵ **Larynx.** Voice: trembling; weak; unequal, now strong and again weak; hoarse; rough; hollow; loss of voice.

❙ Simulating membranous croup; caused by checked or non-appearing eruptions, especially by hives or urticaria.

Laryngeal lining dirty-red or anæmic, with bluish-red patches; indolent, or burning ulcers; laryngeal phthisis.

Sudden catarrh, threatening suffocation at night.

²⁶ **Breathing.** Respiration short and anxious.

Difficult breathing, with much anxiety.

❙ Breathing asthmatic: must incline the chest forward; must spring out of bed at night. θ Asthma.

Air-passages seem constricted, cannot breathe fully.

Dyspnœa increased after coughing, with sensation of constriction of chest or stomach.

❙ Loss of breath immediately on lying down, in the evening, with whistling and constriction in the trachea.

❙ Oppression increased by stormy weather and heavy air; walking quickly; ascending; warm and tight clothing; but especially from changes of warmth and cold.

❙ Wheezing respiration, with cough and frothy expectoration, looking like beaten white of egg.

❙ Great dyspnœa; face cyanotic and covered with cold sweat; great anxiety. θ Emphysema.

Whistling expiration.

²⁷ **Cough.** ❙ Excited by smoky sensation or as of vapors of sulphur in larynx, or by constant titillation in larynx.

Preceded by jerking in hips, which seemed to excite cough.

Cough: when going into cold, open air; especially after drinking; evenings, directly after lying down; has to sit up; afterwards contractive pain in the epigastric region, causing the cough to continue; weakness.

❙ Cough with bloody sputum.

Night cough; must sit up as soon as cough commences; 1 A. M., with gasping for breath.

Deep, dry, unceasing cough; coughs dependent upon asthma, cyanosis, heart diseases; also associated with great exhaustion, collapse, anæmia, nervous irritability.

Expectoration ; frothy saliva ; thick yellow ; green, bitter ; salty ; mucus streaked with blood.

▮ Hæmoptysis after loss of blood ; burning heat all over, especially with pain between scapulæ ; in drunkards or from suppressed menses.

²⁸ **Lungs.**   Tightness of chest, as if bound with a hoop.

▮ Constriction of chest: with great anxiety and restless-ness, evenings ; when going up hill.   ⋈ Lᵗ

Stitches in upper right chest ; in left chest only during inspiration.

Stitching pain in sternum, from below up, when coughing.

▮ Pleurisy with tendency to syncope.

Chilliness in chest, evenings.

Burning in the chest.

▮ Catarrh on the chest, great suffocation ; child tosses about in agony.

▮ Gangrene of the lungs with green, ichorous sputum.

²⁹ **Heart.   Pulse.**   Palpitation ; after suppressed herpes or foot-sweat ; with small, irregular pulse ; strong, visible and audible, chiefly at night.

▮ Palpitation of heart, with anguish, cannot lie on back·; increased by going up stairs.

Heart beats more rapidly and stronger when lying on back.

▮ Angina pectoris ; sudden tightness above the heart ; agonizing precordial pain ; pains into the neck and occiput ; anxiety, oppression ; breathing difficult, faint-ing spells ; least motion makes him lose his breath ; sits bent forward or with head thrown back ; worse at night, especially from 1 to 5 A. M.   Kₗᵗ

▮ Hydropericardium with great irritability, anguish and restlessness ; especially in uræmia, etc.

Pulse : accelerated ; quick and small ; quick and weak ; rapid and weak ; small, very frequent, and irregular, sometimes imperceptible ; thread-like.

³⁰ **Outer Chest.**   Yellow spots on chest.

▮ Stitches and pressing in sternum.

³¹ **Neck.   Back.**   Nape stiff, as if bruised or sprained.

Neuralgic pains on left side of neck.

Drawing pains : between scapulæ ; necessitate lying down ; from small of back to the shoulders.

Stiffness of the spinal column, beginning in the region of the os coccygis.

Loss of strength in small of back.

Bruised pain in small of back.

³² **Upper Limbs.**   Tearing-jerking pain in right shoulder-joint and shoulder.

Pain in the arm of the side on which one rests, at night.

Drawing, jerking and tearing from the tips of the fingers into the shoulder.

Hands and lower half of forearm dark and livid.

Small reddish spot on left elbow-joint, soon forming a blister, becoming in a few hours as large as a hazel-nut and turning black; similar blisters appear on right elbow and next day on left leg.

Trembling of hands.

❙ Ulcers in finger-tips with burning pains.

Tingling in fingers.

³³ **Lower Limbs.** Violent shooting-tearing pain in the hip, thigh, groin and left foot.

Pain back of great trochanter, extending down the thigh, posteriorly, then toward the knee, anteriorly, embracing the patella, down the tibia to the ankle ; pain relieved somewhat by flexion of the knee.

Cracking of knee when walking.

Swelling and pain of knees.

Stiffness of knees and feet, alternating with tearing pains.

❙ Pain as if beaten in knee-joint.

Coldness, especially of knees and feet.

❙ Itching tetters in the bend of the knees.

Cramp in calves.

Drawing pain in legs when resting feet upon the floor, · while sitting.

Swelling of feet, œdematous.

❙ Weakness or weariness of feet, numbness.

Tearing in the heels.

Intolerable itching of feet and thighs.

Toes drawn downwards.

❙ Ulcers on soles of feet and toes.

❙ Sore pain in ball of toes, while walking, as if chafed.

Sensation as if the lower limbs would break down, on going up stairs.

❙ Uneasiness in lower limbs, cannot lie still at night, has to change position of feet constantly or walk about to get relief.

Gressus gallinaceous.

³⁴ **Limbs in General.** Twitching ; trembling; violent starting while falling asleep ; numbness ; lassitude ; ❙ weariness.

Excessive weakness and exhaustion of limbs obliges him to lie down.

Violent tearing in the upper and lower limbs ; cannot rest on the affected side; pain least felt when moving affected part.

³⁵ **Position, etc.** Walking : 3, 20, 26, 33. Ascending : 26, 33. Motion : 2, 3, 5, 23, 24, 34. Moving affected part : 34. Rising up : 3. After rising : 20. Sitting : 20, 23, 27, 33.

Sitting up: 10, 27.   Must sit up: 27.   Sitting bent: 23.
Chest forward: 26.   Stooping: 19.   Leaning: 3.   Resting: 3, 32, 33.   Bending: 23.   Bending knee: 33.   Lying
down: 27, 31.   Lying on back: 19, 29.   Lying on affected
side: 34.   Must lie down: 31, 34.   Cannot lie still: 33.
Must spring from bed: 26.   Rolls on floor: 19.

³⁶ **Nerves.**   Great restlessness, cannot find rest in any position.
Starting when falling asleep.
Hysterical spasms, followed by exhaustion.
❙ Frequent fainting.
Convulsions with opisthotonos; foam at the mouth.
❙ Chorea, uncomplicated cases.
Child lies as if dead; pale but warm; breathless for some
time.
Epileptic convulsions; tetanic spasms.
Exhaustion from the slightest exertion.
❙ After great exertions; climbing mountains, etc.
❙ Very rapid sinking of strength.

³⁷ **Sleep.**   Yawning and stretching.
Frequent startings in and from sleep; awakened by pains,
worse 12 P. M.
Sleeplessness with restlessness and moaning; mal-nutrition; nerves exhausted.
After sleep, feels as if had not slept enough; eyes are
weary; cannot get out of bed.
Dreams: full of care, sorrow and fear; about thunderstorms; fire; of black water and darkness; of death.

³⁸ **Time.**   General aggravation at night, especially after midnight (13 A. M.)
Morning: 20, 40.   Forenoon: 40.   Evening: 6, 26, 27, 28,
40.   Night: 4, 8, 20, 25, 26, 29, 32, 40.   Before midnight: 37.   After midnight: 20, 37.   3 A. M.: I.   11
A. M. and 3 P. M.: 16.

³⁹ **Temperature and Weather.**   Warmth almost always relieves the pain.
General aggravation from cold except headache, which is
relieved by cold washing and cold air.
Cold, damp cellars aggravate or bring on complaints.
Sciatica.
Cold ailment: 20; — water: 10; — washing: 3; — air:
8, 27.   Open air: 2, 3, 4, 8, 40.   Cold: 26.   Room: 2.
Warmth: 4, 8, 10, 20, 26.   Must be covered: 40; —
uncovered: 40.   Change of temperature: 26.   Stormy
weather: 26.   Heavy air: 26.

⁴⁰ **Chill. Fever. Sweat.**   Undefined development of chill
(and heat); either simultaneously, or in alternation.
Shuddering without thirst, worse in open air.
Chill in forenoon, not relieved by anything.

Internal chill, with external heat and red cheeks.

❙ Chill without thirst, followed by heat with much thirst and no sweat; a sweat comes hours afterwards, whereupon ailments increase; liver and spleen swollen. θ Dropsy.

External coldness, with cold, clammy sweat.

During chill (and during heat) aggravation of symptoms which existed previously, but were of slight importance.

Nursing children having no distinct chill must be covered; are very thirsty.

❙ Blue nails and lips during chill.

❙ Internal burning, dry heat; inclination to uncover.

❙ Dry heat, evening and night, with thirst and frequent drinking of but a small quantity at a time.

Excessive heat with small, feeble and very frequent pulse; mouth dry, tongue so dry it is painful to move it; thirst followed by adipsia. θ Typhoid.

Heat at night, as if hot water were poured over one.

Sweat at the end of fever, with cessation of all previous symptoms; sweat relieves the pains; rheumatism.

Sweat in the morning without relief; cold, clammy or sour and offensive smelling.

❙ Sweats on going to sleep; goes off after sweating a little.

Profuse sweat about the knees, at night.

During the sweat unquenchable thirst.

41 **Attacks.** Periodically returning complaints.

Typhus tertianus anteponens.

42 **Sides.** Right: 3, 5, 6, 7, 9, 18, 19, 23, 28, 32. Left: 3, 6, 8, 18, 19, 28, 31, 32, 33. Left to right: 32. Above downward: 19, 23, 32, 33. Below upward: 28, 31, 32, 43. Within outward: 6.

43 **Sensations.** ❙ Burning in internal and external parts.

As if hot water flowed through the blood-vessels, preventing sleep.

Sense of warm air streaming up the spine into the head. θ Preceding epileptic attacks.

44 **Tissues.** Great emaciation, clay-colored face, blue margins around eyes, great weakness of all limbs, want of disposition to do anything and constant inclination to rest.

Muscles lax.

General dropsy, or of thoracic or abdominal cavities.

❙ Post-scarlatinal dropsy; waxy skin. θ Morbus Brightii.

45 **Contact, Injuries, etc.** Touch: 4, 10, 17. Pressure:. 3, 10. 17, 26. Rubbing: 3. Scratching: 46. ❙ Snake-bites.

46 **Skin.** Skin very white and pasty-looking, later yellow, scaly.

Skin dry and scaly.

Blue spots on skin.

Burning, itching, parts painful after scratching.

Very painful black eruption.

❙ Pimples burning violently, causing almost unendurable anguish.

Herpetic eruption itching and burning; eczema, dry desquamation, burning pruritus.

Urticaria, large and very prominent.

Eruption resembling red petechiæ, from the size of a flea-bite to that of a lentil.

❙ Eruption delays or suddenly pales, becomes livid or intermixed with petechiæ; malignant sore throat; dropsy; or eruption well out, but with disproportionate weakness, mild delirium, vomiting, etc.   θ Scarlatina.

❙ Black vesicles causing burning pain.

❙ Variola, asthenic cases; pustules sink, areolæ grow livid; also in hemorrhagic and septic forms.

Ulcer, with high edges; discharges black, coagulated blood.

Ulcer on leg covered with grey crust and surrounded with an inflamed border; burning and painful.   ^

Painful sensitiveness of old ulcers.

Purulent, fetid secretions from eruptions.

Gangrenous aspect of sores.

❙ Carbuncles.

❙ Cancers with burning pain.

Itch-like eruption in bend of knees.

⁴⁷ **Stages and States.**   Hydrogenoid constitution of Grauvogl.

Suits the complaints of drunkards.

⁴⁸ **Relationship.**   Cognates: ❙ *Anthrac.* (carbuncle; anthrax; pyæmia, etc.); *Acet. ac.* (dropsy); *Acon.* (fever, paralysis, sudden chilling); *Apis; Apoc. can.; Baptis.* (sepsis; typhoid); *Bismuth* (vomiting); *Borax* (psoriasis); *Cinchon.* (debility, loss of fluids, dropsy, ague, gangrene ulcers, hæmoptysis, diarrhœa, effects of putrid water, marsh-poisons, etc.); *Carb. an.* (debility, glandular affections); *Carb. veg.* (debility, want of reaction, sepsis, especially ailments from putrid meats, fish or water, etc.); *Calc. ars.* (in epilepsy with heart symptoms); *Camphor.* (collapse, coldness, etc.); *Capsicum* (stomacace); *Crotal.* (blood poisoning); *Cuprum* (cholera, lack of reaction, paralysis, etc.); *Cupr. ars.* (neuralgia of viscera); *Ferrum* (eruption, lienteria, dropsy, chlorosis, neuralgia, etc.); *Graphit.* (chronic eruptions); *Hydrast.* (superior in lupus); *Ipec.* (chills and fever; asthma; catarrh of nose or chest with suffocation, summer complaint, especially in fat children; diarrhœa; vomiting, etc.); *Iris. vers.; Kali bichr.* (often superior in lupus); *Laches.* (in sepsis, etc.); *Mur. ac.; Nitr. ac.* (typhoid states; great debility, ulcers easily bleeding, diphtheria, etc.); *Nux vom.* (better in neuralgia, worse in morning); *Phosphor.; Plumbum* (paralysis, colic, tremors); *Rhus tox.* (mild delirium, ery-

11

sipelas, ophthalmia, scarlatina, typhoid fever, with prostration and involuntary stool; skin symptoms, etc.);
Secal. (cholera, diarrhœa, ulcers, gangrene, etc.); *Sulphur;*
Sulph. ac.; Tabac.; Tereb. (metritis, stupor with dark,
turbid urine, etc.); *Ver. alb.* (coldness, cholera, cholera
morbus, cold sweat.)

| |Complementary to *All. sat.*

❙❙Bad effects from tobacco-chewing; abuse of quinine;
iron or iodine.

Antidotes to *Arsen.* of large doses: **❙❙**sesquioxide of iron;
hydrated peroxide of iron, or precipitated carbonate of
iron; juice of sugar-cane, or honey-water. | |Limewater
in copious draughts, emetics of sulphate of zinc. | |Car-
bonate of potash and magnesia, shaken in oil. |Infu-
· sion of astringent substances. |Large quantities of
diluent drinks.

Of small doses: **❙**Camphor., **❙❙** *Cinchon.,* |❙ *Chin. sulph.,*
❙ *Ferrum, Hepar, Iodium,* **❙❙** *Ipec, Nux vom., Sambuc.,*
Tabac., **❙❙** *Veratr.*

Arsen. antidotes:**❙**Carb.veg.,**❙**Cinchon.,**❙**Ferrum, | |Graphit.,
❙ *Iodium,* **❙** *Ipec.,* **❙** *Laches.,* | |*Mercur.,* | |*Nux vom.,* **❙** *Verat.*
Lead poisonings, and evil effects of alcohol.

ARUM TRIPHYLLUM.

Arisœma triphyllum.   *Araceœ.*

[1] **Mind.** Forgetful.
Absence of mind, giddy.
❙During delirium, boring in the nose; picking at one spot,
or at the dry lips. *θ*Scarlatina. *θ*Typhus.
Wakeful, restless, screaming; delirium part of the time.
Irritable disposition.

[2] **Sensorium.** Vertigo and fulness, with absence of mind.
Light headed, sleepy.

[3] **Inner Head.** Dull headache, upper part feels cold as if open
and without covering.
Headache, pressing on right or both sides, worse from hot
coffee.
Tearing in right forehead and temple.
Stitches over left eye.
Sudden shooting over left eye and occiput.
Tearing, darting, or stitches in temples.

[4] **Outer Head.** Scalp sore to the touch, on the vertex.

[5] **Eyes.** Aversion to light. Obscured sight, as from a veil.

Upper eyelids heavy, with headache.

Tension in the lower lids, as if swollen.

I Quivering of upper lids.

Swelling of the edges of the lids.

Water in the eyes all day, most at the outer canthi.

⁶ **Ears.**   Burning in the right, tearing in the left ear.

Left parotid gland sore to the touch.

⁷ **Nose.**   Coryza, fluent, acrid.

> I Acrid, ichorous discharge, excoriating inside alæ and upper lip.
>
> I Corrosive, yellow, nasal discharge in diphtheria ; nostrils raw.
>
> I Nose moist, but obstructed ; discharge in the morning streaked with blood, during day yellow, thick mucus.
>
> I Nose stopped up, worse left side, must breathe through the mouth ; worse mornings.   θ Scarlatina.
>
> Sneezing, and sleepy, worse at night.
>
> I Nostrils sore, chapped, worse left.
>
> I Drink passes up and through the nose.
>
> I Constant picking at the nose.

⁸ **Face.**   Heat in the face, afternoons, with coryza.

Swollen, bloated face.   θ Scarlatina.

⁹ **Lower Face.**   Lips, nose and face chapped, as after exposure to cold wind.

> I Lips thick, burning, swollen, cracked and bleeding.
>
> I Lips as if scalded, mornings.
>
> I Picks the lips until they bleed; corners of mouth sore, cracked and bleeding, 48.   θ Scarlatina.   θ Typhus.
>
> I Swelling of submaxillary glands, worse left.   θ Scarlatina.

¹⁰ **Teeth.**   Toothache in hollow teeth of left side of lower jaw, towards evening.

¹¹ **Tongue, etc.**   Tongue: cracked, burning, painful ; sore, red, papillæ elevated.   θ Scarlatina.

Root of tongue and palate feel raw.

Sudden glossitis.

¹² **Mouth.**   I Excessive salivation ; saliva acrid.

> I The mouth burns, and is so sore that they refuse to drink, and cry when anything is offered.
>
> I Buccal cavity raw and sore, bleeding.
>
> Putrid odor from the mouth.

¹³ **Throat.**   Constriction in the throat, with sneezing.

Sensation of swelling on the soft palate, when swallowing, with discharge of nasal mucus.

Soreness, burning, and pains in palate, worse when eating or drinking.

> I Throat and tongue very sore, burning pains, putrid ulcers in throat.
>
> I Refuses food and drink on account of soreness of throat.

[14] **Desires. Aversions.** ❘ No appetite; does not want to play; loses flesh; headache; scanty urine.

Desires to drink a little at a time.

[15] **Eating and Drinking.** Worse drinking coffee: 3. Worse drinking or eating: 13.

Headache better after breakfast or dinner.

[16] **Nausea and Vomiting.** Nausea; qualmish; giddy.

[17] **Stomach.** Cramps in the stomach.

[18] **Hypochondria.** Pain in the liver, front then back.

Pain under left short ribs.

[19] **Abdomen.** Rumbling in bowels; flatulency; cutting pains.

[20] **Stools, etc.** Painful urging, with rumbling; tenesmus towards evening.

Fissura ani, with retention of urine.

. Stool: watery, dark brown, with belching; soft, thin, yellow and painless; soft, with tenesmus; at night during sleep.

Burning at the anus.

[21] **Urine.** ❘ Urine scanty or suppressed. θ Scarlatina.

[22] **Male Sexual Organs.** Tearing pain in right testicle during morning; comes suddenly and disappears suddenly.

Smarting at the end of the penis.

[23] **Female Sexual Organs.** Cutting pains in ovaries.

Menstrual blood darker.

[24] **Pregnancy.** Lumps deep in the left mammæ, with aching pains.

Convulsions during dentition, right side lame, quivering of left upper eyelid.

[25] **Larynx.** ❘ Voice hoarse; from over-use of the voice in speaking or singing, worse taking food.

Œdema glottidis.

Voice uncertain, uncontrollable, changing continually.

Mucus in the trachea when coughing.

Loss of voice: after exposure to N. W. wind; when singing.

Must hawk, in the morning; hoarseness more before talking, better afterwards.

Constant pain in the larynx.

❘ Clergyman's sore throat.

[26] **Breathing.** Asthmatic breathing, with chronic catarrh.

[27] **Cough.** Head and breast feel obstructed, full of mucus, without spitting.

Frequent coughing, with much mucus and much spitting.

Burning pain in the lungs when coughing.

Tickling cough from mucus in the trachea; at night after lying down inability to sleep; hoarseness.

[28] **Lungs.** Lungs feel sore.

Soreness in left lung and upper arm, pressing in forehead.

Stitches in right lung and under shoulder-blade.

[29] **Heart. Pulse.** Pulse more frequent.

[31] **Neck. Back.** Stiffness of the neck; with intolerable pressing headache.

Pain as if in atlas and dentoid vertebræ.

Glands of throat or neck swollen.

[32] **Upper Limbs.** Hands stiff and swollen.

[33] **Lower Limbs.** Cramp in the right leg on getting awake in
the morning.

Stinging, pricking or bruised pain in the soles.

[34] **Limbs in General.** Heaviness of the limbs, worse in legs.

[35] **Position, etc.** Better after rising: 20. Rest: 13, 27.

[36] **Nerves.** Lassitude and low spirits.

Right side lame during dentition.

Very nervous.

Greatest weakness or exhaustion.

Spasms of arms and hands; thumbs drawn in.

[37] **Sleep.** Sleepy, yawning and sneezing at 11 A. M.; headache
worse, eyes heavy.

Drowsy in the evening.

❙ Sleeplessness, from soreness of mouth and throat, or from
itching of the skin.

Nightmare.

On falling asleep feels as if she would smother, starts as if
frightened.

[38] **Time.** All day: 7, 13. Morning: 7, 9, 12, 13, 25, 33, 37.
11 A.M.: 7, 37. Afternoon: 8, 40. 4–9 P.M.: 40. Evening: 10, 20, 37. Night: 7, 20, 27, 37. Before midnight:
13. Same hour: 40.

[39] **Temperature and Weather.** N. W. wind: 25.

[40] **Chill. Fever. Sweat.** Repeated chill spreading from the
vertex, with sneezing like after taking a cold, afternoons.

Chills running over the body after much yawning, at the
same hour; on two days.

Flushed, with burning face.

Fever heat very intense. θ Scarlatina.

❙ Typhoid forms of fever: picking the ends of the fingers,
picking the dry lips till they bleed; boring the nose,
restless tossing about the bed, wants to escape, unconscious of what he is doing or of what is said to him;
urine suppressed; great weakness (last stages, probably
with uræmia).

[41] **Attacks.** Sudden: 3. Pains come and goes suddenly: 22.
Same hour: 40.

[42] **Sides.** Right: 3, 6, 7, 18, 22, 24, 28, 31, 33, 36, 37. Left: 3,
5, 6, 7, 10, 18, 23, 24, 28. Both sides: 3. Front to back
(liver): 18.

[43] **Sensations.** Head feels open, as if calvaria were removed.

[45] **Contact, Injuries, etc.** Touch: 4. Pressure: 33.

[46] **Skin.** ❙ Itching. θ Scarlatina.

Desquamation a second or third time, in large flakes. θ Scarlatina.

Little round, red, hard pimples all over the body, legs, arms and face.

[48] **Relationship.** Buttermilk, which •contains *Lactic acid*, antidotes.

Compare: *Amm. mur.*, *Castor.*, *Cepa*, *Kali hydx.*, *Lycop.*, *Mezer.*, *Nitr. ac.*, *Silic.* (nasal discharge), *Arg. nitr.*, *Crocus* (tongue), *Capsic.* (throat), *Caustic.*, *Ferr. phosph.* (hoarseness), *Mercur.* and *Veratr.* (salivation), *Mercur.* and *Bryon.* (lips and corners of mouth).

Concordances: *Laches.*, *Lycop.*, *Ailanth.*, *Arsen.*, *Canthar.*, *Mur. ac.*, *Nitr. ac.*, *Sulph. ac.*, *Hydr. ac.*, *Iodium*, *Phytol.*, *Sanguin.*, *Silic.*, *Sulphur.*

In typhus: compare *Calad.*, *Nitr. ac.*

Arum has in high degree, soreness and cracks in corners of mouth, but *Condurango* must not be neglected for the same site; especially if there is also superficial ulceration of the cornea.

ASAFŒTIDA.

Ferula Asafœtida.   *Umbelliferæ.*

[1] **Mind.** Unsteady and fickle, cannot persevere in anything; wants now one thing, then another, walks hither and thither.

Fits of great joy, with occasional burst of laughter.

Apprehension of dying.

Anxious, sadness.

Ill-humor, irritable mood.

Hysterical restlessness and anxiety.

[2] **Sensorium.** Oversensitiveness, either physical or mental.

Fainting during the height of the paroxysm of colic.

Stupefying tension in the head, mostly left side; worse afternoon or evening; sitting bent forward; after going to bed; better, sitting up.

[3] **Inner Head.** Pressure in sides of head or temples, like from a dull stick, better from touch.

Flying stitch from within outward, in the forehead, temples and sides of the head.

Sensation of swashing and gurgling behind the upper part of the frontal bone.

All the headaches are worse towards evening; in the room, while at rest, sitting or lying. Better when rising or moving about in the open air.

⁴ **Outer Head.** Cold sweat on the forehead.
⁵ **Eyes.** Mist before the eyes.

Sensation of dryness in the eyes.

ı Nocturnal, throbbing pains in and around the eye and head. *θ* Syphilitic iritis.

Sharp pain extending through the eye into the head, upon touching.

ı Extensive superficial ulceration of the cornea, with burning, sticking or pressing pains, from within outwards; rest and pressure relieve.

⁶ **Ears.** Hardness of hearing, with thin, purulent discharge of offensive odor.

⁷ **Nose.** ı Offensive discharge from the nose. Stench from nose.

Unpainful tension over nasal bones, with numbness.

Swelling and inflammation affecting bones, with feeling as if nose would burst.

⁸ **Face.** Flushes in the face.

Small tubercles in the cheeks.

⁹ **Lower Jaw.** Lips puffed up, lower lip and left angle most.

Drawing pains and caries of lower maxilla, with salivation.

¹⁰ **Teeth.** Bluntness of the teeth.

Severe drawing in the lower incisors.

Soreness of the gums.

¹¹ **Tongue, etc.** Greasy taste in the mouth and of the phlegm hawked up.

¹² **Mouth.** Saliva predominantly decreased, except in mercurial caries, when acrid salivation exists.

Burning in the mouth.

¹³ **Throat.** Burning followed by soreness, in the fauces.

Darting stitches, from chest upward towards œsophagus.

Tender feeling in the throat.

ı Sensation of a ball rising in the throat, may cause difficulty in breathing.

Dryness and burning in the œsophagus.

ı Sensation in the œsophagus as if the peristaltic motions were from below upwards; globus hystericus.

¹⁴ **Desires. Aversions.** Desire for wine.

Great disgust for all food.

Beer tastes slimy, aversion to it.

¹⁵ **Eating and Drinking.** After eating: pressure in the stomach, stitches about the lower ribs, tension in the abdomen; squirming and twisting in the bowels; great difficulty in breathing; febrile state.

After drinking: heaviness and cold feeling in the intestines; diarrhœa.

¹⁶ **Nausea and Vomiting.** ı Eructations; smelling like garlic; tasting rancid, sharp or putrid.

ı Flatus passing upwards, none down.

Hiccough-like contractions of the diaphragm.

[17] **Stomach.** Pulsations in pit of stomach, 11 A. M., cause faint feeling.

Sensation of fullness in stomach.

Empty, "gone" feeling in epigastrium.

Pressing, cutting, stitching pain in spells, not regular.

[18] **Hypochondria.** Heat in the spleen and belly.

Violent pressure in scrobiculum towards liver, while sitting.

Stitches as if in the diaphragm, right side.

[19] **Abdomen.** Bellyache, as if the intestines were torn or cut; places in the side sore as if raw, with it a feeling as of something rising from chest to throat; pressure relieves.

Wind colic, with abdominal pulsations; very painful distention of abdomen, rumbling; relieved by passing wind.

[20] **Stool, etc.** Watery stools of disgusting odor; discharge profuse and greenish.

Very offensive diarrhœa, with colic; discharge of fetid flatus.

Obstinate constipation, with abdominal and hemorrhoidal cramps.

Only slime passes, no feces.

[21] **Urine.** Brown and of pungent odor.

Spasms in the bladder, during and after urination.

[22] **Male Sexual Organs.** Needle-like stitches in the penis.

Drawing in the glans, more during the afternoon.

[23] **Female Sexual Organs.** Excited sexual desire.

Menses, too frequent, too scanty and last but a short time.

Labor-like pains in uterine region, with cutting and bearing down.

Bearing down in genitals, worse when riding in carriage.

Uterine ulcer, sensitive and painful.

Leucorrhœa profuse, greenish, thin and offensive.

Swelling and inflammation of the genitals.

[24] **Pregnancy.** Mammæ turgid with milk, like in the ninth month; without being pregnant.

Deficiency of milk, with oversensitiveness.

[25] **Larynx.** Voice weaker, hoarse.

Spasm of glottis, alternating with contraction of fingers and toes.

[26] **Breathing.** Spasmodic tightness of the chest, as if the lungs could not be fully expanded.

Constriction of chest, extending to the throat; hurried breathing.

[27] **Cough.** Irritation to dry cough.

Cough on gaping.

Whooping-cough, even of sucklings, sounding like croup; rattling breathing, anxious and restless, chest and abdomen hot, urine pale.

Hoarse, ringing, short cough, excited by tickling in the trachea, with asthmatic feeling therein; spasmodic contraction of thorax and accumulation of stringy mucus.

[28] **Lungs.** Pressure and burning under sternum often with cough.

Compression of chest, as from a heavy weight.

Pressing stitches in the chest.

Burning in chest, runs through both arms, and through lower limbs down into toes.

Single violent stitches from within outwards, at short intervals; renewed when the chest is touched.

[29] **Heart. Pulse.** Nervous palpitation, with small pulse; from overexertion or suppression of discharges (in women).

Pulse: unchanged; unequal; generally very much accelerated, but small.

Pressure in region of heart as if the heart was too full and expanded, pulse small.

[31] **Neck. Back.** Drawing downwards, in the left side of neck, on motion.

Stitches in the muscles of the back.

Dull pains, or drawing and cutting below the scapulæ.

Burning along the vertebræ, to the left side.

Aching inwardly, along the last dorsal and first lumbar vertebræ.

[32] **Upper Limbs.** Quivering in the shoulder-joint: in deltoid muscle.

Stitches and jerking in the upper arm.

Drawing pain along the upper arm down to the elbow, a fine stitch in the elbow.

Tearing in the forearm down to the tips of the fingers.

When moving the fingers, pain in the forearm.

Tearing stitches followed by burning in the right forearm.

Scraping sensation on the styloid process of the ulna.

[33] **Lower Limbs.** Psoitis if suppuration seems impending.

Caries of the tibia.

Swelling around the ankle, cannot use the foot.

Swelling and caries of the bones of the feet.

Sticking sensation on the ball of the great toe when putting the foot to the ground.

Pain as if a splinter of bone was sticking in the right fibula just above the outer malleolus.   θ After a sprain.

[34] **Limbs in General.** Twitching of muscles of arms and legs.

Pain mostly on the flexor sides of the limbs.

[35] **Position, etc.** Rest: 3, 5. Motion: 31. Sitting: 3, 18. Sitting up: 2. Sitting bent forward: 2. Lying: 3. After lying down: 2. Rising: 3.

Constant change of position.

[36] **Nerves.** Hysteria, with much trouble about throat or œsophagus.

Twitching and jerking of the muscles.

Chorea.

Clumsiness of the body.

[37] **Sleep.** Inclined to sleep.

Sleeplessness at midnight.

About midnight violent pains through left half of body.

[38] **Time.** About 11 A. M.: 17 Afternoon 2, 22, 40. From 3 to 4 P. M.: 40. Evening: 2, 3. Night: 43. Dark till 2 A. M.: neuralgia. Midnight and afternoon: 37.

[39] **Temperature and Weather.** Worse in-doors, better out-doors.

Desire for open air.

Room: 3. Open air: 3.

[40] **Chill. Fever. Sweat.** Crawls run over back, in afternoon.

Chill, coldness and dryness of the skin; also in caries, etc.

Every day between 3 and 4 P. M., coldness and trembling, with unbearable stitches in the head.

Heat in the face, after dinner, with anxiety and sleepiness, without thirst.

Occasional cold, moist skin.

[41] **Attacks.** Intermittent pinching pain in ulcers.

[42] **Sides.** Right: 18, 32, 33. Left: 2, 31, 37. Within outward: 3, 5, 28. Below upwards: 13, 16, 19, 26, 32. Above downwards: 28, 31, 32.

[43] **Sensations.** Numbness with the pains.

Burning or pressing, piercing pain in the muscles.

Crushing pains, worse at night.

Great heaviness of the whole body.

Pain like from splinters.

[44] **Tissues.** Glands hard, swollen, hot and throbbing, with shooting-jerking pains.

Neuralgia of the stump after amputation of the thigh.

Ostitis, caries, bluish redness and swelling of the parts.

Ulcers, with bluish edges, hard, painful to the slightest touch; transparent and thin, very offensive and ichorous pus.

Soft enlargement of bones, also curvature.

Body bloated.

[45] **Contact, Injuries, etc.** Touch: 3, 28, 46. Pressure: 5, 19. Riding in carriage: 23.

[46] **Skin.** Ulcers, with high, hard edges, bluish, etc., sensitive to touch, easily bleeding; pus profuse, greenish, thin, offensive, even ichorous.

Shooting pain around the ulcer.

Ulcers grow black.

Old scars break open and turn black.

[47] **Stages and States.** Phlegmatic temperament.

Scrofulous, bloated, clumsy children.

Venous, hemorrhoidal constitution.

Nervous people.

Syphilitic patients who have taken much mercury.

⁴⁸ **Relationship.** Cognates: *Aurum* (bone diseases; iritis, etc.);
Arg. nitr.; Ammoniacum (family relation); *Castor.; Cinchon.; Caustic.; Conium* (family relation); *Hepar* (sensitive around ulcers; faint with pains); *Ignat.* (hysteria);
Mercur. (syphilis); *Moschus* (hysteria, spasm of lungs,
fainting, etc); *Pulsat.; Thuja; Valer.*

Antidotes to *Asaf.: Pulsat., Caustic., Camphor, Cinchon.,
Mercur., Valer.*

If *Asaf.* has been abused in large doses, electricity may be
useful.

ASARUM EUROPÆUM.

Haselwurz, or asarabacca. HAHNEMANN.   *Aristolochiaceæ.*

¹ **Mind.** Gradual vanishing of thought, like when falling
asleep.

Imagines he is hovering in the air like a spirit, when
walking in the open air.

Stupid feeling in the head, has no desire to do anything.

Great merriness, alternating with occasional momentary
quiet or gloominess.

Tearful sadness and anxiety.

Melancholic irritability.

³ **Inner Head.** Dull headache in the left temple, afterwards
below the parietal bones, lastly in the occiput.

Pressive headache, above the root of the nose; in the temples, particularly the left.

Pressure over greater part of brain, from without inwards.

Drawing headache, as if the temple would be drawn in (at
noon), ameliorated in the open air and when lying down.

Very sensitive compressive headache in the left temple
and behind the ears, more violent when walking or
shaking the head, better when sitting.

Tearing, pulsating pain in forehead, excited by stooping.

⁴ **Outer Head.** Itching, beginning with fine stitches, below
the left temple.

Sensation of coldness at a small spot on the left side of
head, above the ear.

Tension of the scalp; the hair feels painful.

⁵ **Eyes.** Left upper eyelid is somewhat swollen, the eye cannot endure much reading.

Sensation in each eye as if it would be pressed asunder, when reading.

Painful dryness of the eyes.

Watering and burning of the eyes.

⁶ **Ears**. Right auricle hot to the touch.

❙ Oversensitiveness of the nerves, the scratching of linen or silk is insupportable.

Dull roaring of the left ear, like a distant wind-storm; in the right distinct singing.

Diminished hearing of the left ear.

Sensation as if the skin were stretched over the right external ear, with tensive pressure within; worse in cold.

⁷ **Nose**. Discharge of bloody mucus from the nose.

Dry coryza; the left nostril is stopped up.

Tickling in the nose, causing, after unsuccessful efforts, a sneeze, and discharge of clear fluid.

Violent sneezing.

⁸ **Face**. Warmth of the cheeks.

Fine stinging on the right cheek.

Burning-stinging pain on the left cheek.

⁹ **Lower Face**. Dryness of the inner side of lower lip.

Cutting pain, with cramp at the articulation of lower jaw.

¹⁰ **Teeth**. Teeth of the left side feel as if hollow.

Cold feeling in upper incisors like from a cold breath.

Smarting sensation on the gums.

¹¹ **Tongue, etc.** Bread tastes bitter.

Tobacco tastes bitter when smoking.

Burning sensation across the tongue.

¹² **Mouth**. Mucus in the mouth, of a sweetish, insipid taste.

Accumulation of much water in the mouth, with nausea.

¹³ **Throat**. Dryness in the throat, with stitches.

Scraping in the throat.

Tough mucus in throat; is unable to raise it, or hawk it loose.

Swallowing difficult, as from swelling of glands of throat.

¹⁴ **Desires. Aversions.** Loathing of food without any gastric derangement.

❙ Unconquerable longing for alcohol.

¹⁵ **Eating and Drinking.** Early morning hunger.

¹⁶ **Nausea and Vomiting.** Hiccough.

Frequent empty eructations.

Imperfect eructations reaching only to upper part of chest.

Continuous nausea and inclination to vomit (in fauces).

Empty retching; during retchings all symptoms are aggravated, except stupid feeling of head, which decreases.

Vomiting of only a small quantity of greenish, somewhat sour fluid; with great straining, and sensation about the ears as if the head would split.

After vomiting, relief of the head symptoms.

[17] **Stomach.** Pressure in stomach, scrobiculum and abdomen.
Sensation of constriction in the region of the diaphragm.

[19] **Abdomen.** Cutting pain in the upper abdomen, better by passing flatus.

Violent colic and vomiting.

Rumbling and gurgling in the abdomen.

[20] **Stool, etc.** Before stool, cutting in the abdomen and sharp stitches in the rectum, from above downwards.

Stool: whitish-grey, or ash-colored, on the top like bloody mucus; shaggy masses of mucus full of oxyuri.

[22] **Male Sexual Organs.** Violent pain in the left groin, darting through the urethra to the glans, in which a violent smarting, contracted pain remains for a long time.

[23] **Female Sexual Organs.** At the appearance of the menses violent pain in small of the back, which scarcely permits her to breathe.

Vaginal fistula.

[24] **Pregnancy.** Threatened abortion from excessive sensibility of the nerves.

[25] **Larynx.** Stitches and constriction in the larynx.

[26] **Breathing.** Breath very short (night).

Whistling breathing at the beginning of coughing.

Short, jerking breathing on account of stitches and constriction of larynx.

[27] **Cough.** Frequent cough on account of mucus in the chest; mucus rises in the throat, causing difficult breathing, and finally cough, with expectoration.

Inhalation causes irritation to cough, in the throat.

Constant, short hacking cough of consumptives.

[28] **Lungs.** Stitches in right or both lungs during inhalation.

Sharp pressure in the region of the last ribs.

Pain around both lungs, as if constricted by a thin wire.

[29] **Heart. Pulse.** Pulse quick and strong.

[30] **Outer Chest.** Burning sensation, right chest, more external than internal.

[31] **Neck. Back.** Sensation in the muscles of the neck like from a tight cravat, or as if pressed upon by a dull edge.

Burning pain, with stitches in small of back, while sitting.

Tearing pain from crest of one ilium to the other.

Bruised pain in the back.

Dull stitches under the scapulæ.

Laming pains as if bruised in one of the cervical muscles, when moving the head.

[32] **Upper Limbs.** Violent stitch in both shoulders during motion or rest.

Contractive tensive pain in the deltoid muscle, when laying the hand on the table, and while it lies there.

Drawing-laming pain in the left wrist.

Sudden drawing-burning pain from the wrist through the thumb and index-finger.

[33] **Lower Limbs.** Dull pressure in the right hip.

Drawing, tensive pain in head of the left femur.

Severe pain in the hip-joint and in the middle of the thigh, when stepping; the foot feels as if paralyzed, he cannot step properly thereon.

Severe rheumatic tearing stitches in the knees during motion and rest.

Lassitude in the knees.

Drawing in the hamstrings, evenings when lying in bed.

Gurgling sensation in the patella.

Bruised feeling in the left tibia.

Stitches in the sole of the foot.

The little toes pain as if frozen.

[34] **Limbs in General.** Lightness of all the limbs; he does not perceive that he has a body.

Occasional darting and tearing pains in limbs.

[35] **Position, etc.** Rest or motion: 32, 33. Moving head: 31. Shaking head: 3. Rising: 2. Stepping: 33. Walking: 2, 3. Stooping: 3. Sitting: 3, 31. Lying down: 3. After lying down: 40. Lying in bed: 33. Must lie down: 36. Rising to sitting posture: 36. Standing: 33.

[36] **Nerves.** Great lassitude.

Great faintness and constant yawning.

General weary feeling.

So weak and nauseated toward evening, that when he rises to sitting posture he feels as if he would instantly sink down and die; he must lie in bed.

[37] **Sleep.** Frequent yawning.

Great drowsiness by day.

Restless sleep.

Nightly vexatious dreams about humiliations.

[38] **Time.** Early morning: 15. Forenoon: 40. Noon: 3. Evening: 33, 36, 40. Night: 26, 37, 40. Day: 37, 40.

[39] **Temperature and Weather.** Warmth or covering: 40. Open air: 3, 40. Walking in open air:. 2. Cold: 6. Dry, cold weather aggravates rheumatism.

[40] **Chill. Fever. Sweat.** Chill and cold feeling in the forenoon, after eating or drinking, and in the open air, generally with heat of the head.

Great want of vital heat; feels cold continually. θ With vaginal fistula.

Cold feeling, not relieved by covering, or warmth of room.

Heat in the evening, after lying down, particularly in the face and palms of hands.

Alternate flushes of burning heat and coldness.

Sweat increased at night, sour smell; moist profuse in axilla.
Sweats easily, particularly on the upper body.
⁴² **Sides.** Right: 6, 8, 28, 30, 33. Left: 3, 4, 5, 6, 7, 8, 10, 22, 32, 33. Above downwards: 20. Below upwards: 27. Without inwards: 3.
⁴³ **Sensations.** Excessive sensibility of all the nerves; when merely thinking (and this he must do continually) that some one might, with finger-tip or nail, scratch even lightly on linen, or similar material, a most disagreeable sensation thrills through him, arresting momentarily all his thoughts and actions.
⁴⁶ **Contact, Injuries, etc.** Touch: 6.
⁴⁷ **Stages and States.** Nervous temperament, excitable, or melancholic mood.
⁴⁸ **Relationship.** Compare *Cuprum, Nux vom., Phosphor.*
Antidotes to *Asar.: Camphor.*, vinegar, vegetable acids.

AURUM METALLICUM.

Common Gold.   HAHNEMANN.   *Au.*

¹ **Mind.** Weak memory.
Religious mania; prays all the time.
Uneasy, hurried, desire for mental and bodily activity; cannot do things fast enough.
Suicidal mood.
Hallucinations; sees dogs, a hand on the wall, etc., mania.
Apprehensiveness, full of fear; a mere noise at the door makes him anxious.
Melancholy, disposed to weep; imagines he is unfit for this world, that he can never succeed.
Great anguish, coming from the precordial region, driving him from place to place; palpitation.
Weary of life; especially in evening, with longing for death.
Has no confidence in herself, thinks others have none; this makes her unhappy.
Alternately peevish and cheerful.
Contradiction excites wrath.
Mental labor fatigues.
Ailments from grief, disappointed love.
² **Sensorium.** Vertigo: when stooping, as if turning in a circle, goes off on rising; as if drunk, when walking in open air; feels as if he would fall to left side; must lie down; even then for some time it returns on slightest motion.
³ **Inner Head.** Tearing headache deep in the forehead and temples, abating in the open air.

Rush of blood to the head; sparks before the eyes, and glossy, bloated face; worse from mental exertion.

Bruised pain, especially in the early morning or during mental labor, ideas become confused; roaring in head.

Headaches of students, with precordial anxiety and flashes of heat to the head.

Megrim, stitching, burning pains, beating in one side of forehead; nausea, even bilious vomiting.

Fine tearing from the right side of the occiput through the brain to the forehead; worse during motion.

⁴ **Outer Head.** Skull bones painful, as if broken; worse lying down.

Exostoses on the head; boring pains; worse from touch.

Falling out of hair.

⁵ **Eyes.** Objects as if divided horizontally; sees only half of an object, other half as if covered with a dark body.

Tension in the eyes; sees things double or mixed up.

Fiery sparks before eyes: optical illusions in bright colors.

Pupils most frequently contracted.

Cutting pain through the eyes.

Iritis serosa and cornea spotted.

Opacity of the cornea. θ After keratitis.

Eyeballs protrude.

Red sclerotica; burning, stitching, drawing and itching at the inner canthus.

Photophobia, profuse scalding tears on opening the eyes; eyes very sensitive to touch.

Pressive pain in orbit from above downward, within out.

Bones around the eye feel bruised.

Ulceration of the cornea in the course of pannus; pains from within outwards; worse from pressure.

Little blisters turning into crusts on the edges of lids, with some trichiasis.

Eyelids red, suppurating; stinging, prickling, itching; agglutination in the morning; cilia fall out.

⁷ **Ears.** Roaring in the ears; oversensitiveness to noises.

Annoying dryness in ears and nose, with difficult hearing.

Caries of the mastoid process; obstinate otorrhœa.

Burning, prickling, itching; boring pain behind left ear.

Parotids swollen; painful to touch, as if pressed or contused.

⁷ **Nose.** Complaints caused by strong odors.

Sensitive smell; everything smells too strong.

Putrid smell when blowing nose; want of smell.

Ulcerated, agglutinated, painful nostrils, cannot breathe through the nose; crusts in the nose.

Nose feels obstructed as in dry coryza, yet air passes through freely.

Ozæna, excessively fetid discharge; severe frontal headache.

Coryza, thick discharge, like the white of egg; frequent sneezing.

Caries of nasal bones; right nasal bone and adjoining parts of upper jaw painful to touch.

Boring in left side of nasal bone, toward the maxilla.

Burning, itching, stitching, smarting; feeling of soreness in nose, especially when touched.

Mucous discharge from the posterior nares in the morning.

Tip of the nose "knobby," red.   Nose red and swollen.

⁸ **Face.**   Bloated, glossy, worse from mental exertion; cyanotic.

Drawing, deep seated tearing in the left side of the face.

Swelling of one cheek, with drawing and tearing in upper and lower jaws; teeth feel too long.

Inflammation of bones of face; caries of cheek-bones; tearing, boring, burning stitches in the zygoma.

Violent tearing in the malar bone.

Fine eruption on lips, face, or forehead.

⁹ **Lower Face.**   Painful swelling of submaxillary glands.

¹⁰ **Teeth.**   Toothache caused by drawing air into the mouth.

Gums swollen, dark red, sore when touched or when eating; bleed easily.

¹¹ **Tongue, etc.**   Bitter taste; putrid taste, as of spoiled game, between meals.

Loss of taste, with complete immovability of the tongue, which is hard as leather.

Aphthæ on tongue and mouth.

Ulcers on the tongue.

¹² **Mouth.**   Copious saliva; saliva sweetish.

Inside of mouth blistered.

Stench from the mouth; smell like old cheese.

Offensive odor; girls at puberty.

¹³ **Throat.**   Red and swollen tonsils.

Boring in the hard palate; caries of roof, palate and nose.

Stinging soreness in throat only during deglutition.

Difficult raising of phlegm.

Dull, pressive pain, with or without swallowing, in a gland below angle of jaw.

¹⁴ **Desires.   Aversions.**   Hunger, immoderate; relishes his meal, but appetite not appeased.

Immoderate appetite and thirst, with qualmishness in the stomach.

Appetite for milk, wine, coffee.

Aversion to meat.

¹⁶ **Nausea and Vomiting.**   Eructations of gas relieve attacks of palpitation.

Nausea from mental labor.

¹⁷ **Stomach.**   Burning sensation at stomach, with hot risings.

Pressure in region of stomach, at noon.

12

Pressure to the left of the scrobiculum, below cartilages of upper false ribs; worse during expiration.

[18] **Hypochondria.** Burning heat and cutting in right hypochondrium.

Painful accumulation of gas below left ribs, causing stitching pains.

Pressure in hypochondria, as from flatulence; worse after food or drink and motion.

[19] **Abdomen.** Colic, frequent discharge of wind.

Spasmodic contraction of abdomen with great anguish, inclined to suicide.

Tensive pain, as if laced together.

Heaviness in abdomen, with icy coldness of hands and feet.

Ascites from disturbances of abdominal organs.

[20] **Stool, etc.** Passes fetid flatus.

Stools offensive, painful; greyish, ashy.

Nightly diarrhœa, with burning in the rectum.

Hard, knotty or large stools; constipation worse during menses.

Piles with rectal catarrh; costive; external piles bleed during stool.

[21] **Urine.** Constant urging to urinate.

Urine scanty, greenish-brown, in jaundice; clear, gold-colored, in dropsy.

Turbid, like buttermilk; much sediment of mucus.

Urine ammoniacal, decomposes rapidly, smells like the otorrhœa.

Paralysis of the bladder with retention of urine.

Ischuria painful, with pressure in bladder.

[20] **Male Sexual Organs.** Discharge of prostatic fluid from a relaxed penis; settled melancholy, with suicidal mania.

Right testicle swollen, pressive pains when touching or rubbing.

Testes indurated; testes undeveloped; boy pining, depressed, weak.

Itching of the scrotum.

Ulcers on the scrotum; cutting and stinging in perineum.

Inguinal glands suppurate.

[23] **Female Sexual Organs.** Uterus prolapsed and indurated; bruised pain, with shooting or drawing; heaviness in abdomen; after lifting a heavy load; worse at time of menses.

Sterility in syphilitic women; also in the ill-nourished, who are mentally depressed because of their barrenness.

Menses: too late, scanty; preceded by swelling of axillary glands; accompanied by colic, prolapse of the rectum.

Amenorrhœa, with prolapsus uteri and melancholy.

Constant oozing from the vulva.

Thick white leucorrhœa; burning-smarting of the vulva; labia majora red, swollen.

²⁴ **Pregnancy.** Suppressed milk

Palpitation following metrorrhagia after a mole or in childbed, after overexertion.

Labor-pains make her desperate, she would like to jump from the window or dash herself down; often with congestion to head and chest; palpitation.

²⁵ **Larynx.** Voice: nasal; husky, as if he had a cold.

Phlegm deep in the larynx, not easily hawked up.

²⁶ **Breathing.** Dyspnœa: with dull stitches in chest when inspiring; cannot be relieved in any position; takes deep breaths.

ı Asthma from congestion to chest; great oppression at night and when walking in the open air; suffocative fits, with spasmodic constriction of chest; face bluish-red; palpitation; falls down unconscious.

Morning asthma: face cyanotic; light-haired persons; worse after mercury; in wet weather and warm air.

²⁷ **Cough.** With tough yellow sputa on awaking in morning.

Cough from want of breath, at night.

Dry, spasmodic, nervous cough, peculiar to women; periodically, every night from sunset to sunrise.

²⁸ **Lungs.** Shooting pains in chest after attacks of palpitation.

Dull stitches in both sides of chest, with heat in the chest and dyspnœa; increased by inspiration.

Persistent dry catarrh on the chest, early in the morning, on waking; with great difficulty he raises a little phlegm, and this only after rising from bed.

²⁹ **Heart. Pulse.** Frequent attacks of anguish about the heart, with tremulous fearfulness; palpitation with great agony.

Strong beating of heart, with anxiety and congestion to the head, after metrorrhagia; also after exertion.

When riding or walking, palpitation compels him to stop.

Palpitation, with irregular, intermittent pulse; short breathing.

Pain in region of heart, extends down left arm to fingers.

Pains wander from joint to joint, and finally become fixed in the heart; must sit upright; feels as though heart ceased and then suddenly gave one hard thump.

Pulse small, but accelerated.

ı Weak pulse, cardiac asthma, mental depression; great debility.

³¹ **Neck. Back.** Swollen cervical glands.

Tension in neck, as if muscles were too short, even at rest, mostly when stooping.

Spine disease, with gressus gallinaceous.

Pain in small of back as from fatigue.

Tendons of lumbar muscles so painfully stiff, that the thigh cannot be raised; thigh feels paralyzed.

³² **Upper Limbs.** Boring in left shoulder.

Inflammatory- swelling of axillary glands.

Difficult movement of arms; they feel fatigued; forearms feel heavy.

Severe bone pains in right elbow.

Boring in right forearm.

Cramp-like tearing in bones of both wrists.

Palms itch. θ Herpes of the palms.

Boring in finger-joints.

³³ **Lower Limbs.** All the blood appeared to rush from her head into lower limbs; they feel paralyzed, she has to sit down.

Tottering of the knees; stiffness, paralytic feeling; they pain as if firmly bandaged, when sitting.

Right knee becomes weak from walking; drawing when walking or setting foot on floor.

Boring in tibiæ; ankles; dorsum of feet.

Swelling of legs and feet when getting up in the morning, better after walking.

Toes red.

Itching on soles.

³⁴ **Limbs in General.** Limbs go to sleep, numb, insensible on awaking; more lying than moving.

Paralytic drawing in of the limbs in the morning, when awaking; also on getting cold.

Has to seize hold of left arm during attacks of palpitation.

Swelling of periosteum of forearm and thigh bones.

Pain as from bruises in head and limbs, early in bed; mostly at rest; passes off after rising.

³⁵ **Position, etc.** Rest: 31, 34. Sitting: 33. Lying: 34. Must lie down: 2. Walking: 29, 33. Walking in open air: 2, 26. Motion: 2, 3, 18, 34, 36. Exertion: 29. Stooping: 2, 31. Rising: 2, 28, 33, 34, 40. Setting foot on floor: 33. In bed: 37.

³⁶ **Nerves.** In the morning completely exhausted, as if he had not slept at all.

Tremulous agitation, as in joyous hope.

Hysterical spasms; alternate laughter and crying.

When thinking of a motion, he makes small motions without knowing it; when speaking he smiles involuntarily.

Sensation of internal emptiness and weakness of whole body.

Great nervous weakness.

³⁷ **Sleep.** Sobs aloud during sleep; frightful dreams about thieves, with loud screams.

Awake all night, no pain ; no lassitude or sleepiness in the morning.

Sleeplessness after midnight.

Awakened by bone pains, suffering so great he despairs, does not want to live.

Bruised feeling, mornings in bed.

[38] **Time.** Morning: 3, 5, 7, 26, 27, 28, 33, 34, 36, 37, 40. Morning and evening: 27. Noon: 17. Night: 5, 20, 26, 27, 37, 40. Sunset to sunrise: 27. Evening till midnight: 46.

[39] **Temperature and Weather.** Very sensitive to cold.

Generally better growing warm.

Warmth: 26. Room: 46. Cold: 34. Air: 10. Wet weather: 26. Open air: 3, 26, 46.

Many symptoms disappear after washing.

[40] **Chill. Fever. Sweat.** Cold hands and feet; sometimes lasting all night; want of thirst.

Chill lessened after getting out of bed ; shivering in bed ; legs cold as far as the knees.

Coldness of whole body, nausea; chill predominates.

Heat only in face; aversion to uncovering; cold hands and feet.

Heat alternating with chill.

Auric fever : temperaiure raised, pulse frequent, then profuse, lasting sweats, salivation, sore mouth ; profuse urine, or turbid, fetid urine.

Sweat early in morning; mostly on and around genitals.

[41] **Attacks.** Sunset to sunrise: 27. Every three or four days: 3. Every two or three weeks: palpitation. Evening till midnight: 46.

[42] **Sides.** Right: 18, 22, 32, 33. Left: 2, 6, 8, 17, 18, 27, 29, 31, 32, 34. Behind forwards: 4. Without in: 5. Within out: 5. Above downwards: 5.

[43] **Sensations.** Oversensitive to all pain, pains drive to despair, does not want to live.

Susceptible to all sorts of pains; on thinking of them, he imagines he already feels them.

Boring pains, mostly in the bones.

[44] **Tissues.** Violent orgasm; plethora.

Gold, at first, causes a feeling of strength, even of buoyancy; later come depression, sense of illness, etc.

Cancerous ulcers.

Pus yellow, with cheesy flocculi; lumbar abscess.

External parts become black.

Dropsy.

Exostoses of skull and other bones.

Boring in the bones; caries especially after mercury; pains drive to despair; worse at night.

Corpulency; fat about the heart.

Glands painfully swollen; scrofula, ruddy complexion.

⁴⁵ **Contact, Injuries, etc.** Touch: 4, 5, 6, 7, 10, 22. Pressure: 5. Chewing: 10. Seize hold of left arm: 34. Rubbing: 22. Riding in carriage: 29.

⁴⁶ **Skin.** Violent itching, first in the soles of the feet and then over the whole body, from evening till midnight.

Fine papular eruption on the face.

Deep ulcers, affecting the bones; after abuse of mercury.

Small and large blotches, stinging, burning, feeling like hard knots, of a dirty yellow color; less in-doors than in open air.

⁴⁷ **Stages and States.** Women, nervous cough.

Girls at puberty; pre-pubic boys, 22.

Often indicated with old people; weak vision; corpulency; ❙ heart disease.

Scrofula; light haired; sanguine temperament; ruddy complexion.

Syphilitic and mercurial patients; especially advanced cases with melancholy, malnutrition and excessive debility. Syphilis in the strumous after abuse of mercury.

⁴⁸ **Relationship.** After daily use of whiskey, blind.

Antidotes to *Aurum: Bellad., Cinchon., Coccul., Coffea, Cuprum, Mercur., Pulsat., Spigel., Sol. nigr.*

Aurum antidotes: *Mercur., Spigel.*

BAPTISIA TINCTORIA.

Wild indigo.   W. H. BURT.   *Leguminosæ.*

¹ **Mind.** Stupor; falls asleep while being spoken to, or answering.

Confusion of ideas; confused as if drunk.

Cannot confine his mind, a sort of wild, wandering feeling.

Indisposed to think, want of power; mind seems weak.

❙ Body feels scattered about, tosses about to get the pieces together; cannot sleep because cannot get pieces together

Delirium, especially at night, or constant.

Mentally restless, but too lifeless to move.

² **Sensorium.** Head feels heavy, as if he could not sit up.

Frequent fainting; tongue dry, brown in the morning.

Vertigo and weak feeling of entire system, especially of lower limbs and knees.

³ **Inner Head.** Dull, heavy, pressive headache.

Soreness of brain, worse stooping.

Frontal headache: with pressure at root of nose; with feeling of fulness and tightness of the whole head.

Dull pain in anterior lobes of brain and right frontal sinus; afternoon.

Excitement of brain, such as precedes delirium.

Frequent pain in r. temple, sharp pains by spells in both.

Head feels large and heavy; with numb feeling of head and face; stitches or shocks in various parts of head.

Heavy pain at base of brain; pain in base of brain with lameness and drawing in cervical muscles.

⁴ **Outer Head.** Top of head feels as if it would fly off.

Great tightness of the skin on forehead.

Scalp feels sore.

⁵ **Eyes.** Vessels congested, eyes look red, inflamed.

Eyes feel swollen, slight lachrymation, with burning.

Cannot bear light, eyes burn, but do not water. θ Chronic ophthalmia.

Eyeballs feel sore; sore and lame on moving them.

⁶ **Ears.** Dull hearing.

Roaring in ears with mental confusion.

⁷ **Nose.** Thick mucus from the nose.

Dull pain at root of nose.

Sneezing and feeling as after taking cold.

⁸ **Face.** Face: sallow; cheeks yellow, with central deep flush; dark red, with a besotted expression; flushed, dusky; hot and perceptibly flushed.

Burning, prickling of left side of face and head.

Cheeks burn.

Face and whole head feel numb.

Muscles of jaw rigid.

⁹ **Lower Face.** Pain in articulation of lower jaw. θ Typhus.

¹⁰ **Teeth.** Teeth and gums sore; by pressing with the finger, large quantities of blood ooze out.

Sordes on teeth and lips.

¹¹ **Tongue, etc.** Taste: flat, bitter.

Tongue feels swollen, thick, makes talking difficult.

Tongue yellow along the centre; at first white, with red papillæ here and there, followed by a yellow-brown coating in centre, edges being red, shining; dry, brown down centre. See 17, 20. ❙ Cracked, sore, ulcerated.

¹² **Mouth.** Fetid odor; also after mercury.

Putrid ulceration of buccal cavity with salivation; well developed ulcers.

Cancrum oris, copious saliva; gums loose, flabby, dark red or purple, fetid.

Mouth and tongue very dry. θ Fevers.

Stomatitis materna; breath fetid; feeble state.

Saliva rather abundant, somewhat viscid, tasting flat.

¹³ **Throat.** Constrictive feeling causing frequent efforts at deglutition; throat sore, feels contracted.

▌Fauces dark red; dark, putrid ulcers; tonsils and parotids swollen; unusual absence of pain.

Tickling in throat provoking cough; uvula elongated.

Can swallow liquids only; the least solid food gags.

Mucus abundant and viscid, can neither swallow it nor bring it up.

Œsophagus feels as if constricted from above down to the stomach; can only swallow water.

¹⁴ **Desires. Aversions.** Constant desire for water; nausea, want of appetite.

¹⁵ **Eating and Drinking.** All symptoms worse from beer.

After breakfast, dull feeling.

¹⁶ **Nausea and Vomiting,** Pressure at the stomach, belching of large quantities of wind.

Nausea with eructations, followed by painful vomiting.

Feeling as if he would vomit, but no nausea, with severe shooting in left kidney and to the left of the umbilicus.

¹⁷ **Stomach.** Sinking, gone feeling at the stomach, fainting; tongue brown in the morning.

Constant burning distress in epigastrium, severe colicky pains in the umbilical, and especially in the hypogastric region; rumbling in bowels.

Cramp in the stomach, evening.

¹⁸ **Hypochondria.** Pain in liver, from right lateral ligament to gall-bladder; can scarcely walk.

Must stir about, yet motion is painful; pain over gall-bladder.

¹⁹ **Abnomen.** Distress, dull pain in umbilical region.

Distended abdomen; fulness; flatulence, rumbling, feels as if vomiting would relieve; mushy stools.

Sharp, shooting pains in bowels.

Dull aching, distress in bowels.

Right iliac region sensitive.

Abdominal muscles sore on pressure.

Glands of the left groin swollen; painful on walking.

²⁰ **Stool, etc.** Stools: dark, thin, fecal, offensive; soft, papescent, with large quantities of mucus; of pure blood or bloody mucus.

Fetid, exhausting diarrhœa, causing excoriations.

Offensive diarrhœa day and night; child can swallow nothing but milk. See 13.

Dark brown mucus and bloody stools; brown tongue. θ Typhus.

Constipation: hemorrhoids in the afternoon.

Dysentery; rigors, pains in the limbs, and small of the back; stools small, all blood, not very dark, but thick; tenesmus; great prostration, brown tongue, low fever; in the autumn, or in hot weather.

[21] **Urine.**   Shooting pains in region of left kidney.

Urine: scanty, dark red.

Burning when urinating.

[22] **Male Sexual Organs.**   Dull growing in right groin and testicle, also in legs and knee-joints.

ı Orchitis; cannot sleep because he feels as if his body was scattered about the bed.

[24] **Pregnancy.**   Threatened abortion.   θ Typhoid.

Stomatitis materna.

Lochia acrid, fetid; great prostration.

ı Puerperal fever, with typhoid symptoms.

[25] **Larynx.**   Very sore to the touch, swallowing or speaking.

Hoarseness.   Aphonia.

Swelling of epiglottis, mornings.

Increased secretion from the bronchial tubes and fauces, with expectoration of mucus.

[26] **Breathing.**   Oppressed breathing, 6 P. M., with cough, right lung sore, sneezing.

Awoke with great difficulty of breathing; lungs felt tight, compressed; could not get a full breath; must open window and get his face to the fresh air, burning heat of the skin, dry tongue, accelerated pulse.

On lying down difficult breathing, but no constriction of chest, must rise; afraid to go to sleep, fears suffocation.

[27] **Cough.**   Tickling in throat provoking cough.   See 13.

[28] **Lungs.**   Tightness of the chest; constriction.

Pain in right lung; less in the left, with soreness.

[29] **Heart.   Pulse.**   Compass and frequency of the heart's pulsations seem increased; they seem to fill the chest.

Pulse first accelerated, afterwards slow and faint.

[31] **Neck.   Back.**   Neck so tired he cannot hold it easy in any position; sore down the neck.

Cervical muscles stiff, lame.

Back and hips very stiff, ache severely.

Dull lumbar backache, worse walking.

Dull sacral pain, as from pressure, fatigue, long stooping; soon extends around hips and down right leg.

Feels as if lying on a board; changes position often, bed feels so hard, worst part is region of sacrum.

[32] **Upper Limbs.**   Pain in left shoulder, extending down arm.

Feels sore and stiff about shoulders and chest.

Numbness of left hand and forearm, with prickling, worse from movement; sharp darting pains through fingers.

Hands feel large, tremulous.

[33] **Lower Limbs.**   Lower limbs weak, vacillating when walking.

Soreness in anterior portion of thighs, worse after sitting awhile.

Drawing in the hips and calves.

Cramp in calves whenever he moves them.

Left foot numb, prickling.

³⁴ **Limbs in General.** Aching in limbs.

Drawing in arms and legs.

³⁵ **Position, etc.** Motion: 18, 32, 33, 36. Moving eyes: 5. Walking: 18, 19, 31, 33. Must walk: 18, 36. Stooping: 3, 31. Going to bed: 19. Lying down: 26. Wants to lie down: 35. Cannot lie down in one place. Must rise: 26. Position of head not easy: 31. Sitting: 33;— by fire: 40. Parts rested on: 40. Lower jaw dropped; slides down in bed, lies with head thrown back.

³⁶ **Nerves.** Restless, uneasy, could confine himself to nothing; wanted to be moving from place to place, evening.

General weak feeling, but worse of lower limbs.

Great languor; wants to lie down.

Paralysis of whole left side; left hand and arm numb, powerless.

Slides down in bed; feels as if sinking away.

Indescribable sick feeling all over.

³⁷ **Sleep.** Delirious stupor; falls asleep while answering a question or while being talked to.

Afraid to go to sleep, fears nightmare and suffocation. See 26.

Drowsy, stupid, tired feeling; disposition to half close eyes.

Slept well until about 3 A. M., then restless until morning; tosses about.

Restless; does not sleep quietly.

Cannot sleep; head or body feels scattered about the bed.

Restless, with frightful dreams.

Quiet but persistent wakefuless; melancholy.

³⁸ **Time.** Morning: 2, 17, 25, 37. Forenoon: 40. Afternoon: 3, 20. Evening: 17, 36, 40. Night: 1, 40. 3 A. M.: 37, 40. During the day: 40. Day and night: 20.

³⁹ **Temperature and Weather.** Warmth of fire: 40. Open air: 26, 40. Hot weather: 20. Autumn: 20.

Averse to open air. θ Sore throat.

❙Chilly, 10 or 11 A. M., afternoon glowing heat. θ Lung troubles.

⁴⁰ **Chill. Fever. Sweat.** Chilly all day; whole body feels sore; chill over the back while sitting by a fire, forenoon.

Chilly going into the open air; chills over the back and lower limbs; evening.

Whole surface hot and dry, with occasional chills, mostly up and down the back.

Heat at night; burning in the legs preventing sleep.

Limbs feel hot, except the feet, which are cold.

On awaking at 3. A. M., flashes of heat, feeling as if sweat would break out.

Flashes of heat from small of back in all directions; dull, heavy aching, great prostration.

Excellent in phthisis; chills 10 A. M. and 3 P. M.; high fever, drowsiness.

ı ı Typhoid and cerebral forms of fever; ı beginning of typhus when so-called nervous symtptoms predominate.

ı Fever originating from confinement on shipboard, without good care or food.

Early stages, white tongue, red edges; or brown, or yellow-brown down centre; bitter or flat taste; cannot digest food; stools frequent, yellow; gurgling and slight sensitiveness of right iliac region; pulse high; fever tends to increase; parts rested on are sore. θ Typhoid.

Sensation as if there was a second self outside of him. θ Typhoid.

ı Sweat breaks out and relieves; critical sweat on forehead and face. θ Typhus.

Fetid sweat; frequent sweating; also worse from small of back in all directions.

⁴¹ **Attacks.** Pain in spells: 3.

⁴² **Sides.** Right: 3, 17, 18, 19, 22, 26, 28, 31, 40. Left: 8, 16, 17, 19, 21, 28, 32, 33, 36. Above downwards: 13, 31, 32, 43. Up and down: 40. From small of back in all directions: 40.

⁴³ **Sensations.** As if too large: head, hands.

⁴⁴ **Tissues.** Prostration, with disposition of the fluids to decompose.

Stiffness of all the joints, as though strained; rheumatic pains and soreness all over the body.

Discharges and exhalations fetid.

Ulceration of mucous membraees, especially that of the mouth; also with tendencey to putrescence.

⁴⁵ **Contact, Injuries, etc.** Intolerance of pressure; hence must often change position; feels as if bed-sores would form.

Touch: 25. Pressure: 10, 19.

⁴⁶ **Skin.** Burning all over the skin, worse in the face.

Livid spots in the body and limbs; not elevated; of irregular shape.

Eruption like measles urticaria.

Eruption thick on palatine arch, tonsils and uvula; breath fetid; salivation; prostration. θ Variola.

⁴⁷ **Stages and States.** Children; offensive diarrhœa.

Old people; dysentery.

⁴⁸ **Relationship.** Cognates: *Arnic.; Arsen.; Bryon.; Gelsem.* (especially in the malaise, nervousness, flushed face, or drowsiness and muscular soreness in early stages of typhoid); *Hyosc.; Kali chlor.; Laches.; Mur. ac.; Nitr. ac.; Nux vom.; Opium; Rhus tox.*

BARYTA CARBONICA.

Barium Carbonate.   ·   HAHNEMANN.   *Ba Co³.*

Symptoms marked † are from the Acetate.

[1] **Mind.** Memory deficient; child cannot be taught, for it cannot remember; is inattentive.

† Forgetful; in the middle of a speech the most familiar words fail him.

Great mental and bodily weakness, childishness; old people.

Child does not want to play, but sits in the corner doing nothing.

Sadness, dejection of spirits, grief over trifles.

† Dread of men, of strangers; imagines she is being laughed at or criticised, hence so fearful she will not look up.

Solicitude: about his future; † about domestic affairs.

† Irresolute, constantly changing his mind.

Loss of self-confidence; desponding; pusillanimous.

† Sudden ebullitions of anger, but coupled with cowardice.

Thinking of one's complaints makes them worse.

Thinks his legs are cut off and he is walking on his knees.

[2] **Sensorium.** Vertigo: with nausea from stooping; of old people.

Apoplexy: of drunkards; of aged people, who are childish, sensorium not clear, loss of speech, trembling of the limbs.

[3] **Inner Head.** Headache in the evening; every noise, especially male voices, affect the brain painfully.

Headache just above the eyes.

Pressive sticking on the vertex, which extends through the whole head, whenever he stands in the sun.

[4] **Outer Head.** Feeling of tension as if the skin were too tight; forehead and temples.

† Encysted tumor on the scalp.

Right side of the head feels burning hot, but is cold.

Baldness, especially on the crown.

Scalp sensitive on the side on which he is lying, worse from scratching.

Head sensitive to cold.

Crusta lactea, dry scurf, or moist crusts, itching, burning; causes the hair to fall out; cervical glands hard, swollen.

[5] **Eyes.** Weakness of sight caused by old age.

Dim-sighted, cannot read.

Flying webs and black spots before the eyes.

Light dazzles; fiery sparks before the eyes in the dark.

†Quick succession of dilatation and contraction of the pupils; pupil irregular.

Pressure deep in the eyes, worse looking fixedly, or upwards and sideways; better looking downwards.

Opaque cornea; inflammation of the eyes with sensation of dryness; shuns the light.

Lids agglutinated.

⁶ **Ears.** Difficult hearing.

Buzzing and jingling before the ears.

Roaring in the right ear like the sea, at each inspiration.

Cracking in ear when sneezing, swallowing or walking fast.

Itching in the ears.

Tearing with boring and drawing in bones in front of right ear.

Thick crust on and behind the ears; small flat tubercles behind the ears.

Eruption on lobe of the ear.

Right parotid hard and swollen. θ After scarlatina.

⁷ **Nose.** Coryza, nose and upper lip swollen; children with large abdomen.

Frequent nosebleed.

Sneezing causing concussive pain in the brain.

Tormenting dryness in nose; secretion of thick, yellow mucus.

Formation of scabs in the posterior nares and behind the base of the uvula.

Scurfs under the nose.

⁸ **Face.** Face: pale; puffed.

Comedones.

Sensation as if the face were swollen.

Tension as from a cobweb over the face, temples, scalp.

Rough, dry place on the right cheek.

⁹ **Lower Face.** Swelling of the upper lip with burning pain.

Pain in the articulation when closing the jaw.

Indurated swelling of the submaxillary glands.

¹⁰ **Teeth.** After eating some, feels too weak to chew any more.

Toothache in decayed teeth before menses, or from a cold.

Drawing, jerking, throbbing toothache; right teeth feel tense.

Burning stitches in a hollow tooth when touched by warm food; left side.

Gums bleed, are swollen, pale red with a dark red border.

Toothache worse thinking about it; disappears when the mind is diverted.

¹¹ **Tongue, etc.** Paralysis of the tongue; loss of speech.

Hardness on the middle of the tongue, burning when touched; burning sense of excoration at the tip; fissure on the left border, feeling excoriated.

Vesicles on the middle, tip, or under the tongue.

¹² **Mouth.** The buccal cavity feels numb.

Dryness of the mouth early after rising.

Whole mouth filled with vesicles, especially the inside of cheeks.

Saliva runs out of the mouth while asleep, at daybreak.

Intolerable stench from the mouth, unnoticed by himself.

¹³ **Throat.** Smarting in the throat when swallowing, worse from empty swallowing; throat sore to touch.

Liability to tonsillitis after every slight cold, or suppressed foot-sweat.

Tonsils tend to suppurate, especially the right; palate swollen; dark brown urine; sleeplessness.

Chronic induration of the tonsils; sensation as of a plug in the throat; worse swallowing solids.

Sensation in the œsophagus as if a morsal of food had lodged there.

On swallowing, sensation as if the food had to force itself over a sore spot.

Œsophageal spasm, in old people.

¹⁴ **Desires. Aversions.** Hungry, but cannot eat; or, feels as though she needed food, but did not want it.

Thirst, with dryness of mouth, not relieved by drink.

¹⁵ **Eating and Drinking.** Sudden nausea while eating.

Pressure like a stone in the stomach after eating bread; repletion after a little food.

Heaviness of the stomach, nausea, goes off after breakfast.

Soreness in the in stomach as if food passed over sore places.

Cough from eating warm food.

Better from cold diet.

¹⁶ **Nausea and Vomiting.** Eructations: as if air were forcing its way through the stomach, causing a feeling of soreness; sour a few hours after dinner.

Nausea, palpitation and anxiety in the early morning.

Long-lasting nausea.

Water suddenly accumulates in the mouth.

¹⁷ **Stomach.** Pressing in stomach, also after eating.

Sensation of soreness in the stomach.

Pressure as from a stone; better from eructations.

¹⁸ **Hypochondria.** Aching at a small spot in right hypochondrium, when drawing a deep breath, or from pressure.

.¹⁹ **Abdomen.** distended, hard.

Cutting in the hypogastric region at night.

Distention and fulness above the pubes, as if the parts would burst, when lying on the back.

Tension and sensitiveness of the abdominal walls.

²⁰ **Stool, etc.** Scanty, hard or lumpy stool, expelled with difficulty.

Sudden, irresistible urging to stool; soreness in the lumbar region; chills over head and legs: then loose stools, and renewed urging; after taking cold.

Burning and soreness around the anus as if excorioted.

Frequent passage of blood, with distended abdomen.

Crawling in the rectum; expulsion of ascarides.

²¹ **Urine.** Great desire to urinate; cannot retain the urine.

Constant urging, and frequent emissions of urine, every other day; passes much at night.

Dark brown urine; also with the tonsilitis.

²² **Male Sexual Organs.** Diminished sexual ability.

Excoriation between the scrotum and thigh.

Sweat about the scrotum.

²³ **Female Sexual Organs.** Menses scanty, last only one day.

Before the menses: toothache, swollen gums, colic with swelling of the limbs; immediately before leucorrhœa.

During the menses, weight over the pubes; bruised pain in the small of the back.

²⁵ **Larynx.** Feeling as if inhaling smoke or pitch.

Voice imperfect, aphonia; from tough mucus in fauces and larynx; old people.

²⁶ **Breathing.** Oppression, with anguish; in the evening must loosen her dress.

Short breath from fulness in the chest, when ascending a height; stitches in the chest on inspiring.

Suffocative catarrh of old people, with impending paralysis of the lungs.

²⁷ **Cough.** Chronic cough in scrofulous children, with swollen glands and enlarged tonsils; worse after slightest cold.

Cough in the presence of strangers.

Spasmodic cough excited by tickling and roughness in the throat and epigastrium; worse: evening until midnight; lying on the left side; active motion, ascending or stooping; in the cold air; from thinking of it; eating.

Nightly cough, chest full of phlegm.

²⁸ **Lungs.** Sensation of soreness in the chest, when coughing.

²⁹ **Heart. Pulse.** Feels the heart beat.

Palpitation when lying on the left side, with soreness in the region of the heart, great anxiety; renewed by thinking about it.

Orgasm of blood, with anxiety.

³¹ **Neck. Back.** Stiffness in the nape of the neck.

Tension in neck and scapulæ; pain in the loins in cold air.

Stinging pains in the neck.

Chronic torticollis.

Swelling of the glands in the nape of the neck and occiput.

Pain in small of the back.

Tensive pain in the small of the back; worse in the evening; he can neither rise nor bend backwards.

³² **Upper Limbs.** Pains in the arms, with hard, swollen axillary glands.

Pain in the deltoid muscle when raising the arm.

When lying on the arm it goes to sleep.

Tension in small places of the arms.

Fingers numb, as if asleep.

Panaritium, with nightly throbbing and ulceration, from a splinter.

³³ **Lower Limbs.** † Tearing from above downwards in right buttock, periodically increasing and decreasing.

† Drawing pain down entire left leg.

Pain in legs at night, as after excessive walking or dancing.

Has to drag the legs when going up stairs, on account of a lameness in the middle of the thighs.

Severe stitching on thighs.

Tension, as if the tendons were too short, less lying down; worse when standing.

Tremor of the feet while standing, must hold on to something to steady himself.

Soles feel bruised, at night, keeping one awake; better after rising and walking.

Aching lymphatic swelling on the ball of the great toe.

Fetid foot-sweat.

The hard skin on the sole·is painful when walking.

³⁴ **Limbs in General.** Tearing in the limbs, with chilliness.

Stitches in the joints; they feel relaxed.

³⁵ **Position, etc.** Motion: 27. Walking: 17, 33; fast: 6. Dancing: 33. Ascending: 26, 27, 33. Sits in a corner: 1. Stooping: 2, 27. · Cannot rise: 31. Cannot stand: 36. After rising: 12, 33. Rising up in bed: 36. Standing: 33, 36. Standing in sun: 3. Cannot bend backwards: 31. Inclined to lie down: 36. Lying down: 4, 33. Lying on back: 19. Lying on left side: 29. Lying on arm: 32. Raising arm: 32.

❙ Worse lying on painful side.

³⁶ **Nerves.** Nervousness, excessive irritation of all the nerves.

Jerking and starting in daytime.

Prostration, cannot stand, the knees give way.

Weariness, constant inclination to lie down.

Heaviness of the whole body.

General paralysis of old people; loss of memory, childishness, trembling of the limbs; after apoplexy; in old age.

Great weakness, can hardly sit up in bed; if attempted, the pulse immediately becomes quick and somewhat hard, after a while imperceptible.

³⁷ **Sleep.** Talking in sleep (old men).

Awakens often at night; feels too hot; soles of feet feel bruised.

Twitching of muscles of the whole body during sleep.

Ravings of the fancy at night and stupefaction.

On awaking, pressure in limbs; tired, weary limbs.

[38] **Time.** Morning: 12. Early morning: 16. Afternoon: 16. Evening: 3, 26, 27, 31, 40. Evening till midnight: 27. Night: 16, 21, 27, 32, 33, 37, 40. Daytime: 21, 36, 40.

[39] **Temperature and Weather.** Warmth, external: 40. Sun: 3. Warm food: 10, 15. Cold: 27, 31. Cold food: 15. Cold air: 27, 31.

Sensitive to cold air; great liability to take cold, sore throat, cough, diarrhœa, pain in back and loins.

Worse from moistening or washing the diseased part.

[40] **Chill. Fever. Sweat.** Chill and chilliness predominating: often as if cold water were poured over one; better from external warmth; thirst during chill.

Chill from the face or pit of the stomach down the body; or beginning in the feet.

Chill alternating with heat; evening and night.

Frequent flushes during the day; nightly attacks with great anxiety and restlessness.

Anxious sweat.

Debilitating night-sweats.

Offensive sweat of one (mostly left) side.

. Sweat returning every other evening.

Sweat increased by eating.

[41] **Attacks.** Every other day: 21. Every other evening: 40. Increasing and decreasing periodically: 33.

[42] **Sides.** Right: 4, 6, 8, 10, 13, 18, 33. Left: 10, 11, 27, 29, 33, 40. Above downwards: 3, 33, 40. Below upwards: 40. Upper left with lower right.

[43] **Sensations.** Feels "hide-bound;" tension of the skin. Sensation of swelling.

[44] **Tissues.** Tension, shortening of the muscles.

Dwarfish, defective mental and physical growth.

Atrophy, great weakness; face red and abdomen bloated; glands swollen.

Steatoma; sarcoma with burning.

Glands indurated, swollen.

Glandular sequelæ of scarlatina.

Fatty tumors; encysted tumors.

Tearing and tension in the long bones; boring in bones.

Ulcers, fistulous, in glands; mostly glands of neck; feeling of tension.

[45] **Contact, Injuries, etc.** Sensitiveness of part lain on. Touch: 4, 11, 13. Pressure: 18. Rubbing: 46. Scratching: 4, 46.

[46] **Skin.** Pimples on the feet suppurate and spread like ulcers. Ringworms.

13

Skin humid, sore.

Warts.

A small wound, as from a splinter, throbs and ulcerates.

Itching, pricking, burning, here and there; not relieved by scratching or rubbing.

Scratching causes pricking, pimples.

[47] **Stages and States.** Old people; especially when fat.

Scrofulous children; dwarfish; mind and body weak; scurfs on head, ears, nose; eyes inflamed, opaque cornea; abdomen swollen; face puffed; general emaciation.

[48] **Relationship.** Cognates: *Ant. tart.* (paralysis of lungs); *Calc. ostr.* (scrofulosis, coryza, etc.); *Calc. iod.* (large tonsils); *Caustic.* (paretic symptoms); *Conium* (old people); *Dulcam.* (tendency to catch cold); *Fluor. ac.* (old people); *Iodium* (glands); *Lycop.* (tonsils); *Mercur.* (colds, glands, diarrhœa); *Phosphor.; Pulsat.; Sepia* (ringworms); *Silic.* (glands, foot-sweat, etc.); *Sulphur; Tellur.* (ringworms).

Antidotes to *Baryt. carb.: Ant. tart., Bellad., Camphor., Dulcam., Zincum.*

BELLADONNA.

Deadly Nightshade.   HAHNEMANN.   *Solanaceæ.*

[1] **Mind.** Memory lively; remembers things long gone by.

Memory impaired; forgets in a moment what he was about to do.

Absent-minded and forgetful.

Confusion of head, aggravated by movement.

Imagines he sees ghosts, hideous faces, black dogs and various insects.

Delirium; is afraid of imaginary things; sees monsters.

Desire to escape or hide herself.

Weary of life, with desire to drown herself.

Talkative, then mute.

Picking at bedclothes as if looking for something lost, with confused muttering.

Instead of eating, bit the wooden spoon in two, gnawed the plate, and growled and barked like a dog.

Mania, at one time merry, again would spit and bite at those around; thinks himself suddenly rich.

Quarrelsome, during exuberant mirth.

Violent delirium; broke into fits of laughter, then gnashed the teeth; disposed to bite and strike those around.

Starts in affright at the approach of others.

Very excitable mood, easily brought to tears.

Morose and serious.

Anxious and timorous.

Anxious and confused, fears she is about to die.

Fretfulness: nothing seemed right to him; was vexed with himself.

² **Sensorium.** All the senses more acute.

Cloudiness, as if intoxicated.

Blood mounts to the head, which becomes heavy as if giddy.

Weariness of the head.

³ **Inner Head.** Feeling in brain like the swashing of water.

Cold sensation in the brain at the middle of the forehead.

Headache as if a stone were pressing the forehead.

Fulness and pressure at temples and forehead, with pain, making him restless and uneasy.

Pain in head and eyeballs, eyes felt as if starting from their sockets.

Pressive frontal headache so severe, when walking, that the eyes were drawn shut; better when sitting, ceases when lying down, worse rising again or going into open air.

Pressure in head, now here, now there, which occupies each time large areas.

Frequently obliged to stand still in walking, from the violence of the pain in forehead; at every step it seemed as if the brain rose and fell in forehead; pain ameliorated by strong pressure on forehead.

Strong pulsation of blood-vessels of forehead, and pain as if the bones were lifted up.

Violent throbbing in brain from behind forward and towards both sides; the throbbing ends on the surface in painful shootings.

Dull shooting in left temple, from in out.

Severe shooting in right frontal eminence, worse from bending forward, ameliorated by pressure.

Stabbing, as if with a knife, from temple to temple.

Jerking headache, extremely violent on walking quickly, or ascending stairs rapidly; at every step a jolt as if a weight were in the occiput.

Boring, tearing, cutting, shooting pains in various parts of head, generally worse on right side and in forehead, less in occiput.

Pains come on suddenly, last indefinitely, but cease suddenly.

Headache from the heat of the sun.

⁴ **Outer Head.** Head externally, so sensitive that the least contact, even the pressure of the hair, gives pain.

Crampy pain in frontal eminence, entending to zygoma and lower jaw.

5 **Eyes.** Photophobia; worse from artificial light.

Far-sightedness.

Objects appear: double, and seem to revolve and run backwards; inverted.

Bright sparks before the eyes.

Flashes of light before the eyes-

Halo around the light particolored, red predominating; at times light seems broken into rays.

Vision obscured as from a white vapor; pupils dilated.

Deep-seated dull pain in the back of the eye.

Eyes dry; feel stiff; feeling of sand in eyes.

Heat and burning in eyes.

Shooting in the eyes. from within outwards.

Lachrymation.

Spasmodic motion of eyes.

Eyeballs red and prominent.

Conjunctiva covered with red vessels; shooting pains; eyes water.

Yellowness of sclerotica.

Swelling and suppurative inflammation of left caruncula lachrymalis.

Ophthalmia; suddenly appearing, worse right eye; intense photophobia.

Pain in orbits: often feels as if the eyes had been torn out, sometimes as if pressed into the head.

Trembling and quivering of right upper eyelid.

Heaviness of lids.

Lids feel sore, congested and swollen.

6 **Ears.** Extreme sensibility of hearing.

Deafness, as if a skin were drawn over the ears.

Fancied noise awakens; slight delirium on waking.

Tearing in internal and external ear, in a downward direction.

Shooting in internal ear, with hardness of hearing.

Pinching in the ears, first right, then left.

Tearing in right external ear and whole right side of face, downwards.

Swelling of the right parotid gland, with erysipelatous redness and violent shooting pains.

7 **Nose.** Extreme sensibility of smell; odor of tobacco and soot are intolerable.

Frequent sneezing.

Dryness of nose, with dull frontal headache.

Fluent coryza from one nostril only.

Coryza, with offensive smell in nose as of herring pickle, especially when blowing the nose.

Discharge of mucus, mixed with blood, from the nose.

Suppressed catarrh, maddening headache.

Nostrils and corners of lips ulcerated, without pain or itching.

Sudden redness of tip of nose, with burning sensation.

Nosebleed: with congestion to head; in children at night.

⁸ **Face.** Red and hot, or pale and cold; mottled red; swollen and hot.

Sensation of burning heat in whole face, without redness of cheeks; or with marked thirst, body warm, feet cold.

Scraping, itching of forehead.

Neuralgic pains commencing under left orbit and running back to the ear.

Violent shooting in right maxillary joint, extending to the ear; when chewing.

Cutting, tearing pain, mostly right side, shooting from side of the face up to temple, into the ear and down to nape of neck, worse from touch and motion; hard presssure sometimes relieves.

⁹ **Lower Face.** Raw feeling at corners of mouth.

Pustules at borders of lips, with smarting pains.

Severe swelling of the upper lip.

Lips: especially the upper one, crack in the middle; dry and parched.

Sensation as if lower jaw was drawn backwards.

¹⁰ **Teeth.** Dull drawing in upper row, right side, all night.

Toothache some minutes after eating, not during; increases gradually to high degree and as gradually diminishes.

Teeth feel "on edge."

Extremely painful swelling of gums on right side.

Bleeding of gums.

¹¹ **Tongue, etc.** Taste: salty; sour; bitter; pappy; offensive; putrid when eating or drinking.

Bread tastes sour.

Stammering speech.

Paralytic weakness of organs of speech.

Tongue: inflamed and much swollen, papillæ of deep red color; tip and edges light red.

Feeling in tip of tongue as if a vesicle was on it, with burning pain when touched.

Feeling of coldness and dryness of forepart of tongue.

Tongue: white centre with red edges; or two white stripes; covered with white clammy fur, which can be pulled off in strings; dry and furred; covered with much tenacions, yellowish-white mucus.

¹² **Mouth.** Saliva thickened, tenacious, white, clings to the tongue like glue.

Dryness of mouth, with thirst.

Mouth feels hot.

Salivation succeeding the dryness of mouth.

Slimy mouth in morning, when awaking, with pressing headache.

[13] **Throat.** Dryness of roof of mouth, fauces and throat.

Constant urging and desire to swallow; seemed as if he would choke if he did not swallow.

During deglutition, feeling in the throat as if it were too narrow, or drawn together, as if nothing would pass properly.

Throat: feels raw and sore; looks very red and shining.

Fine tearing on inner surface of angle of left lower jaw, in and behind the left tonsil, unaffected by contact; worse when swallowing.

Tonsillitis, worse right side; parts bright red; worse swallowing liquids.

Rapidly forming aphthous ulcers on tonsils; intense congestion; throbbing of the carotids.

Pharynx as if excoriated; scraping; sensation of enlargement with dryness and burning; bright redness or bright and yellowish redness of fauces.

Cervical glands inflame suddenly.

[14] **Desires. Aversions.** Thirst; drinks water, wants lemonade.

Great thirst in evening with watery taste; all drinks are loathsome. Violent thirst at noon.

Desire for lemons (which prove beneficial).

Repugnance to beer, acids, coffee, camphor.

[15] **Eating and Drinking.** Wine aggravates dyspnœa.

After eating: putrid taste in mouth.

After drinking beer, internal heat.

[16] **Nausea and Vomiting.** Violent hiccough.

Hiccoughing eructations; spasm composed partly of eructation, partly of hiccough.

Half suppressed, incomplete eructation.

Nausea in the stomach.

Ineffectual efforts to vomit about midnight, with cold sweat.

Vomiting of mucus; of bile and mucus; of undigested food; watery; can keep nothing down, is pale and weak.

[17] **Stomach.** Painless throbbing and beating at pit of stomach.

Feeling of emptiness in stomach.

Cutting pain in the stomach, worse from motion or pressure.

Hard pressure in stomach after eating.

Distention of epigastrium, with tensive pain in stomach.

Gnawing, pressing, crampy, drawing and wrenching pain in stomach, compels patient to bend backwards, worse after drinking.

Spasm in the stomach like cramp.

Shooting pains in stomach.

Burning in stomach.

Painful pressure in pit of stomach only when walking; compels him to walk slowly.

Hæmatemesis; ringing in ears; red cheeks; feeling of fulness and warmth in stomach.

[18] **Hypochondria.**   Region of liver painful and sore to touch.

Acute pain in region of liver; worse lying on right side; pains go to shoulder and neck; can tolerate no pressure or jar; pit of stomach bloated.

Colic from gall-stones; indurated liver; jaundice.

[19] **Abdomen.**   Distention of abdomen.

During the pain, the transverse colon protrudes like a pad all the way across the abdomen.

Clawing around the navel; better from pressure.

Abdomen distended, hot.

Loud rumbling and pinching in the belly.

Colic, as if a spot in the abdomen were seized with the nails, a griping, clutching, clawing.

Violent cutting pressure in hypogastrium, now here, now there.

Great pain in right ileo-cœcal region, cannot bear the slightest touch, not even the bed-cover.

Feeling as if a hard body pressed from within outwards, at right inguinal ring; the part not feeling hard to the touch; while sitting with body bent forwards.

Fine shooting in left groin.

Tenderness even to slight pressure, especially over ovarian region.

[20] **Stool, etc.**   Pressing in rectum toward the anus.

Voluptuous tickling in lower part of rectum and anus.

Stools: thin, green mucus; frequent, thin; bloody mucus with tenesmus; containing lumps like chalk; clay-colored; chalky white, with granular, slimy mucus; smell sour.

Urging to stool, which is more fluid than usual, but passed in proper quantity.

Involuntary evacuation, paralysis of the sphincter ani.

Bleeding piles; back pains as if breaking.

Spasmodic constriction of sphincter ani.

Mucous membrane of anus seems swollen and pressed out.

Violent itching, at same time constrictive sensation in anus.

[21] **Urine.**   Spasmodic, crampy straining along the ureter, during passage of calculus.

Urine: bright yellow and clear; frequent, copious, pale and watery; first clear, becomes turbid on standing; blood red.

When the urine is heated, almost invariably deposits a cloud of phosphates.

Frequent desire with small quantity.

Involuntary micturition, with paralysis of sphincter and retention with paralysis of bladder.

Vesical region very sensitive to pressure or jar.

Sensation of turning and twisting in the bladder, as if from a large worm, without desire to micturate.

Wets the bed; restless, starts in sleep.

[22] **Male Sexual Organs.** Sexual desire decreased.

Weakness and relaxation of genitals.

Nocturnal emission of semen, during relaxation of penis.

Violent stitches in the testicles which are drawn upwards.

Tearing upwards, in left spermatic cord, evening in bed.

Soft painless tumor on the glans.

Sweating of genital organs.

[23] **Female Sexual Organs.** Pressure downwards, as if all the contents of abdomen would issue through the vulva; worse mornings.

Violent pressing and urging towards the genitals, as if everything would fall out there; worse sitting bent, and in walking; better standing, and sitting erect.

Right ovary much enlarged; stitching, throbbing pains; pains come suddenly and go suddenly.

Clutching or clawing pains, or transient stitches in the uterine region, parts sensitive, cannot bear least jar.

Profuse discharge of hot, bright red blood; sometimes dark, clotted, and of a bad smell; flow of blood between the periods.

Painful menstruation.

Amenorrhœa.

Leucorrhœa; of white mucus; with colic.

Great heat and dryness of vagina.

Climaxis: congestion; axillary glands hard; sudden hot flushes.

[24] **Pregnancy.** Lochia offensive, feel hot to the parts.

Labor-pains: deficient; cease, have only periodical slight pressure on sacrum; amniotic fluid gone; yet os still spasmodically contracted.

Phlegmasia alba dolens.

Appears as if stunned; semi-conscious and loss of speech; convulsive movements in limbs and muscles of face; paralysis of right side of tongue, foam at mouth; renewal of fits at every pain.

Retained placenta, with profuse flow of hot blood, which speedily coagulates.

[25] **Larynx.** Hoarseness; rough voice.

Voice weakened even to complete aphonia.

Speaking is very difficult to him; speaks in a piping tone.

Dryness of larynx.

[26] **Breathing.** Short, hurried, anxious breathing.

Breathing heavy and stertorous.

Difficult respiration.

Asthmatic paroxysm in afternoon and evening, with sensation of dust in lungs.

Asthma in hot, damp weather; worse after sleep.

Quick, short, irregular breathing, alternates with slow, gentle, at times almost imperceptible, breathing; in a child.

[27] **Cough.** Dry cough: from dryness of larynx; from tickling-itching in back part of the top of larynx, evening, after lying down in bed; from sensation of a foreign body in larynx.

Attack of coughing, as if one had inhaled dust; wakens at night; mucous expectoration.

Sensation as if something were in the pit of stomach, which excites cough.

Violent cough about noon, with expectoration of much tenacious mucous.

Cough, with bloody mucous expectoration in the morning; bloody taste in mouth.

Night cough; wakes from sleep.

Attacks of cough ending with sneezing.

Pressing pain in nape of neck when coughing.

Child begins to cry immediately before cough comes on.

Barking cough, waking suddenly, 11 P. M.; face fiery red; crying with cough.

[28] **Lungs.** Noise and rattling in the bronchial tubes.

Pressive pain in chest, with shortness of breath, and at same time between shoulders, when walking or sitting.

Pressure in right chest, causes anxiety.

Constriction across chest, as if pressed inwards from both sides.

Burning in right chest.

Stitches in apex of right lung.

[29] **Heart. Pulse.** Pressure in the cardiac region, which arrests the breathing and causes a sense of anxiety.

Gurgling at the heart, a kind of palpitation, when going up stairs.

Pulse: accelerated, frequently full, hard and tense; large, full and slow; at times small and soft.

Throbbing in the carotid and temporal arteries.

[30] **Outer Chest.** Corroding, gnawing pain beneath the cartilages of last ribs, right side.

[31] **Neck. Back.** Pressive pain externally in neck, when bending head backwards, and when touching the part.

Swelling of glands in nape of neck, with cloudiness of head.

Pressive pain under left scapula, more towards outer side.

Drawing pressure between right scapula and spinal column.
Shooting and gnawing pain in the spinal column.
Stabbing as if with a knife, from without inwards, in the vertebræ.
Drawing, burning and throbbing pain in the spine.
Soreness of last dorsal and first lumbar vertebræ.
Back aches, as if broken.
Cramp-like sensation in left lumbar region.
Curvature of the lumbar vertebræ.
Bearing down on to sacrum.

[32] **Upper Limbs.** Stitching pressure on top of left shoulder.
Heaviness and paralytic feeling in upper limbs.
Violent stabbing, as with a blunt knife, below the head of the humerus, from within out.
Drawing pain on inner side of left upper arm.
Tearing pain in humerus.
Bruised pain in upper arm.
Cutting pain in interior of left elbow-joint when walking.
Sharp shooting externally in left elbow-joint.
Cutting, tearing in lower muscles of both forearms.
Not able to turn the hand easily and freely on its axis (as when dropping from a glass), turns only by jerks; as from want of synovial fluid in wrist-joint; painless.
Painful drawing in the metacarpo-phalangeal articulation of the left middle finger, as if in the periosteum.
Paralytic tearing in the middle joint of right index-finger.
Numbness and prickling in the hands.

[33] **Lower Limbs.** Pain in thighs and legs, as if beaten and as if carious; fine shooting and gnawing along the bones, with violent tearing in the joints; the pain rises gradually from the ankle to hips, necessitates, while sitting, constant motion and shifting of the feet; is milder when walking.
Cramp pain in the gluteal muscles, with tension on bending the body forward.
Cutting stitches in the outer muscles of right thigh, just above knee, only when sitting.
Cramp-like pain in right knee near the patella, towards the outer side when sitting.
Sensation in joints of lower limbs, particularly knees, as if they would give way, especially when walking, and more marked when going down hill.
Burning-stinging in knee-joint, worse at night.
Synovitis of knee-joint; intense inflammation; sense of bubbling as from drops of water.
Dull tearing in the legs.
Tremulous heaviness of legs.
Tearing pressure in middle of the inside of the leg, uninfluenced by motion or contact.

Tension in right tarsal-joint while walking in open air.

Pain in metatarsal bones, as if dislocated.

Boring, digging or shooting pains in soles.

Pain as if bruised in the heel when treading thereon.

[34] **Limbs in General.** Loss of co-ordination of the muscles of both upper and lower limbs, very like the heaviness and helplessness of movement observed in first stage of progressive paralysis of the insane.

[35] **Position, etc.** Disinclination and aversion to work or motion.

Restlessness; he was obliged constantly to move the body to and fro, especially the hands and feet.

Cannot stay long in any position, at one time lies, at another sits, again stands, in all of which he constantly changes his position.

Motion: 2, 8, 17, 20, 21, 33. Walking: 3, 17, 22, 28, 32, 33. Every step: 3. Ascending: 3, 29. Descending: 33. Standing: 22. Sitting: 3, 28, 33; erect 22; bent: 22. Stooping: 2. Backwards: 17. Rising: 3. Lying down: 3, 27.

[36] **Nerves.** Trembling in all the limbs.

Weakness, and tottering gait.

Paralytic weakness of all the muscles, especially of feet.

Great restlessness with sudden startings.

Muscles of face, jaw and limbs, agitated by convulsive twitchings.

Spasm of one and paralysis of other side.

Spasmodic motions of body, generally backwards.

Throws body forwards and backwards, while lying, like constant change from emprosthotonos to opisthotonos.

Convulsions commence in arm. θ Epilepsy.

Clenched the teeth together with such force that they could not be opened.

Stiffness of whole body.

Tetanus, while working in hot sun he became unconscious, jaws fixed, head hot, feet cold.

[37] **Sleep.** Frequent yawning.

Towards evening drowsiness, with yawning; in the morning feels as if had not slept enough.

Sleeps much, yet not refreshed.

Sleep prevented by anxiety.

Sleepy, yet cannot sleep.

Starts as if in affright, during sleep and on awaking.

During sleep: singing and talking loud; moaning.

Vivid dreams, but could not remember them.

Anxious dreams: about murder; street robbers; of danger from fire.

[38] **Time.** Remission forenoon and after 12 P.M.

Morning: 12, 23, 27, 36. Noon: 14, 27. Afternoon: 20, 26.
Evening: 14, 22, 26, 27, 37, 40. Night: 7, 10, 27, 33.
11 P.M.: 27. Midnight: 16. Day or night: 40.

[39] **Temperature and Weather.** Takes cold from having the
hair cut.

Open air: 3, 33.

Worse in sudden changes, from warm to cold.

Better wrapped up warmly in the room.

Spring: boils, etc.

Hot weather: worse from sun; from heat: 3, 20, 26, 36.

[40] **Chill. Fever. Sweat.** Chill in the evening, mostly on
arms, with heat of head.

Internal chill, with external burning heat.

Chill and heat alternating.

Coldness of the limbs, with heat of the head.

Shivering running down the back.

Continuous dry, burning heat, with sweat only on the head.

Internal heat, with anxiety and restlessness.

Heat of forehead, with cold cheeks; of head, with redness
of face and delirium.

Heat predominating; averse to uncovering.

Sweat on the covered parts; with or immediately after the
heat, mostly in face; staining the clothing and of empyreumatic smell; during sleep, day or night; ascending
from feet to head.

Entire want of sweat.

General sweat suddenly occurring and disappears quickly.

[41] **Attacks.** Pains come on suddenly, and after a shorter or
longer duration, cease suddenly.

Sudden attacks of violent cramp-like pain in one side of
chest, or of abdomen, or loin, or one elbow, especially
during sleep, causing one to bend the painful part.

With every labor-pain: 24.

[42] **Sides.** Right: 3, 5, 8, 10, 13, 18, 19, 23, 24, 28, 30, 31, 32, 33.
Left: 3, 5, 8, 13, 18, 19, 22, 31, 32. In out: 3, 5, 19, 32.
Out in: 28, 31. Above downwards: 6, 40. Below upwards: 18, 33, 40. Behind forwards: 3. Front backwards: 8.

[44] **Tissues.** Acts on circular fibres of blood-vessels. On spinc-
ters, as in spasm of os uteri, etc.

Inflammations of serous and mucous membranes.

Pains along the periosteum. Ostitis, traumatic, erysipelatous redness of the part.

Red shining swelling of the joints.

Housemaid's knee, acute symptoms.

Phlegmonous inflammation.

Engorgement of glands; acute swelling.

⁴⁵ Contact, Injuries, etc. Touch: 4, 8, 18, 19, 31. Contact: 33. Pressure: 3, 8, 17, 19, 21. Jar: 21, 23.

⁴⁶ Skin. Painful sensitiveness of skin to contact.

Eruption resembling measles

Heat over whole body, with bluish redness of whole surface.

Skin imparts a burning sensation to the examining hand.

Intense erysipelatous fever, accompanied with inflamed swellings, passing even into gangrene.

Pustules on nape of neck, arms and back.

Red scaly eruption on lower part of body, as far as the abdomen.

Skin scarlet and smooth.

Urticaria during profuse menstruation.

•Jaundice after abuse of peruvian bark or mercury; in complication with stones in gall-bladder.

⁴⁷ Stages and States. Suits plethoric, lymphatic constitutions, who are jovial and entertaining when well, but violent when sick.

Women, children, blue eyes, light hair, fine complexion, delicate skin.

Tuberculous patients; pleurisy.

Young, full-blooded: with fevers and inflammations, when pulse and heat run high, congestions; nervous, delirious, threatened convulsions.

⁴⁸ Relationship. Antidotes to *Bellad.*: of large doses: *Coffea, Hyosc.;* of small doses: *Camphor., Coffea, Hepar, Hyosc., Opium, Pulsat., Vinum.*

Bellad. antidotes: *Acon., Cuprum, Ferrum, Hyosc., Mercur., Plumbum.*

Bellad. is said to be an antidote to Jaborandi.

Vinegar increases headache of *Bellad.*

Bellad. is frequently indicated after *Chamon., Hepar, Laches., Mercur., Phosphor., Nitr. ac.*

After *Bellad.*: *Cinchon., Conium, Dulcam., Hepar, Laches., Rhus, Seneg., Stramon., Valer.,* are frequently indicated.

Complementary to *Calc. ostr.*

BENZOIC ACID.

Benzoic acid. $C_6 H_5, CO, OH.$

¹ **Mind.** Omits words while writing.

Confused head.

Inclined to dwell on unpleasant things.

Child cross, wants to be nursed in the arms.

Anxiety; while sweating.

² **Sensorium.** Vertigo, as if he must fall sideways, mostly in the afternoon.

³ **Inner Head.** Pain and heat in the region of the so-called organs of reverence and firmness.

Head symptoms worse from mental emotions, exposure to a draft of air, uncovering one's self; in the morning on awaking.

⁴ **Outer Head.** Cold sweat on the head.

⁵ **Eyes.** Burning in the eyes and lids.

Throbbing in the eyeball.

Worse reading by artificial light; walking, in the open air.

⁷ **Nose.** Sneezing and hoarseness.

Takes cold in the head readily.

⁸ **Face.** Coppery spots on the face.

Face red, with little blisters.

Burning heat of the face ; or of one side.

Circumscribed redness.

Tension in one side of the face.

Numb feeling in the face.

Symptoms relieved by external heat, pressure, or friction.

Cold sweat on the face.

¹¹ **Tongue, etc.** Taste: bitter; of blood.

Extensive ulceration of the tongue, with deeply-chapped fungoid surfaces.

Tongue coated with white mucus; morning.

¹² **Mouth.** An ulcerated tumor on left side of mouth, upon the soft commissure of the jaws, behind last molar.

¹³ **Throat.** Angina faucium and tonsillaris with the characteristic high-colored, strong urine.

Mouth and throat symptoms relieved by eating.

Heat in the œsophagus, as from acid eructations.

¹⁴ **Desires. Aversions.** Appetite in the evening; lost in the morning ; nausea.

Thirst with sleepiness; evening.

¹⁶ **Nausea and Vomiting.** Loathing sickness at the stomach, pain and discomfort; with gagging.

Vomiting of a salty or bitter substance.

¹⁷ **Stomach.** Weak digestion.

Burning or warmth; pressure in the stomach.

Gastric symptoms increased when walking, especially ascending.

¹⁸ **Hypochondria.** In region of liver constant fine stitching midway in upper portion thereof, not increased by pressure.

Obstruction of the liver.

¹⁹ **Abdomen.** Heat through the abdomen.

Cutting about the navel; tearing bellyache.

Pressure of clothing makes him feel wearied.

20 **Stool, etc.**   Stools copious, watery, greyish-white, like dirty soap-suds; excessively offensive, scenting whole house.

Stool of a strong, pungent smell, like that of the urine.

Putrid, bloody stools.

21 **Urine.**   Sore pain in back; burning in left kindey, with drawing when stooping; dull pain in the kidneys, loins stiff; right knee swollen.

Nephritic colic; urine deep red, of a strong odor.

Irritability of bladder: with muco-purulent discharges, enlarged prostate; with concretions of urate of ammonia; calculus.

Old persons: dribbling of strong-smelling urine.

Dysuria senilis, gravel trifling, irritable bladder.

Urine high-colored; increased specific gravity; hot, scalding; ammoniacal; very offensive in many diseases.

A granular kind of mucus mixed with phosphates in the sediment; urine dark, reddish-brown; acid reaction, or very offensive; fleeting pains in bladder, not when urinating, but at other times; vesical catarrh, from suppressed gonorrhœa, calculi or gout.

White flocculent sediment immediately after voiding urine, composed of phosphate and carbonate of lime, without uric acid; pale, languid; weak loins.

Enuresis nocturna of children; urine strong.

22 **Male Sexual Organs.**   Gleet; urine offensive.

Gonorrhœa suppressed by copaiva, with offensive urine.

23 **Female Sexual Organs.**   Prolapsus uteri with fetid urine.

24 **Pregnancy.**   Gastric derangements when ascending a height.

Retention of urine; infants.

25 **Larynx.**   Slight hoarseness in the morning, sneezing.

26 **Breathing.**   Difficulty of breathing on awaking.

Asthma with inflammatory rheumatic complaints.

Mucous oppression of the lungs.

27 **Cough.**   Dry, constant, hacking cough after suppressed gonorrhœa; cough followed by expectoration of green mucus.

28 **Lungs.**   Pneumonia, asthenic forms, great weakness, difficult breathing increasing every hour.

Stitches in chest, especially on breathing deeply; evening.

Pain about the third rib, right side, midway between sternum and side, increased by breathing.

Pain in left side, about sixth rib, increased by deep inspiration and bending to either side.

29 **Heart.   Pulse,**   Pains change place incessantly, but are most constant about the heart.

Awakens after midnight with violent pulsations of the heart and temporal arteries, 110 per minute; internal but no external heat; cannot go to sleep.

Sense of weakness in the præcordia.

Palpitation while sitting; worse after drinking.

Palpitation worse at night, lying; at times tearing, rheumatic pains in the extremities, relieving the heart.

Pulse accelerated; full; slower and weaker; intermittent.

Gout affecting the heart.

30 **Outer Chest.** Pressure of clothing on chest is annoying.

31 **Neck. Back.** Deep, penetrating pain in posterior part of left side, at about the sixth rib.

Pain right side of back between tenth dorsal vertebra and side.

Dull pain in region of kidneys; stiffness in the loins.

Trembling in the lumbar region.

32 **Upper Limbs.** Tearing pains apparently in the bones.

❙ Ganglion of the wrist.

Fingers swollen; tearing and fine stitching pains in various parts of the limbs.

Red spots on the fingers.

Cold hands, with head symptoms.

33 **Lower Limbs.** Pain in left hip, knee and toes; thence in muscles of calf, and then in the knee; after it has left these parts, it appears in the right thigh and ankle.

Swelling of the right knee, ulcerative pain in the whole leg; with pains in the kidneys.

Pain in the right knee; then in the left.

Cracking or sense of dryness in the knee-joints.

Tearing and stitches especially in the metatarsal-joints of the right great toe.

Pain in right, later in left tendo-achillis.

During the night gout commences in the right great toe.

Gout going from left to right

Cold feet; cold sweat.

34 **Limbs in General.** Gouty concretions.

Nodes on the joints of upper and lower limbs, cracking and kinking on motion.

Tearing, fine stitches in various parts of the limbs.

Syphilitic rheumatism.

35 **Position, etc.** Rest: 4. Motion: 34. Walking: 5, 17, 40. Ascending: 17, 24. Bending to either side: 28. Stooping: 21. Sitting: 29. Lying: 29.

36 **Nerves.** Trembling: with palpitation of heart; in loins. Weariness, lassitude: 4, 21.

37 **Sleep.** Sleepiness, wish dulness of the head.

Awakens: with difficulty of breathing; with palpitation.

Starting up from sleep.

38 **Time.** Morning: 3, 11, 14, 25, 40. Afternoon: 2. Evening: 14, 28. Night: 29, 33, 40. Midnight: 29.

39 **Temperature and Weather.** Heat: 8. Draught of air: 3. Uncovering: 3. Open air: 5.

⁴⁰ **Chill. Fever. Sweat.** Cold hands; feet; back; knees, as from cold wind.

Violent internal heat on awaking.

Sense of heat in œsophagus; stomach ; belly.

Heat: with sweat; with cold in the head; with nightly palpitation.

Sweat while eating; while walking; morning in bed, especially in face.

Cold sweat.

Sweat with itching.

⁴¹ **Attacks.** Periodically: 4.

⁴² **Sides.** Symptoms, in the sick, go fróm left to right, and from below upwards; especially in rheumatism and gout.

Right: 21, 28, 31, 33.   Left: 12. 21, 28, 31, 33.

⁴⁴ **Tissues.** Emaciation.

⁴⁵ **Contact, Injuries, etc.** Pressure: 8, 18, 19, 30.   Friction? 8.   Scratching: 46.

⁴⁶ **Skin.** Itching on various parts, yielding a rather agreeable sensation on being scratched, but leaving a burning.

Slightly elevated, wart-like, round surfaces about the anus, varying from a half to one and a half inches in diameter; with smarting soreness; urine strong-scented and high-colored; after using copavia for chancre.

Syphilitic spots and marks.

⁴⁷ **Stages and States.** Gouty diathesis.

Rheumatic diathesis in syphilitic or gonorrhœal patients.

⁴⁸ **Relationship.** Useful in gout after *Colchic.* fails.

Bad effects from copavia: 22, 46.

BERBERIS.

Bayberry.   *Berberidaceæ.*

¹ **Mind.** Defective recollection and weak memory.

Mental labor, requiring close thinking, very difficult; the least interruption breaks the chain of thoughts.

Indifference and pensiveness, with disinclination to speak.

Everything seems twice as large as natural.

Anxious and fearful.

Fretful humor, with weariness of life.

² **Sensorium.** Vertigo; with danger of falling; when stooping and when rising.

Illusions; in the twilight objects appear twice as large as natural.

³ **Inner Head.** Dulness of the head, like from coryza.

14

Heaviness of the head, particularly when stooping.

Pressure from within outward, particularly in forehead, but also in temples and occiput.

Sensation as if the head were becoming larger.

Tensive pain, also with pressure in the temples and forehead, or with dulness of the whole head.

Stitches in the forehead.

Tearing in the forehead and orbits.

Cold sensation in right temple.

Heat in the head, after dinner and from exertion.

⁴ **Outer Head.** Tension of the scalp and skin of face, as if swollen.

Corrosive itching or stitching on the scalp, changing place from scratching.

⁵ **Eyes.** Pressure in the eyes.

• Violent shooting pains through the eyes into the brain, or from temples to the eyes; sometimes into the arms; also after operation for strabismus.

Tearing in left eye; also in the lids.

Dryness of the eyes, with burning and redness of the conjunctiva.

Sensation of sand between the lids; dryness of internal canthus and sensation as of a foreign body there.

Sticky feeling and white scum on dry eyelids, mornings.

Itching; burning and smarting on the lids, or in the canthi, frequently only on small spots.

. Cold feeling in the eye, like from a cool wind, with lachrymation when closing the eyes.

Quivering of the eyelids when reading by candle-light.

⁶ **Ears.** Beating and fluttering noise in the ear.

Stopped up feeling in the ear, with pressure.

Tearing and stitching in the ears. through the membrana typanani, as if a nail were thrust through, or like from the sting of an insect.

Pimples: nodosities, size of hemp-seed, on the auricle, painful to touch.

Tumor behind the ear, size of a hazel-nut.

⁷ **Nose.** Crawling, smarting or itching in the ears.

Titillating irritation to sneeze.

Drops of blood from the left nostril.

Dryness of the nose.

Obstinate catarrh of left nostril, with secretion, first of yellow water, later purulent white, yellow or green mucus; empyreumatic smell and taste, particularly in morning.

⁸ **Face.** Pale, earthy complexion, with sunken cheeks and hollow, blue encircled eyes.

Tearing and stitches in the cheek and jaw·bones.

Dark red, painful spot on the right cheek.

Sensation as if cold drops were spurted into the face when going into the open air.

Heat and burning of the face, with red cheeks.

⁹ **Lower Face.** Lips bluish on the inside.

Formication in upper lip around mouth and chin.

Burning in lips.

Dryness of lips, with scaling and formation of thin brown scurf on edges.

¹⁰ **Teeth.** Stitches in the teeth, they feel too long or dull.

Tearing in the left molars.

Pain as if the gums were torn, or the teeth pulled out.

Dingy red edges of the gums; small white nodules on gums.

Gums bleed easily.

Ulcer at an upper molar or incisor.

Sore gums during dentition.

¹¹ **Tongue, etc.** Taste: bitter; sometimes sour; of blood.

Tongue smarts when touched.

Slimy furred tongue.

Painful white blisters on tip of tongue.

¹² **Mouth.** Offensive metallic odor from the mouth.

Mouth and fauces dry and sticky, especially in morning, relieved after eating.

¹³ **Throat.** Increased redness of the palate and tonsils; tonsils pain when speaking or swallowing; sticking as from an awl in the throat.

Sensation of a plug in side of throat, with dryness, roughness and scraping; severe pain from empty deglutition.

¹⁴ **Desires. Aversions.** Thirst, with dryness of the mouth.

Great thirst, alternating with aversion to drink.

Appetite either increased or decreased.

¹⁵ **Eating and Drinking.** Before dinner chilliness.

After eating solids, belching for hours, and soreness, continuing the whole night.

¹⁶ **Nausea and Vomiting.** Hiccoughing.

Frequent eructations, alternating with yawning.

Bitter eructation.

Heartburn.

Nausea: before breakfast; after dinner.

¹⁷ **Stomach.** Pressure in the stomach, as if it would burst, also stinging and burning.

Chilliness in the region of stomach, ceasing after vomiting.

Pit of stomach puffed up.

¹⁸ **Hypochondria.** Pressure, also stitching in region of liver.

Colic from gall-stones.

Drawing, tearing in left hypochondrium, with sensation, during inspiration, as if something were torn loose.

Cramp-like contraction in splenic region.

[19] **Abdomen.** Colic-like pains, especially about the navel.

Pressure and tension in the groins, as if a hernia would develop; especially when walking and standing.

Itching, or pressure in the region of the inguinal glands, with pain from touch as if they would swell.

Stitching, tearing or burning in the skin of the abdomen, mostly about the navel.

Rumbling in the bowels.

[20] **Stools, etc.** Watery evacuations.

Large, pappy, free stools, mostly with tenesmus before and after.

Scanty, thin-formed stool, hard or soft.

Hard stool, like sheep's dung, passed only after much straining.

Intense pain before and with stool, as from constriction in the rectum, preventing passage of feces.

Frequent urging to stool.

Hemorrhoids, with itching or burning, particularly after stool, which frequently is hard, and covered with blood.

Soreness in the anus, with burning; pain when touched, and great sensitiveness when sitting.

Pressure in the perineum.

Fistula in ano, with itching there; short cough and chest complaints.

Herpes around the anus.

[21] **Urine.** Burning and soreness in region of kidneys.

Sharp pain in right kidney, near the spine, thence downwards into the bladder.

Tearing, pulsating pain in right kidney.

Stitches from the kidneys to the bladder and urethra.

Cutting pain from left kidney into bladder and urethra.

Pressure and contraction in the vesical region when pressed upon, with burning in the urethra.

Cutting or burning in the urethra, worse when not urinating, frequently more on one side.

Violent urging after urinating, particularly in morning.

Urine: increased and clear, with small slimy sediment, at the beginning and during the exacerbation of complaints; lessened, and with copious slimy sediment, when the complaints abate; warmer, and attended with pain in the lumbar and renal region; dark or bright yellow, or red, with sediment; blood red, speedily becoming turbid, depositing thick mucus and bright red mealy sediment.

Pain in the hips while urinating.

[22] **Male Sexual Organs.** Suppressed sexual desire.

Sensation of weakness and unexcitability in the parts, especially after urinating.

During coition too weak and too short thrill; ejection too soon.

Drawing from right or left testicle to the spermatic cord.

Neuralgia of testes and cords; parts swollen, tender.

Testicle drawn up.

Pains in the external genitals, increased by motion.

Coldness and numb feeling in the prepuce and glans.

Pains in genitals, increased by motion.

Scrotum shrunken, cold, with pressure in the testicles.

[23] **Female Sexual Organs.** Suppressed sexual desire, with long delayed thrill, and frequently, cutting and stitching in the parts during coition.

Menses: too slight, of water blood, or grey mucus; too short; scanty, of black drops or filthy slime.

Acrid leucorrhoea, very prostrating.

Sensation of burning and soreness in vagina.

Vagina painful to touch.

[25] **Larynx.** Hoarseness, with pain or inflammation of tonsils.

Tearing in throat, upwards, particularly left side, with stiffness.

[26] **Breathing.** Oppression, with fluent coryza, mostly at night.

With inhalation, stitching between the shoulders, from the back through the chest.

Shortness of breath when going up stairs.

Obstruction of breath when raising the arm.

[27] **Cough.** Short, dry cough, with stitches in the chest.

[28] **Lungs.** Stitches in and around clavicle, also pulsation and burning.

Pressure behind the left nipple.

Rawness and soreness on the chest, as during a catarrh.

Stitches in the chest; increased by deep inspiration, with short, dry cough.

Tearing in the chest, particularly left side.

Cutting contraction in the chest, to the abdomen, compels one to bend over.

[29] **Heart. Pulse.** Stitches about the heart.

Frequent palpitation.

Slow, weak pulse.

[30] **Outer Chest.** Stitching, pulsating, pressing or tensive pains in the muscles of chest.

Corrosive feeling in the skin.

Pimples on the chest and scapula.

[31] **Neck. Back.** Pain as if bruised or swollen, from right scapula to shoulder-joint.

Tearing in and between the scapulæ.

Tearing in the spine.

Spinal irritation; general hyperæsthesia; pains about kidneys, along false ribs, starting from the spine.

Backache, worse while sitting or lying, mostly in the morning, when awaking.

Bruised pain, with stiffness in small of back ; rises from a seat with difficulty.

Painful pressure and tension in lumbar and renal region, sometimes with sensation of numbness, puffiness, warmth, stiffness and lameness, extending at times into lower limbs.

Constant pulsating stitches in sacrum.

[32] **Upper Limbs.** Gurgling feeling in shoulder, or sensation as of something alive in joint, especially about midnight.

Gurgling feeling in the muscles of right upper arm.

Itching, smarting and burning in the axilla.

Tearing in the shoulder.

Stitches in left upper arm.

Pimple on point of each elbow, much inflamed after rubbing.

Pain the wrist after exertion with the hand.

Tearing along the metacarpal bones.

Tearing in joints of the fingers.

Heaviness and lameness of the arms.

Arms pain as if bruised ; feel weak and lame.

Dingy red marbled spots, with bruised pain.

Lymphatic swelling in the flexors of the arm, with pete-chia-like spots and burning.

[33] **Lower Limbs.** Pain in the thighs, worse from changes of weather, mostly before heavy wind.

Varices, from the groins down the thighs.

Tension in bend of knee, as if the tendons were too short.

Tired, bruised and lame feeling in the knee.

Cramp in the calf of leg.

Tearing pain in the tibia.

Heels pain as if ulcerated, when standing.

Stitches between the metatarsal bones, as from a nail, when standing.

Stitches; burning; itching; smarting; pain and cold feeling in the feet, as if frozen.

Tearing in the balls of feet, painful to step thereon.

Stitches in ball of great toe; in joints of the toes.

Lower limbs pain as if beaten; with heaviness; can scarcely rise from the seat.

Twitching, as from something alive.

Wasting of the lower limbs.

[34] **Limbs in General.** Tearing, also stitching, or throbbing-tearing in the limbs.

[35] **Position, etc.** Affected by the slightest exertion, which also excites breaking out of sweat.

Motion: 22. Raising arm: 26. Walking: 19, 43. As-

cending: 26.   Exertion: 32, 43.   Lifting: 43.   Stretching: 43.   Rising: 2, 31.   Standing: 19, 33, 43.   Stooping: 2, 3.   Sitting: 20, 31.   Lying: 31, 37.

[36] **Nerves.**   Great weakness, like fainting.

Lame feeling all over, with warm feeling in lower part of
back or sacrum.

General relaxation, not inclined to do anything.

[37] **Sleep.**   Sleepiness by day; feels tired, must lie down.

Restless, dreamful sleep, with frequent waking, and congestion of blood to the head.

Difficult awaking in the morning, succeeded by pains in
the head and back, exhaustion, and want of recollection.

Anxious dreams.

[38] **Time.**   Morning: 3, 7, 12, 16, 21, 31, 37, 43.   Forenoon: 40;
11 A. M.; 40.   Afternoon: 3, 16, 40.   Twilight: 1, 2.
Evening: 40.   Night: 15, 26, 40.   Midnight: 32.

[39] **Temperature and Weather.**   Walking in the open air: 43.
Head complaints better in the open air.   Eye complaints
worse in open air.   Changes of weather; heavy winds: 33.

[40] **Chill.   Fever.   Sweat.**   Chill before dinner, with ice-cold.
feet, dry, viscous mouth, without thirst.

Chill from the face and arms to the back and breast, succeeded by heat, with anxiety and oppression of chest,
especially forenoon and evening.

Chill as if in the bones, with warmth of skin.

Coldness of the body, with heat of face, commencing at 11
A. M.; heat and inclination to sweat at night.

With the chill pressure and dulness of the head.

Heat in hands and head in the afternoon.

Transient sensation of warmth at different places.

With the heat, anxiety, oppression of chest, shooting in
the head, thirst, and often sore throat.

Inclination to sweat with the least exercise.

[42] **Sides.**   Right: 3, 8, 18, 21, 22, 31, 32.   Left: 5, 7, 10, 18, 21,
22, 25, 28, 32.   In out: 3.   Above downwards: 21, 28,
31, 34.   Below upwards: 25.   Behind forwards: 26.

[43] **Sensations.**   Great lassitude, increased by walking or
standing.

Unrefreshed, worn feeling; prostration of both mind and
body, in the morning when awaking, also after long sleep.

Exhaustion, even to trembling and shaking of the knees,
also undesirous of occupation.

Faintish weakness after walking in the open air.

Gurgling sensation in the muscles, also with feeling as of
something alive therein.

Pain, with heaviness and powerless of the affected part.

Pains, as from spraining or wrenching, lifting, or stretching.

[44] **Tissues.** In muscles: tension, shooting, tearing, pulsating. gurgling; sensation as of something alive.

Scraping upon the bones.

Cold feeling at the bones.

Varicose veins on many places.

Arthritic and rheumatic affections, particularly with urinary, hemorrhoidal or menstrual complaints.

[45] **Contact, Injuries, etc.** Riding in carriage causes pain in foot.

After riding, faintness.

Touch: 19, 20, 23. Pressure: 21, 46. Rubbing: 32. Scratching: 4: 46.

[46] **Skin.** Burning, smarting, stitching or corrosive itching, which provokes scratching, though it soon returns at the same or some other place.

Boils: hastens suppuration and prevents return.

Red marbled spots: with corrosive or bruised pain; like petechia, with burning, itching and stitching; sensitive to pressure; changing into brown spots.

Running cold, and crawls in the skin.

Swollen varices.

Pimples, usually isolated, sometimes in groups.

Lymphatic swellings.

Jaundice, with pale, tough feces; or with profuse, acrid, watery diarrhœa.

Old yellow spots around the navel peeling off.

Red spot on left eyelid, feels like a mosquito bite, but swelling nearly closes the eye; next day other spots on face, behind the ear, on neck; third day on the chin and nose, with itching and burning; in evening covered with small vesicles, oozing watery fluid.

[47] **Stages and States.** Especially suited where the renal or vesical symptoms are prominent.

[48] **Relationship.** Antidote to *Berber.: Camphor.*

Berber. antidotes: *Acon.*

Pareira Brava is preferable when patient must get on all-fours to urinate; urine contains viscid, white mucus; pains go down into the thighs, rather than into hips as in *Berber.* (Has even relieved heart symptoms, when above are present.)

BISMUTHUM.

Hydrated oxide of Bismuth.   HAHNEMANN. $Bi_2 O_2 OH_2$.

[1] **Mind.** Dulness, heaviness of head.

Solitude is unbearable; desire for company.

Unstable minded: begins now this, again that, holds but a short time to any one thing.

Surly and dissatisfied with his condition, complains.

[2] **Sensorium.** Vertigo, sensation as if the anterior half of the brain were turning in a circle.

[3] **Inner Head.** Pressure and sensation of heaviness in the forehead; at times also in occiput; worse from motion.

Dull, cutting pain in the brain, begins above the right orbit and extends to the occiput.

[5] **Eyes.** Pressure in the right eyeball, from before backwards and from below upwards.

Thickened mucus in both canthi.

[7] **Nose.** Nosebleed, dark blood.

Pressive heaviness at the root of the nose.

[8] **Face.** Earth complexion, blue around the eyes; features changed, as if he had been very sick.

Pressure in the region of the malar bones; better running about and holding cold water in mouth.

[10] **Teeth.** Toothache relieved by taking cold water in the mouth; worse when it becomes warm.

[11] **Tongue, etc.** Taste: sweetish, sour, or metallic, on the back part of the tongue.

Tongue: red; coated white, evenings.

[14] **Desires. Aversions.** Desire for cold drinks in the evening, but no fever.

[15] **Eating and Drinking.** Water is vomited as soon as it reaches the stomach.

Pressure like a load in the stomach after eating.

[16] **Nausea and Vomiting.** Eructations fetid, cadaverous.

Nausea at the stomach after eating or nursing.

Vomiting of bile without effort.

Vomiting: convulsive gagging and inexpressible pain in the stomach; after operations on the abdomen.

Vomits: only at intervals of days when food has filled the stomach; then vomits enormous quantities, lasting all day; all fluids.

[17] **Stomach.** Pressure as from a load in one spot.

Crampy, spasmodic pains in stomach; burning alternating with pressure; pressure in spine, must bend backwards.

Intense malaise in the stomach, with burning; red or white tongue, restlessness, prostration; after blood-letting.

[19] **Abdomen.** Flatulence.

[20] **Stool, etc.** Stools: papescent, foul; watery, cadaverous-smelling.

[21] **Urine.** Copious, frequent, watery.

[22] **Male Sexual Organs.** Seminal emissions, with lascivious dreams.

[23] **Female Sexual Organs.** Menstrual blood dark, pitchy. ·

[27] **Cough.** Sputa dark, bloody or blood-streaked.

[28] **Lungs.** Crampy, pressive pain through the chest, in the region of the diaphragm, when walking.

Boring and burning in the chest; backache.

[29] **Heart. Pulse.** Strong heart-beat.

Pulse contracted, somewhat spasmodic, and at times intermittent

[30] **Outer Chest.** Fine stitches in the centre of the sternum, not affected by breathing.

[32] **Upper Limbs.** Paralytic weariness and weakness in right arm.

Laming, tearing pressure on right forearm; more toward outer side; passes off by motion and touch.

Tearing in metacarpal bones of right fore and middle fingers.

Fine tearing in finger-tips of right hand, particularly under the nails.

[33] **Lower Limbs.** Tearing pain below the external malleolus of right foot, terminating at the tendo-achillis.

Tearing: in the toes; in the heels, more left.

[34] **Limbs in General.** Screwing, boring, tearing pressure in the bones of the hands and feet.

[35] **Position, etc.** Motion: 3, 32. Walking: 28. Running: 8. Must bend back: 17. After rising: 40.

[36] **Nerves.** Restless, moving about; anxiety.

Languor; prostration.

[37] **Sleep.** Cannot get his accustomed morning nap.

Frequent waking at night: as from fright; as from tire.

Restless sleep, through lascivious dreams, sometimes without, more frequently with seminal emission.

[38] **Time.** Morning: 37, 40. Evening: 11, 14. Night: 37. All day: 16.

[39] **Temperature and Weather.** Cold water: 8, 10.

[40] **Chill. Fever. Sweat.** Chill, with deathly coldness of the whole body.

Flushes of heat over whole body, mostly on head and chest, after rising in the morning.

External, dry, burning heat.

[42] **Sides.** Right: 3, 5, 32, 33. Left: 33. Before backwards: 3, 5. Below upwards: 5.

[43] **Sensations.** Sensation of heaviness in internal parts.

[44] **Tissues.**   Has been given in cancer of stomach.
[45] **Contact, Injuries, etc.** Touch: 32. Scratching: 46. After
   operations on the abdomen: 17.
[46] **Skin.**   Ulcers gangrenous, bluish; or dried, parchment-like.
   Corrosive itching aside the tibia and on back of both feet
      near joints, worse from scratching; must scratch till it
      bleeds.
[48] **Relationship.**   Antidotes to *Bismuth.*: *Calc. ostr.*, *Capsic.*,
   Nux vom.
   Bismuth. isomorphic with *Arsen.*, *Phosphor.*, *Antim.*, and
      resembles them in symptoms.

BORAX VENETA.

Sodium Biborate.   HAHNEMANN. $2\,BO_2Na.B_2O._310H_2O.$

[1] **Mind.**   Idles through the afternoon, does not really get at
   work; changes from one work to another, from one
      room to another without keeping to any object.
   Dread of downward motion.
   Great anxiety and sleepiness; anxiety increased until 11 P.M.
   Fretful, ill-humored, indolent and discontented before the
      easy stool, in the afternoon; after it, lively, contented,
      and looking cheerfully into the future.
   Easily startled by unusual sounds.
[2] **Sensorium.**   First, heaviness of head; later, light, clear head.
   Vertigo and fulness in head on ascending a mountain or
      stairs.
   Feels as if pushed from right to left and somewhat forward.
[3] **Inner Head.**   Aching in whole head, with nausea, inclina-
      tion to vomit and trembling in the whole body, at 10 A.M.
   Pressive headache in the forehead.
   Throbbing headache in both temples, or in occiput.
   Tearing; also stitches in the vertex.
[4] **Outer Head.**   Hot head, of infants, with heat of mouth and
      palms.
   Hair becomes entangled at tips and sticks together, can-
      not be separated; if these bunches are cut off they form
      again.
   Sensitiveness of external head to cold, change of weather.
[5] **Eyes.**   Obscuration of left eye, evenings.
   Flickering before eyes in morning, when writing, so that
      he does not see distinctly; there seem to be bright mov-
      ing waves, now from right to left, again from above
      downwards.

Several stitches in succession, in left eye.

Inflammation of left eye at inner canthus, with nightly agglutination.

Inflammation of right eye at external canthus, with irregularity of the lashes; nightly agglutination.

The lashes turn inward toward the eye and inflame it, especially at outer canthus, where the margins of the lids are very sore.

⁶ **Ears.** Very sensitive to the slightest noise, as rumpling of paper, fall of a door-latch, etc.

Difficult hearing, more in the left ear.

Ringing, piping, crackling, drumming, or roaring in ears, more in left.

Stitches in the left ear.

Discharge of pus from both ears.

Inflamed and hot swelling of both ears.

⁷ **Nose.** Bleeding from the nose, morning.

Sneezing causes severe stitch in right side of chest.

Fluent coryza, with much crawling in the nose.

Discharge of much greenish, thick mucus from the nose.

Dry crusts in the nose, re-form if removed.

Boil in the forepart of the left nostril, toward the tip, with sore pain and swelling of tip of nose.

Red and shining swelling of the nose, with throbbing and tensive sensation.

⁸ **Face.** Anxious face during downward motion.

Sickly, pale, earthy color of the face.

Swelling, heat and redness of face, with tearing pain in the malar bone.

Sensation on right side of face, by the mouth, as if cobwebs laid there.

⁹ **Lower Face.** Red inflamed swelling, as large as a pea, on the lower lip, with burning soreness when touched.

Crawling, like insects, on the lips.

¹⁰ **Teeth.** Dull griping in a hollow tooth in wet weather.

Inflamed large swelling on the outer side of gum, which pains severely (gum-boil), with dull pain in a hollow tooth; swelling of cheek and whole left side of face, as far as below eye, where there is formed a watery blister.

¹¹ **Tongue, etc,** Taste: flat and insipid; bitter; food and even saliva taste bitter.

Food has no taste.

Aphthæ on the tongue.

Red blisters on the tongue, as if the surface were eroded; they pain from every motion of tongue, or if anything salt or spiced touches them.

¹² **Inner Mouth.** Aphthæ: in the mouth; on inner surface of cheek, bleeding easily; with great heat and dryness of mouth.

The mucous membrane of forepart of palate is shriveled,
as if burnt, pains especially when chewing.

Mouth very hot.

[13] **Throat.** Palate wrinkled; child cries frequently, when
nursing.

Roughness and burning in throat.

Tough, whitish mucus in the throat, which is loosened
only after great exertion.

[14] **Desires. Aversions.** Longing for sour drinks.

No desire for his smoking tobacco.

[15] **Eating and Drinking.** After eating apples with mutton,
fulness in stomach with peevishness and ill-humor, also
fulness in head.

After every meal flatulent distention.

After smoking tobacco sensation as if diarrhœa would set in.

After eating pears, especially morning or forenoon, pressure in pit of stomach, which disappears on walking.

[16] **Nausea and Vomiting.** Hiccough after eating (also of
infants).

Nausea: in morning; immediately after waking, with inclination to vomit; after drinking water, mucus and
bitter vomit.

Vomiting food and mucus.

[17] **Stomach.** Pain in region of stomach after heavy lifting;
pain extends to the small of back where it is of a
stitching character; so severe that during the night she
cannot turn without pain; better in the morning.

[18] **Hypochondria.** Pressure in left hypochondrium.

Cutting in left hypochondrium on walking rapidly, as if a
hard, sharp, movable piece was there, with sensation in
abdomen as if only hard pieces were in it, and these
were in motion.

Pressure in right hypochondrium.

Cutting in right hypochondrium, extending downwards
across bowels, followed by diarrhœa; evacuation sudden.

[19] **Abdomen.** Flatulent distention after every meal.

Pain in abdomen, as if diarrhœa would set in.

Pinching in abdomen with diarrhœa.

Stitching and pressing pain in groin.

Belly soft, flabby and sunken.

[20] **Stools, etc.** Stools: frequent, soft, light yellow, slimy, with
faintness and weariness; green or brown, diarrhœic;
painless, at first frothy, thin and brown, later cadaverous-smelling, containing bits of yellow feces; colorless
or slimy; green, preceded by crying (infant).

[21] **Urine.** Severe, urgent desire to urinate.

At night must rise several times to urinate.

Desire to urinate, without being able to pass a drop.

The infant urinates every ten or twelve minutes, and frequently cries and screams before the passage.

Hot urine.

Pungent smell of the urine.

Smarting in the urethra after urinating.

[22] **Male Sexual Organs.** Indifference to coition.

[23] **Female Sexual Organs.** Menses too early, too profuse, and
attended with colic and nausea.

Leucorrhœa like the white of egg, with sensation as if warm
water were falling down; leucorrhœa and sterility;
acrid leucorrhœa midway between menstrual periods.

[24] **Pregnancy.** Labor-pains accompanied by violent and frequent eructations.

Milk is too thick and tastes badly; often curdles soon after
it has been drawn.

Constrictive pains in left mamma when child nurses the
right one.

Griping and sometimes stitches in left mamma, and when
the child has nursed she is obliged to compress the
breast with the hand, because it aches on account of
being empty.

[25] **Larynx.** Tearing in larynx extending to chest, exciting
cough.

[26] **Breathing.** Respiration difficult.

Obliged, every few minutes, to take a quick, deep breath,
which is every time followed by a stitch in right side of
chest, with a subdued pain—sigh and slow exhalation.

Shortness of breath after ascending stairs, so that he
cannot speak a word; later, when he speaks, has stitch
in right side of chest.

[27] **Chest.** Hacking and violent cough, with slight expectoration from the chest, of moldy taste and smell.

Musty expectoration, with pain through the chest to back.

Dry, cachectic cough, especially in the morning when
rising and evening when lying down; with stitching
pain in right chest and right flank, relieved by pressure;
washing the chest with cold water affords the most
relief; after drinking wine the pains are aggravated.

Cough with expectoration of white mucus streaked with
blood.

[28] **Lungs.** Tightness in the chest.

Stitches in chest when yawning, coughing or breathing
deeply.

Stitches in right side of the chest in the region of the
nipple, with every paroxysm of cough.

[29] **Heart. Pulse.** Circulation irregular, face bluish, especially around the mouth, nose and eyes, with blue look
of finger-ends and feet; with attacks, during which the
child became prostrate and as if suffocating.

. Sensation as if the heart were on the right side and were
being squeezed.

Pulse somewhat accelerated.

[30] **Outer Chest.** Stitches between the ribs of the right side;
cannot lie upon that side on account of the pain, with
sensitive drawing and obstruction of breathing, has to
catch for breath; if, during sleep, he lies on the painful
side, the pains awake him immediately.

[31] **Neck. Back.** Rheumatic drawing pains in the nape of
the neck, extending to the left shoulder and then into
the scapula; evening, when walking in the open air.

Pain in the back; when walking; as from pressure, when
sitting, or stooping.

[32] **Upper Limbs.** Drawing and tearing pain in and between
the shoulders, so that he cannot stoop.

Tearing and breaking sensation in right wrist.

Burning, heat and redness of the fingers during slight cold,
as if frost-bitten.

Throbbing pain in tip of thumb, day and night, frequently
waking from sleep, at night.

[33] **Lower Limbs.** Erysipelatous inflammation and swelling on
the left leg and foot, after violent dancing, with tearing,
tension and burning in it; increased burning pain when
touched; on pressure redness disappears for a moment.

Pain in the heel as if sore from walking.

Stitches in sole.

Burning, heat and redness of the toes during slight cold,
as if frost-bitten.

[35] **Position, etc.** Restlessness in the body, which does not
permit him to sit or lie long in one place.

Walking: 15, 18, 31, 33. Downward motion: 8. Ascending: 2, 26. Motion of tongue: 11. Sitting: 31. Stooping: 31, 32. Lying on painful side: 30.

[36] **Nerves.** Weakness especially in abdomen and limbs.

Trembling in the whole body, especially in hands, with
nausea and weakness of knees.

[37] **Sleep.** Sleeps more than usual.

Wakes uncommonly early, 3 A.M., cannot fall asleep again
for two hours, on account of heat in the whole body,
especially in the head, with sweat on the thighs.

Child cries out during sleep, as if frightened.

Lascivious dreams, she dreams of coition.

[38] **Time.** Day and night: 32. Morning: 5, 7, 15, 16, 17, 27,
40. 10 A.M.: 3. Forenoon: 15. Afternoon: 1, 40.
Evening: 5, 27, 31, 40. Night: 5, 17, 21, 32. 11 P.M.: 1.
3 A.M.: 37.

[39] **Temperature and Weather.** Symptoms worse in very
warm weather.

Open air: 31. Cold: 4. Change of weather: 4. Wet
weather: 10. Washing with cold water: 27.

40 **Chill. Fever. Sweat.** Chill and chilliness mostly during
sleep.
Chill predominating, especially in afternoon and evening.
Chill and heat alternating.
Chill from uncovering.
Flushes of heat morning and evening.
Hot head, mouth and palms, of infant.
Sweat during the morning sleep.

41 **Attacks.** Every few minutes: 26.

42 **Sides.** Right: 5, 6, 7, 8, 18, 26, 27, 28, 29, 30, 32. Left: 5,
6, 7, 10, 18, 24, 31, 33, 46. Right to left: 5. Above
downwards: 5, 18, 31. Upper right and lower left.

44 **Tissues.** General emaciation.
Parts which are usually red, turn white.

45 **Contact, Injuries, etc.** Touch: 9, 33. Pressure: 24, 27, 33;
of teeth (chewing): 12. Scratching: 46. Lifting: 17.

46 **Skin.** Sensation as if a cobweb were lying upon the skin
of face or hands.
Unhealthiness of the skin; slight injuries suppurate.
Severe itching on the back of the finger-joints, must
scratch them violently. Excellent remedy in psoriasis.
Red papulous eruption on the cheeks and around the skin.
Herpetic eruption on the nates.
Old wounds and ulcers are inclined to reopen and sup-
purate.
Ulcer in the left axilla.

48 **Relationship.** Antidotes to *Borax: Chamom., Coffea.*
Inimical to *Borax : Acetum, Vinum.*

BOVISTA.

Puffball.　　　　　　　HARTLAUB.　　　　　　　*Fungi.*

1 **Mind.** Misapplies words in speaking or writing.
Awkwardness, which makes him drop things from his
hands.
Absence of mind and difficulty in fixing his attention.
Slowness of understanding and comprehension.
Sad, depressed and desponding when alone.
Sensitiveness, great excitability, takes everything amiss.
Moroseness. Ill-humor, aversion to all things.

2 **Sensorium.** Stares vacantly into space.
Vertigo, early in the morning, falls over, losing his senses
for awhile.

³ **Inner Head.** Headache deep in; ɪ sensation as if the head were much enlarged.

Headache at night, worse from sitting up.

Head seems bruised.

Pressing pains in the head.

Headache, right side in the morning; left, evening.

⁴ **Outer Head.** Violent itching of the scalp, especially when getting warm, scratches on forehead until sore; not relieved by scratching.

Scalp tender to the touch.

Falling off of the hair.

⁵ **Eyes.** Inflammation of eyelids, with nightly agglutination.

Eyes dim, without lustre.

Staring at one point.

Blindness of right eye from paralysis of optic nerve.

Objects appear too near.

⁶ **Ears.** Hearing indistinct, misunderstands much that is spoken.

Itching in ears relieved by boring with the finger in ear.

Discharge of fetid pus from the ears.

Boil in the right ear, with pain when swallowing.

Thick oozing scurfs on the ears.

⁷ **Nose.** Scabby nostrils.

Nose stopped up, cannot breathe.

Watery coryza, with dizziness; on blowing the nose drops of blood come out.

Nosebleed during morning sleep, with vertigo.

⁸ **Face.** Alternating red and pale.

Cheeks hot, feel as if they would burst.

Convulsive motions of facial muscles, before asthma.

Pale swelling of cheek after toothache.

⁹ **Lower Face.** Lips cracked, in some places blistered.

Corners of the mouth sore.

Pale swelling of the upper lip.

Stitching like from a needle or splinter, in the lips.

¹⁰ **Teeth.** Scorbutic gums; bleed easily.

Tearing in the lower jaw anterior to the ears; glands under the jaw swollen and throbbing.

Violent drawing-aching in carious teeth, less in the air and in warmth; worse in the evening.

¹¹ **Tongue, etc.** Taste; putrid; bitter.

Stammering, stuttering speech.

Cutting pain in tongue, as with a knife, before asthma.

¹² **Mouth.** Numb feeling in the mouth.

Putrid smell from mouth.

Increased flow of saliva.

¹³ **Throat.** Burning in the throat.

Sore throat, with scratching and burning in œsophagus.

15

Great dryness in throat; when awaking in morning, Tongue feels almost like wood.

Stitching in the throat.

[14] **Desires. Aversions.** No appetite for breakfast, relish for other meals.

Hunger, even after meals.

Longing for cold drink.

No appetite for cooked food, desire for bread only.

[15] **Eating and Drinking.** A little wine intoxicates.

After eating: 16, 19.

[16] **Nausea and Vomiting.** Hiccoughing before and after dinner.

Frequent empty eructatians.

Nausea with shivering all forenoon.

Morning sickness, vomits only water; always relieved by taking breakfast.

[17] **Stomach.** Pressure and fulness in the pit of the stomach; tension in the temples; mental anguish.

Sensation as if a lump of ice lay in the stomach, with pain.

[18] **Hypochondria.** Stitches in region of last rib, either side.

[19] **Abdomen.** Cutting pains around navel.

Griping worse when at rest.

Stitches in the abdomen.

Cutting colic, with coldness, teeth chattering, limbs tremble; worse after stool.

Colic, with bright red urine; relieved by eating.

[20] **Stool, etc.** Disposition to diarrhœa, frequent attacks, each evacuation being followed by tenesmus; diarrhœa before and during menses.

Fruitless urging to stool.

Diarrhœa with cutting pains.

Stools first hard and difficult; last thin, even watery, with much pain in belly.

After stool, tenesmus and burning at the anus: the latter continues long after the watery stool.

Stinking flatus.

Itching in the rectum, as from worms.

Darting from the perineum to the rectum and genitals.

[21] **Urine.** Frequent desire to urinate, even immediately after urination.

Urine: bright red; with violent sediment.

In the urethra, stinging, itching, burning; orifice inflamed, feels glued up; hard node in the urethra.

[22] **Male Sexual Organs.** Seminal emissions.

After coition, reeling and contusion in the head.

Complaints from sexual excess.

[23] **Female Sexual Organs.** Voluptuous sensation in genitals.

Menses: every two weeks much dark and clotted blood;
too late; only at night, or only in the morning.

During the intervals, occasional show of blood.

Burning in the genitals.

Leucorrhœa: like the white of egg, a few days before or after
the menses; while walking; yellow-green, acrid, corrosive, leaving green spots on clothes; thick, slimy, tough.

Painful bearing down in vulva and weight in small of
back, after midnight.

[25] **Larynx.** Hoarseness in the morning.

Roughness in the throat, mornings, with catarrhal speech.

Scratching sensation in the larynx, with viscid phlegm.

[26] **Breathing.** Shortness of breath from every exertion with
the hands.

Oppression of chest, desires to loosen the clothes.

Spasmodic laughing and crying, with asthma, face dark red.

[37] **Cough.** Evening, loose; morning, dry.

Dry cough from tickling in throat.

Cough from tickling in the chest, mornings, after coming
into the room from cold air.

[28] **Lungs.** Stitches in various localities of chest.

[29] **Heart. Pulse.** Palpitation of heart, with tremor of hands.

Visible palpitation, after going up stairs; as if the heart
was working in water; after overexertion.

Pulse accelerated.

[31] **Neck. Back.** Stitches in the neck.

Stiffness of neck in the morning.

Backache, with stiffness after stooping.

Shooting and other pains between shoulders, along borders
of scapula; has to "straighten up" to be relieved.

Intolerable itching at tip of os coccygis; must scratch
until the parts become raw and sore.

[32] **Upper Limbs.** Stitching, boring and tearing pains.

Heaviness and powerlessness in arms and hands; drops
even light things from the hands.

Joints of arms and hands feel disabled and wrenched.

Itching on the arms.

Moist tetter on back of hand.

Whitlow on fingers.

[33] **Lower Limbs.** Sensation of soreness in the hip-joints.

Limbs "go to sleep," cannot stand on them.

Stitching pains in the knees.

Muscles of the calves feel too short, cramp in the morning.

Œdematous swelling of (right) foot even years after a sprain.

Violent stitching in outer malleolus of right foot, with
painfulness of the inner.

[34] **Limbs in General.** Great weakness of the joints.

Sensation: as if beaten; lame, aching; tearing; tension; stitches.

³⁵ **Position, etc.** Rest: 19. Exertion with hands: 26. Over-exertion: 29. Walking: 23. After ascending: 29. ¯On rising: 37. Standing: 33. Must straighten up: 31. Sitting: 3. Stooping: 31.

³⁶ **Nerves.** Rheumatic lameness.

General languor and enervation, particularly in the joints.

Drops things from the hands, as from weakness.

³⁷ **Sleep.** Spasmodic gaping before asthma, morning sweat in bed.

Great drowsiness in afternoon and early in evening.

Night rest disturbed by burning and itching of nettle-rash.

Restless sleep, with many anxious, frightful dreams.

On awaking head aches as from too much sleep; on rising, face pale.

³⁸ **Time.** Morning: 2, 7, 13, 16, 23, 25, 27, 21, 33, 37, 40, Fore-noon: 16. Afternoon: 37, 40. Evening: 10, 27, 37, 40. Night: 3, 23, 37, 40. After midnight: 23.

³⁹ **Temperature and Weather.** Warmth: 4, 10, 46. Hot weather: 46. Coming in room from cold air: 27. Open air: 10. Very sensitive to draughts.

⁴⁰ **Chill. Fever. Sweat.** Chill predominating, even near a warm stove, morning and evening, and even at night, generally with thirst.

Chill, with pains.

Shivering in the evening, spreading from the back; draw-ing pains in bowels.

Heat in evening, daily at 7 P. M.

Alternate shuddering and flying heat, most in afternoon with burning thirst, more with the shuddering.

Sweat every morning, 5–6 A. M.—most profuse on chest.

Sweat in axilla smells like onions.

⁴¹ **Attacks.** Full moon: 46.

⁴² **Sides.** First right, then left: 3. Right: 5, 4, 6, 33.

⁴⁴ **Tissues.** Ebullitions, with much thirst.

⁴⁵ **Contact, Injuries, etc.** Touch: 4. Scratching: 4, 31, 46. Boring in ear: 6.

Unusually deep impression on finger from using blunt instruments (as scissors or knife).

Sensitiveness to touch, pressure with hand is painful.

Cannot bear clothing.

⁴⁶ **Skin.** Urticaria covering nearly the whole body, some blotches nearly two inches in diameter; caused by tar.

Rash, pimples, with burning-itching.

Warts and corns, with shooting pains.

Itching on getting warm, continues after scratching.

Red, scabby eruption on thighs and bends of knees, ap-pears with hot weather and with full moon.

Moist or dry herpes; vesicles forming thick crusts.

Tetter on back of hand; after bright red pimples, rough, dark red, moist spots.

[47] **Stages and States.**   Old maids; palpitation.

Children: stammering.

[48] **Relationship.**   Where *Rhus tox.* seemed to be indicated, but did not relieve; urticaria: 46.

Bad consequence of external application of tar: 46.

Coffee disturbs action of *Bovist.*

Alum. followed *Bovist.* well in rheumatic pains after asthma.

Antidote to *Bovist.: Camphor.*

BROMIUM.

Bromine.   HERING.   *Elementary substance.*

[1] **Mind.**   In evening when alone, felt as if he would see something if he should turn around; as if some one were back of him.

Expects to see something jump around the floor.

Desire for mental labor, preceded by aversion to his own profession.

Crying and lamentations, with hoarse voice.

Great depression of spirits.

Low-spirited and out of humor.

[2] **Sensorium.**   Vertigo: if he puts his foot on a bridge; from sight of running water; worse in damp weather; with nausea and nosebleed; with tendency to fall backwards.

Sensation deep in brain, as if vertigo would come on, or as if he would lose his consciousness.

[3] **Inner Head.**   Headache; heavy pressure in forehead in heat of the sun, passes off when in the shade.

Left-sided headache.

Headache after drinking milk.

[4] **Outer Head.**   Pains in the bones of the head, fore and back part; towards evening in damp weather.

Crawling beneath the skin of the occiput.

Scalp tender; covered with an eruption, with dirty looking and offensive-smelling discharge.

[5] **Eyes.**   Sensitiveness to bright light.

Dilation of the pupils.

Lachrymation of right eye, with swelling of lachrymal gland.

Stitches through left eye.

Throbbing stitches in left upper lid, extending to brow,

forehead and left temple; worse on touching it and from motion; better during rest.

[6] **Ears.** Ringing in right ear. Roaring in ears.

Stitches in the ears. Discharge from the ears.

Throbbing and burning in ears, may be succeeded by burning through whole body.

Hard swelling of left parotid gland, feeling warm to touch.

Suppuration of left parotid, edges of the opening smooth; discharge watery and excoriating; swelling remaining hard and unyielding. θ After scarlatina.

[7] **Nose.** Coryza, with sneezing.

Severe coryza, right nostril stopped up and sore throughout; later the left.

Corrosive soreness on margins of nostrils and under the nose, with stoppage or with scurfs.

Nosebleed, with relief of chest and eye symptoms.

[8] **Face.** Face: pale, or red, or alternately so; bluish tinge turning purplish, with the cough in croup.

Greyish, earthy complexion.

Heat in cheeks, first in right, later in left.

Sensation as of spider-web on face.

[9] **Lower Face.** Boring pain going to the right, or on right side of lower jaw.

Shooting pain on vermillion border of upper lip; afterwards yellow spots, which open and discharge a yellow fluid.

Painless swelling of left submaxillary gland.

[10] **Teeth.** Decayed teeth, sensitive to cold water.

Gums pain in the morning.

[11] **Tongue, etc.** Taste: sweetish; salty; bitter; sour; acrid.

Water tastes salty, in the morning, fasting.

Dry sensation on the tongue.

Burning on the under surface of the tongue.

Stinging in the tip of the tongue.

[12] **Mouth.** Burning sensation in the mouth, œsophagus and stomach.

Mouth dry and parched.

Aphthæ, with affection of the eyes.

[13] **Throat.** Elongation of the uvula.

Scraping in the throat.

Swelling of mucous membrane of fauces and pharynx.

Tonsils swollen, inflamed; constant pain in the throat, swallowing difficult, fluids worse than solids. θ After measles.

Right side of fauces dark red and dry, swallowing painful.

[14] **Desires. Aversions.** Desires for acids, which aggravate the symptoms and cause diarrhœa.

Aversion to the customary tobacco smoking; it causes nausea and vertigo.

Aversion to drinking cold water.

¹⁵ **Eating and Drinking.** After eating oysters, diarrhœa; after acids, diarrhœa.

Gastric symptoms better from black coffee.

Nausea and pains in stomach, better after eating.

After breakfast: 25. After every meal: 20. Drinking milk: 3.

¹⁶ **Nausea and Vomiting.** Hiccough and nausea.

Eructations: empty; tasteless; tasting like foul eggs; with vomiting of mucus.

Nausea and retching, better after eating.

¹⁷ **Stomach.** Pressure in stomach, like from a stone.

Pain in the stomach increased by pressure.

¹⁸ **Hypochondria.** Stitches in the hypochondria; also from right to left.

¹⁹ **Abdomen.** Tympanitic distention of the abdomen and passage of much wind.

Griping and colicky pains.

²⁰ **Stool, etc.** Blind, painful hemorrhoids internally during and after stool; worse from cold or warm water; better from wetting with saliva.

Stools: painless, odorless, like scrapings from intestines; bright yellow, preceded by cutting and rumbling in abdomen; light yellow, slimy mucus; black fecal.

Diarrhœa: after every meal; at night.

Stool: hard, tough, brown and glistening; breaks to pieces like sheep dung.

²¹ **Urine.** Continued desire to urinate, with tickling sensation in tip of urethra.

Dribbling of urine, with burning, after urinating.

Urine: scanty and dark; turbid, and deposits a whitish sediment adhering to the vessel; leaves a red coating on vessel; contains large flakes of white mucus.

²² **Male Sexual Organs.** Increased sexual desire.

Nightly emission.

Hard, painless swelling of left testicle, painful when driving.

Coldness of left testicle.

²³ **Female Sexual Organs.** Dull, constant pain in left ovary.

Hard swelling in ovarian region.

Menses: too early and too profuse; bright red blood; passive flow with much exhaustion; membranous shreds may pass off.

Suppression of menses. θ Scirrhus mammæ.

Headache on appearance of menses.

Violent contractive spasm before or during menses, lasting hours; leaving the abdomen sore.

Loud emission of flatus from vagina.

Vagina painful, as if sore.

[24] **Pregnancy.** Hard, uneven tumor in right mamma, firmly adherent to its surroundings, with lancinating pains, worse at night.

[25] **Larynx.** Cold sensation in larynx, with cold feeling when inspiring, after breakfast; better after shaving.

Larynx painful to touch; constriction in larynx.

Scraping and rawness in larynx, provoking cough.

Contracted sensation internally, in the trachea, or feeling as if the pit of throat were pressed against the trachea.

Sensation of smoothness and emptiness, at a small spot in the larynx.

Voice: husky; hoarse, cannot speak clearly, loss of voice; weak and soft, with raw, scraped feeling in throat.

[26] **Breathing.** Gasping for breath, with wheezing and rattling in larynx, and spasmodic closure of glottis.

Deep, forcible inspiration, is necessary, from time to time.

Difficulty of breathing; cannot inspire deep enough.

Sensation as if the air-passages were full of smoke.

Asthma of sailors, as soon as they "go ashore."

Difficult breathing, must sit up in bed at night. Emphysema, rattling of mucus without choking.

[27] **Cough.** Excited by: tickling in larynx; scraping and rawness in larynx; deep inspiration.

Cough, with sudden paroxysms of suffocation, on swallowing; respiration very short; obliged to catch for breath.

Whooping-cough, with croupish hoarseness of the cough.

Cough night and day, sounds loose, but no expectoration; aggravation from exercise and on entering a warm room.

Sensation of constriction impedes respiration, with dry, tickling cough.

Much rattling in larynx when coughing.

[28] **Lungs.** Affections begin in bronchi and ascend to larynx.

Sensation of weakness and exhaustion in the chest.

Pressure in upper part of chest.

Sharp stitches in right side of chest, especially when walking rapidly.

Cutting pains running upwards. θ Phthisis.

❙ Right lung most affected.

Paralytic drawing pain through left chest, toward scapula and into left arm.

Hepatization of lower lobes in pneumonia.

[29] **Heart. Pulse.** Pulse much accelerated.

Violent palpitation of the heart in the evening, so that she cannot lie on the left side.

Cutting pains running upwards. θ Heart disease.

[30] **Outer Chest.** Pressure below left clavicle.

Tearing in left clavicle.

Stitch pain from mamma to the axilla, cannot bear pressure.

³¹ **Neck. Back.** Stiffness of neck.
Tearing in right lumbar and dorsal muscles, increased by moving these parts.
Sore pain in small of back, unchanged by motion.
³² **Upper Limbs.** Great restlessness and jactitation of arms.
Left arm feels paralyzed.
Weakness of the arms.
Tearing in the arms, especially in hands and fingers.
Icy-cold forearms or only cold hands.
³³ **Lower Limbs.** Pressive bone-pain in left leg.
Boring pains in one or both tibiæ.
³⁵ **Position, etc.** Rest: 5. Motion: 5, 31. Walking: 28.
Riding horseback gives general relief. Exercise: 27, 40.
Exertion: 40. Driving: 22. Must sit up: 26. Cannot lie on left side: 29.
³⁶ **Nerves.** Tremulousness all over; great languor and debility.
³⁷ **Sleep.** Continued yawning with the respiratory troubles; child yawns frequently, and is drowsy.
Awakes unrefreshed; it seems impossible to rise.
Dreams: vivid; of ascending a height; of climbing a steep; of journeyings; of quarrels; of dying; of coffins and funerals.
Jumping up, out of sleep, with whistling breathing.
Starts from sleep with cough, drink relieves it.
³⁸ **Time.** Morning: 10, 11. Evening: 1, 4, 29. Night: 20, 22, 24, 27. Every other night: 40. Day and night: 27.
³⁹ **Temperature and Weather.** Heat of sun: 3. Entering warm room: 27. Damp weather: 2, 4. Warm water: 20. Cold water: 10, 14, 20. Wetting with saliva: 20. "On shore:" 26.
⁴⁰ **Chill. Fever. Sweat.** Chill every other day, with shaking, yawning and stretching, and with cold feet.
Hands cold and moist.
Internal burning heat, like between the skin and flesh.
Sweat on the palms.
Sweat from the least exertion or exercise.
⁴¹ **Attacks.** Periodical pains.
⁴² **Sides.** Right: 5, 6, 7, 9, 13, 24, 28, 31. Left: 3, 5, 6, 7, 9, 22, 23, 28, 29, 30, 32, 33. Right to left: 7, 8, 18. Left to right: 9. Below upwards; 28, 29, 30.
⁴⁴ **Tissues.** Swelling and induration of the glands.
Enlargement of thyroid, in persons with light hair, blue eyes and fair skin.
⁴⁵ **Contact, Injuries, etc.** Touch: 5, 25. Pressure: 17, 30. Shaving: 25.
⁴⁶ **Skin.** Tickling, itching, prickling and stitches in the skin, at various places.

Pimples and pustules.

Boils on the arms and in the face.

[47] **Stages and States.** Acts better, though not exclusively in persons with light hair and blue eyes.

Increased embonpoint.

[48] **Relationship.** *Bromium* follows *Spongia* well, in croup. Antidote: *Amm. carb.*

BRYONIA ALBA.

White Bryony.   HAHNEMANN.   *Curcurbitaceæ.*

[1] **Mind.**   Patient desires to go home.

Great depression and very morose mood, without cause.

Anxiety, worse in room, better in open air; fears not to have the wherewithal to live.

Irritable mood, wishes to be alone.   Very irritable; inclined to fright, fear and vexation.

Obstinate and passionate.   Bad effects from violence and anger.

[2] **Sensorium.**   Pressing outward in frontal region and left eyeball, especially on stooping.

Headache worse by so slight a motion as moving eyelids.

Confusion of head, especially of forehead.

Benumbed, stupid from suppressed eruptions.

Head confused and aching, as after a night's dissipation; does not wish to rise in morning on awakening.

Confusion in head, with drawing in occiput, extending into neck before going to sleep.

Vertigo: as though all objects were reeling; as though the brain were turning around; as if the head were turning in a circle; on rising, or on raising the head; with reeling backward; better from cold.

Great heaviness of head and pressure of brain forwards.

Pressure in the head, as if the brain were too full and pressed outward, mostly when sitting.

Rush of blood to the head.

[3] **Inner Head.**   Headache commences in morning, not on waking, but when first opening eyes.

Pressive pain above left eye, followed by dull, pressive pain in occipital protuberances, thence spreading over whole body; on quick motion, and after eating, pain so severe that it seemed a distinct pulsation within head.

Digging pressure in forepart of brain toward forehead, especially severe on stooping and walking rapidly; walking fatigues him very much.

Tearing across the forehead, then in cervical muscles, then in right arm.

Drawing, tearing pain in right temple, mostly extending to upper molars and muscles of neck.

Throbbing ache on top of head, morning when waking.

Continued stitch deep in the brain, on 'left side, when coughing.

Headache in occiput, extending to shoulders, while lying on the back, in bed, after waking in the morning.

Pressive pain in occiput, drawing down into neck, relieved toward noon.

Headache as though the head would burst, commencing in morning and gradually increasing till evening.

⁴ **Outer Head.**   In the morning the head seems very greasy, with cool head.

Scalp very tender to touch; cannot bear even a soft brush.

Dandruff, rough and uneven.

⁵ **Eyes.**   Very sensitive pressive pain (coming and going) in left eyeball, especially violent on moving the ball with a feeling as if eye became smaller and was retracted within the orbit.

Severe burning and lachrymation of right eye.

Eyeballs so painful that the patient cannot bear to have them touched.

Puffiness of right upper lid.

Painless twitching-drawing together in left upper lid, with a persistent sensation of heaviness therein.

Frequent lachrymation.

⁶ **Ears.**   Intolerance of noise.

Chirping in the head, as from locusts.

Ringing; roaring; humming in the ears.

Swelling, redness, painful sensitiveness and heat of external right ear; at times piercing stitches deep into ear accompanied by swelling and painfulness of right parotid gland.

⁷ **Nose.**   Frequent sneezing.

Nosebleed in morning after rising; less frequently during day; but sometimes during sleep, about 3 A. M.; vicarious: 23.

Fluent coryza, watery or greenish.

Catarrh extending to the frontal sinuses or into chest.

Swelling of tip of nose, with twitching pain in it, and on touch feeling as if it would ulcerate.   Boils.

⁸ **Face.**   Hot, red, soft puffiness of the face.   Erysipelas begins on upper lip and nasal septum.

Face bluish-red, with difficult inspiration.

Pinching pressure in articular cavity of right jaw, more violent on motion.

Twitching, tearing in right malar bone up to right temple, externally, sore to touch.

⁹ **Lower Face.**   Upper lip and nose swollen, red and hot.

Crack in the lower lip.

Lips parched and cracked; he wishes frequently to moisten them.

Lips swollen, rough.

Constant motion of mouth, as if chewing. *θ* In brain affections of children.

¹⁰ **Teeth.**   Teeth seem too long.

Toothache relieved by cold water, aggravated by taking anything warm in mouth.

Tearing, stitching toothache while eating, extending to muscles of neck, aggravated by warmth.

Jerking toothache when smoking.

¹¹ **Tongue, etc.**   Taste: flat, insipid; sweetish; bitter (which cold drinks relieve); offensive, bitter; has no taste for food; when not eating mouth is bitter.

Tongue coated white.

Tongue rough, cracked, and often of a dark brown color.

Dryness of tongue; tip moist.

Several small blisters on tip of tongue.

¹² **Mouth.**   Collection of much soapy, frothy saliva.

Mouth and lips very dry; only momentarily relieved by drinking.

Lower lip dry, burning and sensitive; especially in smokers.

Dryness in mouth, without thirst, or with thirst for large quantities of water.

Offensive smell from mouth, with hawking of offensive, tough mucus, sometimes in round cheesy lumps, the size of a pea.

¹³ **Throat.**   Dryness of throat; dry and raw, on empty swallowing.

A sort of scraping and roughness in the throat posteriorly.

Pain and difficulty on swallowing, as if a hard body was in throat.

Pressive pain in right tonsil.

Slight pain in left tonsil.

Back of throat seems swollen.

Stitch in the throat when swallowing.

Tough mucus in the fauces, loosened by hawking.

¹⁴ **Desires.   Aversions.**   Too great appetite; appetite soon satisfied.

Desires things, immediately, which when offered are refused.

Great desire for oysters and sweets; for coffee.

No appetite for milk; but if he takes it the appetite returns and he begins to relish it; loss of appetite.

Great thirst, desire for large quantities of cold water; also for warm drinks, which relieve.

Great thirst, with longing for wine.

[15] **Eating and Drinking.**   After eating: 3, 16, 17, 20, 27.

Eats little and often.

Drinking: 12, 26, 27.   Wine: 16.

Frequent drinking of cold water relieved the bitter taste and inclination to vomit.

[16] **Nausea and Vomiting.**   Hiccough after eating, and on every shock caused by it pressure in forehead, as if the brain shook from behind forwards.

Eructations after eating; sourish, bitter.

Heart-burn from wine, evenings.

Nausea on assuming an erect position.

Nausea, increased or brought on by the slightest motion; must lie quiet.

Nausea and vomiting in morning when waking.

Vomiting: of solid food, not of drink; of food, immediately after eating; of bitter, musty or putrid liquid, which leaves a similar taste in the mouth.

[17] **Stomach.**   Stomach full, and sensitive to pressure.

Distention of the stomach, and eructations of wind.

Stomach distended, with vomiting after eating.

Feeling of emptiness of the stomach, with distention of the whole abdomen.

Painfulness of stomach after eating oysters and chicken-salad in evening; pain excessive when in motion, perfeet relief from quiet or from eructations of wind or passing wind per anum.

Pressure in the stomach, after eating, like from a stone, makes him fretful.

Epigastric region painful to touch; so sensitive cannot endure the clothes.

Cutting as with knives in epigastric region.

Soreness in pit of stomach when coughing.

Stitching pain in region of stomach, worse from motion, especially from a misstep.

[18] **Hypochondria.**   Tensive pain below false ribs in right hypochondrium, especially sensitive on deep inspiration; even a little flatus causes pain in the liver.

Transient stitches in right hypochondrium, with painful sensitiveness of this region to hard pressure or deep inspiration.

Burning and stitching pain in hepatic region.

Stitches in region of spleen, worse motion.

[19] **Abdomen.**   Griping pains about the navel.

Rumbling and gurgling in the bowels.

Sudden painful cuttings in the intestines, with a feeling

as though one were digging him with the fingers, compelling him to bend double, relieved by profuse pasty evacuations.

Great sensitiveness of abdomen.

Pain in abdomen flying upwards.

Stitches and other pain in the abdomen, which hinder respiration.

[20] **Stools, etc.** Diarrhœa: bilious, acrid stools, with soreness of anus; like dirty water, with whitish granulated sediment of undigested food; urging followed by copious pasty evacuations, with relief of all symptoms excepting confusion of head; mostly at night or after eating; after eating fruit or sour-krout; morning, after getting up, preceded by cutting pains in bowels; burning, worse in warm weather.

Alternation of diarrhœa and constipation.

Obstinate constipation; stools very dry, large and hard; only after much straining.

Stinking flatulence

Aching hemorrhoids.

Hard, black and dry stool, as if burnt, and rather scanty.

[21] **Urine.** Urine: copious and pale; scanty and dark; brown, like beer; red; deposits white sediment.

During motion, some drops of urine pass out of the urethra without sensation.

[22] **Male Sexual Organs.** Increased sexual desire.

Stitches in the right testicle and spermatic cord.

[23] **Female Sexual Organs.** Stitching pain in the ovaries, on deep inspiration.

Severe pain in region of right ovary, like from a sore spot, causing an irritation and dragging, pain extended down to the thighs, while at rest; pain aggravated by touch.

Hemorrhage of dark red blood, with pain in small of back.

Menses: too early, too profuse; blood dark; suppressed, with frequent bleeding of the nose.

Membranous dysmenorrhœa.

Hard black pustule on a swollen portion of left labium.

Dropsy of uterus, the swelling increases during the day and diminishes at night.

[24] **Pregnancy.** After-pains excited by least motion, even taking a deep inspiration.

Lochia too profuse, with burning pain in region of womb.

Suppression of lochia, with sensation as if head would burst.

Drawing or lancinating pains from hip to foot, worse from touch or motion.

Mammæ feel heavy; pale, but hard and painful; tensive burning and tearing pain.

Flow of milk suppressed; scanty secretion of milk.

(Infant) sore mouth; child does not like to take hold of breast, but after mouth becomes moistened it nurses well.

²⁵ **Larynx.**   Voice rough and hoarse.

Tickling in larynx.

Tough mucus in trachea, loosened only after frequent hawking.

²⁶ **Breathing.**   Respiration: impeded; quick and deep, without motion of the ribs, better in cold air and from drinking cold water.

Frequent desire to take a full inspiration, which, however, cannot be done in consequence of a feeling as if there was something should expand but would not.

²⁷ **Cough.**   Hacking, dry cough from the upper part of trachea.

Dry cough: with sticking pain under the sternum; as if coming from the stomach; with a crawling and tickling in pit of stomach.

Sensation as if the head and chest would fly to pieces on coughing.

Cough, with constant crawling, upwards, in the throat, followed by expectoration of mucus.

Cough compels the patient to spring up in bed involuntarily and immediately; or, to press hand on sternum.

Cough worse after eating or drinking, with vomiting of ingesta; worse coming into a warm room.

Nausea excites cough, and coughing often excites vomiting.

Expectoration of mucus streaked with blood.

²⁸ **Lungs.**   Constriction of chest; felt the need of breathing deeply; when attempting to breathe deeply, pain in chest.

Stitch in upper part of chest, through the shoulders, on inspiring.

Chest very sensitive, with stitches in left side, on inspiration.

Sensation of heaviness beneath sternum, extending towards the right shoulder, impeding respiration; deep inspiration was difficult; oppression of right side of chest, with very fine, extremely severe stitches in the right axillary gland.

Stitches in the sternum on coughing; was obliged to hold the chest with the hand.

Sharp pain in left inframammary region; worse during inspiration.

Sharp stitching pain in chest, below right nipple, extending outward, only on expiration.

Short but violent stitches in right side of chest, so that must hold the breath and cannot cry out.

Tearing stitches in left side of chest extend from behind forward, are better during rest, worse during motion and on deep inspiration.

Stitching pain in region of diaphragm, worse from motion or coughing.

[29] **Heart. Pulse.** Oppression in the region of the heart.

Stitching pain in the region of the heart.

Cramp in region of heart, aggravated by walking, raising one's self, or using slightest exertion, even raising arm.

Heart beats violently and rapidly.

Pulse: full, hard, rapid and tense; at times intermittent, with strong orgasm of blood.

[30] **Outer Chest.** Painful spot, as from a bruise, on the second rib of the right side, extending to the sternum.

[31] **Neck. Back.** Pain in nape of back, as after taking cold.

Painful stiffness of muscles of right side of neck, on moving the head.

Dull stitches between the scapulæ, extending from behind forward, in the afternoon while lying.

Pain in the small of the back: which makes walking or turning difficult; as if bruised, when lying on it.

[32] **Upper Limbs.** Painful tension and pressure in the right shoulder, when at rest.

Painful pressure on the top of right shoulder, worse upon touch; on deep breathing it becomes a dull stitching, which extends downwards and outwards to shoulder-joint.

Drawing and tearing pains in the right upper arm.

Swelling of right elbow-joint, with stitches.

Tearing pains on inner surface of forearm, on a line from the elbow to the wrist.

Pain in wrists, as if wrenched or sprained, on every motion.

Fine stitches in wrists, if the hands become warm, and during rest; they do not disappear on motion.

Rather hot pale swelling in last joint of little finger, with sticking in it on moving the finger, or on pressing it.

On writing or taking hold of anything, a sensation as if the finger-joints were swollen and puffed; they are painful on much exertion and on touch.

* Stitching pain in the fingers when writing.

[33] **Lower Limbs.** Legs so weak they scarcely will hold him.

Stabbing pain in the hips.

Great weariness in the thighs, worse going up steps.

Great painfulness of right thigh; the pain comes from the head of femur, extends along the anterior surface of thigh to knee.

Knees totter and knock together when walking.

Pain in right knee, so that in evening he could scarcely walk, and was obliged to keep the leg very quite; inner side of knee very painful to touch.

Pinching, tearing in right calf.

Bruised pain on outer side of left calf, on moving and
turning the foot, as also from touch; during rest a
numb sensation in this place.

Tension in ankles on motion.

Feet are tense and swollen in the evening; pain in feet,
as if sprained.

When walking, a prickling sensation like "pins and
needles" is felt in the soles of the feet, which hinders or
prevents walking.

Hot swelling of the instep, with bruised pain on stretching
out the foot.

Tensive pain on the back of the feet, even when sitting.

³⁴ **Limbs in General.** Heaviness in the limbs; seem like lead.

Weariness and stiffness of limbs, especially the lower.

Rheumatism, with redness and swelling of joints.

Weakness of the limbs obliges him to sit.

³⁵ **Position, etc.** 23, 28, 32, 33. Motion: 39, 16, 17, 24, 28,
32, 33, 36, 44; of eyeball: 5. Walking: 3, 29, 31, 33,
36, 40. Misstep: 18. Exertion: 29, 32. Ascending
stairs: 33. Sitting: 2, 33, 34. Rising: 2, 29, 36.
Stooping: 3. Lying: 31; on back: 3.

³⁶ **Nerves.** Very tired and prostrated; great weariness.

Great weakness and exhaustion, worse from walking.

Sudden prostration, shunning all motion.

Faintness: when rising from bed; from slightest motion.

Spasm developed through repercussion of measles.

³⁷ **Sleep.** Frequent yawning, the whole day.

Much sleepiness during the day.

Sleeplessness on account of uneasiness in the blood and
anxiety; the thoughts crowd upon one another.

Night very restless, disturbed by frightful dreams; frequent waking.

No sleep before midnight, on account of a frequent shivering sensation over one arm and foot, followed by sweat.

Starts in affright before falling asleep.

Motion of the lower jaw, during sleep, as in masticating.

Somnambulism.

Dreams: about household affairs; about business of the
day; of dispute and vexation; anxious.

³⁸ **Time.** Morning: 1, 3, 4, 7, 16, 20, 40, 43. Noon: 3. Afternoon: 31. Evening: 16, 33, 40. Night: 20, 37, 40.
Before midnight: 37. 3 A.M.: 7. Increases morning
till eve: 3. Increases by day, decreases during the
night: 23. Day: 7, 23, 37.

³⁹ **Temperature and Weather.** Better in cold weather and
from taking cold food.

Facial neuralgia relieved by cold applications.

Cold water: 10, 14, 15, 26. Cold air: 26, 40. Warmth:

16

10, 32. Warm weather: 20. Coming into a warm
room: 27. Room: 1, 40. Open air: 1, 40.

Complaints on the first warm days.

⁴⁰ **Chill. Fever. Sweat.** Chill: with external coldness of
body; and chilliness, frequently with heat of head, red
cheeks and thirst; and coldness, mostly in the evening,
and frequently only of the right side ; worse in the room
than in the open air.

Dry, burning heat, mostly only internal, the blood seems
to burn in the veins.

Great aggravation of sufferings during the heat.

Sweat in short spells and only on single parts.

Profuse and easily excited sweat, even when slowly walking in cold open air ; profuse night and morning sweat.

Sour or oily sweat.

⁴² **Sides.**   Right: 3, 5, 6, 8, 13, 18, 22, 23, 28, 30, 31, 32, 33, 40.
Left: 3, 5, 13, 23, 28, 33.   Right to left: 30.   Left to
right: 28.   Behind forward: 16, 28, 21.   Above downward: 23, 24, 32, 33.

⁴³ **Sensations.**   Every spot in the body is painful to pressure;
worse mornings.

Drawing, rheumatic pains in various parts of the body.

Transient drawing and tension in almost all the limbs
and joints.

⁴⁴ **Tissues.**   Dropsical swellings, which gradually increase as
the day progresses, and disappear during the night.

In acute abscess, promotes resorption of pus.

Large abscess at pit of stomach after a blow.

Stitches in the joints, on motion and on touch.

Bone inflamed, sensitive, tense, slightly swollen integuments; in the beginning.

⁴⁵ **Contact, Injuries, etc.**   Touch: 4, 7, 8, 17, 23, 24, 32, 33,
43, 44.   Pressure: 17, 18, 32, 43.   After a blow: 44.

Pain relieved by hard pressure.   θ Facial neuralgia.

⁴⁶ **Skin.**   Yellow skin of the whole body, even of the face.

Red, round, hot spot on the cheek over the malar bone.

Dry, itching eruption over the whole body.

Rash, peculiar to lying-in women and their infants.

Red, elevated, rash-like eruption over the whole body.

Nettle-rash or other eruptions characterized by sensation
of prickling, particularly when the parts are touched.

Slow development of rash in eruptive fevers; or, sudden
receding of rash, with difficult respiration, or inflammatory affections of chest.

Erysipelas when confined to the joints.

When scarlatinal eruption delays, or suddenly recedes;
dropsy, pleuritis or meningitis.

⁴⁸ **Relationship.**   *Bryon.* is frequently suitable after *Acon.,
Nux vom., Opium, Rhus tox.*

After *Bryon.* are frequently indicated *Alum.*, *Kali carb.*,
Nux vom., *Phosphor.*, *Pulsat.*, *Rhus tox.*, *Sulphur.*

Antidotes to *Bryon.*: *Acon.*, *Alum.*, *Camphor.*, *Chamom.*,
Clemat., *Coffea*, *Ignat.*, *Mur. ac.*, *Nux vom.*, *Pulsat.*,
Rhus tox., *Seneg.*

Bryon. antidotes: *Rhus tox.*, *Rhus ven.*, Chlorine.

Conjunctive relation: *Coloc.*

Compare: *Arctium lappa* (muscular pains, dull, heavy,
worse motion; sleepiness, fatigue).

CACTUS GRANDIFLORUS.

Night blooming Cereus.   RUBINI.   *Cactaceæ.*

[1] **Mind.**   Taciturn, unwilling to speak a word, or to answer.
Cries, knows not why; consolation aggravates.
Unconquerable sadness.
Fear of death; he believes his disease incurable.
Hypochondriacal.

[2] **Sensorium.**   Vertigo from congestion; face red, bloated,
pulsation in the brain; madness, anxiety.

[3] **Inner Head.**   Congestion to the brain, bloodshot eyes,
coma, suffocation, flushes in face; fever, from exposure
to sun's rays.
Heavy pain on the vertex, better by pressure, but worse
from talking or strong light.
Pulsation in temples, as if the skull would burst; intolerable at night.
Headache worse right side, caused by excitement, as at
opera; wine; belated dinner.

[5] **Eyes.**   Dimness of the sight; weakness of sight returning
periodically.

[6] **Ears.**   Hardness of hearing from congestion; pulsation in
the ears; noise like running water or buzzing, after
otitis from checked sweat.

[7] **Nose.**   Profuse nosebleed, soon ceasing.

[8] **Face.**   Face: blue; cold sweat; pale; flushed.
Prosopalgia right-sided, chronic; worse from slightest
exertion, tolerable only when lying still in bed; brought
on by wine, music, strong light, or missing dinner at
the usual hour.

[12] **Mouth.**   Fetid breath in the morning.

[13] **Throat.**   Constriction of throat, exciting a constant desire to
swallow.

Constriction of the œsophagus; must drink large quantities to force the fluid into the stomach.

¹⁴ **Desires. Aversions.** Loss of appetite.

¹⁵ **Eating and Drinking.** After eating, weight and distress in the stomach.

After dinner, pulsation (in cœliac axis) behind stomach.

¹⁶ **Nausea and Vomiting.** Nausea in the morning, continues all day.

Acrid, sour fluid, rising into the throat and mouth, making food taste acid.

Vomiting of blood.

¹⁷ **Stomach.** Constrictive feeling at the scrobiculus cordis, extending to the hypochondria, impeding breathing.

Burning; pulsating in the stomach.

¹⁸ **Hypochondria.** Engorgement of liver; acute or chronic from heart disease.

Feeling as of a cord tightly tied around lower part of chest; marking out the attachments of the diaphragm.

Sharp pains shooting through diaphragm and up into chest.

¹⁹ **Abdomen.** Insupportable heat in abdomen, as though something burned him internally.

Wandering pains in the umbilical region, which cease and recur periodically.

²⁰ **Stool, etc.** Morning diarrhœa, preceded by great pain.

Sensation of weight in anus, strong desire for stool, but nothing passes.

Pricking in anus, as from pins, ceasing on slight friction.

²¹ **Urine.** Constant desire to urinate.

Urine: profuse, straw-colored; passes in drops, with much burning; constriction of neck of bladder; suppressed in fever.

Hæmaturia; urination prevented by clots.

²³ **Female Sexual Organs.** Menses too soon; black, pitch-like.

Menstruation with constrictive spasm of uterus; pains agonizing, worse evening; flow scanty, ceases when lying down.

Painful constriction around the pelvis, extending gradually towards the stomach, causing a sensation as of a great blow in the region of kidneys, making her cry out.

Pulsating pain in ovarian regions; pains extend down thighs, return periodically at the same time each day.

²⁴ **Pregnancy.** Inflammation of the mammæ: sensation of fulness in the chest; oversensitive to cold air.

²⁵ **Larynx.** Voice low, hoarse; constriction of the chest.

²⁶ **Breathing.** Oppression of breathing on going up stairs.

Oppression of the chest, as from a great weight, difficult breathing; uneasiness, as if an iron band prevented normal motion of chest.

[27] **Cough.** Spasmodic cough, with copious mucous expectoration.

Cough, with thick yellow sputa, like boiled starch.

[28] **Lungs.** Hæmoptysis, with marked arterial excitement (but less fever and restlessness than *Acon.*); convulsive cough.

Bronchitis, with palpitation of the heart; bronchial catarrh, from overaction of the heart.

Continual rattling of mucus; oppressed breathing; cannot lie in a horizontal position; attacks of anxiety and suffocation.

Pricking pains in chest, bloody sputa; hard, quick, vibrating pulse; sharp, wandering pains in chest and scapular region.

Feeling of constriction in the chest, impeding speech.

Congestion to the chest, which prevents lying down; palpitation; constriction of the chest.

[29] **Heart. Pulse.** Sensation of constriction in heart, as if an iron hand prevented its normal movements.

Pricking pains impeding breathing and movements of the body; oppression; cannot lie on the left side; blue face; pulse quick, throbbing, tense and hard.

Dull, heavy pain, worse from pressure; suffocating respiration; face blue; œdema, especially of the left hand and of the legs to the knees; feet icy-cold; pulse intermittent.

Pains in the apex of the heart shooting down left arm to the ends of the fingers; feeble pulse; dyspnœa.

Endocardial murmurs; excessive impulse; increased precordial dulness, enlarged right ventricle.

Palpitation with vertigo, loss of consciousness, dyspnœa; worse walking, at night, lying on the left side, at the approach of the menses and from any exertion.

Palpitation preceded by rumbling in the stomach.

Palpitation of long standing, caused by an unfortunate love affair.

Irregularity of the heart's action, at times frequent, at others slow; great irritation of the cardiac nerves; enlarged left ventricle.

[30] **Outer Chest.** Sensation of constriction in the middle of the sternum, as if compressed by iron pincers, with difficult breathing; worse from motion.

Rheumatism of the muscles of the chest.

[32] **Upper Limbs.** Formication and weight in the arms.

Œdema of the hands, mostly of the left.

[33] **Lower Limbs.** Restlessness of legs, cannot keep them still.

Œdema of legs, skin shining; dents remain a long time.

[35] **Position, etc.** Motion: 30. Walking: 29. Ascending: 26. Exertion: 8, 29. Lying: 8, 23. Cannot lie: 40; horizontally: 28; on left side: 29.

[36] **Nerves.** General weakness, prostration, great depression, sleepless. Fainting.

[37] **Sleep.** Sleepless without cause; or from pulsations in pit of stomach or in ears.

Delirium at night; on awaking it ceases, but returns in sleep.

[38] **Time.** Morning: 12, 16, 20. Evening: 23, 26. Night: 3, 29, 37. 11 A. M. and 11 P. M.: 40.

[39] **Temperature and Weather.** Exposure to sun: 3, 40. Cold air: 24.

[40] **Chill. Fever. Sweat.** Coldness in back and cold hands.

Chill not relieved by covering; returns the same hour each day; regular paroxysms at 11 A. M. and 11 P. M.

Fever, intermittent, with congestion to head, flushes in face, suppressed urine, pains in bladder, lancinating in heart, violent vomiting; sweat does not appear; after exposure to sun.

Heat after chill, with dyspnœa, headache and thirst; with insensibility till midnight, then shortness of breath and inability to remain lying; followed by profuse sweat, with great thirst.

[41] **Attacks.** Returning periodically: 5, 19, 23, 40.

[42] **Sides.** Right: 3, 8, 29. Left: 32.

Skin symptoms, lower left to upper right; then lower right to upper left.

[43] **Sensations.** Whole body feels as if caged, each wire being twisted tighter and tighter.

[44] **Tissues.** Organic diseases of the heart.

Dropsical affections.

[45] **Contact, Injuries, etc.** Pressure: 3, 39. Friction: 20.

[46] **Skin.** Dry, scaly herpes without itching; appeared first on left inner malleolus, next on outer side of right elbow; then on right inner malleolus, last on outer side of left elbow.

[48] **Relationship.** Antidotes to *Cactus: Acon., Camphor., Cinchon.* Compare: *Acon.* (in hemorrhages, cardiac excitement, etc., but later more anguish and restlessness); *Magnolia grand.* (heart); *Convallaria maj.* (heart).

CALADIUM.

Caladium Seguinum.   •   HERING.   *Araceæ.*

[1] **Mind.** Unconsciousness or coma.

Delirious, unintelligible murmuring.

Aversion to the medicine; required a desperate effort to overcome it.

Mind depressed.

Very carful about his health; apprehensive.

Lascivious ideas.

Restless, cannot control himself after smoking.

After mental exertion, fainting.

Forgetfulness.

[2] **Sensorium.** Vertigo, with nausea, mornings, also with stitches in pit of stomach.

Rocking, dizzy sensation, after lying down and closing the eyes, preventing sleep.

[3] **Inner Head.** Headache, left side, most in forehead and occiput.

Forehead: pressure after smoking; bursting pain; boring.

Drawing in occiput; drawing-tearing up into the head.

Heavy pressing pain after siesta.

Heat rises from below into the head; turns to an internal glowing; periodical heat of head.

[4] **Outer Head.** Left half of head feels as if asleep.

Pimples on the scalp, behind the ear, sensitive to touch.

[5] **Eyes.** Eyes feel too large and are inflamed.

Burning in the eyes.

Eyes close, even while walking in open air, with drowsiness before dinner.

Stitches in the eyes.

[6] **Ears.** Sensitive to noise; the slightest noise startles from sleep.

Earache during the fever.

Burning of upper margin of auricle.

Throbbing and formication around the right ear.

[7] **Nose.** Sudden burning in nose, as from pepper, finally sneezing and fluent coryza.

Discharge of blood and mucus when blowing the nose.

Painful pimples on right side of septum.

[8] **Face.** Heat in the face.

Sensation as if a spider web were sticking here and there.

Flies are attracted to the face and head.

[9] **Lower Face.** Lying with mouth half open, coma, in typhus.

[10] **Teeth.** Drawing: in left molars; from right ear to the teeth.

Boring toothache.

¹¹ **Tongue, etc.** Taste: insipid; herbaceous.

Tongue swollen.

¹² **Mouth.** Burning in the mouth and fauces.

¹³ **Throat.** Scratching sensation in throat as from something sharp, or with dry sensation and much hawking.

Dryness and burning in throat.

Fauces and pharynx dry, not the mouth.

Hawking phlegm and vomiting, after smoking.

¹⁴ **Desires. Aversions.** Thirst and want of appetite, before coma.

Thirstless, even aversion to cold water; drinks only warm drinks.

Drinks hastily on arousing from coma.

Eats, but without hunger.

¹⁵ **Eating and Drinking.** Cold water: 14. Warm drink: 14. Drink: 17. After eating: 26.

¹⁶ **Nausea and Vomiting.** Frequent eructations, of very little wind, as if the stomach were full of dry food.

Nausea, with stitches in the pit of stomach; with hollow feeling in the stomach and faintness.

Acrid, sour vomit, makes the teeth feel too long.

¹⁷ **Stomach.** Fluttering, as from a bird, in the stomach, causes nausea.

Fine, jerking stitches in pit of stomach, which is drawn inwards with each stitch, worse sitting; causes weakness and nausea.

Burning in stomach not relieved by drink.

Cutting, as with glass, in the pit of stomach and in the left flank; preventing sleep after midnight.

Throbbing and heaviness in pit of stomach after walking.

¹⁸ **Hypochondria.** Stitching, pressure and dull pressing jerks in region of spleen.

¹⁹ **Abdomen.** Throbbing mostly above and to right of navel.

Spasmodic cutting below the navel; must bend double.

Abdomen sore to touch, as if beaten, after the cough.

Burning in the hypogastric region.

²⁰ **Stool, etc.** Scanty, putrid-smelling flatus, in the evening.

Stools: soft, yellow; soft, afterwards of thin red blood.

²¹ **Urine.** Sensation of fulness in the bladder, region of bladder sore to pressure.

Stinging deep in the hypogastrium.

Violent pain during urination.

Urine: offensive; with sediment.

²² **Male Sexual Organs.** Sexual desire with relaxed penis, or painful erections without desire.

Impotence, with mental depression.

Glans: very red, covered with fine red points; dry, with desire to rub it.

Prepuce much swollen at the margin, sore and painful.
Parts larger, as if puffed, relaxed and sweating.
Swelling of scrotum.
Pimples on the mons veneris.

[23] **Female Sexual Organs.** Pruritus vaginæ; induces onanism; during pregnancy.

[25] **Larynx.** Larynx and trachea seem to be constricted; impedes deep breathing.

[26] **Breathing.** Breathes in sighing jerks, during unconsciousness and great heat.

Asthma: great oppression, could scarcely get his breath; feels as if mucus would cause suffocation, but without anxiety; attacks after eating, or after siesta; when the rash on the forearm disappears; in alteration with rash on chest.

[27] **Cough.** Sudden and involuntary, caused by an irritation high up in the throat; it is a half cough, half moan.

Cough: weak; toneless; panting, preventing sleep at night.

[28] **Lungs.** Stitches in chest; to left of sternum; in right side with anxiety, better lying on right, worse lying on left side.

[29] **Heart. Pulse.** Pulse: hard and bounding in intermittents; very frequent, hardly to be felt in typhus.

[30] **Outer Chest.** Rash on the chest.

[31] **Neck. Back.** Rheumatic pain between the shoulders; can hardly turn in bed.

Sacral region and back feel bruised, morning when rising.

[32] **Upper Limbs.** Pain in the shoulder, with headache.

Arms "asleep" on waking in the morning.

Pricking in palms, like from pins and needles, has to rub them hard, toward evening, lasting till sleep.

Rash on forearm.

[33] **Lower Limbs.** Furuncle on buttock, pained severely when sitting.

Left knee: throbbing pain when lying, evenings; as if being forced asunder; cracks on stepping and impedes walking.

Sticking and stitching in corns on left little toe.

[34] **Limbs in General.** Limbs weak, cannot get out of bed.

Feels as if beaten in all the joints, heaviness in the limbs, mornings.

[35] **Position, etc.** Walking: 5, 17, 33. Stepping: 33. Rising: 31. Sitting: 17, 33. Can hardly turn: 31. Lying down: 2, 33. Better lying on right, worse lying on left side: 28.

[36] **Nerves.** Lies unconscious; with single jerks, sometimes affecting the whole body.

[37] **Sleep.** Sleep disturbed by every slight noise, even rattling of paper.

Starting in sleep, moaning and groaning.

[38] **Time.** Morning: 2, 31, 32, 34. Evening: 20, 32, 33, 40. Night: 27. Before midnight: 40. After midnight: 17, 40.

[39] **Temperature and Weather.** Open air: 5.

[40] **Chill. Fever. Sweat.** Chill in the evening, with coldness going from the abdomen to the feet and fingers.

Chill after midnight.

Heat only internal, with throbbing in the body.

Heat before midnight, during sleep, passing off quickly on awaking.

Sickly sweat, which attracts the flies very much.

With the breaking out of sweat, amelioration of all the complaints.

[41] **Attacks.** Periodical: 3.

[42] **Sides.** Right: 6, 7, 10, 19, 28. Left: 3, 4, 10, 17, 18, 28, 33. Below upwards: 3.

[43] **Sensations.** Stitches, like with needles, in various parts of body.

[44] **Tissues.** Loss of fluids.

Dryness; inflammation of mucous membranes.

Dropsical swellings.

[45] **Contact, Injuries, etc.** Touch: 4, 19, 46. Pressure: 21. Desire to rub: 22. Must rub: 32. Scratching: 46.

[46] **Skin.** Sudden, violent, corrosive burning, often on small spots, *i. e.*, cheeks, nose, toes, etc.; must touch the parts, but cannot scratch them.

Rash: on chest, alternating with asthma; on the forearm.

[47] **Stages and States.** Lax phlegmatic temperament.

[48] **Relationship.** Antidote to *Calad.: Capsic.*

In poisonings with *Calad.*, the juice of sugar cane.

Ignat. relieves the stitches; *Carb. veg.* relieves rash on arms; *Hyosc.* lessens night cough; *Zingiber* relieves asthma.

Following *Calad.* well: *Acon., Canthar., Sepia, Pulsat.*

Complementary to *Nitr. ac.*

Calad. antidotes: *Mercur.*

CALCAREA OSTREARUM.

Calcium Carbonate. HAHNEMANN. $CaCO_3$.

[1] **Mind.** Forgetfulness.

Misplaces words, and tendency to express himself wrongly.

Thinking is difficult.

Mania-a-potu, with delirious talk about fire, rats, mice and murder.

Disinclination for every kind of work.

Depression and melancholy; tearfulness.

Apprehensive mood; as if some misfortune were about to happen. Shuddering and dread as evening draws near.

Fear seemingly starting from pit of stomach.

ı Fears she will lose her reason; or that people will observe her confusion of mind.

Great anxiety and palpitation of heart.

Irritable without cause; peevishness and obstinacy.

Restless mood, with gloominess and anxiety.

² **Sensorium.** Vertigo: when walking in open air, as if he would reel, especially when turning the head quickly; on going up stairs; worse in the morning, with nausea and vomiting; abdominal congestion; hypertrophy of left ventricle; amenorrhœa gradually developed.

Rush of blood to head, with heat, redness and puffiness of the face; worse from alcoholic drink; worse in the morning when awaking; worse after mental exertion.

Continued dulness of the head, as if too full.

Feeling of fulness in head; dulness and feeling of stupidity.

Heaviness in forehead; worse when reading or writing.

³ **Inner Head.** Frequent one-sided headache, always with much empty eructation.

Stupefying, pressing ache in the forehead, as in vertigo, during rest and motion.

Stitching headache above the left temple.

Headache begins in occiput and spreads to top of head, so severe she thinks the head will burst, and that she will go crazy.

Throbbing headache in middle of brain every morning, lasts all day.

Headache: worse going up stairs, talking or walking, in hot sun or from taking cold; chronic from brain-fag; better from tight bandaging, closing the eyes, vomiting mucus and bile, lying down or pressure with the cold hand.

Icy-coldness in and on the head; also one-sided; congestion alternating with icy-cold sensation.

Headache from overlifting, or other muscular strain.

⁴ **Outer Head.** Large open fontanelles, head large.

Whitish-yellow scales of dandruff; scalp sensitive; hair dry, falls out, on sides of head; head feels cold.

Pimples on the forehead.

Thick scabs, bleeding when picked, itching slightly.

Thick scabs with yellow pus; spreading to the face.

Icy-coldness on the head.

Burning on top of head.

Scratches the head impatiently on awaking or being aroused from sleep.

[5] **Eyes.**   Farsightedness.

Sensitiveness to light; photophobia.

Like a shadow before the eyes, obscuring one side of the object; much dilated.

Dancing wavelets before the eyes which are very annoying.

Ophthalmia: from taking cold; entrance of foreign body; in the newborn; scrofulous.

Opacity of cornea, maculæ, ulcers and fungus hæmatodes; transverse, calcareous band of the cornea.

Interstitial keratitis.

Stitches in the inner canthus.

Stinging pains; worse from candle-light.

Itching in the eyes and canthi.

Sensation of coldness, heat, even burning in the eyes.

Swelling and redness of the eyelids, with nightly agglutination; during the day full of gum, with heat, smarting pain and lachrymation.

Eyes become inflamed and injected at every exposure to cold.

Quivering in the upper eyelid.

Suppurating fistula lachrymalis.

[6] **Ears.**   Hardness of hearing, also after suppression of intermittent by quinine.

Singing and roaring or crackling in the ears.

Cracking in the ears when chewing.

Strange and peculiar noise in the ears when swallowing.

Pulsating in the ears.

Inflammation and swelling of outer and inner ear.

Purulent, offensive discharge from the ears.

Polypus of the ear.

Swelling in front of left ear, painful to touch.

Painful inflammatory swelling of the parotids.

[7] **Nose.**   Impaired smell.

Very offensive smell in nose, as from dung, or rotten eggs.

Severe fluent coryza, with headache.

Frequent sneezing without coryza, or with dry coryza.

Dryness of the nose, or stopped by fetid yellow pus.

Catarrhal symptoms attended with great hunger, a sort of metastasis from the nose to the abdomen, as when the coryza ceases colic sets in.

Sore, ulcerated nostrils.

Bleeding of the nose in the morning.

At night the nose is dry and obstructed, while by day it it moist and free. θ Ozæna.

Nasal polypi.

Swelling of the nose; also at the root.

[8] **Face.**   Face: pale, bloated, blue rings around the eyes; yellow; pale, thin; old, wrinkled, with retarded dentition.

Face feels as if it were swollen.

Rending pains in facial bones.

Moist, scurfy eruption on cheeks and forehead with burning pain; itching and eruption in face, and in whiskers.

⁹ **Lower Face.**   Eruption on the lips and mouth.

Swelling of the upper lip; in the morning.

Pain from right mental foramen along lower jaw to ear, worse cold air, better warmth.

Cracked lips; corners ulcerated.

Painful swelling of the submaxillary glands.

¹⁰ **Teeth.**   Toothache: after drinking cold liquids, or excited by draught or cold; drawing, shooting or boring; during and after menstruation; during pregnancy; worse from warm or cold drinks.

Teeth particularly sensitive to cold air.

Offensive smell from the teeth.

Gums painfully tender; swelling, bleeding.

Difficult dentition.

Fistula dentalis on lower jaw.

¹¹ **Tongue, etc.**   Taste; sour; bitter; offensive.

Difficult, indistinct speech; also in ranula.

Tongue coated white.

Dryness of tongue at night, and morning on awaking.

Swelling of sublingual glands.   Ranula; burning in the mouth.

Burning pain at the tip of tongue, as from soreness; worse from warm food or drink.

Soreness of the tongue, either on the tip, sides, or dorsum; can scarcely talk or eat.

¹² **Mouth.**   Mouth slimy; blisters on the inner surface of cheek and tongue.

Canker sores, especially during teething.

¹³ **Throat.**   Inflammatory swelling of the palate and uvula or tonsils, with sensation as if the throat were contracted when swallowing.

Pain in the throat extending to the ears.

Spasmodic contraction of the œsophagus.

¹⁴ **Desires.   Aversions.**   Great desire for eggs; desire for wine, salt or sweet things.

Ravenous hunger in the morning.

Loss of appetite; but when he began to eat, he relished it.

Will not eat meat; aversion to smoking tobacco.

Great thirst.

¹⁵ **Eating and Drinking.**   After milk, nausea and sour eructations; water-brash.

After meals, heat or flatulency, with nausea; pain in the stomach and abdomen.

¹⁶ **Nausea and Vomiting.**   Eructations: tasting of the food eaten; bitter; sour; of tasteless fluid; of food; burning.

Burning extending to throat. θ Heart-burn.

Nausea: mornings, with qualmishness and shuddering; toward evening, during dentition.

Vomit: sour; of bitter slime; of what has been eaten; black; bloody; of milk in thick curds. θ Dentition.

¹⁷ **Stomach.** Pressing pain in stomach, as if a load or stone were in it, after moderate supper; worse from motion, better lying quiet on back.

Pit of stomach swollen like a saucer turned bottom up; painful to pressure.

Pressing, pinching, or spasmodically squeezing and contracting pains in stomach, particularly after meals, with vomiting of food.

Some forms of gastralgia, with great anguish, with sensation of fixed weight in stomach.

Cutting pain in the epigastrium.

¹⁸ **Hypochondria.** Tight clothes about the hypochondria are unbearable.

Feeling as if laced below the hypochondria, with trembling and throbbing in the epigastric region.

Tightness in both hypochondria.

Pressure in hepatic region, with every step, when walking.

Stitches in hepatic region during or after stooping.

¹⁹ **Abdomen.** Abdomen much distended; hard.

❙ Relieves pain attending passage of biliary calculi.

Frequent severe cramp in the intestinal canal, especially in the evening and night, with coldness of the thighs.

Sensation of pressure or pressing from above downward, or from before backward, in the abdomen.

Peritonitis when the pains are relieved by cold applications.

Feeling of coldness in the abdomen.

Mesenteric glands swollen and hard in children.

Obstructed flatulence.

Writhing, twisting pain in abdomen about umbilical region.

Flatulency and gurgling in right side of abdomen.

Swelling and painfulness of the inguinal glands.

Bearing down in uterine region.

²⁰ **Stool, etc.** Crawling in the rectum, like from worms.

Cramp in rectum, the whole forenoon, a griping and stitching, with great anxiety, was not able to sit, had to walk about.

Stools: frequent, first hard, then pasty, then liquid; thin, offensive, like bad eggs; yellowish, grey, or clay-like, fecal; whitish, watery, worse in the after part of the day, often of sour smell; undigested, hard.

Constipation, stools large and hard; containing undigested food; often with slime.

Stools look like lumps of chalk, in children during dentition.

Discharge of blood from the rectum.

Oozing of fluid from rectum, smelling like herring brine.

Hemorrhoids protruding, painful when walking, better when sitting, cause pain during stool; bleed profusely.

Intense aching and shooting in rectum hours after stool.

Feeling of heaviness in lower portion of rectum.

Great irritability of the anus. Ascarides; itching commencing toward bedtime, and proving very troublesome for hours.

Burning: in the rectum; in the anus.

Hemorrhoids which make even a loose stool painful; they are often painful when walking.

Tendency to diarrhœa and acid stomach, and prolapsus recti; precursory of tuberculosis of lungs.

[21] **Urine.** Frequent urination; also at night.

Urine: very dark colored, without sediment; offensive, dark brown, with white sediment; bloody.

Urinary troubles, from getting the feet wet.

Burning at tip of glans penis.

Burning in urethra during urination.

[22] **Male Sexual Organs.** Sexual desire greatly increased at 3 A. M. Excessive sexual desire, with retarded erection, and too early emission of semen, during coitus; burning and stinging during discharge.

Nocturnal pollutions, which debilitate body and mind.

Inflammation of the prepuce, frænum and orifice of urethra, with a little yellow pus between the frænum and glands.

[23] **Female Sexual Organs.** Metrorrhagia, with leucorrhœa during the climacteric.

Menses: too early; last too long; too profuse.

Discharge of blood between the periods, induced by mental excitement or working.

Membranous dysmenorrhœa.

Suppressed menses: with full habit; after working in water.

Swelling and painfulness of the breasts before the menses.

Stinging in the os uteri.

Aching in the vagina.

Leucorrhœa, like milk, with itching, burning.

Burning soreness in the genitals.

Violent itching and soreness of the vulva.

Inflammation and swelling in the genitals.

Uterus easily displaced by overexertion.

Stinging, burning tubercles on the margin of the labia.

Much sweat about the labia.

[21] **Pregnancy.** Abortus.

Sterility when the menses are too early and copious.

During pregnancy, great fatigue from walking, from feeling of lameness in pelvis.

Alopecia, particularly of lying-in women.

Lochia lasts too long, or has a milky appearance.

Mammæ distended, but milk scanty.

Healthy-looking women with deficient milk, whose children die early with diarrhœa and convulsions, or with hydrocephalus.

Swelling of mammæ, sore to touch; knife-like pains.

Ulcer on the nipple; sore to touch.

Moles and varicose protuberances on the heads of infants.

Muscular weakness of infants.

[25] **Larynx.** Whistling in larynx after lying down, evenings.

Roughness or rawness in the larynx.

Painless hoarseness, mornings; hoarse, as if larynx was lined with mucus.

[26] **Breathing.** Frequent need to breathe deeply.

Shortness of breath on going up the slightest ascent.

Asthma; early in the morning; muscles not rigid; sensation of dust in throat and lungs.

[27] **Cough.** Dry, especially at night; violent, first dry, afterwards with profuse salty expectoration, with pain, as if something had been torn loose from the larynx; with rattling in the chest; in the morning, with yellowish expectoration.

Cough after first sleep, dry at night, loose by day with copious sputum.

Expectoration of a putrid odor; or tastes like ink.

Tickling cough, as from a feather in the throat.

Cough caused by sensation of plug, which moved up and down in the throat.

Cough excited by: inspiration; playing on piano; eating.

Expectoration: of mucus, with sweetish taste; of blood, when coughing and hawking, with rough and sore sensation in chest; of muco-pus that sinks in water, leaving a trail behind.

[28] **Lungs.** Oppression of the chest, as if too full.

Stitches in the left chest on inspiration; cutting through to back.

Stitches in chest and sides of chest, when moving; from deep inspiration, and when lying on the affected side.

Sore pains in the chest, worse during inspiration.

Much mucus in the chest.

Middle of right lung most affected.

Abscesses forming in lungs.

[29] **Heart. Pulse.** Palpitation, with anxiety; also at night, or after meals.

Tremulous pulsation of heart, worse after eating; at night, with anguish.

Pulse full and accelerated, often tremulous.

Much beating in the blood-vessels.

[30] **Outer Chest.** Chest painfully sensitive to the touch, and on inspiration.

Itching on the chest.

Mammary glands pain as if suppurating, especially when touched.

[31] **Neck. Back.** Hard swelling of the cervical glands.

Painless swelling of the glands, in the neck, at the margin of the hair.

Stiff neck with pain extending down into the shoulders on moving it.

Thick strumous tumefaction of the thyroid gland.

Swelling and incurvation of vertebræ of neck and back.

Crawling pain between the scapulæ.

Pain between or in the region of the scapulæ, particularly worse by riding, sneezing, gaping or coughing, or other jarring.

Pain in the sacral region, back and neck, after overlifting, or feeling as if wrenched.

[32] **Upper Limbs.** Stitches in the left shoulder-joint.

The arms feel bruised on moving them or taking hold of them.

The arm goes to sleep if he lies upon it, with pains.

Cramp in the whole of one or the other arm.

Weakness and a kind of paralysis of left arm.

Spasmodic tearing pain on outer side of the forearm.

Pain as from a sprain in right wrist, or as if something had been wrenched or dislocated.

Darting through the wrist-joints.

Trembling of the hands.

Finger-joints much swollen.

Fingers as if dead; numbness of hands.

Felons; hang-nails.

Large painful boil on the first phalanx of fourth finger.

[33] **Lower Limbs.** Painful weariness of the lower limbs, especially of the thighs and feet.

Itching of the thighs.

Sciatic pains caused by working in water.

Swelling of the knees. Rheumatic gout of knee with effusion.

Whitish swelling of leg and foot with sensation of coldness.

Large, red and painful spots on the legs, like erysipelas bullosum.

Legs go "to sleep" in the evening when sitting.

Pain in the calf on walking and stepping.

Cramp: in calves at night, about 3 A. M.; also in hollow of knee when stretching out leg; in sole (left); in toes.

17

Burning in the soles.

Bunions.

Feet feel cold and damp. Foot-sweat makes the feet sore.

³⁴ **Limbs in General.** Weakness and weariness of all limbs.

Paralytic bruised pain in the long bones and in the joints of the limbs, also in the small of back on motion.

³⁵ **Position, etc.** Rest: 3. Motion: 3, 17, 32, 34. Ascending: 23, 26, 36. Walking: 3, 20, 24, 33. Must walk: 20. Every step: 18. Stepping: 33. Exercise: 40. Not able to walk: 36. Could scarcely rise: 31. Sitting: 20, 33. Stooping: 18. Lying: 3; on back; on affected side: 28, 32.

³⁶ **Nerves.** Twitching of the muscles.

Trembling of the body.

Talking produces a feeling of weakness, compelling the patient to desist.

Great weariness, not able to walk.

Children cannot walk; they have no disposition to do so, and will not put their feet down.

Great exhaustion in the morning, unable to go up stairs, or becomes much exhausted from it.

Chorea, sometimes only one-sided, involuntary motions, sometimes falling down; from fright, onanism, or worms.

Epilepsy: before the attack sense of something running in the arm, or from pit of stomach down through abdomen into feet. Causes: fright; protracted intermittent; suppression of chronic eruption. Worse during solstice and full moon.

³⁷ **Sleep.** Inclination to stretch, mornings.

Difficult to arouse on awaking, mornings.

Sleepiness and weariness by day.

Late falling asleep; not until 2 or 3. A. M.

Difficult to get asleep, owing to many involuntary thoughts.

❙ Persistent sleeplessness; so soon as he closes his eyes he sees figures.

Wakes too early; cannot sleep after 3 A. M.

Aroused, as often as he falls asleep, by same disagreeable idea.

Dreams: anxious; frightful; of falling.

Children scream after midnight and cannot be pacified.

³⁸ **Time.** Morning: 2, 3, 7, 9, 11, 14, 25, 26, 27, 36, 37, 40. Forenoon: 20, 40. 2 P. M.: 40. Afternoon: 20. Evening: 1, 19, 25, 33. Night: 11, 19, 21, 22, 27, 29, 33, 37, 40. 2 or 3 A. M.: 37. 3 A. M.: 37. After 3 A. M.: 40. Day: 5, 37.

³⁹ **Temperature and Weather.** Generally better in warmth, worse in cold air.

'Very great sensitiveness to the open air, takes cold easily.
Hot sun: 3. Warm or cold liquids: 10. Warm food or
drink: 11. Draught or cold: 10. Cold air: 40, 46.
Open air: 2, 40. Cold applications: 19.

40 Chill. Fever. Sweat. Takes cold very easily; easily
chilled.

Chill with shivering, mostly in the evening, yet sometimes in the forenoon.

Chills commencing at 2 P. M. Thirst during the chill.

Internal chilliness in the morning, after rising.

Intermittent fever when the chill commences in the pit of
the stomach, like a sort of fixed, cold, agonizing weight,
increasing with the chill and disappearing with it.

Frequent flushes of heat, with anxious palpitation of heart,

Heat followed by chill and cold hands.

Nightly internal heat, especially in the feet and hands,
morning dry tongue.

External heat, with internal chilliness in evening in bed.

Sweat from slightest exercise, even in the cold open air.

Sweat during first sleep. Clammy sweats at night on legs.

Morning sweat. Night-sweats after 3 A. M.

Sweat most profuse on head and chest, and upper part of
body.

Sweat: of the palms; of the feet.

41 Attacks. Some symptoms worse toward new moon.

Worse solstice and full moon: 36.

42 Sides. Right: 3, 32, 46. Left: 3, 6, 28, 32, 33. One-sided:
3, 5, 36. Below up: 3. Above downwards: 36.

43 Sensations. Great heaviness of the body.

General sick feeling.

44 Tissues. Atrophy of the muscles.

Crackling, or crepitation in the joints, as if they were dry.

Cancer of the breast, very sensitive, and painful to touch.

45 Contact, Injuries, etc. Touch: 6, 30, 44. Pressure: 3, 17.
Rubbing: 46.

Parts on which pressure is made get numb quickly.

46 Skin. Dry and shriveled; yellow.

Nettle-rash which always disappears in cool air.

White nettle-rash of children itching intolerably.

Elevated red stripes on the tibia, with severe itching and
burning after rubbing.

Scurfy pimples on border of free edge of lower lip.

Unhealthy, ulcerative skin; even small wounds suppurate.

Moist eruptions behind the right ear.

Ringworms.

Itching over various parts of body.

Many very small warts appear here and there.

Rhagades of hands and fingers of persons who work in lime or water.

[47] **Stages and States.** Fair, plump children.

Leucophlegmatic temperament.

Children; open fontanelles and sutures.

Excessive obesity of young people.

Climacteric: 23.

[48] **Relationship.** *Calc. ostr.* follows well after *Cinchon., Cuprum, Nitr. ac., Sulphur.*

After *Calc. ostr.* may follow: *Lycop., Nitr. ac., Phosphor., Silic.*

Complementary to *Calc. ostr.: Bellad.*

Antidotes to *Calc. ostr.: Camphor., Nitr. ac., Nit. spir. dulc., Nux. vom., Sulphur.*

Calc. ostr. antidotes: *Acet. ac., Bismuth, Cinchon., Chin. sulph., Nitr. ac.*

CALCAREA PHOSPHORICA.

HERING.

[1] **Mind.** Forgetfulness, of what he had done a short time ago.

Writes wrong words, or same words twice.

Difficulty in performing intellectual operations.

Wishes to be at home, and when at home, to go out; goes from place to place.

Involuntary sighing.

Anxiousness. Anxiety: in pit of stomach; of children.

Peevish and fretful children.

Inclined to indignation add anger.

Dulness with every headache; worse from bodily exertion; better from cold washing; from mental occupation.

Feel complaints more when thinking about them.

Ailments: from grief; from disappointed love.

[2] **Sensorium.** Staggering when rising from a seat.

Vertigo: on motion; when walking in open air; worse in windy weather; with costiveness; of old people.

Fulness and pressure, or dulness of head, worse from pressure of the hat.

[3] **Inner Head.** Pressure from the eyes and toward them.

Headache over the forehead, with tearing pains in the arms and hands, most in wrist and right middle finger.

Headache on vertex and behind the ears, with a drawing in the muscles of the neck, to the nape and occiput.

Aching, drawing pains around lateral protuberances of occiput.

Headache of school girls, with diarrhœa.

Headache, worse from change of weather, extending from the forehead to nose; or from the temples to jaw, with some rheumatic feeling from the clavicles to wrists.

⁴ **Outer Head.** Sore pain; drawing, rending, tearing in the skull bones, worse along the sutures.

Skull soft and thin; crackling noise like paper when pressed, mostly in the occiput.

Delayed closure, or re-opening of fontanelles.

Crawlings over the top of head, as if ice were lying over the occiput; head hot; smarting of roots of the hair.

Itching black scurfs; poor crop of hair, or losing the hair.

Ulcers on the top of the head.

Cannot hold the head up; moves it from place to place; head totters.

⁵ **Eyes.** Light, particularly candle or gas-light, hurts the eyes.

Eyeballs pain, as if beaten.

Cool feeling behind the eyes.

Squinting; distortion of eyeballs.

Hot feeling in lids.

⁶ **Ears.** Difficult hearing.

Singing and other noises most in the right ear.

Cold feeling or coldness of the ears.

Aching, pressing, tearing or rending in and around the ears, most behind, or below.

Inner and outer ear swollen, red, sore, itching; hot.

Excoriating discharge from the ears.

Aching sore pain in the region of parotid gland.

⁷ **Nose.** Sneezing, and soreness on the edges of alæ, fluent coryza, forenoon.

Nosebleed; afternoons.

Coryza: fluent in a cold room; stopped in warm air and out-doors.

Point of nose icy-cold.

Nose swollen; nostrils sore.

Large pedunculated nasal polypi.

⁸ **Face.** Pain in face, particularly in upper maxilla, from right to left; extends from other parts, to the face, or vice versa.

Heat in the face.

Face: pale; sallow; yellowish; earthy; full of pimples.

Cold sweat on the face; body cold.

⁹ **Lower Face.** Swollen upper lip; painful, hard and burning.

¹⁰ **Teeth.** Retarded dentition, with cold tumors and emaciation.

Hollow teeth, sensitive to air.

Pain in the canines.

Teeth sensitive to chewing.

[11] **Tongue, etc.** Disgusting taste, on awaking, worse when hawking.

Bitter taste: in the morning, with headache; particularly of wheat bread.

Tongue swollen, numb, stiff, with pimples on it.

Tip of tongue sore, burning, little blisters on it.

[12] **Mouth.** Sore spot inside of the right cheek.

[13] **Throat.** Sore aching in throat; worse when swallowing.

Sore throat, with tickling cough in the evening, worse after going to bed.

[14] **Desires. Aversions.** Hunger at 4 P. M.

Infants want to nurse all the time.

Much thirst, with dry mouth and tongue, during the after part of the day.

[15] **Eating and Drinking.** At every attempt to eat, bellyache.

After meals, more after dinner, headache or drowsiness, weariness, itching; or heart-burn, and other gastric symptoms.

After drinking cold water, cutting in the belly.

Eating ice cream in evening, causes colic.

Juicy fruit, or cider, causes diarrhœa.

[16] **Nausea and Vomiting.** Sour belching and gulping up.

After belching, burning in the epigastrium.

Nausea, rising from the pit of stomach when moving; better at rest; followed by headache and lassitude.

Nausea: from smoking; after coffee.

Vomiturition from hawking phlegm.

Vomiting, with trembling of the hands.

Children vomit, often and easy.

[17] **Stomach.** Indescribable uneasiness in region of stomach.

Sharp cutting, or cramp-like pain, in stomach, with head-ache.

Pressure in the stomach; less during rest.

Stomach feels expanded.

Burning at the stomach, and rising of water into mouth.

Empty, sinking sensation at the epigastrium.

Stomach symptoms worse by taking even the smallest quantity of food.

[18] **Hypochondria.** Throbbing in the right hypochondrium, lessened after belching or passing wind.

Stitches or shooting in region of liver, when taking a deep breath.

Hardness, soreness and pressure in the right side.

Pressure and soreness in the left side.

Stitch in the left side, while breathing.

[19] **Abdomen.** Empty, sinking sensation, around the navel, or in the whole belly.

Motion in belly, like something alive.

Cutting, pinching, sharp colic, followed by diarrhœa.

Burning: in region of navel; in the whole abdomen, rising up into the chest, or into the throat.

Aching soreness, and pain around navel, lessens after passing fetid flatus.

Oozing of bloody fluid from navel of infants.

Aching soreness, cutting, drawing in left groin, later in right.

Abdominal wall: tingling, numb; quivering or aching.

[20] **Stool, etc.** Stitches in the rectum toward the anus or shooting in the anus.

Offensive flatus.

Diarrhœa, during dentition, with much flatus.

Stools: green and loose, sometimes slimy, with children; soft, passed with difficulty, accompanying the headache of school girls.

Pus discharged with the stools, which are extremely offensive.

Hard stool, with depression of mind, causing headache, with old people.

Itching in the anus; most in the evening.

Protruding piles aching, itching and sore; oozing of a yellow fluid.

Small furuncle near anus, to the right, with much pain; cannot sit; has to stand, or lie on left side; discharges blood or pus, and remains a painless fistula.

Fistula in ano, alternating with chest symptoms.

[21] **Urine.** Violent pain in the region of the kidneys, when lifting and when blowing the nose.

Violent pain in the bladder and all neighboring parts.

Shooting in the mouth of the bladder.

Frequent urging to urinate.

Cutting pains in the urethra.

Dark urine.

Large increase of urine with sensation of weakness.

[22] **Male Sexual Organs.** Erection, while riding in a carriage, without sexual desire.

Shooting through the perineum into the penis.

Swelling of the testicles.

Itching of scrotum, with sweating, soreness and pimples.

Scrotum sore, oozing a fluid.

[23] **Female Sexual Organs.** Voluptuous feeling, as if all the female parts were filling up with blood; she feels the pulse in all the parts, with increased sexual desire.

Aching in the uterus.

Drawing pain from right to left, over the pubes, with discharge of some blood; followed by earache, first left, then right.

Menses: too early, blood bright, with girls; too late, blood dark, or first bright, then dark, with women.

Weakness and distress in the region of the uterus, worse during passage of stool and urine.

Leucorrhœa like the white of egg, day and night.

Throbbing, stinging, tickling, sore aching, or pressing, in the genitals, drawing upwards in the symphysis, downwards in the thighs.

[24] **Pregnancy.** Weariness in all the limbs during pregnancy.

Child refuses the mother's breast, the milk tastes saltish.

Milk: acid; watery, thin, neutral.

Mammæ sore to the touch.

Pains and burning in the mammæ.

Nipples aching, sore.

[25] **Larynx.** Hoarseness and cough, day and night.

Must hawk or hem to clear the voice.

Burning at back of tongue, followed by burning in larynx.

[26] **Breathing.** Involuntary sighing.

Breathing more frequent, short and difficult.

Child gets a suffocative attack when lifted up from cradle,

[27] **Cough.** Tubercular cough, with soreness and dryness in the throat.

Cough: with yellow expectoration, more in the morning; with fever, dryness and thirst; from 6 A.M. to 6 P.M.; during difficult dentition; cavities containing pus.

With the cough, stitches in the chest, heat on lower part of chest and upper arm.

[28] **Lungs.** Aching in the chest, with soreness to touch.

Sharp pain about sixth rib, right side; later on the left, about fourth and fifth ribs, coming and going; takes the breath; worse with deep breath, during the day.

Contraction of chest and difficult breathing, evening till 10 P.M.; better lying down, worse when getting up.

[29] **Heart. Pulse.** Palpitation with anxiety, followed by trembling weakness, particularly of the calves.

Feels the beating of the pulse, not frequent but quick; while sitting, feels it in the nape of neck and left chest.

[30] **Outer Chest.** Tearing, pressing and shooting in sternum.

Sore pain on the sternum.

Clavicle sore; first left, then right.

Ulcer over the sternum or clavicle.

[31] **Neck. Back.** Rheumatic pain and stiffness of the neck, with dulness of the head; from slight draught of air.

Cramp-like pain in neck, first one then the other side.

Pains and aches between, and mostly below, the scapulæ.

Violent pain in the region of the kidneys when lifting a weight, or when blowing the nose.

Backache and uterine pains.

Curvature of spine to left, lumbar vertebræ bend forwards.

Violent stitch at a small spot between left ilium and sacrum, from the slightest motion.

Soreness in the sacro-iliac symphysis.

[32] **Upper Limbs.** Hard, bluish lumps, under the arms; oozing and scabbing; after checked itch.

Shooting from clavicle to wrist; worse from change of weather.

Rheumatic pain in upper arm near the shoulder-joint; cannot lift the arm.

Lameness of the arms; formication.

Shootings through the elbows, usually first left, then right.

Aching in the bones of the arm, particularly of thumb.

Pains, as if ulcerated around the nails.

[33] **Lower Limbs.** Nates: feel "asleep;" stinging on small spots; itching; burning; sore spots; oozing scurfs.

Sore pain in the thighs, with aching in the sacral bones.

Pains above the knee.

Knees pain, as if sprained; sore when walking.

Lower limbs "asleep," feel restless, anxious; has to move them.

Pain in the bones, particularly the tibia.

Cramp pain in calves, rending, shooting, warm feeling.

Rending, tearing and shooting in the ankle-joint.

Ulcers on malleolus dexters; edges callous; ichor putrid.

Fistulous ulcer on the ankle.

[34] **Limbs in General.** Feeling of lameness of the flexors, sudden aching of the extensors.

Extensors more affected than flexors.

Aching in limbs, with weariness.

Pains in all joints; most left side; later and less the right.

Pains flying about in all parts of rump and limbs, after getting wet in the rain.

Rheumatism during the cold season, better in the warm.

Rheumatism after every cold.

[35] **Position, etc.** Painful symptoms brought on by moderate motions of single limbs, easier after lying down.

Pains after great exertions, worse when lying down.

Rest: 16, 17. Motion: 2, 16. Exertion: 2. Lifting: 31. Walking: 2, 33. Ascending: 36. Rising: 2, 28. Sitting: 29. Wants to sit: 36. Lying: 28; on left side: 20; worse lying on back, better lying on side: 36.

[36] **Nerves.** Weakness, with other symptoms.

Languor: with diarrhœa; with leucorrhœa; with catarrh; during pregnancy.

Weariness when going up stairs; wants to sit down.

Children do not learn to walk or lose the ability.

Trembling of the arms and hands.

Convulsive starts, when the child lies on its back, cease
when lying on the side.

[37] **Sleep.** Stretching; yawning.

Drowsiness all day.

Disturbed sleep, worse before midnight. .

Dreams: vivid, of late events or last readings; of traveling.

[38] **Time.**   Morning: 11, 27.   Forenoon: 7.   Afternoon: 7, 14.
Evening: 13, 15, 20,.28,40.   Night: 40.   Before midnight:
37.   Daytime: 27, 28, 37.   Day and night: 23, 25.

[39] **Temperature and Weather.**   Warm air: 7.   Open air: 2,
7, 39, 40.   Draught: 31.   Teeth sensitive to air: 10.
Cold room: 7.   Cold washing: 2.   Worse cold season,
better warm: 35.   Change of weather: 3.   Windy
weather: 2.   Getting wet in rain: 35.

[40] **Chill.   Fever.   Sweat.**   Shaking chill, out-doors.

Cold in the lower part of body; face hot.

Heat runs from the head down to the toes.

Dry heat in evening; hot breath; noticeable beating of
heart; mouth and tongue dry without thirst, yawning,
stretching.

Copious night-sweats; on single parts, towards and in thè
morning.

[42] **Sides.**   Right, upper; left, lower; pain in bones.

Right side: 3, 6, 12, 18, 20, 28.   Left side: 18, 29, 31, 35.
Right to left: 8, 23, 28.   Left to right: 19, 23, 30, 32,
35.   Above downwards: 3, 40.   Along sutures: 4.

[43] **Sensations.**   Mostly on small spots.

[44] **Tissues.**   Pains along the sutures or at symphyses.

Non-union of fractured bones.

Curvature of spine to left, lumbar vertebræ bend forward.

Condyles swollen on forearms and lower limbs.

Abscess near the lumbar vertebræ.

Spina bifida.

Large pedunculated nasal polypi.

Incipient mesenteric tabes, with much diarrhœa, fetid,
sometimes lienteric.

Rachitis; fontanelles wide open; diarrhœa, emaciation.

Rheumatic pains in all the joints.

Soreness of tendons when flexing or extending.

Flabby, shrunken, emaciated children.

[45] **Contact, Injuries, etc.**   Sensitive to slight touch.

Pressure aggravates head, chest, belly and limb symptoms.

The place of old injury becomes the seat of new affections.

Every step is felt in the head, or in the sacrum.

Lifting child from cradle: 26.   Riding in a carriage: 33.

[46] **Skin.**   Dry skin; moist on hands.

Skin dark brown, or yellow.

Itching and burning, as from nettles.

Scaling herpes on the lower leg.

Furuncles; ulcers.

Scars from an amputation ulcerate.

[47] **Stages and States.** During dentition: 20.

Children lose flesh; will not stand any more; do not learn to walk.

Girls at or near puberty: 3, 20.

Old people, vertigo; constipation.

[48] **Relationship.** Complementary to *Calc. phosph.: Ruta.*

Sulphur follows well.

Compare with *Calc. ostr., Silic., Fluor. ac., Berber.;* also with *Calc. hypophos.,* which is useful in consumption, with hectic, cavities in lungs, etc., and in severe corneal, crescentric ulcers, when low health prevents healing.

CAMPHORA.

Camphor.   HAHNEMANN.   *Lauraceæ.*

[1] **Mind.** Loss of memory.

Awkwardness.

Delirous, somnolent, with slow fever, at night.

Afraid to be alone, especially at night.

Anxiety, precordial; restless tossing about; palpitation of heart.

Mental excitability.

Thinking about an existing pain causes it to disappear.

[2] **Sensorium.** Feels lighter, as if not touching the ground.

Vertigo: in frequent short attacks; after nausea and retching; and heaviness of head, worse on stooping.

Totters in walking.

Staggers as if drunk.

Vanishing of all the senses, even touch.

Sunstroke or inflammation of the brain arising from exposure to the sun.

Stupor. Fainting. Apoplexy.

[3] **Inner Head.** Rush of blood to the head, with heaviness of head; better from external pressure.

Frontal headache; pressing outward; also left-sided.

Contraction, as if laced together, in the cerebellum and glabella, with coldness all over.

Throbbing, like beats with a hammer, in the cerebellum, synchronous with the pulse; head hot, face red, limbs cool, better standing; mostly with such as were deprived of their usual sexual intercourse.

Pains run from head to tips of fingers, with trembling and uneasiness.

⁴ **Outer Head.** Spasmodic motions of head.

Premature grey hairs.

⁵ **Eyes.** Objects appear too bright, at the same time black spots are seen.

Sparks and fiery wheels, alternating with mistiness.

Letters run together, while reading.

Eyes fixed, staring, turned upwards or outwards.

Eyes closed at first, and later staring, looking upwards.

Pupils contracted, immovable.

Conjunctivæ injected, pupils dilated, lachrymation in open air; lids stiff, sore or tense; quivering of upper lid.

Chronic inflammation of the eyes.

Eyes worse in the sunlight.

⁶ **Ears.** Singing, ringing or buzzing in the ears.

Pain in left ear from dark red pimple, which suppurated in thirty-six hours.

Ear-lobe hot and red.

Yellow blisters around the ear, with erysipelas of the face.

⁷ **Nose.** Fluent coryza, with headache, on sudden change of weather.

⁸ **Face.** Face: red, with warmth of body; bluish and pinched, deathly; pale, with crawlings; pale, distorted and sunken; pale and haggard; pale and livid; cold.

Wild, staring, unconscious look.

Cold sweat on face, with vomiting.

Erysipelatous red cheeks and ear-lobes.

⁹ **Lower Face.** Lockjaw, with coldness and pale surface, (and brownish look of eruption, during partial repercussion, in scarlatina).

Froth or foam at the mouth.

¹⁰ **Teeth.** Teeth seem too long, cutting toothache, which seems to originate from the swelling of a submaxillary gland.

¹¹ **Tongue, etc.** Taste: acute; beef broth tastes too strong.

Food tastes bitter, meat more so than bread.

Speech: feeble, broken, hoarse.

Tongue: cold.

¹² **Mouth.** Saliva, running together, watery.

Coldness in the mouth.

¹³ **Throat.** Heat: on hard palate; in throat; in œsophagus.

¹⁴ **Desires. Aversions.** Neither appetite nor thirst.

Drink pleases, yet has no thirst.

Burning thirst, drinks large quantities without relief.

¹⁵ **Eating and Drinking.** Circulation worse after eating.

¹⁶ **Nausea and Vomiting.** Belching and gulping up the contents of the stomach.

Vomit: bilious; of some blood; mostly sour.

Chronic vomiting, in the morning, of sour mucus.

Watery, slimy vomit. *θ* Summer complaint.

Coldness after vomiting.

Absence of nausea and vomit; body icy-cold. *θ* Cholera.

¹⁷ **Stomach.** Sensation of heat in the stomach.

Coldness in the stomach.

Anguish and burning in œsophagus and stomach.

Pain, as if beaten, or overstretched, in the pit of stomach, with fulness of the abdomen; sensitive to touch. ·

¹⁸ **Hypochondria.** Aching in the anterior part of the liver.

Constrictive pain below short ribs, extending to lumbar vertebræ.

Aching pressure in both hypochondria.

¹⁹ **Abdomen.** Coldness in the upper and lower abdomen, followed by burning heat therein.

²⁰ **Stool, etc.** After taking cold, cutting pain, with a loose discharge of dark brown or black feces, like coffee grounds.

Rice water stools. *θ* Summer complaint.

Diarrhœa, great prostration, cold, yet will not be covered.

Diarrhœa, with colicky pains, with chilliness and sensitiveness to cold air.

Absence of discharges; body icy-cold. *θ* Cholera.

Constipation from inactivity of the rectum.

Urging to stool, and insufficient discharge.

²¹ **Urine.** Urine: scanty, not often; by drops; burning; yellowish-green, turbid, of musty odor; reddish in dropsy. See 23.

Unsuccessful urging to urinate.

Retention of urine: strangury.

²² **Male Sexual Organs.** Want of sexual desire, with weakness of the parts; want of erections; testicles relaxed; impotence.

Gonorrhœa, with constant sticking together of the meatus. Chordee.

²³ **Female Sexual Organs.** Menses increased.

Dropsy of the uterus; red, sometimes greenish urine, deposits a thick sediment; urine passed slowly, bladder being nearly paralyzed, body cold.

²⁴ **Pregnancy.** Labor-pains: weak or ceasing; will not be covered, restless; skin cold.

Suppuration of the mammæ; fine stinging on the nipples.

Newborn children: hard places in the skin on the abdomen and thighs, quickly increasing and getting harder; sometimes with a deep redness spreading nearly over the whole abdomen and thighs; violent fever, with startings and tetanic spasms, with bending backwards.

²⁵ **Larynx.** Voice: hoarse; husky; hollow; weak; uncertain.

Cutting, cold feeling deep in trachea, causes a slight cough.

²⁶ **Breathing.** Quiet; deep and slow; difficult, slow; anxious.
Suffocative oppression.
Asthma, worse from bodily exertion.
Hot breath, with acute eruptions.
Cold breath; also after cold feeling in chest.

²⁷ **Cough.** Dry cough in the forenoon.
Violent dry cough, with hoarseness after measles.
Every inhalation starts the cough.

²⁸ **Lungs.** Mucus in the air-passages.
ची, Influenza, when during the stage of invasion the patient
feels cold and chilly, body and mind seem in a depressed
condition.
Stitches: from the shoulders into the chest; in left side of
chest when walking.
Sensation of coldness, extends from the pit of stomach
over the whole sternum.
Congestion of the chest.

²⁹ **Heart. Pulse.** Trembling palpitation, with anxiety.
Palpitation: with sudden oppression of breathing; with
cold face, limbs and body; with pale face and cold
body; after eating; after waking, with twitches.
Precordial distress, when loudly spoken to; sensation of
severe coldness and irresistible sleepiness.
Pulse: full; weak; not perceptible.
Diminished flow of blood to those parts remote from heart.

³⁰ **Outer Chest.** Fine rash on outer throat and chest.

³¹ **Neck. Back.** Pain in fifth, sixth and seventh cervical
vertebræ; worse from moving the head; better from
pressing the hand thereon.
Painful drawing and stiffness on the side of neck when
walking in open air.
Drawing stitches through and between the shoulder-
blades, extending into chest when moving arms.
Cold feeling, or chilliness in the back.

³² **Upper Limbs.** Convulsive rotation of the arms.
Arms: stiff; powerless.
Painful pressure in right elbow-joint, extends to the hand
when leaning on it.
Hands: tremble; cold; bluish.
Fingers stiff, open, distorted; thumb drawn back at nearly
right angles with its metacarpus.

³³ **Lower Limbs.** Cracking and creaking in the hip, knee,
and ankle-joints.
Drawing, bruised pain in the right thigh, and on inner
side near and below the patella.
Knees give way; tremble.
Cramps in the calves.
Drawing, crampy pain on the dorsum of the feet, especially
on moving them.

Tearing, crampy pain on the dorsum of the feet, extending up the outer side of the calves to the thighs.

Tearing in tips of toes of left foot, and under the nails, when walking.

³⁴ **Limbs in General.** Coldness of the limbs.

Drawing in the fingers, then in the toes.

Rheumatism returns repeatedly, attacking part after part, even internal organs.

³⁵ **Position, etc.** Every motion; 40. Moving, head: 31; arms: 31; feet: 33. Walking: 2, 28, 31, 33. Bodily exertion: 26. Standing: 3. Stooping: 2.

³⁶ **Nerves.** Attacks of malaise.

Trembling of inner parts.

Great prostration.

Easily startled when awake, and then feels throbbing or palpitation.

Spasms of children, with sopor; from suppressed eruptions.

Eclampsia, with anæmia; coldness.

Tetanic spasms of the arms, hands, feet and lower jaw; body stiff, with slight opisthotonos; from suppressed scarlatina.

Epileptic spasm.

Want of bodily irritability; insensibility to touch.

³⁷ **Sleep.** Sleepy in daytime.

Sleep: stupid; deep; unrefreshing.

Dreams: anxious, fearful.

Sleeplessness, alternating with coma.

³⁸ **Time.** Morning: 16. Forenoon: 28. Night: 1.

³⁹ **Temperature and Weather.** Sun: 5. Open air: 5, 31. Cold air: 40. Change of weather: 7. Will not be covered: 20, 46.

⁴⁰ **Chill. Fever. Sweat.** Icy-coldness all over, with death-like paleness of the face.

Great coldness of the surface without the usually accompanying change of color, and at the same time a desire to be uncovered.

Chill, chilliness and sensitiveness to the cold air.

Chill, with shivering and shaking; teeth chattering.

Chill: with anxiety; with unconsciousness; with pale face; with clonic spasm.

Heat, with distension of veins increased by every motion.

Cold, clammy, exhausting sweat.

⁴¹ **Attacks.** Rheumatic attacks remit, go to one part after another.

Attacks come on suddenly.

⁴² **Sides.** Right: 18, 32, 33. Left: 3, 6, 28, 33. Above downwards: 3, 32. Below upwards: 28, 33. Behind forwards: 31.

⁴³ **Sensations.** Sensation of dryness all over the body.
Cramps all over.

⁴⁴ **Tissues.** Soft parts drawn in.
Cyanosis. External parts turn black.
Internal congestions.
Cramps in inner and outer parts.
Cracking of joints.
Stenosis after inflammations.
Dropsy of external parts; less of internal.
Glands inflamed.

⁴⁵ **Contact, Injuries, etc.** Touch: 17, 36. Pressure: 3, 31.

⁴⁶ **Skin.** Dryness of skin, not a trace of sweat.
Blood blisters. Erysipelas. Gangrene. Hard spots.
Sequelæ of measles.
Sudden sinking away of variola pustules.
Measle eruption delays; tetanic rigors; skin cold, bluish;
dysuria.
Scarlatina: with cold, blue, hippocratic face; rattling in
throat; with hot breath, hot sweat on forehead, child
will no be covered.

⁴⁷ **Stages and States.** Irritable,|weakly; blondes most affected.
Sorofulous children are most sensitive to *Camphor.*

⁴⁸ **Relationship.** Antidotes: *Opium, Spir. nitr. dulc., Dulcam.*
Camphor. antidotes: *Canthar., Cuprum, Squilla.*
In most other cases, the smelling of *Camphor.* is not anti-
dotal, but palliative, by producing the symptom "pain
better while thinking of it."
Camphor. aggravates the effect of *Nitrum,* and seems to be
injurious if given after it.
Tea, coffee and lemonade do not interfere.

CANNABIS INDICA.

Indian Hemp. PHILADELPHIA PROVERS' UNION. *Cannabineæ.*

¹ **Mind.** Head feels very heavy, loses consciousness and falls.
Every few minutes would lose himself and then, again
wake up as it were, to those around.
Inability to recall any thought or event, on account of
different thoughts crowding on his brain.
Very absent-minded.
❙Exaggeration of duration of time and extent of space; a
few seconds seem ages; a few rods an immense distance.
Great exaltation of mind; at times with enthusiastic
language.

Sudden transition from one fantasia, when completed, to another; the general character may remain unchanged; after visions of great sublimity, usually follow visions of a quiet, relaxing and recreating nature.

❚ Delirium tremens, trembling, hallucinations; tendency to become furious; nausea; unquenchable thirst.

Hallucinations and fancies innumerable.

Clairvoyance.

Full of fun and mischief and laughs immoderately.

Anguish accompanied by great oppression; better in open air.

² **Sensorium.**   Vertigo, on rising, with stunning pain in back part of head.   Fixed gaze.

Heavy pressure on the brain, forcing him to stoop.

Dulness of head.

³ **Inner Head.**   Dull, drawing pain in forehead, especially over eyes.

Throbbing, aching pain in the forehead.

Jerking in right side of forehead, toward the interior and back part of head.

Aching in both temples, most severe in the right.

Dull stitching in the right temple.

Dull, heavy, throbbing pain through the head, with a sensation like a heavy blow on back of head and neck.

Violent shocks pass through the brain.

Feels as if the top of head was opening and shutting, and as if calvarium was being lifted.   (Like *Act. rac.*)

⁴ **Outer Head.**   Scalp and skin of forehead felt as though tightly stretched over the skull.

Crawling in the scalp, on top of the head.

Soreness of the scalp to touch.

⁵ **Eyes.**   Visual clairvoyance.

Sensitiveness of right eye to light.

Letters run together while reading.

Twinkling, trembling and glimmering, before the eyes.

Injection of vessels of conjunctiva of both eyes.

Jerking at the outer angle of the eye and eyelid.

⁶ **Ears.**   Hearing very acute.

Noise in the ears, as of water boiling.

Periodical singing in the ears during his dreamy spells, ceasing when he came to himself.

Ringing and buzzing in the ears.

Throbbing and fulness in both ears.

Aching in both ears.

⁸ **Face.**   Wearied, exhausted appearance.

Drowsy and stupid look ; also with cold face.

Pale face.

Tense feeling in the facial muscles.

18

Skin of face, especially of forehead and chin, feels as if drawn tight.

⁹ **Lower Face.** Dryness of the mouth and lips.

Lips feel as it glued together.

¹⁰ **Teeth.** Gritting and grinding of the teeth while sleeping.

¹¹ **Tongue, etc.** Every article of food is extremely palatable.

Metallic taste.

Stammering and stuttering.

¹² **Mouth.** Dryness of the mouth, without thirst.

¹³ **Throat.** The throat is parched, accompanied by intense thirst for cold water.

¹⁴ **Desires. Aversions.** Ravenous hunger.

Desire for and dread of water.

¹⁵ **Eating and Drinking.** While eating, his stomach felt swollen and his chest oppressed, as if he would suffocate ; was forced to loosen his clothes.

¹⁷ **Stomach.** Pain in the cardiac orifice, relieved by pressure.

¹⁹ **Abdomen.** Flatulent rumbling in the bowels, at night.

Abdomen feels swollen; relieved by belching.

²⁰ **Stools, etc.** Sensation in the anus, as if he were sitting on a ball; as if the anus and a part of the urethra were filled up by a hard, round body.

Painless, yellow diarrhœa.

²¹ **Urine.** Pain in the kidneys when laughing.

Sharp stitches in both kidneys.

Aching in the kidneys, keeping him awake at night.

Burning in the kidneys.

Urine: loaded with slimy mucus, after exposure to damp cold; pain in bladder and urethra; profuse, colorless.

Urinates frequently, but in small quantity.

Frequent micturition, with burning pain in the evening.

Has to wait some time before the urine flows.

Has to force out the last few drops with the hand.

The urine dribbles out after the stream ceases.

Urging to urinate, but cannot pass a drop.

Burning and scalding, or stinging pain in the urethra, before, during and after urination.

²² **Male Sexual Organs.** Sexual desire excessively increased.

Erections: while riding, walking, and also while sitting still; not caused by amorous thoughts; violent; painful.

Penis relaxed and shrunken.

Uneasiness, with burning sensation in the penis and urethra, accompanied by frequent calls to urinate.

Itching of the glans penis.

²³ **Female Sexual Organs.** Sexual desire increased.

Very profuse menstruation.

Violent uterine colic; nervous agitation, or cold hands and feet.

²⁵ **Larynx.**   Inability to measure the compass and volume of the voice when speaking.

²⁶ **Breathing.**   It requires great effort to take a deep inspiration. Oppression of chest, with deep, labored breathing, worse when ascending.

Feels as if suffocated; has to be fanned.

²⁷ **Cough.**   Rough cough with scraping under the sternum. Hard, dry cough.

²⁸ **Lungs.**   Stitches extending from both nipples through the chest.

²⁹ **Heart.   Pulse.**   Palpitation of heart, awaking from sleep. Pressing pain in the heart, with dyspnœa the whole night. Piercing pain in the heart.

❙ Sensation as if drops were falling from the heart.

Stitches in the heart, accompanied by great oppression; the latter relieved by deep breathing.

Pulse slow (as low as 46); rapid (as high as 160).

³¹ **Neck.   Back.**   Pain across the shoulders and spine, must stoop, cannot walk erect.

³² **Upper Limbs.**   Agreeable thrilling through the arms and hands.

³³ **Lower Limbs.**   Agreeable thrilling, from the knees down. Is unable to walk up stairs on account of almost entire paralysis of limbs, with stiffness and tired aching in knees.

On attempting to walk he experienced intensely violent pains, as if he trod on a number of spikes, which penetrated the soles and ran upwards through the limbs to the hips; worse in right limb and accompanied by drawing pains in calves.

Shooting pains in joints of toes of left foot, worse in great toe.

Aching and stitching pain in the ball of the left great toe.

³⁴ **Limbs in General.**   Paralysis of lower limbs and right arm.

³⁵ **Position, etc.**   Rest gives general relief.

Great desire to lie down in the daytime.

Walking: 22, 33, 36.   Ascending: 26, 33.   Sitting: 22. Stooping: 31.   Rising: 2.

³⁶ **Nerves.**   Thoroughly exhausted after a short walk.

Felt so weak that he could scarcely speak, and soon fell into a deep sleep.

Hysterical catalepsy.

Emprosthotonos, loss of consciousness.

³⁷ **Sleep.**   Excessive sleepiness.

Starting of limbs while sleeping, causing him to wake.

Voluptuous dreams, erections and profuse seminal emissions.

Dreams: of danger and perils encountered; of dead bodies; prophetic; vexatious.

Nightmare every night, as soon as he falls asleep.

[38] **Time.**   Afternoon: 40.   Evening: 21.   Night: 19, 21, 29, 37.

[39] **Temperature and Weather.**   Is not so sensitive to cold as usual.

Damp cold: 21.

[40] **Chill.   Fever.   Sweat.**   Loss of animal heat.

General chilliness.

Coldness of the face, nose and hands, after dinner.

Increased heat of the body.

Profuse sticky sweat standing out in drops on his forehead.

[42] **Sides.**   Right: 3, 5, 33, 34.   Left: 33.

[43] **Sensations.**   An indescribable "queer" feeling pervades the whole body.

Feeling of lightness or buoyancy; as if he was raised from the ground and could fly away.

Sensation as if single parts became larger and thicker.

[45] **Contact, Injuries, etc.**   Touch: 4.   Pressure: 17.   Must loosen the clothes: 15.   Riding: 22.

[46] **Skin.**   Formication or itching on various parts.

Tension in the skin of head and face.

Skin clammy, insensible.

[47] **Stages and States.**   Affects persons of nervous and sanguine temperament most; the bilious nearly as much; the lymphatic but slightly.

CANNABIS SATIVA.

Hemp.   HAHNEMANN.   *Cannabineæ.*

[1] **Mind.**   Says one thing for another when speaking.

Thoughts seem to stand still.

Sadness; despondent in forenoon, lively in afternoon.

Anxious and apprehensive feeling at pit of stomach, with oppression of breath and palpitation.

Makes mistakes in writing.

[2] **Sensorium.**   Vertigo: when standing, with swimming of the head; when walking, with tendency to fall sideways.

Rush of blood to the head, causing heat and flushes.

Violent throbbing, with heat of the head, and fever.

[3] **Inner Head.**   The forehead feels compressed, from the margins of the orbits to the temples; not relieved by bending forward.

Pressure below the frontal eminence, extending deep through the brain to the occiput.

Pressure in the temples.

⁴ **Outer Head.** Sensation as if drops of cold water were falling on the head.

Crawling in the scalp.

⁵ **Eyes.** Alternating dilatation and contraction of the pupils
in the same light.

Sensation of spasmodic drawing, in the eyes.

Pressure from back of the eyes, forwards.

⁶ **Ears.** Ringing in the ears.

Throbbing in the ears.

⁷ **Nose.** Dryness of the nose.

Stupefying pressure, like from a blunt point, on the root
of nose.

Bleeding of nose.

Large pimples on the nose, surrounded by red swelling.

⁸ **Face.** Face pale.

Left cheek red, but not hot; right one pale; pain in a
tooth, right side.

Slight pulsations in various portions of the face, particularly in the left buccinator.

⁹ **Lower Face.** Numbing, compressing pain in left side of
chin, affects the teeth of the same side.

¹⁰ **Teeth.** Pain in hollow teeth.

¹¹ **Tongue, etc.** Loss of taste.

Difficult speech, at times stuttering.

¹² **Mouth.** Dryness of the mouth, throat and lips.

¹³ **Throat.** Burning dryness of the palate, mornings.

Dryness of the throat.

¹⁶ **Nausea and Vomiting.** Eructations: of air; of bitter,
acrid fluid.

¹⁷ **Stomach.** Cramp in the stomach.

Uninterrupted dull stitches, near pit of stomach, just below
ribs.

¹⁸ **Hypochondria.** Dull stitching in the left side, just below
the ribs, when breathing or not.

¹⁹ **Abdomen.** Intestines feel as if bruised.

Painful jerks in the abdomen, moving from place to place,
as if something living were in it.

Pain and pressing outwards in the abdominal ring, as if
the parts would suppurate.

²⁰ **Stool, etc.** Pressure in the rectum and sacral region, as if
the intestines were sinking down and would be pressed
out, while sitting.

Obstinate constipation; sometimes causing retention of
urine.

Constrictive pains in anus, together with a sensation as if
thighs were drawn together, she was obliged to close
them.

²¹ **Urine.** Soreness, and inflammation of kidneys and bladder.

Drawing pain from region of kidneys to inguinal glands, with anxious, nauseous sensation in pit of stomach. .

Long-standing dysuria.

❙Strangury. In typhoid fever.

Burning, smarting in urethra, from meatus backwards; posteriorly stitching while urinating.

Urethra feels inflamed and sore to the touch, along its whole length; during erections tensive pain.

Painless discharge of mucus, more or less profuse.

Burning while urinating, but especially just after

Burning along the urethra, at commencement and at end of urinating.

When not urinating, burning pain in forepart of urethra, which compels him to urinate almost constantly.

Pressure as if to urinate, especially in the forepart of the urethra, when not urinating.

Tearing along the urethra in a zigzag direction.

Jerking stitches in posterior portion of urethra, when standing.

Stream of urine forked.

Urine: white turbid; or red and turbid.

22 **Male Sexual Organs.** Increased sexual desire.

Impotence from sexual abuse.

Frequent erections, followed by stitches in the urethra.

Penis swollen, without marked erections.

Penis painful, as if sore or burnt, when walking.

Burning-stinging of penis.

Piercing pains in penis.

Pressive-dragging sensation in the testicles, when standing.

Great swelling of the prepuce, approaching phimosis.

Dark redness of glans and prepuce.

Light red, lentil-sized spots on the glans.

23 **Female Sexual Organs.** Increased sexual desire particularly in sterile women.

Too profuse menses, with dysuria.

24 **Pregnancy.** Threatened abortion in gonorrhœic patients or occurring from too frequent sexual intercourse.

25 **Larynx.** In morning, tough mucus in lower portion of trachea, cannot be dislodged by coughing and hawking; after hawking and coughing, trachea feels raw and sore; finally, the mucus loosens of itself, and he must hawk it up frequently.

26 **Breathing.** Oppression of breathing, from tensive, pressive pains in the middle of the sternum, which was also sore to touch; sleepiness.

Obliged to breathe deeply; chest oppressed; sensation of apprehension in the throat. .

Dyspnœa and extreme agitation, must sit most of the time.

Wheezing and mucous rales.

27 Cough. Hacking cough, arises from the pit of the throat, with a cool, salty fluid deep in throat, posteriorly.

Cough, with a green, viscid expectoration.

28 Lungs. Sore feeling under the upper part of the sternum.

29 Heart. Pulse. Violent beating of the heart, on moving the body and on stooping, with warm sensation about the heart.

Pulse very weak, slow, frequently almost imperceptible.

31 Neck. Back. Drawing in the neck, extending upwards.

Pain in small of back.

32 Upper Limbs. Rending pressure on shoulder, in attacks.

Coldness and cold feeling of the hands.

Formication and numb feeling in tips of the fingers.

Sudden lameness of the hand, trembling of the hand when attempting to clasp anything.

33 Lower Limbs. Cramp-like, jerking, digging pain in right hip.

Drawing pain in the feet.

34 Limbs in General. Weariness of the limbs.

Neuralgic pains in the limbs.

35 Position, etc. Walking: 2, 22. Moving: 29. Standing: 2, 21, 22. Stooping: 29. Bending forward: 3. Sitting: 20. Must sit: 26.

37 Sleep. Sleepiness.

Uneasy sleep at night.

Dreams disagreeable and frightful; disappointed in everything and is filled with anxiety.

Awoke at night from slumber, with frightful dreams, not knowing where he was.

Vivid, lascivious dreams after midnight.

38 Time. Morning: 13, 25. Forenoon: 1. Afternoon: 1. Night: 37, 40, 43.

39 Temperature and Weather. Worse from warm covering; better when uncovered: 43.

40 Chill. Fever. Sweat. Chill, with thirst and shaking.

Shivering over the whole body.

External coldness of whole body, with exception of face.

Heat only in the face and but slight.

Nightly burning heat.

Sweat wanting; or, only on forehead and neck, at night.

42 Sides. Right: 8, 33. Left, 8, 9, 18. Before backwards: 3. Behind forwards: 5. Below upwards: 31.

43 Sensations. Unendurable fine stitching over the whole body, as from a thousand needle-points, at night, when sweating from warm covering, better when uncovering.

Feels as if hot water were poured over him.

Sensation as if drops of cold water were falling: on the head; from the anus; from the heart.

⁴⁵ **Contact, Injuries, etc.** Touch: 21, 26, 46.
⁴⁶ **Skin.** Itching pimples.
  Vesicles on head and chest filled with serum and sur-
    rounded by red areola; burn when touched.
⁴⁸ **Relationship.** Antidotes to *Cann. sat.*, of large doses: lemon-
    juice; of small doses: *Camphor*.

CANTHARIS.

Spanish Fly.   HAHNEMANN.   *Cantharis vesicatoria.*

¹ **Mind.** Sudden loss of consciousness, face red.   θ Dentition.
  Forgetfulness.
  Confusion of head and pulsation in forehead, in morning.
  Confusion; distraction of mind; inability to concentrate
    thought.
  Furious delirium.
  Irritable, dissatisfied with every one and everything.
  Whining and complaining, with anxious restlessness,
    worse on motion, better lying quiet.
  Paroxysms of rage, with crying, barking and beating; re-
    newed by the sight of dazzling, bright objects; when
    touching the larynx, or when trying to drink water.
  Despondent and low-spirited, says she must die.
  Insolent and contradictory mood, in the afternoon.
  Anxious restlessness.
² **Sensorium.** Vertigo: and staggering; and fainting; while
    walking in the open air, with transient attacks of uncon-
    sciousness; appearance of a fog before the eyes.
³ **Inner Head.** Headache in the forehead.
  Burning in the sides of the head, ascending from the neck,
    with soreness and giddiness; worse morning and after-
    noon; when standing or sitting; better while walking
    or lying down.
  Heaviness in the occiput, with drowsiness and incapacity
    to think; heaviness of the head.
  Inflammation of brain.
  Pains deep in the brain, with constant expression of an-
    guish on the face resembling a sullen scowl or frown,
    with eyes closed; or without expression, if open.
  Painful tearing on the vertex, with sensation as if some
    one were pulling a lock of hair upwards.
  Stitching, tearing or drawing pains in bones of skull.
  Headache from washing or bathing.
⁴ **Outer Head.** Hair falls out when combing.

⁵ **Eyes.** Objects look yellow. Eyes look yellow.
Dimness of sight.
Inflammation of the eyes; from a burn.
Smarting in the eyes.
Eyes protruding; fiery, sparkling, staring look.
Eyes sunken, surrounded by blue rings.
Lachrymation in the open air; must close the eyes; on opening lids, the margins pain as if sore, like raw flesh.
⁶ **Ears.** Ringing, humming or roaring in the ears.
A hot exhalation passes, at intervals, and frequently from the ears.
Tearing in the right ear and right mastoid process.
⁷ **Nose.** Nosebleed early in morning.
Erysipelatous inflammation of the dorsum of the nose, spreading to both cheeks, but more to the right; followed by desquamation.
Secretion of much tenacious mucus from nose, without sneezing; hoarseness and painful hawking of tough mucus from chest; nightly dry, cutting stitches along trachea externally.
Mucus collects in posterior nares, difficult to dislodge.
⁸ **Face.** Expression of extreme suffering.
Death-like look during and after pains.
Face: much swollen and puffy; flushed when stooping; yellow, or very pale.
⁹ **Lower Face.** Dry lips, without thirst.
¹⁰ **Teeth.** Painful red spot, size of a pin's head, over the carious root of an upper incisor; discharges pus from a small opening in the centre, when pressed.
‌ Lockjaw with grinding of the teeth.
¹¹ **Tongue, etc.** Taste: bitter; of pitch; lost.
Gold tooth-plate tastes coppery.
Speech weak and timorous.
Tongue: thickly furred, red at the edges; swollen and thickly coated; at base, in part excoriated, in part covered with blisters; trembling of the tongue.
¹² **Mouth.** Mucous membrane red and covered with small blisters; sore, burning or smarting.
Dryness in the mouth extending into posterior nares.
Burning pain in the mouth, throat and stomach.
Salivation; copious, tasteless; disgusting sweet.
¹³ **Throat.** Burning sensation in throat; throat feels "on fire."
Throat inflamed and covered with plastic lymph.
Throat swollen.
Stinging, dryness in pharynx.
Constriction and intense pain at the back of the throat.
Burning soreness of the throat, which is inflamed.
Aphthous ulcer at the back part of the fauces, covered

with a whitish adherent crust; a similar one on right tonsil.

Swallowing of liquids very difficult.

14 **Desires. Aversions.** Aversion to all kinds of nourishment, particularly in the evening.

Immediately on cessation of pains, patient feels hungry.

Great thirst, with burning pain in throat and stomach.

Thirst, with aversion to all fluids.

Disgust for everything.

15 **Eating and Drinking.** After drinking coffee, sensation of fulness.

Drinking, even small quantities of water, increases the pain in the bladder.

16 **Nausea and Vomiting.** Eructations of sour, frothy mucus, tinged bright red.

Nausea and vomiting.

Vomiting: of the water drunk, also of blood; greenish, offensive; of bile and ingesta; of frothy mucus, tinged bright red; with violent retching and severe colic.

17 **Stomach.** Acute pain in region of stomach and bladder, with such exquisite sensibility that the slightest pressure produces convulsions.

Violent burning pain in stomach; also in pyloric region.

Patient tosses about, as if in despair, with pains in stomach.

Stomach feels as if it were screwed together.

Sensation of fulness extending to chest and abdomen, after taking coffee.

18 **Hypochondria.** Incarceration of flatus under the short ribs.

19 **Abdomen.** Abdomen swollen and tympanitic above; yields a dull sound below. Great distention and tenderness of the belly.

Cutting in the abdomen, as from knives, with burning.

Violent burning pain through the whole intestinal tract, with painful sensitiveness to touch.

Cutting, stitching or burning in the groins.

Abdominal symptoms are apt to be in sympathy or consonance with those in distant parts.

Hard tumefaction above the symphysis pubis, with burning pains in the loins.

20 **Stool, etc.** Violent burning in the anus, after the diarrhœa.

Pain in the perineum, seemingly arising from the neck of the bladder.

Desire for stool while urinating.

Diarrhœa, of blood and mucus.

Dysentery, or diarrhœa, with dysuria; feces red, slimy.

Passage of white, tough mucus with stool, like scrapings from intestines, with streaks of blood; slimy and bloody stools.

Constipation, with retention of urine, or with frequent urination, attended with cutting, burning pains, but little urine being passed at a time.

During stool: colic, pressing, cutting or burning pains in the anus, causing the patient to cry out.

After stool: cutting colic, burning, biting or stinging in anus; chilliness, as if cold water were poured over body.

Passage of pure blood from the anus and urethra.

Cutting in the rectum, partially relieved by discharge of flatus, entirely relieved by stool.

[21] **Urine.** Pain in the region of the kidneys and urging to urinate, steadily increasing in severity.

Constant, dull, painful sensation in region of kidneys, late in evening.

Pain in the kidney extending into the abdomen, the axilla, along the urethra into the bladder.

Paroxysmal cutting and burning pain in both kidneys, the region very sensitive to the slightest touch, alternating with pain in tip of penis; urging to urinate; painful evacuation, by drops, of bloody urine, and at times of pure blood.

Cutting and contracting pains from the ureters down toward the penis; at times the pains pass from without inwards; pressure on the glans relieves pain somewhat.

Heaviness in bladder, feels sore on slightest motion.

Urging to urinate from the smallest quantity of urine in the bladder.

Violent pains in the bladder with frequent urging; intolerable tenesmus.

Violent burning-cutting pains in neck of bladder, extending to fossa navicularis, worse before and after urinating.

With the urging to urinate, stitching pain in forepart of neck of bladder; on continued urging, only a few drops pass.

Urging, worse when standing, and still more when walking; better when sitting.

Fruitless effort to urinate.

Urine passes in a thin and divided stream.

Retention of urine, causing pain.

Urine: turbid and scanty; cloudy during the night, like mealy water, with white sediment; albuminous, containing cylindrical casts, mucus and shreds; looks jelly-like; contains large quantities of pus in vesical catarrh.

Before, during and after urinating, cutting pains in urethra.

[22] **Male Sexual Organs.** Sexual desire: increased; disturbing sleep at night.

Strong and persistent erections, painless and without voluptuous sensation.

Bloody semen.

Erection at night, with contraction and sore pain along urethra.

Painful gonorrhœa with chordee; painful priapism.

Drawing pain in the spermatic cord, while urinating.

Testicles drawn up.

²³ **Female Sexual Organs.** Ovarian region; stitches, arresting the breathing; violent pinching pains, with bearing down towards the genitals; great burning pain.

❙ Inflammation of the ovaries, with cutting or burning.

Swelling of neck of uterus.

Uterine hemorrhage, with great irritation in neck of the bladder.

Menses: too early, too profuse; blood black or scanty, breasts painful.

Amenorrhœa, with fulness and pain in the head.

Violent itching in the vagina.

Swelling and irritation of the vulva.

Pruritus, with strong sexual desire.

²⁴ **Pregnancy.** Vomiting, with violent retching and severe colic and burning at the pylorus.

Promotes (when other symptoms agree) fecundity, expels moles, dead fœtuses and the placenta.

Retained placenta or membranes, usually with painful urination.

Puerperal convulsions: 36.

²⁵ **Larynx.** Voice: hoarse; feeble.

Burning in the larynx; larynx sensitive to touch.

Irritation in larynx, causing short paroxysms of coughing, with hurried and difficult breathing; sometimes with pain in abdomen, or with bloody expectoration.

Burning or biting about the larynx, with contraction, or constriction almost to suffocation.

Profuse catarrh of the air-passages, the mucus being tenacious, with painful hawking and nightly lancinating and dryness in the trachea.

²⁶ **Breathing.** When breathing deeply, and when speaking, she feels as if she dare not exert herself on account of extraordinary dryness or weakness of the respiratory organs; speech therefore weak and timorous.

²⁷ **Cough.** Dry, hacking.

²⁸ **Lungs.** Stitches: in chest, more on right side, or first left then right; in the lower right chest, extending toward the middle of the sternum and axilla.

Burning in the chest.

❙ Exudation within the pleura; dyspnœa, palpitation; scanty urine; tendency to syncope. See 44.

²⁹ **Heart. Pulse.** Anxiety about the heart.

Drawing.pain in the region of the heart.

Stitch in heart followed by a crawling sensation.

❙ Pericarditis with effusion; pulse feeble, irregular; tendency to syncope.

Violent palpitation of heart.

Pulse: very variable, mostly hard, full and frequent, at times intermittent; frequent and small; slow, feeble and scarcely perceptible.

30 **Outer Chest.** Stitches in the sternum.

Burning on the chest.

31 **Neck. Back.** Burning, boring, stitching or lancinating pains in the back, either between or, in the scapulæ, or in the small of the back; sometimes the skin over these parts burns as if a fly-blister were there.

Stiffness in the neck, with tensive pain on stooping.

Drawing, tearing or lancinating pain in the neck; sometimes with burning of the skin over the parts.

Tearing pain in the back, especially mornings.

Pain in the loins, kidneys and abdomen, with such pain on urinating that he could not pass a single drop without moaning or screaming.

Pain in the loins, with incessant desire to urinate.

Lancinations and tearing in the os coccygis, causing him to start.

32 **Upper Limbs.** Tearing and stitching pains in the arms.

33 **Lower Limbs.** Tearing from the right, later left, hip-bone, down to the knees.

Violent pains in the knees.

Knees totter when ascending steps.

Numbness of lower limbs, first of one leg then of the other.

Pain in the soles, as from an ulcer, could not step.

34 **Limbs in General.** Weakness and trembling of the limbs.

Violent pains of various kinds in the upper and lower extremities, first of one leg then of the other.

Tearing in limbs, relieved by rubbing.

35 **Position, etc.** Motion: 1, 21, 40. Walking: 2, 3, 21. Standing: 3, 21. Stooping: 8, 31. Sitting: 21. Lying: 1, 3.

36 **Nerves.** Weakness, prostration, faintness.

Convulsions, with dysuria and hydrophobic symptoms; bright light, drink or sound of falling water, touching the larynx, or painful parts, cause or renew the spasm.

37 **Sleep.** Light sleep; full of wakeful illusions.

Sleeplessness; anxious dreams.

38 **Time.** Some symptoms appear every seventh day.

General aggravation after midnight and during .the day.

Morning: 1, 3, 31. Afternoon: 1, 3. Evening: 21, 40. Night: 7, 21, 22, 40.

39 **Temperature and Weather.** Warm applications relieve pains in knees.

Rays of sun: 46. Open air: 2, 5. Washing and bathing: 3.

⁴⁰ **Chill. Fever. Sweat.** Chill in evening not relieved by external warmth.

Chill, succeeded by thirst without heat.

Chill running up the back.

Cold extremities.

Burning heat at night, which she does not feel.

Burning in the palms and soles.

Heat, with thirst.

Sweat from every movement.

Cold sweat, especially on hands and feet.

Sweat on the genitals.

Sweat smells like urine.

Intermittent fever, every paroxysm being characterized by the Cantharis dysuria.

⁴² **Sides.** Right side: 6, 7, 13, 28, 33. Left side: 29. Left to right: 7, 28. Right to left: 33. Below upwards: 40.

⁴³ **Sensations.** Raw and sore pain in the whole body, internally and externally.

Every part oversensitive, and accompanied by excessive weakness.

Burning, stitching and tearing pains predominate.

⁴⁴ **Tissues.** ❙Inflammation of serous membranes; pleurisy after·*Acon* and *Bryon.*

❙Ulceration and erosion of internal parts; patient lies in a stupor, with occasional twitches of the hands; symptoms of collapse.

⁴⁵ **Contact, Injuries, etc.** Touch: 19, 21, 36, 46. Pressure: 10, 21, 33. Rubbing: 34. When combing: 4.

⁴⁶ **Skin.** Erythema, from exposure to the rays of the sun.

Burning, itching pains.

Erysipelatous inflammation of the skin; forming blisters.

Eczema rubrum.

Ulcerative pain when touched.

Gangrenous ulcers with itching and tearing pains.

Pemphigus.

Itching, as from lice, changing place.

Tearing pain in ulcers.

Burns, before blisters form.

⁴⁸ **Relationship.** Antidotes: *Acon., Camphor., Lauroc., Pulsat.*

Oil increases the pernicious effects of *Canthar.*

Inimical: *Coffea.*

CAPSICUM.

Cayenne or Red Pepper.   HAHNEMANN.   *Solanaceæ.*

[1] **Mind.**   Children become clumsy, awkward; especially with headache.

Taciturn and obstinate.

Haunted by a disposition to suicide.

Homesickness: with red cheeks and sleeplessness; with hot feeling in fauces.

Melancholy or hypochondriasis.

Peevish, irritable, angry; easily offended.

Awakens with fright, screams, and remains full of fear.

After emotions, fever, with red cheeks.

[2] **Sensorium.**   Vertigo, during cold stage of intermittent fever.

Vertigo, with staggering; chills, with anxiety.

Senses obtuse, or increased acuteness of all the senses.

[3] **Inner Head.**   Headache, as if the skull would split, when moving the head, or walking.

Throbbing headache, in one or the other temple.

Pressing frontal headache.

Darting pains in head; worse at rest; better walking.

[4] **Outer Head.**   Head seems too large.

Drawing, tearing pain in the right frontal bone.

Skull feels bruised, on moving the head, or walking.

Itching of the scalp; a sort of biting, burning, itching; better by scratching, but becoming very much worse immediately afterward.

[5] **Eyes.**   Objects appear black.

Dim vision, particularly early in morning; better on rubbing the eyes.

Burning in the eyes, with redness and lachrymation.

Pressing pain in the eyes, as from a foreign body.

Eyes seem large, reddish and protruding.

[6] **Ears.**   Dull hearing, after previous burning and stinging in ear

Catarrhal deafness.

Aching in one or both ears, when coughing.

Tympanum perforated, and cavity filled with thick yellow pus.

Painful swelling behind the ear, very tender to touch; caries of mastoid process.

Tearing pain behind left ear.

Pressive, later an itching pain, deep in the ear.

Ears very hot.

[7] **Nose.**   Influenza, with violent sneezing and discharge of

thin mucus, sometimes with burning, tickling and roughness.

Nosebleed in the morning, in bed; bloody mucous discharge, when coughing.

Collection of thick mucus in the nose and throat.

Tingling, titillation in the nose; tip of nose very hot.

8 **Face.** Cheeks red, not hot, changing with paleness.

Pain in the face, worse from touch in the evening. θ Faceache; pains in a fine line coursing along the nerve.

`Eruption on face or forehead, with corrosive itching.

9 **Lower Face.** Lips: swollen; cracked; smarting.

10 **Teeth.** Gums: hot, burning, swollen, or sensitive; spongy, retracted from the teeth.

Pain in teeth, which seem elongated, but not much worse on biting on them.

11 **Tongue, etc.** Taste: insipid; sour; flat, watery; foul, like putrid water.

When coughing, the air from the lungs causes a strange, offensive taste in the mouth.

Small burning blisters on tongue, painful to touch.

Tongue and inside of lips full of flat, sensitive, spreading ulcers, with a lardaceous centre.

12 **Mouth.** Fetid odor, unbearable, carrion-like.

Saliva: viscid, offensive, copious; salivation during chill.

Burning blisters in the mouth, painful to touch.

13 **Throat.** Uvula elongated, feels as if pressing on something hard.

Small, flat, burning ulcers, in mouth and fauces.

Constriction of the throat, with burning; whitish deposit.

Left tonsil inflamed; right, painful.

Throat inflamed, dark red, burning, pressing.

Soreness, smarting, burning and biting in the throat.

Difficulty in swallowing, tongue furred; haggard look.

Stinging, causing night cough.

Burning, etc., worse between the acts of swallowing.

Continuous stitches in the throat, exciting dry, convulsive cough.

14 **Desires. Aversions.** Appetite increased, alternating with aversion to food.

Thirsty, as the chill comes on.

Intense thirst, abdominal uneasiness, but no tenderness on pressure.

Desire for coffee, but it nauseates.

15 **Eating and Drinking.** Better while eating; worse after.

Food tastes sour.

After eating: burning in the stomach; vegetables cause flatulence.

Water causes purging; shuddering; tenesmus; thin stool; chills.

Nausea, and attacks of suffocation, after coffee, yet desire for it.

Red face immediately after dinner, and the patient must go to stool, during or after which there is burning in the anus.

Drinking: 40.

[16] **Nausea and Vomiting.** Belching, with stitch in the side. Eructations like the fumes of *Capsicum*.

Heart-burn. Water-brash.

Nausea and vomiting, with headache; nervous, spasmodic vomiting.

Vomits phlegm with the chill; vomiting in malignant fevers.

[17] **Stomach.** Accumulation of mucus and acids in stomach. Stomach icy-cold, afterward sensation of trembling or burning in stomach, with occasional pungent eructations.

Deranged stomach, with fever.

Sensitiveness and aching in the region of stomach and duodenum after the colic.

[18] **Hypochondria.** "Catching pain" in the region of the liver, or in lower portion of the right lung, with each cough.

Spleen sensitive, swollen; especially after quinine.

[19] **Abdomen.** Colic around umbilicus with mucous stools, sometimes streaked with blood; every stool is followed by thirst and every drink by shuddering; must go to stool immediately after drinking, passing nothing but mucus.

Burning pains in belly.

Cutting in bowels, as from wind; before stool.

Sore pains in the abdomen and loins.

Hard pushing or sticking sensation in a small spot in the left iliac region.

Abdomen distended; suffocative arrest of breathing or painful pressure in lower part of back.

[20] **Stool, etc.** Stools: frequent, small, with tenesmus and burning in rectum and bladder; bloody mucus, shaggy; greenish, frothy, worse at night; tenacious mucus mixed with black blood.

Diarrhœa with smarting, stinging or burning pains.

Hemorrhoids: burning, swollen, itching, throbbing; with sore feeling in anus; bleeding or blind; with mucous discharge; tenesmus recti et vesicæ with small diarrhœic stools, burning and lancinating pains; profuse flow of blood.

Suppressed hemorrhoidal flow, causing melancholy.

After a drink, must go to stool, but was costive; only a little mucus passed.

[21] **Urine.** Stitches in neck of bladder, when coughing.

Colic, with spasm of bladder.

19

Burning in the bladder.

Frequent unsuccessful desire to urinate.

Tenesmus vesicæ ; strangury.

Burning, smarting, before, during, or after urination.

Discharge from urethra ; purulent ; bloody ; urethra painful to touch ; discharge cream-like.

²² **Male Sexual Organs.** Impotence ; scrotum cold, shriveled.

Painful erections at night ; cream-like discharge from the urethra ; burning, when urinating ; at other times cutting, stinging in the urethra.

Gonorrhœa.

Prepuce swollen.

Testes dwindle ; spermatic cord shriveled.

Crampy pains in testicles, after emissions.

²³ **Female Sexual Organs.** During menstruation : nausea ; pressure in the epigastrium.

Disordered menstruation, with a pushing or sticking sensation in the left ovarian region.

²⁴ **Pregnancy.** During .pregnancy: heart-burn, vomiting ; mucous diarrhœa ; hemorrhoids ; burning in anus.

²⁵ **Larynx.** Tingling, tickling in the larynx.

Hoarseness, nose stopped up, throat feels rough.

²⁶ **Breathing.** Seems as if she could not get the air deep enough into the lungs ; feels obliged to take a deep inspiration, it seems as if it would relieve all symptoms.

Deep breathing, almost like a sigh ; slow breathing.

Painful sensation as if the chest were pressed upon, causing great oppression ; worse on motion.

Asthma : with red face or alternately red and pale ; eructations ; chest feels distended ; wheezing inspiration ; breathing worse when moving about, ascending or walking ; with stiff back.

Sibilant rales mostly left side posteriorly, during inspiration ; spongy sound in expiration ; constant dyspnœa ; oppression at bifurcation of bronchia, better from successful cough.

²⁷ **Cough.** With every explosive cough (and at no other time), there escapes a volume of pungent, fetid air.

Stitches in the suffering parts, with the cough.

Cries after coughing.

Dry, hard, evening cough, with pain in distant parts.

Nervous, spasmodic cough.

Cough in sudden paroxysms, convulses whole body.

Sputum dirty brown, not rusty.

Pains in ears when coughing ; ears and tip of nose hot ; bloody mucus from nose ; eyes protrude with burning and lachrymation.

Cough worse : evening, night ; when lying, until fairly

settled; after sharp winds; dry, cold weather; any
draught, warm or cold; after warm drinks.

²⁸ **Lungs.**   Pain in the chest and back; heat.

. .   Throbbing pain in the chest.

Drawing in one or both sides of the chest, up to the neck.

²⁹ **Heart.   Pulse.**   Pulse: irregular, often intermitting; slow,
intermitting; full, strong, frequent, mostly in evening.

³⁰ **Outer Chest.**   Pains in sternum with sweat, while walking.

³¹ **Neck.   Back.**   Glands of neck painful, swollen.

Jerking, tearing pain in the right cervical glands.

Drawing, tearing pains, in and beside the spine.

Excruciating, tearing pains in the back, extorting cries,
causing him to double up, during the chill.

Pain in sacrum and small of back, with hemorrhoids,
dysentery.

³² **Upper Limbs.**   Drawing, tearing pains in the arms.

Drawing, tearing, and stitching pains from the shoulder
toward the hand and fingers.

³³ **Lower Limbs.**   Shooting-tearing, from the hip to the knee
and foot, especially when coughing.

Pains of various kinds, extending from above downward.

Tensive pain in the knee.

ı Caries of right hip; left leg atrophied and painful.

Cold sweat on upper part of the legs.

Feet cold.

³⁵ **Position, etc.**   Rest: 3. Motion: 26, 40, 44. Moving head:
3, 4.   Walking: 3, 4, 26, 30, 36; in open air: 40.   Ascending: 26. Lying: 27. Desire to lie down: 36. Must
bend double: 31.

³⁶ **Nerves.**   Lack of reactive force, especially with fat people.

Vital forces sunken.   θ Paralysis, gangrene, meteorism,
typhus.

Weak, exhausted.   Staggering when walking.

Great desire to lie down and sleep; does not want to exert
himself in the least.

³⁷ **Sleep.**   Yawning.

Sleepless from emotions, from homesickness, or from cough.

Sleep full of dreams, restless.   Screaming in sleep.

Sensation as if one were falling from a height during sleep.

Many dreams, full of contrarieties.

³³ **Time.**   Remission during day and before midnight.

Morning: 7, 27.   Evening: 8, 27, 29.   Night: 13, 22, 27.

³⁹ **Temperature and Weather.**   Generally better in warmth.

Dreads uncovering, even in hot stage of ague.   Shuns
open air: 47.   Draught: 27, 40.   Open air: 40.   Dry
cold: 27. Sharp winds: 27.

⁴⁰ **Chill.   Fever.   Sweat.**   Skin cool, pulse slow, want of
appetite.

Shivering and chillness after every drink.

Chill begins in back, with thirst, worse after drinking, lessened when walking out of doors.

Chill in the open air, particularly in a draught.

Chill followed by sweat; or by heat, with sweat and thirst.

Chill externally; burning inwardly.

Fever heat, with violent burning.

Heat: followed by chill, with thirst; lessened by motion.

Sweat: violent, copious; lessened by motion.

⁴¹ **Attacks.** Periodicity marked.

Chill spreads gradually until extreme points are reached; then as gradually declines.

⁴² **Sides.** Right; 4, 13, 18, 31, 33. Left: 6, 13, 18, 26, 33. Below upwards: ∠8. Above downwards: 33.

⁴³ **Sensations.** Violent pains at various places; now here, now there; neuralgia of children.

Superficial drawing pains in different parts of the body.

Burning, smarting sensations.

Sensation as if parts would go to sleep.

⁴⁴ **Tissues.** Relaxed fibre; obesity.

Glandular swellings.

Joints: crack; stiff, painful on beginning to move; pain, as if paralyzed.

⁴⁵ **Contact, Injuries, etc.** Worse from touch; skin sensitive, with many internal ailments.

Touch: 8, 21. Scratching: 46.

Seasickness.

⁴⁶ **Skin.** Itching worse from scratching.

Burning in the skin.

Herpetic-like eruption on forehead or face, itching, burning.

Stinging-biting or burning-itching, worse on scalp, face and chest.

Skin bloated, flabby.

⁴⁷ **Stages and States.** Light hair, blue eyes.

Nervous, but full habit.

Phlegmatic; awkward, easily offended; indolent, melancholic; lack of reaction.

Lazy, fat, unclean, dreads the open air.

Children who are always chilly, refractory, clumsy.

Less frequently indicated in persons of tense fibre.

Hemorrhoidal constitutions.

Gouty.

⁴⁸ **Relationship.** Complaints from coffee.

Fevers from, or after abuse of quinine.

Vapor of *Sulphur* or *Sulph. ac.* antidotes feeling as if parts were going to sleep.

Antidotes to *Capsic.*: *Calad.*, *Camphor.*, *Cina*, *Cinchon.*

CARBO ANIMALIS.

Animal Coal.   HAHNEMANN.

[1] **Mind.** Confused, did not know whether he had been asleep or awake; morning.

Desire to be alone; she is sad, reflective; avoids conversation, taciturn.

Alternate cheerfulness and melancholy.

Low-spirited.

Anxiety: apprehensive, after an emission.

Fright in the dark.

[2] **Sensorium.** Vertigo and confusion on sitting up; better when reclining; nausea.

Brain feels as if loose, during motion.

[3] **Inner Head.** Pain in top of head, as if skull had been split or torn asunder; worse during wet weather and at night; must press the head with both hands.

Heaviness: in head at night; weary feet; in the forehead on stooping; especially in cerebellum, worse forenoon, in cold air; better after dinner.

Rush of blood to head; confusion in head.

Throbbing headache after menses; worse in the open air.

[4] **Outer Head.** Skin of forehead and vertex feels tight.

[5] **Eyes.** Dim sight, eyes feel weak.

A net seems to swim before the eyes.

[6] **Ears.** Does not know from what direction sounds come.

Ringing in ears when blowing nose.

Ichorous otorrhœa.

Periosteum behind the ear swollen.

Parotid gland swollen; lancinating pains.

[7] **Nose.** Nosebleed: every morning, preceded by dull feeling in head; preceded by vertigo.

Dry coryza, cannot breathe through nose in morning on waking, and for sometime after.

Coryza, scraping in throat, worse evening, night, and when swallowing.

Fluent coryza, with loss of smell, yawning and sneezing.

Tip of nose: red, painful to touch; skin feels tight, is chapped; little boils inside.

Hard, bluish tumor on end of nose.

[8] **Face.** Face has cachetic appearance; looks earthy.

Heat in face and head, in afternoon.

Erysipelas of face.

Copper-colored eruption.

Acne; young, scrofulous persons.

⁹ **Lower Face.** Shooting and stitches in malar bone, especially left, running towards the ear.

Lips swollen, burning.

Vesicles, or cracks on the lips.

¹⁰ **Teeth.** Teeth loose, sensitive on chewing.

Gums: red, swollen, painful; bleeding.

Gum-boils.

¹¹ **Tongue, etc.** Taste: bitter, especially morning; sour.

Burning on tip of tongue, and rawness in mouth.

Burning blisters on tips and edges of tongue.

Knotty indurations in the tongue.

¹² **Mouth.** Blisters, burning.

Mouth and tongue dry.

Frequent biting of the inside of cheek.

¹³ **Throat.** Mucus in throat, hawking.

Raw sensation in throat and œsophagus, to pit of stomach; not increased by swallowing.

Raw feeling, like heart-burn, better after eating.

¹⁴ **Desires. Aversions.** Ravenous hunger.

No appetite; averse to fatty food.

¹⁵ **Eating and Drinking.** Eating causes: fatigue; distress and burning in stomach; inflation; long-lasting nausea, after meat.

Eating relieves rawness in throat.

After dinner: 3. After eating: 13, 26, 29, 40.

¹⁶ **Nausea and Vomiting.** Eructations tasting of food long eaten.

Heart-burn.

Saltish water runs from the mouth, retching, vomiting, hiccough, cold feet. *θ* Cancer of stomach.

¹⁷ **Stomach.** Spasmodic cramps.

Like a load or weight in stomach on waking, mornings.

Sore feeling in pit of stomach.

Pressing, clawing, griping, burning in stomach.

Faint, gone feeling; also from suckling the child; eating does not relieve it.

Fulness, cold feeling in stomach after slight meal, better laying hand on stomach.

¹⁸ **Hypochondria.** Aching, almost cutting in region of liver, even while lying down.

¹⁹ **Abdomen.** Abdomen greatly distended; much annoyed with flatus.

Painful sensation in right lower abdomen, as if something would be squeezed through.

Feeling in left groin, on sitting down, as if a hard body were lying there; relieved after pressure, by passage of flatus.

Soreness in abdomen while coughing.

Hard buboes, begin to suppurate; or, maltreated cases with callous edges, ichorous, offensive discharge.

[20] **Stool, etc.**   Severe burning in rectum, in evening.

Anus sore; viscid moisture, oozing also from perineum.

Stitches in rectum and anus.

Stool hard, lumpy, scanty.

Unsuccessful desire for stool; passes only offensive flatus; pain in back, and feeling across abdomen as if there was no expulsive power.

Blood passes during stool.

Piles, burn and sting, worse during walking.   Fissura ani with severe burning.

[21] **Urine.**   Frequent desire, urine increased; fetid; sometimes interrupted; more frequent at night.

Inefficient urging, with painful pressure in loins, groins and thighs.

During urination: burning soreness in urethra.

Stitches and lancinating in the abdomen, better from urinating.

[22] **Male Sexual Organs.**   Seminal emissions; parts feel weak; exhausted mentally and bodily.

ı Syphilis; buboes.

[23] **Female Sexual Organs.**   Tearing transversely across the pubes, and then through pudenda, as far as the anus.

Induration of neck of uterus; burning.

Menorrhagia from chronic induration of uterus; also in delicate women, with glandular affections.

ı Burning into thighs; labor-like pains in pelvis and sacrum; slimy, bloody discharge, very weak. θ Cancer uteri.

Menses: too early, too long, not profuse.

During menses: lameness in thighs; pressing in small of back, groins and thighs, unsuccessful desire to eructate, chilly, yawning; the flow weakens her, she can hardly speak; blood dark.

Leucorrhœa: stains linen yellow; offensive; burning, biting; more when walking or standing; causes weak feeling in stomach.

[24] **Pregnancy.**   Nausea, worse at night.

Lochia long-lasting, thin, offensive, excoriating; numb limbs.

Mammæ: darting pains of nursing women, arrest breathing, worse from pressure; hard, painful spots; swollen, inflamed (erysipelatous) during confinement.

ıTumor hard, uneven, skin loose; burning pains; dirty, blue-red spots; pains drawing towards axilla; night-sweat, low-spirited. θ Scirrhus mammæ.

[25] **Larynx.**   Rawness and hoarseness, morning after rising.

Hoarseness, worse evenings; loss of voice during night.

26 **Breathing.** Dyspnœa and anxiety; low-spirited.

Panting and rattling.

Oppression in the morning and after eating.

27 **Cough.** From tickling in the right side of chest, or lying on right side; sputum green.

Severe, dry cough, shakes the abdomen as if all would fall out, must support the bowels; loose rales until something is coughed up; morning on rising and nearly all day.

28 **Lungs.** Sensation of coldness in chest.

Chronic bronchitis, with night-sweats.

Burning (in right side of) chest.

Pneumonia in right lung, suppuration beginning; green sputum.

Pleurisy, lingering; skin livid, emaciation, hectic; or typhoid symptoms.

Sharp burning stitches in chest.

29 **Heart. Pulse.** Palpitation after eating; when singing in church; morning on awaking, must lie still, with eyes closed.

Pulse accelerated, especially evening; beating in blood-vessels.

31 **Neck. Back.** Glands of neck indurated, swollen, painful.

Pressing, drawing and stiffness in lumbar region, as if broken.

Sharp drawing across small of back, sensitive to every step.

Coccyx feels bruised; burning when touched; pain as from subcutaneous ulceration, worse sitting or lying.

32 **Upper Limbs.** Axillary glands indurated.

Arms painful to touch.

Hands and fingers readily go to sleep.

Wrists pain as if sprained.

Hands numb; often with chest affections.

Gouty stiffness of finger-joints.

33 **Lower Limbs.** Stitches in left hip when sitting.

Sweat at night on thighs only.

Painful tension in the calves, when walking.

The foot turns under when walking, as from a weak ankle.

Painful contraction of tendo-achillis.

Pain in heels; feet sore.

Frost-bites; inflamed, burning.

Corns, painful to touch.

34 **Limbs in General.** Bruised feeling, especially during motion.

35 **Position, etc.** Sitting: 2, 19, 31, 33. Motion: 2, 34. Walking: 20, 23, 31, 33. Slight exertion: 40. After rising: 25, 27. Standing: 23. Stooping: 3. Reclining: 2. Lying: 18, 31; on right side: 27. Must lie still: 29.

[36] **Nerves.** Weak, want of energy; head confused; prostration. Easily sprained from lifting even small weights.

[37] **Sleep.** Anxious; frightful visions and restlessness keep him awake.

Sleepy all forenoon; yawning.

Sleep full of vivid fancies; talks, groans, sheds tears.

[38] **Time.** Morning: 1, 7, 11, 25, 26, 27, 29. Forenoon: 3, 37 Afternoon: 8, 40. Evening: 7, 20, 25, 29, 40, 46. Night: 3, 7, 21, 24, 25, 33, 40. Toward morning: 40. All day: 27.

[39] **Temperature and Weather.** Wet weather: 3. Open air: 3. In bed: 40, 46. Aversion to open air.

[40] **Chill. Fever. Sweat.** Chill, especially in afternoon and after eating; evening chill followed by sweat.

Heat always after a chill, mostly at night, in bed.

Sweat generally towards morning, also from slight exertion, even eating.

Night sweat fetid, debilitating, staining yellow.

[42] **Sides.** Right: 18, 19, 27, 28. Left: 9, 19, 33.

[44] **Tissues.** Venous plethora: 47.

Stinging in scars.

Benignant change into ichorous suppurations.

Glands indurated, swollen, inflamed, with lancinating, cutting or burning. *θ* Scirrhus.

Joints weak; easily sprained: 45.

Gummata.

[45] **Contact, Injuries, etc.** Touch: 7, 31, 32, 33. Pressure: 3, 17, 19, 24. Chewing: 10. Lifting: 36.

[46] **Skin.** Itching over whole body; evening in bed.

Erysipelatous swellings, with burning pain.

[47] **Stages and States.** Elderly persons, especially with venous plethora, blue cheeks, blue lips, debility, etc.

Young, scrofulous subjects.

[48] **Relationship.** Antidotes: *Arsen., Camphor., Nux vom., Vinum.*

CARBO VEGETABILIS.

Charcoal.   HAHNEMANN.

[1] **Mind.** Confusion of head, making thinking difficult; morning on waking; he had to make great exertion, as if arousing himself from a dream.

Ideas flow slowly.

Stupor, collapse.

Anxious, as if oppressed, with heat in the face.

Nightly fear of ghosts.

Indifference; heard everything without feeling pleasantly or unpleasantly, and without thinking of it.

Very irritable, excitable and inclined to anger.

Peevish, wrathful.

Restless, anxious; 4 to 6 P.M.

² **Sensorium.** Vertigo : had to hold on to something; also when stooping; from flatulence; venous stasis; especially after a debauch; whirling in head, the whole day.

Fainting after sleep, after rising, or while yet in bed, mornings; belching; caused by debilitating losses, or abuse of mercury.

³ **Inner Head.** Head feels heavy as lead.

Rush of blood to head, nosebleed.

Congestion to head, with spasmodic constriction, nausea and pressure over eyes, feeling of coryza; from overheated rooms.

Painful throbbing in the head, during inspiration.

Pressive headache just over the eyes, with tears; eyes pain on moving them.

Aching and beating over eyes, or in whole head, commencing at nape of neck; worse evening; after a meal, with congestion to head; after a debauch.

Pressure in both temples and on top of head.

Violent tearing in forehead, at a small spot near temple.

Dull headache in occiput; violent pressive pain in lower portion of occiput.

Tearing and drawing in left side of occiput.

Headache like from constriction of the scalp.

⁴ **Outer Head.** Head painfully sensitive to pressure, especially of the hat; worse from taking cold and from getting warm in bed.

Scalp painful to touch.

Hair falls out; worse on back of head; scalp itches in evening when warm in bed.

⁵ **Eyes.** Eyes dull, lustreless, pupils do not react to light.

Shortsighted from overexerting eyes; eyes become weak from overwork or fine work.

Black spots float before the eyes.

Heavy weight seems to rest on the eyes; must make exertion to distinguish letters when reading.

Burning in the eyes.

Hemorrhage from eyes, with congestion to head. θ Whooping-cough.

Muscles of eye pain, when looking up.

Margins of lids itch; morning.

⁶ **Ears.** Ringing in ears; buzzing.

Something heavy seems to lie before the ears; they seemed stopped, hearing not diminished.

Deafness after acute exanthema; abuse of mercury; ears
too dry.

Offensive otorrhœa.

Deficient or badly-smelling cerumen; also with exfoliation
of dermoid layer of meatus.

Left ear hot and red every evening.

Pain from right ear down the neck on turning the head.

θ After itch-like eruptions.

Parotitis, swelling grows hard.

⁷ **Nose.**   Nose pointed; hippocratic face.

Frequent and easy epistaxis; worse at night or in forenoon,
followed by pain over the chest.

Nosebleed: several times daily for weeks; face pale before
and after every attack; after straining at stool; small,
intermittent pulse; after debauch; in old or debilitated
people.

Frequent sneezing, with constant and violent crawling and
tickling in the nose.

Fruitless irritation to sneeze, with crawling in left nostril.

Severe coryza, with hoarseness and rawness on the chest.

Dry coryza.

⁸ **Face.**   Face: very pale; greyish-yellow; greenish; hippocratic.

Cold sweat on face; face cold, tongue cold, contracted.

Cheeks red and covered with cold sweat.   .

Tearing in left cheek; jerking-tearing in right upper
maxilla.

Facial and maxillary bones sore.

⁹ **Lower Face.**   Quivering in the upper lip.

Swelling of upper lips and cheeks, with jerking pain.

Brown, or blackish-looking cracked lips.

¹⁰ **Teeth.**   Drawing and tearing pain in the molars.

Tearing in teeth from hot, cold or salt food; worse when
touched with tongue; whole row too long and tender.

Teeth decay rapidly.

Gums: bleed, also when sucking them; pain as if sore;
recede from (lower) incisors; sensitive when chewing;
gum-boils.

¹¹ **Tongue, etc.**   Bitterness on palate, tongue dry.

Bitter taste before and after eating; salty taste.

Glossitis when tongue becomes indurated.

Tongue heavy, with difficult speech.

Tongue: white; coated with yellow-brown mucus; lead-
colored; blue, sticky, moist; dry, parched, fissured.

Tip of tongue raw and dry; heat in mouth.

Tongue turns black.

¹² **Mouth.**   Mouth and breath cold.

Increase of saliva.

Mouth hot, tongue almost immovable, saliva bloody; edges of gums yellow, indented; gums loose, receding, ulcerated.

Hemorrhage from nose and mouth.

¹³ **Throat.** Scraping, rawness, burning in throat.

Sloughing of some parts of swollen fauces; fetid ichor.

Swallowing, coughing or blowing nose, cause pain in posterior nares and fauces as if sore.

Food cannot be easily swallowed, throat seems constricted, no pain.

Swelling and inflammation of uvula, with stitches in the throat.

¹⁴ **Desires. Aversions.** Want of appetite; eats only dinner; feeling of relaxation and weakness of muscles of limbs.

Longing for coffee; acids; for sweet and salt things.

Aversion to meat and fat things; to milk, which causes flatulence.

¹⁵ **Eating and Drinking.** After eating; acidity in mouth; plainest food disagrees; heaviness, fulness (more after supper), sleepiness; nausea, vomiting; feels as if the abdomen would burst; worse after debauch; from rich living.

After milk, sour eructations.

Dreads to eat because of pains, burning in epigastrium and deep in abdomen.

Gastric symptoms from wine; coffee; too much milk; excessive use of butter, or from rancid butter, from fats in general; fish, especially if tainted; from ice water or different waters; from flatulent vegetables.

Bad effects from abuse of salt or salt meats.

Hot, cold or salt food: 10. Eating or drinking: 27.

¹⁶ **Nausea and Vomiting.** Frequent, empty eructations, also when preceded by pinching in the abdomen.

Pyrosis, great flow of water. θ Catarrh.

Sour or rancid eructations.

Nausea in morning, with qualmishness in stomach.

Vomiting: of blood; of food, in evening; of sour, bilious or bloody masses.

¹⁷ **Stomach.** Aching in pit of stomach.

Burning in stomach, spreading down to small of back and up to the shoulders.

Contractive cramp, also at night, extending to the chest; abdomen distended; must bend double, worse lying down; pain paroxysmal, takes away the breath.

Feels acidity in stomach while lying on the back and when walking; stomach feels very heavy and as if hanging down.

Tense, full feeling; flatulence.

Hæmatemesis; body icy-cold; breath cool; pulse thready, intermittent; fainting; hippocratic face.

Pain in stomach from nursing, or other loss of fluids.

18 **Hypochondria.**   Painful to touch; clothing oppresses him, is unendurable.

Tension, or stitches in region of liver.

Jaundice: after too much or too rich food; from abuse of mercury.

Pressing, pinching in region of spleen; quick, lightning-like stitches; abdomen bloated.

19 **Abdomen.**   Colic from flatulence, abdomen full to bursting; pain worse about bladder, or left of epigastrium; worse from least food; better from passing flatus, or hard stool.

Abdomen distended, better from passing wind upwards or downwards.

Burning, lancinating in epigastrium and deep in abdomen; worse from eating; with anguish, flatulency, diarrhœa.

Abdomen feels as if hanging heavily; walks bent.

Meteorism, with loud rumbling; fetid or odorless flatus.

20 **Stool, etc.**   Acrid, corrosive moisture from the rectum.

Gnawing in the rectum when not at stool; crawling. θ Ascarides.

Flatus, hot, moist, offensive.

Stools: burning, light-colored, fetid, watery, bloody, with tenesmus; covered with filamentous yellow mucus, last part bloody; putrid, cadaverous-smelling, involuntary; dysenteric, terribly offensive; thin, pale mucus; in fragments, tough, scanty, with urging and tingling in rectum, and pressure on bladder and uterus.

Even soft stool passed with difficulty.

Cholera asiatica, stage of collapse.

Hemorrhoids: protrude; blue; suppurating and offensive; with burning; after debauchery; cause dysuria.

21 **Urine.**   Morbus Brightii, from abuse of alcohol.

Blenorrhœa vesicæ; old people.

Urine: reddish, turbid; as if mixed with blood; with red sediment; bloody, with varices of anus and bladder; copious, light yellow, diabetic; milky.

Wetting bed at night.

22 **Male Sexual Organs.**   Onanism during sleep.

Seminal discharge too soon, during coitus, followed by roaring in the head.

Prostatic discharge, while straining at stool.

Swelling of testicles from metastasis of mumps.

23 **Female Sexual Organs.**   Menses: too early, too profuse; blood pale or thick, corrosive, acrid-smelling.

Menorrhagia, burning across sacrum, passive flow.

Leucorrhœa: thin in morning on arising, not through day; milky, excoriating; thick, yellow.

Vaginal fistula, burning pains.

Erectile tumors, blue, hard, pricking.

Varices of vulva, itching of vulva and anus; cause dysuria.

Red, sore places on pudenda; aphthæ; also during leucorrhœa.

²⁴ **Pregnancy.** Labor-pains weak, or ceasing, with great debility; especially after violent disease or great loss of fluids.

Debility from nursing.

Lumps in the mammæ, with induration of axillary glands, and with burning pains, anxiety, want of breath; whining mood.

Brown, foul-smelling lochia.

²⁵ **Larynx.** Deep voice, failing if exerted, no pain.

Hoarseness: and rawness, worse evenings; aphonia mornings; in damp, cool weather; chronic; worse from damp evening air, warm, wet weather, and from talking.

Dingy, purplish, swelling of the lining of the larynx.

Ulcerative pain or scraping and titillation in larynx.

Unusual feeling of dryness in trachea, not relieved by hawking.

²⁶ **Breathing.** Breath cold.

Breathing short, with cold hands and feet.

Desires to be fanned, must have more air.

Difficult breathing, fulness of chest, and palpitation on slightest motion.

Asthma of old people, weakness, trembling; looks as if dying; full of wind, but cannot raise it; better in cold air; worse in morning.

❙Cheyne-stokes breathing in organic heart disease.

Loud, rattling breathing; cough ceases; œdema pulmonum impending.

Great dyspnœa, great anxiety, but not restless; cough in violent spells, watery, profuse expectoration. θ Emphysema.

²⁷ **Cough.** Cough: spasmodic, hollow, in short, hard spells; caused by a feeling as of vapor of sulphur; worse evenning or before midnight; at times dry, painful; at others with purulent, slimy, offensive sputa; with copious sputa night and morning; and vomiting after other symptoms of whooping-cough are gone; with painful stitches through the head; worse going from warm to cold places; motion; walking in open air; after lying down; evening in bed; eating or drinking, especially cold food or drink; talking.

Sputa: yellow-green or purulent; brown, bloody; or less often tenacious, whitish mucus, or watery; of sour or saltish taste; or, of unpleasant odor.

[28] **Lungs.** Burning in chest, as from glowing coals; rawness and soreness.

Congestion to chest and head.

Weak, fatigued feeling of chest.

Burning under sternum; rattling of large bubbles; dyspnœa; cold knees in bed.

Bronchial catarrh, hoarse, mucous rales; chest and ribs feel as if bruised.

Oppressive tearing in the left chest.

Pressive pain in the upper right chest, through to scapula.

Hæmoptysis, burning in chest, paroxysms of violent cough, hoarse; face pale; skin cold; slow, intermittent pulse; wants to be fanned.

[29] **Heart. Pulse.** Palpitation: excessive, for days; after eating; when sitting.

Blood stagnates in capillaries, cyanosis; cold face and limbs, cold sweat; complete torpor; impending paralysis of heart.

Pulse thread-like; weak and small; intermittent.

[30] **Outer Chest.** Brown-yellow blotches on chest.

[31] **Neck. Back.** Cervical glands swollen and painful, especially those near the nape.

Tearing in cervical muscles.

Drawing in nape, up into head, with nausea and rush of water from the mouth.

Rheumatic drawing in back, worse when stooping.

Stiffness of back.

Severe pain in small of back, she was unable to sit; then sensation as of a plug in back, had to put a pillow under it.

Pinching, pressive pain near lowest portion of spine.

Pressive, sore pain beneath the coccyx.

[32] **Upper Limbs.** Burning on right shoulder.

Drawing in the arm on which he is lying at night.

Bruised pain in both elbow-joints.

Arms weary when writing.

Drawing, tearing in left forearm, from elbow to hand.

Tearing: in either wrist; in finger of left hand.

Hands: burn; icy-cold; tip of fingers covered with cold sweat.

Paralytic weakness of fingers when seizing anything.

[33] **Lower Limbs.** Heaviness in the lower limbs.

Severe laming, drawing pain from abdomen down left leg.

Tearing near and beneath left hip, extending to sacrum.

Hip disease, third stage; black, ichorous, offensive discharge; great weakness.

Ulcer on leg burns at night; discharge offensive; skin around mottled, purple.

Left lower leg feels paralyzed.

Toes red, swollen, stinging, as if frosted.

Cramp in soles, evening after lying down.

Tips of toes ulcerated.

[34] **Limbs in General.** Limbs: feel bruised; numb; "go to sleep" when lying on them.

Drawing pain in limbs.

Burning: in limbs; in hands and soles, during menses.

Rheumatic pains, with flatulency.

[35] **Position, etc.** Motion: 26, 27, 37. Moving eyes: 3. Walking: 17, 36, 44; in open air: 27. Sitting: 29, 31, 37. Lying: 3, 17, 27, 33; on back: 17; limbs: 37. Stooping: 2, 31. Must bend double: 17. Must stretch legs: 36.

[35] **Nerves.** Vital force nearly exhausted, cold surface, especially below knees to feet; lies as if dead; breath cold; pulse intermittent, thready; cold sweat on limbs.

Want of nervous irritability, of susceptibility to medicines.

Weary after a short walk.

Faint-like weakness in attacks.

Indolent, weary, in the morning, in bed.

Prostration towards noon, head feels empty, sensation of hunger.

Worse from loss of fluids.

Uneasy feeling in the legs, in the evening, in bed; had to stretch them often.

[37] **Sleep.** Yawning, stretching.

Sleepiness in forenoon while sitting, and when reading; removed by motion.

Sleepy during day; had to sleep before and after noon; at night, sleep full of fancies.

Legs drawn up during sleep, which is restless and disturbed by frequent waking.

Sleepless, from uneasiness in the body; from orgasm of blood.

Does not fall asleep until 1 A. M.

Awakens often from cold limbs, especially cold knees.

Night full of dreams.

[38] **Time.** Morning: 1, 2, 5, 16, 23, 25, 26, 27, 36, 40. Forenoon: 7, 37. Noon: 36. Afternoon: 37. 4-6 P.M.: 1. Evening: 1, 3, 4, 6, 8, 16, 25, 27, 33, 36, 40. Night: 1, 7, 17, 21, 27, 32, 33, 37, 40. Before midnight: 27. After midnight: 37. Day: 2, 37.

[39] **Temperature and Weather.** Worse in changes of weather, especially warm, damp weather.

Warmth: 4. Overheated room: 3. Cold air: 26. Wants to be fanned: 28. Open air: 27. Going from warm to cold: 27. Damp weather: 25.

[40] **Chill. Fever. Sweat.** Shivering in the evening, with weariness and flushes of heat before sleep.

Chill, generally with thirst; mostly evenings, at times left-sided.

Chill with icy-coldness of the body.

Heat, after or independent of the chill.

Flushes of burning heat, evening; generally without thirst.

Hectic fever.

Heat and sweat commingled.

Exhausting night or morning sweats.

Sweats easily, especially about the head and face.

Sweat: profuse; putrid or sour.

[42] **Sides.** Right: 6, 8, 18, 28, 32. Left: 3, 6, 7, 8, 19, 28, 32, 33, 40. Nape to forehead: 3. Above downwards: 6.

[43] **Sensations.** Pains fly all over the body. θ Neuralgia.

Drawing and tearing pains in various parts of the body.

[44] **Tissues.** Sepsis, sunken features, sallow complexion, hectic, typhoid symptoms.

Blood stagnates in capillaries, causing blueness, coldness; ecchymoses.

Anæmia after summer complaint; feeble, pallid, white skin.

Atrophy, body cold, lies as if dead, yet conscious.

Gangrene: humid; senile.

Lymphatic glands swollen, indurated or suppurating; burning pains.

Chlorosis, with itch-like rash and fluor albus; scorbutic gums so weak, can scarcely stand.

[45] **Contact, Injuries, etc.** Worse from overlifting.

Touch: 4, 10, 18. Pressure: 4. Chewing: 10. Grasping anything: 32. Must hold on to something: 2.

Riding aggravates: soreness in limbs; colic.

[46] **Skin.** Nettle-rash.

Dry rash, like itch.

Fine, moist rash, with burning at spots where there is no eruption.

Folds of skin become raw and ulcerated.

Ulcers: varicose; scorbutic; livid, easily bleeding, fetid.

Decubitis in typhus, from decomposition of the blood.

Aneurisms bright red, round, flat, bleeding violently from least wound.

Single, scattered, red spots on the neck.

Itching and soreness in the axillæ.

[47] **Stages and States.** Vital powers low, venous system predominant.

Old people.

Children, after exhausting diseases.

[48] **Relationship.** *Carb. veg.* follows well: after *Sulphur* and *Mercur.*, when itch is dry; after *Veratr.* in beginning of whooping-cough; after *Laches.*, *Kali carb.*, *Sepia*.

After *Carb. veg.*: *Arsen.*, *Cinchon.*, *Droser.*, *Kali carb.*, *Phosph. ac.* are frequently indicated.

20

Ailments from quinine, especially suppression of chill and fever.

Ailments from abuses of mercury, salt or salt meats.

Carb. veg. antidotes: effects of putrid meat or fish, rancid fats; *Cinchon., Laches., Mercur.*

Antidotes to *Carb. veg.*: *Arsen., Camphor., Coffea, Laches., Spir. nitr. dulc.*

CARDUUS MARIANUS.

St. Mary's Thistle. *Compositæ.*

[18] **Hypochondria.** Jaundice; hepatic region painful to pressure; feeling of fulness in right hypochondrium. From hyperæmia of liver, or from duodenal catarrh (several cures).

[20] **Stool, etc.** Bile deficient in the evacuations.

Constipation alternating with diarrhœa.

[21] **Urine.** Coloring matter of bile present in the urine; the latter is scanty, brownish and turbid.

[40] **Chill. Fever. Sweat.** Chills and fever, with above symptoms of jaundice (one marked cure).

CAULOPHYLLUM.

Blue Cohosh. BURT. *Berberidaceæ.*

[2] **Sensorium.** Swimming, a sort of vertigo, with dimness of sight; gulping up a bitter, sour fluid.

[3] **Inner Head.** Headache, pressure behind the eye, dimness of sight; dependent upon uterine derangement.

Severe pains by spells, in the temples, as if they would be crushed together.

[4] **Outer Head.** Rheumatic headaches, especially with females.

[5] **Eyes.** Pressure behind the eyes; profuse flow of tears.

[8] **Face.** "Moth spots" on forehead, with leucorrhœa.

[10] **Teeth.** Teeth all feel sore, elongated.

[11] **Tongue, etc.** Tongue coated white.

[12] **Mouth.** Sensation of dryness in the mouth; heat.

Aphthæ.

[13] **Throat.** Distress in the fauces, which causes frequent inclination to swallow.

[14] **Desires. Aversions.** Great thirst.

Canine hunger, with white coated tongue.

[16] **Nausea and Vomiting.** Empty eructations.

Frequent gulping up of sour, bitter fluid, with vertigo.

Spasmodic vomiting, cardialgia, excessive nausea, spasms of the stomach attending uterine irritation.

[17] **Stomach.** Heat in the stomach; fulness.

Distress in stomach and bowels, with drawing in the right hypochondrium.

Dyspepsia, with spasmodic symptoms.

[19] **Abdomen.** Distention of the abdomen, with tenderness.

Rumbling in the bowels.

Spasmodic and flatulent colic.

Spasmodic action of the muscular tissues of the intestines, from irritation of the motor nerves, or from rheumatism.

[20] **Stool, etc.** Constipation; stool every other day.

Watery stools, great quantity, but no pain; 1 A. M.

Soft stool, very white.

[21] **Urine.** Emission of copious, pale or straw-colored urine.

[22] **Male Sexual Organs.** Every few minutes sharp, stinging pains in the glans penis.

[23] **Female Sexual Organs.** Sensation, as if uterus was congested, with fulness and tension in hypogastric region.

Menses too soon.

Amenorrhœa; spasms, cramps, or great atony.

Painful menstruation, the flow being normal in quantity.

Spasmodic dysmenorrhœa; spasmodic, intermittent pains in bladder, stomach, broad ligaments (groins), even chest and limbs; congestion and irritability of uterus; scanty flow.

Menstrual colic; uterus retroverted.

Irritable vagina, spasmodic, intense pains.

Aphthous vaginitis and spasmodic pains in the uterus.

Leucorrhœa: profuse, mucous; "moth spots" on the forehead; often in little girls.

[24] **Pregnancy.** Threatening abortion, spasmodic bearing down pains; vascular excitement; tremulous weakness; pains severe in back and loins, but uterine contractions feeble; slight flow.

Habitual abortion from uterine debility.

Tormenting, useless pains in the beginning of labor.

Labor-pains short, irregular, spasmodic; patient very weak; no progress being made.

Spasmodic rigidity of the os, delaying labor; pains like needles in the cervix.

Pains become weak, flagging from long protracted labor, causing exhaustion; thirsty, feverish.

Passive hemorrhage after abortion or confinement.

Protracted lochia, oozes passively from the relaxed uterine vessels, great atony.

Suppressed lochia.

After-pains, especially after exhausting, lengthy labor; spasmodic, across the lower abdomen; extend into groins.

[25] **Larynx.** Loss of voice; reflex from uterine disturbances.

[28] **Lungs.** Spasmodic, intermittent pains in chest, with amenia.

[31] **Neck. Back.** Rheumatic stiffness of the nape.

Severe drawing pain in the sterno-cleide-mastoid; drawing the head to the left.

Dull pain in the lumbar region.

[32] **Upper Limbs.** Severe drawing in wrists and fingers.

Rheumatism of wrists and finger-joints, with swelling; cutting in joints when closing hands; pains shift to the nape of neck, with spasmodic rigidity; panting; oppression of the chest; high fever; delirium; nervous excitement.

[33] **Lower Limbs.** Drawing pains in knees, ankles, feet and toes.

All joints crack when walking or turning.

Pain in feet and toes, worse at night.

Pains recur every day.

[34] **Limbs in General.** Rheumatism, especially of the smaller joints.

Constant flying pains in the arms and legs; remain only a few minutes in any one place.

Severe drawing pains in the joints of the arms and legs.

[35] **Position, etc.** Closing hands, cutting: 32. Walking: 33. Turning: 33.

[36] **Nerves.** Chorea at puberty.

Hysterical or epileptiform spasms at puberty, from menstrual irregularities, especially in rheumatic females.

Paraplegia, with retroversion and congestion of the uterus after childbirth; partial loss of sensation; emaciation, anæmia, general debility.

[37] **Sleep.** Sleepless, restless, nervous.

[38] **Time.** 1 A. M.: 20. Night: 33.

[40] **Chill. Fever. Sweat.** Fever high, delirious, nervous excitement, rheumatism.

[41] **Attacks.** Pains are intermittent.

Every day: 33. Every other day: 20. Every few minutes: 22, 34.

[42] **Sides.** Right: 17. Left: 31.

[47] **Stages and States.** Especially suited to females.

CAUSTICUM.

HAHNEMANN.

¹ **Mind.** Weakness of memory; absent-minded.

Inattentive and distracted.

Taciturn, distant; disinclined to work.

Full of timorous fancies, evenings, child fears to go to bed alone.

Great anxiety.

Melancholy mood.   Hopelessness.

Peevish, irritable mood.

Thinking of complaints aggravates them, especially hemorrhoids.

² **Sensorium.** Vertigo: tending forwards and sideways; at night in bed, on rising and on lying down again, or at 11 A.M.; on looking fixedly at an object; better in open air; with weakness in the head and anxiety.   Anæmia.

Dulness of the head.

³ **Inner Head.**   Painless commotion in the whole head.

Pressive pain in right frontal eminence; dull, pressive headache.

Stitches in the temples, worse from sitting or reading.

Throbbing and stitches in the vertex.

Sensation as of an empty space between the forehead and brain.

⁴ **Outer Head.**   Pain at a small spot on the vertex, as if bruised, only on touch.

Tension or itching on the scalp.

⁵ **Eyes.**   Photophobia whole day, constantly obliged to wink.

Flickering or sparks before the eyes.

Sight obscured: as from a gauze before the eyes; as from a mist; momentarily, on blowing the nose.

Perpendicular half sight in cataract; has arrested cataract.

Pain in the eyes, as if sand were in them.

Pressive pain in the eyes, worse from touch.

Constant inclination to touch and rub the eye, which seems to relieve a pressure in it.

Eyes: inflamed; burning, red, dry, stinging.

Smarting and pressure in eyes, which seem heavy; lids red.

Itching of the eyes, especially of the lids.

Inclination to close the eyes, lids seem heavy; even paralysis of upper lids.   ❙Weakness of the recti muscles. Double vision.

Blepharitis, especially if better in fresh air.

Agglutination of the lids.

Lachrymation even in room, though worse in open air.

Corrosive lachrymation, pains shooting, extend up into the head; scrofulous ophthalmia.

Old warts on eyebrows, lids or nose.

⁶ **Ears.** Roaring, or buzzing in the ears.

Words and steps re-echo in the ears; hears with difficulty.

Stitches in right ear, paroxysmal, and in rapid succession.

Feeling of obstruction in ears, with offensive purulent discharge.

Herpes on the ear-lobe.

Meatus dry, with a little brown wax.

⁷ **Nose.** Frequent sneezing.

Fluent coryza, with pain in chest and limbs.

Dry coryza, with stoppage of nose.

Blowing blood from nose, mornings. Profuse nosebleed.

Pimples on the tip of the nose.

Itching of tip and alæ.

Old warts on the nose.

⁸ **Face.** Face: yellow; sickly looking.

Neuralgia: right side; worse at night, chilly, no thirst; drawing pains, extending into cheeks and ear; spasm of muscles and numbness; menses scanty.

Pimples on left cheek, with severe itching. Acne burning after scratching, better washing.

Paralysis of one side of face.

⁹ **Lower Face.** Sensation of tension and pain in the jaws, could only with difficulty open the mouth, and could not eat well,. because a tooth seemed too long.

Arthritic pains in lower jaw.

¹⁰ **Teeth.** Painful looseness and elongation of the teeth. Tooth as if being crowded out of the alveoli.

Teeth painful when chewing.

Pain in sound teeth, or drawing in cold air.

Stitching and tearing toothache.

Swelling of the gums.

Tedious suppuration of the gums. θ Fistula dentalis.

¹¹ **Tongue, etc.** Taste: greasy; of rancid fat; putrid; bitter; as from disordered stomach.

Speechlessness, from paralysis of the organs of speech.

Distortion of the tongue and mouth when talking.

Stuttering, difficult, indistinct speech.

Painful vesicle on the tip of the tongue.

Tongue coated white on both sides, red in the middle.

¹² **Mouth.** Dryness of the mouth and tongue.

Much phlegm in the mouth and throat.

Sore, painful spot on the hard palate.

Swelling inside the cheek; bites it when chewing.

[13] **Throat.** Dryness in throat, posteriorly.

Mucus collects in the throat, cannot be raised by hawking; obliged to swallow it.

Hawking of mucus, with pain in pit of throat.

Rawness in throat, with sensation like heart-burn.

Rawness and tickling in the throat, with dry cough and some expectoration only after long coughing.

Must swallow continually, feels as if the throat were too narrow.

Swelling like goitre, on the throat.

[14] **Desires. Aversions.** Desire for beer.

Thirst for cold drinks; thirst, with aversion to drink.

Aversion to sweet things.

Sits down to the table with some appetite, but can scarcely eat a morsel.

[15] **Eating and Drinking.** Fresh meat causes nausea; smoked meat agrees; bread causes pressure in stomach.

Coffee seems to aggravate every symptom.

[16] **Nausea and Vomiting.** Eructations: frequent, empty; tasting of the food; of food; burning.

Nausea during and after meals.

Sour vomiting, followed by sour eructations.

Vomiting of blood, at night.

[17] **Stomach.** Pain in the stomach in the morning, increased by every quick movement; must lie down.

Cramp in the stomach; pressure in the pit of stomach.

Pinching, clawing in pit of stomach on deep breathing.

[18] **Hypochondria.** Stitches in the region of the liver.

[19] **Abdomen.** Pains in the abdomen, must bend double; worse after the least nourishment or from tightening the clothes.

Colic: in the morning; pain radiates to back and chest.

Stitches in the right side of the abdomen.

Painful distention of the abdomen.

Flatulency, loud rumbling and rolling in the bowels.

Tumid abdomen, in children.

[20] **Stool, etc.** Pressure in the rectum.

Itching and sticking in the rectum.

Frequent, sudden, penetrating, pressive pain in rectum.

Frequent passage of offensive flatus.

Stools: tough and shining; first hard and in pieces, the last soft; knotty, like sheep's dung.

Frequent ineffectual efforts to stool, with much pain, anxiety and redness in face.

The stool passes better standing.

Pulsations in the perineum.

Fissure of the anus, pains worse when walking.

Itching in the anus.

Large, painful pustule near the anus, discharging pus'
blood and serum.

Hemorrhoids: impeding the stool; swollen, itching, stitching, moist; stinging, burning; painful when touched,
when walking, or when thinking of them.

21 **Urine.** Paralysis of bladder from long retention of urine.

Involuntary passage of urine: when coughing, walking
or blowing the nose; at night when asleep.

Diabetes insipidus.

Retention of urine, with frequent and urgent desire, occasionally a few drops or small quantity may dribble
away.

Burning in the urethra when urinating.

Itching of the orifice of the urethra.

Urine: dark brown; turbid and cloudy on standing.

22 **Male Sexual Organs.** Increase of smegma about the glans.

Continuous loss of prostatic fluid; memory weak.

Pressive pains in testicles.

Itching of the scrotum and skin of the penis.

23 **Female Sexual Organs.** Aversion to coitus.

Menses: too early and too profuse, and after ceasing,
a little is passed from time to time for days; smell badly
and excite itching of vulva; only during the day; with
violent pains in abdomen and discharge of large clots;
scanty, with prosopalgia.

Leucorrhœa: profuse, flows like the menses and has the
same odor; only at night and worse then; with scanty
menses.

Soreness in the vulva and between the legs.

Smarting, as from salt, in the pedendum, after urinating.

24 **Pregnancy.** Spasmodic labor-pains. Labor-pains insufficient, irregular; os dilated, but patient has become tired
and fretful.

Milk almost disappeared in consequence of overfatigue,
night-watching and anxiety.

Nipples sore, cracked, surrounded with herpes.

25 **Larynx.** Hoarseness: worse morning and evening, with
scraping in the throat; for several days, could not speak
loud.

Croup, especially when there is a raw sensation in the
larynx. Catarrhal croup.

The laryngeal muscles refuse their service; cannot speak
a loud word. When he tries to raise his voice, it fails
or becomes a squeak.

26 **Breathing.** Arrest of breathing when talking or walking
rapidly, must suddenly catch after breath.

Shortness of breath.

27 **Cough.** Violent, hollow, at times dry, with pain in right

chest; hollow, especially night and morning, with tightly adhering mucus in the chest, and with sensation of soreness on the chest; hacking, from creeping and rawness in the throat; with pain above left hip, and involuntary passage of drops of urine; dry, remaining after pertussis.

Cough worse evening till midnight; from exhaling; drinking coffee; cold air; draught of air; when awaking.

Cough relieved by a swallow of cold water.

[28] **Lungs.**   Soreness in the chest.   ı Burning soreness in a stripe down under the sternum, with cough, etc.

Tightness of chest, must frequently take a deep breath.

Stitches in the chest below the arms, extending to the pit of the stomach, with anxiety.

Rattling in the chest.

[29] **Heart.   Pulse.**   Stitches about the heart.

Palpitation of the heart.

Oppression at the heart, with lowness of spirits.

Pulse excited towards evening, with orgasm of blood.

[39] **Outer Chest.**   Sensation as if the clothing were too tight.

Painful compression of chest from both sides toward the sternum, with oppression of breath and weakness of voice.

Stitches in the sternum from deep breathing or lifting.

[31] **Neck.   Back.**   Stiffness of the neck, could not move head.

Stiffness and pain in neck and throat, with pain in occiput, muscles felt as if bound, could scarcely move the head.

Painful stiffness of back, especially when rising from chair.

Stitches: in the back; in left lumbar region.

Pressing, cramp-like pain in small of back, in region of kidneys.

Dull, drawing pain in region of os coccygis.

Bruised pain in the os coccygis.

[32] **Upper Limbs.**   Pressure on the shoulders.

Dull drawing and tearing in the arms and hands.

Paralytic feeling in the right hand.

Sensation of fulness in the palm when grasping.

Contraction and induration of the tendons of the fingers.

Drawing pains in the finger joints.

Trembling of the hands.

Convulsion of the fingers in writing; writer's cramp.

Warts on tip of the fingers.

Itching on the arms.

[33] **Lower Limbs.**   Soreness high up, between the thighs.

Aching in the hip-joint, as if dislocated.

Bruised pains in the thighs and legs, mornings in bed.

Cramp in the calf, mornings in bed.

Drawing and tearing in thighs and legs, knees and feet, worse in open air, better in warmth of bed.

Cracking in the knees when walking.
· Tension in the knee and ankle-joints.
Tensive pain and stiffness in hollow of knee, when
walking.
Marbled skin of thighs and legs.
Unsteady walking and easy falling, of little children.
Cramp in the feet.
Ball of the great toe: crawling, burning; severe pressive
pain; burning stitches.
Phagedenic blisters and ulcers on the heel.
Sudden cramp in tendo-achillis at night.
Crawling in both soles as from something alive.
Itching on the dorsum of feet.

³¹ **Limbs in General.** Arthritic pains in all the limbs.
Weakness and trembling of all the limbs.
Paralytic weakness of the limbs.
Intolerable uneasiness in the limbs in the evening.

³⁵ **Position, etc.** At night cannot get a quiet position, nor lie
still a minnte.
Partly laid on feels sore, must turn often.
Lifting: 30. Motion: 40, 44. Quick motion: 17. Can
scarcely move the head: 31. Walking: 20, 26, 33, 40.
Standing: 20. Sitting: 3. Must sit up: 37. Rising:
2, 31. Lying down: 2. Must lie down: 17, 37. In
bed: 2, 33, 40.

³⁶ **Nerves.** Weakness and trembling.
Faint-like sinking of strength.
Restlessness of the body.
Hemiplegia after cerebral hemorrhage or softening.
Epileptic attacks during time of puberty, also worse dur-
ing new moon.
Convulsions: with screams, gnashing of the teeth, and
violent movements of the limbs; with feverish heat
and coldness of hands and feet.
Chorea even at night, right side of face and tongue may
be paralyzed.

³⁷ **Sleep.** Yawning and stretching.
Intense sleepiness, can scarcely withstand it, must lie down.
Sleeplessness at night on account of dry heat.
Very uneasy all night, after a short sleep awakened by
anxiety and restlessness, which scarcely allowed ten
minutes quiet in one place; must sit up; involuntary
throwing of the head from side to side, until exhaustion
brought on sleep.
Starting from sleep; many motions with arms and legs,
during sleep, at night.
Dreams: anxious; quarrelsome.

³⁸ **Time.** Morning: 7, 17, 19, 25, 27, 33, 40. 4 A.M.: 40. Even-

ing: 1, 25, 27, 29, 34, 40. 6 to 8 P.M.: 40. Evening,
till midnight: 27. Night: 2, 8, 16, 21, 23, 27, 34, 36,
37, 40. Midnight: 40. Day: 5, 23.

[39] **Temperature and Weather.** Warmth of bed: 33. Room:
5. Open air: 2, 5, 33, 40. Cold air: 27. Cold water:
27. Draught: 27.

[40] **Chill. Fever. Sweat.** Chill and chilliness; predominating frequently with coldness of the whole left side; on
diseased parts.

Much internal chilliness, immediately followed by sweat
without intervening heat; severe internal chill about
midnight.

Shivering beginning in and spreading from the face.

Chill lessened by drinking, and in bed.

Heat from 6 to 8 P.M., heat descending.

Flushes of heat followed by chilliness.

Profuse sweat: when walking in open air; from motion.

Sour-smelling night sweat.

Morning-sweat toward 4 A.M.

[41] **Attacks.** New moon: 36.

[42] **Sides.** Right: 3, 6, 8, 18, 19, 27, 32, 36. Left: 8, 31, 40.

[44] **Tissues.** Rheumatic and arthritic inflammations, with contraction of the flexors and stiffness of the joints.

Tearing, piercing pains at night, compelling motion, but
not thereby relieved.

Emaciation of the feet.

Hemorrhages of very dark blood.

Painful varices, ulcers, or warts; net-like appearance of the
capillaries.

[45] **Contact, Injuries, etc.** Touch: 4, 5, 20, 35. Rubbing: 5.
Tight clothing: 19, 30.

[46] **Skin.** Intertrigo, during teething.

Excessively itching moist tetter on the neck.

Eruption of pimples on the tip of the nose.

Itching: over the whole body; at various parts, especially
on tip and wings of the nose; face; scrotum; back;
arms; palms; dorsum of feet.

Injuries of the skin which had healed, become sore again.

[47] **Stages and States.** Dark hair and rigid fibre most affected.

Children with delicate skin.

[48] **Relationship.** After the abuse of sulphur and mercury in
scabies, *Caustic.* may be indicated.

Antidotes to *Caustic.*: *Asaf., Coffea, Coloc., Nux vom.,
Spir. nitr. dulc.*

Rheumatic contraction of tendons of arms and legs much
increased by *Caustic.*, was promptly relieved by *Guajac.*

Inimicals: Acids, *Coffea, Phosphor.*

CEPA.

Onion.   HERING.   *Liliaceæ.*

¹ **Mind.** Confusion.

Fears she will become distracted, from pain in the suppurations on the fingers.

Very melancholy.

² **Sensorium.** Dulness, pressure, fulness, heaviness in the head, most in occiput, worse evenings, better in the open air, and worse when returning to a warm room.

³ **Inner Head.** Dull frontal headache.

Dull headache, worse evenings.

Like an electric shock, through the head.

⁴ **Outer Head.** Formication in the skull bones.

Prickling sweat on the bald scalp after each meal.

⁵ **Eyes.** Dim and sensitive to light.

Thread-like pain: over the right eye, toward the root of nose; from the cheek towards the eye.

Smarting in the eyes, like from smoke.

Eyes red, itch, and are sensitive to touch, worse left.

Eyes watery, capillaries congested; with coryza.

Shooting pain in right lachrymal duct.

Profuse bland lachrymation.

Smarting of inner surface of upper lids.

⁶ **Ears.** Noises in the ears.

Jerking pains from the throat towards the eustachian tube.

Dulness of hearing.

Earache.

⁷ **Nose.** Epistaxis.

Constant sneezing, with profuse acrid coryza, when coming into a warm room.

Spring coryza; tingling and itching in right nostril.

Every year in August morning coryza, with violent sneezing; very sensitive to odor of flowers and skin of peaches (lasting two or three weeks).

Fluent coryza, headache, lachrymation, cough, thirst, want of appetite, trembling of hands, feverish; worse evenings and in-doors; better in open air.

Profuse, watery, acrid nasal discharge, with bland lachrymation.

Ichor oozing out of the nose. θ Second stage of scarlatina.

Polypus of nose.

⁸ **Face.** Thread-like pains about the face, temples and ears.

Throbbing, drawing, pressing pains, with swelling of cheek.

Face hot.

10 **Teeth.** Toothache with coryza, getting better when the catarrh is worse, and worse when the catarrh ceases.

12 **Mouth.** Dryness of mouth, root of tongue, soft palate and throat.

Bad odor from the mouth or throat.

13 **Throat.** Sensation as of a ball in the throat.

Tough mucus in the fauces and throat.

Numb feeling in posterior wall of pharynx.

14 **Desires. Aversions.** Canine hunger, or may have loss of appetite.

15 **Eating and Drinking.** Bad effects from eating spoiled fish.

16 **Nausea and Vomiting.** Sour eructations.

Belching, with rumbling in and puffing up of abdomen.

Nausea when rising.

17 **Stomach.** Pressure in the stomach.

Pain in the region of the pylorus.

Stomach feels empty, weak.

18 **Hypochondria.** Pressure in region of the liver, with creeping chills along the back ; coldness.

Contracting sensation in the spleen, with stitches while lying.

19 **Abdomen.** Colic ; pain in region of navel, worse sitting ; better walking.

Violent pain in the hypogastrium, to the left, with urging to urinate ; burning micturition.

Annoying pains over the middle of the groin.

Pressure in left inguinal ring.

20 **Stool, etc.** Very offensive flatus.

Diarrhœa after midnight, or toward morning.

Constipation, following intermittents treated by quinine.

Rhagades at the anus.

21 **Urine.** Pains in the region of kidneys.

Region of bladder very sensitive, child screams if the hand is placed there.

Pressing and other pains in region of bladder.

Sensation of weakness or warmth in bladder and urethra.

Copious urine, with other complaints.

Urine red, with much urging and burning in the urethra.

Albuminuria.

22 **Male Sexual Organs.** Increased sexual desire.

After coitus pain in bladder and prostate gland.

Drawing in the spermatic cord.

Burning in the glans.

23 **Female Sexual Organs.** Pain in uterine region.

24 **Pregnancy.** In childbed, panaritia on several fingers, with red streaks up the arm ; pains driving to despair.

25 **Larynx.** Catarrhal hoarseness.

Tickling in throat, with aching in the larynx.

Catarrhal inflammation of larynx.

Pain as if the larynx would be torn when coughing.

²⁶ **Breathing.** Breathing oppressed from pressure in middle of chest.

²⁷ **Cough.** Laryngeal cough, frequently repeated.

Severe laryngeal cough, which compels the patient to grasp the larynx; feels as if the cough would tear it.

Hacking cough from inhaling cold air.

Constant inclination to hack.

²⁸ **Lungs.** Chest laden with mucus.

Pains here and there through the chest

Stitches with burning, in middle of left side of chest, when taking a deep breath.

²⁹ **Heart. Pulse.** Pulse more frequent and full; or, slow and hard.

³¹ **Neck. Back.** Creepings in the back; after sitting, pain under the right shoulder-blade.

Pain in small of back, if the bowels did not move.

³² **Upper Limbs.** Pain in right shoulder-blade when lying in bed.

All the joints feel lame.

Trembling of right hand.

Run-around, pain extends up the whole arm.

Suppuration, after a prick with a needle, under the thumb nail; a red streak up to the elbow.

³³ **Lower Limbs.** Weakness of the hips.

Nettle-rash on the thighs.

Pain above the knees.

Lameness in the knee.

Sore and raw spots on the feet, from friction.

Pain in the great toes.

³⁴ **Limbs in General.** Soreness in the limbs.

³⁵ **Position, etc.** Walking: 19. Rising: 16. Sitting: 19, 31. Lying: 18, 32. Must lie down: 36.

³⁶ **Nerves.** Weak and tired, has to lie down.

Lassitude.

³⁷ **Sleep.** Yawning, with headache and cramp in the stomach.

Restless sleep, drowsy in the morning.

Dreams: of being near the water; of storms at sea, high waves.

³⁸ **Time.** Morning: 7, 20, 37, 40. Evening: 2, 3, 7, 43. After midnight: 20. 2 A.M.: 40. Toward morning: 20.

³⁹ **Temperature and Weather.** Bad effects from getting the feet wet.

Colds, after damp, cold weather and northeast winds.

Cold air: 27. Better in open air, worse in warm room: 2, 7. Spring: 7. August: 7.

⁴⁰ **Chill. Fever. Sweat.** Coldness alternates with heat; during catarrh.

Heat and thirst, with rumbling in the belly.

Heat without thirst, 2 A. M., passes off by daylight, worse again after breakfast.

Sweats easily and copiously.

[41] **Attacks.** Periodic attacks: 45.   Spring: 7.   August: 7.

[42] **Sides.** Right: 5, 7, 18, 31, 32.   Left: 5, 18, 19, 24, 28, 43.

Most symptoms in provings go from left to right; cures symptoms that proceed from right to left.

[43] **Sensations.** Aching through the body.

Neuralgic pains like a long thread; in the face, head, neck and elsewhere; worse evenings.

[44] **Tissues.** Inflammation and increased secretion of the mucous membrane.

Joints ache.

Gangræna senilis, woman, æt. 80 (externally as a salve).

[45] **Contact, Injuries, etc.** Touch: 5, 21.

After hurts and lesions stiffness in back, periodic attacks.

Must grasp larynx: 27.   Rubbing: 33.

[46] **Skin.** Pricking as from pins.

Redness of the skin.

Nettle-rash on the thighs.

Measles.

[47] **Stages and States.** Old age; gangrene.

[48] **Relationship.** Antidotes to *Cepa: Arnic.* against toothache; *Chamom.* bellyache; *Veratr.* colic with desponding.

Phosphor. is complementary.

Cepa is complementary to *Phosphor., Pulsat., Sarsap.*

Calc. and *Silic.* follow *Cepa* well in polypus.

Collateral relations that neither antidote nor follow well: *All. sat., Scilla, Aloe.*

Allium sativum is useful in chronic cough with an abundant mucous expectoration, and sensitiveness to cold air; herpetic diathesis.

CHAMOMILLA.

Chamomile.   HAHNEMANN.   *Compositæ.*

[1] **Mind.** Omits words when writing or speaking.

Confusion of the head, with transient, painful pressure on the eyes, in the afternoon.

Dulness of senses, diminished power of comprehension.

Imagines he hears the voice of absent persons, at night.

Child cries, quiet only when carried.

Whining restlessness; the child wants this and that, which when offered are refused, or pushed away.

Cannot endure being spoken to, or interrupted while speaking, especially after rising from sleep.

Irritable, impatient mood.

Great impatience, everything seems to go slowly.

Peevishness, nothing pleases.

² **Sensorium.** Dulness of senses, with sleepiness, yet cannot sleep.

Vertigo: after eating; staggering, in the morning on rising from bed: with fainting; with dimness of sight when sitting up in bed.

³ **Inner Head.** Pressive pain in both temples, as from strong pressure with the thumbs, forenoon.

Tearing and stinging pain in left side, particularly in the temple, and in and around the eye.

One-sided drawing headache.

Violent stinging pains in left side of head, from the occiput to upper jaw.

Pressing headache, as from a stone in the forehead, hot head, worse evenings.

Intense headache in vertex, like a pressure from within, feeling as if the top of her head were blown off.

Throbbing headache.

Transient attacks of throbbing in one-half of the brain.

Pressure, extending from the vertex to the forehead and temples; worse when thinking of it, from sudden stooping, or from mental exertion.

⁴ **Outer Head.** Head sweats during sleep.

⁵ **Eyes.** Flickering before the eyes when lying down.

Eyes swollen, in the morning; agglutinated with purulent mucus.

Inflammation of the eyes, lids agglutinated in the morning; discharge of blood from the eyes; inflammation caused by exposure to cold, damp atmosphere, or if worse, by every cold change of weather.

Yellow conjunctiva.

Violent pressure in the orbital region; sensation in the eyeball as if it were tightly compressed from all sides, with momentary obstruction of vision.

⁶ **Ears.** Roaring in the ears, as from rushing water.

Stitches in the ear, especially when stooping.

Occasional tearing in the left ear.

Pressing earache in spells, with tearing pain, extorting cries.

⁷ **Nose.** Extremely sensitive to all odors.

Irritation to sneeze, with crawling, dry heat and stopped up sensation; feeling as if coryza would appear.

Coryza: fluent, watery; viscid.

Nosebleed, relieving the confusion of the head.

⁸ **Face.**   Red; or redness and heat of one (left) cheek, other
         pale; pale, sunken, distorted by pain; yellow; bloated.
     Burning in face.
     Left cheek swollen.
     Neuralgia of the face, the pain causes hot sweat about the
         head and extorts screams.
     Gives great relief in ordinary inflammatory and rheuma-
         tic faceache.

⁹ **Lower Face.**   Lips crack and peel.
     Rhagades in the middle of lower lip.

¹⁰ **Teeth.**   Toothache: stitching; digging; gnawing; as from
         taking cold; during or after eating; if anything warm
         is taken into the mouth, especially after coffee; in open
         air; in the room; getting warm in bed; during men-
         struation; most left side and lower teeth; worse at
         night.
     Teeth feel too long.
     Gums red and tender, during dentition.

¹¹ **Tongue, etc.**   Taste: bitter; sour; like rancid fat; putrid.
     Tongue: coated, white; yellowish; or white at the sides,
         red in the middle; red, cracked; coated white, with
         islands on it.
     Burning on the tongue.

¹² **Mouth.**   Fetid smell from the mouth after dinner.
     Heat in the mouth, pharynx and œsophagus to stomach.
     Collection of saliva, of metallic, sweetish taste.

¹³ **Throat.**   Spasmodic constriction of the pharynx.
     Sore throat, with swelling of the parotid gland.

¹⁴ **Desires.   Aversions.**   Thirst for cold water and desire for
         acid drinks.
     Likes to hold the cold water to the mouth, a long time;
         when drinking.
     Aversion to: beer; coffee and warm drinks.
     Want of appetite.

¹⁵ **Eating and Drinking.**   After eating and drinking, heat
         and sweat of the face; after eating, abdomen puffed up.

¹⁶ **Nausea and Vomiting.**   Eructations; sour; constant, empty.
     Fruitless efforts to vomit.
     Nausea and inclination to vomit, and bitter vomiting.
     Inclination to vomit, with diarrhœa and fever during the
         night.
     Vomiting: of bile; of what has been drunk; slimy matter;
         sour.
     Severe vomiting with griping.

¹⁷ **Stomach.**   Pressive pain in stomach and beneath the short
         ribs, which impedes breathing, especially after drinking
         coffee.
     Pressing and cutting in the epigastrium, with anxiety.
     21

Severe painful pressure in the epigastrium makes her toss about in despair.

Stinging pain in pit of stomach.

[18] **Hypochondria.** Stitching pains in the hypochondria.

Stitches in region of liver, with frequent chilliness, after vexation.

[19] **Abdomen.** Griping, tearing colic in region of navel and lower down on both sides, with pain in small of back, as if it were broken.

Feeling of griping and chilliness inside of abdomen, passing downwards into legs as far as the knees.

Colic returns from time to time, flatulence accumulates in the hypochondria, and stitches shoot through the chest.

Wind colic, abdomen distended like a drum, wind passes in small quantities without relief; relieved by applying warm cloths.

Abdomen tympanitic and sensitive to touch.

Constricting pain in the abdomen and back; she kicks, grates her teeth and screams.

Dragging toward the abdominal rings, as if the parts were too weak, and hernia would appear.

❙ Pain in the belly from side to side, just above the navel, corresponding to the transverse colon, commencing in the right and going over to left.

[20] **Stool, etc.** Stools: watery, frequent, preceded by cutting, constricting bellyache, worse in epigastric region; mucous, with colic and vomituritia; bilious, with burning in anus; painful, thin green, consisting of feces and mucus; green, watery, corroding, with colic, thirst, bitter taste and bitter eructations; like chopped eggs, smelling sour; hot, smelling like rotten eggs.

Griping with great ineffectual desire for stool.

Bowels relaxed after "colic;" stools first white then putty-like.

Hemorrhoids: blind; painful, bleeding, burning.

Ulcerating fissures at the anus.

[21] **Urine.** Dragging down the the ureters like labor-pains, with very frequent urging to urinate.

Burning in the neck of bladder when urinating.

Urine: yellow, with flaky sediment; burning in urethra while passing; scanty; turbid, clay-colored soon after passing; turbid, gets thick when standing, sediment yellow.

[22] **Male Sexual Organs.** Violent erections.

[23] **Female Sexual Organs.** Menses: too early; too profuse; offensive.

Drawing from small of back forwards, griping and pinching in uterus, followed by discharge of large clots of blood.

Profuse discharge of clotted blood, with severe labor-like
pains in the uterus; tearing pains in the legs.

Membranous dysmenorrhœa.

Yellow, smarting leucorrhœa.

Burning in the vagina, as if excoriated.

²⁴ **Pregnancy.**   Threatened abortion, with discharge of dark
blood.

Labor-pains spasmodic and distressing; tearing pains
down legs.

Rigidity of the os; scarcely able to endure the pains.

Hour-glass contraction; irritable; thirsty; desire for fresh
air, restless.

Puerperal convulsions, after anger; or has one red cheek,
the other pale.

After-pains very distressing.

Suppression of the lochia, followed by diarrhœa, colic and
toothache.

ı Excessive heat, anxiety, tendency to syncope, red face,
especially redness of one cheek; formation of pus;
puerperal peritonitis.

Mammæ hard and tender to touch; with drawing, rheumatic pains; worse in open air and at night.

Nipples inflamed and very tender; infants' breasts tender
to the touch.

²⁵ **Larynx.**   Sensation of rawness and scraping in the larynx.

Hoarseness, on account of tough mucus in the larynx,
which can only be removed by strong hawking.

Catarrhal hoarseness of trachea, with dryness of eyelids.

²³ **Breathing.**   Oppressed, as if chest were not wide enough.

Short, with rattling.

Threatened suffocation, from repercussion of measle
eruption.

Dyspnœa, constricted feeling at the suprasternal fossa,
with constant irritation to cough.

Asthmatic attack, seemingly produced by an accumulation
of flatus, better from bending the head backwards; in
cold air, and from drinking cold water; worse in dry
weather and from warm diet.

²⁷ **Cough.**   Hoarseness and rattling cough from mucus in the
trachea, especially during winter.

Cough caused by irritation low down in the air-passages,
during the night.

Paroxysms of coughing about midnight, with which something seems to rise in throat, as if she would suffocate.

Constant irritation to cough, beneath the upper part of
the sternum.

Cough particularly at night, with tough, slimy expectoration, tasting bitter.

Cough, with expectoration during day, without at night.
Expectoration bloody, dark, coagulated.

[28] **Lungs.** Constriction in the upper part of chest.

Chest painful when coughing.

Stitches shoot from the abdomen into the middle of the chest, as from flatulence.

Sudden stitches and darts through the chest, extorting screams; dyspnœa taking away the voice and threatening suffocation.

[29] **Heart. Pulse.** Palpitation and faintness.

Pulse small, but tense and accelerated frequently very unequal, and then for a time weak.

[31] **Neck. Back.** Drawing pain in the back.

Pain in the small of the back, especially at night.

Bruised sensation in the muscles of the loins and back.

Small of back feels bruised.

[32] **Upper Limbs.** Pain in the arms, cannot bear the slightest motion.

Stiffness of the arm, tendency to formication when grasping with the hand.

Finger-joints red and swollen.

[33] **Lower Limbs.** Violent drawing, tearing pains, from the left ischium to the os calcis and sole of the foot, with cramp-like tension of the muscles.

Tearing pains from abdomen down into legs. See 23, 24.

Cramp in the calves.

Tearing pain in the feet after a severe chill; must lie down and keep quiet; pain in ankle, worse from every motion.

Redness and swelling around the malleoli.

Heaviness and lassitude in the legs.

Burning of the soles at night; puts the feet out of bed.

[34] **Limbs in General.** Pain in the periosteum, with paralytic weakness.

Drawing and tearing pains in the limbs, worse at night.

Joints sore, as if bruised and tired out; no power in the hands and feet.

Cracking in the joints, especially of the lower limbs, with pains therein, as if bruised.

Aching in all the limbs, with lassitude.

Limbs feel heavy.

[35] **Position, etc.** Inclination to lie down.

Motion: 32, 33. Rising from sleep: 1; from bed: 2. Sitting up in bed: 2. Lying down: 5. Stopping: 3, 6. Must lie down and keep quiet: 33. Tosses about, starts up: 37, 40. Bending head back: 26. Bends backward: 36.

[36] **Nerves.** Child makes itself stiff and bends backwards, kicks with the feet when carried, screams immoderately, and throws everything off.

Convulsions of children: legs moved up and down, grasping and reaching with the hands, mouth drawn from side to side, eyes staring.

Twitching in the eyelid, eyeballs, lips and facial muscles.

Pain in limbs, with weakness, and slow, dragging gait.

General prostration, faintness.

[37] **Sleep.** Yawning and stretching.

Sleep, with half open eyes; sleepy, but cannot sleep.

Sleepless and restless at night.

Scarcely sleeps, and on falling asleep is tormented by anxious, frightening dreams.

During sleep: moaning; weeping and wailing; starting up, crying out, tossing about and talking.

[38] **Time.** Morning: 2, 5. Forenoon: 3. Afternoon: 1, 12. Evening: 3. Night: 1, 10, 16, 24, 27, 31, 33, 34, 37, 46. Midnight: 27. Day: 27.

[39] **Temperature and Weather.** Warmth: 19; of bed: 10. Dry weather: 2, 6. Cold air: 26, 40; damp: 5. Open air: 10, 24. Cold change of weather: 5. Winter: 27. Wants fresh air: 24. Uncovering: 40. Room: 10.

❙ Heat aggravates the pains.

[40] **Chill. Fever. Sweat.** Coldness with thirst.

Chill and shivering, generally of single parts only, with heat of others.

Chill and coldness of the whole body, with burning heat of the face and hot breath.

Chill of posterior part with heat of anterior of body, or vice versa.

Slight shiverings, alternating with heat, creep over the back and abdomen. Shivering when uncovering and from cold air.

Heat and shivering intermingled mostly with one red and one pale cheek.

Burning heat in lightly covered parts, though when not covered almost cold.

Anxious heat, with sweat of the face and scalp.

Long lasting heat, with violent thirst and frequent startings in sleep.

Sweat during sleep, most on the head, usually of sour odor, and with smarting sensation in skin.

Revulsion of, and therefrom entire want of sweat.

[42] **Sides.** Right: 18. Left: 3, 6, 8, 10, 18, 33. Above downwards: 24, 33. Below upwards: 28. Behind forwards: 23.

Symptoms in provings go from right to left; therefore cures from left to right.

[43] **Sensations.** The paralytic sensations are always accompanied by drawing or tearing pain, and the drawing or tearing pains rarely occur without the paralytic or numb sensation in the part.

⁴⁴ **Tissues.** Muscular or articular rheumatism, with great
nervous excitability; also when pains are erratic, worse
knees and ankles; numbness afterwards. They drive
him out of bed and compel him to walk about.

⁴⁵ **Contact, Injuries, etc.** Touch: 19, 24, 46. Wants to be
carried: 1.

⏐ Wounds which suppurate (topically and internally).

⁴⁶ **Skin.** Unhealthy, every injury suppurates.

Exanthema difficult to heal.

Red rash on the cheeks.

Skin inclined to inflammation.

Burning and smarting pain in the ulcer, at night, with
crawling and painful oversensitiveness to touch.

Itching pimples covered with scurfs, and ulcerating around
the ulcer.

Severe itching of the sweating parts.

Skin yellow, jaundiced.

⁴⁷ **Stages and States.** Children. Light or brown hair, ner-
vous, excitable temperament.

Adults; even aged persons with arthritic or rheumatic
diathesis.

⁴⁸ **Relationship.** Antidotes to *Chamom.: Acon., Alum., Borax,
Camphor., Coccul., Coffea, Coloc., Ignat., Nux vom.,* and
especially *Pulsat.*.

Similar to *Tarax.* See 11; *Hepar., Calend.* (suppuration).

Chamom. antidotes: *Coffea, Opium.*

Complementary to *Magnes.*

CHELIDONIUM.

Celandine.   *Papaveraceæ.*

¹ **Mind.** Great absence of mind, forgets what she wants to do
or has done.

Weeping. Sadness.

Fears of becoming crazy.

Anxiety: allowing no rest at any employment; as if she
had committed a crime.

Desponding mood.

Irritability. Ill-humor.

² **Sensorium.** Vertigo; with bilious vomiting and pain in
the liver; with confusion of the head; with stumbling,
as if to fall forwards.

³ **Inner Head.** Pressure in forehead, extending to orbits,
which, on moving the eyes, pain as if sore.

Tensive pain in forehead, as from a band above the eyes.

Pressive pain in right side of head.

Violent pain in left side of head and face.

Heaviness in the occiput, with pressure in left ear.

Coldness in the occiput, rising from the nape; worse when moving; better during rest.

⁴ **Outer Head.** Pain in the temporal bone behind the ear

Trembling of head and limbs.

⁵ **Eyes.** Dazzling spot before the eyes, lachrymation when looking at it.

Misty appearance before the eyes.

Objects appear double.

Contractility of pupils diminished.

Opacity of the cornea.

Aching in the eyeballs; worse moving the eyes.

Tearing pain in left eye, extending to zygoma, teeth, forehead and temple; first relieved by pressure, but soon cannot endure the slightest touch; periodic, evening in bed.

Conjunctiva swollen, dark red, as far as the cornea.

Whites of the eyes dirty-yellow.

Lids swollen, red, could open them but little.

Agglutination of lids in the morning.

Neuralgia of eyebrows and temples.

Pressing pain over left eye, which seems to press down upper lid.

⁶ **Ears.** Loud, distant roaring in the ears.

Sensation of wind rushing out of the ears.

Ears feel stopped.

Long-continued stitch in right external ear, passing off gradually.

⁷ **Nose.** Coryza: dry, nose stopped; fluent, with sneezing.

⁸ **Face.** Expression: anxious, disturbed; sickly.

Face: greyish-yellow; sallow; sunken; yellow, especially of forehead, nose and cheeks.

Right cheek-bone feels as if swollen.

Violent tearing in maxillary antrum.

Flushes of heat in the face.

⁹ **Lower Face.** Dryness of the lips.

¹⁰ **Teeth.** Tearing pains from right ear to right teeth, afternoons.

¹¹ **Tongue, etc.** Taste: bitter; insipid; pappy.

Tongue: slimy, coated white or grey; coated thickly yellow, with red margin, showing imprints of the teeth.

¹² **Mouth.** Bitter water collects in the mouth.

Dryness of mouth.

Bad odor from the mouth.

¹³ **Throat.** Choking, as from hasty swallowing.

Larynx as if pressed upon, impeding swallowing.

Dryness in the throat; hawking up lumps of phlegm.
Tonsils ache.

¹⁴ **Desires. Aversions.** Desire for milk, which agrees.
Fond of vinegar, or sour wine; dislike: to cheese; to meat.
Loss of appetite, with disgust and nausea.

¹⁵ **Eating and Drinking.** All complaints lessen after dinner.

¹⁶ **Nausea and Vomiting.** Hiccough.
Bilious eructations.
Short breath and anxiety, relieved by belching.
Nausea: with heat in stomach; causes great bodily heat.
Heart-burn.

¹⁷ **Stomach.** Pressure, with distention of stomach.
Constriction, tension and sensitiveness in pit of stomach
and right hypochondrium.
Feeling of anguish, in pit of stomach.
Gnawing, grinding pain; better while eating.

¹⁸ **Hypochondria.** Pains from region of liver, shooting toward
the back.
Stitches in region of liver; pressive pain in region of liver.
Left hypochondrium sensitive to pressure.

¹⁹ **Abdomen.** Colic, with nausea and retraction of the navel.
Pain across the umbilicus, as if the abdomen were con-
stricted by a string.
Abdomen distended, feels full and uncomfortable.
Rumbling, gurgling, pinching and cutting in the bowels.
Spasmodic drawing pains in both inguinal regions.

²⁰ **Stool, etc.** Crawling and itching in the rectum.
Frequent discharge of flatus.
Stools: thin, pasty, bright yellow; pasty, light grey; pale,
slimy; mucous diarrhœa, at night; constipated, like
sheep's dung.
Diarrhœa and constipation alternately.

²¹ **Urine.** Spasmodic pain in right kidney and in liver; worse
from 4 to 9 P.M.
Violent pains in direction of ureters, preceding passing of
turbid urine.
Urging to urinate.
Urine: profuse, whitish, foaming; red and turbid; dark
yellow, clear; lemon-yellow, turbid; dark, brownish-red.

²² **Male Sexual Organs.** Frequent erections, even during day.
Pain in the glans.
Drawing pain: in the spermatic cords; in the testicle.
Redness, heat and swelling of scrotum, with small, flat
vesicles, painful to touch, become moist, next day form
dry scales.
Itching and creeping on scrotum and glans.

²³ **Female Sexual Organs.** Menses too late; too profuse; pain
under the right scapula.

Burning in the vagina, recurring each day at precisely the same hour.

²⁴ **Pregnancy.** Longing for unusual articles of food.
Milk diminished.

²⁵ **Larynx.** Feels swollen; feels as if pressed upon.
Hoarseness.

²⁶ **Breathing.** Short and quick breathing, with oppression, which is relieved by a few deep inspirations; with anxiety, as if he must choke.

²⁷ **Cough.** Violent, somewhat spasmodic; dry, in paroxysms; racking, as in consumption, with much expectoration from the lungs, also with pain behind the sternum, especially at night; mornings, with copious mucous expectoration.

²⁸ **Lungs.** Stitches in left chest on inspiring.
Pains in the chest and back.
Oppression of the chest; the clothing seemed too tight.
Spasmodic pressure behind middle of sternum, awoke him at night; extended into the bronchi, with sensation of constriction in them.
Stitches in chest, worse right side.
Soreness in lower ribs, right side.
Deep-seated pain in whole right side of chest.

²⁹ **Heart. Pulse,** Very irregular palpitation of the heart.
Violent palpitation, with tightness of the chest.
Pulse: slow; small and quick; full and hard, though but slightly accelerated toward evening.

³¹ **Neck. Back.** Stiffness: of the neck; of the muscles of right side of neck.
Pain in right cervical muscles, and in region of right clavicle.
Pain in right side of back, with heaviness of occiput, pressure toward the left ear.
Constant pain under the inferior angle of right scapula; may extend into chest or stomach, causing nausea or vomiting.
Pain in the vertebra, worse from motion and pressure, trembling, spasms of limbs; spasmodic myelitis.
Stitches beneath the right scapula.
Pain as though the lower lumbar vertebræ would separate, when bending forwards.

³² **Upper Limbs.** Pain in the right shoulder.
Stiffness in the wrist.
Tearing in tips of fingers.

³³ **Lower Limbs.** Drawing pain in hips, thighs, legs and feet, more right side.
Pain in right knee, with burning and stiffness; worse when moving.

Stiffness of the ankles.

34 Limbs in General. Limbs: feel heavy, stiff and lame; feel paralyzed; cold.

Rheumatism, the least touch anywhere is exceedingly painful; sweat without relief.

❙ Rheumatism worse in the lower limbs, especially in the right tarso-tibial articulation; worse from walking.

35 Position, etc. Rest: 3. Motion: 3, 31, 33. Moving eyes, 3, 5. Walking: 34, 40. Bending forwards 31. Desire to lie down: 37. In bed: 5, 40. After lying down: 40.

36 Nerves. Great debility and lassitude after eating.

Trembling and twitching of the limbs.

Weariness, indolence, indisposed to work.

Tonic spasms in flexors of fingers and toes.

37 Sleep. Drowsiness during the day.

Sleepiness, desire to lie, without being able to sleep.

Restless sleep before midnight.

Sleepless, with headache.

Awakes terrified, by the usual sufferings.

Dreams: of corpses and funerals.

38 Time. Morning: 5, 27, 40. Afternoon: 10, 15. 4–9 P.M.: 21. Evening: 5, 29, 40. Night: 20, 27, 28. Before midnight. 37. After midnight: 40. Day: 22, 23, 37.

39 Temperature and Weather. Renewal of ailments on change of weather.

Open air: 40. Room: 40.

40 Chill. Fever. Sweat. Internal chill: with severe shaking, evening in bed; when walking in open air; passes off in the room.

Chill and coldness of whole body; worse on hands and feet, with distention of the veins.

Right foot icy-cold.

Shivering: without external coldness; running down back.

Internal heat without thirst, evening after lying down.

Burning heat of hands, spreading thence over the body.

Heat: of the head and face; on scapulæ; in hip-joints.

Sweat during sleep, after midnight and toward morning; better after awaking.

41 Attacks. Periodic: 5, 23.

42 Sides. Right: 2, 3, 6, 8, 10, 17, 18, 21, 23, 28, 31, 32, 33, 34, 40. Left: 3, 5, 18, 28, 31. Front to back: 18. Back to front: 31. Above downwards: 21, 40.

45 Contact, Injuries, etc. Touch: 5, 22, 34. Pressure: 5, 18, 31. Clothing seems too tight: 28.

46 Skin. Yellow, yellowish-grey.

Red and painful pimples and pustules on various parts.

Itching of the skin.

Old putrid spreading ulcers.

⁴⁷ **Stages and States.** Spare subjects disposed to abdominal plethora, cutaneous diseases, catarrhs or neuralgia. Blondes.

⁴⁸ **Relationship.** *Chelid.* follows well after *Ledum.*

After *Chilid., Arsen.* will often be useful.

Acids, wine or coffee restrict its action.

Antidotes to *Chilid.: Acon.* removes the aggravation, with excited circulation.

Chelid. antidotes: *Bryon.*

CHININUM SULFURICUM.

Sulphate of Quinine.

¹ **Mind.** Buoyancy, excited state; later despondency.

Feeling of impending evil; anxiety.

Memory "muddled;" lost power of naming substantives.

² **Sensorium.** Whirling in the head like a mill-wheel.

³ **Inner Head.** Violent throbbing headache; vertigo; heat in face; closes eyelids involuntarily from sheer prostration; intermittent type of cerebro spinal meningitis (clinical).

⁵ **Eyes.** Disk and retina very anæmic; disk looks dry.

Dim vision, as from a net, or as from a fog.

Pupils dilated.

Eyes very sensitive to light; lachrymation in the full glare of light.

Bright light and sparks before the eyes. Black spot size of pin's head moves with the right eye.

Intermittent strabismus.

Can see objects only when looking sideways.

⁶ **Ears.** Ringing in the ears; also with deafness. Meniére's disease.

⁸ **Face.** Pale, suffering; sickly.

Puffy face; œdematous.

Aching about left malar bone in the evening.

¹² **Mouth.** Mouth dry.

Tongue white; thick yellow fur on it; yellow at the root; flabby.

Saliva increased.

Taste: pasty, flat; bitter.

Speech disturbed or difficult.

¹⁸ **Hypochondria.** Pain in the region of the liver, shortly before going to bed.

Dull pain in region of spleen, disappears on pressure. Stitches.

20 **Stool, etc.** Dysentery, the fever intermits or the evacuations exhale a gangrenous odor.

21 **Urine.** Deposit of a straw-yellow, granular, or of a brick-red sediment.

29 **Heart. Pulse.** Precordial anxiety; palpitation; or heart feeble, general prostration.

Pulse full and large; weak and trembling.

31 **Neck. Back.** Sensitiveness of last cervical and first dorsal vertebræ to pressure; also of dorsal vertebræ. Third dorsal painful to touch, with oppression of the chest.

34 **Limbs in General.** Weakness; trembling; power of will over limbs seems greatly hampered.

Inflammatory rheumatism, fever remitting or intermitting; joints exquisitely sensitive.

36 **Nerves.** Restlessness, excessive sensibility to touch, noises.

Weakness; trembling; faintness; hunger.

40 **Chill. Fever. Sweat.** ▮ Chill 10–11 A.M. and 3–10 P.M., periodical, anteponing or tertian. Trembling of the limbs; pain in spleen; spine sensitive; face pale; thirst; lips blue; ringing in the ears.

General chilliness, especially on the back.

Extremities, also nose, chin, cold.

Bodily temperature diminished.

Heat intense; fulness of head, face red; great thirst; after going to bed, heat, with frequent yawning and sneezing; delirious. Veins on arms and legs enlarge; skin hot, dry. Pain in spine on pressure.

Flushes of heat, thirst, 4 P.M.

Sweat with thirst; profuse even while quiet, coming on gradually after the heat; profuse also on least motion; soaking sweat mornings in bed; profuse, exhausting, nightly diarrhœa. ▮ Profuse during sleep.

Congestive chills.

41 **Attacks.** ▮ Symptoms return periodically, on alternate days, or antepone.

▮ To be thought of when typhoid fever, eruptive fevers, pneumonia, etc., display intermittent symptoms or become rapidly pernicious.

44 **Tissues.** Suppuration with chilliness; profuse sweat.

Œdema, especially with liver and spleen affections; malaria.

48 **Relationship.** Compare with: *Cedron* (clock-like regularity of symptoms; debility, but of nervous origin rather than from sweating); *Helian.* follows well to prevent return of chill.

CICUTA VIROSA.

Water Hemlock.   *Umbelliferæ.*

[1] **Mind.** Dull and stupid, mental torpor.

Feels as if he was in a strange place, causes fear.

Aberration of mind, singing, performing the most grotesque dancing steps, shouting.

Likes childish toys, jumps from bed in a happy, childish state.

Weeping, moaning and howling.

Answers short. Quiet disposition, contented, happy.

Anxious thoughts of the future; feels sad.

Old men fear long spell of sickness before dying.

Anxiety, excessively affected by sad stories.

Mistrust and shunning of man; despises others.

[2] **Sensorium.** Vertigo: on rising from bed, as if everything moved from side to side, or approached and then receded; reeling; falling on stooping.

Bad effects from concussion of the brain, when spasms set in.

[3] **Inner Head.** Pressure deep in the brain; heaviness in front or back of head.

Rending, cutting pain of one side; thinking of headache causes it to disappear.

Headache in the morning on waking, as if the brain were loose and was shaken on walking; when thinking as to its exact nature, it ceased.

[4] **Outer Head.** Sinking of the head forward when looking at anything, or sitting in apparent sleep; when aroused head was bent forward and stiff.

Jerking and twitching of the head.

Starting, trembling of the head, worse moving the head; with this, single jerks, like electric shocks, worse in the cold; better at rest and from warmth.

[5] **Eyes.** Eyes sensitive to light.

Letters go up and down or disappear; or colors of rainbow around them; objects appear double and black.

Staring at an object, the head inclined forward.

Pupils: dilated in concussion of the brain; contracted in spasmodic affections.

Blue margin around the eyes; eyes sunken.

[6] **Ears.** Oversensitiveness of hearing.

Hardness of hearing, in old people.

Ears very hot, at other times very cold.

Burning, suppurating eruption on and around the ears.

⁷ **Nose.** Nose very sensitive to touch, slight touch causes it to bleed.

Yellow discharge from the nose; yellow scurfs in the nose.

Frequent sneezing, without coryza.

⁸ **Face.** Face: deathly pale and cold; red; bluish, puffed up.

Distortions of the face, either horrible of ridiculous.

Convulsion of the facial muscles.

Dark red pimples on face and hands, come with burning pain, coalesce.

Burning, suppurating, confluent eruptions of the face.

Herpes on the face.

⁹ **Lower Face.** Lockjaw, teeth press firmly against one another.

Yellow scurfs on the left corner of the mouth, discharging yellow scurfs on the left corner of the mouth, discharging yellow corrosive fluid, may extend over the lip, chin and cheek.

Cancer of upper lip.

¹⁰ **Teeth.** Grinding of the teeth.

¹¹ **Tongue, etc.** Swelling of the tongue; white, painful, burning ulcers on edges of the tongue; painful to touch.

Speech difficult; when talking he feels a jerk in the head from before backwards, as if he had to swallow the word, as in hiccough.

¹² **Mouth.** Foam in and about the mouth.

¹³ **Throat.** Inability to swallow.

The throat felt as if grown together, internally; externally painful, as if bruised, on moving, or touching it; eructations from noon till evening.

After swallowing a sharp piece of bone, the œsophagus closes, and there is danger of suffocation.

¹⁴ **Desires. Aversions.** Great longing for charcoal.

Thirst, with inability to swallow.

¹⁵ **Eating and Drinking.** Immediately after commencing to eat, feels satisfied.

Immediately after eating, bellyache and sleepiness.

¹⁶ **Nausea and Vomiting.** Violent hiccough and crying.

Nausea in the morning, and when eating.

Vomiting; of bile; of blood; on stooping, during pregnancy; alternating with tonic spasms, in the pectoral muscles, and distortion of the eyes.

¹⁷ **Stomach.** Sudden shock deep in the pit of stomach causes opisthotonos.

Burning pressure at the stomach and abdomen.

Swelling and throbbing in the pit of the stomach.

Heat in the stomach.

¹⁹ **Abdomen.** Colic, with convulsions, also vomiting.

Distention and painfullness of the abdomen.

Chronic painful hernia.

[20] **Stool, etc.** Frequent liquid stools.

Cholera, when purging ceases, and congestion to brain and chest, turning the eyes, difficult breathing, and other symptoms set in.

Itching in the rectum, with burning pain after rubbing.

[21] **Urine.** Either great quantities of urine, with great urging, or no urine at all.

Involuntary emission of urine, with old men.

Paralysis of the bladder, with great anxiety about it.

[22] **Male Sexual Organs.** Testicles drawn up toward the external abdominal ring.

Sore, drawing pain in the urethra, as far as the glans, obliging one to urinate.

Stitches in the fossa navicularis, with nightly emissions.

[23] **Female Sexual Organs.** Menses delayed.

Spasmodic state, if menses do not appear.

Tearing and drawing in the os coccygis, during menses.

[24] **Pregnancy.** Eclampsia during childbed.

[26] **Breathing.** Oppression, can scarcely breathe; this may arise from tonic spasm of the pectoral muscles.

[27] **Cough.** Cough, with expectoration.

[28] **Lungs.** Great heat in the chest.

Cold sensation in the chest.

[29] **Heart. Pulse.** Trembling palpitation of the heart.

Feels as if the heart stopped beating; and sometimes faint feeling therewith.

[30] **Outer Chest.** Sensation of soreness at the lower end of the sternum.

[31] **Neck. Back.** Pain in the nape, spasmodic drawing of the head backward, with tremor of the hand.

Tension in the muscles of the neck.

Tonic spasm of the cervical muscles.

Tearing, jerking in the os coccygis.

[32] **Upper Limbs.** Complete powerlessness of the limbs, after spasmodic jerks.

Numbness of the fingers.

Veins of the hands enlarged.

Frequent involuntary jerking and twitching in the arms and fingers.

[33] **Lower Limbs.** Painful feeling of stiffness in the muscles of the lower limbs.

Trembling of the left leg.

His legs refused to carry him, and he staggered.

When walking, she does not step properly on the soles of the feet, they tilt inwards.

Gressus vaccinus.

[35] **Position, etc.** Moving head: 4. Moving throat: 13. Rising from bed: 2. Walking: 3, 33. Stooping: 2, 16. Sitting: 4. Rest: 4. Turning head: 31.

³⁶ **Nerves.** · Convulsions, with loss of consciousness, frightful distortions of the limbs and whole body.

Convulsions, with opisthotonos.

Epileptic attacks, with swelling of the stomach, as from violent spasms of the diaphragm; hiccough; piercing cries; redness of the face; trismus; loss of consciousness and distortions of limbs; involuntary urination.

Suddenly becomes stiff and immovable.

Tonic spasm renewed from the slightest touch; from opening the door, and from loud talking.

Somnambulism, fixed gaze, partial loss of consciousness.

Sudden rigidity, with jerks, afterwards great relaxation and weakness, during worm affections.

General prostration.

³⁷ **Sleep.** Soporous condition. θ Cholera.

Frequent waking, with sweat all over; feels invigorated.

Dreams: vivid, about the events of previous day.

³⁸ **Time.** Morning: 3, 16. Noon till evening: 13. Night: 22, 40. Toward morning: 40.

³⁹ **Temperature and Weather.** Great desire for warmth of stove.

Warmth: 4, 40. Cold: 4.

⁴⁰ **Chill. Fever. Sweat.** Chill and chilliness, with desire for warmth and the warm stove.

Chill starts in chest and runs down legs and into arms, with staring look.

Heat slight, and only internal.

Typhoid fever, with vertigo, noises in the ears, deafness; eyes dull, glassy; face pale; violent thirst; meteorism; sopor and silent delirium.

Sweat at night, and in morning hours, most on abdomen.

⁴² **Sides.** Right: 46. Left: 9, 32, 33. One side: 3. Before backwards: 11. Above downwards: 40.

⁴³ **Sensations.** Sensation in many parts, as from a bruise.

⁴⁵ **Contact, Injuries, etc.** Touch: 7, 11, 13, 36, 46.

⁴⁶ **Skin.** Red vesicle on right scapula very painful to touch.

Elevated eruption as large as peas, on both hands, even on the balls of the fingers, with burning pain when touched; later it became confluent.

⁴⁷ **Stages and States.** Old people: 1, 6, 21.

⁴⁸ **Relationship.** *Cicut.* is sometimes indicated after *Laches.*

Antidotes to *Cicut.: Arnic., Opium.*

Tobacco against massive doses.

Cicut. antidotes *Opium.*

Compare with *Cereus serpen.* (pustules in beard).

CIMEX LECTULARIUS.

Acanthia graveolens. WAHLE IN ROME. *Cimicidæ.*

[1] **Mind.** Anxiousness.

Very much vexed, would like to tear everything into pieces.

Disgust at his own sweat.

[2] **Sensorium.** Dulness of the head.

[3] **Inner Head.** Drawing headache, particularly under right frontal bone.

Headache, almost depriving him of power of thinking.

Violent headache, caused by drinking.

[7] **Nose.** Annoying dryness of nostrils.

Sneezing for an hour, at noon.

Fluent coryza, with pressure in frontal sinuses.

[11] **Tongue, etc.** Tongue feels as if scalded; coated whitish.

[13] **Throat.** Pressure and choking in the gullet, during the fever-heat, spreading through the chest, impeding breathing; no thirst, but when drinking to overcome the choking, the water goes down only at intervals, as if the throat was contracted, or feels as if she had swallowed too large a morsel.

Palate and upper gums feels as if scalded.

[14] **Desires. Aversions.** Great hunger after the heat.

Thirst, but afraid to move to get a drink.

Desire to drink, without thirst.

[15] **Eating and Drinking.** After drinking: 40.

[16] **Nausea and Vomiting.** Qualmishness, with the fever.

[20] **Stool, etc.** Constipation, fèces dry and hard, like dog stool.

Hemorrhoidal pains with the stool.

[21] **Urine.** Urine deposits a red coating on inside of vessel.

During the fever, urine very hot.

[23] **Female Sexal Organs.** Hot sensation inside the labia.

[27] **Cough.** Cough, with belching, gagging or vomiting.

Violent cough, with purulent sputum, and with chill and fever in daily attacks.

[29] **Heart. Pulse.** Pulse feeble, intermitting.

[33] **Lower Limbs.** Heaviness in lower limbs.

Hamstrings feel too short, knees are flexed; attempting to stretch them, causes pain in the thighs.

Restlessness of lower limbs, like overfatigue from a long walk.

Knees feel cold, as from a cold wind.

[35] **Position, etc.** Every movement, especially extending a limb, gives tensive pain in the extensor tendons.

22

Suffers thirst rather than move.

Has to sit down; loins or limbs are weary.

36 **Nerves.** Weariness, with inclination to stretch all day.

37 **Sleep.** Irresistible sleepiness.

38 **Time.** Noon: 7.

40 **Chill. Fever. Sweat.** Before the chill, thirst and heaviness in the legs.

Chill, commencing with clenching of hands and violent raging.

Chill, attended with pain in all the joints; sensation, as if the tendons were too short, knee-joints are usually contracted, so that the legs cannot be stretched; chest feels oppressed; must take a long breath, frequently; irresistible sleepiness; hands and feet as if dead.

Chill terminates with a tired feeling in the legs, obliging one to change position constantly.

After the chill, thirst; drinking, however, causes violent headache; tickling in larynx, causing dry, continuous cough, which lasts through the heat; oppression of breathing, heaviness in middle of chest, and anxiety; abstaining from drinking ameliorates all this

Heat with gagging; the œsophagus feels constricted.

Sweat, mostly on head and chest, accompanied by hunger.

Sweat relieves all the other symptoms; during feverish affections.

Musty-smelling sweat, the odor is to him very offensive.

42 **Sides.** Right side seems most affected.

43 **Sensations.** Sensation as if he would creep into his own body, he crouches together as much as he can, with pain in thighs.

CINA.

Wormseed.   HAHNEMANN.   *Compositæ.*

1 **Mind.** Pitiful weeping when awake.

As if frightened, jumps out of bed, sees imaginary objects, screams, trembles, talks hurriedly, anxious; evening and before midnight.

Child does not want to be touched; cannot bear you to come near it; desires many things which it refuses when offered; is not pleased or satisfied with anything; uneasy and distressed all the time.

2 **Sensorium.** Weak, hollow, empty feeling in the head, with inclination to vomit.

[3] **Inner Head.** Stupefying headache, especially in the fore-head, then also in occiput; when walking in open air.

Headache, pain in chest and back, caused by fixing eyes steadily upon some object, as when sewing; worse from pressure.

Dull headache, with sensitiveness of the eyes, in morning.

Intermittent pressure, as from a heavy weight, as if the brain were pressed down on the middle of the vertex; pressure increases and renews the pain.

Drawing from the left frontal eminence to the root of nose, causing confusion of head.

Headaches are anæmic, hence better stooping, though they are worse from mental exertion.

[4] **Outer Head.** Child leans its head sideways, all the time.

Turning the head from one side to the other.

[5] **Eyes.** Can see more clearly for awhile after rubbing the eyes.

On rising from bed, black before the eyes, with dizziness in the head and faintness, totters to and fro; better on lying down; dull headache, with affection of the eyes.

Optical illusions in bright colors.

Pupils dilated.

[6] **Ears.** Dull stitches below the mastoid process.

Cramp-like jerking in the external ear, like earache.

[7] **Nose.** Sneezing, with the whooping cough.

Violent sneezing, with stitches in the temples.

Bleeding of the nose.

Stoppage of the nose, in the evening.

Itching of the nose. ❙ Boring in the nose, with the finger.

Child rubs the nose on the pillow, on the shoulders of the nurse, or with the hands.

[8] **Face.** Pale, with sickly look about the eyes; pale and cold; red.

Dark rings around the eyes.

Pain, as if both malar bones were pressed together with pincers; worse from external pressure.

[9] **Lower Face.** White and bluish about the mouth.

[10] **Teeth.** Grinds the teeth at night.

[11] **Tongue, etc.** Tongue coated brownish-yellow; whitish.

[12] **Mouth.** Much frothy saliva, with rattling phlegm on chest.

[13] **Throat.** Frequent motion, as though swallowing something.

[14] **Desires. Aversions.** Desires many and different things.

Desires for bread; great hunger after eating.

Thirst.

[15] **Eating and Drinking.** On drinking wine, she shudders, as though it were vinegar.

[16] **Nausea and Vomiting** Hiccough during sleep.

Vomiting of mucus.

[17] **Stomach.** Constant pressure in the stomach at night, causing restlessness.

Gnawing sensation in the stomach, as from hunger.

[19] **Abdomen.** Pinching, or cramp-like pressure, transversely across the epigastric region, after a meal.

Boring pain above the navel, passes off when pressing thereon.

Painful twisting about the navel; with a peculiar sickish pressure.

Belly hard and distended.

[20] **Stool, etc.** Diarrhœa after drinking; stools watery, white.

Stool rather hard and black.

Itching at the anus.

[21] **Urine.** Frequent urging, with passage of much urine, all day.

Urine becomes turbid immediately.

[23] **Female Sexual Organs.** Menses too early and profuse.

[24] **Pregnancy, etc.** Child refuses the breast.

[26] **Breathing.** Short, at times interrupted.

Inhalation, broken into two.

Oppression of the chest, the sternum seems to lie too close and the breathing becomes oppressed.

[27] **Cough.** Short hacking cough at night.

Hacking cough, followed immediately by an effort to swallow something.

Violent periodically recurring paroxysms of whooping-cough, excited by sensation as if down were in the throat, or by adherent mucus in larynx; after cough, gurgling sound.

Gagging cough, morning after rising; irritation renewed by inspiration.

Hoarse gagging cough, in the evening.

Rattling cough in spells.

Expectoration: whitish, slimy, rarely somewhat bloody, almost tasteless,, detached with difficulty.

[28] **Lungs.** Stitches in the left side; burning stitches in chest.

Rattling in throat and chest; catarrh, when excessive nervous irritability co-exists.

[29] **Heart. Pulse.** Pulse small, but hard and accelerated.

[31] **Neck. Back.** Drawing-tearing pain down along the whole spine.

Paralytic feeling in nape of neck.

Tearing-jerking pains in the middle of the spine.

Fatigued pain in the loins, as if he had stood a long time.

Bruised pain in small of back, not aggravated by motion.

[32] **Upper Limbs.** Boring, pinching pain in the left upper arm.

Single, small, jerking stitches, now in right, again in left hand.

[33] **Lower Limbs.** Paralytic pain in left thigh, near the knee.
[35] **Position, etc.** Motion: 31. Walking in the open air: 3. Rising from bed: 5. Lying down: 5.
[36] **Nerves.** Trembling of the body, with shivering sensation, while yawning.

Child complains of being always tired.

Twitching of the limbs; jerking and distortions of limbs.

Convulsive attacks at night.

Spasms of children, with throwing arms from side to side.

Epilepsy, with rigidity and full consciousness.

Convulsions of the extensor muscles; the child becomes suddenly stiff; there is a clucking noise, as though water were poured out of a bottle, from the throat down to the abdomen.

Chorea, the distortions often commence with a shriek, extend to the tongue, œsophagus and larynx, continue even through the night.

[37] **Sleep.** Sudden distressing cries in sleep; tossing about in sleep.

Cannot sleep; when falling asleep, starts, screams, turns over, kicks off the bedclothes.

[38] **Time.** Morning: 3, 27. Evening: 1, 7, 27, 40. Night: 10, 17, 27, 36, 40. Before midnight: 1. Whole day: 21.

[39] **Temperature and Weather.** External warmth: 40. Open air: 3.

[40] **Chill. Fever. Sweat.** Chill, with shivering and shaking, even near a warm stove; chill ascends from the upper part of body to the head.

Chill, face pale and cold; hands warm.

Chill not relieved by external warmth, mostly in the evening and with great paleness of the face.

Chill in evening and fever all night. *θ* Nursing children.

Burning heat over the whole face, with redness of the cheeks and thirst for cold drink.

Fever daily at the same hour.

Heat most severe over the head and face; face pale.

Nightly heat; with thirst; with anxiety.

Sweat generally cold, on the forehead, around the nose, and on the hands.

After the sweat (frequently also before the chill) vomiting of food, with canine hunger at the same time.

[41] **Attacks.** Recurring daily at same hour: 40.

[42] **Sides.** Right: 32. Left: 3, 28, 32, 33. Above downwards: 31, 36. Below upwards: 40.

[43] **Sensations.** Dull twinges sometimes like a pinching, at others like a pressure or a blow, or jerk, or again like an itching, at various places, but especially at the posterior portion of the crest of the ilium, on the hip; the places are painful on pressure, as if sore or bruised.

⁴⁵ **Contact, Injuries, etc.** Touch: 1. Pressure: 3, 6, 8, 19, 43. Rubbing: 5, 7. Scratching: 46.

Child wants to be carried.

⁴⁶ **Skin.** Itching unchanged or lessened by scratching.

Furuncles.

Ulcers with scanty discharge.

⁴⁷ **Stages and States.** Dark hair.

⁴³ **Relationship.** Ailments from *Capsic.*, or abuse of *Cinchon.* or *Mercur.*

Antidotes to *Cina: Camphor., Capsic., Cinchon., Pip. nigr.*

Santonine relieves asthenopia from some refractive anomaly.

CINCHONA OFFICINALIS.

Peruvian Bark.   HAHNEMANN.   *Rubiaceæ.*

¹ **Mind.** Chooses wrong expressions, or misplaces them.

Slow train of ideas.

Ideas and projects crowd on his mind, especially in evening.

Fixed idea that he is unhappy, persecuted by enemies.

Delirium after depletion; on closing eyes, sees figures of persons.

Compelled to jump out of bed; wants to destroy himself, but lacks courage.

Inclined to reproach and vex others.

Dislike to all mental or physical exertion.

Low-spirited, gloomy, has no desire to live.

Dread of dogs and other animals at night.

Inconsolable anxiety, even to suicide.

Indifference, apathy.

Ill-humor.

Stubborn, disobedient, longing for dainties; face pale, or at times red; restless all night; children.

Intolerance of sensual impressions.

Nervous irritation.

Worse exerting the mind.

² **Sensorium.** Dulness of head, giddiness, as from sitting up at night and sleeplessness.

❚ Heaviness of the head, fainting, loss of sight, ringing in ears; cold surface. *θ* After hemorrhage.

Vertigo: after loss of animal fluids; from anæmia; head feels weak, can hardly hold it erect; with the chill; on raising the head; with nervous erethism, hysterical excitability; with fainting.

Dulness of the head, as from coryza or intoxication.

Heaviness of the head, increasing vertigo.

³ **Inner Head.**   Intense throbbing heaeache; carotids throb. θ After loss of blood.

Stitches from temple to temple.

Sensation as if head would burst, with sleeplessness; worse from motion or any jar; better in the room and when opening the eyes.

Whole head feels bruised; worse from exerting the mind.

Headache from suppressed coryza; worse in open air, or exerting mind.

Brain feels bruised; worse on moving, even opening his eyes; scalp sensitive; worse at night.

Headache in occiput after sexual excesses or onanism.

Headaches, worse from draught of air, in the open air, slightest touch; better from hard pressure.

Headache from occiput over whole head from morning until afternoon; worse lying, must stand or walk; drives to madness.

Tearing, drawing, oppressive pains, as from load on head.

⁴ **Outer Head.**   Burning in forehead, with hot sweat on it.

Scalp sensitive to touch, roots of hair hurt when hair is moved.

Scalp feels as if the hair was grasped roughly by the hand.

Profuse sweat on head, especially when walking in open air.

⁵ **Eyes.**   Nocturnal blindness.

Worse from light; better in the dark.

Scintillations, or black motes before eyes.

Amblyopia in drunkards; after masturbation, tendency of blood to head.

Pressure in eyes, as from drowsiness.

Letters pale, surrounded by white borders.

Dilated, not very sensitive pupils.

Pressure, as from sand in eyes; photophobia; eyes hot, red; or, dim and faint, as if filled with smoke.

⁶ **Ears.**   Fine ringing in ears, debility.

Hardness of hearing; humming in ears.

Stitches in the ears.

Tearing pains in ears, worse from the least touch; ears red; stitches, with ringing.

⁷ **Nose.**   Smell too acute.

Dry coryza, toothache, lachrymation; much sneezing.

Nosebleed, anæmia; ringing in ears; face pale, fainting.

Habitual nosebleed, especially morning, on rising.

⁸ **Face.**   Face hot, when entering room from open air.

Veins of face distended.

Face: red, during fever; hollow, pale, or livid, with atrophy; pale, blue around the eyes; yellow; earthy; grey; yellow or black; hippocratic.

Neuralgia, periodical attacks; pains excessive, skin sensitive to least touch; part feels weak; face alternately red and pale; pains from left to right; mostly in infraorbital and maxillary branches.

⁹ **Lower Face.** Lips: burning; swollen; dry, hard, cracked, blackish; blackish and shriveled.

Submaxillary glands swollen, painful during swallowing.

¹⁰ **Teeth.** Toothache, veins in forehead and hands distended; throbbing pain.

ı Toothache while infant sucks the breast.

Toothache worse from least contact, moving body, tea, open air, or current of air; better from pressing teeth together.

Toothache during sweat.

Swelling of gums; mouth dry.

¹¹ **Tongue, etc.** Taste: too acute; putrid, morning; bitter in back part of throat; flat, watery.

Food tastes bitter or too salt.

Tongue white; or yellow; thick, dirty coating.

Tongue white, mornings; child restless all night; no appetite for breakfast.

Tongue black, or raw, as if burned.

Burning as from pepper on tip of tongue, followed by ptyalism.

¹² **Mouth.** Salivation day and night, years after mercury, great weakness, especially of stomach.

¹³ **Throat.** Throat feels rough, scraped, producing a sore sensation on swallowing.

Difficult deglutition, as from contration of the œsophagus.

Gangrene of throat.

¹⁴ **Desires. Aversions.** Longs for spirits; sweets; sour, cooling things; roasted coffee.

Children dainty, desire various things without knowing what.

Wants highly seasoned food.

Canine hunger; worse at night.

Voracious appetite. θ Atrophy.

Violent thirst for cold water; drinks little and often.

Loathing of food as if he had overeaten.

Averse to bread; to beer; to butter; to meat; to fat things; to warm food.

Loss of appetite in foggy weather.

Loss of appetite, nausea, desire to vomit.

Aversion to all food, even when thinking of it; dread of labor; drowsy by day; yellow eyes.

¹⁵ **Eating and Drinking.** Worse drinking wine and other liquors.

Worse after breakfast.

Sour eructations after milk.

Gastric symptoms from: eating fish; excessive use of tea; sour wine; new beer; impure water; fruit.

Warm drinks impede digestion.

Worse from smoking.

¹⁶ **Nausea and Vomiting.**   Heart-burn, after milk.

Belching, sour rising.

Eructations taste of the food; or are bitter.

Vomit: sour; blackish; bloody; worse at night.

Frequent vomiting.

¹⁷ **Stomach.**   Pulsations in pit of stomach.

Heavy pressure in stomach, after small quantity of food.

Cold feeling in stomach; constant satiated feeling, yet can eat, but feels worse afterwards.

Fulness in stomach and bowels; flatulence; belching does not relieve.

Slow digestion, food remains long in stomach; especially if eaten too late in day.

Hæmatemesis, great loss of blood, weak, pale, cold hands and feet; stomach very sensitive to touch.

Gastralgia after depletion; acidity; bloating after food or drink; satiety; relieved by motion.

Stomach feels sore, as if ulcerated, cannot bear slight touch.

¹⁸ **Hypochodria.**   Pain in hepatic region, as from subcutaneous ulceration; worse from touch.

Swollen, hard liver.

Colic from gall-stones.

Gastro-duodenal catarrh after loss of fluids or severe illness.

Enlarged spleen.

Aching, stitching pains in spleen when walking slowly; pains extend in direction of long axis of spleen.

¹⁹ **Abdomen.**   Pressing-aching below navel.

Flatulence from excessive tea drinking.

Colic better bending double.

Colic worse at night and after eating.

Colic at a certain hour each afternoon; " 3 months colic."

Abdomen distended, wants to belch.

Abdomen as if packed full, not relieved by belching.

Tympanitic abdomen, pressure as from a hard body; or, spasmodic, constrictive pains from incarcerated flatulence; worse at night or after depletion; also in typhus, worse mornings.

Strangulated hernia; gut black; after operation.

²⁰ **Stool, etc.**   Stools: loose, brownish, painless, with feeling of debility; frothy, painless, diarrhœic, with fermentation in bowels; after sour beer; painless, black; thin, large,

with passage of wind, mornings; offensive, undigested, or white, papescent, at night; yellow, watery, involuntary; cadaverous-smelling, chocolate-colored, worse at night.

Diarrhœa comes on gradully, more and more watery, pale, pinkish, with rapid emaciation.

Constipation: large accumulation; stool difficult, even if -soft; after long purging.

Mocous discharge from the rectum.

Bleeding piles, burning and itching.

Tingling in the anus.

²¹ **Urine.** Frequent micturition.

Burning at orifice of urethra, especially painful from rubbing of clothes.

Urine: turbid, dark, scanty; white turbid, with white sediment; pale, becoming cloudy or depositing a dingy, yellow, loose sediment.

Scanty, greenish-yellow, brick-dust sediment.

Pinkish sediment.

²² **Male Sexual Organs.** Sexual desire; lascivious fancies.

Impotence, with lascivious fancies.

Nocturnal emissions, frequent and debilitating.

Consequences of excessive or long-continued seminal losses; onanism.

Painful swelling of spermatic cord and testicle, especially . the epididymis; tearing in left testicle and left side of prepuce; cramp-like, contractive pain in the testicles, evenings, θ After gonorrhœa.

Contractive pain in urethra.

²³ **Female Sexual Organs.** Ovaritis from sexual excess or hemorrhage, parts very sensitive to slight touch.

Dropsy: of ovaries; of uterus.

Congestion to the uterus, fulness, pressing and heaviness, worse when walking.

Menses: too early, profuse, black clots, with spasm in chest and abdomen; painful.

Metrorrhagia, blood dark, fainting, covulsions.

Discharge of bloody serum, alternating with pus.

Leucorrhœa: instead of menses, with itching; with spasmodic uterine contractions, painful bearing down to vulva and anus; menses increased.

Painful induration in the vagina.

²⁴ **Pregnancy.** Nymphomania of lying-in women.

Abortion; abdomen distended, belching does not relieve.

Labor-pains cease from hemorrhage; cannot have the hands touched.

Uterine hemorrhages, ringing in ears, fainting, cold, loss of sight; discharge of dark clots; uterine spasms; twitches, jerks; wants to be fanned.

Lochia lasts too long; drawing about ovaries; or discharge fetid or cheesy; purulent.

Asphyxia of the newborn; after great loss of blood by the mother.

²⁵ **Larynx.** Hoarse, voice rough, deep from adhering mucus.

Sore sensation in larynx and trachea.

Influenza, with debility, loss of appetite, heat without thirst.

²⁶ **Breathing.** Asthma, looks as if dying; worse autum, wet weather, or after depletion.

Cannot breathe with head low.

Wheezing, whistling inspiration, crowing, rattling, oppressed and painful.

Oppression of the chest; also evenings, lying down.

Nightly suffocative fits; spasmodic cough.

Suffocative catarrh and paralysis of lungs of old people.

Rattling in chest; loud sounds through the nose.

Inspiration slow, difficult; expiration quick, blowing, short. θ Œdema glottidis.

Oppression of chest, as from fulness of stomach; also from continued talking.

Breath cold.

²⁷ **Cough.** With pain in larynx and sternum; with pain througout whole cavity of chest.

Cough causing cutting in left lower abdomen; expectoration difficult, black.

Cough with granular sputum during day or evening, none night or morning.

Dry, spasmodic or suffocative night cough, as from vopor of sulphur, with bilious vomit.

Cough first hollow, dry and painful, later bloody expectoration.

Sputa slimy, whitish.

Coughs worse: lying with head low, or on left side; moving; deep breath, talking, laughing; eating, drinking; evening or after 12 P.M.; lightly touching larynx; least draught; loss of fluids; after being awakened.

²⁸ **Lungs.** Loud, coarse rales, great debility, anæmia; œdema of legs.

Pneumonia after hemorrhages, bleeding or with bilious symptoms; or incipient gangrene.

Pressure in chest, as from violent rush of blood, violent palpitation; bloody sputum; sudden prostration.

Stitches in right chest up to axilla, prevents bending forward and breathing; stitches in left chest; stitches under sternum worse during deep breathing and sudden movements.

Phthisis of drunkards, suppuration of lungs.

Cannot bear percussion or even auscultation, chest so sensitive.

Hæmoptysis: with subsequent suppuration of lungs; stitches in chest worse from slight touch.

²⁹ **Heart. Pulse.** Palpitation: with rush of blood to face, head and redness of face, with cold hands; after loss of fluids.

Pulse: frequent, small, hard; more quiet after meals; feeble, rapid; unequal, intermitting.

³¹ **Neck. Back.** Pressure as from a stone between scapulæ.

Pain in small of back at night, lying on it.

Insupportable pain in small of back, like a cramp, worse from least movement.

Laming, drawing, tearing in back and thighs.

³² **Upper Limbs.** Aching in shoulder-blades and limbs; worse from least pressure; restless, wants to change position.

Spasmadic stretching of the arms, whith clenched fingers.

Hands tremble (when writing).

Veins of hands distended.

Swelling of back of left hand.

One hand icy-cold, the other warm.

Nails blue.

³³ **Lower Limbs.** Hip disease, with profuse suppuration, sweat, diarrhœa.

Pain in the right knee, up to thigh, or down towards the leg; pains worse from contact than from motion.

Legs feel as after a long walk.

Uneasiness in legs, must move them or draw them up.

Hot swelling of right knee, painful to slight touch.

Knees weak, especially when walking.

Rheumatic pains in metatarsal bones, and phalanges, worse from motion and contact.

Swelling of the feet; hot, arthritic.

³⁴ **Limbs in General.** Darting-tearing, worse from contact, especially in hands and feet.

Pains in all the limbs, as if clothing were too tight, after a walk in the open air.

Pains in limbs increasing gradually, worse from slight touch.

Parts around swollen joints very sensitive to least touch; worse at night, parts feel weak.

Heaviness in limbs, especially the thighs.

Limbs pain, especially joints, as if bruised, worse in rest, better moving.

³⁵ **Position, etc.** Rest: 34. Sudden motion: 28. Motion: 3, 10, 17, 27, 31, 33, 34, 36. Walking: 4, 18, 23, 33, 34. Must stand or walk: 3. Wants to change position: 32. Lying: 3, 26; on back: 31; on left side: 27; with head

low: 26, 27. Parts lain on: 36, 40. Raising the head:
2. Bending double: 19.

[36] **Nerves.** Great debility, trembling, averse to all exercise;
nervous; sensitive to pain, to draughts of air; sleepless.

Complaints from loss of animal fluids.

Convulsions: rush of blood to head, throbbing carotids;
from great loss of blood.

Epileptic spasm far apart; deathly pallor; relaxation of
muscles.

Paralysis from loss of fluids; after arsenical poisoning;
onanism.

Numbness of parts on which he lies.

Twitching of limbs.

[37] **Sleep.** Irresistibly sleepy during day and after eating.

Constant sopor or unrefreshing sleep.

Sleepless, aching in head (until 12 P.M.), anxiety on waking, from frightful dreams.

Sleepless from crowding of ideas, making plans.

During sleep: snoring, blowing expiration; moaning,
whining.

Sleep too short, unrefreshing; awakens too early.

Worst sleep after 3 A. M.

On awaking: cannot collect one's senses; vertigo; hunger; sweat; languor; unrefreshed; head hot; oppression of chest.

[38] **Time.** Morning till afternoon: 3. Morning: 7, 11, 19, 20,
27, 40. Forenoon: 40. Afternoon: 19, 40. Evening:
1, 22, 26, 27, 40. Night: 1, 3, 5, 11, 14, 16, 19, 20, 22,
26, 27, 31, 34, 37, 40. 3 A.M.: 37. Day: 27, 37. Day
and night: 12.

[39] **Temperature and Weather.** Room: 3. Entering room
from open air: 8. Warm stove: 40. Draught: 3, 10,
27, 36. Open air: 3, 4, 10, 34. Foggy weather: 14.
Wet weather: 26. Covering up: 40.

[40] **Chill. Fever. Sweat.** Chill preceded by palpitation,
anxiety and hunger.

Chill over the whole body, increased by drinking, thirst
before or after, but not during the chill.

Internal violent chill, with icy-cold hands and feet, and
congestion of blood to the head.

Chill and heat alternating in the afternoon.

Fugitive chills in the back, tendency to sweat on covering up.

In the evening in bed, he cannot get warm.

Wants to be near the stove, but it increases the chill.

Chill most afternoon or evening; less forenoon.

General heat, with distended veins.

Heat of face, with cold body.

Long-lasting heat, which frequently sets in late after chill.

During the heat: thirstlessness or thirst for cold drink only; desire to uncover; aversion to food; or canine hunger; pains in the liver, chest, back, limbs.

Sweat: debilitating, night or morning; profuse; partial, cold, or profuse, with thirst; greasy; on the side on which one lies.

During the sweat, increased thirst.

Revulsion of sweat, and therefrom want of sweat.

Heat of the face, with cold body.

Sweat profuse, morning and night.

Sweat partial, cold; or, profuse, with thirst; sweats easily, especially at night in sleep.

Fever, with dry mouth, burning lips; red face, delirium; chill when uncovered; pains in limbs.

Sweat on side lain on; sweat less after meals.

Suppressed sweat.

Hectic fever, frequent night-sweats, diarrhœa, pallor; skin dry, flaccid; sleepless; nervous; hunger; after exhausting disease, loss of fluids, etc.

Acute fevers, with profuse sweats.

Typhoid fevers: 1, 2, 8, 9, 11, 18, 19, 20, 26, 36, 37.

41 **Attacks.** Worse every other day: congestions; chills; neuralgia.

Autumn: 26.

Worse during increase of moon.

Alternate weakness and feeling of great strength, especially in joints.

Pains in organs, alternate with wandering rheumatic pains.

42 **Sides.** Right: 28, 33. Left: 22, 27, 28, 32. Left to right: 8. Above downwards: 23, 33. Below upwards: 28, 33.

43 **Sensations.** Pain in every joint, bones, periosteum as if strained.

Pains with lameness or weakness of affected parts.

Single parts feel pithy, numb.

44 **Tissues.** Hemorrhages from mouth, nose or bowels; wants sour things.

Glands swollen, hot, painful.

Chlorosis, dropsy, poor digestion; after exhausting diseases or discharges.

Red inflammatory swellings.

Wounds become black, gangrenous.

Muscles lax.

Emaciation, especially of hands and feet; atrophy of children.

Humid gangrene; parts turn black.

Anasarca, ascites in the aged; also from liver and spleen diseases; drunkards.

Caries with profuse sweat.

⁴⁵ Contact, Injuries, etc. Touch: 3, 4, 6, 8, 10, 17, 18, 23, 24, 27, 28, 33, 34, 46. Pressure: 3, 10, 32. Rubbing: 21. Jarring: 3.

⁴⁶ Skin. Skin: dry, flaccid; yellow; of whole body sensitive, even palms of hands.

Ulcers ichorous, sensitive; ichor has a putrid smell.

Ulcers flat, shallow, copious discharge.

Small-pox, pustules black.

⁴⁷ Stages and States. Swarthy persons.

Debilitated, "broken down," from exhausting discharges.

Old women after menopause; pleurisy, dropsy.

⁴⁸ Relationship. Antidotes to *Cinchon.* are: *Aran. diad., Arsen., Carb. veg., Eupat. perf., Ferrum, Ipec., Laches., Natr. mur., Nux vom., Pulsat., Sepia, Sulphur, Veratr,*

Cinchon. is frequently indicated in ailments from *Arsen., Calcar.,Coffea, Helleb., Jodum, Mercur.,Sulphur,Veratr.*

Also in hemorrhages from abuse of *Chamom.*

Complementary to *Ferrum.*

Cinchon. increases the anxiety caused by *Digit.*

Inimical to *Selen.*

Cinchon. antidotes: *Arsen., Ipec.*

Chin. mur. is sometimes preferable for periodical severe pain in or above eye, with chills; iris involved; cornea ulcerated.

In intermittent fever of nervous or hysterical women, compare *Tarent.*

CISTUS CANADENSIS.

Rock Rose.   BUTE.   *Cistaceæ.*

¹ Mind. All mental excitement increases the suffering.

Bad effects of vexation.

³ Inner Head. Headache in the sinciput after being kept waiting for dinner; better after eating.

Headache generally grows worse toward evening and lasts all night.

⁴ Outer Head. Pressing pain at root of nose, with headache.

Pressure in the glabella.

Head drawn to one side by swellings in the neck.

⁵ Eyes. Scrofulous inflammation of long standing; feeling as if something were passing around in eye, with stitches.

Spasmodic piercing pain in the middle of the upper rim of the right orbit, with some headache on that side.

⁶ **Ears.** Watery, bad-smelling pus discharged from the ears; inner swelling of the ears.

Tetters on and around the ears, extending into the external meatus.

Swelling beginning at ear and extending half way up cheek.

Swelling of parotids.

⁷ **Nose.** Cold feeling in the nose.

Frequent and violent sneezing, mostly evening and morning; chronic nasal catarrh.

Left side inflamed and swollen.

Tip of nose painful.

Eczema of the nose.

⁸ **Face.** Flushes of heat in the face.

Vesicular erysipelas.

Heat and burning in bones.

Sharp shooting, intolerable itching and thick crusts, with burning on the right zygoma.

⁹ **Lower Face.** Caries of the lower jaw; with suppurating glands in the neck.

Open, bleeding cancer on lower lip.

Lupus exedens on mouth and nose.

¹⁰ **Teeth.** Twitching, stitching toothache in an upper left decayed molar.

Scorbutic swollen gums, separating from the teeth; easily bleeding, putrid, disgusting.

¹¹ **Tongue, etc.** Dryness of tongue and roof of mouth.

Tongue sore, surface as if raw.

¹² **Mouth.** Inhaled air feels cool to tongue.

¹³ **Throat.** Fauces inflamed and dry, without a dry feeling; tough, gum-like, thick, tasteless mucus is brought up by hawking, mostly morning.

Sore throat from inhaling the least cold air, not from warm air.

Must swallow saliva to relieve the unbearable dryness, especially during the night.

Dryness in the throat, worse after sleeping.

A small dry spot in the gullet; worse after sleeping; must get up and drink; better after eating; throat looks glassy; on the back of throat stripes of tough mucus.

Stitches in throat cause cough; when mentally agitated.

¹⁴ **Desires. Aversions.** Desire for acid food; for acid fruits; but pain and diarrhœa follow after eating them.

¹⁵ **Eating and Drinking.** Eating and drinking relieve dry throat; pain in sinciput less.

After eating: pain in stomach; cold feeling in stomach; After fruit or coffee, diarrhœa.

¹⁶ **Nausea and Vomiting.** Cool eructations.

Frequent nausea.

[17] **Stomach.** Cold feeling in stomach before and after eating.

[19] **Abdomen.** Cold feeling in whole abdomen.

Flatulence and bruised pain in hypochondria; evening and night.

[20] **Stool, etc.** Thin, greyish-yellow, hot stools; squirting out; irresistible urging; worse afterpart of night until noon.

Diarrhæa from coffee, acid fruits; diarrhœa, with goitre.

Discharge of much flatus.

Chronic diarrhœa.

[22] **Male Sexual Organs.** Itching on the scrotum.

[23] **Female Sexual Organs.** Catamenia does not appear, after erysipelas.

[24] **Pregnancy.** Induration and inflammation of the mammæ.

Left mamma inflamed, suppurating, with a feeling of fulness in the chest; sensibility to cold air; scrofulous.

[25] **Larynx.** Inhaled air feels cool, in larynx and trachea.

Chronic itching in larynx and trachea.

Pain in the trachea.

Goitre size of hen's egg; frequent diarrhœa.

[26] **Breathing.** Asthmatic, in the evening after lying down and at night, loud wheezing; sensation as if the trachea had not space enough.

[27] **Cough.** From stitches in the throat; with painful tearing in the throat; the neck studded with tumors.

[28] **Lungs.** Feeling of rawness from chest to throat.

Fulness in the chest.

[30] **Outer Chest.** Hurts when touched.

Pressure on chest.

Small painful Pimples, which bleed easily and heal slowly, across the shoulders and on the breast.

[31] **Neck. Back.** Scrofulous swelling and suppuration of the glands of the throat.

Drawing pains at nape, and each side of spine; headache in the temples.

Scrofulous ulcers on the back.

Burning, bruised pain in the os coccygis, prevents sitting; worse from touch.

[32] **Upper Limbs.** Violent pain in left shoulder and chest; feels as if eructation would relieve it.

Tips of fingers sensitive to cold air.

Tetter on the hands; blisters, oozing after scratching, with hot swelling.

Panaritium.

Hard, thickened places on hands of workmen; with deep, oblique cracks.

[33] **Lower Limbs.** Pains in knee and right thigh, walking or sitting.

23

Tearing in the knees; evening.

Hard swelling around mercurio-syphilitic ulcers on legs.

Piercing pain in the right great toe; evening.

Cold feet.

Swelling of left leg, ulcer thereon ; skin copper-colored.

[34] **Limbs in General.** Bruised pain, as from fatigue.

[35] **Position, etc.** Walking: 33. Lying: 26. Sitting: 31, 33.

[36] **Nerves.** Involuntary drawing and trembling feeling in muscular parts of hands and lower extremities, with pain in the wrists, fingers and knee-joints.

Trembling with the fever.

[37] **Sleep.** Restless at night; pain from flatulence.

Sleeplessness from dryness of throat.

Anxious dreams.

On awaking, pain under the hypochondria.

[38] **Time.** Morning: 7, 13. Evening: 3, 7, 19, 33, 34. Night: 3, 13, 19, 37, 40. After part of night till noon: 20.

[39] **Temperature and Weather.** Cold air: 13, 32, 46.

[40] **Chill. Fever. Sweat.** Chilliness. Chill succeeded by heat, with trembling, accompanied by a quick swelling and great redness of the glands below the ear and in the throat.

Cold feeling: in the abdomen; in the larynx and trachea.

Cold feet.

Heat with thirst, drinks frequently.

In a warm room, skin grows moist; forehead cool externally, with an internal feeling of coolness.

Night-sweats.

Sweats very easily.

[42] **Sides.** Right: 5, 8, 33. Left: 7, 10, 24, 32.

[44] **Tissues.** Glands swollen, inflamed, indurated or ulcerated.

Scrofula.

Old ulcers.

Caries of the lower jaw.

Pains in all joints ; drawing, tearing; worse in evening.

[45] **Contact, Injuries, etc.** Touch: 30, 31. Scratching: 32.

[46] **Skin.** Itching all over the body, without eruption.

Herpetic eruption on various parts.

Scrofula; extremely sensitive to cold air.

Mercurio-syphilitic ulcers, surrounded by hard swelling; on the lower limbs.

[48] **Relationship.** *Bellad., Carb. veg., Phosphor.*, act favorably between repeated doses of *Cistus*.

Sepia cured painfully swollen nose, resulting from *Cistus*.

Drinking coffee after *Cistus* may cause diarrhœa.

CLEMATIS ERECTA.

Waldrebe. STAPF. *Ranunculaceæ.*

[1] **Mind.** Difficulty in thinking.

Fear of being alone, but disinclined to meet even agreeable company.

Low-spirited and fear of approaching misfortune.

Irritable, taciturn, does not want to go out.

Ailment from homesickness or contrition of spirit.

[2] **Sensorium.** Dulness and cloudiness in the head, with tendency to vertigo.

[3] **Inner Head.** Boring pain in the left temple.

Pressive, tensive pain in the forepart of the brain, worse walking than when sitting; with heaviness of the head.

[4] **Outer Head.** Eruption on occiput, extending down the neck; moist, sore, with crawling and stinging-itching; often drying up in scales; itching worse when getting warm in bed; only slight, and but temporary relief by scratching.

[5] **Eyes.** Smarting of the eyes worse when closing them; on reopening them, great sensitiveness to light.

Eyes smart, as if raw, capillaries enlarged, lachrymation; smarting worse when closing the eyes; sensistive to open air, fears to open them; "gets black" before the eyes.

Inflammation of the iris.

Burning and inflammation of inner canthus.

Pustular conjuctivitis, with agglutination of lids in the morning.

Complaints from bright sunlight.

[6] **Ears.** Ringing in the ears, as from bells.

Burning pain on the auricles, with heat.

[7] **Nose.** Violent coryza, with sneezing.

Discharges streaked with blood.

Dryness of nose, with heat.

[8] **Face.** Pale and sickly countenance.

Aching in the right side of face, which is tender to touch; better from smoking, worse when lying on painful side.

Shooting, upward, right side of face to eye, ear and temple.

[9] **Lower Face.** Burning-cutting through the lower lip.

Cancer on the lip; pain in periphery of ulcer.

Vesicular eruption on the lip.

Suppurative pimples on the chin.

[10] **Teeth.** Toothache: stitching and drawing worse at night, better for a short time from cold water, better when drawing in the air, better in open air; worse from warmth

of bed, relieved by cold water; crumb of bread starts aching; worse from smoking tobacco; from syphilitic affections, when mercurialized.

Decayed teeth feel too long; contact extremely painful; free flow of saliva.

Gums of left lower molars pain, as if sore, worse while eating.

[11] **Tongue, etc.** Tongue dry, in the morning, on awaking.

[12] **Mouth.** Breath offensive to others.

[14] **Desires. Aversions.** Long-lasting satiety; can eat, and with relish, yet immediately feels it is too much.

Aversion to beer.

[15] **Eating and Drinking.** After eating, weakness in all the limbs, with pulsation in the arteries.

[16] **Nausea and Vomiting.** Nausea, with weakness in the legs, from smoking tobacco.

[18] **Hypochondria.** Bruised pain in the hepatic region, when touched or bending.

[19] **Abdomen.** Lancinating pains, from belly to chest, aggravated by breathing, also during micturition.

Increased sensitiveness of both inguinal regions.

Swelling and induration of the inguinal gland, with jerking pains.

[20] **Stool, etc.** Frequent stools becoming more and more loose, without abdominal pain.

Constipation.

[21] **Urine.** Vesical neuralgia; the urethra or seminal cord most affected.

Urine frequent but scanty.

Interrupted flow of urine, with burning during, but most at the beginning of micturition, or during the interruptions.

Sharp stitches in the urethra.

Urinary deposit pus-like.

Involuntary flow, by drops, after micturition.

Long-lasting contraction and constriction of the urethra, urine emitted by drops, as in spasmodic stricture.

[22] **Male Sexual Organs.** Sexual desire weak.

Burning in the penis during seminal discharge in coitus.

Right spermatic cord sensitive, testicle drawn up.

Pain in the testicles, drawing to the spermatic cord.

Painful, inflamed and swollen testicles.

Induration of the testicles.

Swelling of the right half of the scrotum; testicle relaxed, hanging down.

Involuntary erections by day.

[23] **Female Sexual Organs.** Menses too early.

Softened scirrhus, with corrosive leucorrhœa and lancinating pains.

[24] **Pregnancy**. Scirrhus of (left) mamma, with stitches in the shoulder or gland, or into the arm, very painful, worse during cold weather, during the night, during increasing moon; edges of ulcer sting.

[25] **Larynx**. Dryness and burning in throat.

[26] **Breathing**. Respiration impeded when ascending a hill, or walking over an uneven road.

[27] **Cough**. Cough usually dry.

[28] **Lungs**. Oppression of the chest.
Aching in the chest.
Left side of chest seems most affected.
Stitching pains in the chest.

[29] **Heart. Pulse**. Sharp stitches in region of heart, from within outwards.
Pulse: unchanged; excited, with throbbing in the veins.

[31] **Neck. Back**. Small of back: burning; pressure in; bruised pain.

[32] **Upper Limbs**. Swelling of the axillary glands.
Pressing or drawing in the muscles of the arms and hands.
Rheumatic pains in the hands.
Arthritic nodes on the finger-joints.

[33] **Lower Limbs**. Scaly herpes on the thighs.
Burrowing, boring or pressive pains on the tibiæ.
Rheumatic pains in the lower limbs.
Violent itching of the toes, evenings, after lying down; sweat between the toes.

[34] **Limbs in General**. Weakness, heaviness, weariness and bruised sensation.

[35] **Position, etc.** Walking: 3, 26. Ascending: 26. Closing the eyes: 5. Bending: 18. Sitting: 3. Lying: 33, 36; on painful side: 8.

[36] **Nerves**. Great debility.
Twitching of the muscles.
Vibratory sensation through whole body after lying down.

[37] **Sleep**. Sleepiness, great desire to sleep during the day, even mornings, early.
Sleeplessness, evening and night.
Uneasy sleep, dreaming and tossing about.
Unrefreshed from sleep, mornings.

[38] **Time**. Morning: 5, 11, 37, 40. Evening: 33, 37. Night: 10, 24, 37, 40. Day: 22, 37.

[39] **Temperature and Weather**. Sunshine: 5. Warmth of bed: 4, 10, 46. Uncovering: 40. Open air: 5, 10. Cold weather: 24. Cold water: 10, 46. Wet pultice: 46.

[40] **Chill. Fever. Sweat**. Chill, with shivering, followed by sweat, without intervening heat.
Shivering from uncovering.
Dry heat, with general hot sensation only at night.

Heat of one side.

Profuse sweat at night, most toward morning, with aversion to uncovering.

[41] **Attacks.**   Increase of moon: 24, 46. Decrease of moon: 46.

[42] **Sides.**   Right: 8, 28, 22. Left: 3, 6, 10, 24, 28. Above downward: 4. Below up: 8, 21. Within outward: 29.

[44] **Tissues.**   Skin and muscles lax.

Hot, painful swelling of glauds.

[45] **Contact, Injuries, etc.**   Touch: 8, 10, 18, 22. Scratching: 4.

[46] **Skin.**   Eruption looks inflamed during the increasing and dry during the decreasing moon; moist eczema, itching terribly; worse from washing in cold water, from warmth of bed, from wet poultices.

Dark, burning, miliary eruption, with violent itching.

Eruption on neck and occiput.

[47] **Stages and States.**   Light hair.

Torpid, cachetic conditions.

[48] **Relationship.**   Has the same impetigo on the neck and occiput as *Petrol.*

Clemat. follows *Silic.* well.

Antidote to *Clemat.: Bryon.* for the toothache.

Clematis vitalba is preferable to the *Clem. erecta* for varices, varicose ulcers.

COCCULUS.

Cocculus Indicus.   HAHNEMANN.   *Menispermaceæ.*

[1] **Mind.**   Stupid feeling in the head.

Slowness of comprehension.

Time passes too quickly.

Thoughts fixed on one unpleasant subject; she is absorbed and observes nothing about her.

Sobbing, moaning and groaning.

Sudden great anxiety.

Vacillating, cannot accomplish anything at her work or finish anything; with contracted pupils.

Very easily affronted; every trifle makes him angry.

Startles very easily.

[2] **Sensorium.**   Vertigo: as from intoxication, or with inclination to vomit, when raising up in bed; must lie down.

Head befogged, generally increased by eating and drinking.

Dulness of the head, as after being drunk.

Sensation of emptiness and hollowness in the head, worse in open air and after eating, better when getting warm in bed.

³ **Inner Head.**   Headache, with nausea and inclination to
vomit.

Headache as if the eyes were being torn out.

Pressing headache from without inwards; or as if compressed by a bandage; or, as if screwed together.

Pressing pain in forehead, from without inwards, with
nausea; aggravated by riding in a wagon; from eating;
drinking and sleeping; from thinking; ameliorated during rest, in-doors.

Violent headache, cannot lie on back of head, must lie on
side; worse least light; noise excites vomiting.

Beating in forehead, evenings, worse before and after eating; also when riding, especially in cold air ; from talking; better in-doors.

Headache in occiput and nape, sensation of opening and
shutting like a door; even in spotted fever.

⁴ **Outer Head.**   Convulsive trembling of the head from weakness of the muscles of the neck; worse in the open air
and after sleeping; from coffee and tobacco; better in
warm room.

Cramp-like pain in left temporal muscle.

⁵ **Eyes.**   Dimsightedness; obscured vision.

Dark spot before the eyes, though objects appear clearly.

Bruised pain in eyes, with inability to open lids, at night.

Pupils: dilated ; contracted.

Eyes protruding.

▮ Eyes closed, with the balls constantly rolling about.

Eyelids inflamed.

⁶ **Ears.**   Sensitiveness of hearing.

Noise in the ears like rushing of waters, with hardness of
hearing.

⁷ **Nose.**   Sense of smell either acute or weak.

Discharge from nose bloody; pus-like.

Worse from strong smells.

⁸ **Face.**   Face: pale; blue around the eyes; sweat in face, cold.

Red cheeks and heat of face, in cold room.

Pressive, benumbing and cramp-like pains in region of
malar bones and masseter muscles; worse opening jaw.

⁹ **Lower Face.**   Pustule below the right angle of mouth, with
tensive pain when touched.

Swollen hard glands under the lower jaw, and nodes on the
forearm, which are painful when stroked.

¹⁰ **Teeth.**   Hollow tooth, pains only when chewing, even soft
food; not when biting with empty mouth.

¹¹ **Tongue, etc.**   Taste: bitter; putrid; sour; offensive; metallic; like sulphur.

Food tastes as though salted too little; tobacco tastes bitter.

Yellow-coated tongue with aversion to food.

Tongue as if paralyzed ; pains at base when protruded.
[12] **Mouth.** Dryness of the mouth, at night, without thirst.

Sensation of dryness in mouth, with frothy saliva and violent thirst.

[13] **Throat.** Dryness in the pharynx.

Pressive pain in the tonsils, worse when swallowing the saliva than when swallowing food.

Burning in the œsophagus, extending into the fauces, with taste of sulphur in the mouth.

A sort of paralysis, preventing swallowing.

Choking constriction in upper part of fauces, with difficult breathing and irritable cough, or disposition to cough.

[14] **Desires. Aversions.** Hunger without appetite.

Thirst with aversion to drink.

Thirstless.

Disgust for beer; aversion to sour things.

Longing for cold drink, especially beer.

[15] **Eating and Drinking.** All symptoms and affections, particularly of the head, increased by eating or drinking.

Coffee aggravates the headache.

[16] **Nausea and Vomiting.** Frequent empty eructations; then she wants to eat.

Nausea which is felt in the head, and inclination to vomit, in morning, can scarcely rise on account of faintness.

Nausea and vomiting when riding in a carriage or getting cold.

Disposition to vomit, with profuse flow of saliva, on getting a chill or taking a cold; also, in connection with headache and pain in the bowels, as if bruised.

Vomit: sour; bitter; of bad odor.

[17] **Stomach.** Violent cramp of stomach; also with flatulency and much saliva; gastralgia.

Contractive pain in the epigastrium, taking the breath.

Painful sensation of fulness in the stomach.

[18] **Hypochondria.** Pain as if beaten in hypochondria.

Pressive pain in the hepatic region, increased by coughing and bending over.

Stitches in hepatic region.

[19] **Abdomen.** Emptiness and sensation of hollowness in the abdomen.

Sensation in abdomen as if sharp stones rubbed together on every movement.

Great rumbling in the bowels.

Spasmodic flatulent colic about midnight, flatus passed without relief; belching relieves; pain severest in epigastric, umbilical and right iliac region.

[20] **Stool, etc.** Contractive pain in rectum, preventing sitting, afternoons. Stool followed by tenesmus recti causing faintness.

Diarrhœa, with sensation in abdomen as of sharp stones rubbing together.

Diarrhœa only through the day, thin, yellowish, without pain.

Incarcerated flatus; obstruction of the bowels.

Hard stool every other day, expelled with great difficulty.

[21] **Urine.**   Frequent desire to urinate, with small discharge.

Watery urine.

[22] **Male Sexual Organs.**   Seminal emissions at night.

Excitement of the genitals, with desire for coition.

Increased sensitiveness of the genitals.

Drawing, sore pain in the testicles when touched.

Itching of scrotum.

[23] **Female Sexual Organs.**   Menses profuse and too often, when rising upon the feet it gushes out in a stream.

Scanty discharge of black blood.

During the effort to menstruate, she is so weak that she is scarcely able to stand.

Leucorrhœa in place of the menses.

Leucorrhœa, like serum, mixed with a purulent, ichorous liquid.

Dysmenorrhœa followed by hemorrhoids. Also with severe cutting in the womb, or sensation as if latter was distended; seasick feeling, flatulent gastralgia.

Painful pressure in uterus, with cramps in chest, nausea and fainting.

[24] **Pregnancy.**   Shivering over the mammæ.

Discharge of bloody mucus from the uterus, during pregnancy.

Spasmodic and irregular labor-pains.

Terrible pain in small of back, with hour-glass contraction of uterus.

Spasms following difficult labor, and brought on by changing the position of the patient.

[25] **Larynx.**   Tightness in the larynx.

Talking aggravates all the symptoms, particularly of head.

[26] **Breathing.**   Obstruction of breath at the throat-pit, as if the throat were constricted.

[27] **Cough.**   Fatiguing cough from oppression of the chest.

Cough increased by indulging the irritation.

[28] **Lungs.**   Contractive tension of right side of chest taking the breath.   Cramps in the chest, also hysteric.

Audible rumbling in the left side of chest, as if from an emptiness, especially noticeable when walking.

[29] **Heart. Pulse.**   Pulse small and spasmodic, often imperceptible, seldom hard, somewhat accelerated.

Palpitation of the heart, from quick motion and mental excitement, with dizziness and faintness.

[31] **Neck. Back.** Painful stiffness of neck when moving it.

Disabling drawing in the small of the back.

Paralytic pain extending over hips; with anxiety and apprehension.

Spasmodic constriction the length of the spine; worse on motion.

[32] **Upper Limbs.** Stitches in the shoulder-joint and muscles of upper arm, during rest.

Stitches in the right upper arm.

Now one hand, and again other, is numb and as if asleep.

Now one hand, and again other, is alternately hot or cold.

[33] **Lower Limbs.** Pain as if beaten in the thighs.

Inflammatory swelling of knee, with transitory stinging pains.

Cracking in the knees when moving.

Lower limbs: nearly paralyzed; paralytic feeling in.

Hot, itching, swelling of the feet.

Cold feet.

Œdema of feet, with paralysis of lower limbs, after a cold.

[34] **Limbs in General.** Involuntary motions of right arm and right leg, cease during sleep.

Here and there in the limbs, a laming-drawing, as if in the bones, continuous or in attacks.

Cracking and creaking in joints; painful stiffness of joints.

Now the hands, and again the feet, "go to sleep," alternately, in short attacks.

[35] **Position, etc.** Rest: 3, 32. Motion: 19. Walking: 28. Moving: 33. Moving head: 31. Quick motion: 29. Slight exertion: 40. Rising on the feet: 23. Raising in bed: 2. Bending over: 18. Change of position: 24. Must lie down: 2. Sitting: 20. Cannot stand: 23, 36. Lying: 3.

[35] **Nerves.** Great lassitude of the whole body, it is an exertion to stand firmly. Feels too weak to talk loud.

Epilepsy in the morning on rising from bed; fever afterwards.

Hysteric complaints, with sadness.

Paralysis of face, tongue or pharynx; paraplegia, with nunbness and tingling.

[37] **Sleep.** ▮ Sleeplessness from night-watching; also from pure mental activity.

Sleep disturbed by excessive anxiety and restlessness.

Sleep aggravates all the symptoms, particularly of head.

Anxious, frightful dreams.

[38] **Time.** Morning: 16, 40. Afternoon: 20, 40. Evening: 3, 40, 46. Night: 5, 12, 22, 40, 46. Evening till morning: 40. Midnight: 19. Day: 20.

[39] **Temperature and Weather.** Cannot bear the cold or
warm (open) air.

Getting cold: 16. Cold room: 8. Cold air: 3. Open
air: 2, 4. Getting warm: 2. External warmth: 40.
Warm room: 4. In-doors: 3, 4.

[40] **Chill. Fever. Sweat.** Chill frequently alternating with
heat.

Internal chill in afternoon and evening; attended with
shivering through whole body, but more in back and
on legs; not relieved by external warmth.

Continuous chilliness, with hot skin.

Dry heat the whole night through.

Flushes of heat, with burning heat of cheeks and cold feet.

Sweat of the body from evening till morning, attended
with cold sweat on the face.

Morning sweat principally on the chest.

Sweats over the whole body from the slightest exertion.

Sweat of the affected parts.

[41] **Attacks.** Every other day: 20.

[42] **Sides.** Right: 9, 18, 19, 28, 32, 34. Left: 28. Without
inwards: 3, 44. Above downwards: 33.

[44] **Tissues.** Emaciation.

Anæmic states.

Gouty pains or cracking in the joints.

Paralysis of inner parts.

Paralytic pain; tearing; soreness; digging; or as if beaten
in the bones.

Glands: burning; pressure from out inwards; hot swelling; cold; stinging.

[45] **Contact, Injuries, etc.** Touch: 9, 22, 46. Stroking affected
part: 9. Riding in carriage or sailing: 3, 16.

[46] **Skin.** Much itching, especially in the evening when undressing, or at night in a feather-bed.

Ulcers very sensitive to touch; pains in thin peripheries.

[47] **Stages and States.** Often indicated with children and
women.

Light hair.

Drunkards.

[48] **Relationship.** Ailments from: *Chamom., Cuprum., Ignat.,
Mercur., Nux vom.*, and from abuse of spirituous liquors.

Useful after *Nux vom.* in gastralgia.

COFFEA.

Coffee. HAHNEMANN. *Rubiaceæ*

[1] **Mind.** Ecstasy, full of ideas; quick to act, no sleep on this account.

Delirium tremens: unsteady running about; imagines he is not at home, with trembling of hands; small, frequent pulse.

Excessive weeping and lamentations over trifles.

Child cries and laughs easily; while crying, it suddenly laughs quite heartily, and finally cries again.

Cries and trembles, does not know what to do.

Cheerfulness.

Fear of death.

Pain seems insupportable, driving to despair.

Bad effects from sudden pleasurable surprise.

[2] **Sensorium.** All the senses more acute, reads fine print easier; hearing, smell, taste and touch acute, particularly also an increased perception of slight passive motions.

Threatening of apoplexy; overexcited, talkative, full of fear, pangs of conscience, aversion to open air, sleepless, convulsive grinding of teeth.

[3] **Inner Head.** Congestion of blood to the head, especially after pleasant surprise; from talking.

Headache from thinking.

One-sided headache, as from a nail driven into the head, worse in the open air.

Headache, as if the brain were torn or dashed to pieces.

Feels and hears a crackling, in vertex, when sitting quietly.

[5] **Eyes.** Reddish; increased visual power.

Pupils dilated.

[6] **Ears.** Hearing more acute, music has a shrill sound.

Aversion to noise; it hurts him.

Crackling noise in the head (one side), synchronous with the pulse; particularly morning and in the open air; better in doors.

[7] **Nose.** Acute, sensitive smell.

Nosebleed: with heaviness of head and ill-humor; during straining at stool.

[8] **Face.** Dry heat of the face, with red cheeks.

Neuralgia of right side of face and head and right eyeball at 1 P. M.

Sweat on the face, with internal chilliness.

[10] **Teeth.** Toothache: stinging, jerking, intermittent aching;

with restlessness, anguish and weeping mood, especially at night and after a meal; aggravated, from hot or warm drink, from chewing, at night; ameliorated when holding ice or ice-cold water in mouth.

[11] **Tongue, etc.** Taste: more acute; sweetish.

[13] **Throat.** Steady pain from side of palate into œsophagus; constant desire to swallow, from sensation as of plug in throat.

Uvula too long, swollen.

Sore throat, worse from cool air

[14] **Desires. Aversions.** Increased hunger, with hurried eating.

Thirst at night wakens him; thirst during the sweat.

Aversion to coffee.

[15] **Eating and Drinking.** Eats and drinks hastily.

Bad effects from wine or liquor drinking.

After eating: 10. Hot or warm drink: 10. Ice or ice-cold water: 10.

[16] **Nausea and Vomiting.** Hiccough, eructations.

Constant inclination to vomit, felt in the throat.

[19] **Abdomen.** Colic: as if the stomach had been overloaded; as if the abdomen would burst; cannot bear the clothes to be tight on the abdomen; exceedingly painful, driving to desperation.

Continuous pinching pain in the iliac regions.

Pressure in the abdomen, as from incarcerated flatulence.

[20] **Stool, etc.** Diarrhœa: watery, painless, all day, from too much care about domestic affairs; during dentition.

Fetid flatus.

[21] **Urine.** Frequent and copious.

[22] **Male Sexual Organs.** Sexual organs much excited without emission of semen, and with dry heat of the body.

Scrotum relaxed.

[23] **Female Sexual Organs.** Menses: too profuse and of long duration; profuse, with coldness and stiffness of body; only during the evening.

Metrorrhagia: large black lumps, worse from every motion, with violent pain in the groins and fear of death.

Leucorrhœa: like mucus, or milky; more while urinating.

Voluptuous itching in the vulva, but parts too sensitive to rub or scratch.

[24] **Pregnancy.** Excessively severe pains from threatened abortion, or labor.

Labor-pains ceasing, with complaining loquacity.

During labor or after-pains, extreme fear of death.

Puerperal fever from mental excitement, frequent crawling, with feverish warmth, tongue moist, no thirst; delirious talking, eyes open, shining; violent abdominal pains, with oversensitiveness, despair, sleeplessness.

²⁵ **Larynx.** Spasmus glottidis, starts from sleep with short inhalation or gasping, with wheezing, cold sweat, blue face; worse when put into the bath.

Larynx as if covered with dry mucus.

Rawness in larynx, with hoarseness, in the morning on awaking.

²⁶ **Breathing.** Oppression of chest; short inspiration; chest heaves visibly.

Asthmatic attacks in morning, wants to move continually.

²⁷ **Cough.** Short; dry, hacking; spasmodic and dry ; at night ; during measles.

Irritation to cough, out-doors.

²⁸ **Heart. Pulse.** Palpitation of heart, violent, irregular, with trembling of limbs.

Pulse more frequent, but less vigorous, even small and weak.

³¹ **Neck. Back.** Laming pain in small of back, while sitting or standing.

³² **Upper Limbs.** Pains extend from the face down the arms, even to finger ends.

³³ **Lower Limbs.** Sciatic or crural neuralgia, in attacks; rending, shooting, increased by walking : relieved by pressure, worse afternoon and night; restless and sleepless at night.

³⁴ **Limbs in General.** Twitching of the limbs.

³⁵ **Position, etc.** Motion: 23. Wants to move: 26. Exercise: 40. Walking: 33. Sitting: 3, 31. Standing: 31.

³⁶ **Nerves.** Physical excitement through mental exaltation.

Great nervous agitation and restlessness.

Convulsions of teething children, with grinding of teeth and coldness of limbs, after overexcitement.

Fainting from sudden emotions.

³⁷ **Sleep.** Sleeplessness: from overexcitement of body or mind.

Quick to act; no sleep on this account.

³⁸ **Time.** Morning: 6, 25, 26, 40. Afternoon: 33. Evening: 23, 40. Night: 10, 14, 27, 33, 40. All day: 20.

³⁹ **Temperature and Weather.** Hot or warm drink : 10. Ice or ice-cold water: 10. Cold air: 13. Cold: 40. Open air: 2, 3, 6, 27. In-doors: 6. Bath: 25.

⁴⁰ **Chill. Fever. Sweat.** Chills running down the back.

Chill increased by exercise.

Internal shivering, with external heat of face or whole body.

Chilly feelings, with internal and external warmth.

Great sensitiveness to cold.

External heat, with shivering in the back, in the evening after lying down. Dry heat at night, with delirium.

Sweat in the face, with internal shivering; slight, morning.

⁴² **Sides.** Without inwards: 2. Above downwards: 32, 40.

⁴⁵ **Contact, Injuries, etc.** Rubbing or scratching: 23. Pressure: 33; of clothes: 19. Chewing: 10. Passive motion: 2.

⁴⁶ **Skin.** Dryness of the skin, but not in febrile diseases.

Excessive sensitiveness of the skin.

Measles, with overexcitability and weeping.

Scarlet rash, with overwhelming pains and lamenting mood.

⁴⁸ **Relationship.** Antidotes to *Coffea: Acon., Chamom., Nux vom., Pulsat.*

Coffea antidotes: *Chamom., Coloc., Nux vom., Psorin.*

Chronic affections from abuse of coffee require: *Chamom., Ignat., Mercur., Nux vom., Sulphur.*

Inimicals: *Canthar., Caustic., Coccul., Ignat.*

COLCHICUM AUTUMNALE.

Meadow Saffron.   STAPF.   *Melanthaceæ.*

¹ **Mind.** Perception entirely lost, unconscious.

Memory weakened.

Can read, but cannot understand even a short sentence.

Intellect beclouded, though he gives correct answers.

Confusion of the head.

Indisposition for exertion of any kind.

Mood usually cheerful; or sad; rarely irritable.

External impressions such as bright light, strong odors, contact, misdeeds of others make him quite beside himself.

Surly, ill-humored, not satisfied with anything.

Pains worse by mental exertion or by emotions.

² **Sensorium.** Vertigo: while siting, after walking; on rising.

³ **Inner Head.** Boring headach, especially over the eyes.

Pressure in the head; especially in the occiput, also deep in cerebellum, excited by mental exertion.

Pressive heaviness deep in the cerebellum, especially on moving or stooping.

Painful rending in left side of head, from eyeball to occiput.

Creeping sensation in the forehead.

⁴ **Outer Head.** Tearing in the scalp, at small spots, particularly on the occiput.

When raised the head falls back, mouth opens wide.

Difficulty in moving the head.

Porrigo favosa, oozing acrid ichor.

⁵ **Eyes.** Violent, sharp tearing pain in and around eyeball.

Drawing-digging pain deep in the orbit, like in sclerotitis.

Inflammation of the eyes, dimsightedness, watering of the eyes, white spot on the cornea.

Soft cataract.

Pupils much dilated, only slightly sensitive to light, or immovable and slightly dilated.

Eyes: half open; sunken, staring.

Pressure and biting in the canthi, with moderate lachrymation.

⁶ **Ears.** Hearing generally acute.

Roaring in the ears; they feel stopped up.

Earache with stitches in the ears.

Tingling of the ears, as after being frosted.

Discharge from ears, with tearing in them. θ After measles.

⁷ **Nose.** Smell morbidly acute; the odor of meat broth causes nausea, and that of fresh eggs nearly fainting.

Sore pain in the septum.

Nosebleed.

Sneezing, also with crawling sensation in the nose.

Long-lasting coryza; discharge thin, tenacious.

Nostrils dry and black.

⁸ **Face.** Doleful, sad expression; sunken; risus sardonicus; cadaverous looking; pale; yellow spotted; cheeks red and hot; covered with sweat.

Œdematous swelling of the face.

Pain and swelling from a decayed tooth; tongue furred.

Tearing and tensive pains in the facial mucles, moving from one location to another.

Drawing in the bones of face or nose, sensation as if they were being rent asunder.

Tingling in the skin of the face, as after being frosted.

⁹ **Lower Face.** Cracked lips.

Thick, brownish coating on lips, teeth and tongue.

¹⁰ **Teeth.** Grinding of the teeth.

Teeth very sensitive when pressing them together.

Teeth feel too long.

Toothache worse from cold; after warm things.

Tearing in the jaws and gums.

¹¹ **Tongue, etc.** Tastelessness of food.

Loss of speech. θ During typhus.

Tongue: bright red; heavy, stiff and numb; projected with difficulty.

¹² **Mouth.** Profuse flow of saliva, with dryness of the throat.

Inflammation of mucous membrane of mouth and throat.

Heat in the mouth, with thirst.

[13] **Throat.** Tickling in the throat, as if coryza were setting in, inducing cough and clearing the throat.

Much greenish, thin mucus in throat, comes sometimes involuntarily into the mouth.

Inflammation and redness of the palate and fauces.

Tonsils inflamed and swollen; here and there spots covered with pus, swallowing difficult.

[14] **Desires. Aversions.** Great thirst, but no appetite.

Aversion to food; loathing the sight and still more the smell of it.

[16] **Nausea and Vomiting.** Nausea, eructations and copious vomiting of mucus and bile.

Frequent copious eructations of tasteless gas.

Nausea, with great restlessness, and on assuming the upright posture, a qualmishness in stomach and inclination to vomit.

Violent retching, followed by copious and forcible vomiting of food and then of bile; better if lies perfectly still.

[17] **Stomach.** Epigastrium extremely sensitive to touch or pressure.

Stomach icy-cold, with colic.

Colic: aggravated by eating; after flatulent food; with great distention of belly; better when bending double.

[18] **Hypochondria.** Pain in right hypochondrium, as from incarcerated flatus.

Anxious feeling in the præcordia.

[19] **Abdomen.** Flatulent distention of the abdomen, with less frequent and less copious stools.

Pressing, tearing, cutting or stitching pains in abdomen.

Tympanitis.

Colic: aggravated by eating; after flatulent food; with great distention of belly; until diarrhœa sets in; better from bending double.

[20] **Stool, etc.** Very offensive flatus in the evening.

Stools: frequet, abundant, watery, with flocculi; yellowish and bloody; scanty, with tenesmus, salivation and copious secretion of urine; copious, frequent, watery, or bilious, often without pain, sometimes with cutting colic; scanty, difficult, of bloody mucus and shreds, with pain in anus, and violent tenesmus; constant ineffectual effort to pass feces; green, watery, very offensive mucus; pass insensibly, involuntarily.

Spasm of the sphincter during or independent of discharge, with a shuddering over the back.

Stools frequent, somewhat bloody, and very fetid; dysentery.

[21] **Urine.** Pain in the region of the kidneys.

More urging and more discharge of urine.

Urine: copious, watery and frequent; dark and turbid,

24

with tenesmus of bladder and burning in urethra; of sour smell and acid reaction; dark, scanty, discharged in drops, whitish sediment; ∎ bloody, almost like ink, containing albumen.

Urine scanty, looking like bits of decomposed blood, with offensive smell.

Urethra hurts while the urine passes, as if raw.

²² **Male Sexual Organs.** Tearing in glands and left spermatic cord.

²³ **Female Sexual Organs.** Menses too early.

²⁴ **Pregnancy.** Feverish restlessness, in the last months of pregnancy.

Nipples dark, brownish-red, protruding; unbearable pain on the slight touch by the child; breasts full, skin hot, pulse strong (lying-in, fourth day).

²⁵ **Larynx.** Voice hoarse, or deeper than usual.

²⁶ **Breathing.** Accelerated and audible; slow; irregular; asthmatic.

Oppression of the chest.

²⁷ **Cough.** Slight cough, with coryza.

Frequent, short, dry cough, from tickling in the larynx.

Night cough, with involuntary spurting out of urine.

²⁸ **Lungs.** Dull stitches in posterior part of the thorax, during expiration.

Violent cutting pain in the chest, interrupting breathing.

Stinging in the region of the heart, with oppression.

Spitting blood, after injuries.

²⁹ **Heart. Pulse.** Violent palpitation, with anxiety.

∎ Heart disease, following acute rheumatism.

Hydropericardium.

Pulse: accelerated and hard, or full and slow; slow and feeble; quick and thready.

³⁰ **Outer Chest.** Stinging and tearing in the muscles of chest.

³¹ **Neck. Back.** Stitching and tension between the scapulæ.

Rheumatic pains in neck and back.

Drawing, tension and stitches occurring, or much aggravated, on motion.

Sudden tearing and shooting in the loins.

Spot on the sacrum feels sore, as if ulcerated; very sensitive to touch.

³² **Upper Limbs.** Rheumatic pains: on the clavicle, shoulders, arms, back and neck, preventing motion of the head; in elbow-joint, forearm, wrist, and ligaments of finger-joints.

Laming pain in the arms, which makes it impossible to hold the lightest thing.

Œdematous swelling of the hands.

³³ **Lower Limbs.** Flying pains in the hips.

Tearing: in the thighs; knee-joints, with swelling; in patella; in tibiæ, calves, ankles, toes, tendo-achillis.

With the pains, weariness, heaviness, and inability to move.
Knees strike together, can hardly walk.
Œdematous swelling and coldness of legs and feet.
Tingling in the toes, like after being frosted.

[34] **Limbs in General.** Numbness of the hands and feet, with
pricking, as if asleep.
Pains in the shoulder and hip-joints; and in all the bones,
with diffiulty of moving the head and tongue.
Tearing pains in the muscles and joints.

[35] **Position, etc.** Exertion: 1. Motion: 3, 4, 31, 32, 34.
Rising: 2, 16. Sitting: 2. Stooping: 3. Bending
double: 17, 19.

[36] **Nerves.** Great weakness, as after exertion.
Sudden sinking of strength; extreme prostration.
Paralytic feeling with the pains.
Paralysis after sudden suppression of sweat, particularly
foot-sweat, by getting wet.

[37] **Sleep.** Comatose state.
Great sleepiness during the day, falls asleep while reading.
At night, sleep disturbed or driven away by pains.
Wakened from sleep by frightful dreams.
Starting, jerking in sleep.
Lying on the back.

[38] **Time.** Evening: 20. Night: 27, 37, 40. Day: 37.

[39] **Temperature and Weather.** Warmth: 40. Cold: 10.
Getting wet: 36.

[40] **Chill. Fever. Sweat.** Chill and shivering, running
through all the limbs; even in the warm room.
Frequent shiverings, running down the back.
Chilliness even near the warm stove, intermingled with
short flushes of heat.
External dry heat the whole night, with violent, unquenchable thirst.
Body hot and limbs cold. θ In typhus.
Sweat wanting. θ In intermittents.
ı Copious sour sweat, suddenly coming and going. θ In
rheumatism.

[41] **Attacks.** Autumn dysentery.

[42] **Sides.** Right: 18. Left: 3, 18, 22, 28. Above downwards: 40. Cures gout going from left to right.

[43] **Sensations.** Shuddering and creeping, in isolated parts,
such as is felt on getting cold from change of weather.
Tearing tensive pains over small parts, at a time; quickly
changing location.

[44] **Tissues.** Acts markedly on the periosteum; synovial membranes of joints, especially small joints; that part of
nervous system which presides over function of voluntary motion.

Stands in close relation to the fibrous tissues; redness, swelling, heat, etc., not tending to suppuration, but easily and quickly changing location; redness paling as disease shifts.

Painful flexion of the joints.

Emaciation. Œdema. Anasarca.

Dropsy of cavities and internal organs, especially hydro-pericardium; hydrothorax; ascites; hydrometra.

45 **Contact, Injuries, etc.** Touch: 1, 17, 24, 31. Pressure: 10, 17. When the head is raised: 4.

46 **Skin.** Skin dry, sweat suppressed, or profuse sweating.

Stitches in the skin.

Tingling here and there, as after being frosted.

47 **Stages and States.** Gout in persons of vigorous constitution. Often indicated with old people.

48 **Relationship.** Antidotes to *Colchic.:* For the affection of the heart, feels as if dying: *Spigel.* Copious draughts of rice water, prevent its action on the bowels. In poison-ings give *Amm. caust.*, a few drops in sugar water.

General antidotes to *Colchic.: Bellad., Camphor., Coccul., Nux vom., Pulsat.*

Colchic. follows well where *Nux vom.* or *Lycop.* has relieved.

COLLINSONIA.

Stone Root.   *Labiatæ.*

3 **Inner Head.** Dull frontal headache, with frequent flying pains in the legs; tearing in the knees.

11 **Tongue, etc.** Tongue yellow along the base and centre; rough, bitter taste.

19 **Abdomen.** Dull distress in the right hypochondrium; cut-ting pains in the hypogastrium; with faintness.

20 **Stool, etc.** Constipation, stool light-colored, lumpy, with hard straining.

Diarrhœa, mucous, bloody; thin, yellow matter, or watery, with violent tenesmus and sharp cutting in the bowels.

ı Hemorrhoids, blind or bleeding; sense of weight in rec-tum, itching, feeling as of sticks or sand; caused by con-gestive inertia of lower bowel. Also for obstinate cases.

22 **Male Sexual Organs.** Varicocele; rectal symptoms decide.

23 **Female Sexual Organs.** Chronic inflammation; retro-flexion or retroversion; prolapsus; when there is pelvic passive congestion, hemorrhoids, etc., ovarian neuralgia, lancinating pains, worse right side.

Pruritus vulvæ; prolapsus uteri or during pregnancy.

[27] **Cough.** Spits dark, tough, coagulated blood, covered with viscid mucus; previously the blood was discharged per anum.

[29] **Heart. Pulse.** Irritable heart, it beats rapidly and irregularly, worse least motion or excitement; periodical spells of faintness; when reflex from pelvic and rectal symptoms (clinical).

[44] **Tissues.** Acts upon the lower portion of the bowels, causing congestive inertia. Reflexly, or by similar drug effect, veins elsewhere are affected; hence its use (like *Arnica*) as a vulnerary, and also its employment in varicocele.

[48] **Relationship.** Compare: *Aloes* (rectal dysentery; latter has more paresis of rectum): *Æsculus* (piles); *Nux vom.*

COLOCYNTHIS.

Bitter Cucumber.   HAHNEMANN.   *Cucurbitaceæ.*

[1] **Mind.** Confusion in the left side of head, with pressing burning pain in the left orbit, temple and nose, on dorsum nasi and in the upper teeth.

   ❙Greatly affected by the misfortunes of others as well as her own.

   Depressed, joyless; disinclined to talk, answer, to see friends.

   Extreme irritability; nothing seems right to him; extremely impatient; every word provokes him.

   Anger, with indignation; also bad effects therefrom, particularly vomiting and diarrhœa.

[2] **Sensorium.** Vertigo, when quickly turning the head, as if he would fall, tottering of the knees.

   Dulness of head and giddiness, at beginning of colic.

[3] **Inner Head.** Pressive frontal headache, worse while stooping, or lying on the back.

   Painful tearing through the whole brain, becoming unbearable when moving the upper eyelid.

   Severe burning, boring pain, on right side of forehead.

   Tearing in the left side of forehead.

   Pressure in both temples.

   Boring stitches in the right temple, disappearing on touch.

   Pressing and dull throbbing in left temple, growing gradually more acute and cutting.

[4] **Outer Head.** Roots of the hair painful.

   Smarting, burning on the scalp, left side.

[5] **Eyes.** Vision obscured.

Painful pressure in the eyeballs, especially on stooping.

Sharp cutting in the right eyeball, with pain in the eyes.

Smarting in the eyes.

Discharge of acrid fluid from the eyes.

6 **Ears.** Roaring and throbbing in both ears, especially the left.

Crawling; itching; stitching; cutting or aching in the ears, relieved by putting the fingers into the ear.

7 **Nose.** Fluent coryza, worse in open air than in the room.

Beating and digging pain, from left side of nose to glabella.

8 **Face.** Face: dark red; or pale, with relaxed muscles and sunken eyes.

Tensive tearing pain, with heat and swelling, especially of left side; worse from touch or motion, better in perfect rest, and from external application of warmth.

Left-sided tearing, or burning and stinging pain, extending to the ear and head; tearing in the cheeks.

Constriction and pressing in the left malar bone, extending into the left eye.

Transient stitches in the upper jaw recurring frequently.

10 **Teeth.** Drawing and twitching toothache.

Beating toothache, first in one, then in another tooth of left side.

11 **Tongue, etc.** Taste: bitter, of food and drink, less frequently offensive or metallic.

Tongue: coated white, or yellow; rough; burning on tip.

Scalded sensation of the tongue.

13 **Throat.** Dryness; rawness; roughness; or scraping in throat.

14 **Desires. Aversions.** Canine hunger, with longing for bread and beer.

Aversion to food, with scraping in the throat.

Diminished appetite, without thirst, still great inclination to drink; succeeded by a putrid taste in the mouth.

15 **Eating and Drinking.** After the least food or drink, diarrhœa.

Potatoes cause bellyache; coffee relieves the colic.

16 **Nausea and Vomiting.** Nausea arising from the stomach.

Vomiting of bitter-tasting, yellow fluid.

17 **Stomach.** Feeling of emptiness in the stomach.

Burning pain in the stomach.

Feeling of fulness in the epigastric region.

Griping in the epigastrium, after each meal, worse toward evening.

Cramp in the stomach at night, relieved by belching.

Pit of stomach very sensitive to touch.

❙ Violent cutting, tearing pains, which from different parts of chest and abdomen, concentrate in the pit of stomach, better from hard pressure and bending double; brought on by vexation and indignation.

[18] **Hypochondria.**   Transient stitches in the hepatic region.
[19] **Abdomen.**   Abdomen distended and painful; tympanitic.
Incarcerated flatus.

❙ Cramp-like pain in both sides of abdomen, worse after pressure, or leaning with belly on a table.

❙ Collection of fat in abdomen since her first confinement.

Severe colicky pains, mostly around the navel; has to bend double, being worse in any other posture; great restlessness and loud screaming on changing position; worse at intervals of five or ten minutes.

❙ Colic so distressing that they seek relief by pressing the corner of a table, or head of bed-post, against abdomen.

Colic-like, spasmodic pain after vexation.

Colic spreading from the navel, better from frequent discharge of flatus.

Isolated, deep stitches, sometimes in left, at others in right flank, apparently connected with the ovaries.

Pain in the groin, like from hernia, and on pressure, sensation as if a hernia were receding.

[20] **Stool, etc.**   Chronic watery diarrhœa mornings, with pain in sides of abdomen.

Dysentery-like diarrhœa, renewed each time by the least food or drink.

Bloody diarrhœa, with violent pain in the bowels, extending down into the thighs.

Frequent urging to stool, with sensation as if the anus and rectum were weakened by long-continued diarrhœa.

Stools : copious fecal diarrhœa, accompanied by great discharge of wind; fluid; after eating, with discharge of flatus and painful feeling in abdomen, better after getting warm in bed; thin, frothy, saffron-yellow, of musty odor ; slimy, bloody, like scrapings of the bowels, with tenesmus during stool ; relief of pain after stool.

Constipation, stools hard; also when caused by cheese.

Painfully swollen hemorrhoids, in rectum and at anus.

[21] **Urine.**   Sudden violent pressure upon the bladder, which was full, passed off suddenly on the emission of flatus.

Abundant urine; frequent desire to pass water, with burning in bladder and stitches; alternating with stitches in the rectum.

Frequent tenesmus vesicæ, with scanty emission.

Urine: fetid; brown; viscid; deposits copious sediment, which becomes jelly-like; faint flesh-colored, with light brown, flocky, unequally translucent sediment, and depositing small, hard, reddish crystals, which adhere to the vessel, and are not easily removed by water.

[22] **Male Sexual Organs.**   Sexual desire strong; with erections.
[23] **Female Sexual Organs.**   Cramp-like pain in the left ovarian region, as though the parts were squeezed in a vice.

Intense boring or tensive pain in ovary, causing her to draw up double, with great restlessness. Deep stitches, worse in left ovary.

Suppression of the menses, caused by chagrin.

Dysmenorrhœa, cramping pains, must bend double, sometimes worse after eating or drinking.

Swelling of labia, with dragging pain and heat to vagina.

Metritis, from indigestion, colicky pains bend her double; cutting, as from knives, in the bowels, great distress, distention of the abdomen; feeling as if the intestines were being squeezed between stones.

May be indicated in some cases of very painful cancer.

24 **Pregnancy.** During pregnancy, frequent attacks of colic, which draws the patient nearly double.

Suppression of the lochia: with violent colic; from anger or indgnation; with tympanitic swelling of the abdomen and diarrhœa.

25 **Larynx.** Frequent tickling and irritation in the larynx.

26 **Breathing.** Asthmatic attacks at night, with slow, difficult breathing, which provokes cough.

Oppression of chest, worse evenings and before midnight.

27 **Cough.** Titillating cough, frequently during the night.

28 **Lungs.** Stitching pains in right or left side of chest.

29 **Heart. Pulse.** Stitches in the cardiac region.

Pulse: generally full, hard and accelerated; less frequently, small and weak. Strong throbbing in all the blood-vessels.

31 **Neck. Back.** Feeling of stiffness in the muscles of the nape, when moving the head. Drawing in the nape.

Violent tensive drawing in the left cervical muscles, worse on motion. Pressure in left side of nape, worse from turning.

Drawing pain, internally, in region of right scapula, as if the nerves and vessels were made tense.

Tensive stitches in the right loin, felt only during inspiration, and most violent when lying on the back.

Painful lassitude in small of back and lower extremities, in the evening.

Pain in the small of the back.

32 **Upper Limbs.** Swelling and suppuration of the axillary glands.

Drawing, lancinating in left shoulder from the face and neck.

Rheumatic pains through the arms.

Pains in the palms, as if the muscles were contracted.

Tearing in joints of left hand.

Tensive pain in left thumb, impeding motion.

Violent drawing pain in the right thumb, like in the tendons, beginning in the ball and passing off at the tip.

[33] **Lower Limbs.** Crampy pain in the affected hip, as though the parts were screwed in a vice; lies upon the affected side, with knee drawn up.

Drawing, twitching, with dull throbbing in region of left hip, and in right loin.

Pain as if the hips were screwed together.

Shooting pain, like lightning, down the whole limb.

Pain in right thigh only when walking, as if the psoas magnus were too short.

Drawing in inner side of left thigh, afternoons.

Drawing pain in right thigh, down to the knee.

Drawing in external condyle of right femur.

Continuous pain in left knee-joint, impeding walking.

Cramp in the left calf.

Drawing, aching in the left foot.

Left foot "goes to sleep."

[34] **Limbs in General.** Tearing or drawing pains in all limbs.

[35] **Position, etc.** Rest: 8. Walking: 33. Motion: 8, 31. Moving the head: 31. Turning the head: 2, 31. Moving the upper eyelid: 3. Stooping: 3, 5. Bending double: 17, 19, 23, 24. Bending the knee: 33. Lying on back: 3, 31. Lying on affected side: 33.

Motion generally relieves drawing, tearing and burning pains.

[36] **Nerves.** Great tendency of the muscles of all parts of the body to become painfully cramped.

Sensation of weakness, of faint feeling.

[37] **Sleep.** Yawning and sleepiness.

Sleeplessness and restlessness, with the pains.

Dreams: disturbing sleep; vivid; anxious.

[38] **Time.** Morning: 20, 26. Afternoon: 33. Evening: 17, 26, 31. Night: 17, 27, 40. Before midnight: 26.

[39] **Temperature and Weather.** Warm applications: 8. Warmth of bed: 20. Open air: 7.

[40] **Chill. Fever. Sweat.** Chill and coldness of the whole body, frequently with heat of the face.

Coldness of hands or soles of the feet, rest of body warm.

Chill and shivering, with the pains.

External dry heat.

Internal sensation of heat, with external flushes.

Sweat at night, smelling like urine, causing itching of the skin.

Sweat principally on the head and extremities.

[41] **Attacks.** Increasing gradually: 3.

[42] **Sides.** Right: 3, 5, 18, 19, 26, 31, 32, 33. Left: 1, 3, 4, 6, 7, 8, 10, 19, 23, 28, 29, 31, 32, 33.

[43] **Sensations.** Rheumatism, with all sorts of pains, with formication and numbness.

⁴⁵ **Contact, Injuries, etc.** Touch : relieves pain in temples, 3 ; in ear: 6 ; increases faceache; stomach sensitive to it. Hard pressure relieves: 17, 19. Pressure relieves, but after is worse.

⁴⁶ **Skin.** Itching; prickling; crawling; formication.
Desquamation over the whole body.

⁴⁸ **Relationship.** *Coloc.* antidotes: *Caustic.*
Antidotes to *Coloc.: Camphor., Coffea, Staphis.*
Large doses are counteracted by tepid milk, infusion of galls, *Camphor., Opium.*
Staphis. is very similar with regard to mind symptoms and pains in abdomen.
Smoking relieves pain in bowels.
In aggravations of colic, give a cup of coffee to palliate, and repeat *Coloc.* if necessary.

CONIUM MACULATUM.

Poison Hemlock.   HAHNEMANN.   *Umbelliferæ.*

¹ **Mind.** Extreme want of memory.
Dulness, difficulty in understanding what he is reading.
Disinclination for business.
Aversion to man, and yet averse to being alone.
Complete indifference.
Hypochondriacal depression and indifference when walking in the open air.
Easily disturbed by trifles, moved to tears.
Morose mood; everything about him impresses him unpleasantly.
Very ill-humored from 5 to 6 P.M.

² **Sensorium.** Vertigo: like turning in a circle, on rising from a seat; worse when lying down, as though the bed were turning in a circle; when turning in bed or when looking around; from motion downwards; when walking ; venous abdominal hyperæmia.

³ **Inner Head.** Headache as if the head were too full and would burst; morning when awakening.
Stitching pain from within outward, in the forehead, mornings, or at noon.
Tearing in the head, must lie down.
Tearing headache, with nausea.
Sensation in right half of brain as of a large foreign body.
Pain in the occiput, with every pulse, as if pierced with a knife.

⁵ **Eyes.** Weakness of sight; also from partial paralysis of
    optic nerve.

Shortsighted.

Objects look red; rainbow-colored; striped, confused spots.

Sluggish adaptation of the eye to varied range of vision.

Weakness and dazzling of the eyes, together with giddi-
    ness and debility, especially of arms and legs; on walk-
    ing, staggering as if drunken.

Aversion to light, without inflammation of the eyes.

Cataract from contusion.

Pupils dilated.

Ulcers on the cornea (right to left); great photophobia, but
    little injection.

Burning of the eyes.

Could scarcely raise the eyelids, they seemed pressed down
    by a heavy weight; disposed to fall asleep.

Burning on inner surface of the lids.

Smarting pain in the inner canthus, with lachrymation.

⁶ **Ears.** Ringing; humming and roaring in the ears.

Painful sensitiveness of hearing, noise startles.

Ears feel as if stopped up, when blowing the nose.

Accumulation of ear-wax, looking like decayed paper,
    mixed with pus or mucus; or blood-red; hard wax, and
    oversensitive to noise.

Stitches in the ears.

Otorrhœa in the scrofulous; inflammation of mastoid cells.

Tumors and boils behind the ears.

Parotid glands swollen and hard.

⁷ **Nose.** Acute sense of smell.

Purulent discharge from the nose; also, hardened crusts.

Epistaxis.

Frequent sneezing.

⁸ **Face.** Earthy, yellow; pale; purple, bloated.

Stinging, tearing faceache, at night.

Moist and spreading herpes, on the face.

⁹ **Lower Face.** ▮ Cancer of the lips, from pressure of the pipe.

Lips and teeth covered with black crusts.

Lips: burning; dry; shooting in the lips.

Blisters, or eruption on the lips.

Submaxillary glands swollen and hard.

¹⁰ **Teeth.** Drawing in a hollow tooth, when eating cold things,
    not from cold drink.

¹¹ **Tongue, etc.** Taste: bitter.

Speech difficult, from lingual paralysis.

Tongue swollen, painful, stiff.

¹³ **Throat.** Pressure in the œsophagus, as if a round body
    (globus hystericus) were ascending from the stomach.

¹⁴ **Desires. Aversions.** Craving coffee, salt, or sour things.

Loss of appetite.

Thirst.

[15] **Eating and Drinking.** Sour rising from the stomach, after eating.

Cold eating: 10. After eating: 17. Cold drink: 10. After drinking: 29.

After taking small quantity of milk, sudden distention or the abdomen.

[16] **Nausea and Vomiting.** Eructations: offensive; frequent, empty; with heart-burn.

Vomiting: violent; of black masses, like coffee-grounds, in clear, sour water; of chocolate-colored masses, sour and acrid.

[17] **Stomach.** Sense of fulness and repletion in the stomach.

Violent pains in the stomach, always two or three hours after eating, but also at night; somewhat better in the knee-elbow position.

Swelling in the region of the pylorus.

Pressing, burning, squeezing pain, extending from the pit of the stomach into the back and shoulders.

Pressure and raw sore feeling at the pit of the stomach.

[18] **Hypochondria.** Stitches in the hepatic region.

Painful tearing in the hepatic region.

Hard swelling of the liver.

[19] **Abdomen.** Swelling of the abdomen.

Stitches extending from abdomen to right side of chest.

Pinching pains in abdomen, as if diarrhœa would set in.

Colic from incarcerated flatus.

Cutting in the abdomen before the emission of flatus.

Very sensitive across the abdomen.

Aching pain in the hypogastric region.

Forcing down feeling in hypogastric region.

[20] **Stool, etc.** Frequent ineffectual urging to stool; or small quantity passed each time.

Stools: undigested, painless; involuntary during sleep; painful, diarrhœic; hard with tenesmus.

Burning in the rectum during stool.

After each stool trembling weakness.

Frequent stitches in the anus.

[21] **Urine.** Pale; white, turbid; with grey or white sediment.

During micturition, flow intermits.

Sharp, lancinating pain in neck of bladder.

Frequent micturition at night.

Immediately after urinating, burning in the urethra, morning.

[22] **Male Sexual Organs.** Sexual desire without erection.

Emissions without dreams: 48.

Discharge of prostatic fluid on every change of emotion, without voluptuous thoughts; with itching of prepuce.

Bad effects from suppressed sexual desire or from excessive indulgence.

[23] **Female Sexual Organs.** Induration and enlargement of the ovary, with lancinating pains.

Stinging in the neck of the uterus.

Induration and prolapsus at the same time.

Fibroids with pricking pains: 48.

Burning, sore, aching sensation in the region of the uterus.

At every menstrual effort breasts become sore and painful.

Pressure from above downwards, and drawing in legs during menses.

Dysmenorrhœa, with shooting pain in left chest.

Menses: suppressed; too late and scanty; preceded by melancholy, followed by acrid leucorrhœa.

Leucorrhœa: thick, milky, with contractive, labor-like colic, coming from both sides; of white, acrid mucus, causing burning.

Before the discharge of leucorrhœa, griping in abdomen.

Indurations of the vulva from injuries.

Severe stitches in the vulva.

Violent itching of the vulva.

Large pimple on the mons veneris, painful to touch.

[24] **Pregnancy.** Terrible nausea and vomiting during pregnancy.

Rigidity of the os uteri during labor.

Cough during pregnancy, worse at night.

❙ Túmors in mammæ, with piercing pains, worse at night, gland abnormally tender.

Hardness of the right mamma, with painfulness to touch, and nightly stitches in it.

Stitches as with needles in the left mamma.

Shriveling of the mammæ, with increased sexual desire.

[25] **Larynx.** Dry spot in the larynx, with almost constant irritation to cough.

Hoarseness.

[26] **Breathing.** Asthmatic paroxysms come on in wet weather; face bluish-red.

[27] **Cough.** Powerful, spasmodic paroxysms, excited by itching and tickling in the chest and throat, or by a dry spot in the larynx, worse at night and when lying down.

Expectoration during the day; difficult; bloody, copious and purulent, sometimes hardened; expectoration, of putrid taste and smell.

Cough: loose, with inability to expectorate; must swallow what is raised; spasmodic, dry, worse evenings and night, very fatiguing.

[28] **Lungs.** Sharp thrusts directly through the chest, from sternum to spine, while sitting.

Violent stitches in right chest about nipple, on every inspiration, while walking, worse from hard pressure with hand.

²⁹ **Heart. Pulse.** Violent palpitation after drinking.

ı Pulse unequal in strength and sometimes irregular in rhythm; insufficiency of the mitral valve.

³⁾ **Outer Chest.** The clothes lie like a weight on the chest and shoulders.

³¹ **Neck. Back.** Stitches in small of back, with drawing through lumbar vertebræ, while standing.

³² **Upper Limbs.** Shoulders feel bruised and sore.

Cracking in the wrist-joint.

Yellow nails.

Itching on the dorsum of the finger.

³³ **Lower Limbs.** Sensation of weakness, even to trembling, in the right thigh, while walking.

Pain in the knee like from fatigue.

Cracking of the knee-joint.

From slight exposure of the feet he catches cold.

Red spots on the calves, turning yellow or green, as from contusion, preventing movement.

³⁴ **Limbs in General.** Trembling.

Difficulty in using the limbs; unable to walk.

All the joints pain as if beaten; unpainful lameness.

³⁵ **Position, etc.** Motion downwards: 2. Walking: 2, 5, 28, 33, 34, 36. Walking in open air: 1. Rising: 2. Standing: 31. Turning in bed: 2. Preventing motion: 33. Inclined to sit: 36. Knee-elbow position: 17. Lying down: 2, 3, 27, 36. Sitting: 28.

³⁶ **Nerves.** Trembling of all the limbs.

Hysteria, advanced cases, thin, wasted, feeble and cold, tendency to syncope.

Sudden loss of strength while walking; inclined to sit down.

Muscular paralysis without spasm.

Exhausted, faint, and as if paralyzed after a short walk.

Sick and faint early in the morning in bed; fainting fits.

³⁷ **Sleep.** Stupid in the morning.

Falls asleep late; after midnight.

Unrefreshing sleep.

Roused from sleep with pain.

Dreams: frightful.

³⁸ **Time.** Morning: 3, 21, 36, 37, 40. Noon: 3. Afternoon: 40. Evening: 1, 27. Night: 8, 17, 21, 24, 27, 37, 40, 47. Day: 27, 47.

³⁹ **Temperature and Weather.** Desire for warmth of sun: 40. Open air: 1. Wet weather: 26.

⁴⁰ **Chill. Fever. Sweat.** Chill and coldness in the morning and afternoon (3 to 5 o'clock).

Chill, with continuous desire for warmth, particularly that of the sun.

Internal chill in morning; with shivering in afternoon.

Great heat, internal and external, with great nervousness.

Heat, with profuse sweat at same time.

Sweat day and night, as soon as one sleeps, or even when closing the eyes; also night and morning, offensive odor and smarting.

[42] **Sides.**   Right: 3, 18, 19, 24, 28, 33. Left: 23, 24. Both sides: 23.   Right to left: 5.   In out: 3.   Above downwards: 23.   Below upwards: 13, 19.   Front backwards: 17, 28.

[44] **Tissues.**   Swelling of the glands, with tingling and stitches; after contuisons and bruises.

Chlorosis, chilliness, excessive faintness, palpitation of heart, pale face, suppressed menses and profuse leucorrhœa.

[45] **Contact, Injuries, etc.**   Touch: 23, 24. Pressure: 9, 28, 30. Contusions: 44, 46.

[46] **Skin.**   Erratic itching on all parts of the boddy.

Tetters: humid, burning, corroding, crusty

Blackish ulcers, with bloody, fetid, ichorous discharges, especially after contusions; spread rapidly.

Petechia, in old persons.

Urticaria from violent bodily exercise.

[47] **Stages and States.**   Old maids.   Old men.

Suited to women with tight, rigid fibre, and easily excited, as well as to those of opposite temperament.

Light haired persons.

Children: marasmus, with frequent sour evacuations, worse during the night, better by day.

[48] **Relationship.**   Antidotes to *Conium: Coffea, Nitr ac. Nitr. spir. dulc.*

Conium antidotes: *Nitr. ac.*

Compare: *Clemat.* (mammæ), *Digit.* (bladder), *Gelsem.* (paralysis), *Secale* (uterine fibroids), *Verbasc.* (emissions without lewd dreams). *Conium* has helped in the dry cough of pulmonary phthisis, when *Hyosc.* and *Drosera* have failed.

CROCUS SATIVUS.

Saffron.   STAPF.   *Iridaceæ.*

[1] **Mind.**   On attempting to write something down, cannot, on account of loss of recollection.

Sings involuntarily, on hearing even a single note sung,

laughs at herself; but soon sings again in spite of her determination to stop.

Changeable disposition: depression and hilarity; or, ill-humor and lively mood, alternating.

Restless, anxious, sorrowful mood.

² **Sensorium.** Vertigo, with confusion.

Congestion of the head, with nosebleed.

³ **Inner Head.** Sudden broad thrust: in the right temple; extending into the brain, causing him to start; above the left frontal eminence, extending deep into the brain.

⁵ **Eyes.** Must wink and wipe the eyes, frequently, as though a film of mucus were over them.

The light seems dimmer than usual, as if obscured by a veil.

Appearance of a spot jumping up and down before sight.

Pupils much dilated.

Feeling as though water were constantly coming in the eyes; only in the room.

Feeling in the eyes, like after much weeping.

Sore burning in the eyes after reading awhile; also dimness, must wink frequently.

Twitching and itching in the upper lid.

Inclined to press lids tightly together from time to time.

⁶ **Ears.** Humming in the ears, causing impairment of hearing, worse when stooping.

⁷ **Nose.** Epistaxis of very tenacious, thick, black blood, with cold sweat in large drops, on the forehead.

Violent sneezing.

⁸ **Face.** Yellowish earthy color of the face.

¹¹ **Tongue, etc.** Tongue coated white, papillæ elevated, better after breakfast.

¹³ **Throat.** Feeling as if the uvula were elongated, during and when not swallowing.

¹⁴ **Desires. Aversions.** Excessive thirst for cold drinks.

¹⁶ **Nausea and Vomiting.** Eructations, tasteless.

Violent heart-burn.

Feeling of nausea in the chest and throat.

¹⁷ **Stomach.** Distension of the stomach and abdomen.

Sensation of fermentation, in the stomach.

Sensation as if something living were jumping about in pit of stomach.

¹⁹ **Abdomen.** Sensation in the abdomen, as if something living were jumping about, with nausea and faintness.

Stitches in the abdomen arresting respiration, with uterine inflammation.

²⁰ **Stool, etc.** Stools contain dark, stringy blood.

Sensitive, dull, long stitch near left side of anus, from time to time.

Crawling in the anus, as from thread-worms.

Intolerable writhing in the anus.

²² **Male Sexual Organs.** Excitement of sexual desire.

²³ **Female Sexual Organs.** Sensation as if the menses would appear, with colic and pressing towards the genitals.

Uterine flow during full or new moon.

Menses profuse and lasting too long, but come at proper time; blood dark, clotted, stringy.

Metrorrhagia of dark, viscid, stringy blood, in black clots, after overheating, straining or lifting, also after abortion or delivery; worse from slightest motion.

²⁴ **Pregnancy.** Lochia dark, stringy.

²⁶ **Breathing.** Offensive sickly odor of the breath.

²⁷ **Cough.** Violent attack of exhausting dry cough, relieved by laying the hand on the pit of stomach.

Cough, with spitting of blood.

²⁸ **Lungs.** Heaviness of the chest, must frequently take a deep breath.

Dull stitches in the left chest.

²⁹ **Heart. Pulse.** Pulse: feverish, accelerated.

Anxious palpitation of the heart.

Palpitation of the heart on going up stairs.

³² **Upper Limbs.** Pain on moving the upper arm, as if the head of the humerus were loose and would easily be dislocated.

Chilblains on the hands and fingers.

³³ **Lower Limbs.** Violent cracking of the hip or knee-joint, when stooping.

Knees give way.

Chilblains on the toes.

Burning and tingling of the feet.

Aching of the soles from standing.

³⁵ **Position, etc.** Motion: 23. Standing: 33. Stooping: 6, 33.

³⁶ **Nerves.** Excessive prostration and weariness in the evening, as from severe physical exertion, accompanied by great sleepiness, with feeling as if the eyelids were swollen; literary occupation relieves.

Jerking in the muscles. Spasmodic contraction of single sets of muscles.

Jumping, dancing, laughing, whistling, wants to kiss everybody.

³⁷ **Sleep.** Sings in sleep.

Dreams: confused; frightful.

³⁸ **Time.** Morning: 11. Afternoon: 40. Evening: 36, 40. Night: 40.

³⁹ **Temperature and Weather.** Room: 5. Overheating: 23.

⁴⁰ **Chill. Fever. Sweat.** Chill in the afternoon, growing worse toward evening, with shivering from the back down the legs; trembling.

25

Thirst, with the chill and heat.

Flushes of internal heat, with prickling and crawling in skin.

Heat, principally of head and face, with paleness of cheeks and thirst.

Heat, with intense redness of face, and distention of blood-vessels.

Violent heat over whole body, chiefly in the head, with redness of the face and great thirst, without much dryness of the mouth; toward evening.

Sweat scant, only at night, and then cold and debilitating.

Sweat only on the lower half of the body.

[41] **Attacks.** New and full moon: 23.

[42] **Sides.** Right: 3. Left: 3, 20, 28..

[43] **Sensations.** Sensation, as of something living, jumping, in various parts.

[45] **Contact, Injuries, etc.** Laying hands on: 27. Pressure: 5. Straining: 23. Lifting: 23.

[46] **Skin.** Prickling and crawling in the skin.

Scarlet-colored spots on the skin.

Scarlet redness of the skin.

Painful suppuration of bruised parts (old cicatrized wounds reopen and suppurate).

[48] **Relationship.** Antidotes to *Croc. sat.: Acon., Bellad., Opium.*

CROTALUS.

[1] **Mind.** Nervous agitation; anxious, pale, with cold sweat.

Excessive sensitiveness; moved to tears by reading.

Irritable, cross, infuriated by least annoyance.

Memory weak; obtuse, stupid, cannot express himself correctly; makes ridiculous mistakes in spelling. Perception diminished.

Mental delusions; awakes struggling with imaginary foes; thinks he is surrounded by enemies or hideous animals.

Delirium, languor, drowsiness, stupor.

Muttering delirium of typhoid. Delirium with wide-open eyes; yellow fever.

Intense restlessness, twitching; delirious with moans.

Delirium tremens, nearly constant drowsiness, but with inability to sleep; also in broken-down constitutions.

Melancholy with timidity, fear; anxiety; weeping; or snappish temper.

Sadness, her thoughts dwell on death continually (*C. Cascarella*).

Marked indifference. See also 46.

[2] **Sensorium.** Vertigo: with faintness, weakness, nervous trembling; with pale face; with falling and loss of consciousness; auditory; cardiac, with soft, weak pulse; anæmic, better resting head; with venous congestion, degraded blood.

Fainting: on assuming an upright position; in attacks; and falling.

Apoplectic convulsions, especially at the onset of some zymotic disease. Apoplexy in homorrhagic or broken-down constituions, or in inebriates.

[3] **Inner Head.** Headache dull, heavy, aching, worse on awaking in the morning; makes mistakes in spelling; accompanied by vertigo, nausea, or malaise.

Dull, heavy, congested feeling in front of brain, worse from intellectual exertion.

Throbbing headache, nausea; before menses.

‖ Severe pain at centre of forehead; dilated pupils; profuse menses.

Neuralgic pains in right eye, on top of head and down back of neck; pressure and heavy pain on top of head.

Dull, heavy pains over the eyes and in sides of nose; nervous depression of spirits.

Headache as if constricted, then sensitiveness of brain, pulsations; with sensitiveness of the heart when lying on the left side.

Dull, heavy, throbbing occipital headache, faint spells; hunger and general trembling: 14.

[4] **Outer Head.** Pustules, boils, carbuncles, slow in their progress, unhealthy or hemorrhagic.

[5] **Eyes.** Vision: dimness when reading; lost, with lethargy and coldness; ptosis; lost, with falling to the ground powerless.

Blood oozes from the eyes; also retinal apoplexy.

‖ Burning in the eyes. Redness with lachrymation.

‖ Pressure and oppression above the eyes.

Neuralgic affection of the eye, as if a cut was made around the eye; sensitive to light.

Sensation of dryness and burning; redness, with a zone around the cornea.

‖ Yellow color of the eyes; also of the whole body.

[6] **Ears.** Hearing: Sensitive to noises. Insensible to noises. Nervous deafness. Meniére's disease: 2.

Blood oozes from the ears.

[7] **Nose.** ‖‖ Epistaxis, especially during diphtheria.

‖ Ozæna of syphilitic origin or following exanthemata; sanguinolent discharge.

Redness or blueness of the point of the nose.

[8] **Face.** Expression: besotted; anxious, pale; of indifference; flushed, excited.

Color: livid, bloated; purple, face tumid; blue around sunken eyes, face chalky; I yellow; flushed; death-like pallor; leaden.

Cold sweat, drawn features, formication, trembling and quivering of lips and eyelids.

Face swollen, puffiness at angles of lower jaw; swelling of parotid and submaxillary glands.

[9] **Lower Face.** Lockjaw. Lips swollen; stiff and numb.

[10] **Teeth.** I Grinds the teeth at night.

Gums swollen, painful, borders reddened; I bleeding; white.

[11] **Tongue, etc.** Tongue red and sore; I yellow; stiff and numb; smooth and red; I swollen and protruded.

Tongue and all around throat feel tied up, he cannot speak.

[12] **Mouth.** Salivation; flow bloody or frothy.

[13] **Throat.** I Dry, with thirst.

Pricking, sensation of constriction in fauces.

Angina tonsillatis; constriction of throat; tongue yellow.

Sudden sore throat as if uvula and velum were swelling, with dry mouth; preceded by palpitation and trembling of heart.

Neuralgic drawing in fauces, worse left side near root of tongue, almost causing choking.

Sensation of swelling of velum, with feeling of mucus in fauces, which must be swallowed or hawked up; or as if uvula hung too low; followed by yawning and headache in one spot to right of vertex.

I Great difficulty in swallowing anything solid.

[14] **Desires. Aversions.** I Insatiable thirst, dry tongue, fever.

I Hungry, trembling, weakness; occipital headache: 2.

[16] **Nausea and Vomiting.** Heart-burn; œsophagus as if full of a rancid fluid.

Eructations sharp, sour; rancid.

Nausea and malaise, anxiety; deathly sickness.

Vomiting: and giddiness; incessant with thirst; of grass-green fetid ejecta; I bilious, with anxiety, palpitation, weak pulse; of blood; I of food, violent.

Ineffectual retching, with feebleness.

[17] **Stomach.** Weight on stomach, tremulous weakness, as from impending evil; soreness, tenderness.

Agonizing pain, restlessness, coldness, weak pulse.

Pylorus constricted; lining of stomach turgid.

I Cannot bear clothes round stomach and below hypochondria.

I Stomach so irritable it can retain nothing.

¹⁸ **Hypochondria.** Tenderness, shooting pains; jaundice; malignant jaundice; also with dark hemorrhages from nose, mouth, etc.; dark, scanty urine.

Stitches in region of liver on drawing a long breath; costive; urine jelly-like and red like blood.

¹⁹ **Abdomen.** Violent pain in the course of the colon.

ı Swelling of the whole abdomen; yellow fever.

Peritonitis, with effusion of bloody serum; especially in septic or zymotic diseases; low temperature.

ı Inguinal glands enlarged; sloughing, unhealthy pus.

Typhlitis; when of low type, red tipped tongue, prostration; no stool, or discharges very offensive.

²⁰ **Stool, etc.** ı Bleeding from the anus and other openings of the body.

Constipation, with congestion to the head and headache.

Vomiting, purging and micturition simultaneously caused by spasmodic contractions, with tenesmus and strangury.

ı Dysenteric discharges of dark, fluid blood; involuntary; great debility and faintness.

Sudden, extreme coldness and blueness; suppressed urine; feeble pulse; liquid, dark discharges (probably useful in cholera).

²¹ **Urine.** ı Albuminuria, in the course of typhoid, diphtheria, etc.; urine smoky, from transuded blood.

ı Urine green-yellow from much bile.

Suppressed or scanty urine.

Urine copious and light colored.

²² **Male Sexual Organs.** Sexual instinct increased with entire relaxation of the penis.

²³ **Female Sexual Organs.** Profuse menses: 3.

ı Dysmenorrhœa; beforehand, pain in hypogastrium and down thighs; flow copious for two days, then lingers on and off for four more; heart weak, feet cold.

Sharp, neuralgic pains, intermittent, from left side of womb to transverse colon, thence cutting across as if from both sides towards centre; thence up to face and temple; with dull frontal headache.

²⁵ **Larynx.** Painful when touched.

Hoarseness, voice weak.

²⁶ **Breathing.** Breathing: anxious; embarrassed, with constriction of throat; jerking; quick, labored, with weak pulse and nervous agitation; slow, labored, imperceptible pulse; difficult as if lungs would not expand.

²⁷ **Cough.** From tickling in throat, suprasternal fossa or trachea; worse from external pressure and on awaking.

Cough with stitch in the left side and bloody expectoration from the lungs.

ı Whooping-cough, debility, face blue or pale, remaining so for a time after paroxysm; epistaxis, puffed face;

frothy, stringy sputum; threatened pulmonary oedema
or paralysis.

| Moderate cough, with expectoration of bloody mucus.

²⁸ **Lungs.** | Oppression in old people, with hydrothorax; in
fever and ague.

Stitch pains in the chest; pleurisy with fever of a remittent type.

²⁹ **Heart. Pulse.** Heart: beats rapidly, but feebly, sometimes
with no pulse at wrist; worse on any exertion, when
breathing becomes affected.

| Palpitation as if heart tumbled about; feeling of trembling of the heart.

Heart tender when lying on left side.

Pulse: frequent, but soon weak; fluttering, trembling;
quick, thready; intermittent, irregular.

³¹ **Neck. Back.** Softening of the spinal cord.

Drawing, tensive pain from right shoulder along neck, as
from a tense tendon, worse from pressure and from
moving arm.

³² **Upper Limbs.** Left axillary glands swollen and tender.

Paroxysms of bruised pains in bones of shoulder.

| Hands "go to sleep," more the left, worse from exertion.

Violent, spasmodic pain in left palm as from a bee-sting.

Oozing of blood from under the nails.

³³ **Lower Limbs.** Legs "go to sleep" and tingle while sitting
or when crossing them.

Drawing suddenly from left hip to foot.

During and after walking feels as if a tendon was drawing
from sole of right foot through bone of leg.

Cramp-like pains in calf, heels, toes.

Sore pain in calf; in sole of foot.

Swelling of the feet every evening.

³⁴ **Limbs in General.** Bruised pain in joints and bones.

Heaviness, as if bones were made of heavy wood.

Numb pain as after cramp, in anterior of fingers and in
toes.

Drawing pains in knee, tibia, back, etc.

Throbbing pains in finger-tips, etc.

³⁵ **Position, etc.** Resting: 2. Walking: 33. Motion: 31.
Sitting: 33. Exertion: 29, 32, 36. Upright: 2. Lying:
3, 29.

³⁶ **Nerves.** Convulsions, trembling of limbs; foaming at the
mouth; violent cries, delirium.

Contraction of flexors.

Great loss of power: | easily tired by slight exertion; | muscles refuse their service; paralysis of one side.

| Tremulous weakness, as from impending evil.

³⁷ **Sleep.** | Sleepless from disproportionate nervous agitation.

Starts in sleep.

    ı Drowsy, but cannot sleep.

    ı Torpor, drowsiness, coma.

    ı Symptoms generally worse after sleep.

    Dreams: of traveling; of quarrels; **ı** of the dead (*C. Cas-carella*).

[38] **Time.** Night: 10. Evening: 33. Morning: 1, 3.

[40] **Chill. Fever. Sweat.** Surface cold, especially extremities. Flushes of heat all over.

    Fever: **ıı** dry skin, dark brown, dry tongue; or, tongue coated yellow with red edges and tip; delirium, low muttering: drowsiness; urine dark, scanty; costive, or fetid, bilious or bloody stools; **ıı** hemorrhagic tendency, oozing of blood from every orifice and even from the pores; skin yellow; vomiting of bile or blood; liver tender; heart weak, fainting, hence in typhoid, bilious remittent, yellow fever, pyæmia, etc.

    ı Malignant scarlatina.

    Sweat cold; sudden attacks of cold sweat.

[41] **Attacks.** Marked periodicity; pains come and go suddenly or re-appear every three months, every year, etc.

[42] **Sides.** Is said to act more on the right side.

[44] **Tissues.** *Crotal.* affects the nerves and the blood; causing dizziness, confusion or deep coma; trembling, tetanic spasms, paralysis; congestion of the various tissues, inflammations of a low type, ecchymoses and effusions into brain, lungs, heart, etc., and into serous cavities; hemorrhages dark, fluid; gangrene, sloughing. It is, therefore, indicated in diseases of an adynamic character, whether caused by previous low states of the system, or by zymotic and septic poisoning, abuse of alcohol, etc. Especially characteristic are evidences of cardiac debility: feeble pulse, sluggish circulation, bluish skin, faintness, general debility.

    Œdema of the whole body. General anasarca.

    Bruised, drawing, or paralytic pains in the bones, worse awaking.

[45] **Contact, Injuries, etc.** **ı** Worse from touch: 17, 18, 29, 33. Pressure: 31.

    ı Stings of insects; **ı** dissecting wounds; ailments from vaccination.

[46] **Skin.** Itching, stinging, all over. Urticaria. Stings of insects.

    • Skin dry, stiff, like thin parchment. Usually dry and cold.

    ı Chilblains, gangrene pending; circulation sluggish.

    ı Skin yellow; jaundice, septicæmia, etc.

    Ecchymoses, purpura hemorrhagica; petechiæ.

    Erysipelas, phlegmonous, phlyctenous or œdematous; skin

bluish-red, low fever; during zymoses or in the enfeebled; also in wounds; more frequent in the face.

Felons, pemphigus, pustules, boils, gangrene, abscesses, etc., when the fever is low, the parts bluish and the discharges scanty, tardy, or dark, fluid, unhealthy; diarrhœa with the gangrene.

Old cicatrices break open again.

Hot swellings, with cold skin and sickly appearance.

Obstinate ulcers, even malignant, with yellow complexion and great indifference.

[48] **Relationship.** Very similar are *Laches.*, *Naja* and *Elaps.;* distinctions, therefore, are mainly relative. *Crotal.* is preferable in fluid hemorrhages, yellow skin (hence in yellow fever with black vomit, etc.), epistaxis of diphtheria. *Naja* has more nervous phenomena. *Laches.* has skin cold and clammy, rather than cold and dry; hemorrhages with charred straw sediment; and more markedly, ailments of the left side. *Elaps* is preferable in otorrhœa, and in affections of the right lung. The Cobra-poison coagulates blood into long strings.

The *Crotal.* poison is acid; the *Viper* neutral. The "Rotten-Snake" causes more sloughing than any other.

Compare also: *Tarent. cub.*, *Arsen.*, *Lauroc.* (tetanus, whooping-coug), *Apis*, *Carb. veg.*, *Silic.* (vaccination), *Camphor.* (in coldness; probably *Crotal.* has more maked genuine collapse, with confused speech, etc.).

Effects modified by: *Ammon.*, *Camphor.*, *Opium*, *Coffea*, *Alcohol*, radiated heat.

CROTON TIGLIUM.

Croton oïl seeds.   HENCKE.   *Euphorbiaceæ.*

[1] **Mind.** Not disposed to work.

Feeling of anxiety, as though some personal misfortune would befall him.

Morose, dissatisfied.

[2] **Sensorium.** Dulness, or heaviness of the head.

Dizziness and faintness, with exhaustion and diarrhœa.

[3] **Inner Head.** Sensitiveness of the head; the weight of the hat causes headache.

[5] **Eyes.** Opacity of the cornea.

Copious lachrymation.

Keratitis pustulosa; with much eruption on the lids and face; with excessive photophobia.

Conjunctivitis pustulosa, eyes feel hot and burning, espe-cially at night; face red and burning; feverish.

6 Ears. Spasmodic, twinging pains, deep within the left ear.

9 Lower Face. Lips dry and parched. θ Cholera infantum.

15 Eating and Drinking. Eating: 20. Drinking: 20. Hot milk: 19.

17 Stomach. Sensation of emptiness in the stomach.

Sinking in the stomach, with sensation of weakness.

19 Abdomen. Abdomen full and distended, with griping pain about the navel.

Unpleasant sensation of emptiness and hunger; rumbling in the abdomen.

Gurgling in the intestines, as though only water were in them, mostly on left side.

Griping about the umbilicus.

Colic better from hot milk.

Swashing in the intestines as from water.

20 Stool, etc. Flatulence, soon followed by urgent desire for stool.

Evacuation sudden, with much flatus.

Stools: yellow water; light brown, covered with mucus, with frequent urging; dark green, or greenish-yellow, liquid; tenacious mucus; watery, mixed with whitish flakes; coming out like a shot.

Diarrhœa worse after drinking; while nursing; while eating; during summer.

Upon pressure at the umbilicus, a painful sensation is felt down to anus, where there is constant pressure outwards.

Dragging in the anus, as if diarrhœa would easily ensue.

Burning in the anus.

Pain in the anus, as if a plug were forcing outwards.

22 Male Sexual Organs. Frequent corrosive itching on the glans and scrotum.

Scrotum shriveled, itching severely, disturbing sleep; bet-ter from scratching, which, however, caused a voluptu-ous sensation.

Corrosive, itching pain on the scrotum, worse while walk-ing; redness of the part. ∎ Eczema scroti worse at night.

Vesicular eruption on the scrotum and penis.

23 Female Sexual Organs. Intense itching of the genitals, re-lieved by very gentle scratching.

24 Pregnancy. etc. Breasts hard and swollen, with pain from nipple to scapula.

Nipple very sore to touch, excruciating pain running from nipple through to scapula of same side, when the child nurses.

26 Breathing. Feels as though he could not expand the lungs.

28 Lungs. Feeling of fulness in both sides of the chest, with burning stitches in left side of thorax and toward both scapulæ.

[35] **Position, etc.**   Walking: 22, 46.

[36] **Nerves.**   Very great debility.

[38] **Time.**   Night: 5.

[39] **Temperature and Weather.**   Summer: 20.

[40] **Chill.   Fever.   Sweat.**   Coldness of the feet, extending as far up as the calves.

[42] **Sides.**   Left: 6, 19, 28, 46.   Before backwards: 54.

[45] **Contact, Injuries, etc.**   Touch: 24, 46.   Pressure: 3, 20. Scratching: 22, 23.

[46] **Skin.**   Red moist spot, exuding an offensive moisture, on left thigh opposite scrotum; it is painfully sore to touch and on walking; troublesome smarting when walking.

Itching and painful burning, with redness of the skin; formation of vesicles and pustules; desiccation of the pustules; desquamation, and falling of the pustules.

Itching pustules. ❙ Itching attending eczema.

[48] **Relationship.**   *Crot. tig.* antidotes *Rhus tox.* poisoning.

CUPRUM METALLICUM.

Metallic Copper.   HAHNEMANN.   *Cu.*

[1] **Mind.**   Saying words not intended, forerunner of apoplexy. Full of erroneous, anxious ideas, one following the other quickly; thinks he is a great military commander.

Weeps often.

Mania: with biting and beating; tearing things to pieces; with anxiety.

Delirium: afraid of every one who approaches him, shrinking from them; tries to escape.

Unconquerable sadness, constant restlessness, as if some misfortune were approaching; fears he will lose his reason.

Paroxysms of anxiety; full of fears.

Changeable mood; children cross and irritable, or indifferent and dull, in brain affections.

❙ Senses less acute. θ Cholera.

❙ Acuteness of senses; oversensitive. θ Whooping-cough.

Restless tossing about.

Mental and bodily exhaustion, from over-exertion of mind or loss of sleep.

[2] **Sensorium.**   Vertigo: with weariness, the head has a tendency to sink forward; worse from motion, better lying down.

³ **Inner Head.** Pain in the head, as if hollow.

Strange tingling pain in the vertex; menses omitting.

Violent continuous headache, increased periodically.

Violent dull headache over the glabella.

Stitches in the temples, with redness of the eyes.

Congestion to brain, with convulsive motions of extremities.

Affections of the brain, in children with catarrhal fever, difficult dentition, or exanthematic diseases.

Exacerbation in brain affections, evenings.

Headache after epileptic attacks.

⁴ **Outer Head.** Tossing about of the head.

❙ Children cannot hold the head up. θ Brain affections.

⁵ **Eyes.** Sight obscured.

Eyes: dim; lustreless; sunken, with blue rings around.

Great itching in the eyes toward evening.

Pressing pain in the eyes.

Bruised pain in the orbits when moving the eyes.

Eyes red, inflamed.

Eyeballs red, move like a pendulum from side to side.

Quick rotation of the balls, with lids closed.

⁶ **Ears.** Difficult hearing.

Boring in and behind ears, pressing pain in front of ears.

Swelling of the meatus externus.

⁷ **Nose.** Sensation of great congestion of blood to the nose.

Nosebleed: on right side only.

Copious fluent coryza.

Stoppage of the nose.

⁸ **Face.** Expression: sad, depressed; of suffering; prostration.

Face: very red, eyelids closed and balls constantly rotating; blue; pale; greyish, dirty; sunken features, pinched; icy-cold.

⁹ **Lower Face.** Mouth firmly closed.

Lips blue.

Froth from the mouth.

¹⁰ **Teeth.** Rending pain from teeth to temples.

Gums ulcerated.

¹¹ **Tongue, etc.** Taste: sweet or sweetish metallic; coppery.

Tongue: red; dry and rough, papillæ enlarged; coated white, yellowish or brown.

Chronic glossitis.

¹²**Mouth.** Frothy saliva, with cough.

Dry mouth. θ In brain affections.

Induration of the salivary gland, with or without fistula.

¹³ **Throat.** Palate red, fauces inflamed.

Tonsils inflamed.

Dull, piercing pain in left tonsil, increased by external touch.

Gurgling noise of the drink passing down the œsophagus.

¹⁴ **Desires. Aversions.** Loss of appetite, great thirst for cooling drink.

¹⁵ **Eating and Drinking.** A swallow of cold water relieves the cough, or vomiting.

Milk brings on water-brash.

¹⁶ **Nausea and Vomiting.** Hiccough: precedes vomiting: begins attack of asthma.

Constant eructations.

Nausea and vomiting after taking cold.

Nausea, vomiting and cramps during catamenia.

Frequent nausea and fearful vomiting, catamenia omitting.

Nausea, vomiting and torpid stool, with brain affections.

Vomiting: in gushes of whey-like fluid; frothy mucus; bilious; bloody.

¹⁷ **Stomach.** Deathly feeling, with pain behind ensiform cartilage.

Pressure in pit of stomach.

Pressure at the stomach, with nausea.

Eructations, rumbling in stomach.

Sensation as of a round ball going to and fro under ribs, with different sounds, worse from fluid food; better from tight clothing or bandage around abdomen, and when lying quiet.

Burning in epigastric region, which is sore to touch.

Sensation as though something bitter were in the stomach.

Sensation as though the clothing were lying too hard on pit of stomach.

¹⁸ **Hypochondria.** Drawing pain from left hypochondrium to hip.

¹⁹ **Abdomen.** Cramps in the abdomen.

Violent colicy, cutting, drawing pains in abdomen; abdomen drawn in; colic not increased by pressure.

Violent spasms in abdomen and upper and lower limbs, with penetrating, distressing screams.

Intussusception of the bowels, with singultus, violent colic, stercoraceous vomiting and great agony.

Big belly, of children.

Inguinal gland swollen.

Spasmodic movements of the abdominal muscles.

²⁰ **Stool, etc.** Constipation, alternating with diarrhœa.

Diarrhœa: profuse, squirting out; much wind passing.

Stools: grey, with flocculent matter in cholera, also masses of whey-like fluid.

Summer complaints of children, with brain affections.

Thread-worms. Round worms.

²¹ **Urine.** Must urinate during the night.

Scantiness or entire suppression of urine.

Urine: acid; straw-colored, after standing turbid, and a reddish. thin sediment adheres to the vessel.

²² **Male Sexual Organs.** Gonorrhœa, with a changeable dis-
charge, now more, again less; orifice of urethra sticking together.

²³ **Female Sexual Organs.** Menses not appearing after the
suppression of foot-sweat.

Before menses spasmodic dyspnœa.

Before or during menses, or after suppression, violent,
unbearable cramps in abdomen, extending up into
chest; causing nausea, vomiting, and sometimes convulsion of limbs and piercing shrieks.

Vaginismus.

²⁴ **Pregnancy.** Spasms during parturition, with violent vomit-
ing; or, with every paroxysm, opisthotonos, spreading
out the limbs and opening the mouth.

Clonic spasms during pregnancy, when attack commences
in one part, as in fingers, or a limb, and gradually
spreads.

ı Most distressing after-pains, particularly of women who
have borne many children.

Cramping after-pains, which often produce cramp in the
extremities.

After confinement, rash and convulsions.

Swelling and induration of the mammæ.

²⁵ **Larynx.** Hoarseness as soon as he breathes dry cold air.

Talking is difficult, voice powerless.

Contraction of the larynx with the cough.

²⁶ **Breathing.** Breathing: whistling; quick rattling; short,
panting; seems to be interupted, in the throat.

Dyspnæa; short, superficial, quick respirations, aggravated by coughing, laughing, bending upper part of
body backwards, walking quickly, or inhaling acrid
vapors.

Violent asthmatic attacks come on suddenly, lasting from
one to three hours, and cease suddenly.

Beginning paralysis of the lungs: indicated by sudden
difficulty of breathing, followed by great prostration.

²⁷ **Cough.** Cough: dry; dry, suffocative, worse nights; even-
ing dry, morning slight expectoration of phlegm, with
dark blood of putrid taste and smell; uninterrupted,
cannot speak a word, discharge of bloody mucus from
the nose; after sea wind; worse inhaling cold air;
taking deep breath; laughing; after eating solid food;
when bending backwards; better by drinking cold water;
with whooping, children get stiff, breathing ceases, spasmodic twitchings, after awhile consciousness returns,
they vomit and recover, but slowly.

²⁸ **Lungs.** Shooting pains in sides of chest, must cry out.

²⁹ **Heart. Pulse.** Anxious feeling about the heart.

Stitches below the heart. Boring pain in region of heart.
Palpitation of the heart.
Fatty degeneration, slow pulse, feeble cardiac action; even
angina.
Pulse: very changeable; thready, tense; small, hard and
moderately frequent.

[31] **Neck. Back.** Glands of the neck indurated.
Paralysis of all muscles of back up to neck; also of limbs;
lower limbs œdematous, but retain their sensibility.

[32] **Upper Limbs.** Anchylosis of the shoulder-joint.
Numbness and lameness of arms.
Twitching in the hands and fingers.
Stitching, rending or drawing pains.
Stiffened and inflamed hands and fingers.
In the bend of the elbow, tetter, with yellow scabs; itch-
ing violently, particularly in the evening.
Little vesicles on tips of fingers, oozing watery fluid.

[33] **Lower Limbs.** Paralysis of lower limbs from psoas abscess.
Twitching in the lower limbs; drawing them backwards.
Lameness of lower limbs, with contraction of the muscles.
Great weakness of the legs, the knees give way.
Spasms and cramps in the calves.
Drawing and digging pain in the calf.
Burning in the soles.
Suppressed foot-sweat.
Icy-coldness of the feet.

[34] **Limb in General.** Cramps in the limbs.
Weariness of the limbs.
Contraction of the joints.
Limbs cyanotic.

[35] **Position, etc.** Tossing about: 1, 4. Head tends to sink for-
ward: 2. Motion: 2. Moving eyes: 5. Walking: 26.
Lying: 2. Lying quiet: 17. Cannot hold head up: 4.
Bending body backward: 26, 27. Body bent forward: 36.

[36] **Nerves.** Weariness of long duration.
Great weakness of the muscles.
Great prostration with nervous excitability, constant rest-
lessness driving out of bed.
Nervous trembling, with very great acuteness and sensi-
tiveness of the senses.
Twitching, jerkings or startings during sleep.
Stiffness of the whole body; body bent forward.
Contraction of muscles and tendons.
Clonic spasms: accompanying brain affections; beginning
in the fingers or toes.
[1] Epileptic convulsions: trembling, tottering and falling
unconscious, without a scream; preceded by drawing
in left arm; aura epileptica; with froth at the mouth,

opisthotonos, limbs abducted; followed by headache; during sleep at night; each new moon; after spasms, turns and twists until another comes.

❙ Eclampsia of children, during dentition.

❙ Child lies on belly and spasmodically thrusts breech up.

[37] **Sleep.**   Sleep heavy, even to comatose state.

Sleepy, without being able to sleep.

Sleep full of dreams.

[38] **Time.**   Morning: 27. Evening: 3, 5, 27, 32. Night: 21, 27, 36, 40.

[39] **Temperature and Weather.**   Dry cold air: 25, 27.

[40] **Chill. Fever. Sweat.**   Feverish sensation, as if a cold wind were blowing out from the skin.

Chill over the whole body, most severe on the extremities.

Chill after every attack of indisposition.

Icy coldness of the whole body.

Skin: moist and cool, particularly extremities; dry, burning hot; warm, dry and withered.

Burning in the soles.

Flushes of heat.

Debilitating, exhausting internal heat.

Cold sweat at night.

Many attacks end in sweat.

Foot-sweat, also suppressed foot-sweat.

[41] **Attacks.**   Periodically: 3.   Coming suddenly, ceasing suddenly: 26.   New moon: 36.

[42] **Sides.**   Right: 7.   Left: 13, 19, 29, 35.   Below upward: 10, 23, 31.   Above downward: 13, 18.

[44] **Tissues.**   Pain in the bones, as if they would break.

Promotes suppuration in swellings.

Inflammation of the cellular tissues.

Caries.

[45] **Contact, Injuries, etc.**   Touch: 13, 17.   Pressure: 19. Tight clothing or bandage: 17.

[46] **Skin.**   Skin: inelastic; dough-like.

Unbearable itching, without eruption.

Measle eruption develops, and day cough ameliorated.

Repercussion of eruption, with convulsions, vomiting or gagging; pale face and twitching of limbs.

Tetters: spreading, oozing; in the bend of the elbow.

Old ulcers.

[48] **Relationship.**   Antidotes to *Cuprum:* sugar or white of egg against massive doses.

Hepar s. c., or potash soap, after poisoning from food containing copper.

If *Cuprum* aggravates, smelling of alcoholic solution of Camphor relieves.

Dynamic antidotes: *Bellad., Cinchon., Conium, Dulcam., Hepar, Ipec., Mercur., Nux vom.*

Veratr. follows well after *Cuprum* in whoo ;ing-cough.

Cuprum is complementary to *Calc. ostr.* in the same forms of disease.

Cuprum ars. ❙ excellent in severe burning, cramping pains within the abdomen (many cases).

CYCLAMEN EUROPÆUM.

Sow-bread.   HAHNEMANN.   *Primulaceæ.*

[1] **Mind.** Dulness of head.

Confusion of head.

Absorbed in deep thought, seeks solitude, thinks about his future.

Melancholy; inclined to cry.

Joyous feeling, alternating with irritability.

Great sadness, as if he had committed a bad act or not done his duty.

Peevish, irritable or morose.

[2] **Sensorium.** Feels as if the brain was in motion when leaning against something.

Vertigo: objects turn in a circle, or about her, or make a see-saw motion; when walking in open air; better in a room and when sitting.

Dizzy, fulness and heat of head.

Dulness of all the senses.

[3] **Inner Head.** Slight pressure in vertex, as if brain was enveloped in a cloth, which would deprive him of his senses.

Violent frontal headache; semi-lateral headache (left).

Stitching, darting or boring pains in temples.

Headache worse in evening or in morning when rising.

Headache relieved by cold water applications.

Congestion of blood to the head.

Increased warmth of head.

[4] **Outer Head.** Tearing, pressing pain externally.

Fine sharp formicating-stinging on scalp, changing place when scratching; worse evenings, at rest; better walking about.

Papulous eruption on scalp.

Head feels bound.

[5] **Eyes.** Now yellow and again green before the eyes.

Fiery specks and sparks before the eyes.

Sight: as if looking through dark blue glass; like mist before the eyes; ❙ dim vision with the headache.

Halo around the light.

Dimness of sight, with fiery sparks before the eyes.

Diplopia. Strabismus.

Dilated pupils; or contracted and dilated alternately.

Eyes sunken and have a weary look.

Left eye drawn toward the inner canthus.

Swelling of upper eyelids.

Dryness and pressure in the lids, as if swollen, with violent formicating stitches therein, and in the eyeball.

Heat in the eyes.

6 Ears. Roaring; humming; or ringing in the ears.

Dulness of hearing, as if cotton was in the ear or something lying before the (right) ear. '

Drawing pain in right internal ear; hearing impaired.

Itching of ears, with increase of cerumen.

7 Nose. Sense of smell diminished.

Frequent sneezing, with itching in the ear.

Dryness of nose.

Fluent coryza (morning).

Pressing pain over the nasal bones.

8 Face. Pale face; rings around eyes; anæmic women.

Pimples soon filling with whiteish-yellow lymph and then shriveling.

Drawing together of forehead.

9 Lower Face. Itching on lower jaw.

Sensation of numbness of upper lip or as of an induration therein.

Dry lips, without thirst.

10 Teeth. Tearing; stitching; boring, in teeth (more right).

11 Tongue, etc. Taste: flat; offensive; putrid; fatty.

Food tastes flat, or is almost tasteless.

Tip of tongue red, with small burning blister thereon, impeding speech and chewing; saliva increased; tongue coated yellowish-white.

Fine stitches on the tongue.

12 Mouth. Saliva increased.

Viscid muscus in mouth.

Heightened redness of mouth.

13 Throat. Dryness of palate, evenings, with thirst and hunger.

14 Desires. Aversions. Little hunger or appetite.

No desire for breakfast or supper; entire loss of appetite.

ı After eating but little, aversion to food, with nausea in throat.

Aversion to bread with butter, to fat.

Thirst during the night, intermittent.

Thirstlessness.

15 Eating and Drinking. After eating: sleepiness; hiccough, rumbling in bowels; digestion weakened.

16 Nausea and Vomiting. Violent hiccough.

26

Eructations: tasting sour; of the food; of a fatty taste.

Nausea after eating or drinking; except from lemonade.

Nausea after fat food.

Nausea and fulness in the chest, with unusual hunger.

Vomiting: of watery mucus; of food; of greenish fluid.

[17] **Stomach.** Stitches in the stomach.

Fulness and pressure in pit of stomach, as after eating too much.

[18] **Hypochondria.** Stitches in region of liver.

Ball-like distention in bowels, on right side below the liver.

[19] **Abdomen.** Full feeling in abdomen.

Distention of abdomen.

Intestines painful to touch.

Stitches in umbilical region; stitches, or pinching in abdomen.

Cramp-like pains.

Running and crawling in bowels, as of something alive.

In left inguinal canal: stitches; itching.

[20] **Stool, etc.** Pressure in rectum or anus.

Heat in rectum, with swelling of the hemorrhoidal veins.

Urging to stool; tenesmus.

Stool; odorless, brownish-yellow, mixed with some mucus.

Watery diarrhœa.

Frequent passage of hard stool.

Drawing, pressive pain in and about the anus and perineum, as if a spot was suppurating; when walking or sitting.

Hemorrhoidal flow.

[21] **Urine.** Urine profuse, watery and frequent.

Frequent urging, with scanty discharge; also seldom and scanty.

Urine dark red, containing much flocculent matter.

[22] **Male Sexual Organs.** Erections at night, without exciting dreams.

Stitches in urethra.

Phimosis.

Prepuce and corona glandis feel sore, from slight rubbing.

[23] **Female Sexual Organs.** Menses profuse and frequent.

Menorrhagia, with stupefaction of head and vision abscured, as from a fog. Flow clotted, black; membranous.

Flow less when moving about; worse in the evening when sitting.

Menses suppressed or scanty, and painful; dread of fresh air.

After menses, swelling of mammæ, with secretion like milk.

[24] **Pregnancy.** ▮Loathing and nausea in mouth and throat.

[25] **Larynx.** Voice weak when reading aloud.

[26] **Breathing.** Oppression of chest, with impeded breathing.
Breathing accelerated.

[27] **Cough.** Suffocative cough, caused by scraping and dryness
in trachea.

[28] **Lungs.** Pressure in the middle of sternum.
Stitches in left side of chest, later in right side.
Stitch about the apex of heart.
Tearing stitches, with oppression and shortness of breath,
during motion and rest.

[29] **Heart. Pulse.** Buzzing in region of heart.
Sensation as of something alive, running in the heart.
Stitches about the apex of heart.
Palpitation.
Pulse: double beat, very rapid; scarcely perceptible.

[30] **Outer Chest.** Pressure in middle of sternum.
Contractive sensation of chest.
Sensation as if air streamed from the nipples.
Mammæ swollen, tension and stitches therein; hard and
painful discharge of milky fluid.

[31] **Neck. Back.** Stiffness of neck, with laming pain.
Drawing rheumatic pain in left side of neck.
Twinges up the back relieved by drawing the shoulders
backwards, aggravated by the reverse.
Deep penetrating dull stitches in region of right kidney,
worse during inhalation.

[32] **Upper Limbs.** Tearing, terminating in a stitch, over the
scapulæ, with laming pain in the arms.
Itching on the shoulder and in the axilla.
Laming, hard pressure in right arm, as if in the perios-
teum and deep-seated muscles; extending to fingers,
impedes writing.
Bruised pain in the elbow-joint, outside; worse from mo-
tion of arm and touch.
Tearing pain in elbow and wrist-joints.
Feels as if she must let fall that which is in the hands.
Cramp-like slow contraction of right thumb and index
finger, the tips approach each other and can only be
extended by force.
Fine prickling between the fingers, ceasing after scratching.
Red blisters, preceded by severe itching on ring and little
fingers, left hand.
Distention of veins on dorsum of hand.

[33] **Lower Limbs.** Rheumatic drawing in left gluteus maxi-
mus near the spine, while sitting; ceases when standing.
Cramp-like pain on right thigh above the popliteal space.
Drawing pain in flexors of leg, seeming to start from hol-
low of knee and draw to tip of the toes.
Itching on right calf, with swelling of blood-vessels.

Pain in the bottom of foot, as if sprained, more at heel.

Burning, sore pain in the heels, when walking in open air; also when standing or sitting.

After walking, toes feel dead.

[34] **Limbs in General.** Limbs feel as if their mobility were impaired.

[35] **Position, etc.** Rest: 4, 28, 44. Motion: 32, 36. Walking: 2, 4, 20, 23, 28, 34, 44. Rising: 3. Standing: 33. Sitting: 2, 20, 23, 33. Bending shoulders back: 31.

[36] **Nerves.** Great lassitude of body, particularly of knees, though spirits may be good.

Enervation of whole body, burdensome to move even a limb.

[37] **Sleep.** Frequent yawning.

Great inclination to slumber, mornings.

Restless sleep, dreams of money.

Nightmare soon after falling asleep.

Sleep disturbed, and toward morning full of dreams; also a pollution.

Goes to sleep late, awakes early, so weary at usual hour for rising cannot get up.

Early awakening, yet so tired and sleepy, cannot arise.

Dreams: lascivious; frightening; vivid.

[38] **Time.** Morning: 3, 7, 37. Forenoon: 40. Evening: 3, 4, 13, 23, 45. Night: 14, 22, 40.

[39] **Temperature and Weather.** Room: 2. Uncovering: 40. Open air: 2, 23, 33. Cold air: 40. Cold water: 3.

[40] **Chill. Fever. Sweat.** Chill forenoon or evening.

With evening chill, great sensitiveness to cold air and uncovering. Chill predominates.

Heat principally of face, but without thirst, succeeds the chill; the hands continue cold a long time.

Sensation of heat through the whole body, particularly in the face and on the hands.

Heat of various parts, but not of the face.

General heat after eating.

Sweat at night during sleep, moderate, of offensive odor.

[42] **Sides.** Right: 6, 10, 18, 31, 32, 33. Left: 5, 19, 28, 29, 31, 32, 33. Left to right: 28. Below upwards: 31. Above downwards: 32, 33.

[44] **Tissues.** Pressive, drawing or tearing pains at parts where bones lie near surface; worse while walking than when at rest.

[45] **Contact, Injuries, etc.** Touch: 19, 32. Rubbing: 22. Scratching: 32.

[46] **Skin.** Itching, leaving a numb sensation.

Papulous eruption.

Bright red spots like burns, on the thighs.

[48] **Relationship.** Antidotes to *Cyclam.: Camph., Coffea, Pulsat.*

DIGITALIS PURPUREA.

Foxglove.   HAHNEMANN   *Scrophulariaceæ.*

[1] **Mind.** Dulness of head as from inebriation, with increased mental activity.

Overworked mind, pulse being weak.

Lascivious fancies day and night.

Tearfulness, low-spirited.

Internal anxiety, like from troubled conscience.

Anxiety, with great fear for the future, worse at 6 P. M.

[2] **Sensorium.** Vertigo: when walking or riding; with trembling; with very slow pulse.

[3] **Inner Head.** Pressure in forehead when exerting mind or thinking of it.

Bores head in the pillow, pulls the hair; shrill cry; vomits easily: urine scanty; cyanotic.

[5] **Eyes.** Diplopia.

Objects appear either green, yellow, or as if silvered.

Chronic inflammation of the conjunctiva.

Yellowish redness of the conjunctiva palpebrarum.

Pupils not very active.

Inflammation of the meibomian glands.

Swelling of the lower lid.

Lachrymation, worse in bright light or cold air.

Agglutination of the lids in the morning.

Both eyes turn to the left.

[6] **Ears.** Sudden crashing noise in the head, on falling asleep; awaking with a frightened start.

Noise before the ears like boiling water.

[8] **Face.** Bluish-red; pale; of death-like appearance.

[11] **Tongue, etc.** Taste: flat, slimy; sweetish, with constant ptyalism.

Talking: 27, 28.

Tongue coated white.

[14] **Desires. Aversions.** No appetite, tongue clean, stomach empty.

[15] **Eating and Drinking.** Eating: 27. Drinking cold things: 27.

[16] **Nausea and Vomiting.** Nausea, as if she would die.

Constant nausea and gagging, with clean tongue, covered with white slime.

Inclination to vomit.

Persistent nausea and vomiting; nausea even after the vomiting.

Vomiting in the morning: of food; of bile.

[17] **Stomach.** Burning in stomach, extending up the œsophagus.

Weakness (sinking) at stomach, feels as if he were dying.

Soreness and bloatedness of the pit of stomach.

¹⁸ **Hypochondria.** Soreness and hardness in region of liver. Jaundice and easy vomiting; pulse slow.

¹⁹ **Abdomen.** Cutting in the abdomen.

²⁰ **Stool, etc.** Frequent desire to evacuate bowels, accompanying urging to urinate; very small, soft stools without relief.

Stools: violent diarrhœa, ash-colored, or very light; delayed, chalky.

Stool in evening, passing great quantities of thread-worms.

²¹ **Urine.** Fruitless effort to urinate.

Constant urging to urinate, with scanty discharge each time.

Feeling of fulness, continuing after urination.

Increased desire to urinate after a few drops have passed, causing patient to walk about in distress, although motion increases the desire.

Constriction and burning as if the urethra was too small; enlarged prostate.

Urine: scanty, thick, turbid, blackish.

Brick-dust sediment in the urine.

Throbbing pain in region of neck of bladder, during straining effort to pass water.

²² **Male Sexual Organs.** Nightly emissions, with great weakness of the genitals; with sadness and despair (Digitaline); after emission sensation of something running out of urethra.

Balanitis, phimosis, with great burning on urinating; dropsy of the prepuce.

Testicle swollen.

Hydrocele.

²³ **Female Sexual Organs.** Labor-like pains in abdomen and back, before the menses.

Leucorrhœa.

²⁵ **Larynx.** Choking when trying to swallow. θ Spasm of the glottis.

Hoarseness early in the morning.

²⁶ **Breathing.** Respiration slow, asthmatic, paroxysm early in the morning, especially in cold weather.

Distressing nausea at the pit of stomach with orthopnœa.

Painful asthma, worse when walking.

²⁷ **Cough.** Hollow, deep, spasmodic cough, excited by roughness and scratching in roof of mouth and in the trachea; morning without, evening with, scanty, yellow, jelly-like mucus, expectorated with difficulty.

Cough worse about midnight and towards morning; from getting heated; from eating; from drinking cold fluids; talking, or walking in the open air.

Expectoration of sweetish taste; sometimes with a little dark blood.

[28] **Lungs.** Peculiar, seemingly rheumatic pains and catarrhal affections of the lungs, with serous exudation.

Passive congestion of the lungs, depending on a weakened, dilated heart.

Desires to lie on the back, lungs constricted; sputum tough or bloody mucus.

Great weakness in the chest, can't bear to talk.

Emphysema, in complication with heart disease, feels better while lying perfectly quiet in the horizontal position.

Moist rales, yet cough dry; pulse thready. θ Senile pneumonia.

[29] **Heart. Pulse.** Violent but not very rapid beating of heart.

Inflammation of the pericardium, with copious serous exudation.

Pulse: small, irregular; slow; extremely slow, particularly when at rest; becomes accelerated, full and hard from every motion; intermitting the third, fifth, or seventh beat.

[32] **Upper Limbs.** Heaviness or paralytic weakness of left arm. The fingers "go to sleep" frequently and easily.

[33] **Lower Limbs.** Swelling and painfulness of the feet.

Paralytic feeling in the limbs.

[35] **Position, etc.** Rest: 29. Motion: 21, 29, 47. Walking: 2, 21, 26, 27. Lying quiet horizontally: 28.

[36] **Nerves.** Great weakness.

[37] **Sleep.** Lethargy, great sleepiness.

Uneasy, unrefreshing sleep.

Frequently startled and awaking, at night.

[38] **Time.** Morning: 5, 16, 25, 26, 27. Evening: 20, 27. 6 P.M.: 1. Night: 22, 37, 40. Midnight: 27. Day and night: 1.

[39] **Temperature and Weather.** Getting heated: 27. Open air: 27. Cold: 40. Cold air: 5. Cold weather: 26.

[40] **Chill. Fever. Sweat.** Chill more internal, with warmth of face, beginning with cold extremities, then spreading over the body.

Chilliness and shivering over the whole back.

Internal chill, with external heat.

Chill, with heat and redness of the face.

Chill and heat in alternation.

Excessive coldness of the hands and feet, with cold sweat.

Great sensitiveness to cold.

Sudden flushes of heat followed by weakness.

Heat of body, with cold sweat of face.

One hand hot, the other cold.

Sweat at night, generally cold and somewhat clammy.

Sweat immediately after the chill.

Sweat: on upper part of body; on the face.

⁴² **Sides.**   Right: 18.   Left: 32.   Below up: 40.

⁴⁴ **Tissues.**   Piercing pains in the joints.

Distended veins on the eyes, ears, lips and tongue.

Flabby, œdematous swelling all over; with fluttering, weak pulse, cold legs.

⁴⁵ **Contact, Injuries, etc.**   Riding: 2.

⁴⁶ **Skin.**   Itching of the skin.

Desquamation.

Jaundice.

⁴⁷ **Stages and States.**   During the climacteric, sudden flushes of heat followed by great debility, irregular pulse; least motion brings on palpitation.

⁴⁸ **Relationship.**   Antidotes of large doses: sweet milk with Fœnum græcum; vegetable acids, vinegar, infusion of galls, ether, *Camphor.*

Of small doses: *Nux vom., Opium.*

Cinchon. increases anxiety of *Digit.*

Compare: *Convallaria, Magnolia grand, Lycop.*

DIOSCOREA VILLOSA.

Wild Yam.   Cushing.   *Dioscoreaceæ.*

¹ **Mind.**   Irritable.   Depressed in spirits: 22.

Calls things by wrong names.

² **Sensorium.**   Dull, confused, dizzy; mouth dry and bitter.

³ **Inner Head.**   Dull pains, worse after dinner.

Sharp pains over the eyes.

Squeezing pains in head; temples as if in a vise; nausea, dry mouth.

⁵ **Eyes.**   Eyes weak, sore, smart; lids gummed together.

Feeling as of a round substance, or as of sticks in the eyes.

⁶ **Ears.**   Pains in the ears, worse blowing the nose.

Pains sharp, or dull, squeezing before and behind ears, extending to the angles of the jaws.

⁷ **Nose.**   Bad smell in nose as if bilious.

Nose stopped up, dry; or watery discharge. (See Throat.)

¹¹ **Tongue, etc.**   White, dry; yellow-white; brown and sore on the tip, worse in the morning.

Bites the tongue; spasmodic closure of the jaw.

Taste: bitter, nasty; rough; or flat, pappy.

¹² **Mouth.**   Dry, yet full of sticky mucus; no thirst.

¹³ **Throat.**   Fauces dry, burning, smarting, sore.

¹⁵ **Eating and Drinking.** After excess in eating, errors in diet, or in tea drinkers, excessive flatulent colic.

¹⁶ **Nausea and Vomiting.** ı Belching large quantities of wind, tasteless, sour, bitter, or like rotten eggs, with only partial relief of pains.

¹⁷ **Stomach.** ı Distress, with frequent sharp pains; must unfasten clothing; distress and burning in the morning; belching relieves.

Hard pain in region of somach.

ı Sharp, cramping pain in pit of stomach, then belching of enormous quantities of tasteless wind; hiccough and discharge of flatus from bowels.

¹⁸ **Hypochondria.** ı Cutting pains in stomach and region of gall-bladder; gastrodynia.

ı Sharp pains in the liver, extending to the nipple.

¹⁹ **Abdomen.** Faintness at epigastrium.

ı Steady, twisting pains in the bowels, worse lower, constantly changing; worse lying down.

ı Griping in the umbilical region; constant dull aching with sharp, cutting pains all through intestines.

ı Rumbling in the bowels; passes large quantities of flatus; severe pains.

ı Constant distress in navel and hypogastric regions; cutting, colicky pains; belching.

ı Colic bends him double; worse lying down; better by stretching, or by rising and walking; a constant pain, worse at intervals. Flatulent spasm.

ı Flatulence after meals; wind colic, but with little or no hepatic derangement.

Pains begin in a small spot and radiate thence upward and downward; may, early in the attack, extend to stomach, liver, spleen or uterus; often the pains jump from place to place, especially to a distant part.

²⁰ **Stool, etc.** Sudden urging to stool, especially early in the morning.

Expulsion of flatus difficult and with violence; often with watery evacuations, but only with partial relief of pains.

Stool in the morning, followed by protrusion of hemorrhoids, with pain and distress.

Sensation as if the feces were hot; hot flatus.

Profuse, thin, yellow stool in the morning; does not relieve pains in bowels; stools offensive, bilious; faintness.

²² **Male Sexual Organs.** Constant excitement of genitals; frequent erections.

Sexual desire diminished.

Emissions during sleep without erections; genitals cold, relaxed; weakness, especially weak knees, afterwards; depressed in spirits.

Pains in the inguinal region extending into the testicles.
Strong-smelling sweat on scrotum and pubes.

[27] **Cough.** Hacking cough from tickling low down in throat.

[28] **Lungs.** Pains in the region of the nipples.
Pains through the lungs to the back and vice versa.
Tightness across upper part of chest; distressed feeling.

[29] **Heart. Pulse.** Sharp pains arresting breathing and motion, with faintness.

[31] **Neck. Back.** Lame and stiff; weakness in small of back.
Dull pain in lumbar region, worse bending the spine; sharp, extending to the testicles.

[33] **Lower Limbs.** ı Pain in right leg from point of exit of sciatic nerve, felt only when moving the limb, or when sitting up.

[34] **Limbs in General.** Sharp pains in various parts of the body and limbs; darting from place to place.
Limbs feel weak, worse at the knees: 22.

[35] **Position, etc.** Pains, except headache, are usually relieved by motion. Stooping, bending: 19, 31. Motion: 29, 33. Lying down: 19. Sitting up: 33. Stretching: 19 Walking: 19.

[36] **Nerves.** Strengthens nerves; later, trembling, languor, faintness, numdness and tingling.
Acts, probably, chiefly upon the nerves, especially upon the solar plexus and upon the spinal nerves, causing pains over the body and in the viscera, also reflex pains

[38] **Time.** Morning: 11, 17; 20.

[39] **Temperature and Weather.** Generaly better in open air.

[40] **Chill. Fever. Sweat.** Chilliness: with bitter mouth; with aching bones, backache, pains in lungs, sore throat, etc.
Cold extremities, feeble pulse, but no fever; with the colic.
Sweats easily, while chilly.

[42] **Sides.** Pains spread; especially from abdomen to distant parts.

[44] **Tissues.** Joints painful; weak, worse knees: 22.

[46] **Skin.** Nails seem unusually brittle.
Itching, burning of various parts.
ı Panaritium, early when pains are sharp and agonizing, or when the picking is felt; nails brittle.

[48] **Relationship.** *Camphor.* seems to increase its effects.
Compare with: *Coloc.* (in latter colic is less continuous, and is better from pressure and bending double).

DOLICHOS.

Cowhage.   JEANES.   *Leguminosæ.*

⁵ **Eyes.** Eyes yellow. *θ* Jaundice.
¹⁰ **Teeth.** Soreness and tenderness of gums, in teething children.
  Gums swollen; neuralgic pains in them, worse at night.
¹³ **Throat.** Pain, like a splinter, near the right tonsil, worse
  when swallowing.
²⁰ **Stool, etc.** ı Constipation during teething or pregnancy.
  ı White stools. *θ* Jaundice.
²⁷ **Cough.** ı On lying down at night.
⁴³ **Sensations.** Neuralgic pains following herpes zoster.
⁴⁶ **Skin.** Violent itching all over body, without any visible
  eruption. *θ* Constipation during pregnancy. *θ* Jaundice.
  Dry, tettery eruption on arms and limbs, resembling zona.
⁴⁸ **Relationship.** In teething affections, if feverish symptoms
  exist, always give a dose of *Acon.* before the *Dolich.;*
  where this precaution has been neglected, convulsions
  have followed the use of even the high potencies.

DROSERA ROTUNDIFOLIA.

Roundleaved Sundew. HAHNEMANN.   *Droseraceæ.*

¹ **Mind.** Mental restlessness; when reading cannot dwell
  long on one subject; must change always to something
  else.
  Anxiety: with flushes of heat; when alone, especially in
  the evening, also when awaking at night; especially
  the evenings, as if it would impel him to commit suicide
  by drowning.
  Very irritable; a trifle will disturb.
  Distrust.
² **Sensorium.** Dulness of the head.
  Vertigo when walking in open air, tendency to fall to left.
  Heaviness of the head.
³ **Inner Head.** Pressive pain in forehead and zygoma, from
  within outward.
  Drawing pain in left side of head.
  Lancinating, tensive, frontal headache, worse from stoop-
  ing.
  Lancinating pain in forepart of brain, worse moving the
  eyes, better from supporting the head on the hands.

⁴ Outer Head. Smarting, burning pain in the scalp.

Sore feeling in skin of right temple.

Itching, gnawing on the forepart of scalp, relieved by rubbing.

Corrosive itching on the scalp.

⁵ Eyes. Farsighted, weakness of the eyes when looking carefully at small things; quivering before the eyes; dazzling; worse from light, daylight or candle-light.

Light gause before eyes; when reading, letters run together.

Pupils first contracted, later dilated.

Severe stitches, from within outward, in the eyes.

⁶ Ears. Difficult hearing, with increased humming before the ears.

Stitches in the ears.

Pain in right internal ear, as if pressed together.

⁷ Nose. Nosebleed.

Frequent sneezing, with or without fluent coryza.

Profuse fluent coryza, particularly in the morning.

⁸ Face. Face puffed and livid.

Cheeks and eyes sunken.

One (left) side of face cold, the other (right) hot, during morning hours.

Heat of face, with cold hands.

Small pustules, here and there, on the face, with fine, stitching sensation when touched.

Prickling, burning pain in skin of cheek below left eyelid.

⁹ Lower Face. Stitching, tearing pain on left inferior maxilla, as in the periosteum.

Lower lip cracked in the middle.

Dryness of the lips and little sense of taste.

Burning in the skin, at right angle of mouth.

¹⁰ Teeth. Cold sensation in the body of an incisor.

Stitching toothache, mornings, after warm drink.

¹¹ Tongue, etc. Food seems tasteless.

Bread tastes bitter.

Taste: bitter, in throat, after eating; putrid.

Small, round, painless swelling in the middle of tongue.

Fine prickings on dorsum of tongue.

Stitching, smarting pain in right side and tip of tongue.

Whitish ulcer on tip of tongue.

¹² Mouth. Smarting pain on inside of left cheek, like from pepper.

Profuse flow of watery saliva.

Water-brash.

¹³ Throat. Rough, scraping, dry sensation on soft palate and in fauces, exciting cough.

¹⁴ Desires. Aversions. Aversion to pork.

¹⁵ Eating and Drinking. Right after dinner, burning, raw feeling.

After eating: 11, 16.   Warm drink: 10.   Drinking: 16, 27, 37.

16 Nausea and Vomiting.   Frequent hiccough.

Eructations tasting bitter or sour.

Nausea after fatty food; worse after midnight till morning.

Vomiting of bile, in the morning; of mucus, or food when coughing; after drinking; especially at night or before dinner.

Worse after vomiting.

17 Stomach.   Contractive tension at pit of stomach, as if everything would be drawn inwards, especially during deep inhalation.

18 Hypochondria.   Painful to touch, and when coughing.

Must support the hypochondria with the hands, when coughing.

19 Abdomen.   Bellyache after sour food.

Stitches in right side of abdomen while sitting.

Dull stitch from right to left across the abdomen, almost taking the breath, while walking.

Stitch from the left loin into the penis.

20 Stool, etc.   Outward pressing pain, independent of stool.

Frequent stool, with colic.

Stools: soft fluid; white, slimy and stinking, with the watery, odorless urine.

With the stool, discharge of bloody mucus; afterwards pains in abdomen and small of back,

After stool, constant inclination to stool.

21 Urine.   Frequent urging to urinate, with scanty discharge, frequently only by drops,

Frequent, profuse urination.

Urine dark and of strong smell.

22 Male Sexual Organs.   Itching stitches in the glans.

23 Female Sexual Organs.   Delay of the first menses.

Menses too late; too scanty.

Blood dark.

Leucorrhœa, with labor-like pain.

25 Larynx.   Voice: hoarse, deep, requires exertion to speak; husky; hollow, toneless.

Epiglottis in constant motion, to and fro.

Constriction of the larynx when talking.

Sensation as from a feather in larynx, exciting cough.

Mucus in the larynx, either hard or soft.

Chest and throat symptoms worse from talking or singing.

The sick involuntarily support the larynx on swallowing or coughing.

26 Breathing.   Oppression, with every word he speaks the throat contracts; not so when walking.

Difficult breathing, worse after midnight.

Sensation as if something in the chest prevented exhalation when talking or coughing.

[27] **Cough.** Whooping, in periodically returning paroxysms; in such frequent succussions that he can scarcely get his breath; with ringing sound; evening after lying down; at night; wakes at 2 A. M.; with drawing in of the abdomen.

During cough: efforts to vomit; vomiting of water, mucus and food; stitches in the muscles of the chest; or, bleeding at nose or mouth.

Cough aggravated: by warmth; drinking; tobacco smoke; laughing; singing; weeping; after lying down; after midnight or in the morning.

Expectoration yellow, bitter, or offensive, also bloody or pus-like.

[28] **Lungs.** Constriction of chest and hypochondria.

Severe stitches in the chest, when sneezing or coughing, must press on chest with the hands, for relief.

Burning sensation in centre of chest.

Violent, oppressive, stitching pain across the chest, passing off during motion.

[30] **Outer Chest.** Stitches in muscles of chest, when breathing or coughing.

[31] **Neck. Back.** Neck stiff and painful on motion.

Pain between the scapulæ drawing to the small of back.

Stitching-tearing from the spine to the anterior spinous process of left ilium, when sitting.

Back pains as if bruised, in the morning.

[32] **Upper Limbs.** Quivering on right shoulder only when at rest. Inclination of the fingers to contract spasmodically, with rigidity when grasping anything.

Coldness of the hands.

[33] **Lower Limbs.** Pressing pain in posterior muscles of thigh, worse from pressure and stooping; could not lie thereon at night, passes off after rising.

Laming pain in right hip-joint and thigh, with pain in the ankle, as if sprained; when walking, must limp.

Occasional single stitches in the middle of left thigh anteriorly.

Fine, cutting stitch in the right calf, coming on when sitting, passing off when walking.

Tearing pain in right ankle, as if sprained, only when walking.

Stiffness of the ankles.

Feet feel chilly, covered with a cold sweat.

[34] **Limbs in General.** Limbs feel as if beaten and are outwardly painful.

All the limbs feel lame.

Gnawing and stitching pain in the bones of the limbs, especially severe at the joints; severe stitches in the
joints; less painful during motion than during rest.

Painful stitching pressure in the muscles of upper and
lower limbs, in every position.

³⁵ **Position, etc.**   Rest: 32, 34, 40. Motion: 28, 31, 34. Moving eyes: 3.   Walking: 19, 26, 33.   Walking in open
air: 2.   Sitting: 19, 31, 33.   Lying: 27, 33; on back:
37.   Rising: 33.   Stooping: 3, 33.   Every position: 34.
Supporting head on hand: 3.

³⁶ **Nerves.**   Torpidity.   Attacks, with numbness.

Weakness of whole body, with sunken eyes and cheeks.

³⁷ **Sleep.**   Frequent yawning and stretching.

Frequent starting from sleep, at night, as from fright; yet
when awake is not fearful.

Frequent waking from sleep.

Sleeplesness.

Snoring when lying on the back, asleep.

Vivid dreams: partly pleasant, partly anxious; vexatious,
over the wrong-doings of others; of thirst and drinking,
awakes, is thirsty and must drink.

³⁸ **Time.**   Morning: 7, 8, 10, 16, 27, 31, 40.   Forenoon: 40.
Evening: 1, 27, 40. Night: 1, 16, 27, 33, 37, 40. After
midnight: 26, 40.   Till morning: 16.   2 A. M.: 27.

³⁹ **Temperature and Weather.**   Open air: 2.   Getting cold:
27.   Warmth: 27.

⁴⁰ **Chill.   Fever.   Sweat.**   Chill, with coldness and paleness
of face and cold extremities.

Chill in forenoon.

Internal chill at night, in bed and during rest.

Chill and shivering when at rest, seems to be too cold
everywhere, even in bed.

Chill during the day, heat at night.

Heat almost exclusively on face and head.

Increased warmth of upper body, evening.

Heat, worse after midnight.

Cold sweat: on the forehead; feet.

Warm sweat at night, particularly after midnight and in
the morning hours, most profuse in face.

Sweat over the whole body, with a cough which brought
on violent retching.

⁴² **Sides.**   Right: 4, 6, 8, 9, 11, 19, 32, 33.   Left: 2, 3, 8, 9, 12,
19, 31, 33.   Right to left: 19.

Within outwards: 3, 5, 20.   Without inwards: 17.   Above
downwards: 31.

⁴⁵ **Contact, Injuries, etc.**   Touch: 8, 18.   Pressure: 18, 25,
28, 33.   Rubbing: 4, 46.   Scratching: 46.   Wiping
with hand: 46.

[46] **Skin.** Prickling, stinging, itching, gnawing in the skin.

Itching generally relieved by scratching, rubbing or wiping with the hand.

Eruption, like measles.

Eruption, with painful soreness or stinging.

[48] **Relationship.** *Sulphur* and *Veratr.* are the most appropriate intercurrents in whooping-cough. *Conium* follows well in dry cough of phthisis.

Complementary to *Nux vom.*

Closely allied to *Ipec.* in affections of the larynx.

Antidote to *Drosera: Camphor.*

DULCAMARA.

Bittersweet.   HAHNEMANN.   *Solanaceæ.*

[1] **Mind.** Cannot find the right word.

Mental confusion, cannot concentrate his thoughts.

Delirium at night, with pain.

Asks for one or another thing, rejecting it when proffered.

Depressed.

Inclination to scold, without being angry.

Restless, quarrelsome.

[2] **Sensorium.** On awaking, morning, dizzy, dark before the eyes, trembling and weakness.

Dulness of senses.

[3] **Inner Head.** Boring, burning in forehead, with digging in brain; worse from motion, even talking; head heavy.

Dull headache, continuous; pain in head, chest and stomach, with great uneasiness, depressed spirits, labored respiration, mental confusion, cannot concentrate his thoughts.

Congestion to head, buzzing in ears, dull hearing; worse from getting feet wet.

Sensation as of a board pressing against the forehead.

Chilliness in cerebellum and over the back, returning every evening; cerebellum and whole head as if enlarged; worse cold; damp weather; worse until 2 P. M.; better lying down.

[4] **Outer Head.** Sensation of chilliness in cerebellum and over the back; feeling as if the hair stood on end; recurs every evening.

Ringworm of scalp; glands about throat swollen.

Thick crusts on scalp, causing hair to fall out.

⁵ Eyes.   Aching in eyes when reading; sight dim; scintillations; worse at rest.

Threatened amaurosis in scrofulous children.

Dim sight, sees as through a gauze.

Ophthalmia; scrofulous, from every exposure to cold.

Paralysis of the upper lids.

⁶ Ears.   Buzzing in the ears.

Dull pains, humming in ears, obtuse hearing.

Earache; nausea; buzzing; worse at night and when still.

Swelling of parotids; also after measles.

⁷ Nose.   Nosebleed, hot, clear blood; pressure above nose;
worse after getting wet.

Coryza, dry; better during motion; worse during rest; renewed by the slightest exposure.

Severe coryza, skin hot, dry; limbs cold, stiff, numb and
painful; general offensive sweat.

Nasal catarrh dry, in a dry atmosphere.

⁸ Face.   Complexion pale, watery or milky.

Face pale, with circumscribed red cheeks.

Faceache and asthma, after disappearance of tetters in face.

Humid eruptions on cheeks.

Face bloated.   θ Dropsy.

Thick brown-yellow crusts on face, forehead and chin;
crusta lactea.

⁹ Lower Face.   Twitching of lips when in the cold air.

Mouth distorted; drawn to one side.

¹⁰ Teeth.   Toothache from cold, especially with diarrhœa;
confusion in head; profuse salivation; teeth feel blunt,
or as if asleep.

Scurvy; from cold.

Receding, spongy gums; ptyalism.

¹¹ Tongue, etc.   Bitter taste.

Itching, crawling on tip of tongue.

Mouth and tongue dry.

Dry, swollen tongue.

Inarticulate speech from a swollen tongue, but talks
incessantly.

Tongue and jaws become lame, if cold air or water chills
him.

Tongue paralyzed from cold.

¹² Mouth.   Saliva tenacious, soap-like; gums spongy.

Increased flow of saliva.

Mouth dry, without thirst.

Stomacace: rheumatic; also after abuse of mercury, with
ptyalism and swollen cervical glands.

¹³ Throat.   Much mucus in fauces.

Tonsillitis, from every cold change.

Pressure, as if uvula were too long.

27

[14] **Desires. Aversions.** Hunger without appetite.
Hunger, after the fever.
Great thirst for cold drinks.

[15] **Eating and Drinking.** Cold drinks: 16.

[16] **Nausea and Vomiting.** Nausea, loss of appetite; cholerine.
Great chilliness during the vomiting.
Vomiting, early in the morning, of tenacious mucus.
Vomiting of greenish, yellow, slimy substances, together
with the liquid drank; after cold drinks.

[17] **Stomach.** Retraction and burning in the epigastric region.

[19] **Abdomen.** Cutting pain above navel.
Colic after a cold; griping, nausea, followed by diarrhœa.
Dropsy of the abdomen.
Swelling of inguinal glands from a cold.

[20] **Stool, etc.** Stools: whitish, watery; with flocculi; slimy,
watery, yellow-green; worse at night, in wet weather;
changeable, white, yellow or green; watery; sour-smelling; nausea, with desire to evacuate.
Diarrhœa: from cold; or, change from warm to cold, especially cold, damp weather; in the morning, profuse
thin stools; of rheumatic origin; during dentition.
Dysentery, from cold, damp weather; increased flow of
saliva; burning, itching of rectum, heat of skin, thirst.

[21] **Urine.** Constant desire to urinate, felt deep in abdomen.
Painful pressing about bladder and urethra, discharge of a
few drops of urine, with mucous sediment.
Urine; scanty, fetid, turbid; on standing, oily, containing
a tough, jelly-like, white or red mucus mixed with
blood; milky; fetid or muco-purulent.
Bright's disease from exposure to cold and dampness.
Retention of urine; stranguiy from a cold or from cold
drinks.
Urine passed involuntarily; paralysis of bladder.

[22] **Male Sexnal Organs.** ı Impotence; herpes on genitals.
θ Herpes præputialis.

[23] **Female Sexual Organs.** Menses suppressed by cold.
Rash before menses.
Menses too late, too short; blood watery, thin.
Mammæ engorged, hard; amenorrhœa.

[24] **Pregnancy.** Suppressed milk, from taking cold.
After weaning, mother has eruptions on the skin.
Herpes on mammæ; nursing women.
Lochia suppressed by cold or damp.

[25] **Larynx.** Rough, hoarse voice; catarrh.
Hoarse after measles.
Influenza.
Trachea full of mucus.

[26] **Breathing.** Labored respiration.

Asthma, with faceache after disappearance of tetters in face.

Asthma humidum, dyspnœa, loose, rattling cough, copious sputa; worse during wet weather.

Oppression of chest, from mucus.

²⁷ **Cough.**   Dry, hoarse, rough cough; or, loose, with copious expectoration of mucus; dull hearing catarrhal fever.

Chronic mucous cough after measles.

Panting cough, like whooping-cough: worse with each deep inspiration.

Expectoration of pure blood.

Cough worse when lying down, from warmth of the room, or deep inspiration; better in the open air.

Whooping-cough: excited by excessive secretion of mucus in larynx and trachea.

²⁸ **Lungs.**   Bronchitis; offensive-smelling night-sweats.

Tuberculosis in scrofulous subjects; also worse in changes from warm to cold; sputa tough, green; cough moderate; stitches here and there in chest; diarrhœa.

Phthisis mucosa.

❙Rheumatic pleuritis and pleuro-pneumonia, with tough, difficult, discolored sputa.

❙Hydrothorax, worse wet weather.

Mucus on the chest, must cough long before raising it; suffocative catarrh.

Hæmoptysis, bright red; tickling in larynx; worse at rest; caused by a cold or loose, protracted cough.

Pain in left chest, as if lung moved in waves.

²⁹ **Heart. Pulse.**   Palpitation at night.

Pulse: small, hard and tense, especially at night; collapsed.

³¹ **Neck. Back.**   Neck stiff, back painful, loins lame, after taking cold.

Spinal meningitis during scarlatina or measles, eruption does not develop.

Myelitis after taking cold during menstruation.

Hyperæmia of the spinal cord.

Drawing pain from small of back down thighs, during rest; stitches when moving, relieved by pressure.

Coldness in small of back.   Sacrum feels cold.

³² **Upper Limbs.**   Herpes on arms and hands.

Exostosis on the arm, from suppressed itch.

Warts on hands.

Sweat in palms.

³³ **Lower Limbs.**   Herpetic eruption on knee.

Exostosis on upper part on right tibia, with bluish-red spots; suppurating lumps.

Swelling of the calf of the leg; scrofula.

Gout in the big toe; first left, then right.

Tingling in the feet.

Erysipelas of feet; skin peels off; itching.

³⁴ Limbs in General. Cold limbs.

Rheumatism after acute eruptions, or when chronic forms. alternate with attacks of diarrhœa.

Pains in the joints on exposure to cold.

Rheumatism after exposure to wet; parts as if beaten,. severe pains when remaining in one position, subside- only when he moves about.

³⁵ Position, etc. Rest: 5, 6, 7, 28, 34. Motion: 3, 7, 31, 34, 44. Lying down: 3, 27. Worse lying on back, better on side. Worse when stooping; better when · erect. Worse when bending diseased part backwards. Worse dancing.

³⁶ Nerves. Great general uneasiness.

Convulsions beginning in the face.

One-sided spasms; speechless.

Prostration, languor.

Paralysis from suppressed eruptions, from cold; paralysis. of upper and lower limbs and tongue; the paralyzed. arm feels icy-cold.

³⁷ Sleep. Falling asleep, evening, starts as if in affright.

During sleep, mouth open, snoring.

Sleep restless after 12 P. M.

Uneasy sleep, confused dreams, frequent sweat; tosses. from side to side.

Sleep worse after 3 A. M.

³⁸Time. Morning: 2, 16, 40; 2 P. M.: 3. Evening: 3, 4, 37, 40. Night: 6, 20, 28, 29, 40. After midnight: 37. 3. A.M.: 37.

³⁹ Temperature and Weather. Warmth: 40, 46. Warm. weather: 30, 28. Warm room: 27. Cold: 34, 44, 46. Cold air: 9, 11. Cold, damp weather: 3, 13, 20, 21, 24, 28, 44, 46. Open air: 27. Dry atmosphere: 7. Wet weather: 26, 28, 34.

⁴⁰ Chill. Fever. Sweat. Chill commencing in or spread-ing from the back, not relieved by warmth; mostly towards evening.

Chill with the pains. Chill with violent thirst.

General dry burning heat all over. Heat and burning in the back.

Heat with delirium, without thirst.

Fetid sweat, with skin diseases; with copious limpid. urine.

Offensive sweat, night and morning, over the whole body; during day more over back, in axillæ and palms.

Sweat suppressed and entirely wanting.

[42] **Sides.** Left: 28. Right: 33. Left to right: 33. Above
  downward: 31.

  ❙ Rending pains, upwards. θ Rheumatism.

[43] **Sensations.** Pains in many parts, as if from cold.
  Bruised feeling.

[44] **Tissues.** Hemorrhages: blood watery, or bright red.
  Skin inactive; mucous surfaces overactive, especially from
    suppressed eruptions by cold.
  Cold swelling of glands, also inflammation and indura-
    tion of cervical and inguinal glands; tensive pain.
  Anasarca after fever and ague, scarlatina, rheumatic fever.
  Dropsy after suppressed sweat, by damp, cold air.
  Scrofula. Exostoses. Emaciation.

[45] **Contact, Injuries, etc.** Pressure: 7, 31. Scratching: 46.
  Touch: 46.

[46] **Skin.** Skin hot, dry.
  Tetter oozing a watery fluid, bleeds after scratching.
  Thick brown herpes, red border; glands swollen.
  Red spots, as if from flea-bites.
  Eruption of itching pustules, ceasing to itch after scab-
    bing over; sensitive to touch; worse washing.
  Impetiginous eczema of scrofulous children.
  Suppressed itch.
  Painful ulcers; discharge scanty.
  Nettle-rash, with much itching; after scratching it burns;
    increases in warmth, better in cold.
  Small furuncles on places formerly injured by concussion.
  Warts, fleshy or large, smooth; on dorsa of hands and on
    the face.
  Retrocession of eruptions, from exposure to damp, cold
    air: 26.
  Skin callous.

[47] **Stages and States.** Phlegmatic, torpid, scrofulous patients,
    who are restless and irritable; take cold in cold changes.

[48] **Relationship.** Abuse of *Mercur.:* ptyalism; glandular
    swellings; canker; bronchitis; diarrhœa; susceptible
    to changes in weather.
  Complementary to *Baryt. carb.*
  Antidotes to *Dulcam.: Camphor., Cuprum., Ipec., Mercur.*
  Incompatible: *Bellad., Laches.*

ELATERIUM.

Squirting Cucumber. *Cucurbitaceæ.*

[16] **Nausea and Vomiting.** Nausea; vomiting of a watery substance, or of greenish, bilious matter, with great weakness.

[19] **Abdomen.** Cutting, griping, pains in the bowels.

[20] **Stool, etc.** ׀ Copious, liquid, frothy or of an olive-green color.

[33] **Lower Limbs.** Shooting, also dull, aching pains in the course of the left sciatic nerve to the instep and toes.

[44] **Tissues.** Causes profuse, watery serum to flow from mucous membranes, especially from the intestinal and gastric.

[48] **Relationship.** Compare: *Croton tig.* (collateral relation), *Secale* (olive-green diarrhœa), *Veratr. alb., Colchic.* (cholera-like symptoms.)

ERIGERON.

Horseweed. BURT. *Compositæ.*

[3] **Inner Head.** Congestion of the head, red face, nosebleed; febrile action.

[16] **Nausea and Vomiting.** Violent retching and burning in the stomach, with vomiting of blood.

[20] **Stool, etc.** Stools: small, streaked with blood; tormina; burning in the bowels and rectum; hard lumps of feces mixed with the discharges.

Hemorrhoids bleeding; with hard lumpy stools; burning in the margin of the anus, it feels as if torn.

[21] **Urine.** Urination painful or suppressed.

Dysuria of teething children; frequent desire, crying when urinating; urine profuse, of very strong odor; external parts (female) inflamed or irritated, with considerable mucous discharge.

[23] **Female Sexual Organs.** Metrorrhagia: with violent irritation of rectum and bladder; after abortion, with diarrhœa and dysuria; with prolapsus uteri.

Very profuse flow of bright red blood; every movement of the patient increases the flow; pallor and weakness.

Leucorrhœa profuse, with spasmodic pains, and irritation of the bladder and rectum.

[24] **Pregnancy.** Bloody lochia returns after the least motion; worse during rest.

[27] **Cough.** Bloody expectoration, incipient phthisis.

EUPATORIUM PERFOLIATUM.

Boneset, Thoroughwort.   HANES.   *Compositæ.*

[1] **Mind.**   Feels at night as if he was going out of his mind.
Moaning with the aching pain.
Anxious countenance.
Desponding, with fever.

[2] **Sensorium.**   Faintness from motion, during the fever.
Whirling around in the brain; early, morning.
Sensation, as if falling to the left.

[3] **Inner Head.**   Headache, with the chill.
Headache and nausea every other morning, when awaking.
Soreness and pulsation on the back part of the head.
Heat on top of the head; distressed feeling.
Throbbing headache during chill and heat.
Headache and trembling during the hot stage of intermittent.
Shooting from left to right side of head.
Sick headache: when first awaking, continuing all day; every other morning.
Pain in occiput after lying, with sense of weight, must aid with hand in lifting head.

[4] **Outer Head.**   Right parietal protuberance sore.
Head drawn spasmodically backwards.   θ Spotted fever.

[5] **Eyes.**   Great aversion to light.
Painful soreness of eyeballs.
Redness of margins of lids, with glutinous secretion from meibomian glands.
Intense pain darting through the eyes, as from needles; eyes not inflammed.
Sclerotica yellowish.

[6] **Ears.**   Buzzing in ears, heat on top of head.

[7] **Nose.**   Coryza, with aching in every bone.
Influenza, with weak pulse, prostration, bones sore; especially with inebriates and with old people.

[8] **Face.**   Sallow, sickly, with intermittent fever; pale, with catarrhs; red, skin dry.
Sudden severe contraction of muscles of right cheek.

[11] **Tongue, etc.**   Tongue covered with white fur, or yellow-coated.   Taste bitter.

[12] **Mouth.**   Paleness of the mucous membrane of the mouth.
Breath smells mouldy, sourish.

[13] **Throat.**   Fauces sore.

[14] **Desires.   Aversions.**   Longs for ice-cream.
Distaste for food.

Canine hunger with or before argue, or after quinine.

Loss of appetite.

Thirst for cold water.

15 **Eating and Drinking.** After drinking cold water: shuddering; vomiting bile.

After eating: violent distressing pains; no ease until all is vomited.

16 **Nausea and Vomiting.** Sick stomach, night before ague paroxysm.

Vomiting; as the chill passes off, or between chill and fever; of bile at the close of hot stage; of bile, with trembling and great nausea, causing great prostration; preceded by thirst.

17 **Stomach.** Distressing pain in scrobiculum during chill and heat.

18 **Hypochondria.** Soreness in region of the liver.

Tight clothing is oppressive.

19 **Abdomen.** Violent colicky pains in upper abdomen, with headache and other pains.

Abdomen full and tympanitic.

20 **Stool, etc.** Considerable griping, worse after stool, with tenesmus.

Emission of fetid flatus, with relief.

Morning diarrhœa.

Frequent green, watery stools.

Constipation, with catarrh.

21 **Urine.** Dark brown, scanty, depositing a whitish, clay-like sediment; profuse, pale, with gout.

Inflammation of meatus urinarius, in a woman.

22 **Male Sexual Organs.** Itching of the mons veneris.

25 **Larynx.** Hoarse; throat dry, sore; can hardly talk; worse mornings, when he gets up.

26 **Breathing.** Difficulty of breathing, attended with perspiration, anxious countenance, sleepiness.

Great oppression of the chest; a full breath hurts; rattling on chest.

Dyspnœa, with hard, dry cough.

Must lie with head and shoulders high.

27 **Cough.** Hectic cough, from suppressed intermittent fever.

Loose cough during apyrexia; also at night, after measles.

Rough, scraping cough, chest sore; must support it with the hands; flushed face, tearful eyes.

28 **Lungs.** Soreness in chest; worse from inspiration.

Pain and soreness behind the sternum; heart feels as if in too small a place.

Oppression in middle of sternum; feels as if something were pressing against his heart; palpitation.

Pain through right nipple, when breathing.

Deep-seated pain in left side and right shoulder.

31 Neck. Back. Intense aching in back and limbs.

Pain in back of neck and between the shoulders.

Aching soreness in the back.

32 Upper Limbs. Stiffness of arms and fingers during chill.

Wrists pain as if broken or dislocated.

Heat in hands, sometimes with sweat.

33 Lower Limbs. Severe pains, like cramps, waken out of
   sleep; cold sweat follows.

Lameness in right hip and lower extremity when walking.

Flagging of muscles of left thigh, as if falling off the bone.

Burning of skin of inside of thighs.

Throbbing in right foot.

Stinging, as from pins in feet; beginning of chill.

Heat in soles of feet in the morning.

Pain in heel, as if stabbed.

Sharp, burning pain in feet, could not keep her shoes on.

Gouty swelling of left big toe; ankles and feet dropsical.

34 Limbs in General. Intense aching in limbs, as if the bones
   were broken; back and limbs ache, as if broken.

Pains all over; left ankle, hip, shoulder; pains come instantly and go away as quickly.

35 Position, etc. Very restless, can't keep still, though there
   is a great desire to do so.

Not relieved by motion. Motion: 2, 40.

Walking: 33. Lying: 3, 26, Cannot raise head: 40.

36 Nerves. During fever, weak, faint, nervous, trembling.

37 Sleep. Yawning and stretching, with intermittent.

Sleepy; difficult breathing.

Profound sleep at noon, yet can hear every sound.

Sleepless, with the fever.

On awaking, headache.

33 Time. Morning: 2, 3, 20, 25, 33, 40. 7–9 A.M.: 40. Noon:
   37, 40. Night: 27, 40. All day: 3.

39 Temperature and Weather. Wants to be warmly covered
   during chill.

Uncovering: 40.

40 Chill. Fever. Sweat. Before chill: thirst; cough the
   night before; pain above right ilium; yawning.

During chill: thirst, head throbs; aching all over, as if in
   the bones; more shivering than the degree of coldness
   warrants; trembling, nausea; moaning with pains.

At end of chill: vomiting bile.

Chill spreads from the back; begins between 7 and 9 A.M.

Chill early morn one day, light chill about noon next day.

Fever preceded by thirst, cannot raise the head; cheeks
   red; throbbing headache; sleep and moaning; trembling, faint from motion; vomiting of bile at end of hot
   stage, followed by slight sweat and sleep.

Skin bathed in sweat; or sweat scanty.

Nightly sweat, with chillines, from moving or uncovering.

Hectic from suppressed ague.

Bilious fever; remittent fever. Dengue.

[41] **Attacks.** Every other morning: Intermittents of any type, but especially the tertian.

Pains come quickly and go quickly: 34.

[42] **Sides.** Inability to lie on left side.

Right: 4, 8, 28, 33, 40. Left: 2, 28, 33, Left to right: 3.

[43] **Sensations.** Sense of numbness, as if the flesh were falling from the bones.

Pains in back, head, chest, etc., the more general and severe, the better adapted.

[45] **Contact, Injuries, etc.** Must support with the hands: 27.

[46] **Skin.** Eruptions develop tardily; especially measles.

Spotted fever; head drawn backwards; limbs ache, feel sore.

Ringworms.

[47] **Stages and States.** Old people.

Inebriates.

[48] **Relationship.** *Eup. perf.* is followed well by *Sepia* or *Natr. mur.*

EUPATORIUM PURPUREUM.

Trumpet Weed.   MRS. H. H. DRESSER.   *Compositæ.*

[1] **Mind.** Stupid, dull.

Sighing.

Depressed, sleepy.

Homesick.

[2] **Sensorium.** Light, dizzy, as though flying round and round; sensation as if falling to the left.

[3] **Inner Head.** Sick headache: dull hammering, beating, stitching, or boring pain in left side of head; pressing from right to left; beginning in the morning and increasing during the afternoon and evening; worse in cold air; better while walking slowly in fresh air.

[4] **Outer Head.** Soreness of scalp.

Sweat on head, profuse about forehead.

[5] **Eyes.** Staring.

Eyes suffused during fever.

Conjunctiva yellow, with the chill.

[6] **Ears.** Crackling in ears, like burning birch-bark.

Ears feel as if filled up.

[7] **Nose.** Fluent coryza; great heat, sneezing.

⁸ **Face.** Face flushed, with fever.
  Shining of the face.
⁹ **Lower Face.** Lips blue; intermittent.
¹¹ **Tongue, etc.** Tongue furred, brown along the centre; bitter,
  pappy taste, with the chill.
  Tongue numb; pricking, stinging pain.
¹³ **Throat.** Choking fulness of throat, must swallow often.
  Pain in left side of throat, causing pain in swallowing;
  before chill.
  Burning as if scalded, in back of throat.
¹⁴ **Desires. Aversions.** Thirst during chill and heat; or
  before chill.
  Wants lemonade or cold drinks during the chill.
  Thirst, with dropsy.
  No appetite.
¹⁶ **Nausea and Vomiting.** Vomiting with the sick headache.
  Great nausea, but no vomit, with the chill.
  Nausea, vomiting with the fever.
¹⁷ **Stomach.** Crampy pain in stomach.
¹⁹ **Abdomen.** Rumbling in bowels.
  Lower belly swollen and hot.
  Colic all over abdomen after voiding urine.
²⁰ **Stool, etc.** Bilious diarrhœa; bowels loose, ague.
²¹ **Urine.** Suppression of urine.
  Incontinence of urine; especially with children.
  Deep, dull pain in kidneys, also cutting pains; chronic
  nephritis.
  Violent dysuria: after a jolting ride during pregnancy;
  from displaced uterus.
  Constant desire to urinate; even after frequent passages,
  bladder still feels full.
  Soreness and pain in the bladder; deep aching; uneasi-
  ness; catarrh.
  Smarting, burning in bladder and urethra on urinating.
  Frequent effort, with passage of but a few drops of urine.
  Urine: very copious; scanty, albuminous; scanty but
  frequent.
²³ **Female Sexual Organs.** Quick, jerking pain in left ovary.
  Heavy pressure above left ovary.
  Numbness, worse in groin.
  Leucorrhœa abundant.
  External genitals feel as if wet.
²⁵ **Larynx.** Hoarseness, with rough voice.
²⁶ **Breathing.** Difficult breathing.
  Grating sensation in chest at every deep inspiration.
²⁷ **Cough.** Hacking cough in the evening. ¡ᵖ
  Cough, with soreness and heat in bronchia.
  Dry, hacking cough in spells, before the attack; ague.

[29] **Heart. Pulse.** Pulse accelerated and full; ague.

[31] **Neck. Back.** Violent cutting in the back.

Neuralgic pains from below upwards, mostly left side of back and hip.

Labor-like pains in the back.

[33] **Lower Limbs.** Legs: numb; weak, tired.

[34] **Limbs in General.** Rheumatic pains changing place, always from below upward.

Pain in arms and legs before chill.

[35] **Position, etc.** Chill aggravated by motion.

Changing position: 40. Walking: 3.

[36] **Nerves.** Restless, tossing, moaning.

Weak, tired, faint with urinary symptoms.

[37] **Sleep.** Yawning; sighing.

Sleep restless, disturbed; ague, with frightful dreams, during the fever.

[38] **Time.** Morning till evening: 27. Night: 40.

[39] **Temperature and Weather.** Cold air: 3. Walking in fresh air: 3.

[40] **Chill. Fever. Sweat.** Chilly when changing position during sweat.

Chill begins in small of the back, and spreads over the body; violent shaking, with comparatively little coldness; bone-pain; thirst during chill and heat.

Nails blue.

Fever protracted, followed by slight sweat, mostly about forehead and head.

Night sweats: hectic.

[41] **Attacks.** Chill at different times of the day.

Every other day.

[42] **Sides.** Left: 2, 3, 13, 31. Right to left: 3. Below upwards: 31, 34.

[44] **Tissues.** Emaciation; accompanying chronic inflammation of the bladder.

[45] **Contact, Injuries, etc.** Jolting ride: 21.

EUPHRASIA.

Eyebright.　　　　HAHNEMANN.　　　　*Scrophulariaceæ.*

[1] **Mind.** Weakness of memory.

Confusion of the head.

Inert hypochondriacal mood, takes no interest in surrounding objects.

[2] **Sensorium.** Vertigo; with heaviness of the head; with tendency to fall.

[3] **Inner Head.** Dull frontal headache.

Violent beating headache.

Headache (in the evening) as if bruised, with coryza.

Stitches in the brain.

Headache, as if the head would burst, with dazzling of the eyes, from sunlight.

[5] **Eyes.** Photophobia: in day and sunlight; worse in the evening; must remain in darkened room; even to spasm of the lids; with swollen, agglutinated lids; thick yellow discharge between the lids.

Pressure in the eyes, on looking at the candle-light.

Pupils much contracted.

Pressive, cutting pain in the eyes, extending to the frontal sinuses.

Stitching pressure in the eyes.

Burning stitches in the eyes.

Dry pressure in the eyes, as if sleepy.

Sensation as of sand in the eyes.

Spots, vesicles and ulcers of the cornea.

Opacity of the cornea.

Sensation as if a hair hung over the eye and must be wiped away.

Catarrhal ophthalmia, with lachrymation and considerable mucous discharge, injection of conjunctiva, phlyctenulæ near the cornea, at the same time coryza and pain in the forehead.

Capillaries of conjunctiva enlarged.

Chemosis, acrid tears and coryza.

Profuse flow of acrid tears, with great sensitiveness to light.

Violent itching of the lids, with catarrhal ophthalmia.

Rheumatic inflammation of the eyes, almost blinding him.

Inflammation and ulceration of the margin of lids.

Pain in the eye, alternating with pain in the abdomen.

Lids swollen.

Inflammation and swelling of the meibomian glands.

[6] **Ears.** Ringing in the ears.

Earache.

[7] **Nose.** Profuse, bland, fluent coryza, with scalding tears and aversion to light; worse evening and during the night, while lying down.

Sneezing, with coryza.

Small red spots, like pimples, on upper right side of nose, twinging, starting pain in the nose.

Pain from right to left over the bridge of the nose; left half of face and forehead, and left eye inflamed; earache.

Flat cancer on right side of nose.

[8] **Face.** Redness and heat of the face.

Rash in the face, itching in the warmth, becoming red and burning when moistened.

Stiffness of the left cheek when talking or chewing, with
sensation of heat, and stitches therein.

⁹ **Lower Face.** Stiffness of the upper lip, as if made of wood.

¹⁵ **Eating and Drinking.** Eating: 27. Tobacco smoke: 27.

¹⁹ **Abdomen.** Frequent colic.

²⁰ **Stool, etc.** Old flat condylomata at the anus, with severe
burning; worse at night.

Pressure in the anus while sitting; even in piles.

²¹ **Urine.** Too often and copious.

²² **Male Sexual Organs.** Genital organs appear drawn in;
pressure above the pubes, evenings.

²³ **Female Sexual Organs.** Amenorrhœa, with inflammation
of the eyes and ulcer on right side of the bridge of nose.

Menses painful, lasting only one hour, time regular.

Menses late, scant and of short duration.

Condylomata, with stitches and itching, especially when
walking.

²⁵ **Larynx.** Catarrhal hoarseness.

²⁷ **Cough.** Cough: on rising in the morning, continuing until
lying down again; can scarcely get breath; tickling in
the trachea, worse from tobacco smoke; better when
eating; from mucous or watery vomiting; came on after
hemorrhoids had disappeared; with severe coryza; eyes
affected; difficult expectoration during the day; interruption of breath; no cough at night; from the smoke
of wood.

³¹ **Neck. Back.** Cramp-like pain in the back.

³² **Upper Limbs.** Sensation in the arms as if they had gone
to sleep.

³³ **Lower Limbs.** Cramp in calf, particularly when standing.

³⁵ **Position, etc.** Lying down: 7, 27. Standing: 33. Walking: 23. Rising: 27.

³⁷ **Sleep.** Sleeplessness after midnight.

Frequent awaking, as from fright.

Usually worse after sleep.

Awakes too late.

³⁸ **Time.** Day: 27, 40. Morning: 27. Forenoon: 40. Afternoon: 40. Evening: 3, 5, 7, 22. Night: 7, 20, 27, 37, 40.

³⁹ **Temperature and Weather.** Generally worse in bed; better
after getting out of bed.

Better out-doors; worse in-doors.

Warmth: 8. Moisture: 8.

⁴⁰ **Chill. Fever. Sweat.** Chill and internal chilliness in
the forenoon; external chill and coldness on the arms,
in the afternoon.

Heat descending.

Attacks of heat during the day, with redness of face and
cold hands.

Sweat often confined to front part of body.

Sweat during sleep at night, of very strong offensive odor, most profuse on the chest.

⁴² Sides. Left side.

Upper right, lower left side.

Right: 7, 23. Left: 7, 8. Right to left: 7. Below upwards: 43.

⁴³ Sensations. Crawling, as from a fly, in one or the other limb, from below upwards in a straight line, afterwards numbness of the part.

⁴⁴ Tissues. Swelling of the cervical glands.

Emaciation.

⁴⁵ Contact, Injuries, etc. Bad effects from falls, contusions, or other mechanical injuries of external parts.

⁴⁶ Skin. Warts.

⁴⁸ Relationship. Antidotes to *Euphras.: Camphor.*, *Pulsat.*

FERRUM.

Iron.   HAHNEMANN.   *Metals.*

¹ Mind. Head confused, muddled; with cold feet and stiff fingers.

Mind confused, cannot collect his thoughts.

Prone to weep or to laugh immoderately; with a choking sensation in throat, as if swollen outside.

Not inclined to talk or study; nervous, restless.

Lively in evening.

Depression of spirits; also after menses.

Excitable, pettish, least contradiction angers.

Proud, self-contented look.

Nervous, hysterical feeling.

² Sensorium. Vertigo: on rising suddenly, things grew black, had to lean against something, or fall; nausea, protration, lethargy; as if balancing to and fro, as when on the water; when walking over water, as when crossing a bridge.

³ Inner Head. Head dull and full, eyelids heavy, apt to sleep, while sitting reading.

Pain over left eye, coming suddenly.

Awaked 3 A.M., with stitches in both temples, which spread gradually over whole forehead, with chilliness.

Throbbing pain in top of head when moving suddenly.

Headache on top of head, as if skull was pushed upwards.

Weight in back of head, from ear to ear.

Congestion to head, pulsating, hummering pains; head sensitive; worse after 12 P.M.; returning periodically; feeling of an iron band around the head; better from external pressure; face red.

Pain in back of head when coughing.

Beating in back of head and neck, gradually extending to sides and forehead, worse stooping or moving.

Headache: occupying left side of head; with coryza; after menses.

Head hot, feet cold.

Writing causes headache to re-appear

⁴ Outer Head. Scalp and hair feel sore; drawing in chest.

Pressure on top of head when cold air touched it.

Slight itching in scalp and cold feet.

⁵ Eyes. At night can see in the dark; hysteria.

Dark before the eyes; giddy.

Letters run together when reading or writing.

Eyes weak, with lachrymation.

Pupils contracted.

Pressure in the eyes as if they would protrude; worse right.

Redness and swelling of both lids.

Inflamed eyes, burning, stinging.

Can scarcely open eyes; lids pressed down.

Suppurating stye on upper lid.

⁶ Ears. Ringing in right ear.

Oversensitive to sounds.

Stitches in the ears in the morning.

Ulcerative pain of the outer ear.

⁷ Nose. Bloody, puruloid, greenish, whey-like, slimy, acrid discharge; cold in head.

Dropping of fluid from posterior nares or frontal sinuses; headache.

Nose continually filled with clotted blood; especially with coryza.

Epistaxis; in anæmic patients subject to ebullitions.

Scabs out of nose, or coughed up every few weeks.

⁸ Face. Face ashy pale or greenish; it becomes bright red with pain and other symptoms.

Blue rings around the eyes, which are dull, lustreless.

Face feels as if swollen and bloated.

Face pale, with red spots.

Face fiery red, veins large; congestion to head.

Yellow spots on face.

Face pale, collapsed, or expressionless, stiff and stupid; pneumonia.

Neuralgia after cold washing and overheating.

⁹ Lower Face. Lips pale, dry.

[11] **Tongue, etc.** Unbearable taste of blood.

Taste like rotten eggs.

Bad taste, mouth dry, tongue coated white.

[12] **Mouth.** Dry in the morning.

Paleness of the buccal cavity.

[13] **Throat.** Like a lump in left side of throat, below the tonsil; worse from empty swallowing; not when eating and drinking.

Throat sore; dull, heavy all day, lively in evening.

Constrictive sensation in throat.

[14] **Desires. Aversions.** Appetite good and bad alternately; with diarrhœa.

Loathing sour things.

Aversion to: meat, which disagrees; beer; hot things.

Appetite for bread.

Appetite lessened or natural.

Thirstless, or unquenchable thirst.

[15] **Eating and Drinking.** Worse from meat; sour fruit.

Solid food seems dry and insipid while masticating.

All food tastes bitter.

After eggs, vomiting.

After fat food, bitter eructations.

Wine agrees, if not acid.

After eating, heat in stomach, nausea.

After least food or drink, especially after meat, spasmodic pressure at the stomach.

Cold water: 20.

[16] **Nausea and Vomiting.** Eructations: sour; foul; burning, relieving burning in stomach.

Nausea: with headache; with nightly diarrhœa; with vertigo.

Vomiting: at midnight, or morning after breakfast; as soon as food is taken.

[17] **Stomach.** Heat and burning in stomach, with momentary, cramp-like pain in splenic region.

Heavy pressure in pit of stomach.

Palpitation in stomach and through œsophagus, as if a nerve was quivering, with an occasional suffocating feeling, as if a valve rose in the throat.

Occasional uneasiness at splenic end of stomach.

[18] **Hypochondria.** Tightness in right hypochondriac region.

Pain in small of back and liver, all day.

Fulness in region of liver.

Liver enlarged, sensitive to pressure.

Spleen large; after intermittents.

Shooting pain in left hypochondrium.

Cramp-like sensation in splenic region.

[19] **Abdomen.** Abdomen hard, distended, but not with flatulence.

28

Rumbling, with pain in small of back and kidneys, and slight urethral soreness when urinating.

Flatulent colic at night; violent rumbling.

Bowels feel sore when touched, as if bruised, or weakened by cathartics.

20 **Stool, etc.** Prolapsus recti; with children.

Straining for stool all day, sick at stomach, disagreeable taste, worse drinking cold water.

Diarrhœa, with undigested food; painless and involuntary during a meal.

Rice-water discharges; cold, with cold, sour sweat.

Stools: watery, with burning at the anus; slimy, with discharge of ascarides; stools with blood and mucus.

Costive: stools hard and difficult, followed by backache.

Itching at the anus at night, from ascarides.

Piles, copious bleeding or ichorous oozing; tearing pains, with itching and gnawing.

21 **Urine.** Pains in bladder.

Slight soreness in urethra.

Involuntary urination at night, and also when walking about by day.

Urine more copious and clear; with relaxation and prostration, making him very nervous.

Urine alkaline.

Hot urine; metrorrhagia.

22 **Male Sexual Organs.** Sexual desire increased.

Impotence.

Seminal emissions.

Gleet, copious, painless, milky.

23 **Female Sexual Organs.** Desire lessened, sterility.

During coitus, insensible; painfulness of the vagina.

Dropsy of uterus; face flushes red.

Sharp pains in abdomen, bearing down in uterus, with aching below it.

Sticking, shooting pains in uterus.

Pains near mouth of uterus when lying down.

Passive flow, dark, grumous. θ Menorrhagia.

Swellings and indurations in the vagina.

Vagina too dry.

Prolapsus of vagina.

Before menses, stinging headache, ringing in ears, discharge of long pices of mucus from uterus.

Menses: too late, long-lasting and profuse; flow watery, or in lumps; preceded by labor-like pains; varices in legs worse; intermit two or three days, then return; uterus displaced; come on with a physical languor and mental depression unfitting her for work; could overcome them by forced exertion. Hysterical symptons after menses; suppressed.

Leucorrhœa mild, milky, or itching, sharp, with soreness.

Much itching of vulva; delicate women, with red face.

²⁴ **Pregnancy.**   Prevents abortion.

Promotes expulsion of moles.

Spasmodic labor-pains.

Uterine hemorrhage with labor like pains, glowing face; flow watery, or containing lumps; pulse full, hard.

²⁵ **Larynx.**   Voice: hoarse; almost extinct.

Roughness of the throat; hoarseness.

²⁶ **Breathing.**   Breath hot.

Dyspnœa increases slowly.   θ Pneumonia.

Difficult inspiration, as from heaviness of the chest.

Breathing dry, loud, anxious; sometimes in children, rattling.

Oppression from orgasm of blood; chest scarcely moves in breathing; nostrils dilated during expiration.

Asthma, worse after 12 P.M., must sit up; better walking slowly about and talking; better uncovering chest; after itch.

Suffocative fits evening, in bed, with warmth of neck and trunk, limbs cold.

Breath fails at end of coughing fit.

²⁷ **Cough.**   Spasmodic, from tickling in trachea; at night, must sit up to raise the sputum; spasmodic, after eating with vomiting of food; after drinking; with stitches and soreness.

Sputa: copious, putrid, purulent greenish or frothy, worse morning; copious when moving; scanty, thin, frothy, with streaks of blood.

Dry, tickling cough, with blood spitting.

Cough, worse from abuse of tea, quinine, brandy, tobacco smoke; loss of fluids.

Hæmoptysis morning and at night; blood bright, coagulated, scanty during slight cough with interscapular pains, heavy breathing; must sit up; better walking slowly about, notwithstanding weakness obliges lying down; palpitation.

Hæmoptysis: of onanists; consumptives; from severe exertion; after loss of fluids; from suppressed menses.

²⁸ **Lungs.**   Shooting-stinging in chest.

Feeling of dryness in the chest.

Slight heaviness in upper part of left lung, making breathing rather difficult; sore feeling below clavicle and left nipple, cannot take a long breath.

Slight, dull, heavy pain across upper part of chest, rendeing breathing uneasy.

Sticking and bruised sensation in the chest.

Constricting spasm of chest.

Flying pains in chest; blood-spitting; persons who flush easily and get epistaxis, dyspnœa, palpitation.

29 Heart. Pulse. Consecutive heart disease; chlorosis.

Hard, strong beating of the heart; pseudo-plethora.

Palpitation, better walking slowly; also in onanists; after loss of fluids; with blood-spitting.

Throbbing in all blood-vessels; soft bellows sound at apex.

Pulse full, hard; increased by exertion.

30 Outer Chest. Drawing in chest and around heart; scalp sore.

31 Neck. Back. Neck: sore as if bruised; stiff.

Neck and shoulder painful when lying on right side.

Constant pains along back, worse in those parts she had to lie on.

Lumbago all night, goes off on rising.

Pain in region of kidneys, with desire to make water.

32 Upper Limbs. Shoulders sore to touch, painful, also arm.

Pinching in right deltoid.

Boring in right shoulder, and from biceps to elbow; worse from motion; better from heat; worse from weight of bedclothes.

Right arm lame.

Irresistible desire to bend arm, with intense pain; drives out of bed, 2 A.M.; better walking slowly about.

Arms nearly rigid.

When writing the hand trembles, does better when writing fast.

Hands cold, stiff, numb; palms hot.

Fingers: stiff, numb, contracted.

33 Lower Limbs. Violent pain in the hip-joint, worse evening until 12 P.M.; must get out of bed and walk about; can hardly put foot to the ground; but pain lessens while walking.

Varicose veins inside of right thigh, then of left.

Numbness of thighs.

Neuralgia, throbbing at night; worse rest; better moving.

Legs feel weak.

Calves weak, as if bruised.

Cramps in calves, worse at rest, especially at night.

Toes contracted.

Shooting-pricking in right instep.

Cramp in soles of feet.

Heel pains.

Feet cold, numb, stiff.

Soles feel hot.

34 Limbs in General. Nightly tearing in arms and legs.

Swelling of hands: also of feet to the ankles.

35 Position, etc. Motion: 3, 32, 33, 40. Walking: 2, 21, 26,

27, 29, 32, 33, 36. Exertion: 5, 23, 27, 29. Stooping: 3.
Lying: 23, 27, 31, 36; on back: 37. Sitting: 3, 37.
Must sit up: 26, 27. Rising: 2. Must bend arm: 32.
Rest: 33.

³⁶ Nerves. Increased bodily irritability; excitable.
Restless, must walk slowly about.
Tired, aching, as from lying long in one position.
Prostration, lethargic dulness, vertigo.
So weak she must lie down.
Paralysis from loss of fluids.

³⁷ Sleep. Falls asleep: from debility; while sewing, sitting and
studying.
Sleepy at night with inability to sleep.
Anxious tossing in bed after 12 P.M.
Can lie only on the back, at night.
Child does not sleep because of itching from ascarides.
Dreams: vivid; confused; unpleasant.
Nightmare.

³⁸ Time. Morning: 6, 12, 16, 27, 40. Morn till noon: 40.
Evening: 1, 13, 26, 33, 40. Night: 5, 16, 19, 20, 21,
26; 27, 31, 32, 33, 34, 37, 40. After midnight: 3, 26,
37. Day: 13, 20, 21, 40.

³⁹ Temperature and Weather. Generally worse in cold, or
wet weather; better in warm air.
Cold air: 4; weather: 44. Cold washing: 8. Overheating: 8. Heat: 32. Warmth of bed: 26. Inclines to
uncover: 40.

⁴⁰ Chill. Fever. Sweat. Chilly every evening: hectic fever.
Frequent short attacks of chilly shivering.
Chill with hot and red face, thirst.
General coldness in evening, in bed, often lasting all night.
Chilly and want of animal heat.
Thirst with chill.
Dry heat, worse towards evening; face red; inclined to un-
cover; better moving or speaking, and after meals.
Sweat profuse, long-lasting, as well by day at every motion,
as at night and morning, in bed.
Clammy, generally debilitating sweat.
Every other (third) day sweat from morn till noon.
Strong-smelling night-sweat.
At times anxious cold sweat (with cramps of different
parts).
Sweat stains yellow, is fetid on going to sleep.
Worse while sweating.
Intermittent fever after abuse of quinine; congestions to
head; veins distended; vomiting ingesta; swelling of
spleen; anæmia masked by pseudo-plethora.

⁴¹ Attacks. Periodical attacks of pain.

Menses intermit.

Every other day: 40.

Pains increase gradually.

⁴² **Sides.** Left: 3, 13, 17, 18, 28, 40, 46. Right: 5, 6, 18, 31, 32, 33. Right to left: 33. Left to right: cramp in feet; pain in lungs.

⁴⁴ **Tissues.** Red parts become white.

Hemorrhages; blood light or lumpy; coagulates easily.

Blood-vessels distended, especially those of head, face, feet. .

Varices.

Pseudo-plethora; congestions, etc., yet anæmic; the face is earthy, flushing easily.

Erethric chlorosis, worse during cold weather.

Dropsy after loss of fluids, abuse of *Cinchon.*, intermittent fever; anasarca.

Glands swollen, with rending, tearing pains.

Bones disposed to soften or bend; fractures unite slowly.

Cracking in joints.

Sudden emaciation; muscles lax, limbs cold; weak digestion.

⁴⁵ **Contact, Injuries, etc.** Touch: 19, 32, 46. Pressure: 18.

Weight of bedclothes: 32.

Skin. Dry skin. *θ* Pneumonia.

Skin pale, yellow, sallow, dirty, withered, flabby.

Yellow-brown spots, sore to touch.

Scarlatina during desquamation.

Skin peels off on shoulders and left hand.

Warts on fingers and backs of hands.

Ulcers pale, œdematous.

⁴⁷ **Stages and States.** Delicate, chlorotic women.

Weak, nervous, yet face is very red.

Sanguine, choleric.

⁴⁸ **Relationship.** Ailments from *Arsen., Iodium, Cinchon.*

Complementary to: *Alum., Cinchon.*

Ferrum, like the sulphates, aggravates syphilis.

Antidotes to *Ferrum: Arsen., Cinchon., Hepar, Ipec., Pulsat.*

FERRUM IODATUM.

Iodide of Iron. · FeI_2.

⁶ **Ears.** ❙ Roaring.

⁸ **Face.** Injected, red.

¹⁹ **Abdomen.** Fulness even after a little food as if she had eaten too much, a sort of upward pressure; stuffed feeling as if she could not lean forwards.

[21] **Urine.** ı Dark colored, depositing a thick white sediment; urine scalds.

[23] **Female Sexual Organs.** ı Constant bearing down as if something was coming away; while sitting feels as if pushing something up; she can touch the cervix uteri (confirmed).

ı Retroversion of the uterus (many clinical cases).

Leucorrhœa like boiled starch; when the bowels move, the discharge is stringy.

Itching and soreness of vulva and vagina; parts much swollen.

FLUORICUM ACIDUM.

Hydrofluoric Acid.   HERING.   *HF.*

[1] **Mind.** Forgetfulness: in his daily employment; of dates.

Aversion to his own family.

Greatly depressed in mind.

Disposition to be exceedingly anxious; better morning than evening.

Apprehensiveness.

Feeling of indifference towards those he loves best; becomes interested and converses pleasantly with strangers.

Uncommon buoyancy of mind, fears nothing and is well satisfied with herself.

Ill-humored.

[2] **Sensorium.** Congestion of blood mostly to the forehead, with dulness in the occiput toward night.

Sensation of weakness, like numbness in head, same in hands.

[3] **Inner Head.** Compressing pain in the temples.

Headache in the occiput, with fulness in the head.

Headache from the nape, extending through the centre of head to the forehead; also dull feeling in the head.

[4] **Outer Head.** Sensation of numbness in the forehead.

Pain along the sutures.

Caries of the temporal bone.

Must comb the hair frequently, it mats so at the end.

Falling out of the hair, new hair dry and breaks off.

[5] **Eyes.** Heaviness above the eyes, with nausea; worse on motion.

Pressure, as if behind the right ball.

Dark spot before eye, worse reading.

Sensation as of a cold wind blowing under the lids (even in a warm room), must bind the eyes with a cloth.

Sensation of sand in the eyes, or as if a fresh wind was blowing on them.

Feeling as if he must wink, as if something was in the eye that could not be rubbed off.

Increased lachrymation.

Itching in the canthi.

Fistula lachrymalis.

⁶ **Ears.** Intolerable itching in both ears. Itching, better momentarily from scratching, but followed by burning.

⁷ **Nose.** Fluent coryza.

Obstruction of the nose.

Posterior nares feel expanded, during a walk.

Red, swollen, inflamed nose.

Itching on right side of nose.

⁸ **Face.** Pale.

Heat in face, wants to wash it in cold water.

Crusta lactea, dry, scaly, itches very much.

Tubercles in skin of forehead and face, suppurating.
θ Syphilis infantum.

¹⁰ **Teeth.** Sensation of: warmth; heaviness in the teeth; roughness of the teeth.

Mouth and teeth coated with mucus in the morning.

Toothache worse from cold drink; or improved until the water becomes warm in the mouth.

Rapid caries of teeth.

Violent pains at the root of the right eye-tooth, with frequent discharge of pus.

Great sensitiveness to pressure on the gum over the right eye-tooth.

¹¹ **Tongue, etc.** Acrid, foul taste from the roots of the teeth.

Tongue always more or less tender, feeling of rigidity in it, with restricted mobility; painful when talking.

Tongue: vivid red at tip and edges, coated yellow in the centre; whitish and dry.

Tongue deeply and widely fissured in all directions, with a large, deep phagedenic looking ulcer in the centre.

¹² **Mouth.** Increased flow of saliva.

¹³ **Throat.** Red blotches, size of half pea, over the palate and sides of cheek, bleeding easily.

Soft palate and uvula intensely red and much tumefied, breath fetid, voice nasal, articulation indistinct.

Accumulation of mucus in the fauces, disturbs sleep.

Throat peculiarly sensitive to cold, slightest exposure resulting in inflammation, with increase of pain and impeded deglutition.

Constriction in the throat, with difficult deglutition; in the morning, hawking of phlegm mixed with blood.

Excessive pain when swallowing.

¹⁴ **Desires. Aversions.** Hunger predominates.

Thirst, craves refreshing drinks. Desires wine.

Aversion to coffee.

¹⁵ **Eating and Drinking.** Warm drinks: 20. Cold drink:
10. Eating: 19. Complaints worse from sweet things.

¹⁶ **Nausea and Vomiting.** Nausea; with general heat; eructations and lassitude.

Bilious vomiting after slight errors in diet; with increased alvine discharges, preceded by tormina.

¹⁷ **Stomach.** Feeling of fulness and pressure in epigastrium.
Feeling of weight in the stomach between meals.

¹⁸ **Hypochondria.** Sensitive to pressure in right hypochondrium.

Pressing pain in region of spleen and left arm.

Pain from spleen to hip.

Pinching in region of spleen.

¹⁹**Abdomen.** Sensation of emptiness in region of navel, with desire to take a deep breath; better from bandaging or eating.

Great tension and dropsical swelling of the abdomen.

²⁰ **Stool, etc.** Frequent passage of flatus and belchings, with constriction of the anus.

Very loose, bright yellow stools, with a quantity of mucus, preceded by considerable griping.

Stools chiefly during the night or early in the morning.

Stools pappy, yellowish brown, fetid, with tenesmus and prolapsus ani.

Bilious diarrhœa worse during day, soon after drinking, especially warm drinks.

Tardy, infrequent and hard slools.

Itching in and around the anus.

²¹ **Urine.** Very frequent discharge of bright colored urine, with increased thirst.

Urine scanty and dark, painful in passing; alkaline.

Whitish or purple colored sediment.

Burning before and after urination, with aching in the bladder.

²² **Male Sexual Organs.** Increased sexual desire in old men, with violent erections at night.

Gleety discharge at night, staining the linen yellow.

Yellow drop from the urethra in the morning.

Dropsical swelling of the penis; also hydrocele.

Oily, pungent-smelling sweat on the genitals.

²³ **Female Sexual Organs.** Menses: too early; too copious; discharge thick and coagulated.

Metrorrhagia with, or in alternation with, difficulty of breathing.

Leucorrhœa acrid: also with itching.

24 Pregnancy. Itching, redness and swelling of right nipple; nipples sore, cracked; congestion to the head.

25 Larynx. Weak voice.

Dryness in larynx and trachea.

Itching in larynx, causing hawking and swallowing.

Soreness and increased irritability in larynx, with impeded respiration and wheezing.

26 Breathing. Difficult breathing, afternoon and evening: 23.

Oppression of chest, better when bending backwards.

Relieves in hydrothorax.

27 Cough. Short, frequent cough, mostly dry, occasionally some whitish, frothy mucous expectoration.

28 Lungs. Upper part of chest seems most affected.

Hydrothorax.

29 Heart. Pulse. Sore pain at the heart.

Small, frequent pulse.

30 Outer Chest. Scaly eruption on the chest and arms.

31 Neck. Back. Pain in the third cervical vertebra.

Rigidity of nape.

Bruised pain in sacrum.

32 Upper Limbs. Pain in right shonlder-joint; shoulder-joints stiffened by rheumatism.

Slight lameness in the right arm.

Rheumatic pains in left arm, from shoulder to elbow, with lameness.

Weakness and numbness of hands.

Constant redness of the hands, especially the palms.

Burning in the hands.

Sharp sticking pain at the root of right thumb-nail.

Acute pricking, as with needles, in the fingers.

Panaritium; ı also simple onychia.

Nails grow more rapidly, crumpled or longitudinal ridges in them.

33 Lower Limbs. Acute stitches in the right hip-bone.

Lameness in the left hip.

Pain in right knee-joint.

Left leg goes "to sleep" easily.

Œdematous swelling up to the abdomen; top of the foot œdematous.

Burning stitches in the soles. Feet hot and burn much.

Soreness between the toes. Soreness of all the corns.

34 Limbs in General. Pain in all the limbs.

35 Position, etc. Motion: 5, 40. Walking: 7. Exercise: 40.

Bending backwards: 26.

36 Nerves. Increased ability to exercise his muscles without fatigue, regardless of the most excessive heat in summer or cold in winter.

Loss of strength.

Sensation of going to sleep of side not laid on.

37 Sleep. Loss of sleep in evening, from crowding of thoughts. Sleeplessness, without inclination to sleep; a short sleep suffices and refreshes him.

Sleep restless and unrefreshing.

38 Time. Morning: 1, 10, 13, 20, 22. Afternoon: 26, 40. Evening: 1, 2, 26, 37, 40. Night: 20, 22, 44. Day: 20.

39 Temperature and Weather. Warm room: 5. Warmth: 46. Heat and cold: 36. Sensitive to cold: 13. Cold: 46. Cold water in mouth: 10. Desire to wash in cold water: 8, 40.

40 Chill. Fever. Sweat. Chill entirely wanting.

General heat, with nausea from the slightest motion, with inclination to uncover, but mostly to wash with cold water.

Clammy, sour and unpleasant-smelling sweat, mostly on upper body, particularly during exercise in afternoon and evening; sweat excessive on palms and feet.

The sweat promotes excoriation and decubitus.

42 Sides. Right: 5, 7, 10, 18, 24, 32, 33, 46. Left: 18, 32, 33.

43 Sensations. Violent jerking, burning pains confined to small spots.

44 Tissues. Diseases of bones, particularly of long bones, suppurate and get better and worse periodically: pains worse at night, with great prostration.

Liver enlarged and indurated.

Varicose veins of the legs; varicose ulcers; nævus, flat.

45 Contact, Injuries, etc. Pressure: 10. Bandaging: 19. Scratching: 6.

46 Skin. Burning pains on small spots of the skin.

Dry cutaneous eruptions; squamous eruptions on the body.

Elevated red blotches; erosions, mucous tubercles.

Nævus on right temple.

Ulcers: painful; worse from warmth, better from cold; with copious discharge, also on legs, worse at ankles, bones diseased.

Old cicatrices become red around the edges, covered or surrounded by itching vesicles, or they itch violently.

47 Stages and States. Complaints of old age, also premature old age, in consequence of syphilitic mercurial dyscrasy.

Weakly constitutions, sallow skin, emaciation.

48 Relationship. After abuse of whiskey, induration of liver; ascites.

Ailments from *Silic.;* also after abuse of mercury.

Fluor ac. follows well: after *Arsen.*, in ascites with diseased liver; after *Kali carb.*, in hip disease; after *Silic.*, in bone diseases; after *Phosph. ac.*, in diabetes (one case),

GAMBOGIA.

Gamboge.   HERRING.   *Guttiferæ.*

[1] **Mind.** Irritable mood.

[2] **Sensorium.** Vertigo during rest or motion, morning when rising.

Heaviness in the whole head, with dulness, sleepiness and pain in the back.

[5] **Eyes.** Violent burning of the eyes and photophobia, evening or afternoon, better from walking in the open air, but returning in the morning.

Violent itching of the eyes in the evening.

Itching at the inner canthi.

Nightly agglutination of lids, burning in morning, photophobia through the day, and frequent stitching pain in eyes.

[6] **Ears.** Ringing in left ear all the time.

[7] **Nose.** Violent chronic sneezing.

Dryness of the right nostril.

[10] **Teeth.** Tearing in all the right molars.

Sensation of coldness at the edge of the incisors.

[12] **Mough.** Dryness of the mouth.

[13] **Throat.** Violent stitches in the right side of the throat.

Pain as from soreness in the throat.

Rawness and burning in throat, causing constant hawking.

[14] **Desires. Aversions.** Thirst after dinner, and especially evenings.

[15] **Eating and Drinking.** After eating: 17, 19.

[16] **Nausea and Vomiting.** Frequent violent empty eructations.

Nausea preceding from stomach, when walking in open air.

Nausea, inclination to vomit, accumulation of saliva in mouth.

Frightful vomiting and purging, with fainting.

[16]**Stomach.** Empty feeling in the stomach and abdomen.

Gnawing in the stomach.

Constant sore pain in the stomach.

Ulcerative pain in the stomach, passing off after eating.

Acute stitches in the stomach.

[19] **Abdomen.** Pinching in abdomen immediately after eating.

Frequent severe pinching in entire abdomen without urging; or, with diarrhœa and burning in anus, with relief of pain.

Rumbling and rolling in the bowels.

Inflation and tension of the abdomen, with pinching in the umbilical region.

[20] **Stool, etc.** Profuse discharge of flatus, especially evening
and nights.

Stools: watery, slimy, undigested, without smell; with
pain in ileo-cœcal region, which is sensitive to touch;
during stool bearing down and colicky pain; prolapsus
ani and cold sweat on the limbs; copious, watery, yellow,
or like curdled milk, of offensive, sickening smell, expelled forcibly; dark green mucus, offensive and corrosive, discharged with a single somewhat prolonged effort;
great relief after stool, as though an irritating substance
were removed from the bowels; profuse, watery, with
colic and tenesmus; diarrhœic, with burning pain and
tenesmus; bloody, dysenteric.

Hard, insufficient stool, with strong urging, pressing and
protrusion of the rectum.

[21] **Urine.** Stitches in the left kidney.

Infrequent urination.

[23] **Female Sexual Organs.** Leucorrhœa.

[28] **Lungs.** Pressure in the middle of the chest.

Pain in the chest as if it were all raw.

[30] **Outer Chest.** Repeated extremely painful stitches in the
sternum.

Weight on the chest, causing sleeplessness.

[31] **Neck. Back.** Repeated gnawing in the os coccygis.

[32] **Upper Limbs.** Pain in the shoulders.

Stitching pains in the upper limbs, come on or are worse
in evenings.

[35] **Position, etc.** Rest: 2. Motion: 2. Rising: 2. Walking
in open air: 5, 16.

The majority of symptoms come on while sitting, and pass
off during motion in the open air.

[37] **Sleep.** Sleepiness, great inclination to sleep.

Sleep broken by anxious dreams.

Anxious, vexatious dreams.

[38] **Time.** The conditions as especially apt to occur toward
evening or at night.

Morning: 2, 5. Afternoon: 5. Evening: 5, 14, 20, 32,
46. Night: 5, 20, 46.

[40] **Chill. Fever. Sweat.** Violent chill, beginning in the
back. Increased heat with anxiety.

[42] **Sides.** Right: 7, 10, 13. Left: 6, 21.

[45] **Contact Injuries, etc.** Touch: 20. Scratching: 46.

[46] **Skin.** Violent itching in various parts of the body, burning
after scratching, worse evenings and nights.

After scratching, burning and ulcerative pain, with swelling and redness of the parts, worse evening and night.

Biting, like from ants, over the whole body, worse evening and night.

GELSEMIUM.

Yellow Jessamine.   WM. E. PAYNE.   *Loganiaceæ.*

[1] **Mind.** Cataleptic immobility, with dilated punils, closed eyes, but conscious.

Delirium in sleep; half waking, with incoherent talk.

Desires to be let alone; irritable, sensitive.

Loqnacity, brilliant eyes, shooting through temples and nasal sinuses; fever.

Depression of spirits; anxiety following a somewhat cheerful, careless mood.

Solicitude about the present.

Fear of death.

Mental exertions cause a sense of helplessness from brain weakness; inability to attend to anything requiring thought.

Complaints from bad or exciting news; from some unusual ordeal.

[2] **Sensorium.** Vertigo, confusion of the head, spreading from occiput over whole head; pupils dilated, dim sight; general depression from heat of sun or summer.

Vertigo, dim vision, fever; seems as if intoxicated when trying to move; worse from smoking.

Giddy, with loss of sight, chilliness, accelerated pulse; dulness of sight or double sight.

When attempting to move, the muscles refuse to obey the will; giddy, confused.

Child dizzy, when carried seizes hold of the nurse, fearing that it will fall.

[3] **Inner Head.** Severe pain in forehead and vertex, dim sight, roaring in ears; head feels enlarged; "wild feeling," alternating with uterine pains.

Hyperæmia of the brain; dull feeling in forehead and vertex, and a fulness in the region of the medulla before spasms.

Fulness in the head, heat of the face, chilliness; pulsation of the caroids; thick speech; brain feels as if bruised; eyeballs feel rew when moving them; double vision.

Heaviness of the head slightly relieved by shaking the head; better after profuse micturition.

Cerebro-spinal meningitis stage of congestion; severe chill, dilated pupils; congestion of spine and brain.

[4] **Outer Head.** Dull, dragging pain in occiput, mastoid and upper cervical regions, extending to shoulders; better quietly resting the head on a high pillow, with eyes half closed; eyes, heavy, sleepy, red.

Pressure on the vertex so great as to extend into shoulders; head feels very heavy.

Cramp-like drawing and tearing, worse from study and exertion, after fever and ague.

Neuralgic headache beginning in upper cervical spine; vertebra prominens sensitive; pains extend over head, causing a bursting pain in forehead and eyeballs; worse at 10 A.M., when lying; with nausea, vomit, cold sweat, cold feet.

Sensation of a band around head above ears; scalp sore.

⁵ **Eyes.** Pupils dilated.

Amaurosis of congestive origin; after apoplexy.

Sees double, when inclining the head towards the shoulder.

Confused vision, eyes look heavy.

Hazy vitreous, very fine.   Increased tension, balls sore.

Serous iritis; serous choroiditis; dull pain to back of head, better from hot applications.

Glaucoma from increased secretion rather than from obstructed excretion.

Detached retina from myopia, severe neuralgia, etc.

Astigmatism.

Eyeballs oscillate laterally when using them.

Eyelids heavy.   Eyes close when looking steadily.

Eyes feel sore in evening, sensitive to light, with lachrymation; lids feel full and congested.

⁶ **Ears.** Sudden transient loss of hearing, rushing and roaring in the ears.

Catarrhal deafness, with pain from throat into middle ear.

⁷ **Nose.** Violent morning paroxysms of sneezing; tingling in nose.

Watery, excoriating discharge; a feeling from throat up into left nostril, like a stream of scalding water; right nostril stopped up; nasal voice.

Coryza in spring and summer weather.

Edges of nostrils red, sore.

Fulness at root of nose; pains extending to neck and clavicles.

⁸ **Face.** Expression heavy, dull, drowsy.

Face: red; yellow, jaundiced; pale, sickly look.

Muscles of face, especially around the mouth, seem contracted, making speech difficult.

Orbital neuralgia in distinct paroxysms, with contractions and twitchings of the muscles on the affected side.

⁹ **Lower Face.** Lips dry; coated with dark mucus.

¹⁰ **Teeth.** Toothache from a cold, or purely nervous; pains from teeth to temple.

Dentition; child frantic, awakens with sudden screams; face deep red; fontanelle pulsates too strongly; pain about ear.

¹¹ **Tongue, etc.** Taste: foul, with blood-colored saliva; bitter. Clammy, feverish, during the sweat.

Tongue: yellowish-white, breath fetid; coated thick, brown; nearly clean; margin red, centre white.

Tongue and glottis partially paralyzed; speech thick, as if drunk, from congestion of base of brain.

Can hardly put tongue out, it trembles so; red, raw, painful, inflamed in the middle.

¹³ **Throat.** Fauces dry, burning, irritated, sore.

Throat feels as if filled up; tonsils inflamed, swollen, mostly in or beginning in the right.

Swallowing causes shooting in the ear.

Dysphagia; paralysis of the organs of deglutition.

Diphtheria, local tingling of parts during the fever; incipient paralysis, impaired vision.

Painful sensation of a lump in œsophagus.

Burning in the œsophagus to the stomach.

¹⁴ **Desires. Aversions.** Little appetite and thirst, but can take food or drink.

¹⁵ **Eating and Drinking.** Wine aggravates, especially the headache and eye symptoms.

Thirst absent or slight.

¹⁶ **Nausea and Vomiting.** Eructations sour.

Nausea, giddiness, headache.

¹⁷ **Stomach.** Cramp in the stomach, better riding and sitting erect,

Feeling of emptiness and weakness in stomach and bowels.

Rumbling and dull pain in the epigastrium, relieved by passage of flatus.

Oppression and fulness in the stomach, worse from pressure of clothing.

¹⁸ **Hypochondria.** Passive congestion of the liver, with vertigo, dim sight and fulness of the head.

¹⁹ **Abdomen.** Sudden spasmodic pain in the upper part of the abdomen, leaving a sensation of contraction and causing him to cry out.

Acute enteritis (catarrhal) during damp weather; warm or cold.

Gnawing pain in the transverse colon.

Wandering, pinching wind colic, less when sitting erect; .more beginning to move, less during continual motion.

Periodical colic, with yellow diarrhœa; evening.

Griping in the lower abdomen, relieved by passing copious bilious stools.

Tenderness in the right iliac region during typhus.

Rumbling in the abdomen, with discharge of wind up and down.

Sensation of soreness of the abdominal walls.

20 Stool, etc. Stools: yellow, fecal; bilious; cream-colored; clay-colored; color of green tea.

Diarrhœa: in nervous persons, subject to nervous chills; after sudden emotions, as grief, fright, bad news, the anticipation of an unusual ordeal.

21 Urine. Copious flow, relieving headache.

Incontinence from paralysis of the sphincter; nervous children.

Alternate dysuria and enuresis; spasms of bladder.

Albuminuria: 24, 36.

22 Male Sexual Organs. Sexual organs irritable, weak; involuntary emissions without erections; spermatorrhœa.

Emission of semen during stool.

Genitals cold, relaxed; dragging pains in the testicles.

Suppressed gonorrhœa; followed by rheumatism or orchitis.

Profuse warm sweat on the scrotum.

23 Female Sexual Organs. Threatened abortion from sudden depressing emotions.

Uterus, as if squeezed by a hand; anteflexion.

Ovarian irritation with the characteristic headache.

Menses suppressed, with congestion to the head; sharp darting, twitching pains in face and head; convulsions (every evening).

Dysmenorrhœa, preceded by sick headache, vomiting; congestion to head; deep red face; bearing down in the abdomen.

Leucorrhœa white, with aching across the lower part of back; heavy fulness in uterine region; amenorrhœa.

24 Pregnancy. During pregnancy: double vision, headache, drowsiness, vertigo, pulsating carotids, small, slow pulse; cannot walk for muscles will not obey; cramps in the abdomen and legs; convulsions with unconsciousness.

Labor-pains gone, os widely dilated, complete atony; drowsy., θ Albuminuria.

Albuminuria, thirstless, erratic pains.

Labor delayed by rigid os; or when pains go from before backward, the uterus seems to go upward. Pains leave womb and fly all over; os rigid.

Sensation like a wave, from uterus to throat, ending with a choking feeling; this seems to impede labor; impending spasms.

Convulsions during labor: 36.

Nervous chills, "chatters," first stage of labor.

25 Larynx. Hoarse in paroxysms, with dry, rough throat; rawness of the chest, catarrh.

Paralysis of glottis.

29

Hawking bloody water.

26 **Breathing.** Slow breathing and slow pulse; heavy, labored; congestion to the chest.

Long crowing inspiration; sudden and forcible expiration; spasm of the glottis.

27 **Cough.** Cough from tickling or roughness of the fauces; hoarse; rawness and soreness of the chest; coryza; bronchial catarrh.

Croupy cough; measles.

28 **Lungs.** Congestive pneumonia, with suffering under the scapulæ, both sides; caused by checked sweat. Short paroxysms of pain superior part of right lung, on taking a deep breath; pulse slow, full.

29 **Heart. Pulse.** Excessive action of the heart.

A peculiar action of the heart, as though it attempted its beat which it failed fully to accomplish, the pulse intermitting each time; worse lying, especially on the left side.

Fears that unless constantly on the move, her heart will cease beating.

Nervous chill, yet skin is warm; wants to be held that she may not shake so. θ Heart disease.

Heart's action: feeble, slow; depressed; hands and feet cold.

Pulse frequent, soft, weak, almost imperceptible; slow and full.

30 **Outer Chest.** Periodical pains in the pectoral muscles.

31 **Neck. Back.** Pains from spine to head and shoulders.

Contractive sensation in the right side of the nape.

Pains in the neck, myalgic, mostly in the upper part of the sterno-cleido muscles, back of the parotid glands.

Congestion of the spine; prostration, languor; muscles feel bruised and will not obey the will.

Locomotor ataxia. Paraplegia.

Dull aching in the lumbar and sacral region; cannot walk, muscles will not obey.

32 **Upper Limbs.** Deep-seated muscular pains in both arms.

Palms hot, dry.

Coldness of wrists and hands.

Arms, weak, numb.

33 **Lower Limbs.** Deep-seated muscular pains in the legs, relieved by motion.

Shooting pains in paroxysms.

Drawing, contracting, crampy pains in the legs, from thighs into toes; worse on motion or walking.

Heaviness, weight; loss of voluntary motion; muscles will not obey the will; calves feel bruised; pain at night.

Feeling when walking, as in a partial luxation of patella.

Coldness of the extremities, especially of the feet, as if in cold water, with anguish and pain in the legs.

[34] **Limbs in General.** Limbs cold, with oppressed breathing; cold hands and feet.

Deep-seated dull aching in the limbs and joints generally; induced by cold, and attended with loss of motion.

Neuralgic pains in the limbs, as a sequel to scarlatina.

[35] **Position, etc.** · Wants to lie still.

Resting on high pillow, head better.

Sitting erect: 17, 19. Walking: 33; in open air: 39. Cannot walk: 24, 31. Moving: 2, 3. Motion: 33. Worse beginning to move, better from continued motion: 10. Fears to remain quiet: 29. Shaking head: 3. Exertion: 40. Lying: 4, 29; with head high: 4.

[36] **Nerves.** Excessive irritability of mind and body; vascular excitement.

Convulsions from reflex irritation; spasms of one leg.

Puerperal spasms, preceded by great lassitude, dull feeling in the forehead and vertex, fulness in the region of the medulla; head feels "big;" heavy, with half stupid look; face deep red; speech thick; pulse slow, full; from protracted labor; rigid os uteri; albuminuria.

Tetanic spasms; jaws locked.

Jactitation of the muscles.

Paralysis of motion; muscles will not obey the will, feel bruised. Tingling, pricking, crawling.

Neuralgia. Acute, sudden, darting pains; shooting, tearing along the tracks of the nerves; especially if aggravated by changes in the weather.

[37] **Sleep.** Yawning, chilly.

Sleeplessness; a wide-awake feeling.

Sleepless from violent itching of face, head and shoulders; sleepless during dentition; face red; also from exhaustion.

As soon as he falls asleep, delirious.

Awakened by headache or colic.

Drowsy, dim sight; a kind of drunken stupor.

Stupor in beginning of fevers; especially with children.

Languid, drowsy, but cannot compose the mind for sleep.

Wakeful or lies in a half awake state, with incoherent talk.

[38] **Time.** Morning: 7. Forenoon: neuralgic headache (10 A.M.). Afternoon: 40. Evening: 5, 19, 23.

[39] **Temperature and Weather.** Worse in damp weather, before a thunder-storm; southeast wind: 19. Heat of sun or summer: 2. Open air: 39. Change of weather: 36.

[40] **Chill. Fever. Sweat.** Chilliness, languid aching in back

and limbs; sense of fatigue, desires to avoid all muscular exertion; every afternoon, 4 to 5 P.M.

Chills begin in the hands; chills running up the back; hands and feet cold,

Feet cold, with heat of the head and face; headache.

Slight occasional moisture; sweat coming gradually and moderately, always relieving the pains.

Sweats freely from slight exertion.

ı Typhoid fever, when so-called nervous symptoms predominate.

Low fevers when pulse is slow, and by lifting or turning the patient, it becomes accelerated.

Eruptive fevers: especially children, tendency to convulsions at the time of the eruption.   Intense fever heat, erethism, but less restlessness than *Acon.;* less violence and suddenness of aggravation than *Bellad.;* languid; asthenic fever; stupor.

⁴¹ **Attacks.**   Fevers remit or intermit.

ı   Periodical attacks.

ꝗᴛˠ Every day at the same hour.

⁴² **Sides.**   Right: 7, 13, 19, 28, 31.   Left: 7   Right to left: 13.
Below upwards: 7, 10, 40.   Before backwards: 24.

⁴⁴ **Tissues.**   Congestions, arterial or venous, with sluggish circulation.

Hemorrhages, blood in drops, crimson.

Affects more the nerves of motion; causes muscular prostration through the nerves.

Catarrhs of mucous membranes; watery mucus, never purulent discharges.

⁴⁵ **Contact, Injuries, etc.**   Pressure: 17.   Riding: 17.

⁴⁶ **Skin.**   Papular eruption, like measles, especially on face.

Skin hot, dry; gastric and nervous fevers.

Erythema, especially in face and neck.

⁴⁷ **Stages and States.**   Young persons; children.

Women.

Nervous persons; excitable.

⁴⁸ **Relationship.**   Antidotes: *Cinchon; Coffea*, salt.

GLONOINUM.

Nitro-glycerin.   HERING. $C_3H_5(NO_2)O_3$.

¹ **Mind.**   Loses senses, sinks down unconscious, congestion alternately to head and heart.

Well-known streets seem strange; way home too long; forgets on which side she lives.

Bright, loquacious, great flow of ideas.

Weeps and shudders between attacks of pain.

Agitation, attempts to run away.

Frantic; attempted to jump from window (with headache).

Fear, throat feels swollen; chest as if screwed together; apprehensive of approaching death; fears she has been poisoned.

² Sensorium. Head felt larger.

Balancing sensation, constant effort to keep head erect.

Vertigo: confusion, faintness, black spots before eyes; worse from stooping or moving head; worse in the open air.

Syncope, nausea, face pale or livid; beating in the head.

Sunstroke: vertigo, violent pain; pale face, feeble pulse; labored breathing, nausea; comatose; or, throbbing in head; face yellowish-red, or livid; eyes fixed; pulse full, slow; tongue coated, no appetite.

³ Inner Head. Tensive pain over eyes and nose, also behind ears, followed by choking sensation about throat.

Headache from below upwards.

Sensation of soreness through whole head, is afraid to shake head; it seems to him as if head would drop to pieces.

Shocks in the brain synchronous with the pulse.

Throbbing: in temples; in vertex; occiput; in whole head.

Dull headache in the forehead, with warm sweat.

Severe pain in forehead, throbbing in the temples, worse from walking.

Dull, pressive pain, worse in occiput and neck; worse from moving head or twisting the neck.

Brain feels too large; bursting feeling; fulness, throbbing of arteries; all the blood seems to be pumped upwards; holds the head with the hands.

Brain as if moving in waves.

Congestion to head, sudden, violent; throbbing felt with every pulse, at every step, or jarring; blood mounts from neck, throat or chest; from occiput toward eyes.

Hemicrania, sees half light, half dark.

Headache with increased secretion of urine.

Headache with red face, accelerated pulse, sweat on face, unconsciousness; better in open air, after sleep, after vomiting.

Cri encephalique.

Headaches worse: from shaking or jarring the head; stooping; bending it backwards; after lying down; when ascending steps; in damp weather; in the sun; while working under gaslight; after overheating, with copious sweat; could not bear touch of hat; cold water (even causing spasms); reading, writing; wine.

Better: from uncovering; in open air.

Headache.

❙ Sunstroke.

⁴ Outer Head. Consequences of cutting the hair.

Rigidity of occipito frontalis.

Head feels too large.

⁵ Eyes. Flashes of lightning, sparks, before eyes.

Objects dance with every pulsation.

Dim sight with vertigo, with fainting, black spots before the eyes.

Pupils contracted. θ Sunstroke.

Pupils dilated; eyes upturned; sunstroke; eyes rolled outwards and up; convulsions.

Eyes injected red, protruding, wild, staring; eyes dull, staring, sunken.

Photophobia.

Sees everything half light, half dark.

Letters appear smaller.

Drawing, pressing, aching, bursting pain; soreness, quivering, twitching.

⁶ Ears. Deafness, ears as if stopped up, deafness followed by blurred vision.

Ringing in the ears, audible pulse.

Throbbing-piercing from within outward, in right ear.

Throbbing: above ears; from occiput to ears.

Sensation of fulness in and around ears.

Ears red.

⁷ Nose. Pains in root of nose, headache extends to nose.

Sudden sneezing; fluent coryza.

⁸ Face. Flushed, hot, especially about the eyes and forehead, with headache; livid, purple; alternately flushed and pale; pale during the heat, in sunstroke, congestions to brain, etc.

Sweat on the face.

Faceache, muscles twitch, even unconsciousness, breathing stertorous; faceache worse in heat of bed.

Masseter muscles affected.

Sudden neuralgic pains from decayed tooth, concentrating in temple; head heavy, but cannot lay it on the pillow.

⁹ Lower Face. Jaws clenched in sunstroke.

Lower lips feel swollen.

Chin feels elongated.

¹⁰ Teeth. Pulsating, throbbing pains, teeth feel elongated; decayed.

Stabbing in gums, worse from hot applications, better from cold.

¹¹ Tongue, etc. Taste: bitter, with nausea; aromatic, sweet, warm, leaves fatty taste.

Tongue: milk-white without coating, violent headache; or, light coating; cannot eat; weak; typhoid; feels swollen, raw; numb, as if burnt; prickling, stinging.

Difficulty in conversing, from diminished power of tongue and confusion of ideas.

¹² **Mouth.**   Saliva increased, slimy.

Froth about mouth.   *θ* Convulsions.

Sensation of soreness and swelling on roof of mouth, with pulsation.

¹³ **Throat.**   Soft palate: dry; feels as if drawn up.

Hard palate, sensitive as if swollen; throbbing; swollen sensation in the fauces.

Throat feels as if swelling; full sensation in both sides of neck.

Constriction at top of larynx; in throat, as if throttled.

Tickling, heat, soreness in ;throat.

¹⁴ **Desires.   Aversions.**   Increased desire to smoke.

Wants cold water; also from dry, parched feeling.

Loss of appetite; sunstroke, etc.

¹⁵ **Eating and Drinking.**   Wine aggravates all symptoms.

Alcoholic stimulants cause delirium, congestions, stupor.

¹⁶ **Nausea and Vomiting.**   Nausea: with the congestions; retching, during sunstroke, and faint feeling; causing sweat, which relieves.

Vomiting: spasmodic, in hydrocephalus; in sunstroke.

¹⁷ **Stomach.**   Pain in stomach; distress in epigastrium; sunstroke.

Stomach and head feel as if he had been out in hot sun.

Gnawing in epigastrium.

Faint feeling at pit of stomach; also, with throbbing there.

Pain in pit of stomach, as if sore, when touched; worse when stooping.

¹⁹ **Abdomen.**   Rumbling in bowels, belching, passing offensive flatus.

Cutting, mostly below the navel (wakens one in morning).

²⁰ **Stool, etc.**   Stools: loose, scanty, with much rumbling; copious, loose, dark, lumpy, with colic, heat in the anus, nausea and sudden urging.

Diarrhœa, with sudden cessation of the menses.

Costive.

²¹ **Urine.**   Abundant, highly albuminous; must rise often at night to pass it; high colored, burning while passing; with red sediment and reddish-yellow slime.

²³ **Female Sexual Organs.**   Instead of menses: congestion to head, face pale; worse in warm room; better when walking in the cold air; diarrhœa; fainting.

Before, during and after menses, or when it does not appear, fulness in the head, throbbing.

At climaxis: flushes of heat, pressure in head, nausea, loss
of senses, vertigo, swelling of feet.

[24] **Pregnancy.**   During pregnancy congestions.
Eclampsia: unconscious; face bright red; puffed; pulse
full, hard; urine copious and albuminous.

[26] **Breathing.** Breathing: heavy, labored, stertorous; oppressed;
from feeling of weight; accelerated; must often breathe
deeply; sighing.

[28] **Lungs.**   Chest feels as if laced.
Sinking feeling in head and chest, as from working in hot
room.
Congestions to chest alternately with head.
Numb sensation moving upwards in chest and down left
arm.

[29] **Heart. Pulse.**   Laborious action of the heart; oppression
frequent pulse.
Pressure in heart as if it was being contracted.
Sharp pains in the heart.
Fulness in the heart.
Anxiety in præcordia; weakness.
Heart's action easily excited; violent palpitation, throbbing
carotids, pulsating headache; worse stooping.
Purring noise in region of heart when lying; pulse intermittent; must have head high; worse when lying on
left side; better on right.
Pulse: accelerated; rises and falls alternately; increased
during headache, motion, walking; quick, small, irreg-
ular, with violent action of heart; low, feeble, in sunstroke.

[30] **Outer Chest.**   Sweat on the chest.
[31] **Neck. Back.**   Nape of neck stiff, with headache,
Sharp cutting across scapulæ.
Hot sensation down the back; burning between scapulæ.
Pain down entire spine; after constriction in chest; shiv-
erings downward.
Old contusions.

[32] **Upper Limbs.**   Arms: nervous, uneasy; heavy, as if circu-
lation was checked; numbness, heaviness following the
throbbing; numbness, weariness in left arm.
Weakness of wrist after headache.
Rheumatic pains in fingers of left hand.
Feels pulse in fingers.

[33] **Lower Limbs.**   Knees give way, thigh weak during headache; left thigh numb.
Limbs relaxed, motionless in sunstroke.
Rheumatism of left knee, deep twinging, pricking; worse
from motion; better from straightening limb.
Could not rise on account of weakness in limbs; headache,
worse when covered.

Cold feet, with nausea, palpitation.

³⁵ Position, etc. Worse from moving, shaking, jarring parts. Walking eases pain in limbs.

Better from general motion.

Walking: 3, 29.　Motion: 29, 33; of head: 2, 3.　Ascending: 3.　Stepping or jarring: 3.　Cannot lay head on pillow: 9.　Must have head high: 29.　Lying: 3, 29.　Worse lying on left, better on right side: 29.　Stooping: 2, 3, 17, 29.　Bending head backward: 3.

³⁶ Nerves. Prostration.

Restlessness in limbs, must rise and walk.

Convulsions; epileptiform, cerebral congestion, scanty or suppressed menses; hands clinched, thumbs in palms, face red, eyes rolled upwards, then sopor; left-sided, with fingers spread; face alternately red and pale.

³⁷ Sleep. Drowsy, yawning; face hot and pale.

Restless sleep; awakens with fear of apoplexy.

Confused dreams.

Difficult to awaken.

³⁸ Time. Worse morning and forenoon; headache, languor, colic.

Worse afternoon and evening; headache, diarrhœa.

³⁹ Temperature and Weather. Warmth: 10.　Warm room: 23.　Heat: 3, 40.　Heat of bed: 8.　Sun: 3.　Cold: 10, 23.　Open air: 2, 3, 23.　Damp weather: 3.

। Children after being out in the winter cold, warm their feet at the fire and fall asleep there.

⁴⁰ Chill. Fever. Sweat. Chill: after getting heated; alternates with sweat; with vomiting; head as if screwed up; intermittent fever.

Warmth general; flushes; waves of heat upwards; fever heat, with quick, small pulse, in sunstroke.

Sweat: relieves; most profuse on face and chest; cold on face during congestions; after sleep.

⁴² Sides. Right: 6.　Left: 32. 33, 36.　Above downwards: 28, 31.　Below upwards: 3, 28, 40.

⁴⁴ Tissues. Congestions, blood tends upwards; vessels pulsate; veins (jugular, temporal) enlarged.

Seeming plethora, rapid deviations in distribution of blood.

⁴⁵ Contact, Injuries, etc. Pain and other sensations following late after local injuries.

Touch: 3, 17.　Holding head with hands: 3.

⁴⁷ Stages and States. Females florid, plethoric; sensitive.

Nervous, sanguine, readily affected.

⁴⁸ Relationship. Antidotes to *Glonoinum: Acon., Camphor., Coffea, Nux vom.*

GNAPHALIUM.

Everlasting. *Compositæ.*

[36] **Nerves.** Intense pain along the sciatic nerve; feeling of numbness occasionally taking place of sciatica, and then exercise on foot is excessively fatiguing. (Confirmed in sciatica.)

Gouty pains in the big toes.

[48] **Relationship.** Compare: *Chamom.*, *Coloc.* When either the genito-crural, or the anterior crural nerve is affected, *Xanthox.* is usually the remedy.

GRAPHITES.

Plumbago. HAHNEMANN. *Carbon, amorphous.*

[1] **Mind.** Forgetfulness; dim recollection of recent events.

Weakness in the head, can scarcely think.

Slow in thought.

Dread of work. Hates work.

Mood: changeable; sad, with thoughts of death; sad and weeping; forlorn; depressed; dejected.

Full of fear in the morning.

Solicitude concerning spiritual welfare.

Great anxiety.

Much inclined to grief.

Hesitates at trifles. Timidity.

Fretful. Ill-humored. Easily vexed. Irritable.

Child impudent, teasing, laughs at reprimands.

Fidgety while sitting at work.

Scientific labor fatigues him.

Thoughts of many things at night prevent sleep.

Ailments from grief.

[2] **Sensorium.** Attacks of dizziness, with inclination to fall forward; feels as if drunken when rising from bed in the morning.

Dulness of the head.

Rush of blood, with feeling of heat in the head.

Vertigo: on looking upwards; in the morning on awaking; in the evening, was obliged to lie down; during and after stooping, with inclination to fall forward; venous stagnation.

Frequently feels faint, with partial loss of senses.

Desolate, empty feeling in the head.

Beclouded feeling in the forehead.

[3] **Inner Head.** Forehead: pressure deep in; drawing; tearing; bursting.

Stinging or stitching pains in the temples.

Throbbing in the sides of the head.

Pressive pain: in the vertex; in the occiput.

Tearing pain in one side of head, in teeth and glands of throat.

Pain as if constricted with a cord, particularly in occiput.

Pain from left temple down the side of the face to the shoulder; face distorted; left corner of mouth drawn inward and downward.

Lancinating pain in right temple.

Violent headache, with nausea, during the menses.

[4] **Outer Head.** Scalp feels bruised.

Sensation as if the skin of forehead were drawn into folds.

Coldness of the scalp.

Burning on the vertex in a small spot.

Sweat on the head when walking in the open air.

Itching on the scalp.

Eczema capitis, of entire scalp, forming massive, dirty crusts, which mat the hair together; scabs sore to touch.

Bald places on the head perfectly smooth and shining.

Circumscribed bald spot on front of head covered with herpes.

Porrigo decalvans.

Hair falls out, even on the sides of the head.

[5] **Eyes.** Intolerance of light; with redness of the white of the eye; hyperæsthesia of eyes, with the vertigo.

Shunning daylight usually more than gaslight; photophobia.

Light dazzles the eyes; sunlight causing lancinating pains in the eyes.

Shortsightedness.

Letters: appear double when writing; run together when reading; sees fiery zigzags around the outside of the field of vision, in the evening, with the eyes open.

Flickering before the eyes.

Sees as through a mist; everything turns black before the eyes when stooping.

Tiredness of the eyes.

Pressing pain in the eyes, morning and evening.

Drawing, extending from the eye up into the head.

Stitches from the temple through the eye to inner canthus, on looking at anything white or red, or at the sun.

Smarting in the eyes, with heat in them.

Burning and aching in eyes; burning pain around the eyes.

Ulcer on the cornea, with a few small vessels running into it; with moist fissured eczematous eruptions.

Pustules on the cornea and conjunctiva, with much lachrymation.

Pustule on the cornea, of reddish appearance, with white halo around it; the corners of lids raw and bleed easily.

Arthritic ophthalmia, with contraction and irregularity of the pupils.

Lachrymation in the open air; also chronic.

Thin, acrid discharge from the eyes; pus-like discharge from the eyes.

Internal canthus: itching; burning; stitches; sore.

External canthus: sore and fissured; fissured and bleed easily.

Heat in the eyes and some pus in the canthi.

Swelling of the eyelids and lachrymal gland.

Heaviness of the eyelids; cannot open his eyes.

Lids: feel dry, rough with itching; edges inflamed or covered with scurf; agglutinated night and morning; œdematous.

Left lower lid hangs down.

Inverted lids (margins); wild hairs.

Styes on lower lid, with drawing pain—may prevent return.

On both eyes hordeola and chalaza in all stages, also wens.

Coldness over the eyes.

Twitchings beneath the eyes.

[6] **Ears.** Music makes her weep.

Reverberations in the ear, even his own words and every step.

Hissing; ringing; rushing; roaring; cracking; or clucking sounds in the ears.

Violent nocturnal roaring, ears feel stuffed at times (dur-the full of moon).

Sounds as of rolling thunder before the ears.

Cracking in the ear: when eating in the evening; on moving the jaw, but only in the morning while lying in bed; when sneezing.

Snapping in the ear after every eructation, as if air penetrated the eustachian tube.

Sensation as as if a skin were before the ears.

At every step feels as if a valve in right ear opened and closed.

Loss of hearing, with dryness of the ears.

Acute pressure in the inner ear, like otalgia.

Stitches in the ears.

Distended capillaries on the membrane of right drum.

[I] Both tympana covered with a white coating, but not perforated.

Lining membrane of meatus red and excoriated.

Thin, watery, offensive discharge from both ears.

Gluey, sticky discharge at the external meatus.

Pus runs out of the ear.

Bad odor from the ear.

Copper-colored nodes on the ears.

Swelling of both ears, with moist eruption behind the ears.

Eczema impetiginoides; began as a moisture behind the left ear, thence spread over the cheeks and neck.

Behind the ears: fissures; scabs.

[7] **Nose.** Sense of smell too acute; cannot bear the smell of flowers.

Smell from the nose as from burned hair.

Loss of smell: with dryness of nose; with coryza.

Nosebleed: in the evening, the afternoon preceding rush of blood to the head and heat of the face; at night; in the morning; with running coryza.

Bloody mucous discharge from the nose.

Frequent discharge of thick, yellowish, fetid mucus from the nose.

Purulent, fetid secretion.

Dryness of the nose.

Sneezing: on opening the eyes; either with dryness of nose or running coryza.

Stoppage of the nose, with secretion of tough, badly-smelling mucus.

Coryza on getting cold.

Excoriation of the nose.

Mucus often forms hard masses or crusts in coryza.

Dry scabs in the nose, with sore, cracked and ulcerated nostrils.

Swelling of the nose.

Red nose, with black pores.

[8] **Face.** Face: pale and haggard; pale and bloated; chlorotic; flushed.

Erysipelas: of both sides of the face, with burning-stinging pain; of the cheeks, preceded by alternating chills and heat; of left cheek, after mal-application of *Iodum* for sore of inner nose; of face, from the smell of wood; commencing on right side and going to left.

Hemiplegia facialis (several cases).

Humid pimples on the face.

Moist eczema on the face.

Rhagades on the cheek, running like radii toward the corners of the mouth; an infiltrated spot on the cheek, is covered with dry scales.

Scabs on the face, skin dry, constipated, large stools.

Freckles.

Hair of the whiskers or beard falls out.
⁹ **Lower Face.** Painful nodules on the lower jaw.
Upper lip: twitching; stinging; swollen; painful pimples.
Corners of mouth ulcerated.
Heaviness in the lower lip.
Formication in the lips during the menses.
Lips chapped.
Swelling of the submaxillary glands painful to touch.
¹⁰ **Teeth.** Pressing pain in the teeth, worse from touch or biting.
Drawing pain in the molars while walking in the wind.
Tearing pain, worse by warmth; renewed by going to bed.
Stinging toothache after cold drink.
Toothache, worse at night.
Painful soreness on the inner side of the gums.
Swelling of the gums and dryness of the mouth.
¹¹ **Tongue, etc.** Taste: sour; salty; bitter; like rotten eggs.
Tongue sensitive.
Tongue coated white.
Whitish, painful ulcer on lower surface of the tongue.
¹² **Mouth.** Rotten odor from the mouth and gums.
Acid, foul odor.
Breath smells like urine.
Saliva increased, much spitting.
Dryness of the mouth in the morning.
¹³ **Throat.** Palate: feels sore; and fauces somewhat reddened.
Violent catarrh of the fauces, with sensation as if tough
  food had to pass over a lump in the throat.
Constant cramp in the throat, causing him to retch, as if
  the food would not go down.
Nightly pains in the throat, like a plug.
Ulcerative pain in the throat.
Roughness and rawness in the throat.
Hawking of phlegm.
Throat seems full of gurgling mucus.
¹⁴ **Desires. Aversions.** Appetite: good; excessive hunger,
  or no appetite, with much thirst, or with fulness of the
  abdomen.
Desire for drink, without thirst.
Aversion to: meat; fish; cooked food; salt.
¹⁵ **Eating and Drinking.** Worse when hungry.
Must eat: 17, 26. After eating: 17, 19, 40; dinner: 37;
  boiled meat: 17. After drinking: 40. Drinking warm
  milk: 17. Cold drink: 10, 17.
¹⁶ **Nausea and Vomiting.** Hiccough after either one or all
  meals.
Eructations: sour; tasting of the food eaten; relieve the
  pressure in the stomach.
Rancid heart-burn after dinner.

Qualmishness: mornings and several hours after dinner.
Nausea: and vertigo; and sweat, with anxiety; like faintness, prevents sleep; with spasm in the throat; with
eructation; with headache; with inclination to vomit;
and sour vomiting; in the morning; after eating.
Vomiting: sour; of food.
Vomiting, purging, and icy-cold sweat, with headache.

[17] **Stomach.** Sickening, painful feeling at the pit of stomach.
Pressure in the pit of stomach, night and morning.
Binding, constricting pain in gastric region.
Sensation of lump in the stomach, with constant beating,
as of two hammers.
Pain in stomach: necessitates eating; better from warm
milk, worse from boiled meat, worse from cold drink.
Nightly pinching pain in the stomach, and rooting pain
in the chest.
Griping in the stomach, with flatulency.
Fulness in the stomach and abdomen.
Periodical gastralgia, with vomiting of the food immedi-
ately after eating.
Chronic gastritis, with thirst, especially after the abuse of
alcoholic drinks.
Chronic catarrh of stomach, with frequent eructations.

[18] **Hypochondria.** Stitches in the right hypochondrium.
Hardness in region of the liver.
Stitches in the left hypochondrium.
Burning in the left hypochondrium, internally, worse
when lying on it.
Cannot bear tight clothing around the hypochondria.
Cutting, bearing down pains in the hypochondria and hips.

[19] **Abdomen.** Cramp in the lower abdomen.
Colic: immediately after eating.
Griping, digging pains in the abdomen.
Pain in the belly, in the left side, when lying on the right,
and vice versa.
Pain below the navel, as if the intestines were torn.
Stitches in the left side of the abdomen.
Burning pains radiating through abdomen, in gastralgia.
Abdomen distended, hard.
Accumulation of serum in the abdominal cavity.
Œdema of external abdomen.
Itching of the abdomen.
Large blisters on raised base, from navel to spine.
Rumbling in the abdomen.
Incarcerated flatus.
Pain in the inguinal regions.
Painful pressing toward the groin and anus.
Herpetic eruption in the groins.

Glandular swelling in the groins.

²⁰ **Stool, etc.** Excessive discharge of flatus.

Stools: rarely diarrhœic and then usually painless; purging and vomiting, with icy-cold sweat; knotty, the lumps being united by mucous threads; sour-smelling; thin, scalding, light brown; brown fluid, mixed with undigested substances, and very fetid; hard, lumpy, with blood and slime.

Constipation: large, knotty feces; chronic, with hardness in region of liver; with dryness of mucous membrane of rectum and fissure of the anus.

After stool there is some mucus remaining about the anus.

❙ Tapeworm.

❙ Fissura ani; severe, sharp, cutting pain during stool, followed by constriction and aching for several hours, worse at night.

Protrusion of rectum, without urging to stool, as if the anus were lame.

Large hemorrhoidal tumors.

Hemorrhoids, with pain on sitting down, or on taking a wide step, as if split with a knife, also violent itching, and very sore to touch.

Hemorrhoids of the rectum, with burning rhagades at the anus.

²¹ **Urine.** Urging to urinate, with scanty discharge.

Frequent urination at night.

Urine: dark brown; becomes turbid and deposits a white or reddish sediment; smells sour.

Stitches or smarting in the urethra when urinating.

Pain in the os coccygis while urinating.

²² **Male Sexual Organs.** Uncontrollable sexual excitement; violent erections.

Impotence, with dislike to coition.

Want of proper sensation during coition.

Almost involuntary emission, without erection.

Nocturnal emissions, with flaccid penis.

Dropsical swelling of the prepuce and scrotum.

Hydrocele (left side), with herpetic eruption on scrotum.

²³ **Female Sexual Organs.** Great aversion to coitus.

Tumor, size of an orange, right iliac fossa, also similar one in left; both hard, round, slightly movable; not painful to pressure, nor producing inconvenience from weight.

Pains from left ovary through pelvis and down the thigh.

Os uteri standing backwards, can only be reached with difficulty.

Pain in the uterus when reaching high with the arms.

Bearing down pain in the uterus to the back, with weakness and sickness.

Painful pressure towards the pudenda.

Menses: too scanty and too pale; too late, with violent colic; blood sometimes dark.

During the menses: heat in abdomen; urging, pressing like labor-pains; hoarseness; lassitude and weakness.

Copious leucorrhœa, before and after the menses.

Profuse leucorrhœa, perfectly white, especially on rising from the bed in the morning, weakness of the back when walking or sitting.

ı Leucorrhœal discharges occur in gushes day or night.

Vesicles or excoriations in the vagina.

Vagina cold.

Œdema of the pudenda.

Excoriations in perineum, vulva and between thighs.

²⁴ **Pregnancy.** Tendency to obesity.

Nipples painful.

Cancer of the mammæ, from old cicatrices, which had remained after repeated abscesses.

ı Hard cicatrices remaining after mammary abscess.

²⁵ **Larynx.** Voice: not clear, in singing; hoarseness in the evening; chronic hoarseness.

Laryngeal region sensitive to touch.

Soreness and roughness of larynx, and tickling cough.

²⁶ **Breathing.** Respiration has dry sound.

Constriction of chest, as if about to suffocate, when falling asleep.

Suffocative attacks waken from sleep, generally after midnight, has to jump out of bed, take hold of something, and must eat something.

²⁷ **Cough.** Cough: caused by deep inspiration; with strangling, red face, watery eyes, straining all over; loose, from tickling deep in the chest; at night.

Expectoration: salty; day and evening.

²⁸ **Lungs.** Cramps of the chest.

Pains in the chest.

Pain in the middle of the chest, with cough, scraping, rawness and soreness.

Stitching pains in the chest.

²⁹ **Heart. Pulse.** Region of heart: constriction; pressure; stitches.

Sensation like an electric shock, from heart toward front of neck.

Strong pulsation of the blood in the whole body, but especially about the heart, increased by every motion.

Palpitation of the heart: with anxiety; with nosebleed.

Pulse full and hard, somewhat accelerated in the morning, slow during day and evening.

³⁰ **Outer Chest.** Stinging in fleshy part of chest.

30

Pimples on the chest.

[31] **Neck. Back.** Pain in nape of neck.

Stiffnesss of back of neck; also, with headache.

Seventh cervical vertebra sensitive, with burning pain; anæmia.

Eruption on the nape, dry, peeling in fine, mealy scales, without itching.

Unpainful swollen glands on side of neck.

Contracting pains in the back.

Weakness in back and loins on walking.

Sacral pains, with sensation of crawling and stitching.

Small of back aches, as if bruised or broken.

Numb pain, from the sacrum down the legs.

Pain in the os coccygis while urinating.

[32] **Upper Limbs.** Shoulder and neck painful.

Rheumatic or burning pains, especially in left shoulder.

Burning pressure beneath the armpit.

Jerking in the arms.

Arms feel "asleep."

Right upper arm sore, tender and swollen.

Herpes circinatus hard to the touch and wrinkled looking, itching terribly, in bend of the elbow.

Left hand becomes numb and like dead, with formication extending up the arm.

Cramp in the hand.

Horny callosities in the hands.

Pain in the thumb-joint, as if sprained.

Gouty swelling of the fingers.

Raw, moist places between the fingers.

Finger-nails thick, exfoliate, or black and rough, matrix inflamed, with soreness, throbbing and numbness; **no** suppuration.

[33] **Lower Limbs.** Excoriation between the legs.

Tearing, or bruised pains in the thighs.

Numbness of the thighs.

Stiff feeling in hollow of knee, as if tendons were too short.

Bruised pain in the knees.

Tetters in the hollow of the knee.

Cramp in the calves.

Restlessness in the legs.

Heaviness of the legs.

Great œdema of the limbs, chiefly the lower, which are very large, with profuse, constant watery exudation from the skin below the knees, epidermis exfoliated.

Ulcers on lower limbs, with acrid pus, dryness of skin and constipation.

Stitches in the heel, when putting it down.

Weakness of feet, cannot walk.

Callous ulcers of the feet.
Stiffness and contraction of the toes.
Gouty tearing in the toes.
Ulcers; or spreading blisters on the toes.
Thick and crippled toe-nails.

[34] **Limbs in General.** Drawing pains in the limbs.
Tearing: in the feet and hands; in all the limbs.
Startings of the hands and feet.
Heaviness in limbs.
Limbs go " to sleep."
Hands and feet: either hot or cold.

[35] **Position, etc.** Stiffness on first beginning to move.
Motion: 29, 40. Stepping: 20, 33. Walking: 31. Walking in open air: 4 ; in the wind: 10. Rising from bed: 23. Must jump from bed: 26. Sitting: 1, 20. Stooping: 2, 5. Must lie down: 2, 27. Lying: 19. Lying in bed: 6. Lying on affected side: 18. Reaching high: 23.

[36] **Nerves.** Cataleptic condition, conscious, but without power to move or speak.
Tremulous sensation through the whole body.
Tired feeling. Lassitude.
Weakness. Exhaustion. Prostration.

[37] **Sleep.** Constant yawning.
Excessively tired and sleepy.
Sleepiness: during the day, must lie down; after dinner.
Light slumber at night.
Wandering fancies at night.
Nightly pains felt in sleep.
Cannot go to sleep till late.
Sleeplessness.
Starting in sleep.
Dreams: vivid; anxious; frightening; horrible; vexatious.

[38] **Time.** Morning: 1, 2, 5, 6, 7, 12, 16, 17, 23, 29, 40. Afternoon: 7, 16. Evening: 2, 5, 6, 7, 25, 33, 40. Night: 1, 5, 7, 10, 13, 17, 20, 21, 22, 27, 37, 40. After midnight: 26.
Day: 37. Day or night: 23. Day and evening: 27, 29.

[39] **Temperature and Weather.** Takes cold easily.
Warmth: 10. In bed: 33. Open air: 4, 5, 40.

[40] **Chill. Fever. Sweat.** Chilliness in the morning, in bed.
Chill and chilliness, most in the evening.
Chill worse after meals, better after drinking, better in open air.
Heat evening and night; also, with restlessness.
Sweats from the slightest motion.
Profuse night-sweat.
Sweat, often on front of body only.
Sweat stains yellow, is sour and offensive smelling, and frequently cold.

Entire inability to sweat.

41 Attacks. Full moon : 6.

42 Sides. Right: 3, 6, 18, 19, 32. Left: 3, 5, 6, 8, 18, 19, 22, 32, 33. Right to left: 8, 23.

43 Sensations. Great sensitiveness of internal parts.

Cramp-like sensations of various parts.

Numbness of various parts.

44 Tissues. Burning pain in an old cicatrix.

Emaciation of suffering parts.

Swelling and induration of the glands.

Œdematous complaints.

45 Contact, Injuries, etc. Touch: 9, 10, 20, 25, 32. Pressure: 18, 23.

46 Skin. Itching over various parts of body.

Violent itching and burning, with eruptions.

Eczema, with profuse serous exudations, in blondes inclined to obesity; also alternating with internal affections.

Itching blotches on various parts of the body, from which oozes a watery, sticky fluid.

Skin is not inclined to heal, ulcerates readily.

Old ulcers, with fetid pus, proud flesh, itching, stinging.

❙ Old scars from ulcers.

Skin dry, inclined to crack.

See: 4, 5, 6, 7, 8, 9, 19, 20, 22, 23, 30, 31, 32, 33.

48 Relationship. Complementary: *Arsen.*, *Caustic.*, *Ferrum*, *Hepar.*

Graphit. is antidoted by: *Acon.* (for the cough), *Arsen.* (for the grief), *Nux vom.*

Graphit. antidotes: *Arsen.*, *Iodum*, *Rhus tox.*

Graphit. follows well after *Lycop.*

GRINDELIA.

Compositæ.

37 Sleep. On falling asleep the respiratory movement would cease, and would not be resumed until awakened by the suffocation resulting. (*G. Squarrosa.*) [Confirmed in Squarrosa and Robusta.]

GUAJACUM.

Guajaci Resina.   HAHNEMANN.   *Zygophylleæ.*

[1] **Mind.** Forgetfulness, especially of names.
   Thoughtless staring: during the morning.
   Disinclination to labor.
   Sad and depressed.

[2] **Sensorium.** Dizziness on rising.

[3] **Inner Head.** Headache across the forehead.
   Violent, sharp stitches in the brain.
   Rheumatic pains in one side of head, extending to face.
   Megrim.
   Attacks of gout in the head.

[4] **Outer Head.** Neuralgia on left side of head and face, extending to neck.
   External headache, with the sensation as if the blood-vessels were overfilled; extends to face and neck. θ Neuralgia.
   Pulsative throbbing in outer parts of head, with stitches in temples; removed for a short time by external pressure and by walking, increased by sitting and standing.
   Perspiration, principally on head and forehead (when walking in the open air.
   Tearing pain in the skull.

[5] **Eyes.** Dilated pupils.
   Swelling of the eyes.
   Sensation of swelling and protrusion of eyes; eyelids appear too short to cover them.
   Hard pimples around the eyes.

[6] **Ears.** Painful dragging and tearing in left ear.
   Violent otalgia, with tearing in the left ear.
   Spasmodic earache.

[7] **Nose.** Pains in bones of the nose.
   Pains from head to nose.
   Nose swollen.
   Fluent coryza.

[8] **Face.** Heat in the face, especially in the evening.
   Face: red and painfully swollen; gets spotted; eyes, nose, cheeks swell; looks old.
   Lancinating and painful stitches in right malar bone and cheek.

[9] **Lower Face.** Dull ache in the left side of jaw.

[10] **Teeth.** Toothache when biting the jaw together.
   . Tearing in the teeth, ending with stitches.

[11] **Tongue, etc.** Food does not taste right.

Thick white fur on tongue.

¹² **Mouth.** Inflammation of the mouth.

¹³ **Throat.** Violent burning in the throat.
Threatened tonsillitis.

¹⁴ **Desires. Aversions.** Violent hunger, in the afternoon and
evening.
Much thirst.
Aversion to milk.
No appetite.
Aversion to all food, could not eat anything.
Desire for apples, which relieves gastric symptoms.

¹⁵ **Eating and Drinking.** After eating without appetite, she
gets sick.

¹⁶ **Nausea and Vomiting.** Frequent empty eructations.
Nausea from sensation of phlegm in the throat.
Every morning vomits a mass of watery phlegm with
great exertion.

¹⁷ **Stomach.** Burning in stomach and abdomen.
Cramp and pain in stomach.

¹⁸ **Hypochondria.** Constrictive sensation in the epigastric
region, with anguish and difficult breathing.

¹⁹ **Abdomen.** Great accumulation of wind in the whole ab-
domen; pinching in abdomen from incarcerated flatu-
lence, receding towards rectum until emitted.
Twitches in abdominal muscles.
I Inguinal hernia.

²⁰ **Stool, etc.** Diarrhœa commencing in the morning; skin
dry, chilly.
Cholera infantum, emaciation; face like that of an old
person.
Costive; hard stool, crumbling; very offensive.

²¹ **Urine.** Continuous urging even after urination, with pro-
fuse fetid urine. See 40.
Stitches in neck of bladder after ineffectual pressure to
urinate.
Cutting in urethra while urinating, as from something
biting passing.

²² **Male Sexual Organs.** Nocturnal emissions without dreams.
Gonorrhœa-like discharge.

²³ **Female Sexual Organs.** I Subacute and chronic ovaritis,
especially in rheumatic women.

²⁴ **Pregnancy.** Chilly crawls over the mammæ.

²⁵ **Larynx.** Violent, spasmodic, inflammatory affection in the
windpipe, most in larynx, with such palpitation of heart
that they could not get out of bed, nor call for help;
feel as if suffocating.

²⁶ **Breathing.** Sudden stuffed feeling in præcordia, like an
arrest of breathing; often attacks her suddenly even at

night in sleep, causing dry cough, frequently repeated
until expectoration appears.

[27] **Cough.** Tight, dry, with burning fever; hot face.

Coughing with copious spitting of phlegm, and later of
stinking pus; coughing up blood.

Dry cough, relieved by detaching and raising a little
mucus; rheumatic patients. See Heart.

[28] **Lungs.** ❙ Pleuritic stitches; left side, worse from breathing
deeply; especially in phthisis pulmonalis.

Intense pain in upper part of chest, from motion of the
head; expectoration of fetid pus.

[29] **Heart. Pulse.** Palpitation.

Sudden stuffed sensation in precordial region like an arrest of breathing; comes suddenly even when asleep,
causing dry cough.

Pulse small, soft accelerated.

[31] **Neck. Back.** Pain from head to neck.

❙ Excessive stiffness of one side of back, from the neck extending to the small of back, when moving.

Contractive pain between the scapulæ.

Chilliness in the back, in the afternoon.

Shuddering and feverish chill in the back.

Aching in the nape of neck, right and left of vertebræ.

Corrosive itching in the back (by day).

[32] **Upper Limbs.** Sharp stitches in the top of right shoulder.

Rheumatic pains in left arm, from shoulder or from elbow
to wrist.

Stitches in the right thumb.

Pain first in knuckles, then in whole hand.

Hands hot.

[33] **Lower Limbs.** Gouty inflammation and abscess at knee,
repeated after a fall, with violent pain and loss of sleep.

Pricking in the nates, as if sitting on needles.

Tension in thighs, especially the right, as if muscles were
too short, with languor when walking; worse from touch,
better when sitting.

Pains begin in middle of thigh or leg and extend to knee.

Tearing, drawing lancinations in leg, from right tarsus to
knee.

Exhaustion in the lower limbs.

Spongoid state of the tibia.

The whole left leg is cramped.

Right leg swollen and contracted, stiff, immovable, drawn
close up to the thigh.

Violent stitches from outside of right calf down to ankle.

[34] **Limbs in General.** Tearing and stinging in limbs.

Pains after abuse of mercury.

Arthritic lancinations, followed by contractions of limbs.

Tearing, pricking pains in the muscles of the extremities, with heat of the parts.

The limbs go to sleep.

Stinging pains in the limbs, worse from the least motion.

35 Position, etc. Yawning and stretching relieves the general ill-feeling.

Walking: 4, 33; in open air: 4. Motion: 28, 31, 34. Standing: 4. Sitting: 4, 33. Lying on back: 37.

36 Nerves. Exhaustion, as after great exertion, especially in thighs and arms.

Immovable stiffness of the contracted limbs.

37 Sleep. Nightly restlessness and sleeplessness.

Nightmare when lying on the back; waking with screams.

On awaking: unrefreshed; everything seems too tight; clothes feel damp.

❙ Frequent awaking from sleep as if falling.

38 Time. Morning: 1, 16, 20. Afternoon: 14, 31, 40. Evening: 8, 14, 40. Night: 22, 26, 37, 40.

39 Temperature and Weather. After a cold, violent pain in limbs.

Can bear no heat, with pain in joints.

Walking in open air: 4.

40 Chill. Fever. Sweat. Internal chilliness through the whole body, followed by heat, most in face, towards evening; without thirst.

Chilliness internally, even near the warm stove, principally in the afternoon and evening.

Burning fever, face spotted; eyes, nose and cheeks swollen; tight, dry cough.

❙ Feeling of heat in the painful limbs; rheumatic cases.

Skin hot, especially on the hands.

Night-sweats, smelling very offensive.

The provers that sweated had no urinary disturbances and vice versa.

The usual general sweat, changes to dryness and chilliness.

41 Attacks. Sudden attacks: 26.

42 Sides. Right: 8, 32, 33, 44. Left: 6, 9, 28, 32, 33. Right and left: 31.

Pains first in left limbs, next day in right.

Above downward: 31, 32, 33. Below upward: 33.

43 Sensations. Pressive, drawing, tearing pains; often ending in a stitch, especially the head pains.

44 Tissues. All excretions are of an unbearable stench.

Rheumatic swelling of joints.

❙ Acts on fibrous tissues.

Aching in the bones, with swelling. θ Syphilis.

Great emaciation.

Contraction of limbs.

Pain in all the joints, even on chest.

Caries and spongious affections of bones; right tibia and tarsal bones spongious, cannot bear the sightest touch.

❙Excretions are all intolerably offensive.

Contractions, with pain from the slightest motions.

❙Joints swollen, painful and intolerant of pressure; can bear no heat.

Pressing pain in bones.

[45] **Contact, Injuries, etc.**   The affected parts are very sensitive to touch.

Cannot bear any pressure, with pain in joints.

Touch: 33.   Pressure: 4; of teeth together: 10.   Effects of a fall: 33.

[46] **Skin.**   Scratching improves.

Itching, tetter-like eruptions.

Appears to promote breaking of abscesses.

[47] **Stages and States.**   ❙Syphilides.

Children; growing pains.

Old women.   ·

Dark hair and eyes.

[48] **Relationship.**   *Guajacum:* has proved useful after abuse of mercury in rheumatism, gout, contraction; antidoted *Caustic.*, which had much increased the contraction of limbs in a rheumatic patient; also antidoted *Rhus tox.*

Nux vom. antidotes *Guajacum.*

Followed *Sulphur* well in cholera infantum.

Compare: *Rhus, Mezer., Rhodod., Phytol., Stillingia, Kali hydr., Mercur.*

HAMAMELIS VIRGINIANA.

Witch Hazel.   HERING.   *Hamamelaceæ.*

[1] **Mind.**   Forgetful.

No desire to study or work.

Depressed in mind; also after emissions, with regretful mind.

Irritable.

[2] **Sensorium.**   Vertigo when stooping.

Swimming sensation on rising.

Nausea and vertigo, with desire to lie down.

[3] **Inner Head.**   Feeling as if a bolt was passing from temple to temple.

Fulness in the forehead, with pressing in the root of the tongue.

Bursting headache on awaking, insupportable on bending downward.

Dulness and fulness in the head all day.

Headache after an emission; depressed in mind.

⁴ Outer Head. Hammering over the left eye, as if he would go out of his mind.

⁵ Eyes. Eyes feel weak, but are less inflamed; painful weakness of the eyes.

Feeling as if both eyes would be forced out of the head, better by pressing them with the fingers, but worse for a few moments afterwards.

Sore pain in the eyes; eyes painful under slight pressure.

Swelling of eyeballs and lids, with bloodshot appearance of the right eye.

Eyes inflamed; vessels greatly injected; caused by a foreign substance, as melted sugar; intense soreness.

⁶ Ears. Deafness in right ear, passes off by noon

Bleeding at the right ear, also nosebleed, which clears her head, relieving her.

Buzzing, ringing in ears.

⁷ Nose. Oversensitive smell.

Bad smell from the nose.

Sneezing spells, watery, excoriating, burning discharge.

Nose feels stopped up.

❙Epistaxis, flow passive, non-coagulable.

⁸ Face. Burning in right cheek.

Occasional shooting pains along the right superior maxillary to malar bone: 10. Muscles feel sore and stiff: 32, 33.

⁹ Lower Face. Lips: dry; sore, cracked.

¹⁰ Teeth. Sharp lancinating along the molar teeth, extending to malar bone; also in temporal region.

Teeth ache, can scarcely sleep, yet not decayed. Pains worse in warm room.

Gums: sore, painful, swollen; bleed easily; passive; dark fluid; ❙after extraction of teeth.

¹¹ Tongue, etc. Metallic taste; tongue coated white.

Scalding sensation on the tongue.

Blisters on the sides of the tongue; canker spots near tip.

¹³ Throat. Severe stinging in uvula, as if it would break, when he coughs.

Dryness of the lips and fauces; must drink large quantities of water to assist deglutition.

Sore throat, worse right side; right tonsil more swollen; reddened, and veins enlarged, varicose.

Sore throat in those predisposed to fulness of the veins, worse in warm, moist air.

Hawks considerably.

[14] **Desires. Aversions.** No appetite for breakfast; consider-
able thirst, relieved by small quantities of water.
Appetite good.
Very thirsty, afternoon, evening; throat dry.
Averse to water, makes him sick to think of it.

[15] **Eating and Drinking.** After eating: nausea, must keep
quiet; eructations; hiccough.
Pork nauseates.

[16] **Nausea and Vomiting.** Eructations after a meal, taste of
the food.
Nausea, eructations and violent hiccough after pork, fol-
lowed by burning in stomach and œsophagus; later,
cramp pains in stomach and chest.
Nausea, vertigo, must lie still to prevent vomiting.
Nausea, headache in frontal bone on waking.
Nausea and inclination to vomit after a meal.

[17] **Stomach.** Hæmatemesis, blood black; sensation of trembling in the stomach, or fulness and gurgling in the
abdomen; feverish by spells; weak, cold, quick pulse,
profuse sweat.
Heaviness at back of stomach; pain in back of stomach,
along the spinal column.
Violent throbbing in the stomach.
Cramp in stomach; after eating.

[19] **Abdomen.** Cramps in stomach and transverse colon two
hours after a hearty dinner.
Flatulence.
Burning in the epigastrium and umbilicus.

[20] **Stool, etc.** Stools: costive; hard, coated with mucus.
Dysentery when the amount of blood is unusually large;
dark, small clots, or patches through the mucus.
❙ Large quantities of a tar-like blood.   θ Typhoid.
Piles bleeding profusely; with burning, soreness, fulness
and weight; back as if it would break; urging to stool.
Itching at the anus.

[21] **Urine.** Increased desire to urinate.
Urine clear, copious.
Scanty, high-colored urine.
Hæmaturia; passive congestion of the kidneys; dull pain
in renal region.
Irritation of the urethra, followed by a discharge and
ardor urinæ.

[22] **Male Sexual Organs.** Emissions at night, without being
aware of it; headache, depression of mind.
Erections: great desire for an embrace.
Severe neuralgic pains in testicles suddenly shifting to
bowels, causing nausea and faintness; profuse cold
sweat on scrotum; capillary stasis.

Orchitis, intense soreness and swelling.

❙ Varicocele.

23 Female Sexual Organs. Dysmenorrhœa, with severe pains through the lumbar and hypogastric region and down the legs; fulness of the brain and bowels, with severe pain through the whole head, causing stupor, deep sleep; varicose veins.

❙ Metrorrhagia, passive flow; anæmia.

Amenorhœa, vicarious bleeding from nose or stomach; costive; varices on the legs.

Leucorrhœa, great tenderness of the vagina; flow bloody.

Vaginismus, intense soreness; prurigo of vulva.

Ovaritis after a blow; diffused agonizing soreness over the whole abdomen; menses irregular; worse at time of menses; retention of urine.

24 Pregnancy. Sore nipples.

❙ Phlegmasia alba dolens.

Varicose veins.

25 Larynx. Hoarse on arising; awoke hoarse.

26 Breathing. When lying, felt a smothering sensation.

27 Cough. Tickling cough, taste of blood on awaking.

Dry cough, severe stitching in uvula, as if it would break.

Expectoration thick, yellowish or greenish-grey, tasting putrid.

28 Lungs. ❙ Hæmoptysis, tickling cough, with taste of blood, or of sulphur; dull frontal headache; tightness of the chest; cannot lie down, because of difficult breathing from congestion; fulness in the head; mind calm.

Stitches in lower part of lungs.

Sensation of constriction across chest, increased by a long or deep breath.

29 Heart. Pulse. Palpitation.

Pricking pain in region of heart and superficial veins of both arms.

30 Outer Chest. Dull, aching pain constantly in muscles of left chest, worse using arms, afternoon and evening.

31 Neck. Back. Sore pain down the cervical vertebræ.

Tearing pains across small of back, with fulness of joints of legs.

Small of back feels as if it would break.

32 Upper Limbs. Bruised feeling in upper arms and shoulder, worse from motion.

Stiffness in arms and shoulders.

Tenderness of the right biceps, increased by pressure.

Stiffness of elbow-joint.

Rheumatic pain, constant aching in the left arm.

Lancinating in the left wrist-joint.

Violent pain in back of right hand to shoulder-joint.

Hands chapped.

Thumb-nail becomes sore, pus discharges after a slight knock.

³³ **Lower Limbs.**   Sore pain in right femur, muscles of thighs sore, as if bruised.

Soreness in femoral vessels in middle of thigh.

Weakness of the knees, afternoon.

Forcible feeling in the varices; veins sensitive, dilated.

³⁴ **Limbs in General.**   Tired feeling in arms and legs.

Rheumatism, with great soreness of the muscles.

³⁵ **Position, etc.**   Motion: 32.   Using arms: 30.   Stooping: 2. Rising: 2.   Desire to lie down: 2.   After lying: 40. Must lie still: 16.   Cannot lie: 28.

³⁷ **Sleep.**   Uneasy, restless morning sleep.

Emissions of semen during sleep.

³⁸ **Time.**   Noon: 6.   Afternoon: 33.   Afternoon·and evening : 14, 30.   Night: 22, 40.

³⁹ **Temperature and Weather.**   Takes cold easily from every exposure; but especially to warm, moist air; subject to varicose veins.

Cold creeps in the open air, chills run up the legs, head stopped up, dull pain over orbit.

Warm room: 10.   Warm, moist air: 13.

⁴⁰ **Chill.   Fever.   Sweat.**   Chilly on going to bed; dreaded an attack of fever.

Chilliness over back and hips, extending down the extremities.

Fever at night; hands hot, burning in eyelids on closing them.

Sweats freely at night, after lying down.

Pulse accelerated; fever.

Pulse 60 to 70 and full.

⁴² **Sides.**   Right: 5, 6, 8, 13, 32, 33.   Left: 4, 30, 32.   Below upward : 32, 39.   Above downward: 40.

⁴³ **Sensations.**   Prickling, stinging: veins, muscles, skin.

Bruised, soreness.

⁴⁴ **Tissues.**   Varicose veins and ulcers, with stinging or pricking.

Venous: congestions; hemorrhages; passive.

Phlebitis; prickling pains.   Hæmorrhagic purpura.

⁴⁵ **Contact, Injuries, etc.**   Pressure: 5, 32.   From a blow: 23.

⁴⁶ **Skin.**   Chilblains always bluish.

⁴⁸ **Relationship.**   Complementary to *Ferrum* (hemorrhages). *Pulsat.* relieved toothache, worse in warm room.   In purpura.

Compare: *Chloral, Sulph. ac., Clem. vitalba.*

HELLEBORUS.

Christmas rose.   HAHNEMANN.   *Ranunculaceæ.*

[1] **Mind.**   Total unconsciousness.

Weak memory.

Diminished power of mind over body; cannot fix ideas; slow in answering, stares unintelligently; muscles do not act properly if the will is not strongly fixed upon their action; as when spoken to, the attention being thereby diverted, she drops things.

Dull, says nothing.

Delirium.

Thoughtless staring.

Constantly picking his lips and clothes.

Much lamenting, moaning.

Involuntary sighing.

Frequent screams in meningitis, or hydrocephalus.

Tries to escape, to throw herself into the river.

Melancholy: silent; during puberty; with anguish.

Homesickness.

Woful, despairing mood.

Indifferent.

Irritable; worse from consolation, does not want to be disturbed.

A noise or shock shortens the attack.   θ Eclampsia.

Thinking about the symptoms lessens them.

[2] **Sensorium.**   Vertigo: with nausea, watery vomit and loose bowels; while stooping, ceasing when becoming erect.

[3] **Inner Head.**   Pressing headache, from within outwards; stupefaction; heavy head; worse from moving head, from exertion; better in the open air.

Stupefying headache, with coryza (4 to 8 P.M.); worse from stooping; better at rest and in the open air.

Shooting pains in the head.   θ Dropsy after scarlatina.

Stupefied; head hot, heavy; boring head in the pillows, chilly; fingers cold.

Dropsy of the brain; post scarlatinal.

Burning heat in head; pale face.

Sensation in occiput, as from a blow.

[4] **Outer Head.**   Sore feeling as if bruised, worse in back part of head; worse on stooping.

Rolls head night and day, moaning.

Throws head back, and from side to side.

Hair falls off, with pricking on scalp, worse on the occiput; face and body œdematous.

Partial sweat on the scalp.

Humid scurf.

⁵ **Eyes,** Photophobia, without inflammation.

Insensible to light. θ Hydrocephalus.

Pupils: contracted; dilated; alternately contracted and dilated.

Nyctalopia.

Eyeballs turned upwards, squinting.

Vacant look, pupils dilated, eyes wide open.

Eyeballs red, glassy.

Eyes sunken, blue edges.

Lids sticky, dry, sensation as if they were pressed down.

Loses hair, from the eyebrows.

⁶ **Ears.** Roaring and ringing in the ears.

⁷ **Nose.** Smell diminished.

Nostrils look as if smoked, sooty.

Nose pointed; nostrils dirty, dry.

Frequently rubs the nose.

Sneezing.

⁸ **Face.** Face: red, hot, but pale; pale, œdematous, distorted; pale, sunken, icy-cold; livid, with cold sweat.

Forehead or face wrinkled.

Stupid expression.

Left-sided neuralgia; parts so tender, cannot chew.

⁹ **Lower Face.** Constant chewing motion.

Corners of mouth sore; steady flow of saliva; upper lip cracked; lips dry, cracked.

White blisters on the swollen lips.

Lower jaw hangs down.

¹⁰ **Teeth.** Grinds the teeth.

Toothache during the chill.

¹¹ **Tongue, etc.** Taste bitter.

Tongue: dry; white, mornings; dry and red in typhus; slightly protruded and oscillating; trembling; numb, insensible; swollen; full of vesicles; pimples on the tip.

¹² **Mouth.** Mouth dry, also palate, with cutting, scraping in palate on moving the mouth to swallow.

Mouth, gums and tongue full of flat, yellow ulcers, with elevated, grey edges; or red, swollen bases; carrion-like odor; salivation; aphthæ.

¹⁴ **Desires. Aversions.** Hunger: child nurses greedily; with disgust for food.

Greedily swallows the cold water; bites the spoon, but remains unconscious. ▮Hydrocephalus.

Thirst: with disgust for drink; but no appetite.

¹⁶ **Nausea and Vomiting.** Nausea, cannot take food, though hungry.

Vomiting of greenish-black substances, with colic.

¹⁷ **Stomach.** Intense burning into the œsophagus.

Fulness and distension of pit of stomach.

Pit of stomach sunken.

Pressing in region of stomach.

Stomach painful when coughing, or walking.

¹⁹ **Abdomen.** Griping, pinching about navel, followed by gelatinous stools.

Gurgling, as if bowels were full of water.

Abdomen swollen, distended, painful to touch.

Ascites: especially after scarlet fever; in scrofulous children.

Excessive colic, weakness, features sunken, face cold, pale, covered with a clammy sweat; pulse thready; thin diarrhœa.

²⁰ **Stool, etc.** Stools: loose, watery; of white mucus, jelly-like, with tenesmus; involuntary.

Feeling as if the intestines had no power to evacuate the feces, during soft stools.

Blenorrhœa of rectum, with spasms of the bladder.

²¹ **Urine.** Spasmodic urging, causing spasms; very little urine passes.

Bladder overdistended; retention of urine from atony of muscular coats.

Urging frequent, with scanty discharge.

After great pressure he passes, with much pain, a few drops of blood.

Passes blood and slime, with burning and stinging.

Suppressed urinary secretion, with dropsy.

Urine: scanty, dark, with floating, dark specks; like coffee-grounds; albuminous, scanty; profuse, passed in large quantities.

²² **Male Sexual Organs.** Desire suppressed; genitals relaxed; no erections.

²³ **Female Sexual Organs.** Suppression of the menses; amenorrhœa from disappointed love.

Uterine dropsy.

²⁴ **Pregnancy.** Puerperal convulsions.

²⁵ **Larynx.** Voice weak, with hydrocephalus.

²⁶ **Breathing.** Sighing.

Chest constricted, gasps for breath, with open mouth; propped up in bed. θ Hydrothorax.

Breathing difficult, with anxiety, worse every evening; must sit up.

²⁷ **Cough.** Dry, worse at night, with gagging; dry, while smoking tobacco.

Tension in region of left short ribs, during cough.

²⁹ **Heart. Pulse.** Pulse: often slower than beating of heart; frequent, soft, intermittent in hydrocephalus; small, wiry, in hydrothorax; almost imperceptible.

31 Neck. Back. Neck rigid in spotted fever.
Cervical muscles stiff.
Cervical glands swollen.
Cramp in spinal muscles. θ Hydrocephalus.
Severe pain down neck, in left side of face and in teeth.

32 Upper Limbs. Arms moving continually, automatically, except when asleep.
Thumb drawn in to the palm.
Boring, sticking in wrist and finger-joints.
Ulceration around the nails.
Humid, painless vesicles between fingers.

33 Lower Limbs. Pricking in the left hip.
Hip and knee-joints stiff.
Boring, stinging in knee and foot-joints.
Legs drawn up, with every attempt to change her position. θ Hydrocephalus.
Legs œdematous.
Humid, painless vesicles between the toes.

34 Limbs in General. Piercing in limbs, with uterine dropsy.

35 Position, etc. Slides down in bed. θ Typhoid.
Lies on the back, limbs drawn up. θ Typhoid.
Worse from bodily exertion.
Motion: 40. Moving head: 3. Exertion: 3. Walking: 17.
Getting out of bed: 40. Must sit up: 26. Erect: 2.
Stooping: 2, 4. Lying down: 40.

36 Nerves. Convulsive twitching of muscles.
Automatic motion of one arm and leg in hydrocephalus.
Convulsions: with extreme coldness; of sucklings.
Epilepsy, with consciousness, followed by deep sleep.
Sudden relaxation of muscles.
Great debility.

7 Sleep. Drowsy, when left alone, he goes to sleep.
Constant somnolence; can be aroused, but not to full consciousness. θ Typhoid fever.
Soporous sleep, with shriek and starts.
Dreams: confused, anxious, cannot be remembered.
During sleep, muscles twitch.

38 Time. Remission during the day.
Worse from evening until morning.
Evening: 26, 40. 4 to 8 P. M.: 3. Night: 27. Toward morning: 40. Night and day: 4.

39 Temperature and Weather. Worse from uncovering; better in warm air, or wrapping up.
Feels better in open air; with sensation as after a long illness.
Cool air: 44. Open air; 3. Averse to uncovering: 40.

40 Chill. Fever. Sweat. Chill spreads from arms; goose-flesh, pains in joints; face hot; drowsy; worse after getting out of bed, and from motion.

31

Burning heat, followed by chill and colic.

Burning heat, with internal chilliness and aversion to drink; can drink but little at a time; evening in bed.

Heat or sweat, with aversion to uncover.

After lying down in bed, heat, generally with sweat.

Sweat: cold, clammy; sticky; less after sleep; relieves; towards morning, temperature unchanged.

⁴²Sides. Left: 27, 31, 33.

⁴³Sensations. Pricking, tearing, pressing pains, running across affected parts.

⁴⁴Tissues. Red parts become white; anæmia.

Loss of flesh; aphthæ.

Dropsy: of brain, chest or abdomen; sudden swellings; anasarca; after scarlatina, nephritis, intermittents, etc. Concomitants: debility, fever, pains in limbs, diarrhœa, suppressed urine.

Stinging-boring, in the periosteum; worse in cool air.

⁴⁵Contact, Injuries, etc. Touch: 19. Chewing: 8.

⁴⁶Skin. Itching unchanged by scratching.

Skin: pale; yellow.

Livid spots on the skin.

Painless ulcers.

Skin peels off; hair and nails fall out.

⁴⁷Stages and States. During dentition, brain symptoms.

Weakly, scrofulous children.

⁴⁸Relationship. Antidotes: *Camphor.*, *Cinchon.*

HELONIAS DIOICA.

Blazing Star. DR. C. B. PARR. *Melanthaceæ.*

¹Mind. Dull, inactive.

Restless, wants to be continually moving about.

Desire to be let alone; conversation is unpleasant.

Dull, gloomy.

Irritable; cannot endure the least contradiction or receive any suggestions in relation to any subject.

Fault finding.

Always better when doing something, when the mind is engaged.

²Sensorium. Pain in the head is increased by stooping, and attended by increased vertigo.

³Inner Head. Fulness and pressure in the forehead or vertex; worse, or renewed, when thinking thereof.

Pressing pain in one or both temples (in a small spot).

Burning in front and top of head, better motion and mental exertion, worse when either is desisted from.

⁸ Face. Pale, earthy.

¹¹ Tongue, etc. Bitter, disagreeable taste, every morning, 5 A.M., on awaking; tongue and fauces dry.

Tongue white. θ Diabetes.

¹² Mouth. Salivation of pregnant women and teething children.

Mouth gets sore; stomatitis materna.

¹⁴ Desires. Aversions. Loss of appetite, eructations, fulness, cramp, and painful congestion of the stomach.

Appetite poor, food tasteless; "bilious;" sleepy during the day.

¹⁶ Nausea and Vomiting. Tasteless eructations; flatulence, each causing nausea.

Nausea at supper.

¹⁷ Stomach. Cramp-like pain in the stomach.

Burning in stomach; burning and aching in spine; eructations.

Irritable stomach, with general dropsy.

¹⁸ Hypochondria. Pain in left side, as if in spleen, which feels as if distended, causing a dull ache.

¹⁹ Abdomen. Motion and rumbling in the abdomen, as if diarrhœa would come on; cramps in the stomach.

Colic-like pains in hypogastric region, off and on all day.

Burning in the lower third of abdomen.

²⁰ Stool, etc. Stool: loose, yellow in the morning; lumps of feces in the evening.

²¹ Urine. Constant aching, extreme tenderness of the kidneys, especially the right.

Burning sensation at the kidneys; can trace their outlines by the burning. At 2.30 P.M., dull heat, and pressure in the vertex, as if skull were too full.

Weariness, languor, weight in the region of the kidneys; mind dull, inactive; afternoon and evening.

Burning-scalding when urinating; desire frequent and urging.

Strangury.

Involuntary discharge of urine after the bladder seemed to be emptied.

Urine: profuse, clear, light-colored; albuminous; diabetic.

²² Male Sexual Organs. Sexual desire and power increased.

Erections unusually strong and frequent.

Impotence.

²³ Female Sexual Organs. Loss of sexual desire and power with or without sterility.

Profound melancholy, deep, undefined depression, with a

sensation of soreness and weight in the womb; "a consciousness of a womb."

Dragging weakness in sacral region, with prolapsus; also at climaxis, with marked debility; profound mental gloom..

Prolapsus uteri and ulceration of the cervix; discharge constant, dark, badly--smelling; flooding on lifting a weight, and on least exertion; face sallow, having an expression of suffering; great vaginal irritation; pain in small of back.

Prolapsus uteri, leucorrhœa; the os protrudes externally.

Uterus low down, fundus tilted forwards; the finger passes with difficulty between the os and the rectum.

Menses too frequent and profuse in women who are feeble from loss of blood. Flow passive; dark, coagulated, offensive.

Amenia, arising from or accompanied by disordered digestive apparatus and anæmia.

Scanty menstrual flow, with heaviness, languor, drowsiness and albuminous urine.

Great uterine hemorrhage all through the proving; pain in back, through to the uterus.

Profuse flooding, with serous leucorrhœa, much uterine and ovarian pain; climaxis.

Leucorrhœa, with atony and anæmia.

Labia and pudendum hot, red, swollen, burning and itching terribly; epidermis every morning falls off in thin, transparent exfoliations. Mucous surface of labia red, swollen, covered with a curdy deposit, like aphthæ.

[24] **Pregnancy.** Threatened abortion; especially in habitual abortion.

Albuminuria during pregnancy: great weakness, drowsiness.

Nipples sensitive, painful, breasts swollen; nipples tender, will not bear the pressure of ordinary dress.

[29] **Heart. Pulse.** Palpitation.

[30] **Outer Chest.** Chest sensitive to the air.

Aching, as if the front of chest had been compressed in a vise.

[31] **Neck. Back.** Burning and heat in the dorsal region, mostly between the lower half of the scapulæ; while sitting reading, at night.

Back aches across the lumbar region; feels tired and weak; burning and tired aching in lumbar and sacral region on sitting down.

Pain about the upper part of the sacrum and pelvis; more severe at night.

Pain in lower part of back, through to uterus; piercing, drawing.

Aching pain in sacrum, also down into each buttock.
[33] **Lower Limbs.** Severe pains in the right hip-joint, worse during motion.

Numbness in feet, going off by motion, only felt when sitting still.
[35] **Position, etc.** Motion: 1, 3, 33, 40. Moving arms: 40. Sitting: 31, 33. Stooping: 2.
[36] **Nerves.** Tired, weary, drowsy.

Languor, unusually tired, yet knows no reason.

Debility. θ After diphtheria.
[37] **Sleep.** Drowsy, heavy. Sleepy during the day.
[38] **Time.** Morning: 11, 20, 23. Afternoon: 21. Evening: 20, 31. Night: 31. Day: 14, 19.
[39] **Temperature and Weather.** Oversensitive to air: 30. Room: 40.
[40] **Chill. Fever. Sweat.** Chill, seemingly radiating from solar plexus all over body, caused by motion of arms.

Flushes of heat pass over him with every movement while in a room.
[42] **Sides.** Right: 21, 33. Left: 8. Below upwards: 33.
[44] **Tissues.** Anæmia, atony, from prolonged hemorrhage.

Dropsy from albuminuria, general debility, uterine atony or after uterine hemorrhage.
[45] **Contact, Injuries, etc.** Pressure of clothing: 24.
[47] **Stages and States.** Women with prolapsus from atony, enervated by indolence and luxury; feel better when the attention is engaged, hence when doctor comes; worn out with hard work, do not care for sleep; so tired, and the strained mucles burn and ache so.

Climaxis.
[48] **Relationship.** Relieves the mental depression resulting from abuse of *Kali brom.*

Relieved prolapsus, caused by *Lilium.*

Collateral relations: *Veratr., Sabad., Colchic.*

HEPAR S. C.

Liver of Sulphur.   HAHNEMANN.   *Sulphurets.*

[1] **Mind.** Great weakness of memory, with the irritability.

Sad mood for hours; must cry vehemently.

Low-spirited, even to thoughts of suicide.

Great anxiety in the evening.

Hypochondriacal.

Oversensitiveness and irritability, with quick, hasty speech.

² **Sensorium.** Vertigo: mornings; when closing the eyes, at siesta; evening, with nausea; when riding in a carriage; when shaking the head.

Fainting from the slightest pains, evenings.

³ **Inner Head.** Boring headache: at the root of the nose, every morning; in right temple, from without inwards; worse from motion or stooping. .

Semi-lateral pressure in the head, as from a plug or dull nail, at night or when waking in the morning; worse when moving the eyes and when stooping.

Aching in the forehead, from midnight till morning.

Lancinating headache, better when walking in open air.

Headache when shaking the head.

Sense of swashing in the head.

Morning headache, worse from every concussion.

⁴ **Outer Head.** Burning-itching on scalp, from forehead to occiput.

Sensitiveness of the scalp to touch, with burning and itching in the morning after rising, after abuse of mercury.

Disposed to take cold, from uncovering the head.

Humid eruptions feeling sore; of fetid odor; itching violently on rising in morning; burning and feeling sore on scratching; scabs easily torn off, leaving a raw, bleeding surface.

Boils on the head and neck, very sore on contact.

Nodosities on the head, sore to touch, relieved by covering the head warmly, and from sweat.

Falling off of the hair, with very sore, painful pimples, and large bald spots on the scalp.

Head bent backward, with swelling below the larynx; violent pulsation of the carotids, rattling breathing.

⁵ **Eyes.** Shunning the light.

Eyes ache from bright daylight, when moving them.

Objects appear to be red.

Sight becomes dim when reading.

Ulcers on the cornea.

Pressure in the eyes as from sand.

Eyes are protruded. θ Croup.

Pressing pain in the eyeballs, feels bruised when touched.

Stitches in the eyes.

Inflammation of the eyes and lids; sore to the touch; lachrymation.

Little pimples surround the inflamed eyes.

⁶ **Ears.** Whizzing and throbbing in the ears, with hardness of hearing; cracking in the ear when blowing the nose.

Darting pain in the ears.

Increase of ear-wax.

Discharge of fetid pus from the ears.

Itching of outer ear.

Scurfs on and behind the ears.

⁷ **Nose.** Sense of smell acute; also with the vertigo.

Nosebleed. θ After singing.

Coryza, with inflammatory swelling of the nose, painful as from a boil; also with cough.

Sore pain on the dorsum of nose, when touching it.

Itching in the nose.

⁸ **Face.** Yellow color of face, with blue rings around the eyes.

Heat and redness of the face.

Erysipelatous swelling of the cheeks in the morning.

Bones of face painful to touch.

Boils very painful to touch.

Eruptions scurfy, and very painful to touch.

⁹ **Lower Face.** Itching around the mouth.

Boils on the lips and chin, very painful to touch.

Sore and smarting pimple on the vermilion border of upper lip.

Middle of lower lip cracked.

Eruption, with sensation of heat in the corners of mouth.

Ulcer at the corner of the mouth.

Itching pimples on the chin.

¹⁰ **Teeth.** Gums and mouth very painful to touch, bleed easily.

Toothache, worse in warm room; when biting teeth together.

Looseness of the teeth.

Hollow teeth, feel too long and painful.

¹¹ **Tongue, etc.** Taste: putrid; metallic; bitter.

Hasty speech.

Tip of tongue very painful, and feels sore.

¹² **Mouth.** Ulcers on gums and in mouth, base resembling lard.

¹³ **Throat.** Scraping in the throat when swallowing.

Hawking up of mucus.

Swelling of the tonsils and glands of the neck.

Scraping sore throat, impeding speech, but not swallowing.

Dryness of the throat.

Stitches in throat, extending to ear, worse when swallowing food.

Sensation as if a fish bone or splinter were sticking in throat.

Sensation of plug in the throat.

¹⁴ **Desires. Aversions.** Longing: for acids; wine; sour and strong-tasting things.

Unusal hunger in the forenoon.

Much thirst.

Aversion to fat.

¹⁵ **Eating and Drinking.** Heaviness and pressure in the stomach, after moderate eating.

[16] **Nausea and Vomiting..** Eructations frequent, odorless and tasteless.

Constant sensation of water rising in the œsophagus, as if she had eaten sour things.

Heart-burn.

Frequent but momentary attacks of nausea.

Attacks of nausea, with coldness and paleness.

Inclination to vomit, with flow of saliva from the mouth.

Vomiting every morning.

[17] **Stomach.** Stomach frequently and easily disordered.

Pressure in the stomach, after moderate eating.

Swelling and pressure in the region of the stomach.

Distention of pit of stomach, has to loosen the clothing.

Burning in the stomach.

[18] **Hypochondria.** Stitches: in region of liver; in region of spleen, when walking.

[19] **Abdomen.** Contractive pain in the abdomen.

Fermentation above the navel, with eructation of hot air.

Colic, with dry, rough cough.

Rumbling in the abdomen.

Swelling and suppuration of the inguinal glands.

[20] **Stool, etc.** Constipation: stools hard and dry; especially with eruption in bend of elbows, or in popliteal space.

Feces not hard, but expelled with difficulty.

Diarrhœic stools: white and fetid, child has a sour smell; sour-smelling and whitish; clay-colored; green, slimy, of sour smell; with tenesmus.

Diarrhœa: worse during the day; after eating, and after drinking cold water.

Dysenteric stools; difficult evacuations of soft stool or of bloody mucus with tenesmus.

Burning in the rectum.

Protrusion of hemorrhoids.

Hemorrhage from the rectum, with soft stool.

Sweat on the perineum.

[21] **Urine.** Dark red and hot; bloody; sharp, burning, corroding the prepuce.

Urine passed tardily and without force, feels as if bladder could not be emptied thoroughly.

Burning in the urethra, during micturition.

Great soreness in the urethra, during micturition.

Inflammation and redness of the orifice of the urethra.

Wetting the bed at night.

[22] **Male Sexual Organs.** Sexual desire increased, erections feeble.

Discharge of prostatic fluid, after micturition and during hard stool, also independent of either.

Itching on the penis, and at the frænum preputii.

Chancre-like ulcers on the prepuce.

Mercurialized chancres.

Secondary syphilis.

²³ **Female Sexual Organs.** Congestion of blood to the uterus.

Menorrhagia, in women with chapped skin and rhagades of the hands and feet.

Discharge of blood with the menses.

Metritis, with burning, throbbing pains.

Uterine ulcers, with bloody suppuration, smelling like old cheese; edge of ulcer sensitive, frequently a pulsating sensation in the ulcers.

Much itching, or little pimples around the ulcer.

Leucorrhœa, with smarting of the vulva.

²⁴ **Pregnancy.** Frequent momentary attacks of nausea.

Mammæ swollen, not sensitive to touch, but she cannot walk up or down stairs.

Cancer of the breast, with stinging, burning of the edges; smells like old cheese.

Little pimples, or smooth ulcers, surround the scirrhus, or principal ulceration.

²⁵ **Larynx.** Hoarseness, roughness in the throat.

Sensitiveness of larynx to cold air.

Wheezing in the larynx, and painfulness of a small spot in the larynx.

Croup: with deep, rough, barking cough, hoarseness or aphony, with slight suffocating spasms; some rattling of mucus, after dry, cold wind; with swelling below the larynx; with great sensitiveness to cold air or water; cough worse before midnight, or toward morning.

²⁶ **Breathing.** Rattling; anxious, wheezing; frequent deep breaths, like after running; anxious, short, wheezing, threatening to suffocate, must bend the head back and sit up.

²⁷ **Cough.** Croupish, hoarse; dry; loose and choking; with bloody expectoration; excites vomiting; whooping, croupish sound, pain in larynx, choking from mucus in larynx, worse in morning.

Cough caused by: limb getting cold; eating or drinking anything cold; cold air; lying in bed; talking; crying; drinking.

After cough: sneezing; crying.

²⁸ **Lungs.** Sensation as of drops of hot water, in left chest.

Soreness in the chest.

Weakness of the chest; cannot talk from weakness.

Spasmodic constriction of the chest, after talking.

Tenacious mucus in the chest.

²⁹ **Heart. Pulse.** Palpitation of the heart, with fine stitches in the heart and left half of the chest.

Pulse hard, full, accelerated; at times intermitting.

31 Neck. Back. Violent pulsation of the carotids.

Drawing between the scapulæ.

Sensation as if bruised, in small of back and thighs.

Stitches and rheumatic pains in the back.

32 Upper Limbs. Suppuration of the axillary glands.

Offensive sweat in the axilla.

Tearing in arms, extending toward the suppuration in breast.

Pain as if bruised in the os humeri.

Encysted tumor at the point of the elbow.

Itching in the palms.

Itching, rough, dry, scaling skin of the hands.

Fingers as if dead.

Tingling in the tips of fingers.

Panaritium.

33 Lower Limbs. Left hip pains as if sprained, when walking in the open air.

Buttock and posterior thighs painful, when sitting.

Bruised pains in muscles of anterior thighs.

Swelling of the knee.

Knee pains as if bruised.

Cramps: in the calves; in soles and toes.

Swelling of feet around the ankles, with difficult breathing.

Pricking in both heels.

Tingling in the toes.

Burning, stinging pains on the toes.

Cracked skin of the feet.

Coldness of the feet.

34 Limbs in General. Drawing pains in the limbs, especially in the morning, when awaking.

Weakness in the limbs; they feel bruised.

35 Position, etc. Motion: 3, 40. Moving eyes: 3, 5. Shaking the head: 3. Walking: 18; in open air: 3, 33; up or down stairs: 24. Sitting: 33; with head bent back: 26. Stooping: 3. Lying in bed: 27, 43.

36 Nerves. Trembling weakness, after tobacco smoking.

Fainting from slight pains.

Spasms after injury, as of pressure on the head; trismus of the newborn: 48.

37 Sleep. Sleepiness during the day, worse toward evening; with frequent, almost spasmodic yawning.

Excess of thoughts prevent sleep, after midnight.

Violent starts, when falling asleep.

Starts from sleep, feeling as if about to suffocate.

Wakes at night, with erection and desire to urinate.

Dreams: anxious; of fire.

38 Time. Morning: 2, 3, 4, 8, 16, 27, 34, 40. Forenoon: 14.

Toward evening: 37. Evening: 1, 2, 40. Night: 3, 21, 40. Before midnight: 25. After midnight: 25, 37. Midnight till morning : 3. Day: 20, 37, 40. Day and night: 40.

39 Temperature and Weather. Warm room: 10. Covering head warmly: 4. Uncovered head: 4. Open air: 40. Cold air: 25, 27. Dry cold winds: 25.

Cold northwest winds.

40 Chill. Fever. Sweat. Chill during the day, alternating with heat and photophobia.

Chill about 6 or 7 P. M.

Nightly chill in bed, with aggravation, of all complaints.

Chill, then thirst; one hour later, much heat, with interrupted sleep.

Great chilliness in the open air.

Dry, burning heat, with redness of the face and violent thirst, all night.

Flushes of heat, with sweat.

Sweats day and night, without relief; or first can't sweat at all, and then sweats profusely; easily by even slight motion.

Night or morning sweat, with thirst.

Cold, clammy, frequently sour, or offensive-smelling sweat.

42 Sides. Right: 3. Left: 28, 29, 33. Without inward: 3.

43 Sensations. Painful sore feeling on the side on which he lies, at night; must change position.

44 Tissues. Caries.

Glands inflame, swell and suppurate.

Rheumatic swelling, with heat, redness and sensation, as if sprained.

Hard, burning nodosities.

45 Contact, Injuries, etc. Touch: 4, 5, 7, 8, 10, 24, 46. Pressure: 10. Scratching: 46. Concussion: 3.

46 Skin. Yellowness of the skin.

Burning-itching on the body, with white vesicles, after scratching.

Humid soreness on the genitals, scrotum, and the folds between the scrotum and the thigh.

Eruptions very sensitive, sore to touch.

Miliary rash in circles.

Itching rash in bends of knees and elbows.

Nettle-rash.

Dry, pimply eruptions.

Eczema, spreading by means of new pimples appearing just beyond the old parts.

Unhealthy skin; slight injuries suppurate.

Ulcers: discharge bloody pus, smelling like old cheese; edges very sensitive, and have a pulsating sensation; discharge corroding.

Stinging, burning of edges of ulcers.
[48] **Relationship.** *Hepar* is frequently indicated after : *Bellad.,*
Laches., Silic., Spongia, Zincum, Arnic.(traumatic spasms).
After *Hepar* are frequently indicated: *Bellad., Mercur.,*
Nitr ac., Spongia, Silic.
Hepar s. c. antidotes: mercurial or other metallic prepara-
tions; also iodine, and particularly the iodide of potas-
sium and cod liver oil.
Antidotes to *Hepar s. c.: Acet ac., Bellad., Chamom., Silic.*

HYDRASTIS CANADENSIS.

Orange root.—Golden seal.   BURT.   *Ranunculaceæ.*

[1] **Mind.**   Forgetful; cannot remember what he is reading or
talking about.
Irritable; disposed to be spiteful.
[2] **Sensorium.**   Feeling as if intoxicated; headache; weakness.
[3] **Inner Head.**   Dull, heavy frontal headache over eyes;
catarrhal.
Sharp cutting in the temples and over the eyes; more
over the left; better from pressing with the hand.
Dull frontal headache, with dull pain in the hypogastrium
and small of back.
[4] **Outer Head.**   Vertex headache every other day, commencing at 11 A. M., with nausea, retching and anguish.
Eczema on margin of hair in front; worse coming from
the cold into a warm room; oozes after washing.
[5] **Eyes.**   Smart, burn; profuse lachrymation.
Opacity of the cornea; scrofulous ophthalmia, with or
without ulceration; thick mucous discharge.
[6] **Ears.**   Roaring in the ears, like from machinery.
Otorrhœa, thick mucous discharge.
Membrana tympani purplish and bulging.
[7] **Nose.**   Tickling, like a hair, in the right nostril.
Coryza watery, excoriating; burning in the nose, more the
right nostril; discharge scanty in the room, profuse out
of door; rawness in throat and chest.
Sneezing, with fulness over the eyes, dull frontal head-
ache, pain in the right breast and down the arms.
The air feels cold in the nose.
Secretion, more from the posterior nares, thick, tenacious.
Nosebleed, left nostril, with burning rawness; followed by
itching.
Soreness of the cartilaginous septum, bleeding when
touched; inner edge of right ala sore and thickened.

Ozæna, with bloody, purulent discharge.

8 Face. Expression weary, dull, skin pale, or yellow-white.

Erysipelatous eruption following flushes of heat.

9 Lower Face. Aphthæ on the lips; tongue swollen.

11 Tongue, etc. Taste: flat; peppery.

Tongue: swollen, shows marks of the teeth; coated white, or with a yellow stripe.

Tongue as if burned or scalded, later a vesicle forms on tip.

12 Mouth. Excessive secretion of thick, tenacious mucus.

Stomatitis after mercury or chlorate of potash; nursing women or weakly children; peppery taste; tongue as if burned, or raw, with dark red appearance and raised papillæ.

13 Throat. Hawking of yellow, tenacious mucus from posterior nares and fauces; rawness of fauces; ulcers in the throat; after mercury.

15 Eating and Drinking. Indigestion from atony of stomach.

Bread or vegetables cause acidity, weakness, indigestion.

16 Nausea and Vomiting. Eructations of sour fluid.

Vomits all she eats, except milk and water. θ Cancer.

17 Stomach. Faintness at the stomach; sinking, gone feeling, with continued violent palpitation of the heart

Stomach actually sunken, weak, faint. θ Marasmus.

Acute, distressing, cutting pains.

Chronic gastric catarrh.

Carcinoma, with emaciation, goneness.

18 Hypochondria. Torpor of liver, with pale, scanty stools.

Liver atrophied. θ Marasmus.

Jaundice, with catarrh of stomach and duodenum.

19 Abdomen. Burning in the region of the navel, with "goneness," faintness, in the epigastrium.

Loud rumbling, with dull aching in the hypogastrium and small of back; worse moving.

Cutting, colicky pains, with heat and faintness; constipation; better after passing flatus.

Cutting in the hypogastrium, extending to the testicles, faintness, after stool.

Sharp pain in the cœcal region.

Sharp pain in the region of the spleen, with dull pain and burning in stomach and bowels.

Dull dragging in groins, cutting pains extending into testicles.

Pains in the groin, as if he had strained himself; clothing uncomfortable.

20 Stool, etc. Fetid flatus.

Stool light colored, soft, acrid; greenish.

Stool lumpy, covered with mucus; constipation.

Hemorrhoids; costive; even a light hemorrhoidal flow exhausts.

Fistula ani.

21 Urine. Dull aching in the region of the kidneys.

Urine: smells decomposed; increased and of neutral reaction.

Catarrh of bladder, with thick, ropy, mucous sediment in urine.

22 Male Sexual Organs. Debility, after spermatorrhœa.

Gonorrhœa, second stage, thick yellow discharge.

Gleet, debility; copious, painless discharge.

Dragging in right groin to testicle; thence to left testicle, thence to left groin.

23 Female Sexual Organs. Leucorrhœa tenacious, ropy, thick, yellow.

Ulceration of the cervix and vagina; leucorrhœa; debility; prolapsus uteri.

Pruritus vulvæ, with profuse leucorrhœa; sexual excitement.

25 Larynx. Scraping in the larynx.

27 Cough. Dry, harsh cough, from tickling in the larynx.

28 Lungs. Rawness, soreness and burning in the chest.

Bronchitis of old exhausted people; thick, yellow, tenacious, stringy sputa.

Phthisis; to relieve the goneness in stomach, emaciation, loss of appetite.

29 Heart. Pulse. Palpitation, with faintness.

Pulse slow during the chill.

31 Neck. Back. Muscles of neck feel sore.

Tired aching across small of back and in limbs: knees ache.

32 Upper Limbs. Pain from head to shoulders, with aching in both, more the left.

Rheumatic pains in elbow, forearms, right shoulder, and first fingers of left hand.

33 Lower Limbs. Pain from right hip to knee, while walking; cannot stand or bear one's weight.

Outer part of left knee aches while sitting, worse when walking.

Legs feel weak; knees weak; aching.

Aching in sole of left foot; no relief from change of position.

Atonic ulcers on the legs.

34 Limbs in General. Limbs tired, ache, with coryza.

Shifting pains in right arm and leg, then left leg.

35 Position, etc. Morning: 19. Walking: 33. Sitting: 33. Change of position: 33.

36 Nerves. Faintness, goneness. Weakness, physical prostration.

❙ Frequent sudden attacks of fainty spells, with profuse

cold sweat all over.   θ Cancerous ulcers on left side of
throat, inside.

[37] **Sleep.**   Awakened by backache and dull pains in navel and
hypogastric region.

Dreams worrisome, restless sleep.

Difficulty in awaking.

[38] **Time.**   Morning or evening: 40.   11 A.M.: 4.   Evening: 40.
Night: 46.

[39] **Temperature and Weather.**   Room: 7.   Out-doors: 7.
Coming from cold air into warm room: 4.   Washing: 4.

[40] **Chill.   Fever.   Sweat.**   Chill morning or evening: chilliness, especially in the back or thighs, with aching;
pulse slow.

Heat in flushes.   Great heat of the whole body.   Constant
dull burning pains all the evening.

Gastric, bilious or typhoid forms of fever, with gastric disturbances, jaundice and great debility following.

[42] **Sides.**   Right: 7, 22, 32, 33, 34.   Left: 3, 7, 19, 22, 32,
33, 34.   Right to left: 22, 34.   Above downwards: 19,
22, 33.   Below upwards: 22.

[44] **Tissues.**   Mucous membranes; secretions increased, tenacious, ropy; erosions.

Muscles greatly weakened; atony.

Marasmus.   Scrofula.   Cancer cachexia.

Cancers hard, adherent, skin mottled, puckered; cutting
like knives; in mammæ.

[45] **Contact, Injuries, etc.**   Pressure of hand relieves the head.

Clothing feels uncomfortable about the groins.

Touch: 7.

[46] **Skin.**   Erysipelatoid rash on the face, neck, palms, joints of
fingers and wrist, with maddening, burning heat, later
skin exfoliates; pains worse at night.

Lupus.

Variola, itching-tingling of the eruption; face swollen;
throat raw; pustules dark; great prostration.

[47] **Stages and States.**   Old people: 28.

[48] **Relationship.**   Antidotes to *Hydrast.*: *Sulphur* (against the
head symptoms and sciatic pains).

Bad effects from *Mercur.*, or the chlorate of potash.

Superior to *Arsen.* in lupus; compare *Kali bich.*

HYOSCYAMUS NIGER.

Henbane. HAHNEMANN. *Solanaceæ.*

[1] **Mind.** Stupor, unconsciousness; does not reply to questions; does not recognize any one. Answers properly but immediately stupor returns.

Makes irrelevant answers.

Inability to think; thoughts cannot be directed or controlled.

Stupid, or illusions of the imagination and senses.

Sees persons who are not and have not been present.

Thinks he is in the wrong place.

Delirium continued while awake. ▮Delirious without apparent heat; the face is pale and the limbs are cold, though the temperature is high.

Delirium: talks of business; complains of imaginary wrongs.

Delirium tremens, with clonic spasms; averse to light and company; visions, as if persecuted.

Insane passion for work.

Indistinct, muttering loquacity.

Silly, smiling, laughs at everything, silly expression.

Cried and laughed alternately, gesticulated lively.

Lascivious mania, uncovers body, especially sexual parts; sings amorous songs.

Cries out suddenly.

Whines, but knows not why.

Muttering, picking at bedclothes.

Plays with his fingers (not picking bedclothes).

Wants to go from one bed to another.

Restless, jumps out of bed, tries to turn away.

Does foolish things, behaves like one mad.

Abuses those about him.

Tries to injure those around him; convulsions after trying to swallow.

Scolds; raves.

Answers no questions.

Cannot bear to be talked to.

Anxious apprehension.

Fears: being left alone; poison, or being bitten; being poisoned or sold.

Makes no complaints; has no wants.

Does not know whether or not to take what is offered.

Jealousy.

Fright, followed by convulsions.

Unfortunate love, with rage and incoherent speech.

Disappointed love, followed by epilepsy.

² Sensorium.   Vertigo, with drunkenness; also from smell of flowers, from gas, etc.

Sudden falling, with a shriek; sopor.

ı Rolls head, stertor, hiccough; concussion of brain.

Apoplexy, snoring; involuntary stool and urine.

Repeated attacks of fainting.

³ Inner Head.   Pain and heat in head, after a meal.

Headache, better walking.

Congestion to head.

Cerebral hyperæmia, delirious, unconscious, blue-red face; red, sparking eyes.

Heaviness, vacant feeling, confusion, severe pain; pains in meninges; pressure in left side of forehead, changing to shooting.

Heat and tingling in head; violent pulsations, like waves, head shakes; worse becoming cold, after eating; better bending head forward, and from heat.

Brain feels as if loose.

Stupor; shakes head to and fro; swashing sensation in brain.

⁴ Outer Head.   Catches cold in head, especially from dry, cold air.

Rolling the head.

Head sinks on one or other side.

⁵ Eyes.   Farsighted, clearsighted; pupils dilated.

Illusions; objects look red as fire, or too large.

Amblyopia; epilepsy.

Double sight.

Night blindness.

Constant staring at surrounding objects, self-forgetfulness.

Eyes protrude.

Eyes red, sparkling, staring; rolling about in orbits; squinting.

Tearing, beating in right eye, which waters and seems projected.

Pupils altered, dilated or contracted; slow respiration.

Eyes open; distorted.

Quivering in the eye.

Spasmodic closing of eyelids; cannot open eyelids. θ Spinal meningitis.

Rending pains in angles of eyes, disappearing when touched.

⁶ Ears.   Buzzing, singing, rusing in ears.   Deafness.

Hard hearing, as if stupefied, especially after apoplexy.

⁷ Nose.   Sense of smell weak, or lost.

Nosebleed, bright red, with salivasion.

Sudden jerks at root of nose.

32

Cramp-pressure at root of nose and malar bones.

Nostrils sooty, smoky.

8 **Face.** Face: flushed; dark red, bloated; cold and pale; distorted; stupid expression; muscles twitch, makes grimaces; bluish, mouth wide open; approaching cerebral paralysis in typhus.

Lockjaw; fully conscious.

9 **Lower Face.** Foam at the mouth.

Lips dry.

10 **Teeth.** Closes the teeth tightly.

Toothache, driving to despair; tearing, throbbing, extending to the cheeks and along lower jaw.

Tearing in teeth as if blood was forced into them, flushes of heat, congestion to head; worse from cold air, morning.

Teeth feel loose when chewing; also, too long.

Intense pain in gums after extraction of a tooth.

Sordes on teeth and in the mouth.

Grating the teeth.

11 **Tongue, etc.** Putrid taste.

Very talkative, or loss of speech.

Tongue: red or brown, dry, cracked, hard; looks like burnt leather; clean, parched; white.

Paralysis of tongue; speech embarrassed.

Tongue protruded with difficulty, can hardly draw it in.

12 **Mouth.** Salivation; saliva saltish; bloody.

Cadaverous smell from mouth, worse morning and evening.

13 **Throat.** Elongated palate.

Throat and mouth dry, parched and red, inability to swallow.

Throat dry, burning; shooting, pricking pains, difficult swallowing, as from constriction; dread of liquids.

Constriction of the throat, impeded deglutition.

Spasmodic contraction of œsophagus after injury; solid and warm food swallowed best; fluids cause spasm; hiccough, nausea, stiff neck.

Difficult to swallow liquids; an attempt to swallow renews spasm.

14 **Desires. Aversions.** Hungry gnawing: 36.

Thirst, drinks but little at a time.

Dread of water.

15 **Eating and Drinking.** After eating: 3, 36. Great thirst: 21.

16 **Nausea and Vomiting.** Hiccough, with spasms and rumbling in abdomen.

Eructations: empty; incomplete; bitter.

Nausea: with vertigo; and vomiting.

Retching and vomiting, with colic, extorting cries.

Vomiting: of food and drink; of blood, with convulsions; of bloody mucus, with dark red blood.

[17] **Stomach.**   Pit of stomach tender to touch.

Cramps in stomach, with loud shrieks, vomiting, convulsions; cramps better after vomiting.

Burning and inflammation of the stomach.

Hæmatemesis, pit of stomach sensitive; dull aching about liver; abdomen bloated.

[18] **Hypochondria.**   Stitches or dull pain in region of liver.

[19] **Abdomen.**   Colic, as if abdomen would burst; presses the fists into sides; cutting, vomiting, belching, hiccough, screaming.

Abdomen distended, sore to touch, tympanitic.

Umbilicus open, urine oozing through.

Enteritis or peritonitis, with typhoid symptoms.

Abdominal muscles sore.

Roseola on abdomen.

[20] **Stool, etc.**   Paralysis of rectum, or sphincter ani.

Frequent urging, with small discharges.

Stool small in size.

Diarrhœa, colicky pains, frequent urging to stool; or sphincter weak, can hardly retain the feces; worse by least mental excitement or trouble.

Diarrhœa of lying-in women.

Yellow, watery stools, involuntary during sleep; old men.

Involuntary stool at night.

Hemorrhoids bleeding profusely.

Constipation, with epilepsy.

[21] **Urine.**   Micturition: frequent, scanty; difficult, from spasmodic or inflammatory condition of neck of bladder; involuntary; has no will to urinate.

Urine: scanty; retained or suppressed; turbid, with muco-purulent deposit; with red, sandy sediment.

[22] **Male Sexual Organs.**   Sexual desire excessive; lascivious, exposes his person.

Impotence.

[23] **Female Sexual Organs.**   Lascivious, uncovers sexual parts.

Uterine cramps, with pulling in loins and small of back; irritable uterus.

Metritis, typhoid state.

Continuous bright red flow, with spasmodic jerkings, great vascular excitement. θ Metrorrhagia.

Pale flow, with convulsions.

Menses preceded by hysterical or epileptic spasms; laughing loud, uninterrupted; profuse sweat and nausea.

During menses, convulsive trembling of hands and feet, headache, profuse sweat; lockjaw; enuresis.

[24] **Pregnancy.**   Painless diarrhœa of lying-in women.

Hemorrhage after labor, after miscarriage; spasms, twitchings of single muscles.

Puerperal spasm, shrieks, anguish; chest oppressed, unconscious.

Children at the breast have singultus.

Umbilicus open, urine oozing through.

[25] **Larynx.** Voice husky, as from mucus.

Constriction of the larynx.

Hysterical aphonia.

[26] **Breathing.** Loss of breath, as from rapid running.

Mucuous rales during stupor or furious delirium.

Rattling breathing.

Oppression of the chest, with internal stinging, worse during inspiration.

[27] **Cough.** Dry, hacking or spasmodic cough, worse lying, better sitting up; worse at night, also, after eating, drinking, talking, or singing; velum palati usually elongated.

Expectoration of saltish mucus, or bright red blood, mixed with coagula.

During cough: spasms of the larynx; painful epigastrium and hypochondria.

[28] **Lungs.** Tight feeling across chest, as from overexertion, running.

Spasms of chest, arrest of breathing, must lean forward.

Exhausted from long talking, body, and especially chest, weak; green sputum, weak pulse.

Stitches in side of chest.

Hæmoptysis, bright red, with spasms, also, in drunkards.

Pneumonia: cerebral symptoms, delirium, sopor; dry, fatiguing night cough, or rattling in chest.

[29] **Heart. Pulse.** Pulse: accelerated, full, hard and strong; rapid, intermitting; slow and small; weak and irregular; small, weak, scarcely perceptible.

Carotids beat violently.

[30] **Outer Chest.** Muscles sore.

Roseola on chest.

[31] **Neck. Back.** Spinal meningitis, with convulsions, jerks of muscles; after injury.

[32] **Upper Limbs.** Arms tremble, especially in the evening and after exercise.

Painful numbness of hands.

Rigor of hands.

Fingers look and feel too thick.

[33] **Lower Limbs.** Cramps in anterior part of thigh.

Swelling of the feet.

Toes spasmodically contracted in walking or going up stairs.

[34] **Limbs in General.** Trembling of arms and hands.

Lancinating pains in almost all joints, especially on motion.

Cold hands and feet.

35 Position, etc. Motion: 34, 40. Walking: 3, 28, 32, 33. Ascending stairs: 33. Exertion: 32. Sitting up: 27, 46. Leaning forward: 28. Bending head forward: 3.

36 Nerves. Throws arms about, misses what is reached for, gait tottering; chorea.

Convulsions after meals: child sickens after eating, vomits or shows distress at the stomach, sudden shriek, and then insensible.

Convulsive jerks; long-lasting spasms.

Angular motions; jerks of single muscles or sets of muscles.

Subsultus tendinum.

Epilepsy. Before the attack: vertigo, sparks before eyes, ringing in ears, hungry gnawing. During attack: face purple, eyes projecting, shrieks, grinding teeth; urination. After attack: sopor, snoring.

Suffocating spells and convulsions during labor.

Convulsions of children, especially from fright.

Restless, turns from one place to another.

Paralysis after spasms, or after diphtheria.

37 Sleep, Stupid and drowsy, or excitable and sleepless.

Falls asleep while answering.

Deep sleep with convulsions.

Constant slumber, with picking.

Sleep, with outcries.

Sleepless, or, constant sleep, with muttering.

Sleeplessness, after violent disease, or with irritable, excited persons.

Lying on back, suddenly sits up, then lies down again.

Starts in sleep, after a fright.

Dreams: anxious; lascivious.

Awakening with screams.

38 Time. Morning: 10. 11 A.M.: 40. Morning and evening: 12. Evening: 32, 40. Night: 5, 20. 27, 28, 40.

39 Temperature and Weather. Worse in the sun: head.

Heat: 3. In bed: 40. Becoming cold: 3. Dry cold air: 3, 4. Cold air: 10.

40 Chill. Fever. Sweat. Chill alternate days, 11 A.M.; cannot bear to be talked to, or hear the least noise.

Chill from feet upwards; shivering, heat of face.

Cold at night, up the back from small of back; cannot get warm in bed.

Whole body cold, with burning redness of face.

Chill, alternating with heat.

Burning heat all over, every evening congestion to head; putrid taste.

Heat, no desire to drink.

Skin burning hot to examining hand.

Congestive chills.

Sweat, mostly on legs.

Sweat: cold; sour; weakening; during sleep.

[41] **Attacks.** Alternate days, at 11 A.M. : 40. Every evening : 40.

[42] **Sides.** Upper right, lower left.

Right 5, 17. Left : 3. Below upward : 40.

[43] **Sensations.** Sensation of pricking all over.

As if blood burned in the veins.

Want of sensation : 46.

[44] **Tissues.** Fulness of the veins; full pulse.

Hemorrhages usually light red.

Obesity. ·

Skin and muscles lax.

[45] **Contact, Injuries, etc.** Touch: 2, 5, 17, 19. After injury: 2, 31.

[46] **Skin.** Skin often pale, with delirium; body hot.

Hot, dry, brittle skin, want of sensation.

Brown or gangrenous spots.

Skin red, or with red rash.

Varicella; vesicles in crops, sleepless; nervous; dry cough, must sit up.

Gangrene, with nervous restlessness; itching around.

Large pustules, clustering from hips to knees.

Ulcers painful, bleeding; bruised feeling on moving the part.

Scarlatina, with marked mental symptoms.

[47] **Stages and States.** Nervous, irritable, excitable.

Sanguine temperament.

Drunkards.

Hysterical subjects.

Old men.

[48] **Relationship.** *Hyosc.* is suitable in: hard hearing after apoplexy. *Bellad.* failing; hæmoptysis of drunkards, after *Opium* or *Nux vom.;* congestive chills, after *Bellad.* and *Opium* fail.

Excessive lasciviousness yields to *Phosphor.*, when *Hyosc.* fails.

Complaints from inhaling ether.

Ailments from *Plumbum*, or abuse of *Bellad.*

Antidotes: vinegar, *Bellad.*, citric acid, *Cinchon.*, *Stramon.*

HYPERICUM.

St. John's Wort.   C. HERING.   *Hypericaceæ.*

¹ **Mind.** Makes mistakes in writing; omits letters; forgets what she wanted to say. Confused.

Increase of intellectual power.

Erotic ideas; brain excited, as after tea.

Sees spirits, spectres. Delirium.

Singing followed by weeping and loud screaming, with gasping for breath.

Great anxiety; also in meningitis.

Melancholy.

Irritable, inclined to speak sharply; slept badly, languid on waking.

Consequences of fright. Removes effects of shock.

² **Sensorium.** Buzzing sensation in vertex at night, as if something living were in the brain.

Sensation as if being lifted up high into the air; tormented by anxiety that slightest touch or motion would make her fall down from this height; with headache. θ After a fall on occiput.

Heaviness and dizziness in the head.

Vertigo at night, with urging to urinate.

Asphyxia after a fall; when jerking or shooting pains appear.

³ **Inner Head.** Dull headache, head heavy; morning.

Burning in the vertex, heat, pulsation (afternoon).

❙ Tearing stitches in brain; beating, mostly on vertex. θ Meningitis.

Sensation as if the head became elongated.

❙ Headache, with sore eyes, after a fall.

⁴ **Outer Head.** Sensation in forehead, as if touched by an icy-cold hand, in afternoon, after which a spasmodic contraction is felt in right eye.

Head hot, carotids throbbing.

Hair moist, rest of body burning hot.

Pressure in left temple, after breakfast.

Fractured skull; bone splintered.

⁵ **Eyes.** Disturbed look, stares at people, eyes fixed; pupils dilated.

Stitches in right eye.

Stye on lower left lid.

⁶ **Ears.** Sensitiveness of hearing; during catamenia.

Shooting through the ear.

Relieves pains of synechia. See 45.

Ears hot; scurf on the ear.

[7] **Nose.** Exceedingly fine sense of smell.

Nose dry, very annoying.

Sneezing, leaving a raw, sore feeling in the throat.

Sore inside the nose, itching; all the time picking nose.

Dryness of left nostril; crusts in it.

[8] **Face.** Expression of suffering.

❚ Face hot, bloated. θ Meningitis.

Cheeks red; erysipelatous redness.

Dull faceache, aching in brows; afternoon, evening; worse at night, disturbing sleep.

Headache extending into zygoma or cheek.

Red eruption on both cheeks, chin and nose; sometimes dry, with thin crusts; sometimes fiery red, oozing yellow drops.

[9] **Lower Face.** Eruption around the mouth and on right ear.

Yellowish-greenish scabs, with cracking and moisture.

Lips dry, feel hot.

[10] **Teeth.** Severe aching in decayed tooth at night; restless, wakeful; better lying on affected side, and keeping quiet.

[11] **Tongue, etc.** Taste: insipid; of blood.

❚ Tongue coated white or yellow; great thirst. θ Meningitis.

[12] **Mouth.** Dry, burning heat in the mouth and on the lips.

[13] **Throat.** Expansion of throat and abdomen.

Sensation as if a worm was moving in the throat.

Hot risings in œsophagus after a fright, or with anxious feelings.

With hemming, some bright, red blood comes up.

[14] **Desires. Aversions.** Desire for warm drinks. θ Meningitis.

Great thirst, white tongue; in morning after heat and delirium.

Desire for wine; for pickles.

Appetite increased morning and evening.

[15] **Eating and Drinking.** Tasteless.

Belching, when drinking water.

Smoking tobacco does not taste well.

After breakfast, headache, eructations, gastric symptoms, pressure in stomach, towards the back; pains in limbs.

After supper, flatulence and diarrhœa.

After eating: 17.

[16] **Nausea and Vomiting.** Eructations: tasteless; bitter; preventing sleep at night.

Nausea, weakness every morning.

Nausea, abdomen distended, cracking pains in bowels, awaking in the night.

¹⁷ **Stomach.** Pain in stomach, nausea and diarrhœa, chill; after eating.

¹⁸ **Hypochondria.** Sticking or dragging in the right hypochondrium.

¹⁹ **Abdomen.** Tympanitic distention of abdomen; relieved by a stool.

Cutting in belly, in region of navel.

Pinching pains, diarrhœa; with catamenia.

²⁰ **Stool, etc.** Loose, bilious, yellow stools evening or morning.

Cholera morbus, slimy stools.

Summer diarrhœa, with eruption of the skin.

Diarrhœa driving out of bed in the morning.

Constipation; violent tenesmus, with discharge of a hard, little ball.

Awakes with distended abdomen, relieved by stool.

Rectum feels dry, morning.

²¹ **Urine.** Nightly urging to urinate, with vertigo.

Urine: much diminished; bloody; turbid; of peculiar odor.

Swelling and hardness of the female urethra, with burning, soreness and sensitiveness; especially if caused by instruments for uterine prolapsus.

²² **Male Sexual Organs.** Sexual functions excited.

Tearing in the genital organs, with the desire to urinate.

²³ **Female Sexual Organs.** Menses: too late, with tension in the uterine region, as from a tight bandage; increased in quantity; three days before their appearance, pinching in the abdomen, diarrhœa, cold feet; headache, wrenching pain over eyes, better in motion; severe backache. Attended by sickening pain in belly, sensitiveness of hearing.

Leucorrhœa, with delayed menses, palpitation, pressure in the small of the back, and heaviness in lower bowels.

Leucorrhœa in a child, milky, but corroding.

²⁴ **Pregnancy.** Labor-pains tardy.

After-pains violent, in sacrum and hips, with severe headache; after instrumental delivery.

²⁵ **Larynx.** Hoarseness, scraping and roughness in the larynx, upper part of pharynx and nares, in a foggy atmosphere.

²⁶ **Breathing.** Spasmodic asthmatic attacks, with changes of the weather from clear to damp, or before storms; after lesion of the spinal cord, by a fall, years before.

²⁷ **Cough.** ı Spells of short, barking cough. θ Meningitis.

Hacking couch, from an irritation in throat, much increased by the heat and cold air.

Dry cough and prostration in the morning.

Whooping-cough, worse from 6 to 10 P. M.

Nervous system much affected.

[28] **Lungs.** Anxiety in the chest, in the forenoon, with short breath, dizziness and bitter belching.

Stinging left chest, worse when moving.

Cutting in the upper right chest, then in lower left.

[29] **Heart. Pulse.** Hard beating of the heart.

Pulse: quick and hard; frequent.

[30] **Outer Chest.** Stitches under the mammæ.

Stinging, burning pain on one edge of left pectoral muscle.

Dull pressure, right chest, from seventh rib down, after breakfast.

[31] **Neck. Back.** Cutting between scapulæ.

Lies on the back, jerking head backward.

❙ After a fall, slightest motion of arms or neck extorts cries; cervical vertebræ very sensitive to touch.

Entire spine tender; paroxysms of pain in different joints, with mania.

❙ Consequences of spinal concussion.

Stinging near edge of right scapula near spine; morning.

Stitches in the small of the back.

Aching pain and sensation of lameness in the small of back.

Violent pain and inability to walk or stoop, after a fall on the coccyx.

[33] **Upper Limbs.** Flying pains, right shoulder.

Cutting under left scapula.

Stitches on the top of the shoulder at every inspiration.

Tension in both arms and in the hands.

Pressure at insertion at of right deltoid.

Numbness in left arm; better from rubbing.

Hard pain running down left median nerve.

Cutting in fleshy ends of fingers.

[33] **Lower Limbs.** Weakening drawing, over the front of legs; shooting pain, as if in the periosteum.

Left leg numb, cold, while sitting.

Articular rheumatism (knees), with great effusion around the joint, with muddy urine looking like the settlings of beer.

Fearful pains in knees, sharp, could hardly touch them.

The feet feel pithy, as if pricked with needles.

Sensation as if the left foot was strained or dislocated.

Lying in bed the feet tingle.

Excruciating pain in bunions (external applications),

[34] **Limbs in General.** Crawling in hands and feet, as if they were numb.

Feeling of weakness and trembling of all the limbs.

Sensation of lameness of the left arm and right foot.

Cannot walk, spine affected.

[35] **Position, etc.** Great dread of motion, would not walk,

screamed when it was proposed to lift her to another place.

Slightest motion of arms or neck extorts cries.

Rest: 10. Motion: 2, 23, 28, 31. Walking: 31, 34. Lying down: 33. Lying on painful side: 10. Sitting: 33.

[36] **Nerves.** Prevents lockjaw from wounds in soles, fingers or palms of hands.

Convulsions from blows upon the head.

Convulsions after every slight hurt or concussion.

Epileptiform spasms after knocking the body against anything.

Jerks in the limbs.

Weariness on awaking; goes off by noon.

[37] **Sleep.** Constant drowsiness.

Spasmodic jerks of the arms or legs on going to sleep; twitchings.

On awaking: weary, better by noon; feels refreshed; bowels distended.

Dreams: with activity, traveling; vivid; distressing.

[38] **Time.** Morning: 3, 14, 16, 20, 27, 31. Forenoon: 28. Noon: 36, 37. Afternoon: 3, 8. Evening: 8, 14, 20, 27. Night: 2, 8, 10, 16.

[39] **Temperature and Weather.** Foggy weather: 25. Changes from clear to damp: 26. Before storms: 26. Cold air: 27.

[40] **Chill. Fever. Sweat.** Shuddering over the whole body, with desire to urinate.

Heat, with delirium, wild staring look, hot head, throbbing of carotids, bright red, bloated face, hair on head moist, burning heat of skin, great oppression and anguish.

Chill followed by heat, with sweat on hands and feet.

[42] **Sides.** Right: 4, 5, 9, 18, 30, 31, 32. Left: 4, 5, 7, 28, 30, 32, 33. Before backward: 15. Upper right to lower left: 28. Left upper and right lower: 34. Above downward: 32.

[43] **Sensations.** Flesh sore all over, bruised.

[44] **Tissues.** Injury to parts rich in sentient nerves; especially fingers, toes, matrices of nails.

Lacerations when the intolerable pain shows nerves are severely involved.

Local congestions: nervous erethism, with or without hemorrhage; great nervous depression following wounds.

Always modifies and sometimes arrests ulceration and sloughing.

Next to the nervous tissues, the joints are affected; all articulations feel bruised.

[45] **Contact, Injuries, etc.** Punctured wounds feel very sore; from treading on nails; rat-bites, etc.; prevents lockjaw.

❙ Wounds from crushing, as mashed fingers, especially tips.

ı Nerves lacerated, pains excruciating.

Relieves pains in old cicatrices.   (See 6.)

Painful wounds before suppuration.

Rheumatism, bunions, corns, etc., when the pains are so disproportionately severe as to show nerves are attacked.

After a fall, asphyxia.

ı After a knock or blow on the head, spasms.   Touch : 31, 33.   Rubbing : 32.

⁴⁶ **Skin.**   Great itching when undressing, most in sacral region.

Skin rough, as if full of small knots.

Pimples on forehead, throat, back, hips.

Tetters, beginning with sore places, and forming hard, yellow crusts, with violent itching.

Smarting eruption, like nettle-rash, on the hands.

⁴⁸ **Relationship.**   Antidotes to *Hyper.: Arsen* against weakness or sickness in the morning ; *Chamom.* for pain in face ; mesmerism ; *Sulphur.*

Cures where formerly *Acon.* and *Arnic.* were given in alternation in wounds.

IGNATIA.

St. Ignatius's Bean.   HAHNEMANN.   *Loganiaceæ.*

¹ **Mind.**   Absent-minded.

Desire to be alone.

Changeable disposition ; jesting and laughing, changing to sadness, with shedding of tears.

Taciturn mood.   Sadness.

Sensitive mood, delicate conscientiousness.

Affectionate disposition, with very clear consciousness.

ı Great grief after losing persons or objects that were very dear.

Anger, followed by quiet grief or sorrow.

ı Children after having been reprimanded or scolded, are sent to bed and get sick.

Ailments from grief, mortification, bad news, or suppressed mental suffering.   Jealousy.

Effects of disappointed love.

² **Sensorium.**   Heaviness of the head.

³ **Inner Head.**   Pressing frontal headache over the glabella, must bend the head forward ; followed by inclination to vomit.

Headache, like a pressure with something hard, on the upper surface of the brain.

Throbbing pain in the occiput, worse when pressing at stool.

Weight at back of head; tendency of the head to incline backward.

Pain with every throb of the arteries.

Pain as if a nail were driven out through the side of the head, better by lying on it.

Headache, worse mornings; from moving the eyes; from noise; from coffee, tobacco, or alcohol; close attention.

Congestion to the head, from being spoken to.

Head feels sore; bruised.

⁴ Outer Head. Trembling and shaking of the head.

Head bent backward, during spasms.

⁵ Eyes. Cannot bear the glare of light; sunlight causes headache.

Flickering zigzags before the eyes.

Dimsighted.

Pain from head into left eye; latter burns and waters.

Pain under the upper lid as if it were too dry.

Sensation as of sand in the eyes.

Acrid tears in the eyes, during the day.

Swelling of the upper lid.

Nightly agglutination of the lids.

⁶ Ears. Roaring in ears relieved by music.

Intolerance of noise; headache from noise.

Sound before the ear, as from a strong wind.

Hard hearing except for speech.

Tugging pains in the ears.

Itching in the ears.

⁷ Nose. Stoppage of one nostril.

Fluent coryza.

Soreness and sensitiveness of inner nose, with swelling.

Nostrils ulcerated.

⁸ Face. Convulsive twitchings of muscles of face.

Alternate redness and paleness of face.

Redness and heat of one cheek and ear.

Face clay-colored and sunken, with blue rings around eyes.

⁹ Lower Face. Twitching of corners of mouth.

Spasmodic closing of the jaws.

Lips dry, cracked, bleeding.

Ulceration of one of the corners of the mouth.

Inside of lower lip painful, as if sore.

Pain in the submaxillary glands, when moving the neck.

¹⁰ Teeth. Jaws feel as if crushed.

Boring pain in the front teeth; soreness in all the teeth.

Toothache, worse after drinking coffee, after smoking tobacco; after dinner; in the evening; after lying down; or in the morning, on awaking; worse in intervals between meals.

Difficult dentition, with convulsions.

[11] **Tongue, etc.** Taste: sour, also of saliva; flat, like chalk.
Food has no taste.
When talking or chewing, bites the cheek or tongue.

[12] **Mouth.** Accumulation of much saliva in the mouth.
Inner mouth inflamed and sore.
Putrid odor from the mouth.

[13] **Throat.** Stitches in the soft palate, extending to the ear.
Inflamed, hard swollen tonsils, with small ulcers.
Stitches in the throat, only between the acts of swallowing.
Sensation as from a lump in throat, when not swallowing.
Choking sensation from the stomach up to the throat.
Throat worse when not swallowing, and when swallowing
liquids; better when swallowing food.

[14] **Desires. Aversions.** Hunger and nausea at the same time.
Feeling of hunger in the evening, prevents sleep.
Desire for various things, but when offered appetite fails.
Appetite for: sour things; bread, particularly rye bread.
Aversion to: tobacco;•warm food; meat; spirituous liquors.

[15] **Eating and Drinking.** Drinking coffee: 10, 21. When
eating: 11, 13, 40. After eating: 10, 36. After eating and drinking: 16. Warm drink: 27. Hasty drinking: 36. Smoking: 10, 16.

[16] **Nausea and Vomiting.** Hiccough: after eating and drink-
ing; from smoking.
Belching, with pressure in the cardia.
Regurgitation of the ingesta.
Gulping up of a bitter fluid.
Nausea, without vomiting; empty retching, better by eat-
ing.
Vomit: bitter; of food.

[17] **Stomach.** ＩSensation of weakness (sinking) in the pit of
the stomach, with qualmishness and flat taste, or sighing,
Spasmodic pains in the stomach; also when better eating.
Periodical attacks of cramps worse at night, from touch;
worse from a change of position; useful during attacks
of gastralgia.
Gnawing, cutting pain in the stomach.
Heaviness and pressure in the pit of the stomach.
Bloated stomach.
Anxious feeling in the præcordia.
Fulness and pressure in epigastrium; distention of hypo-
chondria and pit of stomach, so full she can hardly
breathe.

[18] **Hypochondria.** Swelling and induration of the spleen.

[19] **Abdomen.** Periodical abdominal spasms.
Drawing and pinching in umbilical region.
Colic pains, first griping, then stitching, in one or the
other side of the abdomen.

Flatulent colic.

²⁰ Stool, etc. Diarrhœa: painless, with rumbling of wind;
worse at night and from fright, with great timidity;
with smarting in the rectum.

Fruitless efforts and urging to stool.

Stools large and soft, but passed with difficulty.

Contractive sore pain in the rectum, like from blind hemorrhoids, one or two hours after stool.

Constriction of the anus after stool, worse while standing.

Stitches from the anus up the rectum.

Itching at the anus from seat-worms.

Prolapsus of the rectum, from moderate straining at stool.

²¹ Urine. Sudden, irresistible desire to urinate.

Pressure to urinate, from drinking coffee.

Frequent profuse passage of watery urine.

Burning, smarting, or soreness in urethra during urination.

²² Male Sexual Organs. Sexual desire weak.

Erection during stool.

Contraction of penis, it becomes quite small.

Soreness and ulcerative pain, combined with itching, at
the margin of the prepuce.

Itching around genitals and on penis in evening after lying down; passes off after scratching.

²³ Female Sexual Organs. Menses: too soon; scanty, or
profuse.

Menstrual blood black, of putrid odor, in clots.

Metrorrhagia from chamomile tea.

Cramp pains in uterus, with lancinations, worse from
touching the parts.

Violent labor-like pain, followed by purulent, corrosive
leucorrhœa.

²⁴ Pregnancy, etc. Milk diminished.

After-pains with much sighing.

Puerperal convulsions, commence and terminate with
groaning and stretching of limbs; accompanied with
vomiting.

²⁵ Larynx. Voice: low; trembling; hoarseness from cold.

Sensation of soreness in the larynx.

Constrictive sensation in trachea and larynx.

²⁶ Breathing. Desire to take a deep breath.

Frequent sighing.

Impeded inspiration, like from a weight on the chest.

Oppressed breathing, alternating with convulsions.

Oppression of chest at night, worse at midnight.

Loses breath when running.

²⁷ Cough. Dry, spasmodic cough.

Hollow, spasmodic cough, caused, in evening, by a sensation
as from fumes of sulphur, or from dust in pit of throat;
in morning, from a tickling above the pit of stomach.

The longer the cough, the more the irritation to cough increases.

Cough every time he stands still, after walking.

Cough after warm drink; sleepy after each coughing spell.

Expectoration: in evening, rarely in morning; difficult, in evening; tasting and smelling like old catarrh.

²⁸ **Lungs.** Stitches in the chest, from flatulent colic.

Spasmodic constriction of the chest.

²⁹ **Heart. Pulse.** Palpitation of the heart at night and in the morning, in bed.

Pulse: generally hard, full and frequent, with thrrobing in blood-vessels: less frequent small and slow; variable.

³¹ **Neck. Back.** Stiffness of the nape of the neck.

Painless glandular swellings on the neck.

Pain in the sacrum, also when lying on back, mornings.

Spine disease, with gressus gallinaceus.

³² **Upper Limbs.** Quivering jerks in deltoid muscle.

Pains in joints of arms, when bending them backwards; like from overexertion, or as if bruised.

Numb feeling of arms at night, in bed, with it a sensation as if something living were running in the arm.

³³ **Lower Limbs.** Lancinating, cutting pains in hip-joint.

Ischias: intermitting, chronic; better in summer, worse in winter; beating as though it would burst the hip-joint, accompanied by chilliness, with thirst, flushes of heat, particularly in the face, without thirst.

Knees are involuntarily drawn upwards when walking; gressus gallinaceus.

Convulsive jerking of the lower limbs.

Cracking of the knees.

Heat of the knees, with coldness of the nose.

Heaviness of the feet.

Bruised or stinging sensation in the soles of the feet.

Burning in the heels, at night; when they come in contact, however, they feel cold.

³⁴ **Limbs in General.** Tingling in the limbs.

Pain as if sprained or dislocated, in shoulder, hip and knee-joints.

Single jerks of the limbs when falling asleep

³⁵ **Position, etc.** Moving: the eyes: 3; the neck: 9. Walking: 33. Running: 26. Standing: 20, 27. Head bent backward: 4. Must bend head forward: 3. Bending arms backward: 32. Lying down: 10, 22; on painful side: 3; on back: 31, 36. In bed: 29, 32. Better from change of position.

³⁶ **Nerves.** Trembling of the limbs.

Languor in the limbs.

Spasms of children, preceded by hasty drinking.

Convulsive twitchings, especially after fright or grief.

Convulsions: during dentition, with frothing at the mouth, kicking with the legs; during the commencement of exanthematic fevers; of children after punishment; after fear or fright; return at same hour daily.

Chorea after fright with grief, worse after eating; better lying on back.

Children convulsed in sleep after having been punished.

Paralysis after great mental emotion, and night watching in the sick chamber.

[37] **Sleep.** Spasmodic yawning: with pain in the lower jaw, as if dislocated; so that water runs from the eyes.

Sleep very light, hears everything, even distant sounds, during sleep.

Restless sleep.

Snoring inhalations during sleep.

During sleep of children: chewing motion of mouth and startings (flexors); stamping with feet and grinding of the teeth.

Child awakens from sleep with piercing cries and trembles all over.

Dreams: of one and the same object, the whole night through.

When falling asleep: 34. On awaking in morning: 10.

[38] **Time.** Morning: 3, 10, 27, 29, 31. Afternoon: 10. Evening: 10, 14, 22, 27. Night: 5, 17, 20, 26, 29, 32, 33, 36. After midnight: 26. Same hour daily: 36. Day: 5.

[39] **Temperature and Weather.** From getting heated: 46. External warmth: 40. Draught of air: 46. Open air: 46. Better in the summer, worse in the winter: 33.   KIt

[40] **Chill. Fever. Sweat.** Chill and chilliness, with increased pains.

Chill, with thirst, better from external warmth.

Chill, frequently of only the posterior part of body.

External coldness, with internal heat.

Internal chill, with external heat.

External heat without thirst, with intolerance of external warmth.

Flushes of heat, external.

Continuous quick alternations from heat to cold.

One-sided burning heat of the face.

Fainting during the heat or sweat.

Sweat slight, or only in the face.

Sensation as if sweat would break out, which, however, does not follow.

Sweat when eating; and then often on a small spot on face.

Sweat at times cold, but generally warm and somewhat sour-smelling.

[41] **Attacks.** Periodical: 17, 36.

[42] **Sides.** Left side: 18. One-sided: 40. In to out: 3, 43. Below upwards: 13, 20.

[43] **Sensations.** Oversensitive to pain.

Pressing pains from in to out, as from a hard, pointed body.

Tension in internal parts.

Pain in small circumscribed spots.

[45] **Contact, Injuries, etc.** Generally worse from slight touch; better from hard pressure.

Touch: 17, 23. Scratching: 22, 46.

[46] **Skin.** Great sensitiveness of the skin to a draught of air.

Itching: better from gentle scratching; when getting heated in the open air.

Skin chafed, sore.

Ulcers: painless; discharge scanty.

[47] **Stages and States.** Especially suitable to nervous and hysterical females of mild, but easily excited nature.

[48] **Relationship.** *Ignat.* antidotes: *Zincum.*

Ignat. may be indicated in ailments from *Coffea*, *Chamom.*, brandy, *Pulsat.*, tobacco.

Coccul. removes the decreased sexual power produced by *Ignat.*

Antidotes to *Ignat.*: *Arnic.*, *Camphor.*, *Chamom.*, *Coccul.*, *Coffea*, *Nux vom.*, *Pulsat.*

Inimicals: *Coffea*, *Tabac.*

ILLICUM ANISATUM.

Star-Anise.   Franz.   *Magnoliaceæ.*

[3] **Inner Head.** Pains in the head; less evenings, worse mornings.

[6] **Ears.** Buzzing in the ears.

Ringing in ears, followed by sleep.

Itching over left ear, going off when touching the place.

[7] **Nose.** Acute catarrh.

Watery discharge from the nostrils.

Warm smarting sensation in nose, succeeded by sneezing.

Sharp stitches in tip of nose.

[9] **Lower Face.** Stinging sensation in upper lip, as if blood would press out, better from touch.

Dryness of upper lip, which is drawn closer to the teeth.

Burning in the inner surface of lower lip, with sensation as if it had gone to sleep.

¹¹ **Tongue, etc.**   Rye bread tastes well, smells refreshing.
Tongue covered with aphthæ.
Aphthæ most on edges of tongue.
Edges of tongue folded like little bags.

¹³ **Throat.**   Tough, viscid phlegm from stomach; with old
drunkards.

¹⁵ **Eating and Drinking.**   After eating but little, satiety.
All food, except rye bread, tastes too salty or bitter, yet
appetite is good.

¹⁶ **Nausea and Vomiting.**   Nausea in stomach, extends up
to the chest, then ceases.
Nausea, with gagging and inclination to vomit.

¹⁷ **Stomach.**   Bloating of the stomach; acidity.

¹⁸ **Hypochondria.**   Pain in the splenic region.

¹⁹ **Abdomen.**   Three months' colic; bowels disturbed.
Violent wind colic.
Rumbling in abdomen.

²⁰ **Stools, etc.**   Stools: bilious; compact and dark colored.

²¹ **Urine.**   Retention of urine.

²⁶ **Breathing.**   Old asthmatics.

²⁷ **Cough.**   After coughing, feeling of emptiness.
Frequent cough, with pain.
Spitting blood in small quantities and with pus-like
phlegm, with pain in right chest.
Whitish expectoration.

²⁸ **Lungs.**   Tough, viscous phlegm, with old drunkards.
Pain in region of third rib, about one or two inches from
the sternum, generally on right side, but occasionally
left.

²⁹ **Heart.   Pulse.**   Palpitation, with aphthæ and weakness.

³¹ **Neck.   Back.**   Cramp-like drawing, as from a cold, in the
left side of dorsal vertebræ.

³³ **Lower Limbs.**   Left thigh feels as if broken at the middle,
when sitting, ceases on rising.

³⁵ **Position, etc.**   Sitting: 33.   Rising: 33.

³⁸ **Time.**   Better in the morning; worse, evening: 3.

⁴² **Sides.**   Right: 27, 28.   Left: 6, 18, 28, 31, 33.

⁴⁵ **Contact, Injuries, etc.**   Touch lessons itching and other
sensations in skin: 6, 9.

⁴⁷ **Stages and States.**   Old drunkards, catarrh of stomach.

⁴⁸ **Relationship.**   Old drunkards: 13, 28.
Where *Bryon.* and *Acon.* did not relieve blood-spitting.

IODUM.

Iodine. HAHNEMANN. *The Element.*

[1] **Mind.** Feels constantly as if she had forgotton something.

Fixed, immovable thoughts.

Fear of evil, with overcarefulness.

Shrinking and fear when anyone comes near, particularly the physician (this is not in gout).

Mind very sensitive during digestion, felt like crying.

Melancholy mood, low-spirited.

Irritability and sensitiveness. Excessive excitability.

Must keep in motion day and night, brain felt as if it were stirred up, felt as if going crazy

[2] **Sensorium.** Vertigo: only on left side; with throbbing in head and all over body, tremor at heart, fainting; worse immediately after rising from a seat or bed; or by sitting or lying down after slight exercise.

[3] **Inner Head.** Headache; left side and top, sometimes paralytic feeling of the arms.

Headache, as if a tape or band were tightly drawn around head.

Headache worse: in warm air; when riding a long time in a carriage; from walking fast.

Pressure on a small spot above root of nose.

Throbbing in the head, at every motion.

[5] **Eyes.** Optical illusions in bright colors.

Obscuration of sight.

Like a vail before the eyes.

Protrusion of the balls.

Smarting in the eyes.

Constant tearing pain around right eye; passing backwards from inner canthus to articulation of jaw.

Trembling of the lids.

Dilation of the pupil, with constant motion of the balls.

White of the eye dirty yellow.

Œdematous swelling of the lids.

[6] **Ears.** Sensitiveness to noise.

Hearing first sensitive, then dull.

Buzzing in the ears.

Adhesions in the middle ear.

[7] **Nose.** Sensation as if the alæ were spread wide open and nose dry; loss of smell; in the evening, sneezing.

Dry coryza, becoming fluent in the open air.

Chronic fetid discharge form nose; nose painful and swollen.

[8] **Face.** Face: pale, yellow, or soon changing to brown; sallow, distressed; pale, alternating with red.

Convulsive twitchings of the facial muscles.

Coldness of the face in very fleshy children.

[10] **Teeth.** Toothache, gums swollen and bleeding.

Little blisters form on the gums.

Gums puffed, red, inflamed, painful to touch, and bleed easily.

[11] **Tongue, etc.** Taste: salty; sourish; sweetish, on tip of tongue.

Tongue: dry; brown and dry; thickly coated.

[12] **Mouth.** Mouth filled with mucus on awaking in the morning, with putrid taste, not relieved by washing mouth with water.

Copious, sweet saliva.

Ptyalism; also, that after mercury.

Aphthæ in the mouth.

Ulcers in the mouth, gums red and swollen, receding from the teeth, bleeding slightly, and with small ash-colored painful ulcers; profuse fetid ptyalism.

Thick, brown, croup-like exudation in mouth and fauces.

[13] **Throat.** Swelling and elongation of the uvula.

Inflammation of the throat, with burning pain.

Sensation of constriction (fulness or pressure) in the larynx, with impeded deglutition.

Ulcers in the throat, with swelling of the gland of neck.

Inflammation and ulceration of the œsophagus.

[14] **Desires. Aversions.** Hunger, suffering from it, must eat every few hours; gets anxious and worried if he does not eat.

Eats freely, yet loses flesh all the time.

Alternate canine hunger and want of appetite.

Much thirst: 40.

[15] **Eating and Drinking.** Fasting causes pain in the chest.

Eating: 16, 17; heavy food: 16. Drinking milk: 20.

[16] **Nausea and Vomiting.** Hiccough.

Heart-burn, after heavy food.

Empty eructations from morning till evening.

Sour eructations, with burning therefrom.

Qualmishness, nausea, with spasmodic pain in stomach.

Violent vomiting renewed by eating.

Vomiting: of bile, with violent colic; of milk.

Stomach. Spasmodic pains in stomach, renewed by eating.

Pulsations in the pit of stomach.

Tenderness of the epigastrium.

Stitches in stomach, relaxed feeling, must loosen clothing; milk disagrees; intense thirst.

[18] **Hypochondria.** Region of liver sore to pressure.

Swelling of the spleen, after intermittent fever; vague
pains down to left iliac region.

¹⁹ **Abdomen.**   Swelling and distention of the abdomen.

Incarceration of flatulence in left side of abdomen.

Violent throbbing of the aorta abdominalis.

Swelling of the inguinal glands.

²⁰ **Stool, etc.**   Stools: of watery, foaming, whitish mucus,
always in the morning; copious, papescent; dysenteric, mucous, without feces; whey-like; fatty.

Constipation, alternating with diarrhœa.

Constipation, with ineffectual urging, better after drinking
milk.

Stools hard, knotty, dark colored.

²¹ **Urine.**   Incontinence of urine, in the aged.

Urine: dark, thick, ammoniacal; dark, yellowish-green;
acrid; milky; with a variegated cuticle on its surface.

²² **Male Sexual Organs**.   Bearing down, or twisting, in the
seminal cord.

Swelling and induration of testicles, and of prostrate gland.

Painless swelling of the testicles, with offensive sweat.

²³ **Female Sexual Organs.**   Menses: sometimes too early, at
others too late; premature, violent and copious.

Uterine hemorrhage, renewed after every stool.

Metrorrhagia, with acute pain in mammæ; or, mammæ
dwindle away and become flabby.

Induration and swelling of the uterus and ovaries.

Dropsical affections of the ovaries, with pressing down
toward the genitals.

Dull, pressing, wedge-like pains, from right ovary toward
the uterus.

Leucorrhœa: acrid, corroding the limbs; worse at time of
menses.

Bluish-red nodosities, size of a hazel-nut, in the skin of
both mammæ; dry, black points at the tips.

²⁴ **Pregnancy.**   *Iodum* should not be given during lying-in,
except in high potencies.

²⁵ **Larynx.**   Hoarseness, lasts all day, phlegm in small quantities and tough, constant hemming and hawking.

Tightness and constriction about the larynx, with soreness and hoarseness.

ı Œdema glottidis (may be used by inhalation).

Membranous croup, with wheezing and sawing respiration, dry, barking cough, especially children with dark
eyes and dark hair; child grasps the throat with the
hand, raises large, tough flakes (not stringy exudation);
fever.

²⁶ **Breathing.**   Shortness of breath, palpitation and feeling of
weakness on going up stairs.

²⁷ **Cough.** Dry morning cough, from tickling in the larynx.
Dry cough, with stitches and burning in the chest.
Cough, with expectoration of large quantities of mucus,
frequently blood-streaked.
Expectoration: salty; sourish; grey or white.

²⁸ **Lungs.** Sensation of weakness in the chest.
Sharp, quick, piercing pains.
Tendency to bronchial and pulmonary congestion and
hemorrhage.
ı Hepatization, worse upper part of right lung; high fever,
restlessness, thirst; apathy. Rapid hepatization; tightness across the chest.

²⁹ **Heart. Pulse.** Violent palpitation, worse from the least
exertion.
Sensation as if the heart were squeezed together.
Heart acts tumultuously, with hard, full pulse; or, pulse
small, weak.
Constant, heavy, oppressive pain, in region of the heart.
Pulse: large, hard and accelerated, with orgasm of blood
and beating in the blood-vessels; rapid, but weak and
thread-like; accelerated, by every slight exertion.

³¹ **Neck. Back.** Goitre, with marked hardness.
Swelling and induration of the cervical glands.
Spinal complaints, with gressus vaccinus.

³² **Upper Limbs.** Weariness of the arms, as if paralyzed, in
the morning, in bed.
Painful weakness in the extensors.
Pains in the left elbow.
Coldness of the hands and feet.
Fingers "go to sleep."

³³ **Lower Limbs.** Hot, bright red swelling of the knee, with
inflammation, pricking and burning; aggravated by
touch or pressure.
Violent itching nettle-rash, particularly around the knee;
on outer side of left knee especially.
Œdematous swelling of the feet.
Acrid, corrosive sweat of the foot.
Painful corns.

³⁴ **Limbs in General.** Subsultus tendinum of hands and feet.
Chronic arthritic affections, with violent nightly pains in
the joins, no swelling.

³⁵ **Position, etc.** Motion: 1, 3. Sitting: 2. After rising: 2.
Lying down: 2, 32. Walking: 3. Exertion: 2, 29.
Ascending: 26.

³⁶ **Nerves.** Twitches of muscles.
Trembling of limbs or whole body.
Great debility; sweats, even from talking.
Rapid failing of strength.

37 Sleep. Sleeplessness after midnight.
Restless sleep, with vivid or anxious dreams.
38 Time. Morning: 12, 20, 27, 32, 40. Evening: 7. Night:
34, 40, 44. After midnight: 37. Day and night: 1.
Day: 16, 25.
39 Temperature and Weather. Warm air: 3. Warm room:
40. Open air: 7.
40 Chill. Fever. Sweat. Cold feet, the whole night.
Chill, with shaking, also in the warm room.
Chill, frequently alternating with heat.
Flushes of heat over the whole body.
Internal heat, with coldness of the skin.
I Marked fever, restlessness, thirst, throbbing headache,
circumscribed red cheeks; mind apathetic. θ Pneu-
monia, croup, etc.
Profuse night-sweat.
Debilitating, sour-smelling sweat in the morning hours,
with much thirst.
42 Sides. Right: 5, 18, 23. Left: 2, 3, 18, 19, 32, 33. Right
to left: 23.
44 Tissues. Swelling and induration of the glands.
I Plastic exudations.
Nightly bone-pains.
Arthritic affections of the joints, with effusion and with
great emaciation.
Emaciation.
45 Contact, Injuries, etc. Touch: 10, 33. Pressure: 18, 33.
Riding: 3.
Violent pulsations all over; anguish and dyspnœa; com-
pression of the brain.
46 Skin. Rough, dry skin. Dirty yellow, clammy, moist
skin.
Scars itch, break open, or pimples break out on them.
Nodes.
47 Stages and States. Dark hair and eyes.
Overgrown boys; weak chests.
Scrofulous diathesis.
Aged persons.
48 Relationship. *Iodum* is frequently suitable in ailments
from *Arsen.*, *Mercur.*, *Calcar.* or *Arg. nitr.*
Iodum follows well after *Mercur.*, and is followed by *Kali
bichr.* (croup).
Iodum and *Lycop.* are complementary.
Antidotes to *Iodum:* of large doses, starch or wheat flour,
beat up in water; of small doses, *Ant. tart.*, *Arsen.*,
Bellad., *Camphor.*, *Chin. sulph.*, *Cinchon.*, *Coffea*, *Hepar*,
Opium, *Phosphor.*, *Spongia*, *Sulphur.*

IPECACUANHA.

Root of Ipecac.   HAHNEMANN.   *Rubiaceæ.*

[1] **Mind.** Full of desires, but knows not for what.
   Screams, howls violently.
   Taciturnity, wrapt in thought.
   Ill-humor, despises everything.
   Irascible, restless, angry in suddenly appearing spells.
   Ailments from anger, mortification, or vexation, with
      indignation.
[2] **Sensorium.** Vertigo when walking and when turning.
[3] **Inner Head.** Headache, as if bruised, all through bones of
      head and down into root of tongue: nausea, vomiting;
      better out-door.
   Heat and throbbing in the head, with red cheeks.
   Aching in the forehead; fine stinging pains in forehead.
   Throbbing in the forehead.
   Pains into eyes, with lachrymation.
   Semi-lateral headache, with nausea and vomiting.
   Lancinating in the head.
   Pain in occiput and nape of neck.
[4] **Outer Head.** Open fontanelles; occiput and neck sore.
[5] **Eyes.** Worse from light, especially of a candle.
   Blue and red halo around the light.
   Obscuration of sight; eyes inflammed, red.
   Dilated pupils.
   Red circle around the cornea.
   Scleroticæ yellow.
   Violent inflammation of the sclerotic conjunctiva; che-
      mosis; profuse lachrymation; gushing of tears; nausea.
      Cornea dim, with a number of depressions on it; pus-
      tules.
   Severe shooting pains through the eyeballs.
   Twitching of the eyelids.
[6] **Ears.** Cannot endure the least noise.
   Ears cold, during the febrile heat.
[7] **Nose.** Loss of smell; catarrh, with nausea, epistaxis; stop-
      page of nose.
   Nosebleed; blood bright.
[8] **Face.** Face: pale, bloated; livid; yellow; deathly pale,
      eyes sunken, and with blue margins.
   Periodical infra and supraorbital neuralgia, with photo-
      phobia, lachrymation and smarting eyelids; malarial.
   Convulsive muscular twitchings.
   Rash.

⁹ **Lower Face.** Red skin around the mouth.

Lips blue; during chill.

¹⁰ **Teeth.** Child thrusts its fist into its mouth; screams; face pale; dentition.

Pain in a hollow tooth when biting on it.

¹¹ **Tongue, etc.** Taste: bitter; sweetish, bloody; like rancid oil, when swallowing.

Tongue: clean; yellow or white; grows pale.

Disinclined to talk; tongue dry.

¹² **Mouth.** Saliva increased.

Smarting in the mouth and on the tongue.

¹³ **Throat.** Fauces dry, sore, rough, stinging.

Difficult deglutition.

Pressure in the throat, with pains in the diaphragm.

¹⁴ **Desires. Aversions.** Desire for dainties, sweets.

Averse to all food, no appetite; earthy taste; stomach feels relaxed; nausea.

Thirst.

Thirstlessness.

¹⁵ **Eating and Drinking.** Aggravation: from indigestible substances, lemon peel, raisins, cake, etc., even spasms therefrom; from fruit, salads, pastry, pork, fats, etc.

After any cold drink (also from ice cream) colic, nausea, vomit.

Drinking: 40.

¹⁶ **Nausea and Vomiting.** Empty belching; copious saliva.

Hiccough, with nausea.

Nausea, constant, with almost all complaints; nausea, as if from the stomach.

Nausea and retching from smoking; primary effects of tobacco.

Vomiting: of ingesta; bile; copiously of jelly-like mucus; of blood, or of a pitch-like substance; of a dark colored liquid, with or without blood; of sour fluid; always with nausea.

Vomiting: with thirst, sweat, bad breath; with diarrhœa, colic, distended abdomen; after vomit, sleepy.

Vomiting worse from stooping.

¹⁷ **Stomach.** Violent distress in pit of stomach.

Indescribable sick feeling in the stomach.

Gastric catarrh, from indigestible food or ice-cold things.

Stomach feels relaxed, as if hanging down.

Attacks of clutching pains.

Beating in the stomach.

Dyspepsia every day, or every other day, at the same hour.

¹⁸ **Hypochondria.** Pain in the left hypochondrium.

Diaphragm, as if pressed between two millstones.

¹⁹ **Abdomen.** Griping, as from a hand, each finger seemingly

pressing sharply into the intestines; better during rest, much worse by motion.

With every movement cutting, almost constantly running from left to right.

Flatulent colic, with frequent loose stools.

Cutting about the umbilicus.

Inguinal hernia readily reducible.

²⁰ **Stool, etc.**   Diarrhœa, with pain, causing unceasing screaming and tossing about.

Stools: yellow, painless, fermented; as if fermented, green as grass, with nausea and colic; green mucus; covered with red, bloody mucus; bloody; pitch-like or like frothy molasses; slimy, bloody, offensive, followed by tenesmus.

Autumnal diarrhœa; much griping about navel.

Beginning cholera infantum, nausea, vomiting, colic, diarrhœa; especially in fat, pale children.

Itching at the anus.

Shooting from right kidney to knee.

²¹ **Urine.**   Urine: scanty, dark red; turbid, with red sediment.

Unsuccessful urging to urinate.

Hæmaturia: with cutting in abdomen and urethra; from suppressed itch.

²³ **Female Sexual Organs.**   Prolapsus and hemorrhage at the menstrual period.

Menses too early and profuse.

²⁴ **Pregnancy.**   Hemorrhage from the uterus, blood bright red, profuse, clotted; nausea; breathing heavy, oppressed; stitches from navel to uterus.

Labor-pains spasmodic; cutting across from left to right; nausea; clutching about the navel.

Lying-in: 46.

²⁵ **Larynx.**   Voice hollow.

Laryngismus stridulus.

Rattling in bronchia, when drawing a long breath.

Foreign substances in the windpipe; suffocative attacks.

²⁶ **Breathing.**   Breathing: sighing; quick, anxious.

Breath: fetid, with vomit and sweat; short, as from inhaling dust.

Difficult expiration.

Violent constriction of throat and chest, peculiar panting sound; gasps for air at open window; face pale; worse from least motion; threatened suffocation. θ Asthma.

Loses breath with the cough.

During a catarrh, threatened suffocation, especially if it is suddenly suppressed.

²⁷ **Cough.**   Cough: rough, shaking; dry, from titillation in upper part of larynx; with every breath; with inclina-

tion to vomit; with spitting of blood from the least effort; constant, no phlegm yields, though the chest seems full; strangling, so much mucus seems accumulated in the bronchia; croupy, at night; fat children.

Whooping-cough, with nosebleed, bleeding from mouth, vomiting; loses breath, turns pale or blue, and becomes rigid.

Suffocative evening cough; continuous cough, with sweat on forehead, shocks in the head, retching and vomiting.

Expectoration, mornings, of a light red blood, mixed with mucus; or of ropy mucus, often vomited up.

[28] **Lungs.** Infantile pneumonia; respiration rapid, difficult; surface blue; face pale.

Rattling of large bubbles; fever, but face rather pale; cough and gagging.

Hemorrhage from the lungs; worse from least exertion; frequent hacking, with expectoration of blood-streaked mucus.

Fine rattling noises in chest, spasmodic cough; nausea.

θ Œdema pulmonum.

[29] **Heart. Pulse.** Pulse: large and soft; accelerated, but weak.

[31] **Neck. Back.** Swelling and suppuration in the throat-pit.

Cramp between the scapulæ during motion.

Shooting pains, from right kidney down thigh to knee.

[32] **Upper Limbs.** Coldness of one hand, while the other is hot.

[33] **Lower Limbs.** Sensation in the femur, as if dislocated, on sitting down.

Cramps in the thighs at night.

Convulsive twitchings of legs and feet.

Itching of the calves.

Ulcer, with black base, on the foot.

[34] **Limbs in General.** Pain in back and limbs.

Cold hands and feet.

[35] **Position, etc.** Walking: 2. Turning: 2. Stooping: 16. Motion: 19, 26, 31, 40. Rest: 19. Tossing about: 20. Least effort: 27, 28. Sitting: 33.

[36] **Nerves.** Body rigid, stretched out, followed by spasmodic jerking of the arms.

Tetanic spasms from swallowing tobacco.

Awkward, stumbles against everything.

Convulsions: in whooping-cough; from suppressed exanthema; from indigestible food, etc.

Epileptiform spasms, with shrieks; opisthotonos; face pale, puffed; gastric derangements.

Very weak, averse to all food; nausea; sudden prostration.

[37] **Sleep.** Yawning and stretching.

On falling off to sleep, shocks in the limbs.

Sleep, with half-open eyes; moaning, groaning.

Sleepless.

When deprived of sleep; nausea, languor.

38 Time. Morning: 27. 11 A. M.: 40. Evening: 27. Night: 17, 33.

39 Temperature and Weather. Oversensitive to heat and cold.

Worse in winter and in dry weather.

Worse in warm moist wind, south winds: catarrhs; asthma.

Out of doors: 3, 40. Air at open window: 26. Warmth: 40. Open air: 40. Room: 40.

40 Chill. Fever. Sweat. Chill every other day at 11 A. M.

Coldness of upper part of body.

Chill worse in a warm room or from external heat; lessened by drinking, and in the open air. Vomiting during.

Internal chill, external heat.

Backache, short chill, long fever; heat usually with thirst; headache, nausea and cough; sweat last.

Heat all over, with alternate coldness and paleness of face; cold sweat on the forehead.

Sweat: hot, sudden attacks in the room; partial, cold; on upper part of body; worse by motion; smells sour; stains yellow; increased out of doors; cold, clammy; profuse after quinine.

Intermittent fevers after abuse of quinine; also in beginning of irregular cases, especially if there is much nausea; also like *Natr. mur.*, chill, fever and sweat with frontal headache.

Worse during sweat; better after it.

41 Attacks. Attacks of illness, with loathing of food.

Every day or every other day at same hour: 17, 40. Autumn: 20.

42 Sides. Right: 21, 31. Left: 18. Left to right: 19, 24. Above downward: 31.

44 Tissues. Hemorrhages, bright red.

Plethora, fat children.

Pains as if all the bones were being torn to pieces; with vomiting and pains in the bowels.

Dropsy in internal parts.

Skin and muscles lax.

Chlorosis: menses scanty; skin and mucous surfaces pale, anæmic.

46 Skin. Miliaria rubra, with dyspnœa, colic, nausea.

Miliary rash on forehead, temples, cheek.

Skin itches; he scratches until he vomits.

Rash (of the lying-in).

Eruptions suppressed, or tardily appearing, with oppression of the chest; vomiting and tickling cough.

Erysipelas, the redness leaves too soon, with renewed vomiting.

[43] **Relationship.** *Ipec.* is followed well: by *Arsen.* in cholera infantum, debility, croup, chills, etc.; by *Ant. tart.* in foreign substances in larynx; by *Nux vom., Arsen.* in checked cold; by *Apis* in keratitis.

Antidotes to *Ipec.: Arnic., Arsen., Cinchon., Nux vom., Tabac.*

Ipec. antidotes: *Alum., Arnic., Arsen., Cinchon.,* vapors of copper, *Dulcam., Ferrum., Lauroc., Opium, Tabac., Tart. em.*

Complementary: *Cuprum.*

IRIS VERSICOLOR.

Blue flag.   Kitchen.   *Iridaceæ.*

[1] **Mind.** Low-spirited.

Fear of approaching illness.

Easily vexed.

Cannot fix his mind on his studies. Dulness of mental faculties.

[3] **Inner Head.** Dull throbbing or shooting in right side of forehead; nausea; worse toward evening; from rest, from cold air, or coughing; better from moderate motion.

Tired headache, from mental exhaustion.

Sick headache, eighth day. Begins with blurred vision.

[4] **Outer Head.** Shooting in the temples, mostly the right, with constrictive feeling of the scalp.

[5] **Eyes.** Redness of the conjunctiva, as from a cold; eyes feel dull, with the neuralgia; burning in the internal canthus, with effusion of tears.

[7] **Nose.** Constant sneezing; sharp pains in centre of temples; tickling cough; light, mushy stools.

[8] **Face.** Neuralgia involving supra and infraorbital, superior maxillary and inferior dental nerves; begins after breakfast every morning, with a stupid, stunning headache; copious urine; disposition to stool; burning at the anus

Sunken eyes with blueness around.

[11] **Tongue, etc.** Loss of taste; flat taste.

Tongue feels as if scalded; greasy feeling on arising in morning.

[12] **Mouth.** Burning in mouth and fauces, as if on fire.

Ulcers on the mucous lining of the cheeks.

Salivation after diphtheria, with swelling of the parotids.

Saliva taste greasy, slimy.

[14] **Desires. Aversions.** Loss of taste and appetite.

[15] **Eating and Drinking.** Headache after breakfast; aching in the stomach before breakfast and after a cold drink.

Milk sours and is vomited.

[16] **Nausea and Vomiting.** Eructations tasteless, or of sour food.

Nausea and vomiting of sour fluid that excoriates throat; sour vomit with the headache.

Vomiting: of food, an hour after eating; of bile, with great heat and sweat.

[17] **Stomach.** Great burning distress in epigastrium; can hardly endure it.

Colicky pains every few minutes, in the epigastrium.

Shocks of pain in the umbilical region up to epigastrium; nausea, straining and belching of wind,

Inflammation, burning distress in pancreas, sweetish vomit.

[18] **Hypochondria.** Cutting in the region of the liver.

Pain in right hypochondriac region; worse from motion.

Pains above the chest of the ilium, right side, then left.

[19] **Abdomen.** Colicky pains, intermittent, about the navel, before each spell of vomiting or purging.

[20] **Stool, etc.** Stool: thin, watery, tinged with bile, copious, in a continuous stream; green, undigested; mushy, pappy with fetid flatus; bloody mucus, with great straining; burning in anus and rectum after stool; black, with fever, hot sweat, white tongue, severe headache, despondency; yellow, watery, corrosive.

[21] **Urine.** Scanty, red; burning the length of the urethra after passing it; clear, profuse.

[22] **Male Sexual Organs.** Nocturnal emissions, with amorous dreams; coldness and itching of the parts.

[24] **Pregnancy.** Morning sickness, vomit sour or bitter.

[25] **Larynx.** Dry, tickling cough, smarting-burning in throat.

[27] **Cough.** Short, dry cough, from tickling in the larynx.

[28] **Lungs.** Pain in left side of chest, as if the ribs were pressing against the lungs.

[32] **Upper Limbs,** Pains shift about rapidly in phalanges and metacarpal bones.

[33] **Lower Limbs.** Sciatica, sudden shooting, causing lameness; feels as if (left) hip-joint was wrenched; pain and lameness extend to popliteal space; worse from moderate, better from violent motion.

[34] **Limbs in General.** Shifting pains in right hip, both knees (worse right) and in right foot especially, and first joint of great toe.

[35] **Position, etc.** Motion: 3, 18, 33, 34.

[36] **Nerves.** Faint, weak knees, trembling; sunken eyes; after

protracted or severe sero-bilious stools, as in summer diarrhœa.

[38] **Time.** Morning: 8, 11, 15, 24. Evening: 3. Night: 22, 46. 3 A.M.: 20. Day: 3.

[39] **Temperature and Weather.** Cold air: 3, 13. When covered: 40.

[40] **Chill. Fever. Sweat.** Chills, with sleepiness.

Heat followed by chill, with cold hands and feet.

Chills over the whole body, even when well covered; fever with muttering delirium and bilious diarrhœa.

Skin hot; dry, black stool.

Sweat all over, particularly on the groin.

[41] **Attacks.** Every morning: 8   Every eighth day: 3.

[42] **Sides.** Right: 3, 4, :8, 34, 46. Right to left: 10. Below upwards: 17, 24.

[44] **Tissues.** Excites the secretion of the glands; salivary, pancreatic, intestinal, etc.

Acts powerfully on gastro-intestinal mucous membrane.

[46] **Skin.** Pustular eruption on scalp, face, around mouth.

Irregular patches on knees, elbows and body, with shining scales, the edges slightly raised.

Herpes zoster on the right side of the body.

Fine eruption, showing black points after scratching, great itching at night.

JACEA. (Viola tricolor.)

Pansy.   FRANZ.   *Violaceæ.*

[1] **Mind.** Great dulness of the intellect.

Low-spirited about domestic affairs.

Great indifference.

Bad, morose humor, with disinclination to talk.

Very sensitive and inclined to scold.

[2] **Sensorium.** Vertigo when walking.

Heaviness of the head when raising it, which disappears by stooping.

[3] **Inner Head.** Pressing headache, chiefly in forehead and temples.

[4] **Outer Head.** Scurfs on head, unbearable burning, most at night.

Tinea capitis, with frequent involuntary urination.

Burning stitches in scalp, especially in forehead and temples.

Impetigo of the hairy scalp and face.

Crusta lactea: with violent cough and excessive oppression;
in children recently weaned.

Thick incrustations, pouring out a large quantity of thick
yellow fluid, which agglutinates the hair.

⁵ **Eyes.**   Smarting in the eyes.

The eyelids sink down as from sleepiness.

⁸ **Face.**   Heat of side of face not lain on, evening in bed.

Induration of the skin of the face.

Milk-crust, burning, itching, especially at night, with discharge of viscid yellow pus.

Impetiginous exanthem on the forehead.

Tension in the integuments of the face and forehead.

⁹ **Lower Face.**   Pustular eruption on whole upper lip and
chin; a thick, yellow, friable, semi-transparent incrusta-
tion; acne rosacea on the chin.

¹¹ **Tongue, etc.**   Taste bitter, tongue coated with white mucus.

¹² **Mouth.**   Sensation of dryness, yet with much saliva in the
mouth.

¹³ **Throat.**   Much phlegm in the throat, causes hawking, at
11 A.M.

¹⁵ **Eating and Drinking.**   While eating, hot sweat.

Immediately after eating: dyspnœa, anxious heat.

¹⁸ **Hypochondria.**   Pressing-stinging in the diaphragm.

¹⁹ **Abdomen.**   Cutting pains in the abdomen, with urging to
stool, crying and lamentations, followed by profuse discharge of flatus, with large lumps of mucus.

²⁰ **Stool, etc.**   Stool: soft as if minced; of mucus, with much
flatus.

²¹ **Urine.**   Urging to urinate, with profuse discharge of urine.

Urine: offensive, smelling like cat's urine; very turbid.

Stitches in the urethra.

²² **Male Sexual Organs.**   ▮Involuntary seminal discharges,
with vivid lewd dreams.

Suppression of gonorrhœa.

Venereal ulcers.

Swelling of the prepuce, with itching.

Stitches in penis or pressing in glans; burning in glans.

Itching stitches in the scrotum.

Induration of the testicle, after gonorrhœa.

²⁸ **Lungs.**   Stitches in chest, on ribs, sternum and intercostal
muscles.

²⁹ **Heart. Pulse.**   Oppression and stitches in the heart, on
bending forward when sitting.

Anxiety about heart while lying, with beating like waves.

³¹ **Neck. Back.**   Tension between the shoulder-blades, with
cutting and tingling in the skin.

Swelling and induration of the cervical glands.

³² **Upper Limbs.**   Stitches in the shoulder-joints, elbows, forearms and fingers.

33

[33] **Lower Limbs.** Stitches in the patella, tibia and feet.
Pustulous and ichorous exanthema on the feet.

[35] **Position, etc.** Walking: 2. Raising head: 2. Stooping:
2. Side not lain on: 8.

[36] **Nerves.** Nervous paroxysms after suppressed crusta lactea.

[37] **Sleep.** Yawning.
Goes to sleep late on account of ideas crowding his mind.
The child twitches with his hands in his sleep, with
clenched thumbs, generally dry heat and red face.
Dreams: pleasant or amorous.

[38] **Time.** Forenoon: 40. 11 A.M.: 13. Evening: 8. Night:
4, 8, 40, 46.

[39] **Temperatue and Weather.** Aversion to the open air.
Open air: 40.

[40] **Chill. Fever. Sweat.** Chill or chilliness in the forenoon,
and in the open air.
Dry, anxious heat at night in bed, with red face.
Night-sweat.

[41] **Tissues.** Rheumatism or gout.
Articular rheumatism, with itch-like eruption around the
joints.

[45] **Contact, Injuries, etc.** Worse from pressure on the side
opposite to the unpainful one.
Worse lying on the painful side.
Scratching: 46.

[46] **Skin.** Cutting or stinging in the skin.
Eruption: burning, dry, stinging; violent itching, worse
at night; crusty; scurfy.
Squamous spots on the skin.
Dry scabs over body, exude yellow water when scratched.
Large boils all over the body.
Ichorous ulcers with violent itching.
Burrowing ulcers.
Consequences of suppressed eruptions.
Skin difficult to heal.

[47] **Stages and States.** Scrofulous children.

KALI BICHROMICUM.

Potassic dicromate. DRYSDALE. $K_2\ Cr_2\ O_7$.

[1] **Mind.** Anxiety arising from the chest.
Listlessness, languor; great disinclination for mental or
bodily labor.
Anthropophobia.

Indifferent or low-spirited after the least annoyance, with
distress in stomach.

Ill-humored ; low-spirited.

[22] **Sensorium.**   Vertigo, with nausea, inclination to vomit and
pain in the epigastrium; better in the open air.

Lightness in the head, across the forehead, on stooping;
worse mornings.

Sudden transient attacks of vertigo, when rising from a
seat.

[3] **Inner Head.**   Soon after dinner, a dull, heavy throbbing
above the eyes, as if head would burst; relieved by
lying, or pressing head against anything, or in open
air ; worse stooping or moving about.

Periodic headache with vertigo and nausea, morning
awaking, also in evening; often relieved by pressure,
in the open air, or by eating.

Blindness, followed by violent headache, must lie down;
aversion to light and noise; sight returns with the increasing headache.

In the morning, on awaking, pain in the forehead and
vertex; later extends to the back of the head.

[4] **Outer Head.**   Violent shooting pains from root of nose
along left orbital arch to external angle of eye, with
dim sight, like a scale on the eye; begins in morning,
increases till noon, and ceases towards evening.

Frontal headache: usually over one eye; shooting at intervals in the right temple.

Semi-lateral headache in small spots, or along the course
of a few nerves.

Darting or aching pains on one side; flying pains.

Bones of head feel sore; sharp stitches in the bones.

[5] **Eyes.**   Sight dim, confused: before headache; with vertigo;
with yellow sight.

Photophobia only by daylight; when opening the lids
they twitch.

Catarrhal inflammation, stringy discharge, or scanty secretion, worse mornings on awaking.

On opening the eyes, lachrymation and burning.

Heat and redness in the eyes, with desire to rub them.

Indolent ulcers of the cornea; pale ring around cornea.

Sequelæ of iritis; pains pricking, stinging, wandering;
mostly of the left eye.

True descemetitis; fine punctate opacities on membrane
of Descemet, especially over the pupil.

Conjunctiva red, travered by large vessels; or chemosis
with small spots here and there, like ecchymoses.

White of the eye dirty yellow, puffy, and covered with
yellow-brown points.

Long-lasting dense opacities of the cornea.

Brown spots on the cornea.

Lids agglutinated in the morning; yellow matter in the canthi.

Œdema of the lids; great desire to rub them.

Shooting pains over the eyebrow: 48.

Heaviness of the upper lids on waking; requires an effort to open them.

Lids red, itching, tender; tarsi seem rough, causing a sensation as from sand in the eyes; granular lids.

⁶ **Ears.** Stitches in the left ear and left parotid gland, with headache.

Violent stitches in left ear, extending into roof of mouth, side of head and neck; glands swollen, neck painful to touch.

Thick, yellow, fetid discharge from both ears. *θ* After scarlatina.

Pulsating pains in the ears at night; also stinging; external meatus swollen and inflamed.

Itching of the (right) ear-lobe, waking him.

⁷ **Nose.** Loss of smell.

Fetid smell from the nose.

Burrowing and beating in root of nose; external heat, throbbing; nose swollen and hot; fulness as from something thick; nose dry and heavy as from a weight on it.

Thick, dark red blood from the nose; irregular, small, contracted pulse.

Ropy, tough discharge, often also from the posterior nares; offensive or not. Discharge of tough green masses; or hard plugs.

Coryza fluent, excoriating nose and lip; nostrils sensitive, ulcerated; round ulcer or scabs on the septum; small perforating ulcers on septum.

Spot in the right lachrymal bone is swollen and throbbing; profuse secretion from the nostril.

Coryza, with pressure and tightness at root of nose; distress and fulness from inflammation in frontal sinuses; worse evenings and in the open air; in the morning obstruction and bleeding from right nostril.

Sneezing in the morning; on going into the open air.

Tickling, as from a hair, high up in the left nostril.

⁸ **Face.** Face: pale, yellowish; red, in blotches; flushed.

Expression: anxious.

Bones of face sensitive, painful, as if bruised.

Shooting pain in left upper maxillary bone towards ear; acute infraorbital parts of malar bone.

⁹ **Lower Face.** Digging in the rami of the lower jaw.

Lower lip swelled, chapped.

Ulcerations, with indurated edges and smarting on the mucous surface of the lower lip.

Mumps on the right side.

Parotids swollen; pains from ears into the glands.

[11] **Tongue, etc.**   Taste: coppery; sweetish; sour; bitter, in the morning.

Tongue broad, or with scalloped edges.

▮Sensation of a hair on the back part of the tongue and velum; not relieved by eating or drinking.

Tongue coated thick yellow, edges red and full of small painful ulcers; thick yellow fur toward base in catarrhs of stomach.

▮Tongue dry, smooth, red, cracked; dysentery.

Deep ulcer on edge of tongue; syphilitic ulcers on tongue; deep; stinging.

[12] **Mouth.**   Dryness of the mouth and lips, relieved by drinking cold water.

Saliva: increased, bitter, viscid, frothy; tasting salt.

[13] **Throat.**   Soft palate, slightly reddened; uvula relaxed, with sensation of a plug in the throat, not relieved by swallowing.

▮Œdematous uvula.

Deep excavated sore, with a reddish areola, and containing a yellow, tenacious matter, at the root of the uvula; fauces and palate erythematous, bright, or dark red, or coppery.

Sharp, shooting pains in the left tonsil, extending toward the ear; relieved by swallowing; suppuration of the tonsils.

Ulcers in the fauces; also in the pharynx, discharging cheesy lumps, of offensive smell.

Ulcers on tonsils and throat covered with an ashy slough, dark livid surrounding.

Posterior wall of pharynx is dark red, glossy, puffed, showing ramifications of pale red vessels; on the left of the middle a small crack, exuding blood.

Redness of sound places in mucous membrane of mouth and fauces; tough, stringy nasal discharge; putrid odor; ulcers in the month.   θ Diphtheria.

Throat pains more when putting the tongue out.

Dryness and burning in throat, mornings; often coincident with inability to breathe through the nose.

Burning in the pharynx, extending to the stomach; solids cause pain when swallowed, and leave a sensation as of something remaining there.

[14] **Desires.   Aversions.**   Appetite lost; thirst increased; foul tongue; languor.

Longing for beer; for acid drinks, which increase thirst. Dislike to meat.

15 **Eating and Drinking.** Food lies like a load; sensation after a full meal, as if digestion was suspended.

Pressure and heaviness in stomach, immediately after eating.

Secondary bad effects from malt liquors; especially from lager beer.

16 **Nausea and Vomiting.** Eructations of air, relieving an uneasiness of stomach, as from pent up wind at the great curvature. Fetid eructations.

Nausea, feeling of heat over body, with giddiness, rush of blood to head; worse on moving about, in the morning, at sight of food, after meals, and after stool; excited by drinking and smoking; better by eating and in open air.

Giddiness, followed by vomiting of an acid white mucous fluid, with pressure and burning in the stomach; also in ulcer of stomach.

Vomit: sour, undigested; of bile, bitter; pinkish, glairy fluid; of mucus and blood; of blood, with cold sweat on hands, face hot; of yellow, purulent mucus.

17 **Stomach.** Swelling of the stomach (evening), with fulness and pressure; cannot bear tight clothing; tongue yellow.

Awakens with a start; heat in pit of stomach and spitting of blood; 2 A.M.

Awoke with uneasiness, soreness and tenderness, especially in a small spot towards left of ensiform cartilage; headache in a small spot.

Pains, uneasiness in stomach, alternate with pains in limbs.

Gastric symptoms supersede the rheumatic.

Feeling of coldness in stomach and bowels.

18 **Hypochondria.** Dull pain or stitches in right hypochondrium, especially when limited to a small spot; clay-colored stools; metallic taste; confusion in head.

Stitches in region of spleen, extending into lumbar region, worse from motion or pressure.

19 **Abdomen.** Tympanitis; abdomen feels bloated, followed by eructations.

Gastro-intestinal inflammation, cramps here and there, worse in calves and inner parts of thighs.

Stitches through the abdomen, extending to the spinal column.

Cutting as from knives, soon after eating; colic, alternating with cutting at the navel, during the night.

20 **Stool, etc.** Watery, gushing diarrhœa in the morning;

awakes with urgent desire, followed by violent tenesmus, which prevents her rising; later, burning in the
abdomen, nausea and violent straining to vomit.

Dysentery brownish, frothy, watery, or frequent bloody
evacuations, gnawing about the navel, tenesmus;
tongue smooth, red, cracked.

Clay-colored stools; chronic diarrhœa.

Periodical dysentery every year; early part of summer.

Diarrhœa or dysentery after rheumatism.

Constipation, debility, coated tongue, headache, cold extremities.

Habitual constipation; stools scanty, knotty, followed by
burning and painful retraction of the anus; also periodical costiveness.

Sensation as of a plug in the anus.   Soreness at the anus.

[21] **Urine.**   Pain across the back, with red urine.

Shooting in renal region, small pulse, prostration; suppressed urine.

Continuous desire to urinate during the day.

Frequent discharge of watery urine, of strong smell, awaking him at night.

Scanty, high-colored urine, with copious whitish sediment
and pain in the back.

Scanty urine, with a white film and whitish deposit; mucous sediment.

Painful drawing from perineum into urethra.

Drawing micturition heat in the urethra; burning in
glandular part of the urethra, continuing long after.

After micturition, burning in back part of urethra, with
sensation as if one drop had remained behind, with unsuccessful effort to void it; stitches in the urethra.

[22] **Male Sexual Organs.**   Absence of sexual desire.

Constrictive pain at the root of the penis; morning on
awaking.

Itching in the hairy parts, skin inflames, small pustules
form, of the size of a pin's head.

Chancres ulcerating deeply.

Pricking and itching at the glans penis; ulcers.

Stitches in the prostate when walking, must stand still;
prostatic fluid escapes at stool.

Gleet, with stringy or jelly-like, profuse discharge.

[23] **Female Sexual Organs.**   Menses: too soon, with vertigo,
headache, nausea and feverishness; obstinate suppression of urine or red urine.

Prolapsus uteri, seemingly from hot weather.   Subinvolution of the uterus.

Leucorrhœa yellow, ropy; pain and weakness across the
small of the back, and dull, heavy pains in the hypogastrium.

Soreness and rawness in the vagina.

Swelling of the genitals.

Itching, burning and excitement about the vulva; genuine pruritus.

²⁵ **Larynx.** Hawks copious, thick blue mucus, in the morning.

Early, formative stage of croup; worse 2 to 3 A. M.; the tough mucus strangles him.

Membranous croup; diphtheritic croup; invading larynx, trachea and even the bronchi; voice hoarse, uncertain, cough hoarse, metallic; deglutition painful, tonsils red, swollen; covered with false membrane difficult to detach, with expectoration of tough, stringy mucus; coughs up casts of elastic fibrinous nature; loud mucous rales; wheezing, rattling in aleep; insidious approach; fat, chubby, light-haired children. See 48.

²⁶ **Breathing.** Wheezing, panting on awaking; then cough which forces him to sit up, bent forward.

Slight dyspnœa, as if the mucous membrane of the bronchi was thickened; on rising in the morning.

Tightness at the bifurcation of the bronchi.

Sensation of choking on lying down.

²⁷ **Cough.** Wheezing, with retching and expectoration of tough mucus, which can be drawn in strings to the feet.

Cough excited by: tickling in the larynx; or at the bronchial bifurcation; by oppression at the epigastrium; or accumulation of mucus in the larynx.

Cough, with pain, from mid-sternum through to back; severe stitching, or weight and soreness in the chest.

Cough, worse undressing; morning on awaking; after eating; deep inspiration; better after getting warm in bed.

²⁸ **Lungs.** Pains from back to sternum; or, from mid-sternum darting to between the shoulders.

²⁹ **Heart. Pulse.** Cold sensation about the heart; tightness of the chest; dyspnœa.

Pricking pain in region of heart.

Palpitation, dyspnœa, accelerated pulse, heat, awakens suddenly with a start, 2 A. M.

Pulse irregular, small, contracted, with nosebleed; accelerated; often soft, weak, even fluttering.

³⁰ **Outer Chest.** Dull pain in the right side over a circumscribed spot, worse on inspiration.

³¹ **Neck. Back.** Stiffness of nape of neck on bending head.

Sharp shooting pains, first in left then right renal region, extending down the thighs; worse on motion.

Aching in the back and down the left side into the hip.

Pain in the os coccygis, worse from walking, or touch, and on rising after long sitting.

[32] **Upper Limbs.** Rheumatic pains in both shoulders, worse at night.

Burning pain in middle of forearm, extending to wrist.

Rheumatic pains in elbow and wrist-joints; stinging in the left elbow.

Spasmodic contraction of the hands.

Rheumatic pains in the finger-joints.

Great weakness of the hands.

Bones of the hand as if bruised, when pressed; ulcers on the fingers, with caries.

[33] **Lower Limbs.** Rheumatic pains in hip-joints and knees, on walking or moving; also with restlessness in diphtheria.

Pain in the course of the left sciatic nerve, from behind the great trochanter to the calf; also when better motion; pressure on nerve causes shooting along whole leg.

Pain in the tendons of the muscles of the calf, as if stretched, causing lameness.

Pain in the right hip, extending to the knees.

Heaviness of the legs; aching and weakness in the calves on walking or going up stairs.

Soreness in the heels when walking.

Ulcers on the previously inflamed feet.

[34] **Limbs in General.** Shooting, pricking pains, worse in the morning.

Stiff all over, could hardly move in the morning.

Periodical, wandering pains; also along the bones, generally without localized inflammatory processes.

[35] **Position, etc.** Averse to motion, inclination to lie down.

Motion: 3, 16, 18, 31, 32, 33, 34, 44, 46. Walking: 22, 31, 33. Stooping: 2, 3, 31. Rising from a seat: 2, 31. Cannot rise: 20. Must sit bent forward: 26. Lying: 3, 26.

[36] **Nerves.** Prostration; face pale, cold sweat on face and body.

Weariness in the limbs, as the pains subside.

[7] **Sleep.** Unrefreshing sleep; feels debilitated, especially in the extremities.

During sleep frequent starts, incoherent talk, tossing of the arms.

Awakened: with desire to urinate; by dyspnœa; palpitation; heat; headache.

Worse on awaking: head and chest symptoms especially.

[38] **Time.** Morning: 2, 3, 4, 5, 7, 11, 16, 20, 22, 25, 26. Evening: 4, 7, 25, 33. Night: 5, 6, 19, 21, 32, 46. 2 A.M.: 17, 19, 25. Day: 21. Increasing from morn till noon, decrease from noon till night: 4.

[39] **Temperature and Weather.** Complaints in hot weather: 20, 23, 46. Better from warmth: 27, 40. Cold: 46. Open air: 3, 8, 16. Undressing: 27. Pains worse in winter.

[40] **Chill. Fever. Sweat.** Chilliness in the back, with sleepiness; seeks a warm place.

Chilliness alternating with flushes of heat.

Chilliness with giddiness and nausea, followed by heat, with sensation of coldness and trembling; periodical pains in the temples; without thirst.

Attacks of chilliness from the feet upwards, and sensation as if the skull on the vertex became contracted, in frequently returning paroxysms.

Chill, followed in an hour by heat, with dryness of mouth and lips, which have to be moistened all the time; followed in the morning by great thirst but no sweat. Ill-humor.

Chilliness, especially on the extremities, and flushes of heat alternating with general sweat.

Flushes of heat in the face. Climaxis.

Heat of hands and feet; nausea; pain in the upper part of the abdomen; dryness of the mouth; sleeplessness; followed by sweat of hands, feet and thighs.

Burning heat of the upper part of the body and face, with internal chilliness and violent thirst.

Sweat: on the back, during effort at stool; profuse while sitting quietly; cold on forehead and hands.

[41] **Attacks.** Pains fly rapidly from one place to another, not continuing long at any place, and intermit. __

Periodical attacks: 20

Symptoms alternate.

Gastric symptoms supersede rheumatic.

[42] **Sides.** Right: 4, 6, 7, 9, 18, 30, 33, 46. Left: 4, 5, 6, 7, 8, 13, 17, 18, 29, 31, 32, 33. Left to right: 31. Before backward: 3, 19, 28. Behind forward: 28. Above downward: 31, 33. Below upward: 40.

[43] **Sensations.** Pains in small spots, which can be covered with point of finger.

Pains attack first one part, then reappear in another.

Heavy feeling in many parts.

[44] **Tissues.** Bones feel bruised; caries.

Cracking in all the joints from the least motion.

Rheumatic pains in nearly all the joints.

Diphtheritic formations in nose, mouth, fauces, pharynx, larynx, trachea, bronchi, and even uterus and vagina.

Plastic exudations; ropy, stringy mucus.

Emaciation; anæmia.

[45] **Contact, Injuries, etc.** Desire to rub: 5. Cannot bear clothing tight: 17. Touch: 4, 6, 7, 8, 13, 20, 31. Pressure: 33. Pressure relieves: 3. Rubs the eyelids: 5.

[46] **Skin.** Burning, stinging in the skin. Lupus with much burning.

Skin hot, dry and red.

Violent itching of whole surface; then small pustules form mostly on arms and legs; scabs smart, pain and burn; worse in hot, better in cold weather.

Heat and itching of skin at night, when warm in bed, followed by reddish, hard knots, from size of pin's head to that of a split pea; centre depressed, with a dark scurf; surrounded by an inflamed base.

Dry eruption like measles.

Small pustules over body like small-pox; they disappear without bursting; mostly on face and arms.

Brown spots like freckles on the throat.

Blisters full of serum on the sole of the right foot.

Small pustules on the roots of the nails, spreading over hands to wrists; arm red, axillary glands suppurate; small pustules on the hands secrete a watery fluid when broken; if not touched, fluid thickens into a yellow, tough mass.

Blood-boil on right thigh; right side of spine, near last rib; painful on the least motion.

Ulcers dry, oval: edges overhanging, bright red areola; base hard, corroding; becoming deeper; cicatrix remains depressed.

Scabs on fingers, corona glandis; deep, stinging cicatrices on the hands.

[47] **Stages and States.**   Fat, light-haired persons; fat, chubby children.

[48] **Relationship.**   Ailments from vapor of arsenic; from *Mercur.*, especially *Merc. jod.*

In dysentery, after *Canthar.* has removed the scrapings, *Kali bich.* will sometimes complete the cure.   In croup, useful after *Iod.* has modified fever and ringing cough, and there remain hoarse, barking, cough, tough exudation; general weakness and coldness.   *Ant. tart.* follows well.

Antidotes: *Arsen., Laches.* (croup, diphtheria, etc.), *Pulsat. Cinnabar.* preferable for pains going around orbit.

KALI BROMATUM.

Potassium bromide.

[1] **Mind.**   Imagines she is a devil; cannot sleep; fears to be alone (medicine developed urticaria with relief).

Excited, hands constantly busy; timid, suspicious.

❙ Frightful images at night during pregnancy ; or in children, who awake screaming, unconscious, recognize no one; followed by squinting.

❙ Delirium, with delusions; thinks he is pursued; will be poisoned ; is selected for divine vengeance; that her child is dead, etc.

❙ Delirium tremens, flushed face, horrid illusions.

❙ Melancholy, with delusions; often childish; fits of uncontrollable weeping. Feels as if would go out of his mind. Apathetic, indifferent.

Mentally dull, torpid; perception slow, answers slowly. ❙ Inability to express oneself; ❙ loss of memory; ❙ amnesic aphasia.

Single words forgotten or syllables are dropped.

² **Sensorium.** Vertigo: as if ground gave way; and staggering gait ; with confusion and heat of head, drowsiness, stupor; fainting and nausea followed by sound sleep.

³ **Inner Head.** ❙ Brain irritated, face flushed, pupils dilated, eyes sunken; rolls head; awakes now and then screaming; extremities cold; cholera infantum. See 20, 32, 44.

❙ Active congestion; inflammation before effusion has occurred.

⁴ **Outer Head.** Scalp feels tight, brain numb, confused; difficult walking.

⁵ **Eyes.** Vision: dim, pupils dilated; with heavy lids and invincible drowsiness.

Squinting. See 1.

Hallucinations of sight and sound with or without mania precede brain and paralytic symptoms.

Gaze fixed. Eyes sunken, lustreless.

Vessels of fundus enlarged. Conjunctivæ congested.

⁶ **Ears.** Sounds echo in ears; headache.

Hardness of hearing. Roaring in ears at night synchronous with pulse.

⁷ **Nose.** Smell lessened.

Thick mucus and yellow scabs in nostrils.

⁸ **Face.** Expression: pale, but otherwise appeared as one drunk, with hallucinations, etc.; wearied, anxious; dull, stupefied; imbecile.

Complexion yellow, cachectic.

¹¹ **Tongue, etc.** Tongue: red, dry, enlarged; red, later dry and brown; white, with languor and sleepiness.

Tongue red and tender; gums spongy; diabetes.

Difficult speech; action of tongue disordered; also slow and difficult after waking; stammering.

¹² **Mouth.** Breath fetid; tongue white.

Saliva profuse, with fetid breath.

Taste: foul; lost.

¹³ **Throat.** Dryness.

Uvula and fauces congested, then œdematous.

Dysphagia of liquids (in infants); can swallow only solids.

Anæsthesia of the mouth, throat and pharynx; chronic alcoholism.

¹⁴ **Desires. Aversions.** Thirst intense with dry mouth.

¹⁶ **Nausea and Vomiting.** Sick and giddy.

Repeated retching and emesis.

¹⁹ **Abdomen.** Abdominal spasms, walls retracted, convulsive motions of eyes and limbs; frequent green, watery stools; summer complaint.

Sensation as if the bowels were falling out.

²⁰ **Stool, etc.** ❙ Discharges watery; cholera infantum, especially with cerebral irritation and collapse. See 1, 3, 44.

Constipation; stools dry, hard, infrequent.

²¹ **Urine.** Diabetes, the urine is loaded with sugar.

Profuse, with abundance of phosphates.

Urine scanty; even suppressed in collapse.

Dribbling of urine at beginning of stool.

Incontinence of urine.

²¹ **Male Sexual Organs.** Desire lessened even to impotence.

❙ Seminal emissions, with depressed spirits, dull thought, backache, staggering gait and great weakness.

²³ **Female Sexual Organs.** Has removed ovarian cysts.

Is claimed to be useful in uterine fibroids and subinvolution.

Ovarian neuralgia from ungratified sexual desire; nervous unrest.

²⁷ **Cough.** Paroxysmal, dry, at intervals of two or three hours difficult respiration; followed by a vomiting of mucus or food; worse at night and when lying down.

²⁹ **Heart. Pulse.** Action: lacks energy; sounds seem distant and feeble; slow, fluttering.

Pulse: accelerated, later slower; slow, small weak.

³² **Upper Limbs.** Hands and fingers in constant action, busy (See 1); twitching of fingers.

Trembling of hands during voluntary motion; or, as in delirium tremens.

³⁵ **Position, etc.** Lying down: 27. Motion: 32.

³⁶ **Nerves.** Lessens reflex excitation, hence its antipathic application to epilepsy and kindred affections.

Nervous, busy, must occupy oneself; often in nervous women.

Nervous excitement, irritation and congestion of the cerebral meninges, with mania, etc.

Inco-ordination of muscles; nervous weakness, even paralysis of motion and numbness.

Gait: unsteady, reeling as if drunk, with rolling and

staggering; as one walks with locomotor ataxia. Looks to see if legs are really moving.

Weakness of the extensors of legs and feet.

Languor, disinclined to talk, or use mind or work, indifferent, sleepy, yet by a strong effort of will can act as usual.

General delirium, hallucinations, fancies about being persecuted, ataxia; as in general paralysis.

Restlessness, fitfulness of motion, with giddiness.

[67] **Sleep.** Sleepiness; deep sleep, often broken by a start, though waking is very difficult; confused dreams.

Awakes from a profound sleep, not knowing where he is.

Sleeplessness, especially in anæmic patients, or nervous persons who are exhausted but irritated.

Waking: 11.

[38] **Time.** Night: 1, 6, 27, 46

[39] **Temperature and Weather.** High temperature: 46. Winter: 46.

[41] **Chill. Fever. Sweat.** Lowers the temperature 1° to 2°. Pulse 40. Skin cold, clammy. See 1, 3, 20, 44.

Painful flushings of the face at the climacteric period.

Sweat abundant, viscid; long-lasting and exhausting.

[44] **Tissues.** ▮Muscles irritated, rendered inco-ordinate and then paralyzed.

▮Lowers temperature, with coldness of extremities, hands and wrists icy-cold and wet, cerebral irritation, in cholera infantum. See 1, 3, 20; 40.

Emaciation; weak, pallid.

[46] **Skin.** ▮Acne simplex and indurata; bluish-red, pustular. worse on face and chest; especially in lymphatic constitutions.

Rose-colored, mammilated eruption on the lower extremities; sometimes pustules in centre of patches that become umbilicated, exuding a creamy moisture and forming thick, yellow, scabs.

Slightly elevated, smooth, red patches, like urticaria, but with hardened bases, like erythema nodosum, itching at night in bed and in a high temperature; appear in winter.

Moist eczema of legs with pityriasis of the scalp.

[48] **Relationship.** Compare *Ambr. gris.*, *Hyosc.*, *Gelsem.* (sleepless from nervous exhaustion); *Bellad.* (but latter has sthenic symptoms; *Kali brom.* symptoms of debility, muscular coldness and redness as in collapse); *Opium.*, *Camphor.*, *Camph. brom.* (collapse in cholera infantum).

KALI CARBONICUM.

Potassium carbonate.   HAHNEMANN. K_2O, CO_2.

[1] **Mind.**   Sudden attack of unconsciousness.

At a loss to know how to say what she wishes. θ Puerperal mania.

Absent-minded.

Dulness, confused, stupid, as after intoxication.

Weeps much.

Dread of labor.

Fear of being alone; fears she will die.

Anxiety with fear.

Despondent in the open air.

Peevish, irritable; noise is disagreeable; easily startled, especially if touched.

[2] **Sensorium.**   Giddiness, nausea, pressure in the stomach.

Vertigo when rapidly turning the head or body; evening and morning.

[3] **Inner head.**   Congestion to head, with throbbing and humming.

Forehead: stitches, also in the temples, worse stooping, moving head, eyes or jaw; better raising the head, and from heat; stitches into the eyes and root of nose, with catarrh.

Pressing in the front of head, temples and into the eyes, with heat in face and head. Pressure with photophobia.

One-sided headache, with nausea.

Jerking in head from behind forwards; dark before the eyes; unconscious; better from a drink of cold water.

Headache from riding in a carriage; coughing, sneezing; on awaking from sleep; from coryza.

Pressing pain in back of head.

[4] **Outer Head.**   After being heated, liable to cold from a draught, causing headache, toothache and backache.

Painful tumors on scalp, like blood-boils; worse from pressure and motion, less from heat; itching, as if in bones.

Hair dry, brittle, falling off, mostly from temples, eyebrows and beard; scalp itches and burns morning and evening; oozes if scratched.

[5] **Eyes.**   While reading or looking at a bright light muscæ volitantes; sharp stitches; fog before the eyes.

Bright sparks, blue or green spots before the eyes.

Inclination to stare.

Eyes weak: after coition; after measles; after abortion.

Lachrymation, shunning light; pain deep in eyes.

Corners of eyes ulcerate.

Lids red, swollen; tarsi worse.

Eyelids swollen, also left cheek and upper lip.

Swelling like a bag between upper eyelids and eyebrows.

Enormous bag-like swellings under the eyes. θ Erysipelas.

Eyes sunken.

Sensation of coldness in the lids.

⁶ **Ears.** Roaring, whizzing, crackling noises.

Headache and noises in the ear after a cold drink.

Hearing impaired.

Stitches from within outward; also with drawing behind the ears. θ Otitis.

Right ear hot, left pale and cold.

Discharge of liquid cerumen or pus.

Parotids, especially the right, inflammed, swollen, hard.

⁷ **Nose.** Dull smell; especially from catarrh.

Fluent coryza, excessive sneezing; pain in back, headache and lassitude.

Obstruction of nose, making breathing through nostrils impossible; goes off when walking in open air, but returns in the room; itching in the nose; fetid yellow-green discharge from one nostril.

Dry coryza, with loss of voice, hoarseness; mucus in the throat, sensation of a lump in the throat.

Burning in the nose; sore, crusty nostrils; bloody, red nostrils every morning; external nose red, swollen; stinging pains.

Nosebleed when washing face; every morning at 9 o'clock.

⁸ **Face.** Red and hot; one cheek hot, the other cold; purple, bloated; dark red during cough, otherwise pale; pale; sickly; sallow; grey; yellow.

Face bloated in the morning.

Stinging in the cheeks; tearing stitches from a molar into the forehead, eyes and temples.

❙ Freckles.

⁹ **Lower Face.** Upper lip swollen; bleeding rhagades.

Lips peel, are chapped.

Hard swelling of submaxillary glands.

¹⁰ **Teeth.** Toothache, tearing, lancinating, with pains in facial bones.

Teeth ache only when eating; throbbing; worse when touched by anything cold or warm.

Teeth are loose.

Bad smell from the teeth.

Stitches in the teeth; cheeks swollen, with stinging pains.

¹¹ **Tongue, etc.** Taste bitter; flat.

Tongue swollen, covered with vesicles, the tip burns as if raw, frænum sore.

Tongue white; bad taste.

¹² **Mouth.**   Bad, alkaline smell from mouth; smell like old cheese.

Mouth feels dry, with increased saliva.

Vesicles, painful, burning all over the inner mouth.

¹³ **Throat.**   Crawling in the throat, causing hemming and coughing, and a feeling of tightly adhering phlegm.

Tenacious mucus in the fauces and posterior of pharynx, mornings; difficult to hawk up; sensation as of a lump.

Stinging when swallowing; frequent desire to swallow saliva, but frequently cannot, causing a ckoking.

Pain in the back when swallowing.

When swallowing, the food remains half way, when gagging and vomiting; stricture of œsophagus.

¹⁴ **Desires.   Aversions.**   Desire: for acids; for sugar.   Aversion to rye bread.

No appetite; disgust for food.

Intense thirst.

¹⁵ **Eating and Drinking.**   During eating: sleepy.

After eating: burning from stomach to throat; colic renewed; abdomen distended; stomach replete, especially after soup or coffee; sour eructations; nausea, faintness.

When hungry, feels anxious, nauseated, nervous, tingling; also cough and palpitation, better after breakfast.

Drinking: 26, 27; cold water: 3, 9.   Eating warm food: 27.

¹⁶ **Nausea and Vomiting.**   Eructation sour; nausea.

Sick during a walk, no vomiting, feels as if she must lie down and die.   θ Pregnancy.

Nausea: and loathing; from emotions; with anxiety and faintness.

Retching, vomiting of ingesta and slime; sour.

¹⁷ **Stomach**   Stitches in the pit of stomach; anxiety.

Pressing, tensive pain, awakens at 2 A. M.

Pit of stomach swollen, tense, sensitive to touch.

Deep in the scrobiculum, a lump as large as a fist, sensitive to touch.

Pain in the great cul-de-sac radiating to chest, to back and extremities.   Pains in back and legs after eating.

¹⁸ **Hypochondria.**   Stitches in region of liver, with tension across abdomen.

Swelling of the liver; abscess.

Icterus.

¹⁹ **Abdomen.**   Epigastrium swollen, hard, sensitive; pulsations therein; pains in hepatic and umbilical region, also on both sides of inferior parts of stomach down into bladder and testes.

Cutting, shooting, darting, stitching all over the abdomen.

Tension across abdomen; heaviness, inactivity, coldness.

34

Abdomen distended with wind.

Incarceration of flatus with colic.

20 **Stool, etc.** Unsuccessful desire for stool; rectum feels too weak to expel it.

Stool dry, too large in size; rectum inactive. Feels distressed an hour or two before a passage.

Stools: light grey; frequent, soft, pale.

Painless diarrhœa, with rumbling in abdomen and burning at the anus afterwards. θ Chronic diarrhœa of dyspeptics.

Diarrhœa only by day.

Before stool, anxiety, distressed feeling; white mucous discharge.

After stool: itching about anus; anus feels as if lacerated.

Varices protrude during micturition; blood, then white mucus escapes.

Inflammation, soreness, stitches and tingling, as from ascarides, in the varices.

21 **Urine.** Tensive pain in the left side. Stitches in the region of the kidneys.

Urine: hot, scanty, frequent, sediment red, slimy; blackish, foaming when shaken; with purulent sediment.

Urine flows slowly, with soreness and burning; or profuse, greenish.

After micturition: burning in urethra (also during); prostatic discharge.

22 **Male Sexual Organs.** Sexual desire excessive, with burning sensation or desire deficient.

After coition, weak, especially the eyes.

Copious, painful pollutions, with subsequent painful erections.

Dragging in the left testicle and penis.

Swelling of testes and spermatic cord.

Scrotum feels as if bruised.

23 **Female Sexual Organs.** Stitching pains in and about the uterus; labor-like colic, leucorrhœa; pain like a weight in the small of back.

Nausea, vomiting, stitches through the abdomen; great weakness.

Sore pain in the vagina, during coition.

Menses too early, scanty, pale, of a pungent odor, acrid, covering thighs with an eruption. Flow may be early, and more profuse and long-lasting than usual.

Difficult first menses.

Before menses: sour eructations; swelling of the cheeks; shooting pains over the abdomen; or colicky pains; nettle-rash; increased sexual desire; itching of vulva,

During menses: headache with heaviness; pains in head,

ears, teeth, back; heavy aching in small of back and
down the buttocks; nettle-rash; lassitude.

Menses suppressed, with anasarca or ascites; or every
mouth, sour eructations, etc.; backache compelling her
to sit down.

Yellow leucorrhœa, backache; labor-like pains; itching-
burning in the pudendum (arising from the discharges).

²⁴ **Pregnancy.**   During pregnancy: vomiting; discharge of
coagula.

Abortion impending, with pains from back into buttocks
and thighs; miscarriage at third month.

Consequences of abortion or labor; back weak, sweat, dry
cough, prolonged metrorrhagia.

Labor-pains insufficient; violent backache, wants the back
pressing; bearing down from back into pelvis.

Sharp, cutting pains across lumbar region, or passing off
down the buttocks, thus hindering labor; pulse weak.

Promotes expulsion of moles.

²⁵ **Larynx.**   Aphonia, with violent sneezing.

Scraping, dryness, parched feeling.

Subacute laryngitis with tenacious, glairy mucus.

²⁶ **Breathing.**   Difficult, wheezing breathing.

Dyspnœa, worse from drinking, from motion, cannot walk
fast; arrest of breathing, awaking him at night.

Breathing labored; after paroxysms of cough.

Asthma, must lean forward with head on the table; worse
in the morning.

Dyspnœa, with violent and irregular beating of the heart.

Feels as if there was no air in his chest.

²⁷ **Cough.**   Cough: paroxysmal from tickling in throat, larynx
or bronchi, with dislodgement of tenacious mucus, or
pus, which must be swallowed; spasmodic, with gagging,
or vomiting of ingesta and sour phlegm; tormenting,
gets nothing up, sometimes feels as if a tough membrane
were moving about, but would not loosen.

Cough with sputum of masses of blood and pus.

Cough day and night, dry and teasing; from 3 to 4 A.M.;
with sticking pains at sides of chest; brought on by
eating (warm food), drinking; motion; sitting erect;
lying on the side; or exposure to cold. Better after
breakfast.

Whooping-cough worse 3 A.M.; gagging and vomiting; ·
inflammation of the lungs; swelling between upper lids
and eyebrows.

²⁸ **Lungs.**   Spasms of the chest.

Chest feels weak, faint from walking fast.

Pain through lower third of right chest to back.

Pressure in middle of chest, with gulping of watery phlegm; stricture of the œsophagus.

Pressure, heaviness, anxious feeling.

Pain as if lower lobe of right lung was adhering to ribs.

Phthisis; acts on lower part of right lung; faint spells; sputum contains pus globules, blood and albumen.

Pneumonia, with stitches through right chest, hepatic inflammation; right lung hepatized; worse when lying on right side.

Infantile pneumonia, much rattling both sides; during resolution.

Pleurisy, stitches in the left chest, with violent palpitation; dry cough, worse 3 A.M.

²⁹ **Heart. Pulse.** Crampy pains, as if heart was hanging by bands; burning.

Palpitation in spells, taking his breath.

Heart's beat intermits; heart's action irregular; tumultuous or weak.

Stitches about the heart and through to scapula.

Systolic murmur; stitch pains; second tick loud from pulmonary stagnation. θ Endocarditis.

Ebullitions, with heat from abdomen to head; pulsations all over.

Insufficiency of mitral valves.

Pulse: rapid mornings, less so evenings; unequal, irregular; intermitting; slow and weak.

³¹ **Neck. Back.** Back of neck stiff; shooting pains through the chest; uvula elongated.

Neck feels large, clothing tight; congestion.

Swelling of cervical glands.

ı Backache; while walking she feels as if she must give up and lie down; after confinement, abortion, metrorrhagia, etc.

Sharp stitching pains awaken him 3 A.M., he must get up and walk about; lumbago.

Pulsations in the back.

Backache, as if broken; or as if pressed in from both sides, with labor-like colic and leucorrhœa.

Gnawing in the os coccygis.

³² **Upper Limbs.** Pain, as from blows, under right shoulder, when moving or touching it.

Axillary glands swollen, painful.

Stitching-tearing extending into finger.joints.

Weakness in arms, mornings; arms feel numb, cold; goes to sleep when lain on.

Hands and arms covered with purplish spots.

Weakness with cramps in hands and fingers; paresis.

Finger-tips go to sleep early in the morning.

Palms itch; vesicles form.

[33] **Lower Limbs.** Crampy tearing in hip-joint and knee; bruised pain when moving and when sleeping; coxalgia.

Dull pains in side of knee, when walking or extending leg.

Difficulty in the knees on going down stairs, and still more on going up.

Nightly rheumatic pains.

Burning and stinging in the legs.

Profuse fetid foot-sweat.

Feet heavy, stiff.

Swelling and redness of the soles; chilblains.

Swelling of feet to ankles; feet cold.

Stitches in the painful and sensitive corns.

[34] **Limbs in General.** Jerks the limbs, especially when the feet are touched.

Limbs: tired; cold.

Puffiness; hands and feet cyanotic.

[35] **Position, etc.** Motion: 4, 26, 27, 32, 33. Moving head: 3. Walking: 7, 16, 26, 28, 31, 33. Ascending or descending: 33. Exercise: 40. Turning: 2. Sitting erect: 27 Leaning forward: 26. Stooping: 3. Raising head: 3· Lying: 40; on side: 27; on right side: 28.

[36] **Nerves.** Twitching of the muscles. Parts laid on feel bruised and "go to sleep;" sweat, faintness.

Spasms seem to pass off with frequent eructations. θ Puerperal convulsions. Spasms, with full consciousness.

Paresis; trembling.

[37] **Sleep.** Yawning. Drowsy by day and early in evening.

No sleep; gastric ailments.

During sleep: starting; limbs twitch; gnashing the teeth; crying.

Aroused by asthma.

Awaken between 2 and 4 A.M., with nearly all ailments, especially those of throat and chest.

Horrid dreams, with frequent awaking and desire to urinate.

[38] **Time.** Morning: 2, 4, 7, 8, 13, 26, 29, 32, 40. Noon: 40. Evening: 2, 4, 29, 37, 40. Night: 26, 33, 40, 46. 2–4 A.M.: 17, 27, 28, 37. Day: 20, 37, 40. Day and night: 27.

[39] **Temperature and Weather.** Heat: 3, 4, 10. Room: 7. Open air: 1, 7, 40. Draught: 4. Cold: 27. Washing the face: 7.

[40] **Chill. Fever. Sweat.** Frequent shuddering during the day.

Chilly in the morning; also about noon; begins toward evening, relieved near the warm stove and after lying down; after the pains; increased out-doors.

Potash lowers the bodily temperature.

Heat, yawning, pain in chest and head, pulsations in abdomen, 9 A.M. and 5 P.M.

Internal heat, external chilliness.

Chill and heat, with dyspnœa.

Evening fever; chilly with thirst, then heat without thirst; with violent fluent coryza; later slight sweat, with sound sleep.

Constant chilliness, violent thirst from internal heat; hot hands; loathing of food.

Chill and fever, with oppression of breathing, constriction of chest, pain in region of liver, thirst worse during chill.

Sweat: mostly on upper parts; after eating; easily excited by exercise during the day. Night-sweats, with cough; after pneumonia. Sweat all night without relief.

[41] **Attacks.** Paroxysms recur every two or three hours. θ Asthma.

[42] **Sides.** Right: 6, 28, 32. Left: 5, 6, 21, 22, 28. Within outward: 9. Behind forward: 3.

[43] **Sensations.** Feeling of emptiness in the whole body, as if it were hollow.

[44] **Tissues.** ı Anæmia, with great debility, skin watery, milky-white; muscles weakened, especially the heart; hence weak pulse is a general characteristic.

Obesity.

Disposition to phlebitis.

Tumors with sticking like needles.

Paresis.

Dropsy of old people.

[45] **Contact, Injuries, etc.** Cannot bear to be touched; starts when touched lightly, especially if on the feet.

Touch: 1, 17, 32, 34. Pressure: 4, 24, 32. Scratching: 46. Riding in carriage: 3.

[46] **Skin.** Skin, dry, itches; better from scratching.

Erysipelas.

Herpetic spots on face.

Yellow, scaly spots over abdomen: or around the nipples.

Burning, itching herpes; moist after scratching.

Ulcers bleed at night.

[47] **Stages and States.** Suitable for the aged; rather obese; lax fibre.

Dark hair.

After loss of fluids, or of vitality, especially in anæmic persons.

[48] **Relationship.** In amenorrhœa, after *Natr. mur.* failed.

Complementary to *Carb. veg.*

Kali carb. is frequently suitable after: *Bryon.*, *Lycop.*, *Natr. mur.*, *Nitr. ac.*

After *Kali carb.* are frequently indicated: *Carb. veg.*, *Phosphor.*

Antidotes to *Kali carb.*: *Camphor.*, *Coffea*, *Spir. nitr. dulc.*

Kali sulph. (clinically proved to be good in loose cough and rattling on chest.

KALI IODATUM.

Potassium iodide.   HARTLAUB.

[1] **Mind.** Talkative, disposed to jest; vehement, quarrelsome. Starts at every noise.

Excitation as if intoxicated; also after mercurialization.

[3] **Inner Head.** Hyperæmia in scrofula; also in weak or tubercular patients; hammering in the forehead; head feels inflated; anxious, restless sleep.

Headache and heaviness in head (5 A.M.); better after rising.

Pains in sides of head, as if screwed in; better in open air.

Lancinating and dartings over left eye and in left temple.

[4] **Outer Head.** Violent headache, hard humps on the cranium.

Scalp feels as if ulcerated, when scratching it.

Falling out of hair. θ Syphilis.

[5] **Eyes.** Iritis syphilitica after abuse of mercury; aqueous cloudy; ciliary injection bright, angry looking; pains worse at night.

Irido-choroiditis, especially syphilitic.

Pustules on the cornea; no photophobia, pain, or redness.

Chemosis.

Burning in the eyes; they secrete a purulent mucus.

Œdema of the eyelids, with lachrymation.

Periostitis of orbit, syphilitic or not.

[6] **Ears.** Boring pain in the ears; darting in the ears (right); rachitic children, head tender.

[7] **Nose.** Violent epistaxis, after mercury.

From the least cold, violent, acrid coryza; bloated eyelids, stinging in the ears, red face, white tongue; violent thirst; alternate heat and chilliness; headache; dark, hot urine; abuse of mercury.

Nose red, swollen; discharge acrid, watery; tightness at the root of the nose. θ Syphilis.

[8] **Face.** Swelling of face and tongue, especially after mercury.

Darting and stinging in the face. θ Coryza.

[10] **Teeth.** Feeling as of a worm crawling at roots of the teeth.

Gums swollen; decayed teeth; gum-boils.

Grumbling in teeth and face; copious saliva; thirst; violent darting into ears; abscess of antrum.

Teeth feel elongated.

[11] **Tongue, etc.** Rancid tase in mouth, after eating or drinking.

Bitterness in mouth and throat, going off after breakfast.

Burning of the tip of tongue; vesicles on tip of tongue.

[12] **Mouth.** Irregular ulcers, looking as if coated with milk.

Viscid, saltish saliva during pregnancy.

Bloody saliva, with sweetish taste in the mouth.

[13] **Throat.** Uvula swollen and elongated; mucous membrane as if œdematous.

Goitre (sensitive to contact).

Submaxillary glands swollen, suppurating.

[14] **Desires. Aversions.** Food tasteless.

Excessive thirst day and night.

[16] **Nausea and Vomiting.** Hiccough.

Gulping up of large quantities of air.

[17] **Stomach,** Phlegmasia of the stomach (and intestines).

Burning in the pit of the stomach.

[19] **Abdomen.** Sudden painful bloating of the abdomen or about navel, followed by diarrhœa.

Cutting and burning around umbilicus.

[20] **Stool, etc.** Stools scanty, hard, difficult.

Serous mucus from the rectum.

Diarrhœa and tenesmus, with pain in small of back, as if in a vise; after mercury.

[21] **Urine.** Morbus Brightii, with gout or mercurio-syphilis; granulated kidney.

Painful urging to urinate; also when it disappears when menses come.

Urine: copious, frequent, pale and watery; red as blood.

Urine increased, with unquenchable thirst.

[22] **Male Sexual Organs.** Sexual desire diminished; testes atrophied.

[23] **Female Sexual Organs.** Menses late and more profuse than usual; menses suppressed.

Before menses, frequent urging to urinate; during menses, thigh feels as if squeezed; pains go into the thighs; chilly, heat in the head.

Leucorrhœa watery, acrid, corrosive, with biting in the pudendum.

Discharge of mucus from the vagina.

Atrophy of the mammæ.

[24] **Pregnancy.** Galactorrhœa.

[25] **Larynx.** Nasal, catarrhal voice.

Hoarseness, with pain in chest, cough, oppression of breathing and pain in both eyes.

Awakens with choking, can scarcely breathe; choking spells, œdema of the larynx.

Rough feeling in the trachea, compelling hawking.

[26] **Breathing.** No air enters the lungs, epigastrium sunken; face livid; laryngeal obstruction.

[27] **Cough.** Suffocative cough, larynx swollen.

Cough dry; hawking; later copious, green sputum.

[28] **Lungs.** Stitches through sternum to back, or deep in chest, while walking.

Phthisis pituitosa, with purulent sputum; exhausting night-sweats and loose stools.

Pneumonia in the beginning when the disease localizes itself; also with so extensive hepatization, as to cause cerebral congestion and serous exudation; face red, pupils large; urine suppressed; one side as if paralyzed.

Œdema pulmonum, with pneumonia; or secondary to Morbus Brightii; sputum like soapsuds, green.

²⁹ **Heart. Pulse.** Palpitation, worse while walking.

Darting pains in the heart, when walking; after abuse of mercury; after repeated endocarditis.

Pulse accelerated; frequent.

³¹ **Neck. Back.** Small of back feels as if in a vise: also with darting pains in meningitis; after abuse of mercury.

Bruised pain in lumbar region, worse sitting bent; stitches. θ Bright's disease.

Pain in the os coccygis, as from a fall.

³² **Upper Limbs.** Left shoulder feels bruised.

Tearing in shoulder and ear.

³³ **Lower Limbs.** Gnawing in hip-bones; darting in left hip at every step, forcing him to limp.

Tearing in right thigh and knee, awakens him at night, worse lying on affected side or back. θ Sciatica.

Knee doughy, spongy, no fluctuation; skin red in spots and hot; gnawing, boring or tearing, worse at night, must often change position; white swelling.

Pain as if bruised in the left instep.

Ulcerative pain in heels and toes.

³⁴ **Limbs in General.** Tearing, darting pains; periosteum attacked; jerks or contractions of the tendons; emaciation; worse at night, lying on suffering part; from mercurialization or syphilis; rheumatism; gout.

³⁵ **Position, etc.** Walking: 28, 29; in open air: 39 Rising: 3. Sitting bent: 31. Rying on back or affected side: 33. Must change position: 33, 36.

³⁶ **Nerves.** Subsultus tendinum, or contraction of muscles and tendons.

Restless moving about.

Paralysis. See spinal meningitis.

³⁷ **Sleep.** Sleepless, restless; horrid dreams.

Weeping during sleep.

³⁸ **Time.** Morning: 3. Evening: 40. Night: 28, 33, 34, 40. Day and night: 14.

³⁹ **Temperature and Weather.** Irresistible desire to walk in the open air, it does not fatigue.

Open air: 3. Cold: 7. Warmth: 40.

⁴⁰ **Chill. Fever. Sweat.** Chilly, with thirst (4–7 P.M.); or all night, with shaking and frequent waking; can get warm in bed, but not from heat of stove.

Chill from lower part of back upward and through the whole body; 6–8 P.M.; with sleepiness.

At times chilly, with dry skin; at others profuse sweat.

Flushes of heat, with dulness of the head.

Intermittent fever; thirst with the chill; chill not lessened by warmth; mouth dry; anasarca; scrofula.

⁴¹ **Sides.** Right: 6, 33. Left: 5, 32, 33. Front backward: 28. Below upward: 40.

⁴⁴ **Tissues.** Purpura hemorrhagica.

Scrofula.

Emaciation and loss of appetite.

ı Synovitis.

Distends all tissues by interstitial infiltration : œdema; enlarged glands; tophi; exostoses; swelling of the bones, etc.

Dropsy from pressure of swollen glands.

Secondary syphilis, especially after abuse of mercury or combined with scrofula; buboes, chancres, with hard edges, thin, corrosive, or curdy pus; deep-eating ulcers.

Roseola. Rupia. Rheumatism; pains in bones; necrosis; exostoses; all worse at night.

Glands: swollen, goitre, bronchial, submaxillary, ulcerating, atrophied.

⁴⁵ **Contact, Injuries, etc.** Scratching: 4.

⁴⁶ **Skin.** Itching herpes on the face.

Papulæ worse on face, shoulders and back; dry throat.

Pustulous eruption often umbilicated and leaving scars.

Small boils on face, head, neck, back and chest, leaving scars.

⁴⁸ **Relationship.** After abuse of mercury.

Against abuse of iodide of potassium, *Hepar s. c.*

Kali chlor. compares in albuminuria.

KALMIA LATIFOLIA.

Mountain Laurel.   HERING.   *Ericaceæ.*

¹ **Mind.** In a recumbent posture, the mental faculties and memory are perfect, but on every attempt to move, vertigo.

Anxiety with the palpitation.

Toward evening and the next afternoon very cross.

² **Sensorium.** Vertigo: with headache, blindness, pains in the limbs and weariness; while stooping and looking down, with aching of the face. θ Neuralgia.

A cracking in the head frightens him, it ends like a sound in ears like blowing a horn.

³ **Inner Head.** Headache internally, with sensation when turning, of something loose in head, diagonally across top.

Sensation of heat in the head in the morning.

Pain in the forehead in the morning when waking, after rising, and then increasing.

Pressing pain on a small spot on the right side of the head.

The headache is worse in the evening and in the open air.

A shuddering without coldness commences with cracking; as if surcharged with electricity.

Pain over the right eye; giddiness; eyes weak and watery.

Dulness in the head; headache; backache.

Aching in the forehead, followed by rending in bones of right or left side of face; or, shooting downward into eye-teeth; or, moving backward down the neck and outwardly on both sides; succeeded by pain in left shoulder; or rending in bones of legs to feet.

⁴ **Outer Head.** Neuralgia each afternoon, becoming worse at night; pain from back of neck up over scalp to top of head and temples, also affecting face, mostly on right side. Parts tender to touch; pain shooting; sometimes in spots; better cold; worse heat.

Facial pains after zoster.

Menses regular but painful.

⁵ **Eyes.** Everything is black before the eye when he looks downward; with nausea and eructations of wind (in the morning).

Dull, weak eyes.

Pressure in the right eye (evening); also above right eye.

Sensation of stiffness around the eyes and in the eyelids

Stitches in the eyes (ears, fingers, feet).

Itching in the eyes, and when rubbing them they sting.

The eye symptoms are worse in evening and in open air.

⁶ **Ears.** Stitches in and behind the right ear; in neck and thighs (at night).

Sound like blowing a horn.

⁷ **Nose.** Coryza, with increased sense of smell; with sneezing, dulness, headache and hoarseness.

Tearing in root of nose and nasal bones, with nausea.

⁸ **Face.** Face red, with the throbbing headache.

Anxious expression of countenance. θ Rheumatism of heart.

Flushing of the face, with vertigo. θ Neuralgia.

Prosopalgia, right-sided; pains rending; agonizing; stupefying or threatening delirium.

Face at night itches.

Roughness of cheek (during every summer).

⁹ **Lower Face.** Lips swollen, dry and stiff (morning).

Cracked lips, with dry skin.

Stinging in jaw-bones.

¹⁰ **Teeth.** Teeth tender, with neuralgia of face and head.

Pressing pain in the molars, late in the evening.

¹¹ **Tongue, etc.** Bitter taste, with nausea, less after eating.

Tongue white, dry.

Stitches in the tongue.

Tongue sore, left side; hurts when talking in the evening.

¹² **Mouth.** Tingling in salivary glands, immediately after eating, with sense of fermentation in œsophagus and copious salivation.

Sublingual salivary gland inflamed.

¹³ **Throat.** Throat feels swollen.

Sensation as if a ball were rising in the throat.

Sensation of dryness in throat, with difficult deglutition and thirst.

Great dryness of throat, with aching pains; the dryness causing frequent cough. θ Chronic syphilitic sore throat.

Pressure in the throat; stitches in the eyes and nausea.

¹⁵ **Eating and Drinking.** After eating: feels better every way.

After eating: 11, 12. Drinking wine: 16.

Pains relieved by food. θ Neuralgia.

¹⁶ **Nausea and Vomiting.** Nausea, everything becomes black before the eyes, with pressure in the throat, incarcerated flatulence, oppression of breathing, and rheumatic pains in limbs.

Wine relieves the vomiting.

¹⁷ **Stomach.** Pressure in the pit of the stomach, like a marble; worse when sitting in a stooping position, better when sitting erect, with the sensation as if something would be pressed off below the pit of the stomach.

Eructations of wind. θ Angina pectoris. θ Gastralgia.

Crampy pain with eructation of wind, palpitation. θ Gastralgia.

Pit of stomach sore to touch.

¹⁸ **Hypochondria.** Pains in the region of the liver.

¹⁹ **Abdomen.** Incarcerated flatus, with nausea.

Sensation of weakness in the abdomen, extending to the throat; relieved by eructation.

Sudden pains in paroxysms, across abdomen above umbilicus, from lower border of liver, downward toward the left, then ceasing in right side; worse from motion, better when sitting up; abdominal neuralgia.

²⁰ **Stool, etc.** Stool like mush; easily discharged, as if glazed. followed by pressure on the rectum.

Diarrhœa, with dulness, dizziness, weariness, nausea and bellyache.

²¹ **Urine.** Frequent micturition of large quantities of yellow urine

ı Albuminuria; also with pains in lower limbs.

²³ **Female Sexual Organs.**   Menses eight to twenty-four days too soon; during menses pain in limbs, loins, back and interior of thighs.

Suppressed menses with severe neuralgic pains throughout the whole body.

Leucorrhœa yellowish; one week after menses; symptoms are prominent then.

²⁵ **Larynx.**   Pressure as if some one squeezed the throat with thumb and finger.

Noise as from spasm in the glottis when breathing.

Hoarse with coryza.

²⁶ **Breathing.**   Difficult and oppressed breathing; the throat feels swollen; nausea.   θ Rheumatism.

Oppressed and short-breathed, which obliges him to breathe quickly, involuntarily.

ı Dyspnœa and pain.   θ Angina pectoris.

²⁷ **Cough.**   Cough caused by scraping in the throat.

Expectoration easy, smooth, grey; tasting putrid and saltish.

Frequent cough caused by dryness in the throat: 13.

²⁸ **Lungs.**   Pain in the chest as from a sprain.

Shooting through chest above heart, into shoulder-blades; with pain in left arm.

²⁹ **Heart. Pulse.**   Wandering, rheumatic pains in region of heart; shooting pains above heart through to scapula.

When articular rheumatism has been treated externally, and cardiac symptoms ensue.

When the pains suddenly leave limbs and go to heart.

ı Hypertrophy and valvular insufficiency, or thickening after rheumatism.

Severe pain in cardiac region, with slow, small pulse.   θ Hypertrophy with dilatation and aortic obstruction.

Paroxysms of anguish about the heart, dyspnœa, febrile excitement; rheumatic endocarditis, with consequent hypertrophy and valvular disease.

ı Attacks of angina pectoris.   θ Fatty degeneration of heart.

Palpitation, dyspnœa, pain in limbs, stitch in lower part of chest; right-sided prosopalgia.

Palpitation up into throat, after going to bed; trembling all over; worse lying on left side; better lying on the back; anxiety.

ı Palpitation.   θ Gastralgia.

Pressure like a marble from epigastrium toward the heart, with a strong, quick heart-beat.   Every beat has a strumming, as if it would burst, along sternum to throat.   The third or fourth beat is harder, and is followed by an intermission.

Pulse slow, weak; arms feel weak; pulse scarcely perceptible, limbs cold.

▮ Slow, small pulse. θ Hypertrophy of heart.

▮ Pulse slow and feeble. θ Angina pectoris.

▮ Remarkable slowness of the pulse, 48 in the minute.
θ Neuralgia.

▮ Quickened but weak pulse. θ Rheumatism of heart.

▮ Pulse only slightly accelerated and in many instances
slow. θ Acute rheumatism.

³⁰ **Outer Chest.** ▮ Pleuritis falsa in winter season.

³¹ **Neck. Back.** ▮ Pain proceeded from the neck, which was
tender to the touch. θ Neuralgia.

Violent pain in the upper three dorsal vertebræ, extending
through the shoulder-blades.

Sensation of lameness in the back, evening in bed.

▮ Shooting, stabbing pain from the heart through to the
left scapula, causing violent beating of the heart.
θ Rheumatic affection of heart.

Constant pain in spine, sometimes worse in lumbar region,
with great heat and burning.

Muscles of neck sore to touch and on moving them.

³² **Upper Limbs.** ▮ Pain from the neck down the right arm to
the little or fourth finger. θ Neuralgia.

Pain in the right shoulder; also in deltoids, worse in right.

Stitches in the lower part of the left shoulder-blade.

Rheumatic pains in the arms (right).

Cracking in the elbow-joint.

Stitches in the hands.

The hands feel as if they had been sprained.

Pain in the left wrist, causing the hand to feel paralyzed.

Erysipelatous eruption on hands and extending further.

Weakness in the arms; the pulse being slow.

³³ **Lower Limbs.** Tearing pain from hip down leg to feet.

Stitches externally on knee; in feet, soles, toes, left big toe.

Sensation of weakness in the calves.

The feet feel sprained.

³⁴ **Limbs in General.** The rheumatism often attacks the
heart, and generally goes from the upper to the lower
parts; pains shift suddenly.

The rheumatic pains are mostly in the upper arms and
lower parts of legs; and are worse when going to sleep.

³⁵ **Position, etc.** Recumbent posture: 1. Motion: 1, 19, 31,
44. Stooping: 2. Turning: 2. Sitting stooped: 17;
erect: 17, 19. Lying on left side: 29; back: 29. In
bed: 31. Ascending stairs: 36. Exertion: 36.

Pains worse on the least motion. θ Acute rheumatism.

▮ Pains worse by sitting bent, yet a feeling as if to do so
was necessary, but relieved by sitting or standing
upright. θ Gastralgia.

³⁶ **Nerves.** Weariness in all muscles.

Shuns all exertion, can hardly go up stairs.

❙ Weakness the only general symptom with neuralgia.

Weary and giddy, with the diarrhœa.

Trembling, thrilling, strumming with palpitation.

³⁷ **Sleep.** Restless sleep, turns often.

While sleeping he stands up and walks about; talks in sleep.

Dreams: racking his brains; fantastic: of murder.

³⁸ **Time.** Morning; 1, 3, 5, 9. Afternoon: 4. Evening: 1, 3, 5, 10, 11, 31. Night: 4, 6, 8.

Pains worse during the early parts of the night, or soon after going to bed. θ Neuralgia. θ Acute rheumatism.

³⁹ **Temperature and Weather.** Open air: 3, 5. Cold air: 40. Cold: 4. Heat: 4. Winter: 30. Summer: 8.

Pains are felt from a sudden chill or exposure to a sudden wind. θ Acute rheumatism. θ Neuralgia.

⁴⁰ **Chill. Fever. Sweat.** Chilliness, with coldness; shaking chill in cold air; chills run over the back.

Febrile excitement. θ Endocarditis.

General heat; heat with burning and pain in back and loins.

Cold sweat.

⁴¹ **Attacks.** Pains change places. θ Rheumatism.

❙ Pain occurring at irregular times, continuing for no definite period, coming suddenly or gradually and leaving as uncertainly. θ Neuralgia.

Pains paroxysmal in right arm. θ Neuralgia.

Every summer: 8.

⁴² **Sides.** Right: 3, 4, 5, 6, 8, 18, 19, 32. Left: 3, 11, 19, 28, 29, 32, 33. Diagonally: 2. Above downward: 3, 19, 33, 34. Before backward: 3. Below upward: 4.

Neuralgia of head, ear or face, generally on the right side.

Pains shift about from joint to joint, more when they begin in the upper limbs, and then in the lower. θ Acute rheumatism.

Pains move downward; head; bones of face; from ear to arm; down spine; down leg; arm to fingers.

Pains move upward; neck over head; ball in throat; lower limbs, then upper.

⁴³ **Sensations.** Pains attended with amount of stiffness in right arm. θ Neuralgia.

Pains of a sticking, tearing, pressing character, or shooting in a downward direction.

❙ Sometimes attended with numbness or rather succeeded by numbness of the part affected. θ Neuralgia.

⁴⁴ **Tissues.** Acute rheumatism, going from joint to joint; violent fever; pains intense; ankles most painful and swollen; worse from the least movement.

ɪ Joints hot, red, swollen.   θ Acute rheumatism.
⁴⁵ **Contact, Injuries, etc.**   Touch: 4, 17, 31.   Rubbing: 5.
   Neck tender to the touch.   See 31.
⁴⁶ **Skin.**   Pricking sensation in the skin, with moderate sweat.
   Dry skin.
   Erysipelatous, inflamed eruption on hand (similar to the
      eruption caused by *Rhus tox.*) with oppressed breathing.
   Eruption like itch.
   Red, inflamed places here and there, exceedingly painful,
      as if furuncles would form.
⁴⁸ **Relationship.**   *Kalmia* follows *Spigel.* well in heart diseases.
   Antidote: *Bellad.* helped throbbing head; erysipelas.
   With symptoms indicating *Diosc.*, in gastralgia it had a
      marked beneficial action.

KOBALTUM.

The Element.   HERING.   LIPPE.

¹ **Mind.**   Great exhilaration of spirits, vivacity and rapid
      flow of thoughts.
   Desire for study.
   Indisposed to mental and physical labor; low-spirited;
      thinks too little of himself.
   All mental excitement increases the sufferings.
² **Sensorium.**   Dizziness; dulness; feeling as if head grew
      large (during stool).
³ **Inner Head.**   Pain in the forehead, with uneasiness in the
      stomach.
   Frontal or occipital pain, worse from stooping.
   Dull, pressive pain in temples.
   At every jar, feels as if top of head would come off.
   Frontal headache, with pain back of eyes.
   Headache in morning, with beating and sore aching all
      over.
   Headache when getting up from sitting.
⁴ **Outer Head.**   Great itching in the hairy scalp, in the beard
      and under the chin, burning when scratching.
   Sore pimples along edge of the hair back of head.
⁵ **Eyes.**   Dim vision; darting pains in the eyes when writing,
      with feeling when opening the lids, as if little strings
      were holding them together and snapping.
   Flickering before eyes when reading; letters looked
      blurred.
   Darting, shooting pains in eyes, from bright light.

Eyes ache at night.

Lachrymation and pain from cold air; sensation as if sand were under the lids.

Smarting in lids when using eyes.

6 **Ears.**   Aching, humming in left ear.

Stinging through left ear from roof of mouth.

7 **Nose.**   Putrid, sickish smell before the nose.

Watery discharge, with sneezing.

Nose feels obstructed.

Left nostril feels dry; filled with scales, with itching.

9 **Lower Face.**   Peeling of lips, with soreness and bleeding.

Disposition to keep the jaws tightly closed.

Large boils, very painful, on chin and left lower jaw.

10 **Teeth.**   Pain in hollow teeth, they feel too long; gums swollen, tender, feel as if ulcerated; worse from cold air.

11 **Tongue, etc.**   Flat taste; bad taste, with belching in the morning.

Tongue coated white; cracks across the middle.

12 **Mouth.**   Pricking, sticking in roof of mouth, extending to left ear.

Constant watery secretion, with frequent swallowing.

13 **Throat.**   Soreness, with rawness when hawking.

Dryness and soreness, mornings.

Hawking up thick, white mucus, which fills throat, in morning.

Feeling of fulness, from stomach to throat.

14 **Desires.   Aversions.**   Diminished appetite, especially for supper.

15 **Eating and Drinking.**   After eating: 16, 17, 19.   After drinking coffee: 21.

16 **Nausea and Vomiting.**   Hiccough after eating, with soreness in pit of stomach.

Belching of wind, morning, and after stool.

Rising of sour or bitter water, with pain in stomach; afterward, dryness in throat.

Qualmishness, with fulness of the stomach.

Nausea, with pain in forehead.

17 **Stomach.**   Pain in stomach and abdomen after eating, with feeling of great uneasiness; must move about.

Stomach feels as if it contained undigested food.

Fulness in stomach, extending to throat, with qualmishness.

Soreness in stomach when inspiring deeply, or from hiccough.

18 **Hypochondria.**   Shooting, stitching from region of liver down into the thigh.

Sharp pain in splenic region, worse when inspiring deeply.

19 **Abdomen.**   Abdomen feels empty about the umbilicus.

35

Cutting before stool.

Rumbling in abdomen.

Fulness in abdomen after a light meal.

Colic at 5 A.M., followed by large stool and tenesmus.

20 **Stool, etc.** Urgent desire for stool while walking, worse when standing; stool profuse, watery, spouting.

Stool large, soft, with tenesmus and aching in sphincter ani; severe colicky pain in lower part of abdomen; tenesmus after stool; during stool, dizziness.

Costiveness and looseness alternate.

Feces like hazel-nuts, with dulness in head.

Pressure in rectum.

Constant dropping of blood from anus (stools not bloody).

21 **Urine.** Albuminuria.

Frequent discharge of small quantities of urine.

Increased secretion of pale urine, frequent urination in the morning, after drinking coffee.

Scanty urine, with greasy pellicle; yellow flocculent, or red sediment, and strong pungent smell.

Smarting in end of urethra, during micturition.

Burning in the urethra.

22 **Male Sexual Organs.** Frequent nocturnal emissions, with lewd dreams; only partial, or no erections; impotence.

Severe pain in right testicle, better after urinating.

Yellow-brown spots on the genitals (and abdomen).

25 **Larynx.** Stitches in the anterior part of the larynx.

26 **Breathing.** Frequent sighing.

On taking a deep inspiration, stitches in the chest, soreness in the stomach and pain in the spleen.

27 **Cough.** Cough, with soreness in throat and rawness when hawking.

Short, hacking cough, with expectoration of bright red blood, which seemingly comes from the larynx.

Expectoration of thick, tough mucus, mixed with blood; with fulness and pressive pains in larynx; scratching, rawness and burning in throat, and a disposition to keep jaws tightly closed; worse from pressure, empty deglutition and cold water.

Copious expectoration of sweetish, frothy, white mucus, with lumps in it.

28 **Lungs.** Deep stitches in lower part of chest, mostly left side, from deep inspiration.

31 **Neck. Back.** Pain, between the shoulders, in the lumbar region and small of the back.

Aching pain in the small of the back, or in the spine; worse when sitting, better on rising, walking or lying down.

Backache, with seminal emissions.

Pain along the spine, and from the sacrum down through the legs into the feet, worse while sitting.

[32] **Upper Limbs.** Aching in the wrist-joints, with occasional stitches.

[33] **Lower Limbs.** Shooting into the thigh from the liver.

Excessive weakness of the knees.

Foot-sweat, mostly between the toes, smelling sour or like sole-leather.

Flushes of heat along the legs.

Stitches in the legs.

Jerks in the limbs when falling asleep.

Trembling of limbs, especially legs; aching when sitting.

Pricking, as of needles, in the feet.

[34] **Limbs in General.** Bruised pain in all the limbs.

Stitching in the arms and legs.

[35] **Position, etc.** Stooping: 3. Must move about: 17. Walking: 20, 34. Standing: 20. Sitting: 31, 33. Rising: 3, 31, 37. Lying down: 31.

[37] **Sleep.** Distressing drowsiness in the evening.

Disturbed, unrefreshing sleep.

Wakeful: can do with less sleep.

On rising, pain in head and small of back.

Lewd dreams; emissions, only partial, or no erections.

[38] **Time.** Morning: 3, 11, 13, 16, 19, 21, 40. Noon till 2 P.M.: 4. 4–5 P.M.: 40. Evening: 37. Night: 5, 22.

[39] **Temperature and Weather.** Cold air: 5, 10. Cold water: 27. Warmth of bed: 46.

[40] **Chill. Fever. Sweat.** Chilly from 11 to 12 A.M.; headache, with nausea and languor from noon to 2 P.M.; then fever and sweat.

Chilliness, with yawning, from 4 to 5 P.M.; feels dull and weak, with aversion to mental exertion.

Flushes of heat; with sweat; along the legs.

[42] **Sides.** Right: 18, 22, 33. Left: 6, 7, 9, 12, 18, 26, 28. Below upward: 17. Above downward: 18, 31, 33.

[45] **Contact, Injuries, etc.** Jarring: 3. Scratching: 4, 46. Pressure: 27. Touch: 10.

[46] **Skin.** Much itching all over, when getting warm in bed.

Pimples on shoulders, pit of stomach and buttocks; bleed easily when scratched.

KREOSOTUM.

A product of distillation of wood tar. WAHLE.

[1] **Mind.** Stupid feeling in the head, with vacant gaze; neither seeing nor hearing.

Frequent vanishing of thought.

Frequent failure of thought.

Weakness of memory. Forgetfulness.

Confounding ideas. Also in puerperal metritis, with putridity.

Thinks herself well.

Sorrowful mood, inclined to weep, or longing for death; music and similar emotional causes impel him to weep.

Anxious, apprehensive mood.

Ill-humor. Moroseness. Peevishness, ill-temper.

Obstinacy.

Excited condition.

Ailments from emotions.

[2] **Sensorium.** Vertigo, mornings, in the open air, with staggering like from drunkenness, must hold on to something; passes off in the room.

Roaring in the head.

Painful dulness of the head, as after a carouse.

[3] **Inner Head.** Headache after a carouse

Pain pressing outward in forehead.

Heaviness or pressure in various parts of the head, with sensation as if the brain would force through forehead.

Throbbing and beating in forehead from left side of head.

Tearing, drawing and jerking pains.

Occipital headache; much pain and soreness.

Chronic periodic headache in forehead, piercing pain; wheals or swellings on the scalp.

Dull feeling in head as from a board across the forehead.

Headache, with sleepiness.

[4] **Outer Head.** Eruptions on forehead, as with drunkards.

Scales accumulate in large indurated masses and fall off freely.

Falling off of the hair.

Sensibility of scalp to touch, and when the hair is combed.

[5] **Eyes.** Dimsighted: as if looking through gauze; as if something was floating before the eyes, obliging to wipe them constantly.

Staring, dull, lifeless and stupid look.

Itching and smarting sensation in eyes, on edges of lids; worse rubbing them.

Suggilation on the conjunctiva of right eye.

Heat in the eyes with ulceration. Burning heat, with tears, worse by bright light.

Discharge of hot, acrid, smarting tears.

Slight inflammation of the meibomian glands.

Eyes sunken, with blue rings around.

Eyes protruding.

Chronic swelling of eyelids and their margins.

Agglutination of eyelids.

⁶ **Ears.** Hard hearing.

❙Roaring in the head; also humming and difficulty of hearing before and during menses.

Stitches in ears.

Heat, burning, swelling and redness of left outer ear, proceeding from a pimple in the concha, with stiffness and pain in left side of neck, shoulder and arm.

Itching in the ears.

Humid tetter on the ears, with swelling of cervical glands and livid grey complexion.

⁷ **Nose.** Offensive smell before the nose, with loss of appetite; stinking, in the morning, when awaking.

Nosebleed, with heaviness and throbbing in forehead.

Thin, bright red blood from both nostrils.

Catarrh, fluent or dry, with much sneezing.

Chronic catarrh with old people.

Epithelial cancer on right ala nasi.

Lupus on the nose, left side.

Frequent sneezing, with dry, nasal catarrh.

⁸ **Face.** Sick, suffering expression.

Old looking children.

Complexion: earthy; pale, green, with swelling of cervical glands; pale, bloated; coppery appearance.

Face cold, of pale, bluish tinge, especially on temples and around the nose and mouth.

Flushes of heat, with circumscribed redness of the cheeks.

Face hot, cheeks red, feet cold.

Acne in the face.

❙Burning pains; worse talking or exertion, better lying on the unaffected side; nervous, excitable

⁹ **Lower Face.** Peeling off and cracking of cuticle of upper lip.

Wants to moisten the lips frequently, without being thirsty.

Tumor, size of a pea, on lower lip, with acrid, watery ichor, making the surrounding parts sore.

¹⁰ **Teeth.** Drawing toothache, extends to temples and ears.

Bad odor from decayed teeth.

Toothache: extending to the temples and to the left side of face; drawing, extending to inner ear and temples.

Teeth wedge shaped.

Very painful dentition; teeth begin to decay as soon as they appear; dark specks on teeth, commencing decay.

Gums: bluish-red; inflamed, on upper left side.

Swelling of the gum over a tooth which was not quite through, causes convulsions.

Gums bleed readily, scorbutic, spongy and ulcerated.

Bleeding of gums and nose, blood dark, quickly coagulating.

[11] **Tongue, etc.**   Bitter or flat taste.

Everything eaten tastes bitter.

Tongue: dry; with mucous coating.

[12] **Mouth.**   Putrid odor from the mouth.

[13] **Throat.**   Pressure on the right side when swallowing.

Scraping in throat, with roughness and dryness.

Small round bluish-red spots (petechiæ) on the throat.

Scratching sensation in the throat.

[14] **Desires. Aversions.**   Greedy drinking and vomiting.

Great thirst.

Keen appetite, especially for meat; craves smoked meat.

Aversion to meat, vomits after it.

Loss of appetite.

[15] **Eating and Drinking.**   Water, after it is swallowed, tastes bitter.

Worse from eating cold food.

Better from warm diet.

Dares not remain fasting.

Great desire for spirituous drinks, with weakening leucorrhœa.

Stomach aches, from acid food.

[16] **Nausea and Vomiting.**   Belching and hiccough, especially when sitting up, or being carried.

Belching: sour; empty; after dinner, with throwing off of frothy saliva, and with scraping roughness in throat.

Nausea, during pregnancy; constant inclination to vomit with doing so.

Vomiting: of undigested food two or three hours after eating; with dimness of vision; of everything eaten.

[17] **Stomach.**   Tension over the stomach and scrobiculum, tight clothing is intolerable.

Painful hard spot, at or to the left of the stomach.

[18] **Hypochondria.**   Stitches in the region of the liver.

Bruised pain in region of liver, with sensation of fulness; must loosen the clothes.

Constriction of the hypochondria, cannot tolerate tight clothing.

Pressure in region of the spleen, painful on pressure.

Feeling of fulness, as if he had eaten too much.

[19] **Abdomen.** Ulcerative pain in abdomen.

Pain in region of umbilicus.

Abdomen distended and tense, like a drum, without being hard or painful.

Abdomen not distended, but hard.

Burning in the bowels.

Labor-like pains in abdomen, with drawing in upper abdomen extending to small of back, and pressing toward the lumbar vertebræ, with flushes of heat in face, palpitation of heart, frequent pulse and ineffectual urging to urinate, finally small quantities of hot urine are passed; after paroxysm chill and discharge of milky leucorrhœa.

Sore pain in abdomen during deep inhalation.

Painful sensation of coldness in abdomen; icy-coldness in epigastrium; dyspepsia.

Violent abdominal spasms, worse in the groins.

[20] **Stool, etc.** Cramp-like pain in rectum during stool.

Stools: watery, or papescent, dark brown, putrid evacuations, containing undigested food; greyish or white, chopped, very fetid; frequent greenish, watery; cadaverous-smelling.

Ineffectual, painful urging to stool.

Constipation, stool hard and expelled only after much pressing.

Constriction in case of uterine cancer.

[21] **Urine.** Frequent urgency to urinate, with copious, pale discharge.

Diminished secretion; though drinking much; frequent urging, especially at night, must rise, though but small quantity passes.

Urine: chestnut brown; clouded; reddish, with red sediment; depositing white sediment; colorless; fetid.

Wets the bed at night, wakes with urging, but cannot retain the urine; or dreams he is urinating.

Prepuce bluish-black with hemorrhage and gangrene (topically); syphilis.

[22] **Male Sexual Organs.** Burning in genitals and impotence during coition, with swelling of penis the next day.

[23] **Female Sexual Organs.** Menses: too early, too profuse and too protracted; succeeded by an acrid-smelling, bloody ichor, with itching and biting in the parts; more or less pain during the flow, but much aggravated after it; flow intermits, at times almost ceasing, the recommencing. (See Ears.)

Before menses looks swollen as if pregnant.

Metrorrhagia: dark and offensive, with fainting; pulseless; offensive-smelling in large clots.

Painful urging toward the genitals.

Bearing down and weight in pelvis; also sensation as if something was coming out the vagina; worse by motion.

Leucorrhœa: putrid, acrid, corrosive, stains clothing yellow, stiffens like starch; mild or acrid, causing much itching; milky, after coccygodynia; worse between the menses, or for a few days before menses; great weakness.

Deep in pelvis, violent burning sensation, with constant whining and moaning.

Fundus of uterus swollen and sensitive to pressure.

Orifice of uterus wide open, almost everted, its inner surface like cauliflower; ulcerative pain in cervix uteri.

Scirrhus of vagina, painful to slight touch.

During coition: violent pain, preceded by anxiety and trembling; burning in the parts, followed next day by discharge of dark blood.

Hard lump on neck of uterus, with ulcerative pain during coition.

Corrosive itching within the vulva, with sorenes and burning after scratching; burning and swelling of the labia; violent itching between the labia and thighs.

Soreness and smarting between labia and in vulva.

24 **Pregnancy.**   Nausea during pregnancy; ptyalism.

Vomiting before breakfast of sweetish water, breakfast and dinner retained.

Vomiting after supper.

Metrorrhagia threatening abortion (third month—blood black).

Tightness across the pit of stomach.

Very offensive, excoriating lochia; repeatedly almost ceasing, only to freshen up again.

Lochia blackish, lumpy and very offensive.

Stitches in the mammæ.

Dwindling away of the mammæ, with small, hard, painful lumps in them.

Mammæ hard, bluish-red and covered with little scurfy protruberances, from which blood oozes whenever the scurf is removed.

25 **Larynx.**   Scraping and roughness in the throat; also with hoarseness, ceasing in the motning, after sneezing.

Rough, hoarse speech.

Perichondritis of the larynx, septic form, with softening and degeneration affecting the mucous membrane of larynx, and particularly that of the œsophagus.

26 **Breathing.**   Shortness of breath, with sensation of heaviness in the chest and frequent desire to take a deep breath; chest feels bruised, as if beaten; pain as if sternum were being crushed in; nervous asthma.

Difficult breathing, with anxiety; oppression of chest.

[27] **Cough.** Whistling, dry; evening, in bed; caused by crawling below the larynx, or, as if in the upper bronchi, with dyspnœa; dry, spasmodic, in the morning, causing retching; with escape of urine; with easily detached white expectoration; scraping, with profuse, thick, yellow, or white mucous expectoration.

After every coughing spell, copious purulent expectoration.

Periodical blood-spitting, with greenish-yellow, pus-like sputa.

Expectoration of black, coagulated blood.

Frequent blood-spitting, severe pains in chest, afternoon fever and morning sweat.

Fatiguing cough with old people, copious sputa, thick, yellow or white.

[28] **Lungs.** Stitches: in left chest, just over the heart; across the chest, during the morning till noon; first in left, then in right chest; in the right chest, interrupting breathing; also under the scapula.

Pains in chest, better from pressure.

Anxious feeling of heaviness in chest.

[29] **Heart. Pulse.** Anxiety at the heart.

Stitches: over the heart; in the heart.

Pulsation in all the arteries, when at rest.

Pulse; small, weak and quick; soft, quick and trembling; small and hard, slow.

[30] **Outer Chest.** Chest pains as if bruised, particularly the sternum, and especially on pressure or from inspiration; also extending to clavicles and cervical muscles.

Pain as if the sternum or the whole chest were pressed in.

[31] **Neck. Back.** Glands of neck swollen.

Pain in back at night; worse when lying.

Pain as if small of back would break; worse during rest, better from motion.

Pain in small of back and in sacral region, like labor-pains, urging to urinate and ineffectual desire for stool.

Spasmodic drawing from behind forward, also into the genitals, or down into the thighs.

Continuous burning in the small of back.

[32] **Upper Limbs.** Scapulæ as if bruised.

Stitches in arm, from the shoulder-joint through to the fingers, which feel as if asleep, without power or feeling.

Pain as if bruised when touched on inner side of upper arm.

Pain in elbow-joint, as if the tendons were too short.

Slightly elevated red blotches on left forearm.

Pain in the ulnar muscles, extending to little finger; cramp-like in left arm; drawing, with lameness, in right.

Fingers become white and insensible, especially in the morning after rising.

Pain in left thumb, as if sprained.

Cracking of the skin of the hands.

[33] **Lower Limbs.** Pain in left hip-joint, as if it were luxated, with sensation as if the leg was too long when standing.

Bruised pain on crest of ilium: as if from a heavy burden, or after running; stitches from the same through the abdomen; pain in the same and in the lumbar vertebræ in the morning, as if tired.

Tingling or buzzing sensation in lower limbs.

Pain as from an ulcer in the whole leg.

Boring pain in hip-joints, alternating with numbness and loss of sensation in the whole thigh.

Sensation as if the knee-joint would suddenly give away.

Alternate swelling of the knee-joints and wrists, with sensation of numbness and rigidity of the limbs.

Œdematous, white swelling of both feet.

Stitches in the right ankle and left heel.

Ulcerative pain in soles; burning-itching in soles.

Cold swelling of the feet.

[34] **Limbs in General.** Pain in all the limbs, as if beaten, or as after a long walk.

Skin on the extremities dry and rough.

Lassitude of all the limbs; heaviness, with tired sleepiness.

[35] **Position, etc.** During repose, a sensation as if all parts of the body were in motion.

Rest seems to increase the pains.

She dares not keep quiet for a long time after getting up from sleep.

Inclination for motion.

Sitting up: 16. Resting: 29, 31, 36, 40. Lying: 31. Motion: 31, 36. Standing: 33. Exertion: 36.

[36] **Nerves.** Great debility.

Faintness in the morning, when rising earlier than usual.

Fatigue from the least exertion; also as from too long a foot journey.

Prostation, with sleeplessness.

Spasms during dentition; swelling over a tooth not quite through.

Great restlessness and excitation of the whole body, worse in repose than during motion.

[37] **Sleep.** Great drowsiness, with frequent yawning.

Sleeplessness, worse before midnight.

Child moans constantly, or dozes with half-open eyes; or is cross, sleepless; during dentition.

Tosses about all night, without any apparent cause.

Starting, when scarcely fallen asleep.

Laughs aloud during sleep.

Dreams of crying; of falling from a height; of being out in a snow-storm; of being poisoned; of bright fire; of very dirty (clothes) wash.

Generally better after sleep.

[38] **Time.** Morning: 2, 7, 24, 25, 27, 28, 32, 33, 36, 40. Afternoon: 27. Evening: 27, 37, 46. Night: 21, 31, 37, 46.

[39] **Temperature and Weather.** Generally better from warmth.

Many symptoms are aggravated in the open air, from growing cold and in cold weather; from washing or bathing with cold water.

[40] **Chill. Fever. Sweat.** Transient chill without thirst.

Chill, predominating when at rest.

Shaking chill, with severe flushes of heat in the face, red face and icy-cold feet; after the chill, thirst.

Chill, with great bodily restlessness.

Chill, alterating with heat.

Coldness of face and hands.

Heat mostly in the face.

Flushes of heat, with circumscribed redness of the face.

Sweat scant and only during the morning, with heat and redness of the cheeks.

[41] **Attacks.** Intermittent: 23, 24. Periodical: 27. Boring pain, alternating with numbness: 33.

[42] **Sides.** Right: 5, 7, 13, 18, 28, 32, 33. Left: 6, 10, 17, 18, 19, 28, 29, 32, 33. Left to right: 28. Above downward: 19, 31, 32. Below upward: 30. Before backward: 19. Within outwards: 3.

[43] **Sensations.** Loss of sensation.

[44] **Tissues.** Hemorrhages; small wounds bleed much.

Hemorrhage and fetid stools. θ Typhus.

Excoriation of mucous surfaces.

Rheumatic pains in joints, also stitches, most of hip and knee; when with numbness of whole limb as if asleep.

Numbness, loss of sensation.

Rapid emaciation.

[45] **Contact, Injuries, etc.** Touch: 4, 23, 32, 33. Combing: 4. Being carried: 16. Pressure of clothing: 17, 18. Pressure: 18, 23, 28, 30. Scratching: 23.

[46] **Skin.** Itching: toward evening so violent as to drive one almost wild.

Wheals like urticaria.

Large, greasy-looking, pock-shaped pustules, over the whole body; skin tense, shining, deep red, with a greasy moisture.

Eruption, dry as well as moist, in almost all parts of the body, especially on the backs of hands and feet, in the palms, in the ears, in the popliteal region, and on the knuckles of hands, with much itching.

Old ulcers, painful, putrid.

Skin remarkably pale.

⁴⁷ **Stages and States.** Very tall for her age; blonde; delicate.

Dark complexion, slight, lean.

Complexion livid, disposition sad, irritable.

Old-looking children, hard to awaken.

Often indicated for old women.

⁴⁸ **Relationship.** *Kreosot.* is followed well by *Sulphur.* also by *Arsen.* (in cancer).

Antidotes to *Kreosot.: Nux vom.* against the violent pulsa-tions in every part of body; *Acon.* against the vascular irritation.

After *Carb. veg.* it disagrees.

LACHESIS.

Surukuku. HERING. *Ophidia.*

¹ **Mind.** Thinks herself under superhuman control.

Completely insensibility.

Memory weak; makes mistakes in orthography.

Quick comprehension; mental excitability, with almost prophetic perceptions; ecstasy.

Delirium, fears she will be damned.

Delirium at night, muttering, drowsy, red face; or slow, difficult speech and dropped jaw.

❙ Mania, with great loquacity, frequently jumping from one subject to another.

❙ Mania after overstudying.

Delirium tremens, worse after sleep; cannot bear pressure of neckcloth; loquacious.

Delirium from overwatching, overfatigue; loss of fluids; excessive study.

Thinks she is dead, and that preparations are being made for her funeral; thinks herself pursued by enemies; fears the medicine is poison.

Loquacity, with mocking jealousy; frightful images.

Talks, sings, whistles, makes odd motions.

Proud; jealous, suspicious.

Peevish, disposed to be morose or to quarrel.

Suicidal mood, tired of life.

Great sadness and anxiety, worse in morning on awaking.

Dread of death, fears to go to bed. Fears being poisoned.

² **Sensorium.** Vertigo: from looking at one and the same object; from walking in the open air (at climaxis); from suppressed erysipelas; with pale face; migraine.

Head heavy like lead, worse about occiput. with vertigo.

Rush of blood to the head, after spirituous liquors; from suppressed or irregular menses.

Blowing expiration, cannot bear neck touched; left-sided apoplexy, especially if after mental emotions, or abuse of alcohol.

Severe pains all over the head, so giddy he could not stand; could not see the letters, fell against the wall.

³ **Inner Head.** Frontal headache, faint on rising.

Headache over eyes and in occiput, morning, on rising.

Pressing, bursting pains in temples, better when lying down.

Temporal nerves pain, vertigo, pale face; throbbing temples.

One-sided headache; pains intense, extend to neck and shoulders, with stiff neck; paralytic tongue.

Tearing on top of head from within outward. See Face.

Weight and pressure on the vertex.

Burning of the vertex, at the menopause.

Beating headache with heat, worse on the vertex and right side, or over the eyes, preceding a cold in the head, with stiff neck.

Feeling in back of head as if pressed asunder.

Headache in the sun, glimmering sight.

Throbbing in the head from least movement; congestion.

⁴ **Outer Head.** Purplish swelling; delirious talk when closing the eyes. θ Erysipelas.

ı Tumors which perforate the skull.

Hair falls off, worse during pregnancy; averse to sun's rays.

⁵ **Eyes.** Oversensitive to light.

ı Amblyopia, with lung or heart affections.

Feels, when throat is pressed, as if eyes were forced out.

Whites of the eyes yellow. Redness of the eyes.

ı Retinitis apoplectica.

Ulcers on the cornea.

Severe pain in and above the eyes.

⁶ **Ears.** Sensitiveness to sounds; rushing and thundering in the ears.

Hardness of hearing, with want of wax; dryness in the ears; numbness about the ear and cheek (left).

Ear-wax too hard, pale, and insufficient.

⁷ **Nose.** Nosebleed, dark; with amenorrhœa; typhus, etc.; blowing of blood, mostly in the morning.

Coryza preceded by headache; discharge watery, with red nostrils, herpes on the lips.

Relieves paroxysms of sneezing in hay asthma.

Nasal mucous membrane swollen; sneezing.

Pus and blood from the nose.

Vesicular eruption about the nose.

Nose red externally; nose filled with scabs; discharge of pus and blood; mercurio-syphilis; also in drunkards.

8 **Face.** Flushes of heat in drunkards.

Expression of pain with sopor.

Features distorted.

Livid, grey complexion, with abdominal complaints or ague.

Face pale, with fainting; dizzy with headache.

Yellow complexion, with vermillion redness of the cheeks, or with small red blood-vessels shining through the skin. Syphilis.

Red face, as in apoplexy; bloated red face, with headache, pains in the limbs, stomach, etc.

Erysipelas of the face, with burning and itching, worse after siesta; with hammering headache.

Neuralgia, left side, orbital; rising of heat to the face before, and weak feeling in the abdomen after, the attack.

9 **Lower Face.** Lower jaw hangs down. θ Coma.

Lips dry, cracked, bleeding.

Lower lip swollen.

10 **Teeth.** Decayed teeth pain when biting; after sleep; after abuse of mercury. Decayed teeth crumble.

Cheek swollen, skin tense, hot and crisp, as if it would crack; periodontitis.

Gums bluish, swollen, bleeding, worse from warm drinks.

11 **Tongue, etc.** Sour taste, everything turns sour.

Difficult speech, tongue heavy, cannot open mouth wide.

ı Puts the trembling tongue out with great difficulty. θ Diphtheria, etc.

Tongue: trembles when protruded, or catches behind the teeth; swollen, coated white; papillæ enlarged; dry, red, cracked at the tip; red tip and brown centre; mapped, dry, black and stiff.

Blisters, mostly about the tip.

Talking: 26.

12 **Mouth.** Bad odor from the mouth.

Saliva abundant, tenacious.

Sore mouth in the last stages of phthisis.

Sensation on roof of mouth as if the mucous membrane were peeling off.

13 **Throat.** Uvula elongated; fauces purplish and swollen, or ulcerated.

Feeling of a lump in the throat; suffocative sensation; on swallowing, the lump descends, but returns at once: 48.

When swallowing fluids, they escape through the nose; worse when swallowing saliva, less from liquids, and even relieved by solids.

Much phlegm in the fauces, with painful hawking.

▮ Pain and soreness begin on left side of throat. θ Tonsilitis. θ Diphtheria.

Constriction of the throat; feels as if tied; worse from the
least external pressure; suffocating spells, worse during
or awaking from sleep.

Tonsils swollen, worse the left, with a tendency to the
right; inability to swallow, threatening suffocation; or,
on swallowing, pain shoots into the (left) ear; cannot
. bear anything to touch the neck.

Diphtheritic patches in the throat, spreading from left to
right; fetid breath; worse after sleep; great debility,
feeble pulse; clammy sweat; headache and faintness.

▮ Aggravation by hot drinks; liquids pain more than
solids while swallowing. θ Tonsillitis. θ Diphtheria.

▮ Excessive tenderness of throat to external pressure.
θ Tonsillitis. θ Diphtheria.

Ulcers in the throat; worse in wet weather; after mercury; from syphilis; ulcers extend up into posterior
nares; throat so dry, he awakens choking; soft palate
full of cicatrices, with greenish-yellow ulcers between;
pains shooting; fetid breath.

¹⁴ **Desires. Aversions.** Appetite gone.

Thirst insatiable, with disgust for drink.

Desire for oysters; for wine and liquors; for coffee, which
agrees.

¹⁵ **Eating and Drinking.** After eating: gnawing in stomach
better, but returns in a few hours. θ Cancer of stomach.

After eating: vertigo, languor; gagging and suffocating;
dyspnœa; stomach puffed; eructations; flushes of heat.

After acids, symptoms worse.

Worse from alcoholic drinks (except the snake-bite).

Warm drink: 10, 13. After drinking: 13, 16.

¹⁶ **Nausea and Vomiting.** Eructations, which relieve.

Everything sour; heart-burn.

Nausea after drinking.

Nausea in attacks, weakness, dyspnœa, palpitation, cold
sweat.

Vomiting: of food; of bile; of mucus; with copious saliva.

¹⁷ **Stomach.** Pit of the stomach painful to touch.

Dyspepsia, worse as soon as he eats; costive; weak digestion, especially after mercury.

Gnawing pressure; relieved after eating, but returning as
soon as the stomach is empty.

¹⁸ **Hypochondria.** Acute pain in the liver, extending towards
the stomach.

Liver complaints at the climaxis; after ague; pain as if
something had lodged in the right side, with stinging.

Cannot bear any pressure about the hypochondria.

Contractive pain in the region of the liver.

Ulcerative pain about liver; inflammation and abscess.

[19] **Abdomen.** Painful distention, flatulence; can bear no pressure.

Burning like fire in hypogastric and lumbar region.

Cutting in right side of abdomen, causing fainting attacks.

Swelling in cœcal region; must lie on the back with limbs drawn up. θ Typhlitis.

Abdomen hot, sensitive; painfully stiff from loins down the thighs; pus formed. θ Peritonitis.

[20] **Stool, etc.** Thin, offensive stools.

Stools: watery, light yellow, fecal; dark, chocolate-colored, cadaverous-smelling; of decomposed blood, looking like charred straw; mixed blood and slime; worse at night, after acids; during warm weather.

Painful straining, with discharge of croupous exudate.

Diarrhœa and constipation in alternation.

Costive, ineffectual urging; anus feels closed. Stools offensive, even if formed.

Beating in the anus, as from hammers.

Tormenting urging, but not to stool.

Wants to pass stool, but the pain is so increased thereby, he must desist.

Rectum prolapsed and tumefied.

Piles protruding or strangulated, or, with stitches upward at each cough or sneeze; worse at climaxis, or with drunkards.

Itching at the anus; worse after sleep.

[21] **Urine.** Stitches from kidneys through the ureters.

Urine: almost black; frequent, foamy, dark.

Ineffectual urging to urinate; burning when it does pass.

Feeling as of a ball rolling in the bladder or abdomen, when turning over.

Discharge of offensive mucus during micturition; catarrh of bladder.

[22] **Male Sexual Organs.** Sexual excitement.

Onanism, with epilepsy.

Buboes indurated or with fistulous openings and hectic; after mercury.

Indurated foreskin, after chancres.

[23] **Female Sexual Organs.** Sexual desire. θ Nymphomania.

Swelling, induration, neuralgia, suppuration, etc., of left ovary.

The uterine region feels swollen, will bear no contact, not even of the clothing; bearing down pains.

Uterine and ovarian pains, relieved by a flow of blood.

Pains like a knife thrust into the abdomen.

Uterus feels as if the os was open.

Menses scanty, feeble, but regular; blood lumpy, black or acrid.

Before menses: desire for open air; vertigo, nosebleed; labor-like pains, worse in left ovarian region; bruised feeling in the hips; all better when the flow begins.

Leucorrhœa copious, smarting, stiffening the linen, staining it greenish.

Redness and swelling of the external parts (with discharge of mucus.)

Suitable at the meniopause: flashes, hot vertex; metrorrhagia; fainting.

²⁴ **Pregnancy.** Lochia fetid; urine suppressed; face purple; unconscious; abdomen swollen. *θ* Puerperal fever.

Milk thin, blue; she awakens always sad, despairing.

Lancinating pains in the mamma, pains down the arm; breast bluish, with blackish streaks.

Fungus hæmatodes, frequently bleeding.

²⁵ **Larynx.** Hoarseness, rawness and dryness; larynx sensitive to touch.

Aphonia in phthisis; sputum tough and green.

Impending croup (during diphtheria), awakens suffocating, grasps the throat; fears he is dying.

Larynx externally sensitive to the least touch, which causes suffocation, feeling of a lump in the throat.

Croup, when the patient is worse after sleep; or, seemingly sleeps into the croupy spell.

Suddenly something runs from neck to larynx, stopping the breathing, it awakens him at night. *θ* Spasmus glottidis.

²⁶ **Breathing.** Asthma, worse from covering mouth or nose, or touching the throat, or moving the arms; on awaking; after eating or talking; better sitting up bent forward.

Chest feels constricted.

In the morning when sitting up quickly, the breathing becomes slow, difficult, whistling.

Chest stuffed; short cough, with scanty, difficult expectoration.

Asthma during scabies, if the itching ceases.

²⁷ **Cough.** Gagging, persistent cough, from tickling in the throat under the sternum, or in the stomach; worse on falling asleep or during the day; from change of temperature; after alcoholic drinks.

Has to cough hard and long before he can raise.

Expectoration scanty, difficult, watery, saltish, must be swallowed again; or is accompanied with straining and vomiting.

❙ Spitting large quantities of ropy mucus. *θ* Diphtheria.

36

Cough from ulcers in the throat.

Cough, with slimy, bloody sputum.

❙ After a long, wheezing cough, suddenly spits up profuse, frothy, tenacious mucus.

²⁸ **Lungs.** Oppressive pain in chest, as if full of wind, better from eructations.

Pain in the chest as from soreness.

Burning in the chest.

Stitches in the (left) chest, with dyspnœa.

Pneumonia, hepatization, mostly of left lung; great dyspnœa on awaking.

Useful when tubercles follow pneumonia.

Dropsy of the chest; awakens with suffocating spells; liver swollen; scanty, dark urine; palpitation. θ After scarlatina.

²⁹ **Heart. Pulse.** Palpitation, can bear no pressure on throat or chest; must sit up or lie on the right side; numbness of the left arm, fainting, anxiety.

Pericarditis, dropsy, diphtheritic patches in the throat, after scarlatina.

❙ Restless, trembling; anxiety about the heart; hasty speech; suffocation on lying down; weight on the chest; heart feels constricted. θ Rheumatism of the heart.

❙ Cyanosis neonatorum.

Pulse: small, weak and accelerated; unequal; intermittent; alternately full and small.

³¹ **Neck. Back.** Stiff neck, moves jaw with great difficulty; tearing from nape of neck up either side, to top of head.

Pain in the small of the back, with constipation.

Pain in the os coccygis, when sitting down, feeling as if sitting on something sharp.

³² **Upper Limbs.** Left shoulder and arm weak and lame, worse when lying on the arm.

Soreness of the right shoulder, worse when lying on it.

Axillary glands swollen.

Garlic-like smell of the sweat in the axillæ.

Tingling-prickling in the left hand.

Trembling of the hands. θ In drunkards.

Rheumatic swelling of index-finger and wrist; worse after sleep.

Panaritium, bluish swelling; even necrosis, with fistulous openings, or erysipelas; stinging-pricking pains.

Numbness of the finger-tips (morning).

³³ **Lower Limbs.** Contraction of psoas muscle, after abscess.

Sciatica, left-sided; pain as from a hot iron; worse after sleep.

Uneasiness in the lower limbs.

Contraction of the hamstrings, after a popliteal abscess.

Stinging-tearing in the knees, with swelling.

Aching pain in the shin-bones.

Flat ulcers on legs, with thin, offensive discharge, and
bluish areolæ.

Caries of the tibia.

Lacerating, jerking, rheumatic pains in the legs, as soon
as he falls asleep.

Swelling of the feet, worse after walking. θ During pregnancy.

Tingling in the toes.

Rhagades of the toes.

Gangrenous ulcers on the legs and toes.

³⁴ **Limbs in General.** Erysipelas of the legs or arms; surface
bluish, glossy, swelling, impending gangrene.

Bluish swelling of the joints, after sprains.

Dark bluish swelling of cellular tissue, on hands, arms,
legs; very sensitive; impending gangrene.

Nightly burning in palms and soles.

Limbs stiff or curved, after mercurialization.

³⁵ **Position, etc.** Motion: erysipelas excited by too much
walking; relieves the periodical sufferings.

Walking in open air: 2. After walking: 33. Moving the
arms: 26. Turning over: 21. On rising: 3. Must sit
up: 29. Sitting: 31. Sitting bent forwards: 26. Lying
down: 3, 29, 32. Must lie on back: 19. Lying on right
side: 29.

³⁶ **Nerves.** Crawls on the floor, spits often, hides, laughs, or is
angry; spasms.

Epilepsy comes on during sleep, from jealousy, onanism,
loss of fluids.

Spasms of the legs.

Awkward gait; left side weak; gressus gallinaceus.

Paralysis, left-sided; after apoplexy, or cerebral exhaustion.

Trembling all over; exhausted, faint.

❙ Fainting, with pain in heart, nausea, pale face, vertigo.

³⁷ **Sleep.** Sleepy day and night; sleeps well unless the cough
annoys him.

Children toss about, moaning, during sleep.

Restless sleep, with many dreams and frequent waking.

Persistent sleeplessness; sleepless in the evening, with
talkativeness.

Awakens at night and cannot sleep again.

❙ The mind worse after sleep.

³⁸ **Time.** Morning: 1, 3, 7, 26, 32. Afternoon: 40. Evening
37, 40. Night: 1, 20, 25, 34, 37, 40. Day: 27. Day
and night: 37.

³⁹ **Temperature and Weather.** Worse from the sun's rays: 3,
4. Worse during Spring and Summer; or from ex-

tremes of temperature, debility: 20. Change of temperature: 26. . Wet weather: 13. Desire for the open air: 23. Worse in the open air: 2. Warmth: 44. Warm room: 40. Hot drinks: 13.

⁴⁰ Chill. Fever. Sweat. Chill: runs up the back to head, often on alternate days; abates in the warm room; with chattering of the teeth, desires external warmth.

Wants to be held, or to be pressed down during chill.

After icy-cold calves, shaking chill with warm sweat; then strumming through limbs, intermingled with flushes of heat.

Spasms during every paroxysm, in nursing children.

Chill at night, flushes of heat by day.

Heat, particularly on the hands and feet, in the evening.

Burning in the palms and soles, evening and night.

Heat at night, as from orgasm of blood, throat sensitive.

Internal sensation of heat, with cold feet.

Profuse sweat. with most complaints; sweat about the neck after the first nap; phthisis.

Sweat cold, stains yellow; or bloody, staining red.

Intermittent fever recurs every Spring, or after suppression in the previous Fall by quinine; worse in the afternoon, 2 P.M.; face red, headache, feet cold; talking during hot stage; excessive burning and rending pain during relapse into bilious intermittent after quinine.

⁴¹ Attacks. Periodical attacks: every fourteen days, every Spring: 40.

⁴² Sides. Right: 3, 18, 19, 32. Left: 2, 6, 8, 13, 23, 28, 29, 32, 33, 36. Left to right: throat and ovarian symptoms; also 44. Below up: 40. Within outwards: 3.

⁴³ Sensations. Neuralgic pains change locality, with palpitation.

Tearing pains; prickling; pulsating.

⁴⁴ Tissues. Blood dark, non-coagulable; small wounds bleed much.

Affected parts bluish.

Gangrene.

Ulcers sensitive to touch; ichorous, offensive discharge; many small pimples surround them; areolæ purple; better from warmth.

Dropsy from liver and spleen diseases; after scarlatina; urine black, legs œdematous, first left, then right.

Cellulitis, with burning and blue color of skin.

⁴⁵ Contact, Injuries, etc. Touch: 2, 13, 25, 26, 44. Pressure: 1, 13, ▮29.

▮The greatest sensitiveness, even to touch of edge of bed-clothing on throat, common bed-covering on abdomen.

⁴⁶ Skin. Itching of the whole body, burning; yellow or purplish blisters; scabies.

Miliary eruption; rash appears slowly or turns livid or black; comatose.

Bullæ dark from bloody serum within.

Carbuncles, with purple surroundings and many small boils around them; must rise at night and bathe to allay burning; also when suppuration is tardy and systemic weakness obtains.

Malignant pustule.

Scars redden, hurt, break open and bleed.

Bed-sores, with black edges.

[48] **Relationship.** Followed by *Arsen., Bellad., Carb. veg., Caustic., Conium, Mercur., Lycop.*

Tarent. cub. compares well in carbuncles; the pains are atrocious.

Follows: *Arsen., Bellad., Mercur., Nitr. ac., Hepar.*

Complementary to *Lycop.*

Antidotes: *Arsen. Bellad.*, heat, alcohol, salt.

Compare: *Lact. ac.* in lump or fulness in throat like a puff-ball, not better swallowing, keeps swallowing frothy mucus; constricted feeling low in throat with nausea.

LACHNANTES TINCTORIA.

Red root.   HERING. LIPPE.   *Hæmodoraceæ.*

[1] **Mind.** While dozing through day, sees images.

Loquacious delirium, brilliant eyes, circumscribed red cheeks.

Loquacity, afterwards stupid and irritable.

Became excited over a trifle.

Restless while perspiring.

[2] **Sensorium.** Giddy, with sensation of heat in chest and around the heart.

Dizzy, with sweat and boiling, bubbling in chest and region of heart.

[3] **Inner Head.** Tearing in forehead from left to right side.

Pain in forehead, with general heat, alternating with crampy pain in chest; at last tearing in nose and shoulders.

Tearing in the temples.

Head feels enlarged and as if split open with a wedge from outside inward; body ice-cold, skin moist and sticky; cannot get warm even under a feather bed, face yellow; whines with the pain; head burns like fire, with much thirst.

Vertex feels enlarged and extended upward.

Tearing in the vertex.

Headache until 10 A.M.

Headache pressing the eye outward.

Head feels heavy.

Headache worse toward noon, she becomes more giddy; in the evening, pricking headache.

⁴ **Outer Head.** Draws skin of forehead upward, worse left side.

Sensation as if hair was standing on end, worse on occiput.

Scalp very painful, even to touch.

Red pimples on forehead, become larger and suppurate.

⁵ **Eyes.** Looking intensely, sees gray rings fixed to the spot.

If he looked at a spot for some time, it became quite dark; so also if he reads any length of time.

Moving head quickly, sight becomes obscure.

All symptoms leave while walking about; after sitting down obscuration of sight returns.

Eyes brilliant, face red.

Pupils very large.

Violent lachrymation and burning of eyes, with sensation of dryness; morning.

Compression of left eyeball from below upward.

Pressing as from dust in eyes, with discharge of white mucus.

Eyebrows and lids drawn upward so that he looks with fixed eyes.

When closing eyes, upper lids twitch visibly, worse when closing them tightly.

⁶ **Ears.** Almost complete deafness, etc., during acute disease.

Singing in right ear when walking in open air.

Tearing in the ears.

Crawling in right ear while eating.

Crawling in left ear, better boring with finger, but immediately returning and feeling as if something had closed the ear.

Itching in left ear and soreness in right.

⁷ **Nose.** Burning on right side of root of nose.

Nose bleeds profusely, blood pale.

⁸ **Face.** Yellow face.

Circumscribed red face, 1 to 8 A.M., violent delirium, eyes brilliant. θ Pneumonia.

Redness of the face.

Face swollen, with redness and blueness under the eyes.

Pale, sickly countenance; face and lips light blue; eyes dull, feel thick and cold.

Tearing in temples down into cheeks.

Tearing, pressing in left cheek toward eyes.

Sensation as if something was crawling over face.

⁹ **Lower Face.** Lips red.

Swelling and tension of the lips.

¹⁰ **Teeth.** Upper incisors and eye-teeth feel as if loose, with sensation of soreness, worse when touching with the tongue and closing teeth.

Teeth ache after eating.

¹² **Mouth.** Sensation as if mouth were sore and thick.

¹³ **Throat**. Great dryness of the throat, worse on awaking during the night, with much coughing.

Roughness of the throat, with pricking pain when swallowing; continually increasing dryness of throat, with sleeplessness, followed by hoarseness.

Sensation of swelling in left side of throat; when he swallows he feels an itching in the spot.

¹⁴ **Desires. Aversions.** Much thirst.

Aversion to meat.

¹⁵ **Eating and Drinking.** Drinking coffee, pain in all the teeth.

After eating: teeth pain.

Frontal headache better after supper.

¹⁶ **Nausea and Vomiting.** Hiccough in bed.

Rising of sweetish water, with nausea.

Sudden qualmishness in stomach.

Qualmish about navel, when walking in open air.

¹⁷ **Stomach.** Full feeling in the stomach.

Rolling of wind in stomach.

Beating, in pit of stomach, as from a pulse, as if a hammer was beating on an ulcerated spot.

¹⁹ **Abdomen.** Cutting upper part of abdomen from left to right.

Twirling and twisting in upper part of abdomen, two inches above navel.

Fermentation and rumbling.

Much flatulency in abdomen during pneumonia nervosa.

Sensation of heat through the abdomen, feels as if the bowels would be moved; an evacuation relieves head.

²⁰ **Stool, etc.** Frequent desire to evacuate without result.

Evacuation, with much flatulency and pressing.

Continuous stitch in the anus; morning.

²¹ **Urine.** Pressing on the bladder when urinating.

During the night some drops flow from the urethra, coloring the shirt red.

²² **Male Sexual Organs.** Violent burning in left half of scrotum, drawing toward the right ride.

Tingling and itching of and around scrotum.

Sweat and itching of scrotum and penis.

²³ **Female Sexual Organs.** Menses: early, profuse, bright .red; or mixed, viscid blood and mucus; sense of swelling of abdomen, it feels as if it was boiling.

²⁵ **Larynx.** Hoarseness.

Burning in right side of larynx.

²⁶ **Breathing.** Feels hot and oppressed in the chest, with mild sweat all over; dizzy.

²⁷ **Cough.** Dry, as from the larynx; sputa blood-streaked. θ Pneumonia.

Cough worse in bed, also from sleeping.

²⁸ **Lungs.** Stitches like knives in quick succession, in right side of chest below mamma while at rest and when moving, in afternoon.

Severe pain in chest with the cough, delirium, circumscribed red cheeks, fever worse 1 to 2 A. M. θ Typhoid pneumonia.

Stitches in left side of chest.

Full feeling in chest, must inhale deeply.

²⁹ **Heart. Pulse.** Stitches in heart, with anxiety.

Feels hot in chest and around heart.

Boiling and bubbling in chest and cardiac region.

While lying, feels beating of heart to his head.

Trembling of heart, with great debility.

Pulse 110, small, thin, hard. θ Pneumonia.

³¹ **Neck. Back.** Pain and stiffness in neck, going over whole head and down the nose, then as if pinching nostrils together.

When turning neck or bending head backward, pain in nape as if from dislocation.

Stiff neck, head drawn to one side. θ Diphtheria, scarlatina.

Sensation as if a piece of ice was lying on the back between the shoulders, followed by a chill, with gooseflesh all over.

Burning in region of left kidney, deep, extending towards right side.

Burning in spine four inches above small of back.

Burning in os sacrum, 4 P. M.

³² **Upper Limbs.** Tearing in upper part of arm, beginning at elbow-joint, where it pains most up into the shoulder.

Tearing in elbow-joints at times upwards and then downwards.

Tearing in knuckles of middle fingers of right hand.

Left index-finger drawn crooked.

³³ **Lower Limbs.** Small pimples around left gluteus, discharging a watery fluid when scratched open.

Tearing in left knee; when walking.

Tearing in right tibia.

Tearing from knees to ankles.

Cramps in calves when lying in bed.

Tearing in right big toe, awakening from sleep.

Cramps in feet during the night.

Burning in the feet.

[31] **Limbs in General.** Tearing pains.

Burning of palms of hands and soles of feet.

[35] **Position, etc.** Moving: 28; head: 5. Walking: 5, 33; in open air: 6, 16. Rest: 28. Sitting: 5. Lying: 29, 33. Bending head backward: 31.

[36] **Nerves.** Sensation of great weakness, as from loss of fluids.

[37] **Sleep.** Somnolency, during day, sees images.

Sleepiness, with yawning, eyes feel so heavy she cannot keep them open.

Sleepless, feverish, circumscribed red cheeks.

Sleepless, with increasing dryness of throat.

Wakeful at night without feeling weak.

Restless sleep followed by sweat.

Feverish, distressing dreams (following cramp in left foot during night).

Awakens: 2 A.M. with cramp in her breast extending from right to left; after awaking and stretching; a shock followed by chilliness and goose-flesh all over.

[38] **Time.** Morning: 3, 5, 20, 40. Noon: 3. Afternoon: 28, 31. Evening: 3, 40. From 6 to 12 P.M.: 40. Night: 8, 13, 21, 33, 37, 40, 46. After midnight: 37, 40. Day: 1, 37.

[39] **Temperature and Weather.** Open air: 6, 16.

[40] **Chill. Fever. Sweat.** Body icy-cold.

Hot flat-irons relieve the coldness.

Flushes alternately, with chilliness.

Evening fever, worse 6 to 12 P.M.; face red, worse upper part.

Dry heat, feet burn; restless tossing, with much rumbling in abdomen.

Burning heat, face red, worse on right side; followed by circumscribed redness of the cheeks, also worse right side.

Feverish, with somnolency.

General heat, with sweat on the forehead.

Fever with delirium, red cheeks, eyes brilliant; worse 1 to 2 A.M.

Sweat with dizziness.

Sweat after 12 P.M., after a restless sleep.

Skin cold, damp and clammy.

Morning sweat.

[42] **Sides.** Right: 6, 7, 22, 25, 28, 32, 33, 40. Left: 4, 5, 6, 8, 13, 22, 28, 31, 32, 33. Left to right: 3, 6, 8, 19, 22, 31. Right to left: 37. Without inward: 3. Within out: 3. Below upward: 5, 32. Above downward: 8, 32.

[43] **Sensations.** Twitchings of muscles here and there.

Tearing pains.

Tingling.
Burning in various parts.
[44] **Tissues.** Hemorrhages.
[45] **Contact, Injuries, etc.** Touch: 4.   Boring with finger: 6.
[46] **Skin.** Itches, burns all night, worse after scratching.
Red pimples.
Sensation in skin, as if an eruption would appear.

LAUROCERASUS.

Cherry Laurel. M. MUELLER, HARTLAUB, WAHLE. *Amygdaleæ.*

[1] **Mind.** Loss of consciousness, with loss of speech and motion.
Insensibility and complete loss of sensation.
Dulness of the senses.
Weakness of mind and loss of memory.
Inability to collect one's idea.
Fear and anxiety about imaginary evils.
[2] **Sensorium.** Stupefaction, with vertigo.
Vertigo: with disposition to sleep; worse in the open air.
[3] **Inner Head.** Stupefying pain in the whole head.
Pulsation in the head, with heat or with coldness.
Congestive headache; pulse depressed.
Sensation of looseness of the brain, as if it were falling
into the forehead, when stooping, without pain.
Feeling of warmth in middle of forehead, then coolness as
from a draft of air.
The brain feels contracted and painful.
Stitches in the head.
[4] **Outer Head.** Sensation of coldness in the forehead and
vertex, as if a cold wind were blowing on it, descending
through the neck to the back; worse in the room, better
in the open air.
Itching of the hairy scalp.
[5] **Eyes.** Objects appear larger.
Sensation of a vail before the eyes.
Eyes; staring, wide open; lightly closed; distorted.
Pupils dilated, immovable.
[6] **Ears.** Hardness of hearing.
Tingling in the ears.
Itching in the ears.
[7] **Nose.** Nose feels stopped up; no air passes through.
[8] **Face.** Sunken, with livid, grey-yellow complexion; blue
with gasping; bloated; idiotic expression of face.
θ Chorea.

Twitching and convulsions of the facial muscles.

Titillation in the face, as if flies and spiders were crawling over the skin.

Eruption around the mouth.

⁹ **Lower Face.** Lockjaw.

¹¹ **Tongue, etc.** Tongue: dry, rough; dry and white; cold; or numb as if burnt.

Left side of tongue stiff and swollen, with loss of speech.

¹² **Mouth.** ❙ Foam at mouth. θ Epilepsy.

Dryness in the mouth.

¹³ **Throat.** ❙ Spasmodic deglutition. θ Chorea.

Impeded deglutition.

Spasmodic contraction in the throat and œsophagus.

The drink he takes rolls audibly through the œsophagus and intestines.

¹⁴ **Desires. Aversions.** Disgust for food, during pregnancy.

Violent thirst, with dry mouth.

Entire loss of appetite, with clean tongue.

¹⁶ **Nausea and Vomiting.** Hiccough.

Nausea in the stomach and vomiting of the ingesta.

Eructations tasting like bitter almonds or prussic acid. θ Pregnancy.

❙ Vomiting of food. θ Cough.

¹⁷ **Stomach.** Violent pain in stomach, with loss of speech.

Burning (or coldness) in the stomach and abdomen.

Contractive feeling in the region of the stomach, and cutting pain in the abdomen.

¹⁸ **Hypochondria.** Sticking pain in the liver, with pressure.

Region of liver distended, pain as from subcutaneous ulceration, or as if an abscess would burst.

Indurated liver; atrophic nutmeg liver.

¹⁹ **Abdomen.** Pinching about the umbilicus.

Colicky pains in afternoon, and tearing pains in vertex at night.

Sensation like the falling of a heavy lump from just above the umbilicus to the small of the back; produced by talking or overexertion, also with spasmodic pains in cardiac region.

²⁰ **Stool, etc.** Diarrhœic stools; with tenesmus; of green liquid mucus, with suffocative spells about the heart, forcing her to lie down; involuntary.

Constipation, stools hard, firm, and passed only with much straining.

Ineffectual urging to stool, with emission of flatus only.

²¹ **Urine.** Suppressed urine. θ Cholera.

Retention of urine, as from paralysis of the bladder; or, urine is voided slowly.

Involuntary urination.

The urine deposits a thick, reddish or mahogany-colored
sediment, with floating, jelly-like flocks.

Itching in the forepart of the urethra.

Acid urine, corroding the labia.

[22] **Male Sexual Organs.** Gangrene of the penis.

[23] **Female Sexual Organs.** Menses: too early and too profuse; blood thin; with nightly tearing in the vertex.

Burning and stinging in and below the mammæ.

[25] **Larynx.** Scraping in the larynx, with increased secretion
of mucus; hoarseness.

Spasmodic constriction of the trachea.

Laryngismus stridulus; heart affected.

[26] **Breathing.** Slow, feeble, moaning or rattling; slow, feeble,
almost imperceptible; panting; very difficult.

Dyspnœa, with sensation as if lungs would not be sufficiently expanded, or as if pressed against the spine.

Spasmodic oppression of the chest.

Gasping for breath; suffocating spells; he clutches at his
heart; palpitation.

[27] **Cough.** Short, titillating; dyspnœa; from heart disease, as
stenosis of the valves; cannot lie down; whizzing, with
sensation as if the mucous membranes were too dry;
worse towards evening, from motion, stooping, eating
and drinking, or warmth; with copious jelly-like sputa,
dotted with bloody points.

Whooping-cough, dry, whistling, no sputum; impending
paralysis of the lungs.

[23] **Lungs.** Spasm of chest. Threatening paralysis of lungs.

Pleurisy of drunkards; pulse soft, but quick.

[29] **Heart. Pulse.** Heart's action irregular, pulse slow.

Stitches in region of heart.

Beating, fluttering sensation in region of heart; gasps for
breath; sometimes has slight dry cough.

Palpitation of the heart.

Cold, moist skin; convulsions of muscles of face; pulse
scarcely perceptible.

Apoplexy.

Pulse extremely irregular; at times small and slow, often
imperceptible; at others somewhat accelerated; seldom
full and hard.

Cyanosis neonatorum.

[39] **Outer Chest.** Pain in every external part of the thorax on
moving it.

Burning in the chest on taking an inspiration.

[31] **Neck. Back.** Painful stiffness in left side of neck, and
nape of neck and small of back.

Pressure in nape of neck, particularly in open air, compelling him to bend head forward.

Severe pain in sacral region, extending to pubis.

32 Upper Limbs. Pressure on right shoulder or in shoulder-joint.

Pains as from lameness, also stitches, in right shoulder.

Stitch in both elbows.

Pain, as if sprained, in the right wrist-joint.

Distention of the veins on the hands.

Rough, scaly skin between the fingers, with burning when touched by water.

33 Lower Limbs. Pain, as if sprained, in the left hip-joint.

Sticking in the left knee.

The feet go to sleep (when crossing the legs or sitting).

Ulcerative pains in the lower part of the heels.

Stiffness of the feet after rising from the seat.

ı Cold, clammy feet up to the knees. θ Chorea.

34 Limbs in General. Ends of fingers and toes enlarged, knob-like.

Stinging and tearing in the limbs.

Painless paralysis of the limbs.

35 Position, etc. A little exercise produces a gasping for breath and increased blueness; cyanosis.

Motion: 27, 30. After rising from seat: 37. Stooping: 3, 27. Must lie down: 20. Cannot lie down: 27. Must bend head forward: 31. Lying down: 27. Cannot keep still: 36.

36 Nerves. Want of energy of the vital powers and want of reaction, especially in chest affections.

Rapid sinking of the forces; long-lasting faints.

Epilepsy.

Clonic spasm of all the limbs, with paralytic weakness.

Chorea, with constant jerks, cannot keep still; speech indistinct, gets angry when not understood; gasping; emaciation; after fright.

Gasping before, during and after spasms; bluish skin.

Apoplexy, with paralysis.

37 Sleep. Irresistible sleepiness, especially after dinner and in the evening.

Deep, snoring sleep; soporous condition.

38 Time. Afternoon: 19, 40. Evening: 27, 37, 40. Evening till midnight: 40. Night: 19, 40.

39 Temperature and Weather. Warmth: 27, 40. Open air: 2, 4, 31. Room: 4. Water: 32.

40 Chill. Fever. Sweat. Chill and external coldness.

Cold, moist skin. θ Apoplexy.

Chill, coldness and shivering in the afternoon and evening, not relieved by external warmth.

Chill, alternating with heat. Want of natural animal heat.

Heat after the chill, from evening till midnight.

Heat descending the back.

Sweat generally during and after heat, till toward morning.

Sweat after eating.

[42] **Sides.**   Right: 32.   Left: 11, 31, 33.   Behind forward: 31. Above downward: 40.

[43] **Sensations.**   Painfulness with the ailments.

Acts on brain and spine, especially upon the medulla oblongata; hence characteristic tetanic spasms of the upper part of the body, gasping breathing, etc.

[48] **Relationship.**   Antidotes to *Lauroc.: Camphor.*, *Coffea*, *Ipec.*, *Opium.*

LEDUM PALUSTRE.

Marsh tea.   HAHNEMANN.   *Ericaceæ.*

[1] **Mind.**   Desire for solitude.

After nightmare, fears to go to sleep, lest she die.

Inclines to be out of humor and angry; vehement.

Dissatisfied; hates his fellow-beings.

[2] **Sensorium.**   Vertigo: as from intoxication, especially when walking in open air; feels dull after eating; head inclined to fall backward.

[3] **Inner Head.**   Stupefying headache, causing dulness.

Raging, pulsating headache.

Pressing headache, with distress, when head is covered.

Headache, as if something was gnawing in her temples, occiput and ears.

Head affected after getting wet.

[4] **Outer Head.**   The least covering to the head is intolerable.

[5] **Eyes.**   Photophobia, with severe pain on attempting to open lids.

Pupils dilated.

Pressure (or dull pain) behind eyeballs, as if they would be pressed out.

Ecchymoses of the conjunctiva.

Nightly agglutination of eyes, with inflammation or pain.

Burning on border of lids and feeling of sand in eyes.

Lachrymation: the tears are acrid, and make the lower lids and cheeks sore.

[6] **Ears.**   Ringing, or roaring in the ears, as from wind.

Hardness of hearing: (right ear) as if the ear were obstructed by cotton; after cutting the hair; after chilling the head.

[7] **Nose.**   Long-lasting nosebleed; afterward sore in upper part of nose, with violent burning; blood pale.

[8] **Face.** Pimples and blood boils on the forehead.
Face: alternately pale and red; bloated.
Scaly, dry herpes in the face, burning in the open air.
Glandular swelling under the chin.
Tetter-like, crusty eruption around nose and mouth, with
itching, smarting and burning.

[11] **Tongue, etc.** Stinging on the forepart of the tongue.
Bitter taste in the mouth.

[12] **Mouth.** Offensive breath.

[13] **Throat.** Sore throat, with fine stinging pain, worse when
not swallowing.
Sensation as from a lump in the throat; when swallowing
the pain is stinging.
Malignant sore throat.
Great heat in throat, when moving in the open air.

[15] **Eating and Drinking.** After eating: hurriedly, contracting pain in breast-bone; pressure in stomach after a
small quantity of food; feels dull.

[16] **Nausea and Vomiting.** Sudden running of water from the
mouth; water-brash.
Nausea when spitting.

[19] **Abdomen.** Sensation of fulness in upper part of abdomen.
Colic every evening.
Pain as if diarrhœa would set in, from the umbilicus to
the anus, with loss of appetite and cold feet.
Pain in the loins after sitting.
Ascites.

[20] **Stool, etc.** Constipation; the stool is mixed with blood.
Diarrhœa, stool mixed with mucus and blood; great want
of animal heat.
Sore, itching, smarting, humid spot between anus and
coccyx.

[21] **Urine.** Frequent or diminished, or increased in quantity.
Stream of urine often stops during its flow.
Itching, redness, discharge of pus.
Burning in urethra after urinating.

[22] **Male Sexual Organs.** Inflammatory swelling of the penis;
the urethra is almost closed.
Increased sexual desire.
Nightly emission bloody.

[23] **Female Sexual Organs.** Menstruation too early and too
profuse; the blood is bright red; absence of vital heat.
Profuse leucorrhœa; pale face; copious urination, even at
night.

[24] **Pregnancy.** Milk-leg.
During last months of pregnancy an indescribable pain,
like a gnawing stiffness, in sacrum and hip-bone, down
over the whole thigh, worse when standing.

[25] **Larynx.** Tickling in larynx, with hæmoptysis.

[26] **Breathing.** Spasmodic, double inspiration, with sobbing, as after hard crying.

Oppressed quick breathing; oppressed painful breathing.

Suffocative arrest of breathing and opisthotonos previous to coughing

Oppressive constriction of chest, worse from motion and walking.

[27] **Cough.** Hollow, racking, spasmodic, from tickling in larynx; before cough he loses his breath; after cough, dizziness, staggering; double, sobbing inspiration.

Expectoration after 12 P. M. and in the morning, fetid purulent, or bright red, foaming blood.

[28] **Lungs.** Congestion to the chest, with hæmoptysis.

Burning soreness in the chest; soreness under the sternum.

Stitches in the chest.

Suppuration of the lungs.

Hæmoptysis alternating with rheumatism.

[29] **Heart. Pulse.** ‖Pushing or pressure inward at left edge of sternum; palpitation; also in hemorrhage.

Pulse full and quick.

[30] **Outer Chest.** Eruption, like varicella, on the chest and upper arms, with desquamation.

Red spots and rash, with smarting-itching on chest.

Pain on and in the breast-bone, or below it.

The chest hurts when touched

[31] **Neck. Back.** Painful stiffness of the back and loins when rising from a seat.

Sticking in the shoulder when lifting the arms.

[32] **Upper Limbs.** Severe stitch in shoulder, when raising arms.

Painful throbbing in the right shoulder.

Painful pressure in left or both shoulder-joints, worse from motion.

Rheumatic pain in the joints of the arms.

Tremor of hands when seizing anything, and when moving hands.

Itching rash on the wrist-joint.

Gouty nodosities on the hand and finger-joints; drawing pain fram hands upward.

Perspiration in the palms of the hands.

Panaritium, from external injuries.

[33] **Lower Limbs.** Pressure in right hip-joint, worse from motion.

Rheumatic pains going from below upward, joints pale, swollen, tense, hot; with stinging, drawing pains; worse from warmth of bed and bed-covering, from motion, and in the evening before 12 P.M.

Affected limb cooler than rest of body.

Gout, worse in the feet; gouty nodosities on the joints; fine tearing in the toes.

Synovitis of knee, effusion; constant chilliness.

Swelling of the feet and up to the knees.

Tremor of the knees (and hands) when sitting or walking.

Pain of the soles of the feet, as if bruised, when walking.

Intense itching of top of feet and of the ankles, worse after scratching, much worse in warmth of bed.

Pinching, grasping pain in the left hamstrings, worse at night, with night-sweat and frequent urination; drawing pain from upper part of calf to the popliteal space, cannot lie on left side.

Ball of great toe painful, swollen, soles very sensitive; tendons stiff.

[34] **Limbs in General.**   Rheumatism begins in the lower limbs and ascends.

Heat of hands and feet, evenings.

Long-lasting warm sweat of the hands and feet.

[35] **Position, etc.**   Motion: 26, 32, 33.   Walking: 26, 33; in open air: 2, 13.   Sitting: 19, 33.   Standing: 24.   Lifting the arms: 31, 32.   Rising from a seat: 31.   Exertion: 40.   Cannot lie on left side: 33.

[36] **Nerves.**   Anxiousness and fainting spells.

[37] **Sleep.**   Sleepiness as from intoxication, during the day.

Sleeplessness at night: with restlessness and fantastic illusions as soon as closing the eyes; with restless tossing about.

Talking in her sleep; nightmare, throat feels swollen, sense of suffocation.

[38] **Time.**   Morning: 27, 40.   Forenoon: 40.   Evening: 19, 33, 34, 40.   Night: 5, 22, 23, 33, 37.   Before midnight: 33.   After midnight: 27.

[39] **Temperature and Weather.**   Cannot bear heat of bed or stove; especially on account of burning and pain in the limbs.

Warmth: 33.   Covering: 3, 4, 40.   Open air: 8, 46. Chilliness: 6.   Cutting hair: 6.   Getting wet: 3.

[40] **Chill. Fever. Sweat.**   Coldness, want of animal heat.

Chilliness, thirst, sensation as of cold water pouring over the parts; chilliness morning and forenoon.

Shivering over the back, with heat of the cheeks, without redness, no thirst, cold hands.

General coldness, with heat and redness of the face.

Parts cold to touch, but not to the patient himself.

Heat, no thirst; on awaking covered with sweat, with general itching.

Burning in hands and feet in the evening.

Heat and sweat in alternation.

37

Night-sweats putrid or sour, with inclination to uncover; itching.

Sweat, mostly on the forehead, from the least exertion.

⁴² **Sides.** Right: 6, 32, 33. Left: 29, 32, 33. Below upward: 32, 33, 34.

⁴³ **Sensations.** Numbness and formication of the limbs.

⁴⁴ **Tissues.** Emaciation of suffering parts.

Œdematous swellings of the whole body.

⁴⁵ **Contact, Injuries, etc.** Touch: 30. Taking hold: 32. Scratching: 33.

Splinters, external injuries cause panaritium. See 32.

A misstep causes the sensation of concussion of the brain.

⁴⁶ **Skin.** Purple (bluish) spots over the body, like petechiæ.

Dry, violently itching herpes, burning in the open air.

Blood-boils.

Dry skin, want of perspiration.

Scurfs, on dry, small nodules, often renewed.

Punctured wounds; stings of insects, especially of mosquitoes.

⁴⁷ **Stages and States.** Pale, delicate women, who are always cold.

⁴⁸ **Relationship.** Ailments from abuse of alcoholic drinks.

It is an antidote to bee-stings; and also for the prostration following abuse of *Colchic.*

LEPTANDRA.

Culver's root.   HALE.   *Scrophulariaceæ.*

¹ **Mind.** Desponding; drowsy; with hepatic derangement.

³ **Inner Head.** Constant dull frontal headache; worse in temples, with aching in umbilicus.

⁵ **Eyes.** Smarting and aching in the eyes.

¹¹ **Tongue, etc.** Tongue, yellow or black down the centre.

¹⁶ **Nausea and Vomiting.** Nausea, with deathly faintness on rising.

Vomiting of bile, yellow tongue, shooting pains about the liver, black stools.

¹⁷ **Stomach.** Weak sensation at the pit of stomach.

Great distress in the stomach and small intestines, with immediate desire for stool.

Burning, aching; in stomach and liver, worse from drinking water.

¹⁸ **Hypochondria.** Dull aching in liver, worse near gall-bladder.

Burning distress in back part of liver and in spine.

Jaundice, with clay-colored stools.

[19] **Abdomen.** Rumbling and distress in whole bowels, especially in hypogastrium, with black stools.

Constant dull aching in the umbilical region.

Sharp, distressing pains between navel and epigastrium.

[20] **Stool, etc.** Stools: black, tarry, bilious, undigested, followed by great distress in the liver; mushy, with weak feeling in the bowels; greenish, muddy spouting out like water; worse morning as soon as he moves; from meat or vegetables.

After stool, griping, but no straining,

[21] **Urine.** Red, with dull aching in the lumbar region.

[23] **Female Sexual Organs.** Menses suppressed or retarded; liver affected.

[29] **Heart. Pulse.** Soreness in the cardiac region.

Pulse slow and full.

[31] **Neck. Back.** Sore, lame feeling in the small of the back.

[32] **Upper Limbs.** Pain in the right shoulder and arm.

[35] **Position, etc.** Moving: 20. On rising: 16.

[38] **Time.** Morning: 20.

[40] **Chill. Fever. Sweat.** Chilly along the spine and down the arm.

Shivering, or dry, hot skin; limbs cold and numb; tongue black down the centre. *θ* Bilious fever.

LILIUM TIGRINUM.

Tiger Lily.   W. PAYNE.   *Liliaceæ.*

[1] **Mind.** Ideas not clear, they become more so if he exerts his will; makes mistakes in speaking and writing; cannot apply the mind steadily.

Depression, dulness of intellect and thirst always precede the severe symptoms.

Crazy feeling on top of the head; wild feeling in head, with confusion of ideas.

I Disposed to curse, to strike, to think of obscene things; as these mental states came, uterine irritation abated.

I Hurried manner; desire to do something and yet feels no ambition.

Listless, inert; yet don't want to sit still; restless, yet don't want to walk.

I Low-spirited, can hardly keep from crying.

▮ Tormented about her salvation. θ With uterine complaints.

▮ Apprehensive: as from impending disease or calamity; fears he has heart disease; she fears she is incurable; often with moderate or subacute uterine or ovarian inflammation.

Fear of insanity.

Irritable, impatient.

² **Sensorium.** Vertigo, especially when walking; feeling as if intoxicated; staggering forward; forgetful.

Faint feeling, fear of falling; worse in close warm room, better in fresh air, though he is then chilly.

Faint in a warm room and when standing, with cold sweat on back of hands and on feet. θ Prolapsus uteri.

³ **Inner Head.** Dull frontal headache: worse over left eye, or alternating from side to side.

Wild feeling in head as though she would be crazy, with pain in right iliac region.

Heavy feeling in the head, with morning diarrhœa.

Drawing hot pain through head and eyes, relieved by frequent sneezing, 10 P. M.

Fulness of the head, with pressure outward as if contents would be forced through every aperture.

Shooting in right temple passing over to the left, with a dull, heavy sensation in whole front of head; dim sight; pain in eyes, extending to head.

Dull, pressive aching, from the left temple to occiput; paroxysmal.

⁵ **Eyes.** Blurred vision: after seminal emissions; with prolapsed uterus.

▮ Hypermetropia. Presbyopia.

Muscæ volitantes.

Eyes full of water; face flushed and hot, pricking in skin of forehead.

Eyes painful; sensitive to light.

Intense pain in eyes, extending back into head; dim sight.

Sharp pains over the eyes.

⁶ **Ears.** Rushing sound in both ears.

⁷ **Nose.** Frequent sneezing, 10 A.M., relieving a severe, burning headache and pain in eyes.

⁸ **Face.** Pain in right side of face, right nostril stopped.

Heat and bloated feeling of face and head.

Chilly feeling in face in the forenoon; afternoon fever, congestion to chest; face and forehead flushed and hot; pricking in the forehead.

¹¹ **Tongue, etc.** Taste of blood; congestion to chest.

¹⁴ **Desires. Aversions.** Loss of appetite.

Aversion: to bread; to coffee.

Craving for meat.

Voracious hunger, seemingly along the spine and up to occiput, not appeased by eating.

Thirst, drinks often and much.

Thirst recurring before severe symptoms.

[16] **Nausea and Vomiting.** Nausea: constant, with sensation of a lump in stomach, moving at every deglutition; when thinking of coffee; with morning diarrhœa; with pressure in vagina and pain at top of sacrum.

[17] **Stomach.** Fulness, disturbed feeling, upward pressure, after eating.

Stomach distended, with frequent eructations and escape of flatus per anum.

Hollow, empty sensation in stomach and bowels.

[19] **Abdomen.** Dragging down of whole abdominal contents, extending to even organs of chest; must support the abdomen.

Bloated abdomen after a meal, continuing after a diarrhœic discharge.

Abdomen distended, with moving of flatulence, better from passing wind up and down.

Abdomen sensitive to pressure or jarring.

Abdominal walls sore, previous to stool.

Sensation as if diarrhœa would come on, passing off by urinating.

Bloated feeling in region of uterus, extending to hips.

Abdomen distended and sore after menses cease.

Empty feeling of abdomen and stomach.

Weak, tremulous feeling, extending to anus.

Skin of abdomen feels stretched and stiff.

[20] **Stool, etc.** Morning diarrhœa, stools loose, bilious; dark, offensive, very urgent, can't wait a moment. Stool preceded by griping pains or great urging, with pressure on the rectum; followed by smarting, burning of anus.

Tenesmus and great desire for stool, but every effort resulted only in voiding a little urine.

Escape of flatus, with great distention of stomach and frequent eructations.

Hemorrhoids after delivery, sore to touch, itching; bearing down at stool as if all would protrude through vagina.

[21] **Urine.** Frequent urination through the day; with dull headache moving from sinciput to occiput, finally settling in left temple.

Frequent urging, with acrid smarting after every discharge; urging worse towards morning.

Continuous pressure in region of bladder, constant desire to urinate, with scanty discharge; smarting in urethra and tenesmus.

If desire is not attended to, feeling of congestion of chest.

Urine: milky, scanty; increased and dark; hot, like boiling oil.

²² **Male Sexual Organs.**   Desire increased.

Lascivious dreams and emissions, followed by: irritability, difficulty in fixing one's mind, selecting wrong words.

²³ **Female Sexual Organs.**   Sexual desire increased; obscene.

Ovaries: Burning, stinging, cutting, grasping in ovaries (left); pains extend across hypogastrium, to groin, down leg; bearing down when standing; sensitive to pressure; ovary swollen to nearly size of child's head.

Bearing down in uterus, pains in left ovary and left mamma.

Menses: scanty, flow only when moving about; dark, thick, smelling like the lochia; on second day after time to menstruate, cutting in bowels, limbs clammy; followed by profuse, bright yellow leucorrhœa, excoriating the perineum.

Severe neuralgic pains in uterus, could not bear touch, not even weight of bedclothes or slightest jar; anteversion.

Aching over the pubes, with pain in knees.

Bearing down in uterine region, as if everything would be pressed out; relieved by pressure with hand against vulva.

Bloated feeling in region of uterus; pelvic organs feel swollen; aching apparently around, not in, the uterus.

Intermittent sharp pain across lower bowels.

Burning from groin to groin, with morning stool.

Intermittent labor-like pains in lower part of back, with a thin, acrid, excoriating leucorrhœa, leaving a brown stain; worse afternoon until 12 P.M.

Pressure on anterior wall of rectum.

Voluptuous itching in vagina, with feeling of fulness of parts; stinging in left ovarian region.

With the bearing down: low-spirited, weeping, apprehensive; irritable; opposite and contradictory mental states; urgent desire for stool; anorexia; faint in close room and when standing; frequent, scanty, burning urine; pain in sacrum; bloated feeling in abdomen; limbs cold, clammy.

²⁴ **Pregnancy.**   Delayed post-partum recovery (subinvolution); lochia lasts too long, is profuse, excoriating; dragging pains; smarting in urethra after urination; fears an internal incurable disease.

Cutting in left mamma through to scapula; sighing; short breath.

Cramp-like pain in left mamma, shoulder and fingers.

²⁶ **Breathing.**   Breathing oppressed, with oppression in lower part of chest; worse 4 A.M.

Short, oppressed breathing; sighing; frequent desire to take a long breath.

Feeling of compression and weight.

Chest feels as if too full of blood; slight relief from sighing; oppressive heat, must go into open air; worse in close room; with taste of blood, faint feeling; weak heart-beat, blurred sight, fear of falling.

[28] **Lungs.** Full feeling in chest, with distended abdomen.

Coestricted sensation in left side of chest, extending to right, with sharp pains running up to throat, clavicle, left axilla and scapula; better from changing position.

[29] **Heart. Pulse.** Heart feels as if squeezed in a vise.

Heart feels as if grasped, with pain and heaviness of left mamma to scapula.

Heart as if violently grasped, then suddenly released; and so on alternately.

Constrictive pain about heart, extending through to scapula.

Heaviness in region of heart.

Palpitation worse from lying on either side.

Fluttering, general faint feeling, hurried and forced feeling about the apex; better sitting still.

Fluttering: awakens her at night; with cold hands and feet covered with cold sweat; with sharp, quick pain in left chest.

Conscious pulsations over whole body, and out-pressing in hands and arms, as if blood would burst through the vessels.

[31] **Neck. Back.** Dull pain in nape of neck, with feeling of constriction.

Pain in back and left scapula, seemingly from left mamma.

Pain in dorsal vertebræ, as if the back would break.

Cold feeling in back.

Dull, heavy pain and great weakness in small of back.

Dull pain in lower back and sacrum.

Sensation of pulling upward from tip of coccyx.

[32] **Upper Limbs.** Dull pain in left shoulder.

Drawing pain in left shoulder and neck; stitching in left mamma.

Right hand and arm stiff and painful during the night, abating 8 A. M.

Arms and hands stiff and hot, as if parched.

Stiffness of the fingers almost like paralysis; difficult to guide the pencil.

Pricking in fingers almost like paralysis; difficult to guide the pencil.

Pricking in fingers and hands; sensation of an electric current, first in fingers of left, then of right hand.

[33] **Lower Limbs.** Pain in right hip, extending down the thigh.

Boring; soreness; stitches; or drawing pain in right hip-joint.

Grasping pain in knees.

Heavy aching in knees.

Trembling of knees, abdomen, back and hands

Dull, heavy pains from knees to toes, moving suddenly from place to place.

Legs ache; cannot keep them still; worse when giving up control of herself, as as when trying to go to sleep.

Burning, beginning in soles and palms, thence over body; worse in bed, constant desire to find a cool place.

[34] **Limbs in General.** Burning in palms and soles.

Limbs cold, clammy, more when excited or nervous.

Whole body feels bruised and sore, even pressure of cloth-ing is painful; hands and feet as if pounded; soles sore, worse when stepping.

[35] **Position, etc.** Worse walking, yet pains so much worse after ceasing to walk that he must walk again.

Changing place: 33. Walking: 2, 23, 36. Stepping: 34. Changing position: 28. Standing: 2, 23. Sitting still: 29. Lying: 29.

[36] **Nerves.** Weak, trembling, nervous.

Nervous system irritable.

Aimless hurry and motion; walks to and fro; cannot be amused by thinking or reading.

[37] **Sleep.** Sleepy before bedtime.

Inability to sleep, worse before midnight.

Restless sleep: with wild feeling in head; with frightful, laborious dreams; everything seems too hot; with semi-nal emissions, dull headache, palpitation; with mam-mary pain.

[38] **Time.** Morning: 3, 7, 16, 20, 21, 23. Forenoon: 8. After-noon: 8, 23, 40; till midnight: 23. Night: 29; till morning: 32. Before midnight: 3, 37. 4 A. M.: 26. Day: 21.

[39] **Temperature and Weather.** Close warm room: 2, 23, 26. In bed: 33. Open air: 2, 26, 40. Desire for cool place: 33.

[40] **Chill. Fever. Sweat.** Chills run downwards: with vio-lent beating of heart; with congestion to chest and burn-ing heat all over; with constriction about heart.

Chilly when in cool, open air; yet otherwise better.

Great heat and lassitude in afternoon, with throbbing all over.

[42] **Sides.** Right: 3, 8, 32, 33. Left: 3, 21, 23, 24, 28, 29, 31, 32. Right to left: 3. Left to right: 28, 32. In out: 3. Front backward: 3, 5, 21, 24, 29, 31. Below upward: 14. Above downwards: 33, 40.

[43] **Sensations.** Pains in small spots.

Shifting pains.

Pressing out, as if blood would burst through the vessels.

Throbbing, as if in all blood-vessels.

⁴⁵ **Contact, Injuries, etc.** Touch: 20, 23. Pressure: 19, 23, 34. Jarring: 19, 23.

Cannot walk on uneven ground.

⁴⁸ **Relationship.** Antidotes *Helon.* (anteversion); *Nux vom.* (colic.)

LITHIUM CARBONICUM.

Lithia.　　　　　　　　HERING.　　　　　　　　*Alkali.*

¹ **Mind.** Difficulty in remembering names.

Disposed to weep about his lonesome condition.

Anxiety, hopeless, all night.

³ **Inner Head.** Early on waking, headache in vertex and temples after sudden cessation of menses.

Heaviness in sinciput, worse in frontal eminence.

Pain and heaviness over the brows, worse toward evening.

Headache ceases while eating, but returns and remains until food is again taken.

Pain in left temple.

Throbbing headache.

Confusion of the head.

Pressure in right side of forehead.

⁵ **Eyes.** Black motes before eyes; sensitive eyes after using them by candle-light.

Vision uncertain; right half of objects invisible; second day of menses; pain over eyes.

Sunlight blinds him.

Eyes: pain as if sore; pain as from grains of sand; feel dry and pain after reading.

Throbbing and drawing deep in right eye and around it

Stitches in right eye.

⁶ **Ears.** Earache, left side from the throat.

Pain behind left ear, in bone, extending toward the neck.

⁷ **Nose.** Swollen, red, worse right side; internally sore and dry; shining crusts form.

Nose obstructed above, worse in morning and forenoon.

Mucous discharge in evening.

Dropping from nose in open air.

⁸ **Face.** Pain right side from root of tooth that has been sawn off, extending to temple; next day same on left side from throat to ear.

¹⁰ **Teeth.** Teeth feel numb, dull and loose, cannot bite on them.

¹³ **Throat.** Sore throat in evening, right side.

Sore throat, pain into ear.

Solid lumps from choanæ and fauces, worse morning and forenoon.

¹⁵ **Eating and Drinking.** After fruit: diarrhœa.

¹⁶ **Nausea and Vomiting.** Acidity of stomach.

Nausea with gnawing in stomach, fulness in temples, headache.

¹⁷ **Stomach.** Gnawing in stomach.

Fulness in pit of stomach; cannot endure slightest pressure of clothes.

¹⁸ **Hypochondria.** Pressure in hepatic region.

Violent pain in hepatic region, between ilium and ribs.

Sticking pain in left hypochondrium.

¹⁹ **Abdomen.** Feels swollen, as if distended with wind.

Violent pain across upper part of abdomen.

Pain in left abdominal ring, like a pressing from within outward.

²⁰ **Stool, etc.** Stools soft, light, yellow, in the morning; offensive at night; stinking flatus in evening. Worse after fruit or chocolate.

²¹ **Urine.** Flashes of pain in region of bladder, more toward the right, before passing water; pain extends into spermatic cord after urinating.

Tenesmus vesicæ with micturition; in the evening, while walking.

Quick, strong tenesmus, with sensitive pain in middle of urethra.

On rising to urinate, a pressing in cardiac region, not ceasing until after urinating; morning.

Urine: strong, scanty, dark, acrid; pain when passed, emission difficult; with dark, reddish-brown deposit; turbid, with mucous deposit; profuse, with uric acid deposit.

Frequent, copious urination disturbing sleep.

²¹ **Male Sexual Organs.** Erection after urination at night.

Gonorrhœa, with alternate hemorrhage and discharge.

Burning in urethra.

Pain in testes, and when sitting, stitches in penis.

²³ **Female Sexual Organs.** Menses: late, scanty; cease suddenly, and headache comes on.

²⁶ **Breathing.** On inspiring the air feels cold, even into lungs.

Constriction of chest when walking in open air after breakfast, then expectoration of much mucus, by hawking, seemingly from middle of sternum.

²⁷ **Cough.** Violent, in quick shocks, evening while lying;

must rise; no sputa; irritation to cough, starts at a small spot posteriorly and inferiorly in throat.

²⁸ Lungs.   Pressure in middle of chest from within outward towards both sides.

²⁹ Heart.   Pulse.   Violent pain in region of heart, as she bent over the bed; morning after rising.

ⅼ Valvular deficiencies, worse from mental agitation, which cause a fluttering and trembling of heart.

Sudden shocks in cardiac region.

Rheumatic soreness in cardiac region.

Pains in heart before and at time of urinating; also before and at time of menses.

³¹ Neck.   Back.   Sore feeling right side near the spine, on a small spot; worse from pressure; morning on rising.

Prostrate feeling in sacrum at night.

Stitch in sacrum.

³² Upper Limbs.   Pain near point of right pectoralis major on margin of right shoulder.

Burning stitch in ball of hand in the left thumb.

Itching, throbbing, sensitive pains, in all fingers, worse second and third of left hand, as if in the bones; it extends from hands to finger-ends, only during repose; better on pressure, when grasping and during motion.

Left middle finger painful through and through.

Soreness at margin of nail, with redness and pain.

³³ Lower Limbs.   Itching-burning pain in small spot on right hip, then on thigh, then on little toe; all on external aspect of limb; also, internally on left thigh and knee.

Occasional rheumatic pains.

Knees weak, with pain, worse going up stairs.

Feet, ankles, metatarsus, toes, especially at border of foot and sole, as if gouty.

Ankle-joints pain when walking.

³⁵ Position, etc.   Going up stairs: 33.   Motion: 32.   Walking: 21, 33; in open air: 26.   Sitting: 22.   Lying: 27.   After rising: 29, 31. Stooping: 29. During repose: 32.

³⁶ Nerves.   Prostration of whole body, especially knee-joints and sacrum.

Paralytic stiffness in all the limbs and in whole body.

³⁷ Sleep.   Anxious, restless at night.

Sleep disturbed by pains in sacrum and feet.

Awakened by offensive diarrhœa, tenesmus vesicæ, erections, which subside on urinating.

³⁸ Time.   Morning: 3, 7, 13, 20, 21, 29, 31.   Forenoon: 7, 13.   Evening: 3, 7, 13, 20, 21, 27.   Night: 1, 20, 22, 31, 37.

³⁹ Temperature and Weather.   Open air: 7.   Cool air inspired: 26.

⁴⁰ Chill.   Fever.   Sweat.   Cold feet, soles worse; then sudden heat beginning in soles and extending over whole body.

General feeling of heat in the body; sweat on back of hands.

Copious sweat.

⁴² **Sides.** Right: 3, 5, 7, 8, 13, 18, 21, 32, 33. Left: 3, 6, 8, 18, 19, 32, 33. Within outward: 28. Below upward: 40.

⁴⁴ **Tissues.** Bones, joints, muscles, whole body sore as if beaten.

Arthritis.

⁴⁵ **Contact, Injuries, etc.** Pressure: 17, 31, 32. Grasping with the hand: 32.

⁴⁶ **Skin.** Itching and burning.

Skin rough as a grater, harsh, dry; barber's itch.

Ringworm, dry, itching.

Rough rash over body. θ Secondary syphilis.

Milk crust.

LOBELIA CŒRULEA.

Great Blue Lobelia.   JEANES.   *Lobeliaceæ.*

¹ **Mind.** Much depressed, tearful, unhappy.

Bad effects from grief.

³¹ **Neck. Back.** ❘ Pain or aching in posterior aspect of spleen.

LOBELIA INFLATA.

Indian Tobacco.   JEANES.   *Lobeliaceæ.*

¹ **Mind.** Desponding: sobbing like a child.

Apprehension of death and difficulty of breathing.

² **Sensorium.** Vertigo: and deathly nausea; as if starting from left eye.

³ **Inner Head.** Headache, with slight giddiness.

Dull, heavy pain passing around forehead, from one temple to the other, just above the eyebrows.

Pressing outward in both temples.

Pains through the head in sudden shocks.

⁴ **Outer Head.** Chilliness in left side of head, commencing in ear, with feeling as if the hair would rise on end.

Pressing pain on left side of occiput, worse at night and from motion.

Drawing upward, in a narrow stripe, from right side of throat to behind the ear.

[5] **Eyes.**   Hemiopia.

Pressure on the upper half of eyeballs.

[6] **Ears.**   Sudden shutting up of the right ear, as if stopped by a plug, at 2 P.M., only relieved while boring with his finger in the ear.

[7] **Nose.**   Nosebleed.

Tip of nose very cold.

[8] **Face.**   Neuralgia of left side of face and temples, with retarded menses.

Flushes of heat, or heat of the face.

Sweat on the face with the nausea.

Chilly feeling in left cheek, near ear, extending to lower jaw.

Cyanosis.   *θ* Emphysema.

[10] **Teeth.**   Dull, pressing pain in last left molar, with same sensation in temples.

[12] **Mouth.**   Flow of clammy saliva in the mouth (with nausea).

[13] **Throat.**   Burning in throat; dryness of fauces, spitting at intervals.

Tough mucus in fauces, causing frequent hawking.

Dryness and pricking in throat, not diminished by drinking.

Sensation of a lump in pit of throat, impeding deglutition.

Sensation as if œsophagus contracted from below upward.

[14] **Desires.   Aversions.**   Loss of appetite, with acrid, burning taste in the mouth.

No appetite for dinner.

[15] **Eating and Drinking.**   After breakfast: pressing outward, in both temples; itching in left canthus.

Faint, weak at stomach from excessive use of green tea or tobacco.

Food and drink: 16.   After eating: 18, 19.   After drinking: 40.

[16] **Nausea and Vomiting.**   Hiccough: with profuse flow of saliva; in the evening, followed by drowsiness.

Frequent empty eructations, with flow of water into mouth.

Frequent gulping up of a burning, sour fluid.

Acidity in stomach, with contractive feeling in pit of stomach.

Incessant, violent nausea.

Nausea, with profuse perspiration and copious vomiting.

Heart-burn and running of water from the mouth.

Vomiting, with cold perspiration of the face.

Nausea and vomiting during pregnancy, with profuse running of water from the mouth; morning sickness.

Nausea disappearing very suddenly.

Nausea in last stages of phthisis pulmonalis.

Nausea worse at night and after sleeping; relieved by a little food or drink.

Chronic vomiting, nausea, profuse sweat; but with good
appetite; brick-bust sediment in the urine.

[17] **Stomach.** Heat or burning in the stomach.

Sensation in stomach: of weight; as of a lump; as from
undigested food.

Feeling of weakness of stomach, or in pit of stomach, extending through the whole chest and lower down to
umbilicus.

Bruised soreness from pit of stomach through to back,
after cramp in stomach.

Sensation of oppression at epigastrium, as if the stomach
was too full; worse on pressure.

[18] **Hypochondria.** Fulness and pressure in hypochondria
after eating.

Pinching in abdomen, near the edge of liver.

[19] **Abdomen.** Pain in the abdomen, worse after eating.

Rumbling in bowels and passage of flatus downward.

Sudden sharp pain in left side of abdomen.

Abdomen distended, with shortness of breath.

Tympanitis.

[20] **Stool, etc.** Stool: soft, but passed with great exertion;
green, soft; frequent, loose during day, with great
obtuseness of the head.

Discharge of black blood after stool.

Bleeding piles; copious hemorrhage.

[21] **Urine.** Sticking pain in the region of the right kidney.

Urine increased or diminished.

Urine of a deep red color, depositing a copious, red sediment.

Brown sediment.

[22] **Male Sexual Organs.** Smarting of the prepuce.

Sensation of weight in the genitals.

Aching pain in the urethra.

[23] **Female Sexual Organs.** Menses too early, too profuse.

Violent pain in sacrum; sense of great weight in genitals.

[24] **Pregnancy.** Morning sickness: 16.

With every uterine contraction violent dyspnœa, which
seems to neutralize the labor-pains; rigid os uteri.

[25] **Larynx.** Oppression felt in the throat-pit. 'θ Spasmodic
asthma.

Sensation of fulness in trachea, as if arising from chest,
causing a few short coughs, followed by warmth in
forehead.

Peculiar sensation, between tickling and acrid feeling in
larynx; two short coughs; feeling of narrowness.

[26] **Breathing.** Sensation of a foreign body in the throat, impeding the breathing and swallowing.

Dyspnœa and asthma, with sensation as of a lump in the
pit of the throat, immediately above the sternum.

Contraction of chest, with deep inhalations.

Want of breath, hysterical.

Impossibility of deep inspiration; extreme dyspnœa.

Short inhalation, and long, deep exhalation.

Inclination to sigh, or to get a very deep breath; deep inspiration relieves the pressive pain in the epigastrium.

Asthma, worse from exertion, with a disordered stomach, especially a feeling of weakness in the pit of stomach; asthmatic attack often preceded by prickling all over, even to fingers and toes.

[27] **Cough.**   Cough: with vomituritio; with pain in stomach; short, dry; only a single one, from a feeling of narrowness of chest.

Whooping-cough, violent, racking; seemingly from deep in chest, in paroxysms of long continuance; followed by expectoration of ropy mucus, adhering to pharynx.

Cough, with sneezing, gaping and flatulent eructations.
θ Bronchitis.

[28] **Lungs.**   Pressure on the chest; left chest above the nipple.

Spasmodic contraction of diaphragm.

Pain in chest, with the breathing, while sitting after dinner; disappears when moving about.

Pain in lower chest, most left side.

Burning feeling in chest, passing upward.

[29] **Heart. Pulse.**   Slight, deep-seated pain in region of heart.

Sensation of weakness and pressure in epigastrium, rising to the heart.

Sawing sound about heart, with violent pains, diarrhœa and vomiting.

Short sensation, as if heart would stand still; deep in, above heart, a pain.

Pulse: frequent, but small, weak, in evening; slower than usual.

[30] **Outer Chest.**   Repeated quivering in muscles of left ribs toward spine.

Pressure on lower portion of sternum, left side.

Tension in left chest, from nipple to arm-pit.

Pain behind the sternum.

[31] **Neck. Back.**   Swelling and pain on left side of neck.

Rheumatic pain between the scapulæ.

Dull pressure between the shoulder-blades.

Pain under the right shoulder-blade, worse when bending forward.

About noon a burning pain in back, as if in posterior wall of stomach.

Extreme tenderness over sacrum; cannot bear slightest touch; cries out if any attempt is made to touch the part; sits up in bed, leaning forward.

[32] **Upper Limbs.** Lame feeling in left upper arm.

Rheumatic pain in right shoulder-joint, goes to left upper arm and around elbow-joint.

Fine crawling stitches, inside of right deltoid.

Pain in right deltoid, on a place size of palm of hand, sore to touch.

A sharp shooting pain in an old scar of the right ring-finger.

Sweat of the palms of hands, back of hand is dry and cool; tips of fingers feel very cold; while walking out in the coldest winter weather, but remaining the same in-doors.

[33] **Lower Limbs.** Inflammatory rheumatism in the right knee; swelling and extreme pain.

Painful stiffness in knees, as after a long march.

[34] **Limbs in General.** Shooting pain through whole body, down into tips of fingers and toes.

[35] **Position, etc.** Motion: 4. Walking: 28; in cold air: 32. Exertion: 26. Sitting: 28. Sits leaning forward: 31. In-doors: 32.

[36] **Nerves.** Weakness; feels too weak to stretch out her hand to do anything.

[37] **Sleep.** Gaping, followed by crawling in the nose and sneezing; then gaping and belching of wind.

Wakened early by very impressive dreams; arm amputated, wounded by a shot, etc.

[38] **Time.** Nearly all symptoms disappear in the evening.

Morning: 16. Evening: 16. Night: 6. Day: 20.

[39] **Temperature and Weather.** Cold washing: increases or causes pain; causes difficult breathing.

[40] **Chill. Fever. Sweat.** Chills down the back, with heat in stomach; general shivering.

Thirst before chill; shaking chill and coldness increased after drinking.

Heat, with thirst and sweat.

Flushes of heat.

Heat, with inclination to sweat, particularly in the face.

Sweat, with heat, or after heat has lasted for some time.

Sweat, after heat, with sleep.

Copious night-sweats.

Cold sweat.

[42] **Sides.** Right: 4, 6, 21, 31, 32, 33. Lift: 2, 4, 8, 10, 15, 19, 28, 29, 30, 31, 32. Right to left: 32. Below upward: 4, 13, 28. Within outward: 3.

[45] **Contact, Injuries, etc.** Touch: 31, 32. Pressure: 17. Boring finger in ear: 6.

[46] **Skin.** Prickling-itching of the skin all over the body.

[48] **Relationship.** Useful in morning sickness, after *Ant. tar.* and *Ipec.* fail.

Antidote: *Ipec.* (?)

LYCOPODIUM.

Club Moss.　　　　HAHNEMANN.　　　　*Lycopodeaceæ.*

[1] **Mind.**　Unconscious.

Weak memory; confused thoughts; mixes up letters and syllables, or omits parts of words in writing.

Uses the wrong words for correct ideas.

Absent-minded, thinks he is in two places at the same time.

Dread of men, wants to be alone; also in children; or, dread of solitude, with irritability and melancholy.

Imperious manner; scolds; commands.

Weeps all day, cannot calm herself. Sad, or cheerful and merry.

Loss of confidence in his own vigor.

Doubts about one's salvation.

Anxious as if about to die; even prepares final messages.

Satiety of life, particularly mornings in bed.

Indifferent, taciturn.

Sensitive, even cries when thanked.

Vehement, angry, headstrong.

After a fright, liver complaints.

[2] **Sensorium.**　Vertigo when drinking.

Stupefying headache, with heat in the temples and of the ears; mouth and lips dry; worse from 4 to 8 P. M., when rising up or on lying down.

Impending cerebral paralysis; somnolence, staring eyes; dropped jaw.

[3] **Inner Head.**　Stitches in the temples, mostly the right, from within outward.

Pain in the temples, as if screwed together; worse during menses.

Pressing headache on the vertex; worse from 4 to 8 P. M., and from stooping; followed by great weakness.

Tearing in the forehead or right side of the head, extending down to the neck, with tearing in the face, eyes and teeth; worse on raising one's self, better on lying down.

Tension in the head.

Headache after breakfast.

Headache worse from warmth of bed, getting warm while walking, and from mental exertion; better from the open, cold air, and uncovering the head.

[4] **Outer Head.**　Eruption, beginning on the back of the head; crusts thick, easily bleeding, oozing a fetid moisture; worse after scratching, and from warmth.

38

Pityriasis in spots on the scalp.

Hair falls off after abdominal diseases; after parturition; with burning, scalding, itching of the scalp, especially on getting warm from exercise during the day.

Hair becomes grey early.

⁵ **Eyes.** Sparks before the eyes in the dark.

Photophobia.

Night blindness, with black spots before the eyes.

Sees only the left half of an object distinctly.

Arrested cataract (with chronic dyspepsia).

Eyes, hot, dim, wide open, fixed, and insensible to light.

Obscuration of sight, as from feathers before the eyes.

Conjunctiva looks like a piece of raw flesh; copious discharge of pus; lids puffed out by the pus.

Stitches and soreness in eyes, evenings, when looking at light.

Eyes inflamed, canthi itch, lids red and swollen; troublesome pain if they get dry.

Granular eyelids, dry, with smarting.

Pustules and styes on the lids, more toward inner canthi.

Much mucus in the eyes, with smarting pain.

⁶ **Ears.** Oversensitiveness of hearing.

Roaring, humming and whizzing in the ears; hardness of hearing.

Otorrhœa purulent, ichorous; after scarlatina; with impaired hearing.

Sensation as if hot blood rushed into the ears.

Polypus of the ears.

Humid, suppurating scurfs on and behind the ears.

⁷ **Nose.** Oversensitiveness of smell.

Nose stopped up, especially at the root; breathes with open mouth and protruding tongue. θ Diphtheria.

Snuffles, child starts out of sleep rubbing its nose.

Catarrh of nose and frontal sinuses; discharge yellow and thick; frontal headache, yellow complexion.

Violent coryza, nose swollen; discharge acrid, excoriating; posterior nares dry.

❙ The ichorous discharge from nose begins in right nostril. θ Scarlatina. θ Diphtheria.

Scurf in the nose.

Fan-like motion of the alæ nasi.

⁸ **Face.** Silly expression. See 11.

Copper-colored eruptions on the forehead.

Face: pale, with circumscribed red cheeks; early, yellow, with deep furrows, blue circles around eyes, blue lips.

Flushes of heat in the face.

Spasmodic twitching of the facial muscles.

Œdema of the face.

Eruption on the face, humid, suppurating. Freckles.

⁹ **Lower Face.** Lower jaw hangs down, especially during sleep; or with stupor in exhausting fevers.

Eruption around the mouth; corners of the mouth sore.

Swelling of lower lip. Swelling of submaxillary glands.

Large ulcer on the vermilion border of the lower lip.

¹⁰ **Teeth.** Teeth excessively painful to touch; front teeth loose or as if too long. Teeth yellow.

Toothache, with swelling of the cheek; relieved by the heat of the bed and warm applications.

Gums bleed violently when touched. Gum-boils.

Fistula dentalis.

¹¹ **Tongue, etc.** Taste: sour; bitter; fatty.

❙Tongue is darted out and oscillates to and fro. θ Angina. θ Tonsillitis.

Convulsions of the tongue.

Tongue: heavy, trembling; stiff, with indistinct speech and dryness, mornings; red, dry; becomes black and cracked; painful and swollen in places; tubercles.

❙Tongue distended, giving patient a silly expression. θ Angina. θ Diphtheria.

Vesicles on the tip of the tongue, feeling scalded and raw.

Ulcers on and under the tongue.

¹² **Mouth.** Mouth and tongue dry, without thirst; mouth dry and bitter, in the morning.

Putrid smell from mouth, especially in morning when awaking.

Saliva dries on palate and lips, becoming tough. Saliva tastes saltish.

¹³ **Throat.** ❙Pain and soreness begin on right side of throat. θ Angina. θ Diphtheria.

Fauces brownish-red; diphtheritic patches spreading from right tonsil to left, or descending from the nose; worse from cold drinks and after sleep.

❙Swelling and suppuration of tonsils, going from right to left.

Chronic enlargement of the tonsils.

Hawking of bloody mucus, or of hard, greenish-yellow phlegm: feeling as of a hard body in the œsophagus.

Pharynx feels contracted, nothing can be swallowed.

¹⁴ **Desires. Aversions.** Desire for: sweets; oysters, which disagree.

Aversion to: coffee; tobacco smoke; boiled, warm food; bread (rye); meat.

Canine hunger; the more he eats, the more he craves; head aches if he does not eat.

Hunger, but a few mouthfuls fill him up; constant feeling of satiety.

Thirst with disgust for drink; at night drinks little but often. Want of thirst.

¹⁵ **Eating and Drinking.** After eating: sudden repletion; irresistible drowsiness; followed by weariness; pressure and tension in the liver, especially after satifying one's appetite; constantly spitting food; palpitation of heart.

Eating or drinking: 16, 27. Eating: 29. Drinking: 2. Warm drink: 13. Cold drink: 16.

❙ Aggravation by cold drinks (except water in some cases). θ Angina. θ Diphtheria.

¹⁶ **Nausea and Vomiting.** Everything tastes sour; sour eructations. Frequent belching without relief.

Heart-burn, water-brash. Hiccough.

Nausea: in pharynx and stomach; mornings fasting; in the room, passing off in open air; in the morning and when riding in a carriage; after cold, not after warm drinks (in chills).

Vomits: food and bile; coagulated blood; sour substances; dark greenish masses after eating or drinking.

¹⁷ **Stomach.** Pressure in scrobiculum.

Sensation of twisting, crawling and emptiness in the stomach, with yawning.

Fulness in stomach and bowels; pit of stomach sensitive to contact or tight clothing.

Gnawing, griping in the region of the stomach.

Perforating ulcer; worse sitting bent, better walking about and when warm in bed.

¹⁸ **Hypochondria.** Region of the liver sensitive to contact; sore aching as if from a shock. Backache: 31.

Tension in region of liver. Tensive aching, worse bending body or pressure of hand.

Nutmeg liver, atrophic form.

Hepatitis, chronic forms; abscesses; fan-like motion of the alæ nasi; one hot, one cold foot.

Violent gall-stone colic.

Tension in the hypochondria, as from a hoop.

Tension as from a cord marking the diaphragmatic attachments; cannot stretch or stand upright.

Rumbling of wind in the splenic flexure of the colon.

¹⁹ **Abdomen.** Sensation of something moving up and down in stomach and bowels.

Pressure on hypochondrium causes pains in epigastrium and vice versa; chronic duodenitis.

Spasmodic contraction in the abdomen.

Colicky pains in the right side of the abdomen, extending into the bladder, with frequent urging to urinate.

When turning on to the right side, a hard body seems to roll from the navel to that side. θ Ascites.

Peritonitis with hepatitis and diaphragmitis.

Ascites from liver affections, after abuse of alcohol.

Abdomen distended; feet cold; indurations.

Accumulation of flatulence, which becomes incarcerated; pressure upward, with full feeling, also downward on the rectum and bladder.

Great fermentation in the abdomen; rumbling, croaking, rattling; also with colic and discharge of much flatus.

Brown spots on the abdomen.

Hernia (right side); crural hernia, females.

Renal colic in (right) ureter to bladder; red sand in urine.

Skin of the abdomen is painfully sensitive.

²⁰ **Stool, etc.**   Stools: pale, putrid; thin, brown; mixed with hard lumps; thin, yellow or reddish-yellow fluid.

Constipation: stools hard; ineffectual urging from a contraction of the sphincter ani; after stool feeling as if much remained unpassed, or great distress in the rectum; much flatulence.

Stitches in the rectum.

Itching and tension at the anus (in the evening in bed).

Continued burning pain in the rectum.

Varices protrude; painful when sitting.

Discharge of blood, even with soft stool.

Itching eruption at the anus, painful to touch.

²¹ **Urine.**   Severe backache, relieved by passing urine.

Bearing down over the bladder, frequent desire to urinate; pains worse lying down, especially at night; better from horseback riding.

Turbid, milky urine, with an offensive, purulent sediment; dull pressing in region of bladder and abdomen, disposition to calculi.   θ Cystitis.

Urging to urinate, must wait long before it will pass.

Incontinence of urine.

No urine secreted.

Urine: scanty, dark red, albuminous with strangury; deposits a red, sandy sediment; frequent and copious at night, scanty by day; pale.

Hæmaturia, from gravel or chronic catarrh.

Stitches in the neck of the bladder and anus at same time.

Before passing water, the child screams with pain; red sand on the diaper.

Jerking, cutting in the urethra after urinating.

²² **Male Sexual Organs.**   Impotence: penis small, cold and relaxed; also from poisoning with chlorine; after onanism.

Erections feeble; during and embrace falls asleep.

Excessive and exhausting pollutions.

Soreness between the scrotum and thigh.

Itching of inner surface of the prepuce; yellowish tumor behind the corona glandis.

²³ Female Sexual Organs. Nymphomania.

Cutting across the hypogastrium, right to left; ovaries diseased, right to left; ovarian tumors, ovarian dropsy.

Sensation of pressure through the vagina when stooping.

Physometra; wind discharged from the vagina.

Dropsy of the uterus.

Menses profuse, protracted; flow partly black, clotted, partly bright red or partly serum; with labor-like pains, followed by swooning.

Before the menses, sad, chilly, abdomen bloated.

Menses suppressed, also from fright—delay of first menses.

Leucorrhœa: in starts; milky; blood-red, worse before the full moon; corroding.

Increased discharge of blood from the genitals during every passage of hard or soft stool.

Vagina dry; burning in vagina during and after coition.

Occasional sharp pains running around the labia.

Varices of the genitals. Erectile tumors. Polypi.

Dry, pediculated, painless condylomata.

Inflammation of the external genitals.

²⁴ Pregnancy. Disposition to miscarriage; moles.

During the labor-pains she must keep in constant motion; with weeping; labor-pains run upward.

Nipples sore, fissured, or covered with scurf; bleed easily; stitches and burning.

Hard, burning nodosities in mammæ; with stitching pains.

²⁵ Larynx. Hoarseness; feeble, husky voice; dryness in the windpipe.

Hoarseness remaining after croup; loose cough by day, suffocating spells at night.

²⁶ Breathing. Short, in children, worse during sleep and from every exertion.

Oppression of breathing, worse walking in the open air, with weakness. Dyspnœa, worse when lying on back.

Whizzing breathing in the daytime, with sensation of too much mucus in the chest; loud rattling.

²⁷ Cough. Dry, day and night, with painfulness of the region of the head and stomach; from irritation in the trachea, as from fumes of sulphur.

Sputa are: thick yellow, purulent; greyish-yellow or dirty; fetid pus or mucus streaked with blood; green in the morning; tasting salt.

Cough worse: from 4 to 8 P.M., on alternate days, from exertion, stretching the arms out, stooping and lying down, when lying on the (left) side; from eating and drinking cold things; in the wind or in the warm room. Better lying back or sitting up.

²⁸ Lungs. Continuous pressure on the chest; raw feeling internally; tearing under clavicles, tension.

Catarrh on the chest, of infants; rattling on the chest, which seems full of mucus.

Pneumonia, with raising of mouthfuls of mucus at a time, of a light rust color, stringy and easily separated.

Neglected pneumonia; especially with continuing hepatization and purulent sputum. Typhoid pneumonia.

Stitches in the left chest, also during inspiration.

Paralysis of the lungs.

Hydrothorax.

²⁹ **Heart. Pulse.** Hydropericardium.

Trembling, palpitation; pulsating-tearing in region of heart.

Pulse unaltered; accelerated only after eating or in evening.

Sensation as if the circulation stood still; or, ebullitions of blood.

ı Acceleration of the pulse with cold face and feet.

³⁰ **Outer Chest.** Brownish-yellow spots on the chest.

³¹ **Neck. Back.** One side of the neck stiff and swollen.

Large clusters of red pimples around the neck, with violent itching; cervical glands swollen.

Burning as from hot coals between the scapulæ.

Pain and stiffness in the small of the back (at night.)

Stitches in the small of the back, especially when rising from stooping.

Pain in small of back as if it would break; with hard stool and colic as if intestines would burst.

Pain in the small of the back, extending into the thighs.

ı Pain in back and right side, from congestion of liver: 18.

Pain in the sacral region, worse rising from a seat.

³² **Upper Limbs.** Axillary glands swollen; fetid sweat in the axillæ.

Rheumatic tension in the right shoulder-joint.

Tearing pains in the shoulder and elbow-joints during rest, not in motion; tearing from neck to elbow; also in whole arm; in hands only while in bed.

Pain in the bones of the arms at night.

Weakness of the arms when at work; and conversely they feel powerless, yet he can work: 36.

Arms and fingers go to sleep easily.

Twitching in the arms and shoulders.

Pain as from a sprain in the right wrist-joint.

Great dryness of the hands, especially of the palms.

Panaritium; with gastric affections.

³³ **Lower Limbs.** Rheumatic tension in left hip.

Coxalgia, with violent jerks of the limbs; child awakens cross or with a scream.

Knee: swollen and stiff; swollen, with sweating; white swelling.

Pain as from contraction in the calves when walking (cramp), cramp in the toes.

Oozing of water from sore places in œdematous legs.
θ Ascites.

Old ulcers on legs, with nightly tearing, burning and itching.

Varicose veins on the legs.

Œdema of feet; also when œdema rises till ascites form.

Swelling of the soles; they pain when walking.

Profuse, fetid foot-sweat; with burning of the soles.

I One foot hot, the other cold, or cold, sweaty feet.

Feet feel as if dead or asleep.

Stitches in the big toe of the right foot (in the evening.)

[34] **Limbs in General.** Drawing, tearing in limbs at night and on alterate days; worse at rest; muscles and joints rigid, painful, with numbness; finger-joints inflamed; also with arthritic nodes; swelling of the dorsa of feet; rheumatism; worse in wet weather; better in warmth.

Fissures on the hands; also on the heels.

[35] **Position, etc.** Motion: 24, 32. Walking: 3, 17, 26, 33. Exertion: 26, 27. Exercise: 4. Stretching: 18, 27. Rising: 2, 3, 31. Rest: 32, 34. Lying: 2, 3, 21, 27; on left side: 27. Sitting: 20; bent: 17. Stooping: 3, 23, 27. Standing upright: 18. In bed: 32.

While at rest debility is mostly felt, yet averse to exercise.

Worse on beginning to walk (stiffness); better continuing to walk; child wants to be carried.

[36] **Nerves.** Formication of affected limbs.

Pains drawing, tearing, worse at night; muscles and joints rigid; sensation of torpor in affected part.

Involuntary alternate extension and contraction of muscles.

Spasms, with screaming, foaming at the mouth, unconsciousness; throwing the arms about; cardiac anguish; imagines he will die.

Causes depression of nearly all functions.

Great emaciation and internal debility.

Paralysis.

[37] **Sleep.** Sleepy during day, wakeful at night, mind too active.

Comatose state; often with fevers and exanthemata.

Child sleeps with half open eyes and throws its head from side to side, with moaning.

Soporous in typhoid and exanthematous fevers; impending paralysis of the brain.

Sleep restless: at ease in no position; cries out, starts; has anxious dreams; jerks of the limbs.

Sleep uneasy: wakes often, quite awake at 4 A.M.; anxious, awakes often and cannot soon sleep again.

I On awaking: cross, kicks, scolds; ora wakes terrified, as if dreaming; feels unrefreshed; hungry when awaking at night.

³⁸ **Time.**   Morning: 1, 11, 12, 16, 27.   ❙ From 4 to 8 P. M.:
generally worse, afterward better, except the debility;
also 2, 3, 27, 40.   Evening: 5, 20, 29, 33, 40.   Night: 5,
21, 25, 27, 29, 31, 32, 33, 34, 36, 37, 40, 44, 46.   Day: 1,
25, 26, 27, 37, 46.

³⁹ **Temperature and Weather.**   Generally inclination for the
open air.

Warmth: 3, 4, 10, 17, 27, 34.   Open air: 3, 26.   Uncovering: 3.   Wind: 27.   Wet weather: 34.

Cold drinks: 13.

Aggravation from moistening the diseased parts.

⁴⁰ **Chill.   Fever.   Sweat.**   Chill from 4 to 8 P. M., with numb
hands and feet, icy-cold at 7 P. M.; feels as if lying on
ice; on awaking from a dreamy sleep, covered with
sweat; afterward violent thirst; one-sided (left); chilly
all over at 9 A. M., even heat of stove won't warm.

Nausea and vomiting, then chill, followed by sweat, without intervening heat; or sour vomiting between chill
and heat; chill followed by bloated face and hands.

Flushes of heat over the whole body, mostly toward evening; with frequent drinking of small quantities at a
time; constipation and increased micturition.

Heat, with red cheeks, alternating with chilliness; hectic
fever (with suppuration of the lungs).

Heat, with inclination to uncover.

Sweat: from the least exertion; cold, sour, bloody, or offensive, smelling like onions; clammy at night, often with
coldness of the face.

Old, broken-down cases of malaria; chill; sweat greasy.

Typhus: with stupefaction; murmuring, delirium, subsultus tendinum; meteorism; constipation.

⁴¹ **Attacks.**   Faintish at certain hours in the day; worse every
fourth day (pain from hip to foot).

Full moon: 23.   Alternate days: 27, 34.   Worse in the
Spring.

⁴² **Sides.**   Right: 3, 7, 19, 32, 33.   Left: 5, 18, 28, 33.

Right to left: throat, chest, abdominal and ovarian
symptoms.

Within outward: 3.   Above downward: 3, 13, 19, 31.   Below upward: 24.

⁴⁴ **Tissues.**   Emaciation and debility from loss of fluids; upper
parts wasted; lower limbs swollen.   θ Ascites.

Glandular swellings.

❙ Bones inflamed, mostly the ends; nocturnal bone-pains.
Sensation as if void of marrow.   ❙ Softening; caries.

⁴⁵ **Contact, Injuries, etc.**   The whole body feels bruised.

Touch: 10, 17, 18, 20, 46.   Pressure: 17, 18.   Scratching:
4.   Riding: 16, 21.

Soft parts feel painful to touch or pressure.

46 Skin. Skin dry and hot, especially that of the hands.

Biting-itching when becoming warm through the day.

Dark red blotches here and there.

Flesh in ridges, as if struck with a stick.

❙ Urticaria, chronic cases.

Eruptions: humid, suppurating; full of deep rhagades; breeding lice; itching violently; intertrigo, raw places readily bleeding.

❙ Vascular tumors. ❙ Nævus maternus.

Blood-boils. Boils which do not mature, but remain blue.

Ulcers: bleed and burn when dressed; tearing and itching at night, burning when touched; fistulous, with hard, red, shining, everted edges, and inflammatory swelling of the affected parts; bleeding easily.

47 Stages and States. Often in old women; also persons of keen intellect, but of feeble muscular development; lean and predisposed to lung and hepatic affections.

43 Relationship. Complementary to *Iodum.*

Lycop. follows well after *Calcar* or *Laches.*

After *Lycop.* are frequently indicated: *Graphit., Laches., Ledum, Phosphor., Silic.*

It is rarely advisable to begin the treatment of a chronic disease with *Lycop.;* it is better to give first another antipsoric remedy.

Lycop. antidotes *Cinchon.*

Antidotes to *Lycop.: Acon., Camphor., Caustic., Chamom., Graphit., Pulsat.,* also coffee.

LYCOPUS VIRGINICUS.

Bugle Weed. *Labiatæ.*

1 Mind. Increased mental and physical activity in evening. Slight obtusion of intellect, with dull aching through sinciput. Lessened power of concentration.

2 Sensorium. Vertigo, tends to stagger to right. See 16.

3 Inner Head. Headaches frontal, then occipital; over eyes and in frontal eminences (see 10); pains are aching, pressive, pressing out, congestive; are often succeeded by labored heart or cardiac depression, and are accompanied by intellectual obtuseness.

5 Eyes. Feel weak, as if system was overfatigued. Eyes feel full and heavy; pressing outward, with pressure in front of head.

Dull pain in left supraorbital region.

Neuralgic pain in right supraorbital region and left testicle.

¹⁰ **Teeth.** Toothache in right lower molars, then subacute pain, first in left then in right frontal eminence, in right molar, then right temple, then left molar, then left temple, again to right molar, then to loins, with frontal oppression.

¹¹ **Throat.** Rawness at back of palate, right side, extending to left.

Burning in spot in soft palate, following headache.

¹⁶ **Nausea and Vomiting.** Nausea from back of fauces, relieved by eructations that taste of tea and drug; succeeded by persistent giddiness while sitting, and staggering while walking. See 2.

Nausea and faintness.

¹⁸ **Hypochondria.** Lugging pain in spleen.

Tenderness in left hypochondrium.

¹⁹ **Abdomen.** Flatulence and rumbling.

Aching in inguinal canals, worse walking, better upward pressure; also with pain in testicles. Bearing down as from hernia.

²⁰ **Stool, etc.** Severe colic, followed by profuse, forcible diarrhœa. Stools shining, dark brown, offensive. Tenesmus, with first part of semi-solid movements.

Increased action of bowels aggravated the diarrhœic symptoms; could have a passage at any time, but sphincter under perfect control.

²¹ **Urine.** Tenderness in the bladder.

Bladder feels much distended when empty, with dull pain in left lumbar region.

Urine 1012 to 1020. Deposits mucus, epithelial cells, oxalate of lime, spermatozoa.

²² **Male Sexual Organs.** Neuralgic pain in testicle, with supraorbital pain. Acute aching in same while sitting, 1 P. M., or with occasional darting pains, changing to right then to left, after rising.

Acute pain in testes, from right to left, then right, then both, recurring and lasting whole evening, with aching in inguinal canal.

▮ Sharp darting through the left testicle.

²³ **Female Sexual Organs.** Menses intermit for ten or twelve days; last from half an hour to six hours.

Metrorrhagia.

Vagina hot, os uteri engorged and swollen. •

Puffing of parts on and around pubes and vulva, with dilated condition of vagina.

²⁵ **Larynx.** Constriction in larynx, 7 P. M.

[26] **Breathing.** Oppressed, with sighing breathing, 7 P. M.; wheezing; dyspnœa, as from bronchial cold, accelerated during exercise, especially when going up stairs.

[27] **Cough.** Cough, with hæmoptysis, and feeble, weak heart-action; deep, violent in evening and night, without awaking; renewed by change to cold weather and by cold winds.

Expectoration pale, sweetish, unpleasant-tasting, at times difficult, renewed same as cough.

[28] **Lungs.** Sense of constriction across lower half of thorax, impeding respiration, with subacute pain; worse lying on right side.

[29] **Heart. Pulse.** Constrictive pain, tenderness; marked sense of constriction.

Sensation of pressing outward in cardiac region.

Rheumatoid aching in precordial region and at apex, followed by pains in left wrist, inner side of right calf, and in subclavicular region, and again in left wrist and region of apex.

Labored action of heart; oppression. Palpitation and cardiac distress, worse morning and evening, and when thinking of it.

Tumultuous and forcible beating of the heart.

Acute darting pains in heart, with intermissions of pulse and heart-beat.

Heart-beat more distinct on right sternum. First sound replaced by a blowing sound of mitral regurgitation heard upwards in clavicular region, and particularly between scapulæ; second sound pointed, short, sharp.

Heart-beat slow and weak. Diminished blood-pressure; pulse: 48, 58, weak, compressible.

Pulse: many symptoms increase and decrease according to the weakness or strength of the heart's action.

[30] **Outer Chest.** Myalgic pains, worse morning awaking, ameliorated when he lies on the right side.

Heavy aching in cervical region.

[31] **Neck. Back.** Severe aching down spine, more from friction, passing off after rising, morning.

Congestive pain in nape, with severe continuous dorsal and lumbar pain, worse lower left side.

Rheumatoid pains: scapular muscles, lower dorsal region; from apex of heart by friction to left subscapular region, then to mid-dorsal, and later to apex.

Severe continuous aching in lumbar region.

Flying pains in muscles, with persistent aching in loins and occiput, worse on movement.

[32] **Upper Limbs.** Rheumatoid pains, forearms and wrists, with trembling of hands.

[33] **Lower Limbs.** Rheumatoid pains: knees, legs and thighs, wandering to back, slight lameness and unsteady gait.
Left leg feels shorter than right and so sounds when walking.

[35] **Position, etc.** ·Weak, yet restless change of position.
Sitting: 16, 22. Movement: 24. Walking: 2, 16, 19, 33. Exercise: 26. Ascending: 26. Lying on right side: 28, 30. After rising: 31.

[36] **Nerves.** Restless activity, notwithstanding the nausea, giddiness, etc.
Vital depression; hence the mental depression, tremulousness, etc.
Faintness; slight nausea, walking in' open air.
Faintness, with cardiac depression.

[37] **Sleep.** Restless, full of dreams.
Wakeful on retiring, though fatigued.

[38] **Time.** Worse, generally, mornings and evenings: 1, 25, 26, 27, 29, 30, 31.

[39] **Temperature and Weather.** Cold weather: 27. Cold: 44.
Cold winds: 27. Warmth: 44. Open air: 36.

[41] **Attacks.** Worse on alternate days.

[42] **Sides.** Pains pass from left to right, usually; then they cease or return to left. Right: 2, 3, 10, 13, 22, 29, 33, 46. Left: 3, 10, 13, 18, 22, 29, 31, 33, 46.

[43] **Sensations.** Aching, pressing, rarely darting, stitching pains. Pressing outwards: 3, 29. Flying pains.

[44] **Tissues.** Lowers temperature.
Lessened tonicity of blood-vessels, with consequent congestions. Heart muscle weakened.
Rheumatoid pains; erratic but returning to original location. Better from warmth; worse from cold air and movement.

[45] **Contact, Injuries, etc.** Pressure: 19. Friction: 31.

[46] **Skin.** Prickings as if bitten by insects. Troublesome urticaria, especially on left forearm and right leg, before retiring.

[48] **Relationship.** Compare *Digit.* (latter has slow and strong pulse; or, more characteristically, pulse weak and quickened by least movement; faint, nauseated feeling at pit of stomach); *Cactus; Spigel.* (intermittent pulse); *Kalmia* (slow pulse; rheumatoid pains); *Magnol. grand.; Hamam.* (testicular pains).
Antidotes: *Acon.,* port wine and warmth relieved pains from cold; electric current, slight achings (galvanism failed).

MAGNESIA CARBONICA.

Magnesium carbonate.   HAHNEMANN. $Mg\ CO_3\ 3H_2\ O.$

[1] **Mind.**   Uneasiness, with trembling of hands and absence of mind.

Anxious and warm through the whole body, especially in the head, while eating warm food.

Trembling, anguish and fear, as if some accident would happen; all day, relieved after going to bed.

Sad mood with indisposition to talk.

Much worse from talking or mental exertion.

[2] **Sensorium.**   Vertigo: when kneeling; when standing, as if everything were turning around; in the evening.

[3] **Inner Head.**   Pressure in the forehead.

Pressing headache, from mental exertion and when among many persons.

Violent darting headache after vexation (1 to 10 P.M.).

Lancinating headache early in the morning after rising.

Pulsating sensation in the forehead.

Congestion of blood to the head, especially when smoking.

Heat in the head and hands, with redness of the face, alternating with paleness.

[4] **Outer Head.**   Bruised sensation of the vertex.

Pain on the top of the head, as if the hair were pulled.

Dandruff on scalp, itching during wet and rainy weather.

Falling off of the hair.

[5] **Eyes.**   Black motes before the eyes.

Lenticular cataract

Obscuration of the cornea.

Swelling of the eyeball.

Dryness of the eyes; or, profuse lachrymation.

Inflammation of the eyes, with redness, burning, stinging and obscuration of sight, or dimsightedness.

Agglutination of lids in morning, with pressure in eyes.

[6] **Ears.**   Whizzing, fluttering and buzzing in the right ear, with hardness of hearing.

Dulness of hearing.

Inflammation of ears, with external redness and sensation of great soreness.

[7] **Nose.**   Bleeding from nose in morning, more from right side.

Vesicular eruption in the nose, with pressing pain.

Dry coryza and obstruction of nose, waking one at night.

[8] **Face.**   Face: pale, earthy; alternately red and pale.

Tension of face, as if the white of an egg had dried on it.

Nightly tearing, digging and boring in the malar bone,

insupportable during rest, and driving one from one place to another. Swelling of the malar bone, with pulsating pain.

Hard nodosities, bloatedness and swelling of the face.

⁹ **Lower Face.** Herpetic eruption around the (lower part of the) mouth.

Hard, little nodosities in both corners of the mouth.

¹⁰ **Teeth.** Beating and stinging in the teeth after eating.

Toothache: while riding in a carriage, worse in the cold; at night, compelling one to rise and walk about, the pain is insupportable while at rest; during pregnancy; mostly burning, tearing, drawing, twitching, or great ulcerative pain, with twitching in the fingers and feet.

Teeth feel too long.

Ailments from cutting the wisdom teeth.

Looseness of the teeth, with swelling of the gums.

Slow eruption of the teeth.

Burning vesicles on the gums, on the inside of the cheeks, tongue, lips and palate, they bleed from least contact.

¹¹ **Tongue, etc.** Taste: bitter; sour.

Frequent, sudden stammering speech.

¹² **Mouth.** Dryness of mouth, especially at night and in the morning.

Bloody saliva.

¹³ **Throat.** Stinging pain in the throat when talking and swallowing.

Burning in the throat and palate, with dryness and roughness, as if scraped by an awl.

Frequent rising of mucus in the throat (morning), with roughness and dryness of the fauces.

Soft, fetid tubercles, of the color of peas, are hawked up.

¹⁴ **Desires. Aversions.** Violent thirst for water, especially in the evening and at night.

Desire for: ꟷ meats; bread; acid drink.

¹⁵ **Eating and Drinking.** When eating: 16. After eating: 10. Eating warm food: 1.

¹⁶ **Nausea and Vomiting.** Eructations sour; sour taste and sour vomiting.

Much loathing, without desire to vomit.

Nausea and vertigo while eating, followed by retching and vomiting of a bitter, salt water.

¹⁷ **Stomach.** Constrictive pain in the stomach.

Ulcerative pain in stomach, with great sensitiveness to pressure.

¹⁸ **Hypochondria.** Hardness and stitches in hepatic region.

¹⁹ **Abdomen.** Pressing, spasmodic, contractive, colicky pains; relieved by green stools.

Colic, followed by leucorrhœa. Cutting about navel, better from emitting flatus.

Great heaviness in the bloated abdomen.

²⁰ **Stool, etc.** Stools: grass-green, or like the scum on a frog pond; sour, frothy; or with white, floating lumps, like tallow.

Colic before stool.

Lienteria of sucklings; the milk passes undigested.

Costive; frequent ineffectual urging, with small stools, or only flatus; stitches in the anus.

Ascarides and lumbrici.

²¹ **Urine.** Urine: increased, pale, watery, or green; with white sediment.

Involuntary urination while walking or rising from a seat.

Burning-smarting during urination.

²² **Male Sexual Organs.** Sexual desire diminished; erections wanting.

Discharge of prostatic fluid when passing flatulence.

Inguinal and scrotal hernia.

²³ **Female Sexual Organs.** Menses: late, scanty; stop in the afternoon; flow acrid, dark, pitch-like; preceded by coryza and obstructed nostrils, by labor-like pains, cutting in the abdomen, sore throat, weakness, chilliness, backache; profuse and too early, flowing more at night and at first on rising, also between uterine pains.

Leucorrhœa acrid, white, mucous, preceded by colic.

²⁷ **Cough.** Cough: spasmodic at night; from tickling in the larynx; sputum, mornings and during the day, yellow, thin or tough mucus, or dark blood, tasting saltish.

²³ **Lungs.** Oppression of chest, with sensation of constriction.

Sensation of soreness in chest or in the region of heart.

³¹ **Neck. Back.** Stiffness in the neck.

Pain in the back and small of back at night, as if broken.

Sudden piercing in the coccyx; a violent pain, as if the spine were bent back.

³² **Upper Limbs.** Pain as from dislocation in the shoulder-joint when moving it.

Rheumatic pain in shoulders (at night), with tingling down to fingers; pain prevents least movement of arm.

The skin of the hands become chapped.

Spreading blisters on the hands and fingers, with stinging.

Red, inflammatary swelling of the fingers.

Heat of the fingers (in fever).

³³ **Lower Limbs.** Restlessness in the legs.

Drawing pains in the legs and feet.

Itching of the buttocks, with red spots after scratching.

Painful swelling in the bend of the knee.

Knees painful in walking, the feet when lying in bed.

Cramp in the calves (at night).

Burning spot on the tibia.

³⁴ **Limbs in General.** Rheumatic pains in the limbs.
³⁵ **Positions, etc.** Always worse after long walks.
Tired feeling, especially in the feet and when sitting.
Walking: 21, 33, 36. Must walk: 10, 43. Kneeling: 2.
Standing: 2, 36. Rising 23; from a seat: 21. Cannot
move the arm: 32. Rest: 10. Lying: 33. After lying
down: 40.
³⁶ **Nerves.** Epileptic attacks; while standing or walking he
frequently falls down suddenly, with consciousness.
³⁷ **Sleep.** Sleepiness during the day.
Sleeplessness, from nightly oppression in the abdomen.
Unrefreshing sleep, more tired in the morning than he
was when lying down in the evening.
Awakes about 2 to 3 A. M., and cannot fall asleep again.
Anxious dreams, with starts and crying out in sleep.
³⁸ **Time.** Morning: 3, 5, 7, 12, 27, 37. Evening: 2, 14, 37, 40.
1 to 10 P. M.: 3. Night: 12, 14, 23, 27, 31, 32, 33, 37, 40.
After midnight: 27. Midnight till morning: 40.
³⁹ **Temperature and Weather.** Inclination for open air.
Averse to uncovering, with fever heat.
Worse in cold weather; better in warm air, but worse from
warmth of the bed.
Cold: 10. Change of temperature: 43. Draught: 43.
Wet weather: 4.
⁴⁰ **Chill. Fever. Sweat.** Chill and chilliness, with external
coldness in the evening and after lying down, slowly
going off; followed by heat; chilly in bed as if dashed
with cold water.
Chill: running down back; lessened by out-door exercise.
Great internal heat, at night, restless, yet aversion to uncovering.
Heat, one (right) sided; heat mostly forenoon, often with
sweat on the head.
Sweat greasy, stains yellow; sour putrid-smelling.
Sweat, with thirst, after 12 P. M. till morning.
⁴¹ **Attacks.** All her symptoms are aggravated every third
week.
⁴² **Sides.** Right: 6, 7, 40. Left: 43.
⁴³ **Sensations.** Neuralgic pains, shooting like lightning, worse
on left side; worse in a draught, from changing of temperature, from touch; must get out of bed and walk the
floor.
⁴⁵ **Contact, Injuries, etc.** Predominantly worse from press-
ure; body painful.
Touch: 10. Scratching: 46. Riding: 10.
Worse when riding.
⁴⁶ **Skin.** Itching and great dryness of skin; itching lessened
by scratching.
39

Large, stinging nodosities under the skin.

Painful, small, red herpes, they scale off afterward.

Spreading blisters.

Small blood-boils (lower legs), with headache and yellow tongue.

⁴⁷ **Stages and States.** Nervous, irritable temperament.

Often indicated with children.

⁴⁸ **Relationship.** Complementary to *Chamom.*

Antidoted by *Chamom.* (neuralgia); *Rheum* (abdominal complaints).

It may antidote *Acet. ac.* in overdoses.

Compare: *Ipecac.* (nausea and grass-green stools), *Coloc.* (cutting, griping, better after stool).

MAGNESIA MURIATICA.

Magnesium chloride. HAHNEMANN. $Mg\ Cl_2$.

¹ **Mind.** Disinclined to talk, prefers solitude.

Tearful, inclined to weep.

Anxious in the room, relieved in the open air.

Worse from mental exertion.

² **Sensorium.** Heaviness in the head, with reeling, as if one would fall down.

Vertigo in the morning on rising, during dinner, going off in the open air.

Sensation of dumbness in the forehead, the head feels dull; worse in the morning when awaking and when lying; better from exercise in the open air, and when wrapping head up warmly.

Congestion of blood to head, with painful undulation and whizzing, as of boiling water on the side upon which one rests.

³ **Inner Head.** Every six weeks, pain in forehead and around the eyes; feels as if the head would burst; must lie down; worse from motion and in the fresh air, better from strong pressure.

Tearing and stitches in the temples, with great sensitiveness of the vertex, as if the hair were raised by pulling.

Compressive sensation in head, from both sides, with a hot feeling, and with beating in forehead when pressing upon it.

⁵ **Eyes.** When looking into the light, lachrymation and burning of the eyes.

Yellow color of the scleroticæ.

Eyes inflamed, with violent burning and redness of the scleroticæ.

Tinea ciliaris, pimples on the face coming and going; worse after supper and in a warm room; also in women before menses.

⁶ **Ears.**   Hardness of hearing and deafness, as if something were lying before the ear.

Pulsation in the ear.

Itching of old herpes behind the ears.

⁷ **Nose.**   Coryza, with dulness of the head and loss of smell and taste; discharge of yellow fetid mucus.

Discharge of acrid, corrosive water from the nose; nose obstructed at night.

Redness and swelling of the nose or of the alæ.

Sore pain and burning in the nostrils.

Scurf in the nostrils painful to touch; ulcerated nostrils.

⁸ **Face.**   Pale, yellowish complexion.

Severe cramp-pains in the bones of the face.

Eruptions on the face and forehead; worse nights, in warm room and before menses.

⁹ **Lower Face.**   Large vesicles on the margin of vermilion border of the lower lip itching, afterwards burning.

¹⁰ **Teeth.**   Toothache, almost insupportable if the food touches the teeth.

Sensation as if the upper cuspidati were elongated.

Painful swelling and easy bleeding of the gums.

Slow dentition, with distended abdomen and constipation.

¹¹ **Tongue, etc.**   Feels burnt; mouth feels scalded.

Rhagades in the tongue, with violent burning.

Tongue coated white, early in the morning; or, tip and edges clean, large, flabby and yellow. θ Liver indurated.

Taste: absent; bitter; sour at night.

¹² **Mouth.**   Sensation of roughness of inner side of upper lip when touching it with the tongue.

Dryness of the mouth and throat, without thirst.

Accumulation of water in the mouth.

¹³ **Throat.**   Dryness and roughness of throat, with hoarse voice.

Rising as of a ball from the stomach to the throat, relieved by eructation.

ꟾ Continual rising of a white froth into the mouth.

Difficult hawking of thick, tough (or blood mixed) mucus.

¹⁴ **Desires. Aversions.**   Hunger: but knows not for what; followed by nausea.

Appetite for sweets.

Violent thirst (3 A. M.).

Loss of appetite.

¹⁵ **Eating and Drinking.**   Eating: 17. During dinner: 2, 28.

After supper: 5.

¹⁶ **Nausea and Vomiting.** Regurgitation while walking.

Eructations: tasting like onions; relieve: 36.

Nausea: and faintness, succeeded by coldness and weakness in the stomach; frequent, with accumulation of water in mouth; in the morning after rising.

Eructations, water-brash; stomach and liver sensitive: 18.

¹⁷ **Stomach.** Throbbing in the pit of stomach.

Eroding pains in the stomach, going off after eating and coming on again at the end of digestion.

¹⁸ **Hypochondria.** Pressing pain in liver, when walking and touching it, worse when lying on right side; liver hard and enlarged.

¹⁹ **Abdomen.** Tearing in abdomen; tearing stitches in loins.

Tingling stitches in the abdominal muscles.

Colic in the evening, extending to the thighs, followed by fluor albus; hysteria.

Colic at I A.M., had to lie crooked; could not endure covering.

Abdomen tense, sore as if bruised, sensitive to touch.

²⁰ **Stool, etc.** Stools: in large, hard lumps; crumbling at verge of anus; abdomen distended; knotty, like sheep's dung.

ꙮ Absence of desire for stool; atony as with the bladder.

Much pressure to stool; passage scanty or only flatus.

Diarrhœa of mucus and blood.

Feces covered with mucus and blood.

²¹ **Urine.** Frequent desire to urinate day and night, with scanty discharge.

ꙮ Urine can only be passed by bearing down with the abdominal muscles.

The urine pale yellow, followed by burning in the urethra.

Numbness in the urethra.

²² **Male Sexual Organs.** Frequent erections; early in the morning, with burning in the penis.

After an embrace, burning pain in the back.

Itching on the genitals and on the scrotum, extending as far as the anus.

Scrotum relaxed.

²³ **Female Sexual Organs.** Bearing down in ovarian region.

Uterine diseases complicated with hysterical complaints.

Uterine spasms extending to the thighs.

Suppressed menses.

Menses black, clotted; profuse and early or late, with violent pains, which are worse in back when walking, and in thighs when sitting; pale face, debility, nervous excitement.

Menstrual pains are relieved by having the back pressed.

Scirrhus induration of the os uteri.

Leucorrhœa immediately after every stool, or after uterine spasms; followed by metrorrhagia.

[21] **Pregnancy.** The labor-pains are interrupted by hysterical spasms.

[25] **Larynx.** Hoarseness, with roughness and dryness in the throat; in the morning after rising.

Tingling in the larynx.

[27] **Cough.** Dry cough evening and night, with burning and soreness in the chest.

Spasmodic cough at night, with tickling in the throat.

Bloody expectoration brought on by sea-bathing: 28.

[28] **Lungs.** Sudden heaviness on the chest, with oppression of breathing, at dinner.

Tension and constriction of the chest.

Congestion of blood to chest from bathing in the sea: 27.

[29] **Heart. Pulse.** Stitches in the heart, arresting the breath.

Palpitation of the heart while sitting, going off on motion.

Pulse accelerated, with ebullitions while sitting.

[31] **Neck. Back.** Swelling of cervical glands.

Pain as from bruises, above and in small of back and both hips, with sensitiveness of parts to touch; also during menses.

Contractive, spasmodic pain in the small of the back.

Stitches, tearing and burning in the small of the back.

[32] **Upper Limbs.** Rheumatic pain in the shoulder-joint, extending down the arm to hands; worse from motion.

Tearing pains in the shoulders, arms, wrists and hands.

The arms "go to sleep" when awaking in the morning.

[33] **Lower Limbs.** Sensation of great fatigue in the legs, even while sitting.

Heaviness in the legs.

Twitching, tearing in the hips.

Restlessness and tense feeling in thighs, must move legs for relief.

Pressing pain in the knees.

Cramps in the calves at night.

Burning in the soles, evenings.

Foot-sweat.

[34] **Limbs in General.** Much weakness in the limbs; uterus displaced.

Paralytic drawing and tearing in the limbs.

[35] **Position, etc.** Inclination for motion.

Most of the symptoms appear while sitting, and are relieved on motion and by exercise.

When stretching, the stomach hurts.

Motion: 3, 29, 32, 33. Walking: 16, 18, 23. Exercise in open air: 2. Rising: 2, 16. Lying: 2; on right side: 18. Must lie down: 3. Lying crooked: 19. Sitting: 23, 29, 33.

[36] **Nerves.** Hysterical and spasmodic complaints.

She has many spasms day and night, with great sleeplessness.

Great weakness, from a sea-bath.

Weakness of the body, as if coming from the stomach.

Fainting fits at dinner, nausea and trembling, relieved by
eructations.

³⁷ **Sleep.** Sleepiness during the day, with yawning and sluggishness.

Goes to sleep late; sleeplessness on account of nightly
heat, with thirst.

Restlessness of the body as soon as she closes the eyes;
evening in bed.

Shocks through the body at night, while waking.

Sleep unrefreshing; tired in the morning.

Anxious, frightful dreams, with talking and crying out
during sleep.

³⁸ **Time.** Aggravation from evening till morning; pains.

Morning: 2, 11, 16, 22, 32. Evening: 19, 40. 4 to 8 P.M.:
40. Evening till midnight: 40. Night: 7, 11, 33.
After midnight: 19. Midnight till morning: 40. Day
and night: 21, 36.

³⁹ **Temperature and Weather.** Warm room: 5. Room: 1.
Wrapping head up warmly: 2. Covering: 19, 40. Open
air: 1, 2, 3, 40. Sea-bathing: 28, 36.

⁴⁰ **Chill. Fever. Sweat.** Chill even near the stove; worse
from 4 to 8 P.M.: lessened in the open air or in bed;
chill followed by heat, evening until 12 P.M.

Evening heat, thirst; sweat only on the head; averse to
uncovering.

Sweat, with thirst, from 12 P.M. till morning; averse to
uncovering.

⁴¹ **Attacks.** Every six weeks: 3.

⁴³ **Sensations.** General sensation of soreness, with great sensitiveness to noise.

⁴⁴ **Tissues.** Swelling of the glands.

⁴⁵ **Contact, Injuries, etc.** Better from pressure.

Worse when riding on horseback.

⁴⁶ **Skin.** Blood-boils.

Formication over the whole body.

⁴⁷ **Stages and States.** Women: especially hysterical, with
uterine affections.

Children, especially during dentition.

⁴⁸ **Relationship.** Antidote to *Magn. mur.*: *Chamom.*

MANCINELLA.

Manzanillo.   G. BUTE.   *Euphorbiaceæ.*

[1] **Mind.** Sudden vanishing of thought, forgets from one moment to the next what she wishes to do.
Reluctant answering.
Everything becomes irksome.
Aversion to work.
Fear of getting crazy.

[2] **Sensorium.** Stupefying vertigo.

[3] **Inner Head.** Sharp stitches, particularly in the temples.
Headache, with impatience.
Headache, caused by candle-light.

[4] **Outer Head.** Itching of the scalp.
Hair falls out.

[5] **Eyes.** Burning in the eyes from candle-light.
Burning of eyelids, only when closing them.

[6] **Ears.** Redness and heat of the ears.

[8] **Face.** Heat rising to the face, and soon thereafter painful itching, stitching and burning, continuing the whole day; next morning face swollen; toward noon vesicles, size of small pin-head, and filled with a yellow fluid, form; next day they remove through desquamation.
Pale, yellowish face.
Bashful appearance.

[9] **Lower Face.** Large number of small vesicles on the chin.

[11] **Tongue, etc.** Very bitter taste in the mouth.
Tongue coated white, except on several sharply defined clean spots.

[12] **Mouth.** Unendurable burning and prickling in the mouth, not relieved by cold water.
Whole mouth and tongue covered with small vesicles.
Increased flow of saliva.
Offensive yellow saliva.
Offensive smell from the mouth.
Blister, size of a hazel-nut, on the palate.

[13] **Throat.** Great elongation of the uvula.
Heat in pharynx and down the œsophagus, without thirst.
Great dryness of the throat.
Choking sensation rises in the throat when speaking.
Angina following scarlet fever.
Periodical thrusts (as if electric) in upper part of the throat, waking from sleep.
Yellowish-white ulcers on the tonsils, with violent burning pain.

Tonsils swollen.

Great swelling, and suppuration of the tonsils, with danger of suffocation; whistling breathing.

14 **Desires. Aversions.** Thirst for cold water, but is prevented from drinking by the choking sensation rising from stomach.

15 **Eating and Dinking.** Can only take liquid food, on account of soreness of the mouth.

From drinking water, aggravation of the bloatedness and painfulness of the region of stomach.

Cold water: 12. Drinking water: 19.

16 **Nausea and Vomiting.** Ineffectual desire to eructate.

Inclination to gagging, with nausea.

Excessive nausea.

Continual choking sensation, rising from the stomach as from pressure of wind, with weakness and palpitation of heart.

Repeated green vomit.

Sour, greasy vomit, with aversion to water; on the vomit floats a white mass like coagulated fat.

Vomiting of food, followed by severe colic and profuse diarrhœa.

17 **Stomach.** Pain in region of stomach.

Bloatedness and painfulness of region of stomach, with nervous fever.

Sensation as of flames rising from the stomach.

Sensation as if the stomach drew together in a lump, and then suddenly opened again.

Swelling in pit of stomach.

18 **Hypochondria.** Pain in the left hypochondrium.

Rumbling in the left side when bending to the right.

19 **Abdomen.** Pains in the abdomen, through the bowels, after drinking water.

Intestinal colic: with fainting; with constipation and diarrhœa in alternation.

20 **Stool, etc.** Fulness of the rectum, with a hollow feeling in stomach.

Profuse diarrhœa, with colic and vertigo.

Many bloody stools, with colic, inclination to sleep and vertigo.

Greenish stools, without blood.

Diarrhœa, with burning in the abdomen and anus.

Diarrhœa in alternation with constipation.

21 **Urine.** Tired feeling in region of kidneys, with inclination to rub the parts, and with frequent stretching backward of body.

Sensation of weakness and as if bruised, in region of the kidneys.

Urine: brown; whitish clouded, on standing.

²² **Male Sexual Organs.**   Increased sexual desire.

²³ **Female Sexual Organs.**   Pale menstrual flow.

²⁵ **Larynx.**   Nasal tone.

²⁶ **Breathing.**   Whistling breathing.

During breathing: rattling in left chest; loud rumbling in abdomen; severe pain in middle of sternum, worse from pressure.

²⁷ **Cough.**   Violent cough and painful stitches in trachea from slightest exertion.

Cough, worse at night.

Expectoration relieves the oppression of chest.

²⁸ **Lungs.**   Oppression of the chest.

Rattling in the left chest.

²⁹ **Heart.   Pulse.**   Palpitation of the heart and weakness.

Pulse weak and somewhat accelerated.

³⁰ **Outer Chest.**   Stitches in the middle of the sternum.

³¹ **Neck.   Back.**   Painful stiffness in the neck, especially after sleep, could scarcely move the neck.

Painful stiffness of small of back.

³² **Upper Limbs.**   Painful stiffness of the finger-joints.

Hands as if too thick, "asleep," and heavy.

Clumsiness of the hands.

Hands icy-cold.

³³ **Lower Limbs.**   Quivering and jerking in the legs in attacks.

Trembling of the legs.

Stitches under the heel, from without inward.

Burning and dry feeling in the soles.

Desquamation of the soles, at the end of the fever.

Large vesicles, especially on the soles.

³⁵ **Position, etc.**   Slight exertion: 26.   Bending to the right: 18.   Frequent stretching backward: 21.

Must lie down; the pulse is irregular, limbs cold, great anxiety.

Must lie down on account of the (moderate) fever and violent headache.

³⁷ **Sleep.**   When awaking, hands "asleep" and heavy, and feel as if too thick.

After sleep: bitterness in mouth; great dryness in throat; could scarcely move the neck.

³⁸ **Time.**   Noon: 8.   Night: 27.   All day: 8.

³⁹ **Temperature and Weather.**   Throws off covering: 40   Wants to cover: 40.

⁴⁰ **Chill.   Fever.   Sweat.**   Chilly, icy-cold hands and feet.

Flushes of heat, with sensation as if flames rose from out region of stomach, on account of which threw off the covering.

Burning heat, with inclination to cover himself, in bed.

Burning heat, with thirst.
Cold sweat.
⁴² **Sides.** Left: 18, 26, 28. Below upward: 8, 13, 14, 16, 17, 40. Without inward: 33.
⁴³ **Sensations.** Unnatural lightness, as if flying in the air.
Stitches in various parts of the body.
⁴⁵ **Contact, Injuries, etc.** Pressure: 26.

MANGANUM ACETICUM.

Manganese.   HAHNEMANN.

¹ **Mind.** Constant whining, moaning, or groaning.
Silent, reserved, peevish.
Ill-humored, vexed over trifles.
Low-spirited.
² **Sensorium.** All the senses less acute.
Head feels heavy, it seems larger.
³ **Inner Head.** Congestion of blood to the head, with throbbing in head; better in the open air.
Pressing, boring headache in the temples, extending towards eyes and forehead, going off on bending forward, returning on sitting up, or on bending head backwards.
Stitches (like needles) and darts in left side of forehead.
Jarring of the brain, from motion of the head.
Drawing, stinging or tensive headache in open air, better in-doors.
Headaches arising in room, better in open air, or vice versa.
⁴ **Outer Head.** Cold feeling at a small spot on the vertex.
⁵ **Eyes.** Shortsighted.
Pupils much dilated or contracted.
Burning in eyes and dimsightedness during the day.
Pressure in the eyes when reading by candle-light.
Burning heat and dryness of the eyes.
Eyelids swollen and painful to touch.
⁶ **Ears.** Whizzing and rushing in the ears.
Croaking sound in the right ear when walking.
Dull hearing: relieved by blowing the nose; worse during cold and rainy weather.
Fulness of the ears, with difficult hearing and cracking when blowing the nose or swallowing.
Sudden stitch pain in the deaf ear.
Drawing cramp in the muscles in the region of the left mastoid process, so that he had to incline his head to the right side.

ı Swelling of left parotid, with a reddish hue.   θ Typhus.

⁷ **Nose.**   Coryza dry, with complete obstruction of nostrils; crampy pain at the root of nose; worse in wet, cold weather.

Nose sore to the touch, worse in the evening.

⁸ **Face.**   Twitching stitches from the lower jaw to the temples, when laughing.

⁹ **Lower Face.**   Face pale, sunken.

Eruptions and ulcers at the corners of the mouth.

Dry, parched lips, with shriveled skin, without thirst.

Clear vesicles on the upper lip.

¹⁰ **Teeth.**   Smarting toothache, made insupportable when anything cold touches the tooth.

Violent toothache suddenly going from one place to another up in ears.

¹¹ **Tongue, etc.**   Oily taste in the mouth.

Burning vesicles on the left side of the tongue.

Nodosities on the tongue; warts.

¹² **Mouth.**   Smell from the mouth as of clay or earth (early in the morning after rising).

¹³ **Throat.**   Sore; as if excoriated, with cutting pains, independent of swallowing; palate and lips dry, worse in the open air; when swallowing, stitches into both ears; worse when coughing, with husky voice; feet and ankles swollen.

Throat dry, scratching, feeling as if the trachea was closed with a leaf.

¹⁴ **Desires.   Aversions.**   Aversion to food from a feeling of satiety.

Thirstlessness.

¹⁵ **Eating and Drinking.**   While eating: pressing in stomach and abdomen, more from cold food, especially in weakly females.

After eating: cramp pain in jaws; pain in rectum (after dinner).

¹⁶ **Nausea and Vomiting.**   Rising from stomach, like heartburn.

¹⁷ **Stomach.**   Burning in stomach, extending to chest; sometimes with great restlessness.

Pressing soreness in the epigastrium.

¹⁸ **Hypochondria.**   Pressure in the hypochondria.

¹⁹ **Abdomen.**   Warm contraction extending from middle of abdomen to chest, with nausea.

Cutting in region of navel when taking a long inspiration.

When walking, sensation as if bowels were loose and shaking about.

Abdomen distended, bloated.

²⁰ **Stool, etc.**   Passes much flatus.

Stool yellow, granular, with tenesmus and constriction of anus.

Costive, stool seldom, dry, knotty, difficult.

21 **Urine.**   Desire to urinate frequently; cutting in middle of urethra between micturition.

Urine profuse.

Sediment violet, earthy.

22 **Male Sexual Organs.**   Sensation of weakness in genitals, with burning and drawing in spermatic cords, extending to glans.

Itching in interior of scrotum, which cannot be relieved by pinching and rubbing.

23 **Female Sexual Organs.**   Menses too early and too scanty; bearing-down pains, great weakness, but tardy or absent flow.

Discharge of blood between periods, and pressing in genitals.

25 **Larynx.**   Hoarseness: with coryza; with tickling cough; rough speech in early morning or in open evening air.

Voice not clear, as from phlegm, worse mornings.

26 **Breathing.**   Breath hot and burning, with disagreeable heat in chest.

Pain in second left rib, from talking.

Pains in head, ears, arms, stomach, worse from breathing talking, or laughing.

27 **Cough.**   Causes darting in parietal bones; dry, incessant from irritation mid-sternum; better lying down.

Dry cough from loud reading, with painful dryness, roughness and constriction of larynx.

Sputum of greenish or yellow lumps, easily raised in morning; or difficult, of tough mucus.

Reddish phlegm.

Bloody expectoration.

28 **Lungs.**   Stitches in chest and sternum, running up and down.

Beating in the chest.

Warm contraction extending from middle of abdomen to chest, with nausea.

Bruised pain in upper chest when stooping, better by raising head.

29 **Heart.   Pulse.**   Palpitation of the heart, strong, irregular, trembling, without abnormal sounds.

Sudden shocks at the heart and in left side of chest from above downward.

Pulse very uneven and irregular, sometimes rapid, sometimes slow, but constantly soft and weak.

31 **Neck.   Back.**   Red, swollen streak on left side of neck.

Stiffness of the nape of the neck.

Tearing in whole spinal column, from above downward.
Pain in small of back on bending backward.

³² **Upper Limbs.**   Pain as from a sprain in shoulder-joint.
Rheumatic pains extending from shoulder to fingers.
Gnawing and boring in humerus, as if in the marrow.
Tension in the elbow-joint, as if too short.
Tensive pain in the joints of the arms and wrists.
Rhagades in the bends of the fingers.
Hands when closed or stretched feel swollen.
Chronic swelling and suppuration of the little finger.

³³ **Lower Limbs.**   Tension, drawing stitches in the thigh.
Twitching of muscles in legs from least exertion.
Trembling and unsteadiness of the knees.
Tearing in the knees.
Tension and stiffness in the legs.
Inflammation and swelling of the ankle, with stitches extending to the lower leg.
Burning of the soles of the feet.
Rawness between the toes.
Excruciating pains in left big toe, worse at night and from touch, must change his position.
Rheumatism in feet; cannot bear weight on heel.

³⁴ **Limbs in General.**   Rheumatism shifts from joint to joint, generally crosswise; red, shining swellings; worse from touch or motion, or at night; drawing as from shortening of tendons.

³⁵ **Position, etc.**   Motion: 34; of head: 3.   Walking: 6, 19.
Exertion: 33. Must change position: 33. Sitting up: 30.
Rising from bed: 43. Raising the head: 28. Stooping: 28.   Bending forward: 3.   Bending backward: 31.
Bending head back: 3.   Lying: 27.

³⁶ **Nerves.**   Weakness and trembling, especially of the joints.

³⁷ **Sleep.**   Much yawning.
Feels sleepy early in the evening.
Many vivid dreams, which are well remembered.

³⁸ **Time.**   Worse at night; pains in joints, bones, etc.
Morning: 12, 25, 27. Evening: 7, 24, 37, 40, 43. Night: 33, 34, 40, 43, 44. Day: 5.

³⁹ **Temperature and Weather.**   Worse in hot, foggy weather.
Open air: 3, 13, 25. In-doors: 3.   Cold, rainy weather: 6, 7.   Cold things: 10.

⁴⁰ **Chill. Fever. Sweat.**   Chill generally in the evening, shooting headache, icy-cold hands and feet.
Shaking chill, with heat of the head, stinging in forehead, continuing after chill.
Sudden flushes of heat in face, on chest and over back.
Heat and sweat, with moderate thirst.
Sweat profuse, with short, anxious breathing.

Night-sweats; itching, often only on the neck and lower legs.

⁴² **Sides.**   Right: 6.   Left: 3, 11, 26, 29, 31, 33.   Above downward: 29, 31, 32.

⁴³ **Sensations.**   Burning over whole body; in evening when rising from bed.

Unbearable pains in bones and periosteum, like a digging, worse at night; also digging in joints.

⁴⁴ **Tissues.**   Inflammation of bones, with nightly, insupportable, digging pains.

▮All the bones, particularly in lower limbs, sensitive to touch.   θ Typhus.

Inflammation of joints, with digging pains at night.

Inflammatory swellings and suppuration.

⁴⁵ **Contact, Injuries, etc.**   Every part of the body feels extremely sore when touched.

Touch: 5, 7, 33, 34, 45.   Rubbing and pinching: 22.

⁴⁶ **Skin.**   Rhagades in bends of joints, with soreness.

Itching in hollow of knee and on shin, worse sweating.

Itching on palms, with red spots; lips sore.

Burning in small, red spots, on chest, arms, hands and feet, accompanying rheumatism.

⁴⁸ **Relationship.**   Antidote to *Mangan.: Coffea.*

MARUM VERUM.

Teucrium marum verum. E. STAPF.   *Labiatæ.*

¹ **Mind.**   Great mental excitement and loquacity.

Irresistible desire to sing.

Indolence, physical and mental.

Great sensitiveness and excitability.

Irritable mood at and after dinner, with pressure in forehead.

² **Sensorium.**   Dulness and dizziness.

³ **Inner Head.**   Pressing pain over eyes, worse on stooping.

⁴ **Outer Head.**   Skin of forehead sensitive to touch.

⁵ **Eyes.**   Look as after weeping; smarting in canthi and redness of conjunctivæ.

Profuse smarting tears in the open air.

Upper lids red and puffy.

⁶ **Ears.**   Hissing sound when passing hand over ear, when talking or forcibly inspiring through nose.

Fine ringing in right ear when blowing nose, squeaking, as if air was forced through mucus.

Otalgia, with lancinating pain.

Dry herpes, with white scales, on and behind the ears.

⁷ **Nose.** ❙ Nasal polypus.

Tingling in the nose, frequent sneezing, followed by coryza.

Large, irregular pieces discharged from the nose; foul breath. Ozæna.

⁸ **Face.** Frequent sensation of flushes of heat, but with paleness.

Burning, itching rash on forehead and upper part of face, worse in the evening and from warmth.

⁹ **Lower Face.** Deep furrow, on either side of under lip, with elevated edges.

¹⁰ **Teeth.** Violent tearing in roots and gums of right lower incisors.

¹² **Tongue, etc.** Mouldy taste after hawking mucus.

Smarting, as from pepper, at root of tongue. .

¹² **Mouth.** Much mucus and saliva.

¹³ **Throat.** Tearing and scraping in fauces, worse left side.

Stinging or pressing, hindering swallowing.

¹⁵ **Eating and Drinking.** After eating: 40. After dinner: 1.

After nursing, jerking hiccough and empty belching.

After drinking, cutting colic.

¹⁶ **Nausea and Vomiting.** Gulping of bitter tasting food.

Vomits dark green masses; hiccough, with a stitch through stomach to back.

¹⁷ **Stomach.** Anxious oppression, or empty feeling and rumbling in the stomach.

¹⁹ **Abdomen.** Dull pressing, as from incarcerated flatulence.

²⁰ **Stool, etc.** Diarrhœa, with crying and emaciation in children.

Ascarides, with creeping and itching and nightly restlessness; worse from warmth of bed.

²¹ **Urine.** Increased secretion of pale urine.

²³ **Male Sexual Organs.** Sexual desire decreased.

Pressing, drawing sensation from abdomen into cords and testicles.

²⁵ **Larynx.** Dryness, causing hawking; hissing sound when inhaling.

²⁶ **Breathing.** Stitches in right chest when inhaling; catarrhal asthma, especially in the aged.

Sensation of oppression (without affecting the breathing).

²⁷ **Cough.** Dry, short, from tickling in upper part of trachea, which is worse from coughing.

³² **Upper Limbs.** Burning in the finger-tips. θ Panaritium.

³³ **Lower Limbs.** ❙ Ingrowing toe-nails (right great toe), with ulceration; better moving.

³⁴ **Limbs in General.** Rheumatic pains mostly in bones and joints, worse evenings, better moving.

Limbs go to sleep, with tingling, when sitting.

[35] **Position, etc.** Motion: 33, 34. Sitting: 34. Stooping: 3.
[36] **Nerves.** Nervous, irritable, trembling.
[37] **Sleep.** Restless sleep, excited; also from ascarides.
[38] **Time.** Morning: not refreshed. Noon: debility. Evening:
8, 34, 40. Night: 20.
[39] **Temperature and Weather.** Warmth: 8, 20. Open air: 5.
Desire to exercise in the open air, which does not fatigue.
[40] **Chill. Fever. Sweat.** Chilliness: from want of animal
heat; after eating or from talking about unpleasant
things.
Increased heat and exaltation in the evening, with great
loquacity.
[42] **Sides.** Right: 6, 10, 26. Left: 13.
[45] **Contact, Injuries, etc.** Touch: 4.
[46] **Skin.** Sensation as from flea-bites.
Rash, burning, itching.

MEPHITIS.

Skunk. HERING. *Mustelidæ.*

[1] **Mind.** Fancies so vivid they unfit for mental labor.
Talkative, as if drunk; excited, with heat of the head.
Angry about trifles, or imaginary things.
[2] **Sensorium.** Vertigo sitting, stooping, turning in bed.
Numb and dull, with sensation as if head became enlarged, with ill-humor and nausea.
[3] **Inner Head.** Fulness in head, worse on vertex, worse
studying.
Headache while riding in a carriage.
Heaviness and pressure in back part of head, as if fingers
were pressing on it.
[5] **Eyes.** Inability to read fine print.
Letters become blurred, he is unable to discern them, they
run together.
Weakness of sight, generally with headache and pain in
eyes.
Pain in eyes: when turning them in certain directions;
as from a foreign body; as from overexertion.
Stitches in eyes as from needles.
Stinging and itching in eyes, evenings and mornings.
Inflammation of eyes and lids, especially right side.
Redness of the conjunctiva.
Heat and burning of the eyes.
[6] **Ears.** Fetid discharge from ears.

Erysipelas of the ear, with itching, heat, redness and blisters.

⁷ **Nose.** Dry nose; bleeding from the nose.

Fluent coryza, cough and soreness in chest.

⁸ **Face.** Bloated face.

¹⁰ **Teeth.** Sudden jerks in roots of teeth; strumming toothache.

¹¹ **Tongue, etc.** Coppery taste in the mouth.

Talking: 27.

¹⁴ **Desires. Aversions.** Wants every dish very much salted.

¹⁵ **Eating and Drinking.** After eating: 27. Drinking: 27.

¹⁶ **Nausea and Vomiting.** Nausea, with emptiness in the stomach, and sensation as if the head were distended.

¹⁷ **Stomach.** Pressure in the stomach, and colic.

¹⁸ **Hypochondria.** Rheumatic pain in region of liver.

²⁰ **Stool, etc.** Thin, infrequent.

²¹ **Urine.** Difficulty in urinating all day; stream interrupted.

Frequent micturition, with clear urine.

Urine is turbid in the morning, after evening fever.

²² **Male Sexual Organs.** Warmth of the genitals at night.

Itching of the scrotum.

²³ **Female Sexual Organs.** Burning leucorrhœa.

Soreness of genitals and swelling of labia.

²⁵ **Larynx.** When drinking or talking, liability to have something get into the larynx.

²⁶ **Breathing.** Asthma: as from inhaling vapor of sulphur; in sleep; of drunkards.

Inhalation difficult, exhalation almost impossible; or barking.

²⁷ **Cough.** After drinking, talking or loud reading; spasmodic, hollow or deep, with rawness, hoarseness and pain through chest; with suffocative feeling when inhaling; cannot inhale; vomits all food some hours after eating; convulsions; worse at night and after lying down; in the morning it is loose, with some expectoration.

²⁸ **Lungs.** Pains in chest (last left short rib) when touching it; more when coughing and sneezing.

³¹ **Neck. Back.** Stitches in the spinal column during motion.

Pain in the back and all the limbs, with lameness.

Tension and pain in right side of neck.

³² **Upper Limbs.** Rheumatic pains in arms, relieved on motion.

Restless in left arm, with insensibility.

Trembling of arm when leaning on it.

Painful twitching of the left hand.

³³ **Lower Limbs.** Rush of blood to the legs at night.

Rheumatic pains from hips to feet; arthritic pain in heel.

Legs restless as if becoming insensible; knees feel bruised.

Spasmodic pain in left foot.

40

Stitches in the feet.

Pain in big toe as if being pinched off.

Corns, with pain and burning.

35 Position, etc. With slightest manual work sweat breaks out.

Motion: 31, 32. Turning in bed: 2. Sitting: 2. Stooping: 2.

36 Nerves. Convulsions.

Inclination to stretch with disinclination to do anything. Restlessness.

37 Sleep. Frequent yawning; lachrymation.

Sleepy during day, even in company.

Cannot sleep the whole night.

Awakens early and feels refreshed.

Awakens at night with congestion to legs.

Night walking, open eyes, angry face.

Hair on head rises, cannot be made conscious.

Vivid dreams, which he recollects.

Asthma during sleep; not waking; continues after he has waked up.

38 Time. Morning: 21, 27, 37, 40. Evening: 21. Morning and evening: 5. Night: 22, 27, 33, 37. Day: 21, 37.

39 Temperature and Weather. Cold: colic worse.

Feels less chilly in cold weather; feels pleasant after ice-cold washing.

40 Chill. Fever. Sweat. Cold feeling predominates; evening chilliness, with desire to urinate, colic as if diarrhœa would set in.

Increased warmth, especially in the morning.

42 Sides. Right: 5, 31. Left: 28, 32, 33.

43 Sensations. Strumming through the body; anxiety.

Feels as if threads had been drawn through head and trunk.

Wandering pains with pressure to urinate.

45 Contact, Injuries, etc. Touch: 28. Riding: 3.

MERCURIUS.

Quicksilver.   HAHNEMANN.   *The Element.*

[1] **Mind.** Memory weak; mind obtuse; drowsy.

Anxiety and restless change of place; ebullitions, sweat; apprehensive; imaginary fears; fears he will lose his mind; worse evening and night; wants to go abroad; tries to flee from the house.

Homesickness.

Delirium and other mental derangements of drunkards.

Hurried speech.

Continuous moaning and groaning.

Irritable, quarrelsome; or, taciturn and indifferent.

Suspicious, distrustful mood.

Imbecility; does foolish, mischievous, disgusting actions.

Sensorium. Fainting after sweetish rising in the throat, followed by sleep.

Vertigo: as if in a swing; after stooping; when lying on the back; with headache and nausea; everything turns black.

Dull and stupid feeling, with dizziness.

³ **Inner Head.** Burning in head, especially in left temple; worse at night lying in bed, better on sitting up.

Head feels as if in a vice, with nausea; worse in the open air, from sleeping, eating and drinking; better in room.

Tension over forehead, as if in a hoop; worse at night in bed; better after rising and from laying the hand on it.

Inflammation of brain, with this hoop-like feeling; burning and pulsation in forehead; worse at night, better after riding.

Congestion to the head.

Head feels as if it would burst, with fulness of the brain.

Head feels as if it was getting larger.

Severe pains in forehead, top of head and occiput; stitches through the head.

Dulness in forehead, stitches through temples; aching and weariness in nape of neck.

Tearing in head; heat and sweat; worse at night, in warmth of bed; better toward morning and while lying quietly.

⁴ **Outer Head.** Hydrocephalus; body bathed in sweat.

Sutures open, large head; precocious mental development; dirty color of the face; sour night-sweat.

Exostoses on the hairy scalp, with feeling of soreness when touched; worse at night, in bed.

Scalp: tense; painful to touch; worse when scratching, which causes bleeding; eruption, pustular, fetid, with yellow crusts; erysipelatous; worse on the forehead; hair falls out, mostly on sides and temples.

Lacerating, tearing and stinging in the bones of the skull.

Fetid, sour-smelling, oily sweat on the head; on the forehead it is icy-cold; with burning in the skin; worse at night, in bed, and after rising.

Great chilliness, with contractive, tearing pain of the scalp, extending from forehead to neck.

⁵ **Eyes.** Black points before the eyes.

Vanishing of sight for a few moments.

Much worse from heat and glare of fire.

Lachrymation profuse, burning, excoriating; discharges muco-purulent, thin, acrid; burning, tearing, sticking pains in and around eyes; worse at night; pimples on the cheeks.

Ulcers of the cornea, vascular and surrounded by greyish opacity; pus between the corneal layers, onyx.

Iritis, syphilitic; pains around the eye, on foreghead and temples; worse from touch at night; throbbing, shooting pains in the eye. Hypopion.

Lids: spasmodically closed; thick, red, swollen, erysipelatous; sensitive to cold, heat and to touch; raw, excoriated; burning, as from fiery points; margins ulcerated, scabby.

Ciliary blepharitis, caused by working over fires or forges.

[6] **Ears.** Hardness of hearing; sounds vibrate in the ears; obstruction momentarily better after swallowing or blowing the nose; external meatus moist.

Internal and external ear inflamed, with stinging, tearing pains; purulent discharge, green, offensive, or thin, sanious; glands swollen.

Boils in the external canal; also fungous growths.

Constant cold sensation in the ears.

[7] **Nose.** Nosebleed: when coughing and during sleep; blood hangs in a dark, coagulated string.

Coryza: fluent, corrosive, with much sneezing; nostrils bleeding, scurfy; nose red, swollen, shining; worse from damp weather; at night; from either cold or warm air; not relieved by sweat.

Greenish, fetid pus from the nose; nasal bones swollen.

[8] **Face.** Pale, yellow, earthy; red and hot cheeks; pale and sunken; pale, doughy, full.

Yellow, dirty scurf, with fetid discharge, itching and bleeding when scratched.

Tearing in the face; lacerating pains, salivation; from cold or caries of the teeth.

Swelling of one (right) side of face, with heat and toothache.

Pimples with bluish-red areolæ; no itching.

[9] **Lower Face.** Lips: dry, cracked, ulcerated; black; burning pimples, with yellow crusts.

Mumps on the right side; pale swelling.

Lockjaw from glandular swellings, with stinging pains.

Caries of the jaw.

[10] **Teeth.** Teeth feel loose, fall out.

Toothache from caries; or when the dentine is inflamed; returns in damp weather or evening air; pains tearing, lacerating, shooting into face and ears; worse from warmth of bed, from cold or warm things; better from rubbing the cheek.

. Gums painful to touch, swollen, receding from the teeth; edges whitish; bleeding; fetid odor from the mouth; ulcers with dark red edges.

Pulsating toothache worse at night; gum-boil.

[11] **Tongue, etc.** Taste: bitter; sweetish; saltish; putrid or slimy.

Loss of taste.

Speech quick, stuttering. Complete loss of speech.

Tongue: dry, hard, coated black; red and dry; red, with dark spots and burning; moist, with intense thirst; moist and covered with mucus; thickly coated, dirty yellow, with foul breath; swollen, flabby, takes imprint of teeth; inflamed, indurated or suppurating, with pricking pains.

Ranula, with ptyalism and sore gums.

[12] **Mouth.** Inflamed, with burning, aphthous ulcers; copious, fetid, ropy salivation; scorbutic gums; large blisters in the mouth.

Much slime collects in the mouth.

Ptyalism; saliva fetid or tastes coppery.

Ulceration of the salivary glands.

[13] **Throat.** Uvula swollen and elongated.

Erysipelatous inflammation of the throat.

Painful dryness of throat, with mouth full of saliva; rawness, roughness and burning in throat.

Angina, with stinging pains, worse from empty swallowing, at night and in the cold air.

Tonsils dark red, or greenish-red, studded with ulcers; stinging pains in fauces; quinsy, only after pus has formed to hasten maturing.

Syphilitic ulcers in the throat and mouth.

Glands swollen.

[14] **Desires. Aversions.** Canine hunger, even after eating.

Excessive hunger, but relishes nothing.

Loss of appetite.

Thirst violent, burning, especially for beer and cold drinks.

Desire for milk; for sweets, but they disagree; for beer; for liquid food.

Aversion to meat; to wine and brandy; to coffee; to greasy food.

[15] **Eating and Drinking,** Worse from spirituous liquors; coffee; cold drinks.

After eating and drinking: 3.

[16] **Nausea and Vomiting.** Acrid, bitter, putrid or rancid eructations, worse at night.

Regurgitation or vomiting of food; bitter vomit.

Nausea, with sweet taste in the throat, vertigo, heat and headache.

[17] **Stomach.** Pressure in stomach; it hangs down heavily
even after light, easily digested food.

Stomach: burns, is swollen and sensitive to touch; hard
and tense.

Weak digestion, with continuous hunger.

The stomach feels replete and constricted.

[18] **Hypochondria.** Region of the liver: sensitive; cannot lie
on the right side; swollen, hard, from induration of the
liver; stinging, stitching or passive pains.

Jaundice: with violent rush of blood to the head; bad
taste; tongue moist and furred, yellow; soreness in the
hepatic region; from gall-stones; with duodenal catarrh;
in the newborn; sweat stains linen yellow.

[19] **Abdomen.** Tense, hard, swollen and sensitive; fulness and
tenderness across the epigastrium and hypochondria.

Colic from cold, from the evening air, from worms.

When lying on the right side, the intestines feel bruised.

Enteritis, lancinating pains; bloody, slimy stools; sweat,
without relief.

Hard, painful, hot swelling in the ileo-cœcal region.
θ Typhlitis.

Peritonitis, with purulent exudation, especially with
typhlitis.

On walking, bowels shake as if loose.

Inguinal glands swollen or suppurating.

[20] **Stool, etc.** Stools: undigested, pitch-like, tenacious; yellow,
dark green, mucous and bloody; sour, excoriating the
anus; clay-colored and offensive; slimy, bloody, preceded by anxiety, trembling, faintness; colic; tenesmus;
after stool, tenesmus, a "cannot-get-done" feeling, followed by chilliness.

Blood before, during and after, even a hard, stool.

Constipation, stool tenacious or crumbling, discharged
only with violent straining; constant, ineffectual urging,
worse at night.

Ascarides and lumbrici escape freely.

Prolapsus ani after stool; also, if rectum is black and
bleeding.

Large bleeding varices, which suppurate; hemorrhage
after micturition.

[21] **Urine.** Region of bladder sore to touch; urine passes in a
thin stream or in drops, and contains blood and pus.

Urine passed involuntarily.

Urging to urinate, with copious flow; desire sudden,
irresistible.

Frequent, rapid urination with scanty discharge, often
followed by mucus.

Urine: dark red and turbid; sour and pungent; mixed

with blood, white flakes and pus; flesh-like lumps of mucus.

Hæmaturia, with violent and frequent urging to urinate.

Gonorrhœa, with phimosis or chancroids; green discharge, worse at night.

²² **Male Sexual Organs.**   Lascivious excitement, with painful nightly erections.

Pollutions, sperm mixed with blood; chilliness; sallow face; constipation.   After emissions burning pain in back and icy-cold hands.

Ulcers in the glans, with cheesy base; chancroids.

Children scratch and pull at the genitals all night.

Testicles swollen, hard, shining.

Sweat on genitals; soreness between scrotum and thighs.

Glans and prepuce inflamed; phimosis.

²³ **Female Sexual Organs.**   Menses too profuse; with either sterility or easy conception; with anxiety and colic.

Amenorrhœa, with congestions and ebullitions.

Deep, sore pain in the pelvis, dragging in the loins; abdomen weak, as if it had to be held up; prolapsus uteri et vaginæ; feels better after coitus.

On the os uteri: excrescences, bleeding; deep ulcers, with ragged edges.

Inflammation of the vagina, and still more of the external genitals, with rawness, smarting and excoriated spots.

Itching of the genitals, worse from contact of the urine.

Leucorrhœa smarting, corroding, causing itching; purulent, containing lumps, always worse at night.

²⁴ **Pregnancy.**   Expels moles.

Pain in the mammæ at every menstrual period, as if they would ulcerate.

Milk in the breasts, instead of the menses.

Milk scanty, or spoiled, child refuses it; mastitis.

Mammæ swollen, hard, with sore pains, ulcerated nipples, suppuration of the mammæ.

²⁵ **Larynx.**   Hoarse, rough voice; burning, rawness in the larynx; fluent coryza and sore throat.

²⁶ **Breathing.**   Short-breathed on ascending or walking.

Asthma, from fumes of arsenic; better from tobacco smoke and in the cold air.

Dyspnœa (sensation of spasmodic contraction when coughing or sneezing).

²⁷ **Cough.**   Violent, racking; worse at night, as if the head and chest would burst, sometimes with vomiturition; in two paroxysms, from tickling in the larynx and upper part of the chest; only at night or only by day; with acrid, yellowish mucus, at times mixed with coagu-

lated blood and tasting putrid or saltish; with shortness
of breath and salivation; not allowing him to utter an
audible word; worse at night, in the night air, when
lying on either side.

Bloody sputum in tuberculosis.

[28] **Lungs.** Burning in the chest, extending to the throat.

Acts on lower part of right lung; stitches through to back.

Rush of blood to the chest.

Stitches in the chest, through, from the right scapula;
pneumonia, with bilious symptoms.

Sensation of dryness in the chest.

Suppuration of the lungs after hemorrhages, or after
pneumonia.

[29] **Heart. Pulse.** Weakness at the heart, as if life was ebbing
away; awakens with trembling at the heart, and agitation as if frightened.

Palpitation, with fear; worse at night.

Pulse: full and accelerated, with erethism; frequent at
night, slower by day, when slow it is weak and trembling; imperceptible, with warmth of the body.

Orgasm, with trembling from slight exertion.

[31] **Neck. Back.** Rheumatic stiffness and swelling of neck.

Goitre becomes softened.

Glands inflamed, swollen, with pressing pains and stitches.

Bruised sensation of the scapulæ, back and small of back.

Stinging pains in small of the back, with sensation of
weakness.

Violent pains in spine, worse from motion. θ Meningitis.

Pain the sacrum, as after lying on a hard couch.

Tearing in coccyx, better by pressing hand against the
abdomen.

[32] **Upper Limbs.** Red and hot (arthritic) swelling from the
elbow to the wrist.

Dorsa of the hands raw, denuded; cracks on the joints;
burning, stinging pains.

Moist, itch-like eruption on the hands, with nightly itching; bleeding rhagades.

Nails drop off.

[33] **Lower Limbs.** Tearing in hip-joint and knee, worse at
night; or, with pulsating pain; beginning suppuration.

The child's legs are clammy and cold, worse at night.

Ulcers on legs, which bleed easily and become putrid,
spongy and bluish.

Cold sweat on the feet.

[34] **Limbs in General.** Arms and thighs sore to touch, can
hardly move them.

Twitching of arms and legs.

Rheumatic and arthritic pains, tearing, stinging; worse at

night in the warm bed; with profuse sweat, which gives
no relief; œdema of the affected parts, especially of feet
and ankles; joints swollen, pale or slightly red.

Must move the parts because of uneasiness or of drawing-
tearing pains

[35] **Position, etc.** Motion: 31. Walking: 19, 26. Ascending:
26. Changing place: 1. Exertion: 29, 36, 40. Lying:
3; on back: 2; on right side: 18, 19; on either side:
27. After lying down: 40. Sitting: 3. Stooping: 2.
After rising: 3, 4, 40.

[36] **Nerves.** Convulsions, with cries, rigidity, bloated abdomen,
itching of the nose and thirst; worse at night.

Contraction of joints.

Great weakness, with ebullitions and trembling from the
least exertion.

Legs paralyzed.   θ Spinal meningitis.

Limbs stiff, but can be moved by others; paralysis.

Paralysis agitans.

Formication beginning in hands and feet, pains in thumbs,
elbows, feet; then trembling, muscular contractions.

[37] **Sleep.** Sleepy during the day; sleepless at night, from ebullitions of blood and anxiety; also from embarrassed
portal circulation, with beating at pit of stomach.

[38] **Time.** Remission during the day.

Morning: 3, 40. Evening: 1, 10, 19, 40. Night: 1, 3, 4,
5, 7, 10, 13, 16, 20, 21, 22, 23, 27, 29, 32, 33, 34, 36, 37,
40, 44, 46. Toward morning: 40. Day: 27, 29, 37.

[39] **Temperature and Weather.** Worse in wet weather, and
in the cool evening air.

Worse in the Fall, with warm days and damp, cold nights.

Cold or warm: 7. Warmth of the bed: 3, 4, 10, 34, 40,
46. Averse to uncovering, even of the hands, also: 40.
Open air: 3. Evening air: 10, 19, 27. Cold: 5, 7, 8,
10, 13, 26. Cold or warm air: 7. External heat or
cold: 46. Room: 3. Heat: 5, 7, 10, 46. Damp
weather: 7, 10.

[40] **Chill. Fever. Sweat.** Chill: in the morning when rising,
but more generally in the evening after lying down, as
from cold water poured over one; not relieved by the
warmth of the stove; at night, with frequent urination;
alternating with heat, often only on single parts; internal, with heat of the face.

Heat: in bed, and chill when out of bed; after midnight,
with violent thirst for cold drinks; anxious, with sensation of pressing together of the chest, alternating with
chill; with aversion to uncover.

Sweat: profuse at night; toward morning, with thirst and
palpitation; from exertion, even when eating; evening

in bed, before falling asleep; sour, offensive, or cold, clammy, oily, and causing burning in the skin; with all pains, but giving no relief, even aggravating the weakness; stains linen yellow.

Complaints often increase during sweat.

Hectic fever, especially of children. Irritative fevers.

Intermittent fever: evening chill; heat and violent thirst, or thirst toward morning; during sweat palpitation and nausea; sweat fetid or sour.

Contra-indicated in typhoid fever, except for marked icteroid or scorbutic symptoms.

⁴² **Sides.** Right: 8, 9, 18, 28. Above downward: 4.

⁴¹ **Tissues.** Blood coagulates easily.

Throbbing or pricking-stinging in the veins.

Erysipelatous inflammation, especially about the joints.

Excessive emaciation.

All discharges are acrid.

Œdema of face, hands and feet, with amenia.

Ascites, from organic lesions of liver; anasarca after scarlatina.

Glandular swellings, with or without suppuration.

Bone diseases, worse at night.

Suppuration, especially if too profuse.

⁴⁵ **Contact, Injuries, etc.** Touch: 4, 5, 10, 17, 18, 19, 21, 34. Pressure: 3, 31. Rubbing: 10. Scratching: 4, 8, 22.

⁴⁶ **Skin.** Skin chafed, sore.

Eythema first on thighs; at times vesicles that suppurate and spread rapidly.

Skin dirty yellow, rough and dry; jaundice.

Itching all over, worse at night, when warm in bed.

Scabies, if some of the vesicles become pustular.

Herpes surrounded by a border of large scales.

Herpetic spots and suppurating pustules sometimes running together; forming dry and scaly spots, or crusts, and acrid discharges.

Ulcers superficial, flat, readily bleeding; base lardaceous; worse from heat of bed and hot or cold applications, with clean-cut but irregular edges.

Boils, after pus has formed.

Primary and secondary syphilis; round, coppery-red spots shining through the skin.

Zona like a girdle, from the back around the abdomen; much itching and tendency to suppurate.

Variola in stage of maturation; with dysenteric symptoms.

⁴⁸ **Relationship.** *Mercur.* is often indicated after *Bellad., Hepar, Sulphur* (as an intercurrent), *Laches.*

After *Mercur.* are indicated: *Bellad., Cinchon., Dulcam., Hepar., Nitr. ac., Sulphur.*

Mercur. and *Silic.* do not follow each other well.

Antidotes: *Hepar, Kali hydr., Nitr. ac., Aurum, Mezer., Carb. veg., Sulphur, Iodum, Guajac., Dulcam, Cinchon., Staphis., Ferrum, Bellad., Laches.*

Ailments from: *Arsen.* or copper vapors, *Aurum, Antimon., Laches., Bellad., Opium, Cinchon., Dulcam., Mezer., Sulphur, Calcar.*

Merc. præc. rub. preferable in sycosis, also in squamous syphilides, *Merc. nit.,* in pustular syphilides, and *Merc. biniod.,* in tubercular.

Plantago maj. rivals *Merc.* in toothache: caries, tooth feels long and sore; boring, digging pains worse by contact, in cold or in heat; better lying in moderately cool room. Ciliary neuralgia reflex from pains in decayed teeth. Earache, twinging, sharp pains with pain in teeth.

Merc. dulcis is preferable when there is catarrh of the eustachian tube and pharynx; closure of the tube.

MERCURIUS CORROSIVUS.

Corrosive sublimate.   BUCHNER.   *Hg Cl.*

¹ **Mind.** Stares at persons who talk to him, and does not understand them.

Weakness of the intellect.

Mind sluggish, with torpid digestion.

Anxiety, preventing sleep.

² **Sensorium.** Vertigo, with coldness, cold perspiration; with deafness, when stooping.

³ **Inner Head.** Violent temporal headache.

Heaviness of the head.

Stitches in the forehead.

⁴ **Outer Head.** Swelling of the head and neck.

⁵ **Eyes.** Objects appear smaller; or, double vision.

Pupils contracted and insensible.

Excessive photophobia and acrid lachrymation.

Phlyctenulæ, deep ulcers on the cornea; discharges ichorous, acrid, making the surrounding parts sore; pimples around the eyes like small boils.

Iritis, especially if syphilitic; pains severe, worse at night.

Retinitis albuminurica, also with tearing at the eyebrow, bones tender.

Hypopion occurring in abscess of the cornea or iritis.

Ophthalmia neonatorum, with acrid discharges; caused by syphilitic leucorrhœa.

Posterior synechiæ; causes them to soften.

Lids: œdematous, or erysipelatous; red, excoriated; edges swollen, burning, smarting; edges covered with thick crusts or pustules; spasmodically closed.

6 Ears. Inflammation, with stitches in the ear.

Discharge of fetid pus from the ear.

7 Nose. Swelling and redness of the nose.

Fluent coryza; loss of smell.

Ozæna, discharge from the nose like glue, drying up in the posterior nares; perforation of the septum.

Nose stopped up and at the same time runs; rawness, smarting in the nostrils.

8 Face. Swelling and turning up of the upper lip; dark red, swollen lip.

Face and cheeks swollen, hard, red, bloated.

Paleness of the distorted face.

ı Œdematous swelling of the face, paleness; albuminuria.

Yellow color of the face.

10 Teeth. Looseness of the teeth; they pain and fall out.

Gums swell; covered with a false membrane; gangrenous; bleed freely.

11 Tongue, etc. Lips and tongue, whitish and contracted.

Tongue coated with thick white mucus, or dry and red; papillæ, elevated, strawberry-like; coated white, swollen and stiff.

Swelling of the tongue, with ptyalism.

12 Mouth. Sensation as if the mouth was scalded.

Taste in the mouth, metallic or salty.

Mouth dry, with unquenchable thirst.

Exudations on mucous membranes, extending to tonsils.

Ulcers (phagedenic) in mouth, throat, or on gums, with fetid breath.

Ptyalism, with salty taste; saliva bloody, yellowish, tough, acrid.

Painful burning in the mouth, extending to the stomach.

Discharge of albuminous mucus from the mouth.

Buccal cavity and lips covered with aphthæ; on the lips they are surrounded by vesicles, which burn.

13 Throat. Uvula swollen, elongated, dark red.

Throat intensely inflamed, preventing swallowing and causing suffocation.

Tonsels swollen and covered with ulcers.

Pricking in the throat as from needles.

Retching and vomiting on attempting to swallow.

14 Desires. Aversions. No appetite.

16 Nausea and Vomiting. Vomiting: of albuminous matter; of tough, or stringy mucus; of green, bitter substances; of bile; of blood; like coffee-grounds, with coagulated blood; of pus.

[17] **Stomach.** Distension and soreness of the pit of stomach, not permitting the least touch, even of clothing.

Burning, gnawing, darting pains in the stomach.

[18] **Hypochondria.** Stitches as if in the middle of liver.

[19] **Abdomen.** Bloated abdomen, very painful to least touch.

Cutting below the navel.

Bruised pain in the abdomen.

Pain and distention in colon, especially transverse portion.

[20] **Stool, etc.** Stools: yellow, green, bilious, followed by slime and blood; with tenesmus and insupportable, cutting, colicky pains; after stool, burning and tenesmus of rectum and bladder; worse in Fall; worse after midnight.

Painful bloody discharges, with vomiting.

Constipation.

[21] **Urine.** Tenesmus of the bladder; urine suppressed.

Urine: increased; scanty, hot, bloody; passed in drops with great pain; scanty, brown, with brick-dust sediment.

Filaments, flocks or dark flesh-like pieces of mucus in urine.

❙ Albumen in urine; after diphtheria or in Morbus Brightii.

Gonorrhœa greenish, worse at night; burning, smarting, urination.

Paraphimosis.

[22] **Male Sexual Organs.** Violent erections during sleep.

Fine painful stinging in left testicle.

When the chancre assumes a phagedenic appearance and secrets a thin, ichorous pus.

[23] **Female Sexual Organs** Menses too early and too profuse.

Leucorrhœa, pale yellow; smelling sweetish.

[25] **Larynx.** Hoarseness or aphonia; burning and stinging in the trachea, tightness across the chest.

Larynx and epiglottis pain when swallowing food; pain worse when depressing tongue; cutting in throat, as from a knife.

[26] **Breathing.** Respiration slow; interrupted, sighing.

Excessive dyspnœa; palpitaton.

[28] **Lungs.** Hæmoptysis.

Stitches in chest, through the thorox (right, lower side.)

[29] **Heart. Pulse.** Palpitation of the heart in sleep.

Pain in the precordial region.

Pulse small, weak, intermitting, sometimes trembling.

[31] **Neck. Back.** Glands of neck hard and swollen.

Pains in head, back and limbs; kidneys affected.

Lies on the back with knees up; Pott's disease.

[32] **Upper Limbs.** Arm up to the shoulder much swollen, red and covered with vesicles.

Rheumatic pains in left shoulder and shoulder-blade.

The deltoid muscle feels relaxed.

[33] **Lower Limbs.** Stitches in the right hip-joint.

Sensation as if the legs had "gone to sleep."

The muscles of the thigh and calf feel relaxed.

Cramps in the calves. θ Dysentery.

The feet are icy-cold.

³⁴ **Limbs in General.** Coldness in the extremities, they look purple; with small spasmodic, frequent pulse.

Paralysis of the upper and lower extremities.

³⁵ **Position, etc.** Motion: 40. Stooping: 2, 40. Rising: 40.

³⁶ **Nerves.** Convulsive twitchings of muscles of face, arms and legs, and convulsions of limbs; convulsive contractions.

Trembling.

³⁷ **Sleep.** During sleep, violent hiccough.

Somnolence.

When trying to go to sleep, violent starts.

Sleeplessness on account of vertigo; on account of anxiety.

³⁸ **Time.** Morning: 40. Evening: 40. Night: 5, 21, 40. After midnight: 20.

³⁹ **Temperature and Weather.** Worse in the open air: 40.

⁴⁰ **Chill. Fever. Sweat.** Chilliness: from the least movement and in the open air, generally with colic; in the evening; especially on the head, at night in bed.

External heat, with yellow skin.

Burning, stinging heat in the skin.

Heat when stooping and coldness when rising.

Sweat at night, or fetid toward morning.

Cold sweat, often only on the forehead; or, general cold sweat; with anxiety.

⁴¹ **Attacks.** Autumn: 20.

⁴² **Sides.** Right: 28, 33. Left: 22, 32. Above downward: 12.

⁴⁴ **Tissues.** Buboes.

Swelling of glands.

Necrosis of the upper jaw.

Drawing in the periosteum, with heat in the head; inflammation of the periosteum. Swelling and tenseness, rapid progress of disease. θ In osteo-myelitis.

General anasarca; face red and swollen. θ Morbus Brightii.

⁴⁵ **Contact, Injuries, etc.** Worse from touch: 17, 19.

⁴⁶ **Skin.** Burning and redness of the skin, with the formation of small vesicles.

Grey color of the nails,

Severe and stubborn eczema of the sweating parts of the body exposed to the fumes of the poison.

Condylomata.

Rash of secondary syphilis.

Ulcers which perforate or become phagedenic.

⁴⁸ **Relationship.** *Merc. subl.* antidoted by *Silic.*

MERCURIUS IODATUS FLAVUS.

Protoiodide of mercury.   AMERICA PROVER'S UNION.

[1] **Mind.**   Lively, talkative, good-natured.

Destructive mood.

Anxiety, low-spiritedness, etc., retard the action of remedy.

[2] **Sensorium.**   Dizzy: when reading; when rising from a chair.

[3] **Inner Head.**   Shooting pains in the temples.

Dull headache over the eyes, with pain at the root of nose.

Throbbing pain in the forehead or temples.

Dull, heavy aching at the base of the brain; with 11: 48.

[5] **Eyes.**   Generally, excessive photophobia.

Black motes before the eyes; opacities of the vitreous.

Throbbing, aching, nightly pains.

Keratitis, with ulceration commencing at the corneal margin; with 11.

[6] **Ears.**   Sudden, sharp pains in the ear.

Throbbing, boring, from within outward, deep in left ear.

[7] **Nose.**   Septum nares sore; sharp pains.

Much mucus descends into the throat, causing hawking; spots in nose feel sore; constant inclination to swallow.

[8] **Face.**   Dull aching and soreness in bones of the face; also in jaws.

[10] **Teeth.**   Molar teeth feel too long; worse bringing them together.

Grinding and drawing pains in teeth; wants to press them together.

Stiffness of the jaws.

[11] **Tongue, etc.**   Tongue coated: thick yellow at the base; bright yellow at the back part, tips and edges red (with many affections).

[12] **Mouth.**   Mouth, lips and tongue dry and sticky.

[13] **Throat.**   Throat dry, with frequent, empty swallowing.

Easily detached patches on the inflamed pharynx and fauces; ∎ worse on the right tonsil; salivary glands much swollen; fetid discharge; with 11.

Much tenacious mucus in throat; hawking causes gagging.

Sensation of a lump in the throat.

[14] **Desires.   Aversions.**   Appetite variable; disgust at seeing food.

Excessive thirst; occasionally for acid drinks.

[16] **Nausea and Vomiting.**   Nausea, faintness, with dizziness and suffocation about the heart.

[17] **Stomach.**   Weak, empty feeling at the stomach, nausea.

Bruised, burning pain at the stomach.

Cutting pains, with nausea and inclination to vomit.

[18] **Hypochondria.** Stitches in region of liver, better by pressure with hand; pains about liver, right side of chest and back; soreness under right scapula, worse motion and at night.

[19] **Abdomen.** Hardness of the abdomen, as from flatulence.

Burning at the umbilicus, as from a hot coal.

Faint, sick feeling in the hypogastrium before stool.

Indolent bubo.

[20] **Stool, etc.** Cutting, colicky pains, followed by diarrhœa, or discharge of fetid flatus; stools thin, light brown, frothy.

Frequent urging to stool.

Black discharges, with or without blood.

Stools tough, like putty, with much straining.

[21] **Urine.** Copious, dark red; scanty.

[22] **Male Sexual Organs.** Copious seminal emissions, preceded by lewd dreams.

Hard chancre (given at once it prevents secondary symptoms).

Painless chancres, with great swelling of inguinal glands, not disposed to suppurate.

[23] **Female Sexual Organs.** Yellow leucorrhœa, especially with children.

[24] **Pregnancy.** Morning sickness.

[25] **Larynx.** Loss of voice, hoarseness.

[27] **Cough.** Loose, rattling cough, bronchi loaded with mucus; sputum copious and yellow.

[28] **Lungs.** Stitches through the right side of the chest.

[29] **Heart. Pulse.** Sharp pains at the heart.

Sudden spasmodic action of the heart.

Pulse weak, irregular and labored.

[31] **Neck. Back.** Neck stiff; soreness in occiput, worse when lying.

Sharp pains in the back.

[32] **Upper Limbs.** Arms stiff and sore, worse when moved.

Arms and hands numb.

[33] **Lower Limbs.** Weariness in the legs, tingling.

Dull, boring pains in the legs, worse at night.

Heavy, laming pains in the calves, with pain in left knee-joint.

Lame feeling in the feet.

[35] **Position, etc.** Exercise generally relieves.

Motion: 32. Rising: 2. Lying: 31.

[36] **Nerves.** Very tired feeling; especially of the limbs.

Faint feeling, worse in church.

[37] **Sleep.** Sleeplessness until 1 A.M.

Dreams are frightful.

[38] **Time.** Night: 5, 33, 37, 46.

39 **Temperature and Weather.** Sensitive to the cold air.
The open air relieves unpleasant sensations.
Worse: in cold, damp weather; in Spring.
40 **Chill. Fever. Sweat.** Chills, with trembling all over.
42 **Sides.** Right: 13, 18, 28. Left: 6, 16, 33. Within outward: 6.
44 **Tissues.** Glands swollen, indurated.
45 **Contact, Injuries, etc.** Pressure: 10, 18.
46 **Skin.** Hard papulæ over the body.
Itching, pricking all over, worse at night.
Bright red, fine eruption on chest and abdomen.
Milk crust in children of syphilitic taint.

MERCURIUS IODATUS RUBER.

Biniodide of mercury. AMERICAN PROVER'S UNION. *Hg* I_2.

1 **Mind.** Dulness of head during coryza; better walking in open air.
Delirium, with increased fever; with ulcers on fauces and tonsils.
Cheerful in evening, after pleasant things happened; merry; though head is worse.
Low-spirited, disposed to cry.
Ill-humor and bad taste on waking in morning.
2 **Sensorium.** Vertigo, during grippe; things seem to reel around her.
3 **Inner Head.** Sensation as if bound by a tight cord, in frontal region.
Beating, throbbing from right of sinciput to vertex.
Headache, with grippe.
Pressure over the eyes.
Headache worse afternoon and evening; dull, stolid.
4 **Outer Head.** Pains in bones of head, chiefly occipital.
Small pustules on the head.
Pannus and old granular eyelids.
5 **Eyes.** Eyes inflamed, burn, water; catarrh; bright light irritates.
6 **Ears.** Hearing dull; better evenings; ears close for a few moments at a time; coryza.
Earache in right ear.
Itching in ears.
Ear-wax increased.
Swelling of parotid and neighboring glands.
7 **Nose.** Coryza and dull hearing, better getting warm by walking.

Right side of nose hot, swollen with coryza.

Much sneezing, with running from the nose.

Whitish-yellow, or bloody discharge; affection of posterior nares, with raw sensation; nasal bones diseased; turbinated bones swollen.

Hawks mucus from posterior nares.

Crusty eruption on wings of nose.

8 Face.   Aching in left cheek and eye.

Scabs on the face, right side.

9 Lower Face.   Pain in jaws and temples.

Eczema rubrum on chin.

10 Teeth.   Gums swollen, toothache, glands swollen; boil in the mouth, sleepless; alternately melancholic and cheerful; in periodic spells.

11 Tongue, etc.   Taste: slimy on awaking; bitter; metallic.

Tongue dry, wants to wet the mouth.

Scalded feeling on tongue (one hour after breakfast), small blister on point.

Tongue furred, with grippe.

Aphthæ on the tongue.

12 Mouth.   Profuse saliva, mouth full; teeth of lower jaw ache; metallic taste.

Soreness of middle of inside of left cheek.

13 Throat.   Hawks much; spits a tough, white phlegm.

Sensation of a lump in throat, with disposition to hawk it out; hawked up a hard, greenish lump.

Sticking in the throat.

On waking, throat sore; feels scalded, worse during empty swallowing.

Left tonsil swollen; fauces dark red; ▮ diphtheritic patches, submaxillary glands painfully engorged.

Slight superficial ulcers in the throat, in patches.

Difficult deglutition, with ulcers in the throat.

Tonsils suppurating.

Worse from empty swallowing. θ Diphtheria.

Velum long, seemingly causing the cough; left tonsil inflamed.

14 Desires. Aversions.   Desire to drink but small quantities.

Inclination to have the food more salted.

15 Eating and Drinking.   Heart-burn after dinner.

16 Nausea and Vomiting.   Loud and bitter belching.

Nausea and sore throat.

Nausea and sinking at the stomach, or in the epigastrium, with a general sick feeling.

Nausea while passing a diarrhœic stool.

18 Hypochondria.   Aching and full feeling in right hypochondrium.

Sudden cutting pain in the region of the liver.

Heavy, painful feeling in region of liver, pancreas and spleen.

¹⁹ **Abdomen.** Distended abdomen about the navel, with pain at that part on pressure.

Colic, followed by stool·

Uneasy sore feeling all over bowels.

²⁰ **Stool, etc.** Stool copious, yellow-brown, somewhat watery and coated with mucus, and slightly bloody; preceded by griping and colicky pains; urging and slight tenesmus remained afterwards.

Inveterate piles.

²¹ **Urine.** Increased flow of urine.

Frequent desire to urinate, she cannot hold her water for a moment.

Urine: thick and dark when passing; red.

Ulcers in the bladder.

²² **Male Sexual Organs.** Sexual desire, particularly on going to sleep.

Nocturnal emissions.

Sensitiveness of right testicle and cord.

Hard, red swelling of front of prepuce and painless, hard chancre in the centre.

❙Sarcocele of left testicle.   θ Syphilis.

❙Bubo, discharging for years.   Indolent chancre.

²⁵ **Larynx.** Complete loss of voice.

Hoarse and husky shortly after getting a little wet in an evening shower.

Patches of inflammation livid, purple; thin, offensive discharge.

Swelling of bronchial glands; subacute processes arising from the influence of cold or atmospheric variations.

²⁷ **Cough.** From elongated uvula; with sore throat; with a little loose, whitish, slimy sputum.

Grippe, with fever, headache, giddiness, furred tongue; sweat in bed.

Profuse yellow sputa.

²⁸ **Lungs.** Awoke from a transient feeling of great soreness in whole breast.

Constriction across the chest.

Catching pain under right breast, oppressing the breathing.

²⁹ **Heart. Pulse.** Sharp cutting pain in chest and sticking pain in the heart.

³⁰ **Outer Chest.** Sticking in muscles of ribs, left side, after walking out during thawing weather.

³¹ **Neck. Back.** Swollen glands on neck, with toothache, scarlatina, etc.

Spine sore or painful.

³² **Upper Limbs.** Rheumatic pains in shoulder-joint.

Axillary glands suppurate.

Dull, aching, strained sensation in middle of os humeri, as if about to break.

Rheumatic pains, soreness, stiffness in left arm, worse by motion.

Palm of left hand cracked, horny, several oozing rhagades.

33 Lower Limbs. Aching pains from hip to ankles, as though she had walked many miles, felt more in the bones.

Weakness of knee-joints.

Pains from calves up to the sacrum.

Insupportable pain and aching in legs toward evening, better on moving.

Violent tearing in soles; feet swollen, sore to touch, worse around ankles; after washing the floor.

34 Limbs in General. Rheumatic pains, now here, now there, mostly muscular; alternately in arms and hands, legs and feet; violent pain like otalgia in left ear.

35 Position, etc. Motion: 32, 33. Walking: 30; in open air: 1.

36 Nerves. Weary, especially with rheumatic pain in forearm; bruised feeling.

37 Sleep. Drowsy 8 P.M.; also deep sleep every afternoon.

Toothache on going to sleep.

Insomnia, with ulcerated throat.

Restless from 12 P.M. till morning, with constriction in diaphragm.

Dreams: of swimming; gunning; traveling; lascivious.

On awaking: ill-humor; dull head; slimy taste; throat sore; pain in chest.

33 Time. Morning: 1. Afternoon: 3, 37. Evening: 1, 3, 6, 25, 33, 37. Night: 40. Midnight till morning: 37.

39 Temperature and Weather. Getting warm walking: 7. In bed: 27. Getting wet: 25. Cold, wet weather: 30. Cold on changes of weather: 25. After washing a floor: 33.

40 Chill. Fever. Sweat. Chilly at bedtime.

Intense shivering, followed by feverishness; chilly, followed by flush over face.

Flush of heat and feeling of being tickled.

Fever, with grippe.

Sweats at night in bed. θ Grippe.

Copious night-sweats; hot sweat.

After scarlatina, ulcers in fauces.

42 Sides. Right: 3, 6, 7, 9, 18, 22, 28. Left: 8, 13, 22, 30, 32, 34. Above downward: 33. Below upward: 33.

45 Contact, Injuries, etc. Touch: 33, 46.

46 Skin. Small fissures and cracks.

Hard papules here and there.

Hunterian chancre (given at once, it prevents secondary symptoms).

Pustules, inflamed base, sore to touch; itching slightly, scab over, but pus oozes.

Syphilitic ulcers.

Lupus.

[48] **Relationship.** *Mercur. bi-iod.* follows well after *Bellad.* in scarlatina.

Merc. præc. rub. is preferable for leaden heaviness in occiput, with otorrhœa.

MEZEREUM.

Daphne mezereum.   E. STAPF.   *Thymelaceæ.*

[1] **Mind.** Easily confused, unable to recollect; thinking is difficult.

Restless when alone, longs for company.

Apprehensiveness felt at the pit of stomach, as when expecting unpleasant news.

Hypochondriacal, with low spirits and weeping.

Indifference to everything and everybody.

Angry at trifles: is soon sorry for it.

Irresolute.

[2] **Sensorium.** Head feels dull, or as if drunk; better after meals.

[3] **Inner Head.** Headache in temples and sides of head after exertion and from talking much.

Violent headache with great sensitiveness to the least contact after slight anger.

Headache with dulness, worse in the open air.

Headache relieved by stooping.

Sensation as if the upper part of the head were pithy.

[4] **Outer Head.** Head covered with a thick, leathery crust, under which pus collects and mats the hair. ·

Elevated, white, chalk-like scabs, with ichor beneath; breeding vermin.

Burning, biting, itching on scalp, worse on vertex; scratching changes locality; but increases the itching, sore boils follow, worse at night and when lying down.

Cranial bones pain, are swollen and sensitive to cold or contact; worse from motion and in the evening; caries; itching, burning of scalp.

Scalp numb, with drawing pain, generally only on one side; worse from cold, contact, and in the evening.

Hair covered with scurf, hair comes out in handfuls; scalp and face itch violently, worse when warm; white scales; desquamation; pityriasis.

⁵ **Eyes.** Staring at one spot; vacant look.

Inclination to wink.

Dryness in the eyes, with pressure in them; they feel too large.

Annoying twitching of the muscles of left upper lid.

Lachrymation, with smarting in the eyes.

Ciliary neuralgia, especially after operations on the eye.

⁶ **Ears.** Feels as if too open, and as if air were pouring into them; or, as if the tympanum were exposed to the cold air, with a desire to bore with the fingers into the ear.

Chronic diffuse otitis.

Itching behind the ears, scratching causes small elevations, when scratched off the spots feel sore.

⁷ **Nose.** Ineffectual irritation to sneeze.

Sneezing: with coryza; with sore pain in the chest.

The sense of smell diminished, with dryness of the nose.

Twitching (visible) on the root of the nose.

Fluent coryza, soreness of and scabs in the nose; soreness and burning of the upper lip.

Constant excoriation of the nose.

⁸ **Face.** Grey, earthy complexion.

Face swollen, burning pains, confluent vesicles; nares closed; erysipelas bullosum.

Child continually scratches the face, which is covered with blood; face and forehead hot and red; restlessness; irritability; itching worse at night; it tears off the scabs, leaving spots, on which fat pustules form. The ichor from scratched face excoriates other parts.

Prosopalgia, left-sided; from over eye to eyeball, cheek, teeth, neck and shoulder; lachrymation; conjunctiva injected, parts sensitive to touch.

Neuralgic pains come quickly, and leave the part numb, worse from warmth.

Intolerable nightly burning pains in abscess of the antrum of Highmore; periosteum more affected than the bones, with dull, crampy pain referred to malar bone, with anguish, pale face, chilliness or cold sweat.

Facial muscles drawn tense.

Frequent, troublesome, muscular twitchings of the right cheek.

⁹ **Lower Face.** Honey-like scabs about the mouth.

Neuralgia of inframaxillaris.

Chin covered with elevated, white scabs.

¹⁰ **Teeth.** Boring and stinging toothache, which extends to malar bones and temples; chilliness.

The teeth feel dull and elongated.

The teeth decay suddenly, on the side, above the gums.

The tartar on teeth becomes rough.

Toothache worse at night; when touched with the tongue; better with mouth open, and from drawing in air.

[11] **Tongue, etc.**   Thick, white coating on the tongue, with large, red, elevated papillæ; middle fissured.

Dark redness of the fauces; burning dryness even into larynx; worse every winter; syphilis.

[12] **Mouth.**   Burning in the mouth and throat.

Saliva almost always increased.

Breath smells like rotten cheese.

[13] **Throat.**   Dry feeling in throat; some difficulty in swallowing; constant chilliness, even in bed.

Burning of the pharynx and œsophagus.

Constriction of the pharynx, the food presses on the part during deglutition.

Sensation as if the posterior part of the throat were full of mucus, the same after hawking.

[14] **Desires.   Aversions.**   Canine hunger noon and evening. Wants ham fat; coffee, wine.

Appetite poor.

[15] **Eating and Drinking.**   Beer tastes bitter, causes vomiting. Generally worse from wine.

After meals: 2.   Eating: 17; or drinking: 27.

[16] **Nausea and Vomiting.**   Nausea in throat and stomach; vomit bitter, sour; slimy.

[17] **Stomach.**   Burning and uneasiness in stomach; relieved by eating; canine hunger at noon and evening.

[18] **Hypochondria.**   Dull pain in region of spleen; hardness and swelling with pressive pain.

[20] **Stool, etc.**   Many discharges of fetid flatus, more before stool.

Stool: soft, brown, sour, fermented; contains glistening bodies; undigested; worse in the evening; also from suppressed eruption.

During stool prolapsus recti; anus becomes painful and constricted about the fallen rectum.

Painful constriction, tearing and drawing at the anus, perineum and through urethra; fissure of anus.

Stool dark brown, hard balls, much but painless straining.

[21] **Urine.**   Sticking in the kidney and pain as if torn.

In morning and forenoon frequent and copious discharges of pale urine.

Secretion of urine diminished.

Urine becomes flaky and has red sediment.

Hæmaturia preceded by crampy pain in bladder.

[22] **Male Sexual Organs.**   Violent erections and increased sexual desire.

Testicles swollen.

Painless swelling of scrotum.

Heat and swelling of the penis.

Fine, prickling stitches in penis and at summit of glans.

Discharge of watery mucus; stinging and titillating through the whole urethra and perineum; urethra sore to touch. θ Gonorrhœa.

²³ **Female Sexual Organs.** Menses: too soon, profuse and long-lasting; scanty, with leucorrhœa and prosopalgia.

Uterine ulcer, with smarting, burning, or prickling sensation; discharge albuminous, sometimes tinged with blood.

Leucorrhœa, like the white of an egg; corroding.

²⁵ **Larynx.** Voice failing or interrupted.

Burning and dryness in the trachea, with hoarseness.

²⁶ **Breathing.** Dyspnœa, as if from adhesions, or contraction of lungs.

On stooping, chest feels too tight.

Desire to take a long breath.

²⁷ **Cough.** Spasmodic, caused by irritation from larynx to chest; sputa in the morning, of yellow, viscid mucus, tasting saltish, or like an old catarrh. θ Whooping-cough.

Cough worse: evening until 12 P.M., or day and night, with tension over thorax; when eating or drinking anything hot, must cough until food is vomited; from beer.

²⁸ **Lungs.** Stitches in right side of chest, worse drawing a long breath.

Cramp-like contraction over both chest and back.

²⁹ **Heart. Pulse.** Pulse full, hard, accelerated evenings; at times intermittent; frequent mornings, slow evenings.

³¹ **Neck. Back.** Pain from stiffness of nape and external cervical muscles.

Rheumatic pains in scapular muscles; they feel tense and swollen, preventing motion.

³² **Upper Limbs.** Pain in shoulder-joint, as if it would be torn asunder.

Sore feeling in the right axilla.

Right hand cold, left warm; or, both cold.

Trembling of the right hand.

Finger-ends powerless, cannot hold anything.

Hands "go to sleep."

³³ **Lower Limbs.** Twitching pain from hip-joint to the knee.

Right hip-joint feels sprained on walking.

Pain in the hip, the leg is shortened.

Cracking in the right knee, when rising in the morning.

Drawing pains, sensation of internal heat of limb, surface being cool; better in open air.

The legs and feet "go to sleep."

Stitches in the toes of the right foot.

Pain in the periosteum of the long bones, especially the

tibiæ, worse at night in bed, and then the least touch is
intolerable; worse in damp weather. θ Syphilis.

[35] **Position, etc.**   Motion: 4, 31.   After exertion: 3.   Stooping: 3.   Rising: 33.   Lying: 4.

[37] **Sleep.**   Great inclination to sleep, from debility.

Sleep disturbed by violent pain in the face.

Awakens after midnight, from vivid dreams and with
nightmare; worse on awaking.

[38] **Time.**   Morning: 21, 27, 29, 33.   Forenoon: 21.   Noon :
14.   Evening: 4, 14, 27, 29.   Night: 4, 8, 10, 27, 33,
46.   After night: 37.   Day and night: 27.

[39] **Temperature and Weather.**   Better walking in the open
air; yet sensitive to cold air or to cold washing in the
morning.

Better wrapping up the head and keeping in a dark room.
θ Prosopalgia.

Warmth: 4, 8, 40.   In bed: 13, 33, 46.   Cold: 4.   Open
air: 3, 33, 40.   Damp weather: 33.   Drawing air in
mouth: 10.   Winter: 13.

[40] **Chill. Fever. Sweat.**   Chill from upper arms to back
and legs.   Chill of single parts as if dashed with cold
water.

Chill even in warm room, drowsy; lessened out-doors;
thirst; back of the mouth dry; much saliva in forepart; cramp in the chest, an asthmatic constriction and
oppression.

Hands and feet cold, nails blue, hot sensation on small
spot on top of head.

External coldness, great thirst, no desire for warmth, no
dread of open air; no subsequent heat.   Chill lessened
by heat.

Heat in bed, mostly in head, one-sided (left) heat.

Burning of internal parts, with external chilliness.

Intense heat, after chill, with sleep.

Sweat during sleep, following the chill.   Skin dripping
with cold sweat.

[42] **Sides.**   Right: 8, 28, 32, 38.   Left: 5, 8, 18, 32, 40.

[44] **Tissues.**   Emaciation of face, or of diseased parts.

Joints feel bruised, weary as if they would give way.

Cystic osteoma, burning pains, swelling; worse at night.

Bones inflamed, swollen, especially shafts of cylindrical
bones; caries; after abuse of mercury; feel distended.

Soreness and burning in bones of thorax.

[45] **Contact, Injuries, etc.**   Touch: 3, 4, 8, 10, 22, 33, 43.
Scratching: 6, 8, 46.   Boring with finger: 6.

[46] **Skin.**   Roughness and scaling here and there; skin of hands
rough and dead.

Violent itching, worse in bed, from touch; burning and
change of place after scratching.

Eczema itching intolerably, copious serous exudation.

Ulcerative eruption on finger-joints, itching most at night.

Brownish miliary rash on chest, arm and thighs.

Vesicles form a brownish scab.

Pruritis senilis, intolerable itching.

Ulcers, areolæ sensitive; easily bleeding; painful at night; pus under scabs; burning vesicles around ulcers.

Scabs thick, lamellated, like rupia, bloody secretion beneath; worse on parts devoid of fat.

Neuralgia and burning after zona.

Vesicular erysipelas.

Scurf-like fish-scales on back, chest and thighs and scalp.

[47] **Stages and States.** Phlegmatic temperature.

[48] **Relationship.** Antidotes to *Mezer.: Calc. carb.* (headache); *Nux vom.* (neuralgia of eye); *Mercur.*

Mezer. is frequently indicated against bad effects of *Mercur.; Nitr. ac.; Phosphor.;* spirituous liquors.

MILLEFOLIUM.

Yarrow.   HARTLAUB.   *Compositæ.*

[1] **Mind.** Anxious, with pain in the heart.

Melancholy, sadness.

Much excited, with pains in pit of stomach.

[2] **Sensorium.** Stupefied, intoxicated.

Confused, dull, especially evenings, knows not what he is about nor what he ought to do; seems constantly as if he had forgotten something.

[3] **Inner Head.** Congestion to head; when stooping in evening; at night a stream from chest to head, like a gust of wind, with nosebleed.

Slight throbbing in arteries of head and face.

Fulness in head after siesta.

Dull pain in vertex.

Sensation in right side of head as if screwed together.

Hemicrania.

Violent headache, so that he strikes head against the bedpost or wall; twitching of eyelids and frontal muscles.

Occipital headache: dull toward evening.

Piercing or thrusts in head, vertex, over eye, occiput, side of head.

Headache worse; stooping; on awaking.

[5] **Eyes.** Like a mist before eyes, not near the eyes, but at a distance.

Eyes brilliant.

Inward piercing, pressing in eyes to root of nose and sides of forehead.

Sensation of too much blood in eyes.

Spots on the eyes.

Fistula lachrymalis; lachrymation and discharge from the eyes.

⁶ **Ears.** Noise in left ear causes her to start with fright; later, when laughing, sensation as of cold air passing out.

Sensation as if the ears were stopped up, after dinner.

Darting in left ear.

⁷ **Nose.** Nosebleed: in congestions to the chest and head; excessive.

Piercing pain from eyes to root of nose.

⁸ **Face.** Sensation of heat as if blood was rising to the head.

Tearing: in face to temples; from right lower jaw to ear, then teeth; contortions of face.

¹⁰ **Teeth.** Rheumatic toothache, with diseased gums.

Gum-boil.

¹² **Mouth.** Thirst, mouth dry.

Putrid sore mouth; stomacace, ulcerated gums.

¹³ **Throat.** Uvula relaxed; also tonsils; asthenic catarrh.

Rough feeling in the throat.

Dull piercing pains, right, then left-sided.

Ulceration of the throat; pain in left side of throat when swallowing.

¹⁷ **Stomach.** Painful gnawing and digging in stomach as from hunger.

Pain in stomach as if empty, mornings after waking.

Sensation of fulness in the stomach.

Cramp in stomach, with sensation as of a liquid moving from stomach to intestines, toward anus.

Great pain in pit of stomach, from suppressed variolous pustules; pain after confluent variola.

¹⁸ **Hypochondria.** Pain in region of liver, at beginning of cartilage of twelfth rib; also below.

Piercing in right lower ribs.

¹⁹ **Abdomen.** Wind colic in the hysterical or hypochondriacal; colic during menstruation.

Incarcerated hernia.

Ascites.

²⁰ **Stool, etc.** Bloody dysentery, tenesmus; during epidemics of dysentery; bloody flux after much exertion.

Violent colic, bloody diarrhœa during pregnancy.

Chronic blenorrhœa from atony of mucous membranes; great pain.

Hemorrhoids; profuse flow of blood.

Ascarides.

Offensive flatus.

[21] **Urine.** Pain in region of left kidney, then bloody urine. Involuntary micturition.

Urine bloody; blood forms a cake in the vessel.

Catarrh of bladder from atony.

Stone in bladder, with retention of urine; bloody urine.

Pus-like discharge, after lithotomy.

[22] **Male Sexual Organs.** Want of ejaculation when cohabiting. Gleet.

Swelling of penis and testicles.

[23] **Female Sexual Organs.** Menses: suppressed, with pain in stomach; epilepsy; cough, with bloody sputum; excessive flow, lasts too long; also with colic pains.

Uterine hemorrhages after great exertion.

Leucorrhœa of children from atony of vaginal mucous membrane.

[24] **Pregnancy.** During pregnancy, cramp-like affections.

Barrenness, with too profuse menses.

Lochia too copious.

Lochia suppressed; violent fever, no milk, convulsive twitchings; great pains.

Nipples sore.

[27] **Cough.** With frequent spitting of bright blood; oppression of chest, palpitation; in phthisis; in suppressed hemorrhoids; suppressed menses; checked lochia.

Repeated bronchorrhagia; especially in phthisis; or after a fall.

Blenorrhœa of the lungs.

[28] **Lungs.** Oppression of chest, frequent blood-spitting; piercing pains, stinging, bruised feeling; worse under left shoulder-blade. *θ* Phthisis pulmonalis.

[29] **Heart. Pulse.** Excessive palpitation and bloody sputum.

Ebullitions from coughing blood.

Pulse accelerated and contracted.

[32] **Upper Limbs.** Fine piercing pain in left scapula, in breathing when standing.

Left arm frequently feels as if going to sleep.

Hot hands.

[33] **Lower Limbs.** Right tendo-achillis pains as after a blow or sprain.

First left, then right foot goes to sleep; disappearing on walking.

Hot feet.

[34] **Limbs in General.** Piercing pains, drawing, tearing.

[35] **Position, etc.** Stooping: 3. Exertion: 23. Standing: 22. Walking: 33.

[36] **Nerves.** Convulsions during teething; after labor.

[37] **Sleep.** Yawning, without any weariness.

Congestion from chest to head, like a stream, while asleep.
Falls asleep late, unrefreshed in morning.

38 Time. Morning: 17, 37.   Evening: 2, 3.   Night: 3.

40 Chill.   Fever.   Sweat.   Chilliness, with pains in kidneys.
Fever from suppressed itch.
Colliquative sweats.

42 Sides.   Right: 3, 8, 18, 33.   Left: 6, 13, 21, 28, 32.   Right to
left: 13.   Left to right: 33.   Below upward: 3.   Above
downward: 17.

44 Tissues.   Congestions.
❙ Hemorrhages florid.
Painful varices during pregnancy.
Mucous discharge from atony.

45 Contact, Injuries, etc.   Wounds which bleed profusely;
especially from a fall.
Sprains; effects of overlifting or overexertion.

46 Skin.   Countless vesicles, size of a pea, offensive secretion.
Stomachic pains from suppressed small-pox.

47 Stages and States.   For the aged; atonic; for children and
women.

48 Relationship.   *Millef.* is said to antidote *Arum mac.*
Coffee drunk after *Millef.* causes congestion to head.
Erechthites is a rival of *Millef.* in bright red epistaxis and
in hæmoptysis.
Sen. aur. is excellent in hæmaturia; renal pains with
nausea.

MURIATICUM ACIDUM.

Hydrochloric acid.   HAHNEMENN.   *HCl.*

1 Mind.   Unconsciousness.   Moaning.
Taciturnity.   Introverted and quiet.
Sitting quiet, sad and silent, with anxious care about the
future.
Irritable, disposed to anger and chagrin.   Peevishness.
Restlessness, frequently changing position.

2 Sensorium.   Vertigo: worse moving the eyes; slightly worse
walking, though this relieves headache; with tottering
gait.
Dizzy, nauseated, 1 A.M., worse lying on right side or back
Heaviness in occiput, with obscure sight, worse with effort
to see; also, with swollen glands.

3 Inner Head.   Headache in spells regularly every day, from
9 A.M. until 1 P.M.; begins with soreness over left eye,

then in eyeball and left half of nose, forehead and temple, to back of head.

Headache, as if the brain were torn or beaten to pieces; worse moving the eyes or sitting up in bed; better from moderate exercise.

Headache, as if the brain were clasped by a hand and was being twisted and torn.

Steady, sharp pain in back part of head, with a heavy feeling, as if occiput were filled with lead.

Headache from walking in open air, especially in cold wind.

Distant talking causes headache.

⁴ **Outer Head.** Stiff and sore: in occiput, worse when touched; on left side of head and down spine, worse in lying.

Tearing in the right parietal bone.

Heat on top of head.

Feels as if hair were standing on end.

⁵ **Eyes.** Perpendicular half sight.

Obscured sight; pain in occiput.

Pupils contracted.

Itching, smarting in canthi.

Lids red, swollen.

Stitches out of the eyes.

Worse from light, better in the dark.

⁶ **Ears.** Hardness of hearing; loud cracking sounds during the night; no cerumen; dryness, peeling off in scales; worse right ear.

Distant sounds cause headache; sound of voice unbearable.

Want of feeling in the internal meatus.

Tingling, humming, whizzing in the ear.

Beating or knocking in the ear.

Otalgia, with pressing pain.

Tingling, creeping, cold pain, running from ears up to top of head, sharp boring in temporal regions.

Dark ear-wax, with buzzing.

⁷ **Nose.** Long-lasting nosebleed.

Nosebleed. θ Whooping-cough.

Coryza thin, acrid, making parts sore.

Coryza, with thick yellow discharge.

Discharge of thin pus from nose, excoriating the parts.

Nose stopped up.

⁸ **Face.** Heat in face, glowing red cheeks when walking in open air; no thirst.

Sudden red face, with coma. θ Scarlatina.

Red pimples on forehead, cheeks and around mouth, whole face red; every summer.

Scabs on face, forehead, temples.

Pimples; freckles.

⁹ **Lower Face.**   Lower jaw hangs down.

Pimples around the mouth form a scurf.

Burning lips.

Bloated lower lip; feels heavy, burns.

Pain below left half of lower lip, from 4 P.M. till midnight.

¹⁰ **Teeth.**   Toothache (pulsating) from cold drinks; toothache, with earache.

Tingling toothache; better from warm applications.

Gums swollen, bleeding, ulcerating.

Teeth rise from their sockets.

¹¹ **Tongue, etc.**   Everything tastes sweet.

Taste acrid and putrid, like rotten eggs, with ptyalism.

Tongue heavy as lead, hinders talking; feels lame, sore.

Tongue dwindles.

Tongue sore, bluish; contains deep ulcers: with black bases and vesicles.

¹² **Mouth.**   Stomacace of nursing children; patch on right side of tongue, large and irregular, but very deep; fetid breath.

Stomatitis, with extreme dryness, swollen gums, great adynamia.

Foul breath.   θ Scarlatina.

Mouth as if glued up with insipid mucus; much saliva.

Salivary glands tender, swollen.

¹³ **Throat.**   Rawness and smarting of fauces; burning.

Dry throat, with burning in the chest.

Dark, bluish-red fauces in scarlet fever: 46.

¹⁴ **Desires. Aversions.**   Excessive hunger and thirst.

Aversion to meat.

Morbid longing for alcoholic drinks.

Thirst: 40.

¹⁵ **Eating and Drinking.**   Hiccough (before and after dinner).

Better after drinking.

After eating: worse; diarrhœa.

Cold drinks: 10.

¹⁶ **Nausea and Vomiting.**   Eructations: bitter, putrid.

Vomiting, with belching, coughing; involuntary swallowing; gulping up of contents of stomach into œsophagus, sometimes going down again.

¹⁷ **Stomach.**   Empty sensation in stomach extending through whole abdomen, but no hunger; weak feeling in the stomach from 10 A.M. until evening.

¹⁸ **Hypochondria.**   Pressing and tension in the hypochondria.

¹⁹ **Abdomen.**   Fulness and distention of abdomen, from small quantities of food.

Rumbling and feeling of emptiness.

Cramps in abdomen.

❙ Hernia.

20 Stool, etc. Stool: difficult, as from inactivity of the bowels; too thin, but round; thin, watery, involuntary, while urinating; greenish in typhoid.

Dysentery, blood and slime separated.

Diarrhœa, with much wind; worse morning and evening; with intolerable anal itching, not relieved by scratching; smarting and burning in anus.

As soon as he begins to move, strong urging compelling haste; stools profuse, dark, brown, greenish, gelatinous; followed by dragging, heavy sensation in abdomen.

Piles, suddenly, in children; protruding, reddish-blue, burning; too sore to bear the least touch.

Prolapsus ani while urinating.

21 Urine. Frequent and scanty urination.

Frequent and profuse urination.

Slow emission of urine; bladder weak; must wait a long time before urine will pass; has to press so that anus protrudes.

Urine involuntary.

Urine red, violent; milk-like.

Burning, cutting, while urinating; straining in urethra afterwards.

22 Male Sexual Organs. Organs weak, penis relaxed.

Impotency; desire weak.

Watery, bloody gleet.

Scrotum bluish-red.

Itching of scrotum, not relieved by scratching.

Margin of prepuce sore.

23 Female Sexual Organs. Pressing on genitals, as if menses would appear.

Menses too early and profuse; dejection of spirits, silent, as if she would die; colic; sore piles.

Ulcers on genitals, with putrid discharge, much sensitiveness and general weakness.

Cannot bear least touch, not even of sheet on the genitals.

Leucorrhœa, with backache, sore anus from piles.

24 Pregnancy. Puerperal fever.

25 Larynx. Hoarseness: with sore feeling in the chest; with whooping-cough.

26 Breathing. Breathing deep, groaning; moaning; deep sighing.

Breathing seems to come from the stomach.

Short breath, with rattling after drinking, talking or coughing.

Dyspnœa and constriction of chest. *θ* Whooping-cough.

Oppression across the chest (evening).

27 Cough. Rough, with rattling in chest, followed by cramp in the stomach; short breath; with heat in the face.

Whooping-cough; after the attacks, audible rumbling, gurgling down the chest.

Whooping-cough excited by tickling in chest; in afternoon and evening without, in morning, with a slight dislodgment of a yellow or watery mucus of a fatty taste, and which must be swallowed; sometimes with expectoration of dark blood.

28 Lungs. Stitches in chest, and at heart, when taking a long breath and on violent motion; burning stitches.

Tension and pain on the sternum.

Bursting pain in chest; pain as if beaten.

29 Heart. Pulse. Palpitation of the heart felt in the face.

Stitches in heart.

Pulse slow and weak, sometimes intermitting; slow during day, more frequent at night.

31 Neck. Back. Pressing pain in back, as from a sprain, or as if he had stooped long.

Pressing, drawing, tired pain in lumbar region.

Os coccyx pains.

32 Upper Limbs. Heaviness of the arms, especially forearms.

Scabby eruption on back of hands and fingers.

Numbness, coldness and deadness of fingers at night.

Swelling and burning of tips of fingers.

Itching of palms.

33 Lower Limbs. Wavering gait from weakness of thighs.

Pain in right thigh, with itching in anus.

Œdematous swelling of lower limbs, with shooting pain.

Lower limbs darker colored.

Putrid ulcers on lower extremities, with burning around them.

Cold feet.

Blue feet. θ Scarlatina.

Chilblains (the acid in rum applied externally).

Swelling, redness and burning of tips of toes.

34 Limbs in General. Tearing pains in limbs during rest, better from motion.

All the joints as if bruised.

Pressive drawing in upper arms and knees.

35 Position, etc. Changes position frequently: 1, 40. Moving eyes: 2, 3. Effort to see: 2. Walking: 2, 3, 8. Lying on right side or back: 2, 4. Rising up: 3. Rest: 34, 36. Sitting: 36.

36 Nerves. Prostration and drowsiness all day; she wants to lie about.

Great debility; as soon as he sits down his eyes close; the lower jaws hang down; he slides down in bed.

Paralysis generally one-sided.

Paralyzed tongue and sphincter ani.

42

[37] **Sleep.** Sleepy during day, going off as soon as one moves about.

Sleepless before 12 P.M., delirious tossing, sliding down in bed.

Restless after going to bed, could not sleep before 12 P.M.; groaning, snoring, talking in sleep.

Worse on awaking.

[38] **Time.** Morning: 27, 40. 9 A.M. till 1 P.M.: 3. 10 A.M. till evening: 17. Morning and evening: 20. Afternoon and evening: 27. 4 P.M. till midnight: 9. Evening: 26, 37, 40. Night: 6, 29. After midnight: 2. Night and morning: 40. Day: 29, 36, 37.

[39] **Temperature and Weather.** Aversion to open air: sensitive to cold, damp, stormy, windy weather.

Cold air: 3, 8. Warmth: 10. Every summer: 8. In bed: 40, 46. Wants to uncover: 40, 46.

[40] **Chill. Fever. Sweat.** More chill than heat.

Chill awakens him in the morning.

Evening chill, with coldness in back, external warmth and burning face.

Shivering all over, with hot cheeks and cold hands.

Chill and heat without thirst; rarely, there is thirst in cold stage.

Internal heat, wants to uncover; bodily restlessness.

Heat at night, with palpitation of the heart.

Burning, mostly in palms and soles.

Sweat during first sleep, until 12 P.M., worse head and back.

Night and morning sweats.

Cold sweat on the feet, evening in bed.

Worse when sweating; taciturn; wants to uncover.

Intermittent fever, with periosteal pains.

Typhus: stupid sleep; while awake unconscious; loud moaning; lower jaw dropped; tongue shrunken, dry, like leather; involuntary stools while passing urine; sliding down in bed; bleeding from anus; pulse intermits every third beat.

[41] **Attacks.** Regularly every day from 9 A.M. till 1 P.M.: 3.

[42] **Sides.** Left: 3, 4, 9. Right: 6, 12. Below upward: 6.

[43] **Sensations.** Loss of bodily irritability.

Tearing and stitches through whole body.

[45] **Contact, Injuries, etc.** Touch: 4, 20, 23, 46. Scratching: 20, 22.

[46] **Skin.** Painful putrid ulcers (lower legs), with burning at their circumference.

Eruption of pimples, forming scurfs on forehead, outer ear, lips, hands or back of fingers; itching when getting warm in bed.

Blood-boils, pricking when touched.

Ulcers painful, deep, putrid; covered with scurf.

Black pocks.

Scarlatina: redness intense and rapidly spreading; eruption scanty, interspersed with petechiæ; skin purplish.

[47] **Stages and States.** Black eyes, dark hair.

[48] **Relationship.** Follows well after *Rhus*, *Bryon.*

Mur. ac. antidotes: *Opium.* Cures the muscular weakness following excessive use of opium.

Antidotes to *Mur. ac.* Large doses: carbonate of soda, potassa, lime or magnesia; also, sapo medicinalis. Small doses: *Camphor.*, *Bryon.*

MYRICA CERIFERA.

Wax Myrtle. *Myricaceæ.*

[1] **Mind.** Pleasant exhilaration, succeeded by depression and pressure about the head.

Despondent, dejected, irritable.

Deficient concentrativeness. Dull, drowsy state.

[2] **Sensorium.** Vertigo: with dulness and drowsiness; with rush of blood to head and face, on stooping; with nausea.

[3] **Inner Head.** Awakes with pains in forehead, temples and small of back.

▮ Dull, heavy feeling over and in eyes; drowsiness; jaundice.

[5] **Eyes.** ▮ Congested and yellow.

Feel dull and heavy; also on awaking.

[8] **Face.** Color: ▮ yellow, jaundiced.

Fulness, with heat and throbbing, especially after being out in open air.

[11] **Tongue, etc.** ▮ Thick, yellowish, dark, dry and crusty coating on the tongue, rendering it almost immovable.

Taste: ▮ bad, foul, he cannot eat because of it; bitter, nauseous.

[12] **Mouth.** ▮ Adhesive coating over buccal membrane; dry, scaly crusts on roof of mouth, that water scarcely moistens or dissolves.

▮ Mouth dry, thirst, water relieves only partially and temporarily.

[13] **Throat.** ▮ Stringy, much detached with difficulty; offensive, tenacious mucus in nose and throat.

▮ Pharynx dry, sore as if it would crack, impeding and finally obstructing deglutition.

▮ Slim, glutinous, frothy mucus in the pharynx, even

gargling scarcely detaches it; it causes a disgusting taste, preventing eating.

¹⁴ **Desires. Aversions.** Hunger, yet full feeling as after a hasty meal.

ⅼImagines he cannot eat, hungry, but when food reaches pharynx it is expelled because of a horrid nausea from mucus there.

Loss of appetite, loathing of food.

¹⁷ **Stomach.** Fulness and pressure.

Weak, sinking feeling.

Indescribable feeling of distress in the epigastric region.

¹⁸ **Hypochondria.** ⅼJaundice: fulness of hepatic region and of the upper abdomen; drowsiness, debility; stools mushy, clay-colored. See 5, 8, 11, 21, 46.

¹⁹ **Abdomen.** Griping pains, rumbling, urging to stool, passing only flatus.

Weak, faint feeling as if diarrhœa would ensue.

²⁰ **Stool, etc.** Passes very offensive flatus.

Stools loose, mushy, with tenesmus and cramp-like sensation in the umbilical region.

Stools light yellow; or ⅼmushy, clay-colored; jaundice.

²¹ **Urine.** Urine beer-colored, with yellowish froth; pinkish-brown sediment; scanty.

²⁹ **Heart. Pulse.** Impulse increased, but pulse sixty; pulse feeble, irregular.

³¹ **Neck. Back.** Dull aching, dragging on waking; lassitude, headache.

³⁵ **Positions, etc.** Stooping: 2.

³⁶ **Nerves.** Slight nervous excitement and restlessness; but soon followed by a sick, debilitated sensation that is most characteristic.

³⁷ **Sleep.** Drowsiness, vertigo; semi-stupor.

Restless, or sleeps soundly until towards morning; awakes generally feeling worse.

³⁹ **Temperature and Weather.** Open air: 8, 40.

⁴⁰ **Chill, Fever. Sweat.** Chilliness on going out of doors, slight aching in lumbar region.

Excited, feverish feeling, alternating with chilliness; warm sensation along spine, then chill and gentle sweat.

Face hot and flushed.

⁴⁴ **Tissues.** Catarrh of mucous membrane; mouth, pharynx, bile ducts, etc.

Muscular lameness, lassitude, depressed spirits.

Seems to affect the system profoundly, and has proved curative in low states with or without jaundice, when, with necessary debility, there is a viscous state of the mucous membranes, characterized by scanty, tenacious, crust-forming secretions on the tongue and in mouth and pharynx.

[46] **Skin.** Yellow, jaundiced appearance; itching as from flea-bites.

[48] **Relationship.** Compare: *Digit.* (jaundice), *Chelid.*, *Podoph.*

NATRUM ARSENICATUM.

Sodium arseniate.   GOURBEYRE. $Na_3\ As\ O_4\ 12H_2\ O.$

Hom. Mat. Med. Club of Allegheny Co., Pa.

[1] **Mind.** Nervous restlessness.

Cannot concentrate mind; dull, listless. Forgetful.

[2] **Sensorium.** Confused feeling; head heavy, dull.

Feeling of heat and fulness in whole head.

[3] **Inner Head.** Dull aching in frontal region on awaking in morning; severe during day; indisposed to study or speak.

Aching across brow over orbits and in eyeballs.

Fulness in forehead, with throbbing in top of head.

Every motion jars the head.

[5] **Eyes.** Vision weakened from his condition of health; objects blur when he looks at them for a short time; eyes sensitive to light.

Eyes soon tire and pain when he reads or writes.

Feels as if must close lids to protect the weak eyes.

Lids disposed to close; cannot open them as wide as usual.

Blood-vessels of balls and lids much congested, whole orbital region swollen. Œdema of orbital region, especially of supraorbital.

Congestion of conjunctiva from least exposure to cold or to wind. Conjunctiva dry, painful.

Eyes smart as from wood smoke. Smarting and lachrymation on going into open air.

❙ Inner surface of (lower) lids granular.

❙ Lids agglutinated on awaking, mornings; edges chronically inflamed.

Aching through and over brows and orbits and in temples on awaking.

❙ Eye symptoms worse in the morning.

[7] **Nose.** Smell defective or lost.

❙ Patient feels stuffed up (nose and chest; clinical).

Nose constantly stopped up, worse at night and in morning; must at night breathe with mouth open.

❙ Nasal discharge yellow, tough; hawks it also from posterior nares. Mucus drops from posterior nares.

❙Pieces of hardened, bluish mucus flow from nose, after which mucous membrane feels raw.

❙Dry crust in nose, when removed blood follows.

Nasal mucous membrane thickened, can inhale air, but difficult to exhale.

❙Compressive pain at root of nose and in the forehead; catarrh.

⁸ **Face.** Flushed and hot; feels puffed.

Malar bones feel large, as if swollen.

Swollen, œdematous, more orbital region, worse mornings on awaking.

⁹ **Lower Face.** Corners of mouth fissured; also indurated.

Muscles of mastication stiff, painful to move jaw.

¹¹ **Tongue, etc.** Furred; coated yellow; deep red, corrugated, anterior part fissured; large, moist, fissured, flabby.

¹³ **Throat.** Fauces: dry on swallowing and on inspiration, worse A.M., and after a cold. Fauces and pharynx look red and glassy.

❙Tonsils, fauces and pharynx purplish and œdematous; patched with yellow mucus. θ Diphtheria.

Uvula, tonsils and pharynx thickened; surface irregular, swollen, purplish-red, covered with yellowish-grey mucus, which is hawked out.

¹⁴ **Desires. Aversions.** Appetite excessive.

Drinks often, but little at a time; very thirsty but worse drinking.

¹⁶ **Nausea and Vomiting.** Belching and sour eructations.

Nausea, worse from cold drink of water. Vomits large quantities of sour water, worse after eating.

¹⁷ **Stomach.** Feels sore, warm things cause a sensation of burning, and can be felt entering stomach. Moderate dinner lies heavy; feeling of fulness.

Epigastrium tender; worse just below ensiform.

Sinking sensation in epigastrium, with dull feeling in supraorbital and frontal regions.

¹⁹ **Abdomen.** Gas forms rapidly, worse only when bowels move, colic from flatus and before stool.

²⁰ **Stool, etc.** Alternate relaxation and constipation.

Stool: thin, soft, dark, followed by burning at anus; yellowish, watery; copious, painless; hurries him out of bed in A.M., preceded by colic, relieved after. Weak and nervous, hands tremble: 44.

²¹ **Urine.** Dull aching in kidneys, with profuse natural colored urine.

Sore feeling in region of bladder, worse urinating.

Urine: copious, frequent, clear; heat precipitates phosphates; contains a few epithelial scales, a cast, fat globules.

[22] **Male Sexual Organs.** Dull cutting along Poupart's ligaments, followed by sickening sensation in left testicle as
from a blow, testicle very sensitive while pain lasts.

[25] **Larynx.** Mucus scanty, dark, slate-colored and detached
with difficulty.

Roughness, causing hemming, with spasmodic cough.

During morning irritation in bronchi, with slight cough.

[26] **Breathing.** Respiratory sound very indistinct, especially in
lower lobes; percussion normal.

❙ Lungs feel as though smoke had been inhaled.

[27] **Cough.** Dry, hacking from an uneasy feeling and soreness
beneath cartilages right of fourth and fifth ribs, worse
any exertion.

❙ Dry cough, with feeling of tightness and oppression in
middle and upper third of chest.

[28] **Lungs.** Feeling of fulness, oppression and soreness, worse
during exertion and on full inspiration.

Lungs feel full and clogged, worse behind sternum and
from larynx to epigastrium.

Sharp, quick pain below seventh rib, anteriorly.

Supraclavicular regions sore on pressure.

[29] **Heart. Pulse.** Can feel the heart-beat through chest
distinctly.

❙ Oppression about heart on least exertion. θ Diphtheria.

Sounds heard through nearly every part of chest.

Pulse: irregular, variable in volume, slower than usual.

[31] **Neck. Back.** Neck stiff and sore.

Severe pain between scapulæ; he inclines forward for
relief; worse inspiration, it passes gradually around in
front to ninth and tenth ribs.

Soreness at lower cervical vertebræ down to joints of and
under both scapulæ.

[32] **Upper Limbs.** Neuralgic pains from axilla to little finger.

Rheumatic aching in right arm, worse in shoulder and
wrist.

Light, flying pains in fingers, palms and forearm.

[33] **Lower Limbs.** Feel heavy. Weary feeling from ilium
down outer side of thighs to knees, as from too much
exertion. Bruised feeling along left crural nerve, worse
continued motion.

Aching anteriorly down legs, until restless, uneasy feeling
is produced.

Pains shooting from acetabulum to knee, worse moving
about.

Pain, cramp-like, at junction of heads of gastrocnemius
muscle, extending downwards. Cramp in plantar surface of right foot.

[34] **Limbs in General.** Neuralgic pains recur frequently.

Joints feel stiff. Pains erratic, worse in joints and on left side.

[35] **Position, etc.** Motion: 4, 9, 33. Exertion: 27, 28, 29, 33. Quiet: 36.

[36] **Nerves.** Restless, nervous, cannot sit still without great effort.

Feels tired all over; desire to remain quiet.

[37] **Sleep.** Drowsy, heavy.

Restless sleep, when aroused wakes nervously as in affright.

[38] **Time.** Morning: 3. ❙Eyes worse: 5, 7, 8, 13, 20, 25. Day: 3. Night: 7.

[39] **Temperature and Weather.** More susceptible to cold. Cold: 5, 44. Cold water: 16. Open air: 5. Warm from exercise: 46.

[40] **Chill. Fever. Sweat.** Chilly, disposed to wrap up or get near fire.

Chilly at night, then burning, dry heat. Skin hot and dry.

Surface cool, covered with cold, clammy sweat (clinical in diphtheria).

[42] **Sides.** Pains show preference for left leg.

[44] **Tissues.** Mucous membranes affected: sensitive to cold air, dust, etc., they give him cold or aggravate existing cough, etc. Symptoms of subacute gastritis, chronic diarrhœa, nasal catarrh, etc.

Œdema.

Marked emaciation after previous increase in embonpoint.

[45] **Contact, Injuries, etc.** Jarring: 3. Pressure, etc.: 17, 22, 27, 28.

[46] **Skin.** Squamous eruption, scales thin, white and when removed leave skin slightly reddened. If scales remain, they cause itching, worse when warm from exercise.

[48] **Relationship.** Compare: *Arsen.*, *Lycop.*, (stuffed catarrh), *Kali bich.* (nasal catarrh).

NATRUM CARBONICUM.

Sodium carbonate. HAHNEMANN. $Na_2\ CO_3\ 10H_2\ O.$

[1] **Mind.** Inability to think, or to perform any mental labor; the head feels stupefied if he tries to exert himself.

Difficulty in grasping and connecting thoughts, when reading or listening.

Aversion to man and society.

Sadness; depression of spirits; hypochondriacal mood.

Irritable, excitable mood.

Avarice.

Maliciousness.

Restlessness, with attacks of anxiety, especially during a thunder-storm.

Anxiety, trembling and sweat during the pains.

In the evening, restlessness of body, unless he exerts himself mentally.

Affected by playing on piano for short time, with painful anxiety in chest, trembling of body and weariness; must lie down.

² **Sensorium.** Vertigo: from drinking wine, or from mental exertion.

Dulness of the head when at rest or when in the sun.

³ **Inner Head.** Head feels too large.

Tension and obstruction in head, as if forehead would burst.

Frontal headache when turning the head rapidly.

Shooting pain in left frontal eminence, to left lower occiput.

Stitches in the head and out of the eyes.

Pulsating headache in the vertex every morning.

Tearing pain in forehead, returning at certain hours of day.

Stupefying and pressing headache in forehead, with nausea, eructations and dimness of sight, in evening; worse in room.

Headache from the sun.

⁴ **Outer Head.** Pains on the head at certain hours of the day.

⁵ **Eyes.** Black spots before the eyes when writing.

Dazzling flashes before the eyes, on awaking.

Sensation as of feathers before the eyes.

Dim eyes; has to wipe them constantly.

Cannot read small print.

Stitches in the eyes from within outward.

Ulcers on cornea.

Dermoid swellings on conjunctiva.

Inflammation of eyelids, with photophobia.

Heaviness of the upper eyelids.

⁶ **Ears.** Sensitive to noise.

Hard hearing, as if the ears were closed up.

Otalgia, with sharp, piercing stitches in ears.

⁷ **Nose.** Loss of smell and taste, with coryza.

Coryza fluent; violent sneezing; worse at night, when nose is obstructed; worse from least draught of air, or any change of clothing; worse on alternate days; better after sweat.

Thick yellow, or green discharge; nose stopped at night.

Hard fetid clots, from one nostril; nostrils ulcerated, high up.

Humid herpetic eruptions and ulcers on nose, around mouth and on lips.

Peeling off of dorsum and tip of the nose, painful when touched.

Red nose, with white pimples on it.

[8] **Face.** Pale face, with blue rings around the eyes, swollen eyelids.

Burning heat and redness of face, cheeks swollen.

Bloated face.

Yellow blotches on forehead and upper lip.

Freckles in face.

[9] **Lower Face.** Lips swollen and tettery; burning rhagades on lower lip.

[10] **Teeth.** Digging, boring toothache, especially during or after eating sweetmeats or fruit.

Great sensitiveness of the lower teeth.

Nightly pressing toothache, with swelling of lower lips and of gums.

Toothache lessened by smoking.

[11] **Tongue, etc.** Bitter or metallic taste in mouth.

Dry tongue and dislike to talk.

Stuttering on account of heaviness of the tongue.

Burning about tip of tongue, as if it were cracked.

[12] **Mouth.** Saliva generally increased.

Flat ulcers and blisters inside of mouth, burning and painful when touched.

Slight redness of mucous membrane of mouth and fauces, with rawness and scraping; desire to hawk and hem; mucus collects at night, and is hawked up in morning.

Dry mouth and throat, with inclination to drink.

[13] **Throat.** Throat and œsophagus feel rough, scraped and dry.

Accumulation of mucus in throat, and in posterior nares.

Throat painful when swallowing and gaping.

[14] **Desires. Aversions.** Incessant thirst: great desire for cold water a few hours after dinner.

Increased and ravenous hunger in forenoon, from sensation of emptiness in stomach.

Aversion to milk, and diarrhœa from it.

[15] **Eating and Drinking.** Bad effects from a cold drink while overheated.

After milk, diarrhœa.

Cold drink: 18. Drink: 12. Milk: 20. Eating: 19, 20.

After eating: hypochondriacal; weak digestion; pressure in stomach; eructations; distress and tenderness, with palpitation (may also follow abuse of soda-crackers).

[16] **Nausea and Vomiting.** Continuous qualmishness and nausea.

Vomiting of bile, bitter.

[17] **Stomach.** Gnawing and pressure in stomach, better from eating.

Pit of stomach sensitive to touch and when talking.

[18] **Hypochondria.** Stitches in left hypochondrium; worse after drinking very cold water.

Stitches in hepatic and splenic regions (chronic hepatic (inflammation).

[19] **Abdomen.** Colic, with constriction around stomach; or, contraction of navel and hardness of integuments of abdomen.

Hard, bloated, swollen abdomen.

Accumulation of flatus; loud rumbling; swellings here and there as from incarcerated wind.

Flatus changing place and causing pain.

[20] **Stool, etc.** Passes much sour-smelling or fetid flatus; feces escape.

Yellow stools: soft or watery, with violent, sudden urging and tenesmus; watery, yellow, discharged with a gush; worse from milk or after eating, and from taking cold; spotted with blood.

Frequent ineffectual urging to stool, alternately with liquid stools; weak digestion.

Burning and cutting in anus and rectum during and after stool; sexual excitement; costive.

Tape-worm with stool; itching-creeping in anus.

[21] **Urine.** Frequent, urgent, with scanty or profuse discharge.

Urine involuntary at night.

Urine dark yellow, fetid, sour or like horse's urine; deposits a mucous sediment.

Burning in urethra during and after micturition.

[22] **Male Sexual Organs.** Increased sexual desire (priapism).

Inflammation, swelling and easy excoriation of prepuce and glans penis.

Heaviness and drawing in testicles.

The testicles feel bruised.

Prostatorrhœa after urinating and after difficult stool.

[23] **Female Sexual Organs.** Pressure in hypogastrium as if everything would come out; also with indurated cervix uteri and ill-shaped os.

Menses too early and long-lasting; preceded by drawing in nape of neck and headache; accompanied by tearing headache, distended abdomen in morning, relieved by diarrhœa; nervous, cannot bear music; worse in a thunder-storm.

Leucorrhœa thick, yellow, putrid, ceasing after urinating.

[24] **Pregnancy.** Expels moles, prevents false conception.

Labor-pains weak, or accompanied with anguish and sweat, with desire to be rubbed.

[25] **Larynx.** Hoarseness, with roughness of the chest, coryza, chilliness and scraping, painful cough.

[26] **Breathing.** Dyspnœa and shortness of breathing, from tension of the chest.

[27] **Cough.** Violent, dry cough worse when entering a warm room; short, with rattling on chest; with rumbling, incarcerated flatus; with salty, purulent, greenish sputum.

[28] **Lungs.** Stitches in the chest.

Burning, soreness in right chest; loose cough but no sputum; coldness between scapulæ.

[29] **Heart. Pulse.** Painful cracking in region of heart.

Violent, anxious palpitation of heart when ascending, and and at night when lying on left side.

Burning and distress along the spine with palpitation; thinks he has heart disease.

Pulse excited at night with ebullitions.

[30] **Outer Chest.** Chilliness in one (left) side of thorax.

[31] **Neck.   Back.** Cervical glands swollen; also goitre with pressing.

Stiffness of the neck.

Cracking in cervical vertebræ when moving head.

Stitches in small of back while sitting.

Tingling (formication) in back.

[32] **Upper Limbs.** Rheumatic pain of shoulder, arms and elbows, with weakness of arms.

Twitches and twitching sensation in arms and fingers on taking hold of anything.

Cutting pain in hands.

Trembling of hands, morning.

Contraction of fingers.

Swelling of hands in afternoon.

Warts painful to touch.

Tetter on dorsa of hands; skin dry and chapped.

[33] **Lower Limbs.** Tearing and bruised pain in right hip.

θ Dysmenorrhœa.

Heaviness of legs and feet, with tension in them when sitting or walking.

Tension in bend of knee; the muscles are shortened.

Cramp of the calves.

Blotches (as in lepra) on the legs.

The lower legs are swollen, inflamed, red and covered with ulcers.

Cutting pain and cramps in feet.

Swelling of feet and soles of feet, with stinging in them when walking or stepping on them.

Easy dislocation and spraining of ankle; the ankle is so weak that it gives way; foot bends under when stepping on it.

Black ulcerated pustule on the heel.

Ulcer on the heel, arising from spreading blisters.

Smarting and soreness between the toes.

Swelling, tearing and soreness in (big) toes, preventing sleep.

Blisters on the points of the toes, as if scalded.

Boring, drawing and stinging in the corns.

Cold feet.

[35] **Position, etc.** Most symptoms appear while sitting and go off on motion, pressing and rubbing.

Moving head: 31. Turning head: 3. Playing on the piano: 1. Walking: 33. After exertion: 40. Rest: 2. Sitting: 31, 33. Must lie down: 1.

[36] **Nerves.** Great debility from any exertion.

Twitching in the muscles and limbs.

Contractions of muscles, hands, bends of knees, neck, etc.

[37] **Sleep.** Sleepiness during the day. Falls asleep late at night.

Awakes too early in the morning.

During sleep: starts, twitches; vivid dreams, violent erections and sexual excitement; restless, with ebullitions, palpitation and nightmare.

Anxious, confused dreams.

[38] **Time.** Remission before midnight.

Aggravation in the forenoon.

Morning: 3, 12, 23, 32, 37, 40. Forenoon: 14, 40. Afternoon: 32. Evening: 3, 40. Night: 7, 10, 12, 21, 29, 37, 40. Day: 37, 40.

[39] **Temperature and Weather.** Great liability to take cold; aversion to the open air.

Thunder-storm: 1, 23. Draught: 7. Sun: 2, 3. Warm room: 3. Entering a warm room: 27.

[40] **Chill. Fever. Sweat.** Cold and chilly all day, worse in forenoon; hands and feet cold, head hot, or hands and feet hot, with cold cheeks.

Slight evening chilliness, dulness of head; then heat and sleep.

Heat, with general sweat.

Flushes of heat from the nose down the back; irritability; averse to uncovering.

Sweat profuse from every exertion; anxiety.

Burning sweat on the forehead where the hat presses.

Night-sweat, alternating with dry skin.

Morning-sweat.

Cold, anxious sweat.

[41] **Attacks.** Worse during full moon.

Returning at certain hours: 3, 4. Alternate days: 7.

[42] **Sides.** Right side, particularly upper right, lower left side.

Right: 33. Left: 3, 18, 29, 30. Within outward: 3, 5.

⁴⁴ **Tissues.** Emaciation, with pale face, dilated pupils; dark urine.

Swelling and induration of the glands.

⁴⁵ **Contact, Injuries, etc.** Generally better from touch.

Cutting pain, burning and stinging in wounded parts.

Touch: 7, 12, 17, 32. Taking hold of anything: 32.

⁴⁶ **Skin.** Ulcers, with swelling and inflammatory redness of affected parts.

Herpes, with yellow rings, or suppurating

Formication under the skin. Itching all over as from fleas.

Warts ulcerate.

Skin dry, rough and chapped.

⁴⁸ **Relationship.** *Natr. carb.* follows *Sepia* well.

Natr. carb. antidotes *Cinchon.*

Antidotes to *Natr. carb.*: *Camphor, Spir. nitr. dulc.*

Soda sulphite is preferable for yeast-like vomiting, when the tongue is pallid, dirty and broad.

NATRUM MURIATICUM.

Common Salt.   HAHNEMANN.   *Na Cl.*

¹ **Mind.** Difficulty of thinking; absence of mind; memory and will weak.

Distracted, knows not what to say. Awkward in talking, with absent-mindedness.

Sad, weeping; consolation aggravates, with palpitation and intermittent pulse.

When trying to comfort him, he becomes enraged.

Hurriedness, with anxiety; with fluttering at the heart.

Likes to dwell on past unpleasant occurrences.

Hypochondriacal; tired of life.

Gets angry at trifles; hateful, vindicative.

Joyless, indifferent, taciturn.

Religious melancholy.

² **Sensorium.** Weariness in the head.

Empty feeling in the head, with anguish.

Vertigo: when rising from bed in the morning; periodical, with nausea eructations, colic and trembling limbs; nausea and headache; sometimes as if a cold wind were blowing through the head.

³ **Inner Head.** Bursting headache; beating or stitches through to neck or chest; face red; nausea, vomiting.

Violent jerks and shocks in the head.

Throbbing, as from little hammers; awakens with the headache every morning; worse from reading or talking.

Severe headache, maniacal paroxysms, blasphemous; weak; tongue dry; very thirsty; intermittent pulse; caused by getting wet.

Headache from sunrise till sunset, worse at midday; right eye congested; worse from light.

Heaviness in back part of the head; draws eyes together.

Pain, like a nail driven into the left side of the head.

Pressing headache from both sides, as if in a vise.

Rheumatic tearing from the root of the nose to the forehead; nausea, vomiting; vanishing of sight.

Headache in school-girls.

Headaches are worse in the morning on awaking, moving the head or the eyes; mental exertion; warmth; better from sitting still or lying down, and from sweat.

⁴ **Outer Head.** Cold sensation on the vertex; scalp sensitive; spasm of the eyelids.

Hair falls out if touched; mostly on forepart of head, temples and beard; scalp very sensitive; face shining, as if greasy.

Liability to take cold in the head.

Scalp feels constricted: worse talking and in the open air; better sitting or lying.

Dandruff alternating with catarrh and loss of smell.

Scabs on the head and in the axillæ; eczema raw, oozing a corroding fluid, destroying the hair.

Impetigo, worse on boundaries of hairy scalp, especially about nape of neck; eruption glutinous, with thin gummy scabs; skin sore and red.

⁵ **Eyes.** Fiery, zigzag appearance around all objects.

Double vision; or sees only one-half of an object.

Retinal images are retained too long.

Asthenopia, particularly muscular: ∎ drawing, stiff sensation in muscles of eyes when moving them; letters and stitches in sewing run together; aching in eyes when looking intently; often caused by general muscular weakness, or spinal irritation.

Lids heavy when using them.

Amblyopia and amaurosis; pupils contracted, dependent on menstrual disorders in the chlorotic.

Blepharitis, ulcers on cornea when there is smarting, burning; feeling of sand in eyes, mornings; ∎ acrid, excoriating tears; photophobia marked with spasmodic closure of lids.

Ciliary neuralgia, pain above (right) coming on and going off with the sun.

Sharp pain over (right) eye on looking down, with throbbing headache; worse in the evening.

❙Morbus Basedowii, palpitation, short-breathed on least exertion.

Internal recti weak.

❙Stricture of lachrymal duct, fistula and blenorrhœa of lachrymal sac.

Affections of the eyes maltreated with lunar caustic.

⁶ **Ears.** Buzzing, humming or ringing in the ears.

Hardness of hearing.

Painful cracking in the ear, when masticating.

Pulsation and beating; or stitches in the ear.

Discharge of pus from the ears.

Itching behind the ears.

⁷ **Nose.** Loss of smell and taste, especially with catarrh.

Nosebleed when stopping, or when coughing at night.

Liable to catch cold; coryza fluent, alternately with stoppage of the nose; posterior nares dry, with hawking in morning; spasms of sneezing each morning, or ineffectual attemps.

In catarrh, when the secretion is clear mucus.

Nose sore, interior of wings swollen; scabs in the nose.

Left-sided inflammation and swelling of nose; painful to touch.

Nose on one side feels numb.

⁸ **Face.** Face: yellow; pale; livid; swollen; also wan, pasty.

Heat in the face.

Prosopalgia recurring periodically, especially after checked ague; face sallow; great thirst.

Cheek-bones pain as if bruised, when chewing.

One cheek (left) red (afternoon and night).

Skin of face shining, as if greasy.

Itching and eruption of the face (crusta lactea).

Ulcer on the (left) cheek.

Whiskers fall off.

⁹ **Lower Face.** Lips dry, cracked, with rhagades or bleeding scabs; humid sores in the commissures; upper lip swollen.

Crack in the middle of the lower lip.

Blisters like pearls about the mouth; especially in intermittent fevers.

Lips tingle, feel dumb.

Eruptions and ulcers on the chin.

Submaxillary glands swollen.

¹⁰ **Teeth.** Sensitive to air or touch; molars pain when chewing.

Pain, drawing, tearing from teeth to ears and throat, after eating and at night; cheek swollen.

Decayed teeth feel loose, burn, sting and pulsate.

Gums sensitive to warm and cold things; swollen, bleed easily; are putrid.

Epulis.

ı Fistula dentalis.

¹¹ **Tongue, etc.** Taste: saltish, with dry tongue and anorexia; bitter; putrid or sour, while fasting; water tastes putrid.

Loss of taste. θ Catarrh.

Complains much of dryness of tongue, which is not very dry.

Tongue heavy, difficult speech; children slow in learning to talk.

Mapped tongue; looks like ringworm on the sides.

ı Sensation of a hair on the tongue.

Herpes on the tongue, from sea-bathing.

Burning at tip of tongue.

One side of tongue numb and stiff.

Ranula.

Talking: 3, 4, 25.

¹² **Mouth.** Mouth, lips, and especially the tongue dry.

Feels dry but is not.

Blood-blisters on inside of upper lip.

Sore places in mouth very sensitive, even to liquids.

ı Vesicles and ulcers in mouth and on tongue, smarting and burning when touched by food.

Saliva bloody; salivation.

¹³ **Throat.** Feels very dry, yet he constantly hawks transparent mucus.

Mucous membrane looks glazed, but is not granulated.

Sensation of a splinter sticking in the throat.

Feeling as of a plug in throat, with chronic sore throat.

Uvula elongated; muscles so weak "food goes down the wrong way;" also, in post-diphtheritic paralysis.

Only fluids can be swallowed; solids reach a certain point and then are violently ejected.

¹⁴ **Desires. Aversions.** Excessive hunger; canine hunger, especially for supper, with weak body and depressed mind.

Longs for salt or bitter things; wants oysters, fish, milk.

Loss of appetite.

Aversion: to bread, of which she was once fond; to coffee.

Unquenchable thirst, worse evenings.

¹⁵ **Eating and Drinking.** Better on an empty stomach worse after breakfast; feverish; while eating, sweat on the face.

After eating: empty eructations, nausea, acidity in the mouth, sleepiness, heart-burn, palpitation; epigastric pressure and heart radiating upward to the chest.

Bad effects from acid food, bread, fat and wine.

¹⁶ **Nausea and Vomiting.** Acid eructations and malaise, after eating. Water-brash; heart-burn, with palpitation.

Nausea in the morning; weak after even agreeable food.

43

Vomiting first of food, later of bile; oppression of stomach.

¹⁷ **Stomach.** Pit of stomach feels bruised when pressed, with swelling.

Clawing in pit of stomach; cramp, better from tightening clothes.

Great weakness in stomach by spells.

Red spots on pit of stomach.

¹⁸ **Hypochondria.** Dull, heavy aching and distention about liver after eating, lessening as digestion advances.

Stitches in liver; tension; liver inflamed, swollen; skin yellow, earthy. Bending to left causes stiffness in liver.

Stitches and pressure in region of spleen; spleen swollen.

¹⁹ **Abdomen.** Abdomen swollen; rumbling and incarceration of flatus.

Colic, with nausea, relieved by emission of flatus.

Burning in the intestines.

²⁰ **Stool, etc.** Wants to pass wind, but knows not whether flatus or feces escape.

Diarrhœa: chronic, watery; with fever, dry mouth, thirst; also, if worse as soon as he moves about; much fetid flatus; tendency to hang-nails; green, bloody, watery or brownish, mostly during the day; with infarcted scybala.

Involuntary stools.

Alternate constipation and papescent stool.

Constipation from inactivity of the rectum.

Stool hard, difficult or crumbling; anus contracted; anus torn, bleeding, smarting, burning afterward; stitches in rectum.

Passes blood with stool.

Dryness and smarting of rectum and anus.

Hemorrhoids, with stinging pains; moisture oozes from the anus; herpetic eruption about the anus.

²¹ **Urine.** Tension and heat in the renal region.

Frequent or sudden desire to urinate, cannot retain urine; copious flow.

Polyuria, thirst for large quantities of water.

Urine passed involuntary when walking, coughing or laughing.

Has to wait long for urine to pass, especially if others are near him.

Urinal sediment like brick-dust.

Urine dark, like coffee.

During urination, stitches in bladder, smarting, burning in urethra; smarting and soreness in vulva.

After urination, burning and cutting in urethra.

Hæmaturia.

²² **Male Sexual Organs.** Excessive irritability of the sexual instinct, but with physical weakness.

Shortly after coitus, pollution.

After sexual excesses, paralysis.

Erections in the morning, without sexual excitement.

Gleet-like discharge of clear mucus.

Scrotum relaxed, flabby; buttocks emaciated in infants.

Itching, soreness and moisture between scrotum and thighs; pus-like smegma on the glans.

Itching and crawling sensation at the corona glandis.

[23] **Female Sexual Organs.** Averse to coitus, which is painful from dryness of the vagina. Burning, smarting during coitus; anæmic women with dry mouth and dry skin.

Sterility, with too early and too profuse menstruation.

Uterine cramps, with burning and cutting in the groins,

Every morning pressing and pushing toward the genitals. must sit down to prevent prolapsus.

Prolapsus uteri, with aching in lumbar region, better lying on back; also, with cutting in urethra after micturition.

Menses too late and scanty, or too early and profuse.

Before menses: anxious, sad, qualmish; sweetish eructations in the morning; headache; eyes heavy; palpitation. During menses: headache; sadness; colic. After menses: headache.

Dysmenorrhæa, with convulsions (salt sitz-bath).

First menses delayed; amenorrhœa.

Leucorrhœa, acrid, greenish; in morning, transparent, after colicky pains; causes itching; with yellow complexion.

Itching of the external parts, with falling off of the hair.

[24] **Pregnancy.** Labor progresses slowly, pains feeble, seemingly from sad feelings and forebodings.

[25] **Larynx.** Voice weak; exhausted by talking.

Hoarseness, throat sore, dryness in the larynx.

Accumulation of mucus in the larynx (in the morning).

[26] **Breathing.** Breathing, anxious, oppressed; short on walking fast; better in open air and when exercising arms.

Attacks of suffocation.

Breath hot.

[27] **Cough.** Cough from tickling in the throat, or pit of stomach; sputum in morning of yellow or blood-streaked mucus, with bursting pain in forehead, and shocks or beating as of hammers; involuntary urination; stitches in the liver; tears stream down the cheeks.

Cough worse from rapid motion deep inspiration; lying in bed; becoming warm in bed; empty swallowing, drinking; sour food.

Catarrh, with clear, transparent mucus.

Cough, with sputum of bloody mucus.

Dry cough, with rattling on the chest; also with long uvula, worse lying.

[28] **Lungs.** Sensation and pain in chest, as from tension.

Stitches in chest and sides, short breathed, especially during a long inspiration.

Pain like a cutting cramp through left chest to scapula.

[29] **Heart. Pulse.** The heart's pulsations shake the body; also with aching as if a pressure came from abdomen and compressed heart.

Palpitation: anxious, with morning headache; when moving or exerting one's self; when lying on the left side; on going to sleep and on awaking.

Fluttering of heart, with a weak faint feeling, worse lying down.

Irregular intermission of beating of heart and of pulse; worse lying on left side.

Pulse: at times full and slow, at others weak and rapid; intermits every third beat.

[31] **Neck. Back.** Stitches in neck and back part of head.

Painful stiffness of neck.

Throat and neck emaciate rapidly, especially during summer complaint.

Cervical glands sore when coughing; scabs in the axillæ.

Spine oversensitive; tension and drawing; pains better lying on something hard; weak, nervous; fluttering of the heart.

In small of back pain as if bruised, as if lame; stitches, cutting, pulsation.

Feeling in the sacral region as if beaten.

[32] **Upper Limbs.** Sensation of lameness and of a sprain in the shoulder-joint.

The finger-joints move with difficulty.

Involuntary movements of the hands.

Trembling of the hands when writing.

❙Skin of the hands, especially about nails, dry, cracked; hang-nails.

Warts in palms of hands.

Sweaty hands.

[33] **Lower Limbs.** Pain in hip as if sprained, with stitches.

Drawing pain in right thigh, extending to knee.

Tension in bends of limbs, painful contraction of the hamstrings.

Twitching of muscles of thighs.

Drawing pain in knees when sitting.

Stitches in left knee.

Pain as if the knees and ankles were sprained.

Tension in the calves.

Restlessness in the legs, must move them constantly.

Great heaviness: of the legs; of the feet.

Herpes (in the bend of the knee).

Legs feel as if paralyzed, especially the ankles.

Legs hurt after least exertion; tarsal joints feel bruised.

Lame feeling of ankle-joint, while sitting or walking.

Veins of the feet distended.

Cramp-like stitching pain in right foot.

Feet emaciated.

Big toe red, with tearing and stinging on walking or standing.

Burning of the feet, or great coldness.

Suppressed sweat of the feet.

Stitching pains in the corns.

[34] **Limbs in General.** Weakness of the arms, heaviness; also of the knees and feet.

Sensation as if the limbs had gone to sleep.

Tingling in limbs, especially on tips of fingers and toes.

Cramps in the arms, hands and calves.

Limbs feel weak and as if bruised, worse in morning after rising.

Swelling of the right hand; also of the feet.

Cracking of joints on moving them; stiffness; arthritic swellings.

[35] **Position, etc.** Walking: 21, 26, 33. Must move legs: 33. Motion: 3, 5, 20, 26, 27, 29, 33, 34. Does not want to move: 36, 37. Exertion: 5, 29, 33, 40, 46; of arms: 26. Writing: 32. Rising: 2, 34. Standing: 33. Stooping: 7. Sitting: 3, 4, 23, 33. Lying: 3, 4, 23, 27, 29, 31; on left side: 29; on back: 23, 31.

[36] **Nerves.** Chorea, jumps up high, regardless of things around; jerks of the right side of head; after fright.

Hysterical debility; weakness in the morning in bed.

Prostrated, knows that he is weak and does not want to move.

Useful for congenital malformations caused by contractions of the muscles (externally with friction).

Pains make tears come into the eyes.

[37] **Sleep.** Frequent yawning and stretching; aversion to motion; sleepy, but cannot sleep.

Sleepy by day, sleepless at night.

Somnambulism.

Sleepless; from depressing events; from gnawing grief.

Awakens often: with pains causing dyspnœa and one-sided paralysis; with fright, violent headache, sweat, erethism, throbbing of the arteries.

Dreams: vivid; of robbers in the house, and will not believe the contrary, until search is made; of burning thirst; starts and talks in sleep, tosses about.

Unrefreshed in the morning.

[38] **Time.** Morning: 2, 3, 5, 7, 16, 22, 23, 25, 27, 29, 34, 36, 37.
10 to 11 A.M.: 40. Morning till noon: 40. Noon: 3.
Afternoon: 8. Evening: 5, 14. Night: 7, 8, 10, 37.
Day: 20, 37.

[39] **Temperature and Weather.** Warm in bed: 27.
Heat of stove unbearable.
Headache.
Ailments worse at the seaside.
Worse in heat of sun (feel exhausted); worse in Summer.
Inclination for the open air, and to wash in cold water.
Sea-bathing: 11, 48. Warmth: 3, 10, 27. Cold: 10. Open
air: 4, 10, 26. Dampness: 40. Getting wet: 3.

[40] **Chill. Fever. Sweat.** Chill predominates, mostly internal; hands and feet icy-cold.
Chill from morning until noon; ulcers around the mouth;
nursing children.
Flushes of heat with violent headache; chilliness over the
back, and sweat in the axillæ and on the soles of feet.
Chill 10 to 11 A.M., beginning in feet or small of back;
blue nails; thirst; bursting headache; nausea and
vomiting; sometimes stupefaction.
Heat, with increased headache and thirst, unconsciousness;
or obscuration of sight and faintishness.
Sweat relieving headache and other pains; though it
weakens.
Apyrexia: stitches about liver; great languor; emaciation; sallow complexion; urine muddy, with red, sandy
sediment; loss of appetite; fever-blisters.
Intermittents after: abuse of quinine; living in damp regions, or near newly turned ground.
Sweats easily from any exertion.
Sweat sour, weakening.

[41] **Attacks.** Periodical: 2. Sunrise to sunset: 3, 5. Summer: 31.

[42] **Sides.** Right: 3, 5, 33, 34, 36. Left: 3, 7, 8, 18, 28, 29, 32.

[44] **Tissues.** Varices.
Tendency to dryness, or to erosions of mucus membrane;
secretions acrid, scanty; smarting, burning at edges of
mucous surfaces.
Emaciation even while living well.

[45] **Contact, Injuries, etc.** Sprains (externally and internally).
Touch: 4, 7, 10, 12. Pressure: 17, 31.

[46] **Skin.** Itching and pricking in the skin.
Skin suffused, but no rash; tongue burned as from con-
tinned use of salt; scarlatina.
Large red blotches, itching violently.
Stinging rash over the whole body; nettle-rash after
violent exercise.

Tetter in bends of joints, oozing of an acrid fluid; crusts with deep cracks; scaly eruption on flexor surfaces.

Skin dirty-looking, withered; chlorosis.

Blood-boils.

[48] **Relationship.** *Natr. mur.* antidotes: nitrate of silver, quinine, bee-stings.

Complementary to *Apis*, followed by *Sepia*.

Antidoted by *Spir. nitr. dulc.*, *Phosphor.* (abuse of salt in food); *Arsen.* (bad effects of sea-bathing).

In dry mucous membranes, similar to: *Alum.*, *Graphit.*

NATRUM SULFURICUM.

Glauber Salts.   SCHRETER. $NaOSO_3 + 10Aq.$

[1] **Mind.** Inability to think.

Cheerfulness, happy mood; after stool.

Depressed; tearful; music makes her sad.

Satiety of life; must use all self-control to prevent shooting himself.

Irritable, worse mornings.

[2] **Sensorium.** Vertigo after dinner; then heat from body toward head, becoming more violent until sweat breaks out on forehead.

Muddled feeling, dulness.

[3] **Inner Head.** Pressure in forehead, particularly after meals; as if forehead would burst.

Pressure in forehead and coronal region after sunset, with heat on top of head; relieved by pressure of hand; during quiet and while lying down; worse when thinking.

Heaviness in the head.

Hot feeling on top of head.

Irritation of brain after lesions of the head.

Headache while reading, makes him feel hot and sweat.

Brain feels loose and, when stooping, as if it fell toward left temple.

Jerk in head, throwing it toward the right.

[4] **Outer Head.** Creeping in scalp of vertex.

Scalp sensitive; hair is painful on combing it.

[5] **Eyes.** Sight dim; eyes weak; watering.

Sensitiveness of eyes to light, with headache.

Large, blister-like granulations, with burning tears.

Burning in right eye, burning lachrymation, dim sight; worse near the fire; also morning and evening; burning of edges of lids.

Lids heavy, as if leaden, pressing in eyes while reading in evening.

Itches on edges of lids in the morning.

⁶ **Ears.** Ringing in ears, as of bells.

Piercing pain in right ear inward; sharp, lightning-like stitches in the ear; worse going from cold air into warm room, worse in damp weather, living on wet ground, etc.

Earache, as if something were forcing its way out.

Heat in right ear, evening.

⁷ **Nose.** Nosebleed during menses stops and returns often.

Nose stopped up; sneezing and fluent coryza.

Ozæna syphilitica beginning with ulcers in fauces; no fetor.

Itching of wings of nose, inducing rubbing.

⁸ **Face.** Pale, wan.

Itching of face.

⁹ **Lower Face.** Burning pain in corner of mouth at night; lips burn like pepper.

Upper lips dry, skin peels off.

Vesicles on the lips.

Pimple on chin, burns when touched.

¹⁰ **Teeth.** Throbbing toothache, with great restlessness; worse from warm, but intolerable to hot drink.

Toothache lessened by cool air.

Gums burn like fire.

¹¹ **Tongue, etc.** Taste unpleasant, slimy and tongue coated with mucus.

No taste, mornings; mouth feels rough, numb.

Blisters, with burning pain, on tip of tongue.

Tongue, red.

¹² **Mouth.** Roof of mouth sore to touch.

Burning in mouth, as from pepper; mouth dry, thirst, gums red.

Much saliva after meals.

¹³ **Throat.** Palate burns as if skin was broken, during menses.

Blisters on palate; better from cold things.

Dryness of throat, no thirst.

Throat sore, feeling of contraction when swallowing saliva; soreness is worse by talking or when swallowing solids.

Tonsils and uvula inflamed and swollen; ulcers on tonsils.

Tearing down the throat.

Mucus in throat, at night; hawks salt mucus in morning.

¹⁴ **Desires. Axersions.** Loss of appetite and great thirst.

Disgust for bread, of which she was formerly fond.

Great desire for ice, or ice-cold water.

Thirst in the evening.

¹⁵ **Eating and Drinking.** Vegetables, fruit, pastry, cold food, or drink, and farinaceous food causes diarrhœa.

Hot drinks: 10. Cold things: 13, 14. Eating: 16. Before
  meals: 17. After meals: 3, 12.

[16] **Nausea and Vomiting.** Hiccough in evening; after eating
  bread and butter.

Constant rising of sour water.

Nausea, vomiting first a sour, then a bitter fluid.

Vomiting, with colic.

[17] **Stomach.** Squeamishness in stomach before meals.

Boring in stomach as if it would be perforated; or, burning, pinching in the morning after rising; better after
  breakfast.

Beating pain in stomach, with slight nausea.

Full feeling in stomach and into chest, difficult breathing,
  evening in bed.

[18] **Hypochondria.** Cannot bear tight clothing about waist.

Stitches in region of liver and sensitiveness when walking
  in open air.

Region of liver sensitive to touch, stepping, deep breathing or sudden jar; aching, piercing pain.

Must lie on back, pain when twisting either way.

Pain in left hypochondriac region or above on last ribs;
  also with cough and purulent sputum.

Stitches in left hypochondyium while walking in open air.

[19] **Abdomen.** Pain of a dead, heavy character going through
  from abdomen to back.

Burning in abdomen; bruised pain in bowels; griping
  relieved by kneading the abdomen.

Pinching in bowels, with pain in forehead off and on.

Abdominal flatulency; much rolling and rumbling; incarcerated, especially on right side; collects at night,
  causing a great pain. Inflammation at right groin;
  typhlitis.

Feeling of fulness.

Piercing pain in right flank, with nausea. Pain as if
  distended.

[20] **Stool, etc.** Stool: scanty, slimy, light red or bloody, forcibly and suddenly expelled; half liquid, often painless,
  occasionally involuntarily while passing flatus, or urine;
  or, during sleep; yellow, fluid, soon after rising in the
  morning; in a gush; watery, with much flatus; flatulent
  colic; wind incarcerated, right side.

Diarrhœa worse in wet weather; in morning; after farinaceous food; also in cold evening air.

Hard, knotty stools, streaked with blood, accompanied
  and preceded by smarting in the anus; often with
  scanty menses.

Difficult expulsion of soft stool.

Emission of fetid flatus in large quantities.

Constant uneasiness in bowels and urging to stool.

Knotty, wart-like eruption on the anus and between the thighs; sycosis.

²¹ **Urine.** Piercing in both groins, with urging to urinate; afternoon while walking out-doors.

Pinching around navel while sitting, with urging to urinate, pain going into the groin.

Urine burns when passing; it passes in small quantity.

Sediment yellow-red; in morning, yellow-white.

²² **Male Sexual Organs.** Desire excited in evening; also morning, with erections.

Gonorrhœa; sycosis.

Itching of genitals.

²³ **Female Sexual Organs.** Inflamed, swollen and covered with vesicles of the size of lentils, filled with purulent matter.

Scanty menses; knotty stools.

Menses too late; blood acrid, making thighs sore; lumps of coagulated blood; flows freely when walking.

Before menses: nosebleed.

²⁴ **Pregnancy.** Six weeks after confinement, violent fever.

²⁵ **Larynx.** Hoarseness, with fluor albus.

²⁶ **Breathing.** Short breath when walking, gradually relieved by rest.

Great dyspnœa, desire to take deep breath during damp, cloudy weather.

After sunset, oppressed feeling in chest and feeling of a ball in throat, with tendency to cry; like hysteria.

❙ Asthma with young people from a general bronchial catarrh; afterwards with every change to damp weather.

²⁷ **Cough.** Frequent, with some sputum, stitch in left side of chest, short breathed if coughing while standing; dry, with soreness in chest, rough feeling in throat, particularly at night; had to sit up and hold chest with both hands; loose, from tickling in throat; morning; with purulent sputum and pain about last ribs, left side.

²⁸ **Lungs.** Stitching pain running up from abdomen to left side of chest.

Sycotic pneumonia, inexpressible agony; slowly coagulating blood.

Piercing pain in left chest.

³⁰ **Outer Chest.** Swelling of the ribs, near the sternum.

Spasmodic motion of muscles, worse left side.

Sycotic exanthema every Spring.

³¹ **Neck. Back.** Throat and neck swollen, knotty lumps, distressing pressure on windpipe.

Soreness up and down spine and neck.

Piercing as from knives, between scapulæ, while sitting in the evening; also in middle of sacrum.

Bruised pain in small of back.

Violent suppurative pain in small of back at night, so that she can only lie on her right side; better in morning after getting up.

Itching on back when undressing.

Pain in sacrum, cannot lie on either side.

[32] **Upper Limbs.** Swelling and suppuration of axillary glands.

Piercing in left axilla, on humerus, back of hand, palm of right hand, fingers under the nails.

Tingling in arms and hands; they feel as if paralyzed.

Furuncles on right forearm.

No strength in hands; flexors pain when grasping anything.

Hands tremble on awaking, later when writing.

Panaritium, especially if pain is better out of doors; patient pale, sickly; weary and dull head, worse mornings; caused by living in damp regions, damp walls, etc.

[33] **Lower Limbs.** Piercing pain in left hip, belly and small of back, only during rest.

Pain on right hip-joint; worse from stooping, rising from a seat, or moving in bed.

Suddenly when walking, unbearable stitch in left hip, cannot walk.

Left hip-joint pains as after lying a bad position; difficult to sit down or get up; awakes him at night; can bear any one position only for a short time.

Stabbing in left hip (after a fall).

Pain from hip to knee.

Ulcers on outer part of thigh.

Legs hot, burn to knees, evening and next morning.

Piercing in soles, in heels.

Itching on or between toes, after undressing.

Œdema of feet.

[35] **Position, etc.** Rest: 3, 26, 33. Motion: 18, 33. Writing: 32. Stepping: 18. Walking: 23, 26, 33; in open air: 18, 21. Rising: 33. After rising: 17, 20. Standing: 27. Stooping: 3, 33. Sitting: 21, 27, 31. Lying: 3; on right side: 31; on back: 18.

Has to sit up and lean forward with asthma.

[36] **Nerves.** Prostration; tired, weary, especially knees.

Exhaustion, with the colic.

Chorea, with retarded stools, tetanus of left side; trembling of right, gesticulating convulsively.

[37] **Sleep.** Drowsiness in forenoon, especially when reading or writing.

Soon after falling asleep, starting as in a fright.

Restless, sleepless.

Heavy, anxious dreams; constant waking, with unpleasant, fantastic dreams.

He may lie down earlier or later, after four or five hours
he gets awake with an attack of asthma.

[38] **Time.**   Morning: 1, 5, 11, 13, 17, 20, 22, 27, 31, 32, 33.
Forenoon: 37.   Afternoon: 2, 21.   Evening: 3, 5, 6,
14, 16, 17, 20, 22, 26, 31, 33, 40.   Night: 9, 13, 19, 27,
31, 33, 40.

[39] **Temperature and Weather.**   Going from cold to warm
place: 6.   Cold air: 10.   Open air: 32.   Wet weather:
20, 26.   Damp place: 32.   Uncovering: 46.

[40] **Chill. Fever. Sweat.**   Internal coldness, with yawning
and stretching.

Chills: with icy-coldness and goose-flesh, 4 to 8 P.M., during catamenia, towards evening, without thirst; evening in bed could not get warm all night; up the back,
with chattering of teeth and shaking, without external
coldness.

Chilly in bed and shaking chills out of it, thirst increased,
pulse accelerated.

Hot feeling on top of head.   Sudden flashes toward evening.   Increased warmth of body and restlessness.   Violent fever after confinement.

Sweat: without thirst; at night; in face; on scrotum.

[41] **Attacks.**   Attacks come on suddenly.
Every spring: 30.

[42] **Sides.**   Right: 3, 5, 6, 19, 20, 32, 33, 36, 46.   Left: 3, 18, 27,
28, 30, 32, 33, 36.   Before backward: 19.   Below up-
ward: 28.

[43] **Sensations.**   Sore across the bowels, sides and back.

[44] **Tissues.**   Cracking of joints; knees stiff; pain in bones;
sycosis.

[45] **Contact, Injuries, etc.**   Touch: 9, 12, 18.   Combing hair:
4.   Pressure: 3, 19, 27.   Tight clothing: 18.   Scratching: 46.

[46] **Skin.**   Eczema moist and oozing profusely; secretion more
watery than viscid.

Itching while undressing.

Blisters here and there.

Jaundice.

Sycosis. Leukæmia.

Wart-like, raised, red lump all over the body.

Between scrotum and right thigh, small scabs, itching relieved by scratching; also on forehead, scalp, neck,
chest; sycosis.

[47] **Stages and States.**   Old women, hereditarily inclined to
looseness of bowels.

Sycosis.

❙ Hydrogenoid constitution.

NICCOLUM.

Nickel.   *The Element.*

¹ **Mind.** Quarrelsome; very fretful humor.

Anxiety on moving, as if sweat would break out.

Apprehensive; despondent.

² **Sensorium.** Confused, as after intoxication, in the morning.
Heaviness in forehead, sense of reeling.

Vertigo: on rising in the morning, as from weakness;
with nausea and inclination to vomit.

³ **Inner Head.** Heaviness, fulness; feels as if brain was cut
to pieces on stooping; stupefied sensation.

Head feels thick, dull, in the morning, as from loss of
sleep.

Tearing in the head and in the left eye.

Stitches here and there, worse when stooping.

Pressure on the vertex as with a hand.

Headaches return every two weeks, and are usually better
in the open air.

⁵ **Eyes.** Vision dim, eyes red and sensitive; after exertion,
especially in the evening, eyes give out and burn.

Burning in the eyes, worse morning on waking; better
after washing. Lids agglutinated.

⁷ **Nose.** Violent sneezing without coryza.

Stoppage of the nose, cannot breathe through it; worse at
night.

Redness and swelling of the tip of the nose.

⁸ **Face.** Sensation as if swollen, it seems heavy.

Right side red and swollen with the sore throat.

¹⁰ **Teeth.** Gnawing in a right lower molar; sour, offensive
water exudes on sucking the teeth.

Teeth feel loose and elongated.

¹¹ **Tongue, etc.** Stiff, making talking difficult.

¹³ **Throat.** Right tonsil swollen; sticking on swallowing, as if
in the uvula.

Spasmodic choking and constriction.

¹⁴ **Desires. Aversions.** Averse to meat.

Thirst, worse in the evening.

Generally better after eating.

¹⁶ **Nausea and Vomiting.** Eructations bitter, sour, or empty.

Hiccough every evening.

Nausea, dull head; sour eructations, also mornings after
rising.

¹⁷ **Stomach.** Burning. Pressure, better from soup or from
eructations.

Empty, fasting sensation, but no hunger.

[19] **Abdomen.** Bloated abdomen.

Pinching at the navel and tension in the back before dinner.

Violent cutting in abdomen, followed by soft stool.

[20] **Stool, etc.** ׀ Diarrhœa and tenesmus after milk.

Diarrhœa of yellow mucous stools, expelled with great force and much flatus.

Stool, even if soft, evacuated with great pressure.

[21] **Urine.** Urine increased, with burning during micturition.

[23] **Female Sexual Organs.** Menses early, with pain in abdomen and small of back; or, oftener, late and scanty, with colic, backache, burning in the eyes and great debility.

Vomiting and colic after suppressed menses.

Leucorrhœa profuse, worse after urinating and after the menses.

[25] **Larynx.** ׀ Hoarseness returns annually (in one case with the nausea, intolerance of milk and weak eyes, memtioned above); also after exposure to wind.

[27] **Cough.** ׀ Cough violent at night, must sit up and hold the head.

Cough from tickling in the throat, worse evening after lying down.

[31] **Neck. Back.** Cracking in the cervical vertebræ on moving the head.

Fine stitches and feeling of tension in nape of neck on motion.

Stitches in the small of the back.

Painful gnawing in small of back.

[32] **Upper Limbs.** Left shoulder as if sprained or dislocated, better from violent motion.

[33] **Lower Limbs.** Pain as from weariness in the legs, pressing towards the groins, diarrhœa; during menses.

[34] **Limbs in General.** Tearing in scapulæ, down the arms, in hips and down the legs.

Left arm and leg feel as if would fall asleep; afternoon, sitting. Hands and feet feel heavy, better by motion.

[35] **Position, etc.** Motion: 1, 31, 32, 34. Stooping: 3. Walking: 37, 45. Exertion: 5. Sitting up: 27, 34. Lying: 27.

[36] **Nerves.** Literary men and others who suffer from periodical. nervous headaches, who are weak, with asthenopia, weak digestion, constipation; worse in the morning on awaking.

Feels sick and feverish, as if a severe illness was impending.

[37] **Sleep.** Yawning, drowsiness.

Restlessness, heat, frequent waking, better walking about.
³⁸ Time. Morning: 2, 3, 5, 16, 36, 40. Evening: 13, 27.
Night: 7, 27.
³⁹ Temperature and Weather. Generally better in open air:
3. Washing: 5. Wind: 25. Warmth of stove: 40.
⁴⁰ Chill. Fever. Sweat. Chilliness predominates. Shivering in the back, better warmth of stove. Shivering
and heat alternately.
Heat followed by chilliness.
Sensation of heat all over with anxiety and prostration.
Sweat in the morning in bed; or after midnight.
⁴¹ Attacks. Periodicity, annually: 25; every two weeks: 3.
⁴³ Sensations. Tearing in various parts.
Stitches here and there over body after lying down.
⁴⁴ Tissues. Catarrhs: 7, 13, 20, 25, 27.
⁴⁵ Contact, Injuries, etc. Uneasiness, heat, everything hurts,
must rise from bed and walk about.
⁴⁶ Skin. Itching, not better from scratching, after which pimples appear. Fine burning, stinging, biting.
⁴⁸ Relationship. Compare *Kobalt.*, *Ferrum*, *Zincum*, *Nux
vom.* (literary men, morning symptoms), *Arsen.* (annual
hoarseness.

NITRIC ACID.

Nitric Acid.   HAHNEMANN. $H\,NO_3$.

¹ Mind. Weak memory, aversion to mental exertion.
Taciturn.
Sadness, despondency.
Anxious about his disease, with fear of death; fear of
cholera.
Vindicative; attacks of rage, with curses and maledictions.
Nervous, excitable, especially after abuse of mercury.
² Sensorium. Felt dizzy, dull, stupid.
Vertigo, morning, must lie down.
Congestion to head, with much heat in it.
³ Inner Head. Head sensitive to rattling of wagons over
paved streets, or to stepping hard.
Pressing from without; tension extending to eyes, with
nausea; worse from noise; better on lying down or from
carriage riding.
Stitches in head, compelling one to lie down; disturbing
sleep.
Piercing in temples.

Violent throbbing, hammering on left side of head, coming gradually, towards morning, and going off about breakfast time.

⁴ **Outer Head.** Pain in skull, with sensation as if constricted by a tape; worse evening and night; better from cold air and while riding in a carriage.

Head very sensitive, even to pressure of the hat; worse in the evening and on part lain on.

Head feels hot.

Inflammatory swellings on scalp, suppurating or becoming carious; worse from external pressure, or when lying thereon.

Red pimples, some brownish, on anterior border of hair and on temples.

Humid, stinging eruption on vertex and temples, down also to whiskers; bleeding easily when scratched, and feeling very sore when lain on.

Single, burning, moist sores on scalp.   θ Syphilis.

Hair falls off, with humid eruptions, paining as from splinters; or, when touched; nervous headaches, debility and emaciation.

⁵ **Eyes.** Black spots before the eyes.

Very sensitive to light.

Double vision; shortsightedness.

Pupils dilated and dim.

Eyes inflamed, after syphilis or abuse of mercury.

Iritis, which continually relapses; also old cases spoiled by mercury.

Pressure and stinging in the eyes.

Spots on the cornea.

Staphyloma, as a preventive.

Eyes dim, sunken.

Region of eyes painful, sore to the touch.

Herpetic pannus.

Eyelids swollen, hard, livid.

Paralysis of upper lids.

Fistula lachrymalis.

Flow of irritating tears, after injury of the eye.

Dermoid swellings of the eyes.

⁶ **Ears.** One's speech echoes in the ears.

Beating, humming in the ears.

Cracking in the ears when masticating.

Hardness of hearing, from induration and swelling of tonsils; after abuse of mercury.

Eustachian tubes obstructed.

Terribly offensive, purulent otorrhœa.

Throbbing in the ears.

Auditory canal nearly closed.

Caries of mastoid process.

⁷ **Nose.** Disagreeable smell on inhaling air.

Nosebleed, mornings; black, clotted; also when weeping; blood acrid.

Sneezing during sleep.

Nose obstructed with day coryza, or with dropping of water; wings of nose swollen, burning.

Fetid, yellow, nasal discharge.

Ozæna, with ulcers.

Corroding nasal discharge.

Stitch in the nose as from a splinter.

Tip of nose red, scurfy.

Condylomata on nose.

Large, soft protuberances on alæ, covered with crusts. θ Syphilis.

Dirty, bloody mucus from posterior nares.

Green casts from the nose every morning.

⁸ **Face.** Pale, eyes sunken.

Dark yellow about eyes, with red cheeks.

Swelling of the cheeks.

Bloated around the eyes on waking early.

Rash over the face and forehead, small pimples.

Suppurating pustules, with broad, red circumferences, forming crusts. θ Syphilis.

Comedones.

Freckles.

⁹ **Lower Face.** Swollen lips.

Under lip dry, cracked.

Margin of mouth covered with sores and blisters.

Corners of mouth ulcerated.

Painful swelling of submaxillary gland.

¹⁰ **Teeth.** Pulsating, stinging in teeth, evening in bed and all night, after abuse of mercury.

Teeth feel elongated.

Teeth become yellow or loose.

Pain in hollow teeth.

Gums white, swollen, bleeding.

¹¹ **Tongue, etc.** Taste: bitter, after eating; sour, with burning in the throat.

Tongue: sensitive, even mild food causes smarting; white, dry, mornings; coated green, with ptyalism; dry, fissured.

Deep, irregular-shaped ulcers on the edge of the tongue. θ Syphilis.

Ulceration of tongue, with tough, ropy mucus.

Tongue white, with sore spots.

¹² **Mouth.** Cadaverous smell from the mouth.

Saliva fetid, acrid, makes lips sore.

44

Saliva bloody.

Mucous membrane of mouth, swollen, ulcerated; with pricking pains, especially after abuse of mercury.

Tumor in the mouth, with a streak down the neck.

[13] **Throat.** Palate, tongue, inside of gums sore, with stinging pain and ulceration of corners of mouth.

Stitches in the throat, dry coryza, hoarseness.

Tonsils red, swollen, uneven, with small ulcers thereon.

Dry throat, heat; gums sore.

Diphtheritic membrane on tonsils and fauces; extending to the nose; terrible fetor, intermittent pulse; swollen parotids.

Pricking as from a splinter in the throat; worse when swallowing.

[14] **Desires. Aversions.** Longing for: fat; herring; chalk; lime; earth.

Averse to meat and bread.

Loss of appetite.

Thirst violent in morning. θ Tuberculosis, suppuration of lungs.

[15] **Eating and Drinking.** During and after eating, sweat. Chokes while eating.

After eating; fulness in stomach, debility from least exertion, heat, palpitation; heavy weight in stomach.

Fat food causes nausea and acidity.

Milk disagrees.

[16] **Nausea and Vomiting.** Much nausea, cannot take food; vomits occasionally.

Nausea, with heat in the stomach, extending to the throat.

Nausea better from moving about or carriage riding.

Bitter and sour vomiting, with much eructation; vomits yellow mucus.

[17] **Stomach.** Stitches in the pit of the stomach.

Pain in cardiac orifice on swallowing food.

Burning distress.

[18] **Hypochondria.** Chronic derangement of the liver; icterus.

Liver enormously enlarged; clay-colored stools.

Spleen large after yellow fever.

[19] **Abdomen.** Awakened at midnight, with crampy pains in small intestines; chilly; pain more if he moved.

Incarcerated flatulency in upper part of abdomen, worse morning and evening.

Abdomen distended with flatulence, very tender.

Cutting-pinching, worse in the morning in bed.

Gurgling in left side of abdomen; cold feet; fetor oris.

Pain in abdomen when walking; must bend over; pain settles in ileo-cœcal region; dull sore, tender.

Inguinal hernia; also of children.

Burning over whole abdomen, 2 to 3 P. M.

Stinging soreness when touched.

Swelling and suppuration of inguinal glands.

Inflamed buboes.

²⁰ **Stool, etc.** Desire for stool, but little passes; feels as if it stayed in the rectum and could not be expelled.

Ineffectual urging to stool; colic.

Stools hard, preceded by great pressure, followed by mucous discharges.

Burning in rectum towards the perineum, with ineffectual urging; straining without stool; diphtheritic dysentery.

Sero-croupous discharge, with much straining.

Stools: bloody, with tenesmus; of mucus; putrid, mucous; undigested; loose, much flatulence, rumbling; of yellow-white fluid; loose mornings; green, slimy, acrid diarrhœa.

Hemorrhage bright red, not clotted; faint from least motion; ulcers in ileo-cœcal region.

Piles: old, pendulous, ceased bleeding, but pain when touched, worse in warm weather; slimy, fissured; bleed after every stool.

Fissures in rectum; tearing, spasmodic symptoms during stool; lancinating after, even after soft stools.

Moisture about the anus.

²¹ **Urine.** Cold when it passes; scanty, dark brown, smelling strong like horse's urine; turbid, looks like remains in a cider barrel.

While urinating, smarting-burning in urethra.

Hæmaturia; urging after, and shuddering along the spine, during urination; blood flows actively.

Incontinence of urine.

Spasms of the urethra; rectal fissure.

Ulcers in urethra; bloody, mucous or purulent discharge.

²² **Male Sexual Organs.** Sexual desire too strong.

No desire; want of erections.

Painful spasmodic erections at night.

Hard, brown nodules on scrotum, suppurating.

Brown-red spots, peeling off on discharging.

Gonorrhœa, with chancres, or warts.

Small blisters on orifice of urethra and inner surface of prepuce, forming chancre-like ulcers. θ Gonorrhœa.

❙ Ulcers deep, fistulous, irregular, ragged; edges often raised, lead-colored; bleed easily when touched. θ Syphilis.

❙ Secondary syphilis; 4, 5, 7, 13, 33, 46.

❙ Phimosis.

❙ Chancres after mercury, especially with exuberant granulations.

❙ Condylomata.

Falling off of the hair from genitals.

²³ **Female Sexual Organs.** After coitus, mucous lining of
genitals itches voluptuously; excrescences on uterus.

Pressing down in hypogastrium and small of back, as
though everything would protrude; pain down thighs;
abdomen feels swollen.

Uterine hemorrhage from overexertion of body.

Menses: early, irregular, scanty, and like muddy water;
early and profuse; aching from the thighs; urine offensive.

During menses eructations, cramp-like pain in the abdomen, as if it would burst.

Profuse, brown, offensive discharge between the irregular
menstruations. θ Cancer uteri.

Leucorrhœa: of ropy mucus; of green mucus; of flesh-
colored; acrid, brown, offensive.

Stitches up the vagina, or from without inward, when
walking in the open air.

Itching, swelling and burning of vulva and vagina.

Excrescences on cervix uteri.

²⁴ **Pregnancy.** Metrorrhagia after abortion or confinement.

Hard nodes in mammæ.

Atrophy of the mammæ.

²⁵ **Larynx.** Hoarseness: with coryza; from long talking;
scratching and stinging in throat.

Large, broad condylomata in the larynx.

²⁶ **Breathing.** Awakens often all stopped up with mucus, must
expectorate before he can breathe easily.

Loses her breath and speech, she is so weak. θ Uterine
displacement.

Intermittent breathing.

Short breath, panting during work.

²⁷ **Cough.** Dry, barking, from tickling in larynx and pit of
stomach: worse at night, also in day when lying down.
Sputa of blood mixed with clots during the day.

Cough: dry, sputum is raised with difficulty; in the morning, followed by greenish-white casts, as if from air-cells.
θ Secondary syphilis.

Sputa are yellow, acrid, bitter; sour, offensive.

ı Empyema, with considerable muco-purulent sputum.

²⁸ **Lungs.** Uneasiness in chest.

Congestion to chest, with anxiety, heat and palpitation.

Cramp-like pains in chest.

Stitches in chest, right side.

Chest sore when coughing or breathing.

Soreness at lower end of sternum.

Pain suddenly abates, yet pulse becomes smaller and
quicker. θ Pneumonia. θ Pleurisy of old or cachetic
people.

Lungs attacked, rattling breathing, loose cough; sputum
brown, bloody; pulse irregular. θ Typhus.

Threatened paralysis of the lungs. θ Typhus.

²⁹ **Heart.   Pulse.** Palpitation and anguish, on going up stairs.

Pulse: irregular; one normal, followed by two small, rapid
beats; fourth beat intermits; alternate hard, rapid and
small beats.

³¹ **Neck.   Back.** Swelling of cervical and axillary glands.

Stitches in and between scapulae; neck stiff.

Pain in back and small of back; from cold.

Neuralgic pains up the back, particularly left side.

³² **Upper Limbs.** Aching in right shoulder and arm; arm feels
bruised; at times she cannot raise it.

Rheumatic pains mostly in forearms and fingers.

Numbness, trembling, tingling, of right forearm.

Swelling of finger-joints, stinging pains.

Hands go to sleep in the morning.

Numerous large warts on back of hand.

Herpes between fingers.

White spots on nails.

³³ **Lower Limbs.** Hip as if sprained, with limping.

Pain across both buttocks.

Rheumatic pains in legs and feet.

Soreness along the periosteum on the tibia.

Pain in patella, impeding walking; stiffness and stitches
in knees.

Violent cramp in calf; at night and when walking after
sitting.

Itching of shins, bleeding when scratched; small scabs
form.

Foul-smelling foot-sweat.

▮Chilblains on the toes.

³⁴ **Limbs in General.** Limbs restless in evening.

³⁵ **Position, etc.** Motion: 19, 20, 32, 40. Stepping hard: 3.
Walking: 16, 19, 23, 33. Sitting: 33. Must bend over:
19. Overexertion: 23. Lying: 3, 27, 40.   Must lie
down: 2, 3.   Part lain on: 4.

³⁶ **Nerves.** Excessive physical irritability.

Hysteria.

Twitchings in various parts.

Great weakness; trembling; shocks on going to sleep; depressed in spirits.

Great debility, heaviness and trembling of limbs, especially in the morning.

³⁷ **Sleep.** Drowsy all day from debility, with vertigo.

Difficulty of going to sleep.

Shocks on dropping to sleep.

Pains felt during sleep.

Sleeps badly latter part of night.

On awaking feels as if he had not slept enough.

³⁸ **Time.** Morning: 2, 3, 7, 8, 11, 14, 19, 20, 32, 36, 30. Afternoon: 19, 40. Evening: 4, 10, 19, 34. Night: 4, 10,
22, 27, 33, 40. Midnight: 19. After midnight: 37.
Toward morning: 3, 40. . Day: 27, 37.

³⁹ **Temperature and Weather.** Pains on change of temperature or weather.

Warm weather: 20. In bed: 40. Open air: 46. Cold
air: 4. Cold: 31. Uncovering: 40.

⁴⁰ **Chill. Fever. Sweat.** Chill afternoon and evening, and
after lying down.

Continuous chilliness.

Chilly, with internal heat.

Chilly morning in bed after previous heat.

Awakens at midnight chilly; worse from uncovering or
moving; later hot, prickling all over as from needles.

No thirst during cold or hot stage.

Heat on hands and face.

Heat dry, internal at night, wants to uncover.

Heat in flushes, with sweaty hands.

Heat, with sweat and debility after eating.

Sweat sour, offensive, like urine. Sweat on soles of feet
makes them sore.

Copious night-sweats.

Chill afternoon; then short heat over whole body; afterward profuse sweat over whole body.

Intermittent fever: chill afternoon while in open air, followed by dry heat when in bed, accompanied by all
sorts of fancies while in a state of half waking, without
sleep; sleep and sweat only come on toward morning.
Chronic cases, liver diseased, patient anæmic; general
cachetic condition.

⁴² **Sides.** Right: 18, 28, 32. Left: 3, 18, 16, 31. Without
inward: 3, 23.

⁴³ **Sensations.** Pricking as from splinters.

Gnawing here and there as from ulcers forming.

⁴⁴ **Tissues.** Hemorrhages bright, profuse; or dark.

Putrid decomposition.

Emaciation.

Cracking in the joints.

Glands inflamed, swollen, suppurating.

Caries.

⁴⁵ **Contact, Injuries, etc.** Touch: 4, 5, 19, 20, 22, 46. Pressure: 4. Scratching: 4, 33. Carriage riding: 3, 4, 16.

⁴⁶ **Skin.** Skin dry.

Skin dark, dirty; brown-red spots.

Burning hot skin; fine miliary rash. θ Scarlatina.

Itching nettle-rash in open air.

Blood-boils.

Carbuncles.

Rhagades, deep, bleeding.

Frost-bites, itching; inflamed from slight degree of cold; skin cracked.

Ulcers bleed when touched; stinging pains; feeling as of a splinter; edges hard, everted and irregular; exuberant granulations; after mercury or in secondary syphilis.

Condylomata moist, like cauliflower, hard, rhagadic, or in thin pedicles.

47 Stages and States. Dark complexioned and old people.

48 Relationship. *Nitr. ac.* follows well after: *Calc. carb., Hepar, Kali carb., Natr. carb., Pulsat., Sulphur, Thuja.*

After *Nitr. ac.*: *Calc. carb., Pulsat., Sulphur,* are frequently indicated.

Nitr. ac.: complementary to *Calad.*

Antidotes to *Nitr. ac.*: *Calc. carb., Hepar, Mercur., Mezer., Sulphur.*

Nitr. ac. relieves ailments from: *Calcar., Digit.,* abuse of mercury.

Inimical: *Laches.*

NITRUM.

Saltpetre.   HARTLAUB.   *K NO₃.*

1 Mind. Difficulty of thinking in morning, with warm face; forehead hot.

Anxiety, with sweat; afternoon, also till evening.

Ennui, melancholy, weeping mood.

Timid, sensitive.

Out of humor.

2 Sensorium. Drowsy, dulness of head.

Vertigo: mornings; forgets what he is about to say.

Fainting fits, with vertigo, morning when standing, better while sitting; afterward obscuration of sight.

3 Inner Head. Headache, causing eyelids to close, worse stooping, when head hangs down.

Congestion, throbbing, deep in brain.

Stinging pain in the head.

Stupefying morning headache, as after free indulgence in intoxicating drinks.

Constrictive pain in back of head; parts feel as if stiff, forcing to bend head backward; better tying up hair.

Headache after eating veal, or drinking coffee; better riding in open air.

4 Outer Head. Hot spots on the head.

Headache on top of head, as if hairs were pulled.

Scalp sensitive to touch.

Constrictive pains on head, face, eyes, etc., all concentrating at the root or tip of the nose.

5 Eyes. Transitory blindness.

Rainbow colors around light; colored wheels before eyes.

Burning in eyes, lachrymation and aversion to light, especially in the morning; after washing in cold water.

6 Ears. Deafness from paralysis of auditory nerve; tingling in ears.

Stitches in ears, worse at night, and when lying on affected side.

❙ Ulceration of ear-ring hole.

Tension behind the ear.

7 Nose. Loss of smell, with coryza; husky voice; mucus passes through posterior nares into fauces.

Mucous polypus.

Nosebleed; tip of nose inflamed, sore; blood acrid, like vinegar.

Bones of nose sore to touch; nose swollen internally, with scurfs.

8 Face. Pale face.

Red cheeks, tension, while the headache grows worse.

Tensive pains in cheeks, redness; increased throbbing in head, apparently in middle of brain.

Tearing in facial bones.

Pricking, then burning in skin.

10 Teeth. Toothache, 3 A.M., worse from cold things; feels as if air was rushing in and out of decayed tooth.

Gums red, swollen, bleed easily.

11 Tongue, etc. Repugnant taste all day.

Sour taste in throat; morning on arising.

Tongue burns at its tip, as if cut; burning pimples.

Tongue coated with white mucus.

12 Mouth. Fetid odor from mouth.

Mouth slimy.

13 Throat. Feels choked, as if closed, at night, can scarcely breathe.

Stinging during deglutition.

Sore throat day and night, with inflamed velum palati and uvula.

Hawks sweetish, tough mucus; afternoon; throat rough, as if scraped.

Cutting pains, with impeded deglutition.

14 Desires. - Aversions. Appetite strongest, evenings.

Violent thirst, but no appetite.

Want of appetite, with increased hunger.

[15] **Eating and Drinking.** Cannot drink, has not breath enough.

After veal: headache, colic, diarrhœa.

[16] **Nausea and Vomiting.** Gulps up bitter water, relieving nausea.

Nausea: cold sensation from throat to stomach; choking sensation; faintness; bruised headache; burning eyes; especially at night.

Vomits mucus, with blood.

[17] **Stomach.** Cold feeling; or, burning in stomach; inflammation.

Sharp, sticking pains, so severe he was scarcely able to breathe.

Spasms in stomach, with flatulent colic.

Pressure and gnawing in scrobiculum.

Faint-like weakness in scrobiculum.

[19] **Abdomen.** Violent colic, right side most; worse after veal; incarcerated flatulence; evening.

Stitching pains in abdomen; lower limbs cold; affected parts feel numb, as if made of wood. θ Peritonitis.

Complaints in abdomen, worse from holding the breath.

[20] **Stool, etc.** Stools: watery, thin, fecal; bloody; soft, with colic.

Diarrhœa from eating veal.

Stool hard, like sheep's dung, with tenesmus.

[21] **Urine.** Bright's disease, with pain in small of back, bruised, crampy or burning; diminished urine.

Dysuria and frequent desire to urinate, with pain and heat; after abuse of cantharides; after stimulating injections; condiments; onanism; gonorrhœal extension; cold; turpentine.

Frequent miscturition and discharge of much pale urine, with reddish clouds.

Mucous sediment; salts increased; specific gravity 1030-1040.

[22] **Male Sexual Organs.** Increased desire; if ungratified pains, tension in testes and cords.

[23] **Female Sexual Organs.** Menses suppressed.

Menstrual blood black as ink; colic, pain in small of back, burning in groins; legs feel weak, numb, as if made of wood.

White leucorrhœa, with lameness in small of back.

[25] **Larynx.** Tightness in larynx, during respiration.

Aphonia.

Hoarseness, roughness and scraping in larynx; yellow phlegm.

Tension and cutting in larynx, impeding deglutition.

²⁶ **Breathing.** ｜Cannot drink, for want of breath; has to take drink in little sips.

｜Little children take hold of the cup or glass with both hands and take greedily one sip after another.

Paroxysms of difficult and rapid breathing, evening and night, less in morning; oppressed breathing on ascending stairs.

Asthma, cannot lie in horizontal position.

Terrible attacks of asthma, with violent gasping and suffocation.

Abdominal respiration.

²⁷ **Cough.** Awakens at 3 A.M., with violent, stupefying headache; in open air; worse ascending, or when holding breath; with cutting and stitches in chest; expectoration of coagulated blood; after hawking mucus.

Hæmoptysis at full moon.

²⁸ **Lungs.** Dull tightness and constriction of chest; as if lungs were constricted from the back.

Stitches on drawing a long breath, worse lying, coughing; dyspnœa, great anxiety. θ Pneumonia.

Annoying feeling of heaviness in chest like a great load, pressing the thorax together; dyspnœa to suffocation. θ Pneumonia.

The dyspnœa is very great compared with the apparent slight congestion or hepatization.

Suppuration of lungs, with profuse (colliquative) sweat.

²⁹ **Heart. Pulse.** Palpitation on rising, or moving about quickly, with heat of the face and oppression of chest.

Congestion to chest.

Palpitation audible, with dyspnœa; worse lying on the back, or right side.

Pulse: generally full, hard, accelerated; slow, morning; frequent afternoon and evening.

³¹ **Neck. Back.** Painful throbbing in one of the cervical vertebræ.

Pain like a blow in small of back, on awaking; cannot turn.

Cramp-pain in small of back.

Small of back feels bruised.

Pressure and burning in back, relieved by motion.

³² **Upper Limbs.** Rheumatism of shoulder, worse at night; hands and fingers feels as if swollen.

Stitches in shoulder, elbow, hand, finger; worse at night.

Paralysis (rheumatic).

Numbness and tingling of hands.

Finger-joints stiff, tense.

³³ **Lower Limbs.** Rheumatic pains.

Legs feel weak, paralytic, after a short walk.

Numbness, tingling of feet.

Toes contracted.

³⁴ **Limbs in General.** Rheumatisms, with stitching pains at night.

Parts feel as if made of wood.

Numbness and tingling disappear, and articular pains set in.

³⁵ **Position, etc.** Motion: 29, 31, 36, 40. Walking: 37. Ascending: 26, 27. Exertion: 40. Stooping: 3. Rising: 29. Standing: 2. Sitting: 2, 36. Lying: 6, 26, 28, 29, 40.

³⁶ **Nerves.** Spasmodic painless jerkings of fingers and other parts.

Debility of limbs and body, with heat in face, burning spots in forehead; worse sitting; better moving slowly about.

Paralysis of limbs.

³⁷ **Sleep.** Drowsy all day, also when walking.

Restless sleep; light morning sleep; nightmare.

Sleepless after midnight.

On awaking, sour taste; cough, pain in small of back.

³⁸ **Time.** Morning: 1, 2, 3, 5, 11, 20, 26, 29, 37. Afternoon: 1, 13, 29, 40. Evening: 14, 19, 26, 29, 40. Night: 6, 13, 16, 26, 32, 34. After midnight: 37. 3 A.M.: 10, 27. All day: 11, 20, 37. Day and night: 13.

³⁹ **Temperature and Weather.** Generally worse from warmth of stove.

Better from warm weather.

Worse during wet, cold weather.

Cold things: 10.

Worse while perspiring; better after.

Washing in cold water: 5. Open air: 3, 27.

⁴⁰ **Chill. Fever. Sweat.** Chill and coldness in afternoon and evening, increased from motion, passing off when lying.

Chill, with subsequent sweat, not intervening heat.

Evening chill, with the pains.

Coldness, with thirst; afternoon.

Head feels hot, forehead burns.

Slight heat, evening; heat at night without thirst and without subsequent sweat.

Debilitating sweat from least exertion.

Night-sweat, most profuse on legs; morning-sweat, most profuse on chest.

⁴¹ **Attacks.** Full moon: 27.

⁴² **Sides.** Right side, particularly upper right, lower left.

Right: 19.

⁴³ **Sensations.** Sensation as if parts, or whole body were of wood.

Formication in hands and feet, afterwards in tongue.
Constrictive feeling in many parts.

⁴⁴ **Tissues.** Hemorrhages of bright red blood.
Inflammation of stomach and intestines.
Sudden swelling of body, neck, thighs.

⁴⁵ **Contact, Injuries, etc.** Touch: 4, 7.
Rubbing, scratching relieves.
Riding: 3. Scratching: 46.

⁴⁶ **Skin.** Pricking like needles, then burning; worse in face.
Burning vesicles filled with yellow serum; scratching,
they burst.
Small pustules.
Small, scurfy spots on the head (scalp) itching.

⁴³ **Relationship.** Antidotes to *Nitrum: Nitr. spir. dulc.*
Camphor increases the pains.
Nitrum relieves strangury after abuse of *Canthar.*, turpen-
tine, and abuse of condiments.

NUX MOSCHATA.

Nutmeg.   HELBIG.   *Myristicaceæ.*

¹ **Mind.** Stupor and insensibility; unconquerable sleep.
Unconsciousness, after mental excitement, especially just
before menses; thoughts vanish, with fainting.
Gradual vanishing of thoughts, when reading, inclined to
fall asleep.
Memory weak.
Gives answers wholly irrelevant to the question put to him.
Uses wrong words, during headache.
Surroundings seem changed; fanciful, dreamy images;
does not recognize the known street.
Short time seems very long to her.
Delirium, violent vertigo, strange gestures, loud, improper
talk, sleeplessness.
Delirium tremens, slowness of senses, imaginary fancies;
awakens and knows not where he is; laughter, with
stupid expression.
Laughter, everything seems ludicrous, talks loudly to
herself.
Changeable mood, now laughing, again crying.
Weeping mood, gloomy; fears to go to sleep.
Fickle, irresolute.
Slow action: of senses; of will.
From overtaxing mind: sleepy, gastric ailments, hysteria.

[2] **Sensorium.**   Vertigo: as if drunk, staggering; reeling when
  walking in open air; swimming in head; weak, limbs
  numb, feels as if floating in air.

[3] **Inner Head.**   Apoplexy; softening of the brain.

  Pulsation of the arteries and daily headache; throbbing,
    pressing pain, confined to small spots, worse in left
    supraorbital ridge.

  Painless pulsating in head, fears to go to sleep.

  Head feels full and as if expanding.

  Headache, going from left to right.

  Brain as if loose, with wabbling on motion, as if it struck
    the sides of head; sleepiness; worse after a meal; from
    cold; better from warmth, except from the warmth of bed.

  Severe tearing in occiput, toward nape of neck.

  Headaches are worse: from washing; getting wet; wet, or
    damp, cold weather; change of weather ; riding in a
    carriage; from wine; after eating, especially after break-
    fast; from a little overheating; from suppressed erup-
    tions; before menses; during pregnancy.

[4] **Outer Head.**   Temples sensitive to touch and from lying
  on them; worse wet, cold weather; better from warmth.

  Head drops forward, while sitting.

  Convulsive movement of head from before backward, so
    that talking and swallowing are almost impossible.

  Worse from shaking the head.

[5] **Eyes.**   Objects look: larger; very distant; or vanish, red.

  Motes before the eyes.

  Worse from light, from exerting vision; better in dark.

  Blindness, then fainting.

  Momentary blindness; grasps head, it feels so strangely.

  Staring.

  Pupils dilated and immovable or contracted, with sensa-
    tion of fulness in eyes.

  Eyes dry, she could hardly shut them, green-blue rings
    around them.

  Pterygium.

  Lids heavy, stiff; feels sick, faint.

[6] **Ears.**   Hearing oversensitive; buzzing in ears.

  Ears as if stopped up.

  Tearing in ears; stitches in left ear, worse moving jaw.

[7] **Nose.**   Oversensitiveness of smell.

  Nosebleed, blood usually dark, black.

  Sneezing, nose internally dry, stopped up, must breathe
    with mouth open. Catarrh worse in cold, damp weather.

[8] **Face.**   Burning, constricting, stinging over right eye; face
  red, swollen; lips and jaw compressed; speech difficult.

  Foolish, childish expression.

  Looks thin; suffering expression; blue around eyes; deadly
    pale, worse in damp air.

Eyes dull, heavy looking; distressed look.

Spots, freckles.

⁹ **Lower Face.** Lips chapped.

¹⁰ **Teeth.** Pain in front teeth during pregnancy; stinging, tearing; worse during cold, damp weather, from washing; from touch or sucking teeth, better from warmth.

Gums bleed; scurvy.

¹¹ **Tongue, etc.** Taste: earthy; chalky; bitter; as after salted food.

Tongue: paralyzed; child, though old enough, cannot talk, as if it were difficult to move the tongue; dry feels as if gone to sleep or leather-covered; no thirst; dry at night, or on awaking; coated white, or yellowish, dotted with red papillæ.

¹² **Mouth.** Mouth and throat dry, no thirst.

Saliva lessened; like "cotton."

Water from mouth before menses.

Bad smell from the mouth; tongue white.

Aphthæ of children.

¹³ **Throat.** Difficult swallowing, from paralysis of muscles of deglutitition.

Sore throat, hoarseness; scratching, dryness.

Pain along eustachian tube, as from a foreign body lodged there; before a shower.

¹⁴ **Desires. Aversions.** Appetite and hunger increased; bulimia.

Loss of appetite.

Thirstlessness.

¹⁵ **Eating and Drinking.** After eating: 3, 19, 23, 26, 27. After drinking: 19, 20, 27. After drinking wine: 3, 21, 29. After drinking boiled milk: 20. After drinking beer: 21.

¹⁶ **Nausea and Vomiting.** Hiccough.

Nausea and water-brash: with inclination to sleep; while riding in a carriage; during pregnancy.

Vomiting: spasmodic; during pregnancy; from irritation of pessaries; and acid stomach; flatulence.

¹⁷ **Stomach.** Heat and burning in stomach.

Fulness in stomach, impeding breathing.

Weak digestion, especially in the aged.

Irritation of stomach, from overtaxed mental powers.

Can only digest highly seasoned food.

Cramps in stomach.

¹⁸ **Hypochondria.** Spasmodic pain from right to left hypochondrium, then in a circle in lower part of abdomen; followed by diarrhœa.

"Livergrown," in children.

Enlarged liver; bloody stools; weight about liver; pressure as from a sharp body or stones; swollen feeling.

Diaphragm hurts with inhalation.

Diaphragmitis, oppression of chest, like a pressing load, dry cough, loss of breath; from getting wet.

Enlarged spleen; loose bowels.

Stitches in spleen; must bend double.

[19] **Abdomen.**   Weight in upper part of abdomen; lower part tense.

Cutting, pinching in epigastrium and naval.

Colic immediately after eating and worse after drinking; during day, with dry mouth and thirstlessness; better from hot wet cloths.

Abdomen enormously distended

Sore navel, even ulcerated.

Umbilical hernia.

Cutting, pinching about navel, better from pressure; flatulency, diarrhœa.

Crampy, forcing down pains in bowels and anus.

[20] **Stools, etc.**   Stools: soft, but expelled with difficulty, rectum inactive; like chopped eggs, undigested; loss of appetite, sleepy; bilious, slimy; putrid, bloody; thin, yellow' copious, offensive.

Stools worse at night, exhausting, associated with sleepiness, fainting; worse from cold, damp weather; summer heat; from cold drinks; during dentition; during pregnancy, with sluggish flow of ideas; from boiled milk.

Worms; cutting bellyache, sleepiness.

Alternate hard and soft stools.

Hemorrhoids protrude.

[21] **Urine.**   Renal colic.

Tenesmus of bladder.

Pain from stone in bladder or gravel.

Burning, cutting in urethra, when passing water.

Dysuria, with urging to stool; after dinner and supper, or exertion of body; also, with uterine complaints.

Strangury, from beer or wine; also, in hysteria.

Urine: has a violet odor; is scanty and high colored.

[22] **Male Sexual Organs.**   Inclined to coitus, but genitals are relaxed.

Seminal emissions.

[23] **Female Sexual Organs.**   Sterility.

Spasmodic labor-like pains.

Great irritability of pelvic viscera, worse during menses, when ovaries and uterus are swollen and sensitive to pressure.

Flatulent distention of uterus.

Uterus displaced; mouth and throat dry; sleepy, faint; abdomen enormously distended after a meal; pressure in back outward.

Sensation of a lump in left lower abdomen; anteversion.

Relieves pain and vomiting caused by pessaries.

Prolapsus uteri et vaginæ; sterility; leucorrhœa.

Menses: irregular in time and quantity; flow generally dark, thick; bearing down in abdomen, with drawing in limbs; pains from small of back downward; limbs feel weak, ache; pain in small of back as if a piece of wood was lying crosswise and being pressed out; pain in uterus at the outset; tension in hypogastrium; unconquerable drowsiness; profuse, with fainting, drowsiness; mouth dry; hysteric laughing, worse in open air; scanty or suppressed, from fright; from debility; a cold; overexertion; in hysteria; cramp low down in abdomen, constriction in the bowels; sharp stitches in left lower abdomen, worse when sitting.

Leucorrhœa in place of menses; awakens with dry tongue.

[24] **Pregnancy.** During pregnancy: worse from fright, anger, etc.; nausea and vomiting; difficult stool; dyspnœa, with upward pressure; fainting; drowsiness; skin dry, cold; abdomen sensitive.

Threatened abortion; hysterical females, disposed to fainting; fears she will abort.

Labor: pains false, weak; or, spasmodic, irregular, drowsy, faint spells, the pains being too weak.

Eclampsia: head jerked forward; especially hysterical women, who easily faint and suffer from great languor in back and knees; drowsy before and after spasms.

After delivery: flatulence, with labor-like pains; uterus remains uncontracted; anteversion.

Mammæ too small.

[25] **Larynx.** Voice uncertain, bleating.

Hoarseness, worse walking against the wind.

Feeling of dryness in larynx:

Phthisis laryngea.

[26] **Breathing.** Breath short after eating; sudden loss of breath.

Dyspnœa, with feeling of weight in the chest.

Chest as if too narrow, after cold washing.

Constrictive feeling in muscles of chest.

[27] **Cough.** Dry, with sudden loss of breath; barking; hacking during pregnancy; excited by scratching in throat, crawling in upper part of windpipe; caused by: getting warm in bed; standing in water, bathing; getting overheated; living in cold, dark places; loose after eating, dry after drinking.

Sputa are bloody, dark; slimy, saltish; must swallow the loosened phlegm.

[28] **Lungs.** Weight, pressure on chest, worse on falling asleep at night, or waking from a siesta.

Stitches in chest, tightness, spitting of blood.

Full feeling in upper part of chest, preventing a deep breath.

29 Heart. Pulse. Violent action of heart.

Palpitation: fainting, followed by sleep; hysteric, with weak, small pulse, and changing irregularity in heart's beat.

Feels as if her head would burst and her heart be squeezed off.

Trembling, fluttering of heart, as from fright.

Pulse: small, weak; nun's murmur in carotids; frequent, trembling, accelerated after wine; intermits, the intervals so long that they excite fear of death.

31 Neck. Back. Drawing in muscles of neck, from draft of damp air.

Pains now in back, now in sacrum, knees very tired; worse during rest; lumbago.

Pains along the spine.

Backache, while riding in a carriage.

Pain in small of back and weakness of legs, as from a blow.

Small of back and knees feel weak.

Tabes dorsalis.

32 Upper Limbs. Felt as if all the bood had rushsd to her hands, as though a string were about the arms.

Hands feel cold, as if frozen, with tingling under nails, on entering warm room.

33 Lower Limbs. Legs tired, as after a long journey, must move legs from place to place.

Right knee pains as if wrenched or sprained on moving, and especially going up stairs.

Heaviness and coldness in legs.

Feeling in calves, as of a blow.

Cramps in feet internal burning.

Boring in big toe, after lying down. θ Gout.

34 Limbs in General. Wandering, digging, pressing pains, confined to small spots; lasting but a short time; soon returning.

Muscular rheumatism, from protracted exposure to cold and damp; fugitive, drawing pains; worse in repose from cold, damp air and cold wet clothes; better from warmth.

35 Position, etc. Motion: 3, 33. Exertion: 21, 23, 36. Must move: 33, 36. Walking: 2, 25, 36. Ascending: 33. Bends double: 18. Shaking head: 4. Moving jaw: 6. Rest: 31. Lying: 4, 33. Sitting: 4, 23.

36 Nerves. Staggers in walking; falls often.

Fatigue, feels as if he must lie down, after least exertion; sleepy; chilly, pale face.

Disposition to faint; also, from the pains even when slight.

Restless, must move about.

Spasms of children, with diarrhœa.

Unconscious, rigid, slow, heavy breathing; then writhing in clonic spasms; opisthotonos.

Epilepsy, with consciousness.

Catalepsy.

Hysteria; exhausted from least effort.

Paralysis; with cramps and trembling; of tongue, eyelids, œsophagus.

37 Sleep. Complaints cause sleepiness; irresistibly, drowsy; sleepy, muddled, as if intoxicated; coma, lies silent, immovable.

Restless sleep, from congestion to heart or head, with uterine complaints.

38 Time. Morning: 40. Evening: 40. Night: 11, 20, 28. Day: 19.

39 Temperature and Weather. Warmth: 3, 4, 10, 27, 34. Warm room: 32, 40. Warmth of bed: 3, 27. Summer heat: 20. Hot wet cloths: 19. Cold: 3, 27. Damp, cold weather: 3, 4, 7, 8, 10, 20, 31, 34, 40, 46. Washing or getting wet: 3, 10, 18, 26, 27. Cold wet clothes: 34. Uncovering: 40. Open air: 2, 23, 24. Before a shower: 13.

40 Chill. Fever. Sweat. Chilliness: with pale face in open, especially damp, cold air; from uncovering; better in warm room.

Chilly in the evening, with great sleepiness; chill and somnolency predominating.

Sensation of coldness in the feet, with heat in the hands.

Congestion, ebullitions.

Heat in face and on hands forenoon, with hypochondriac mood, dry mouth and throat, without thirst; drowsiness, coma.

Want of sweat; skin cool, dry.

Sweat: red or bloody; with drowsiness; with shunning to be uncovered.

Intermittent fever, sleepy, tongue white rattling breathing, occasional bloody sputum, little thirst, even during heat.

41 Attacks. Daily: 3. Every winter: 46.

42 Sides. Left: 3, 6, 18, 20, 23. Left to right: 3. Right: 8. 18, 20. Right to left: 18. Within outward: 23. Above downward: 23. Below upward: 24. Behind forward: 24.

44 Tissues. Bleeding from inner parts.

Dryness of inner parts.

Want of blood, anæmia.

Marasmus of little children.

Dropsy of outer parts.

45 Contact, Injuries, etc. Soreness of all parts on which one lies; tendency to bed-sores.

Touch: 4, 10, 24.　Pressure: 19.　Riding in a carriage: 3, 16, 31.

⁴⁶ Skin.　Sensitive, especially to cold, damp air.

Skin cold, dry, not disposed to sweat.

Chilblains, every winter.

Ulcerations of the skin, painful; with hysterical patients.

Blue spots on skin.

Irregular red scaling patches, on face and neck during congestions, at time of menses.

Complaints from suppressed eruptions.

⁴⁷ Stages and States.　Children and women mostly; also, for the aged.

⁴⁸ Relationship.　Conjunctive relations: *Laurus*, *Sassaf.*, *Camphor*.

Disjunctive relations: *Lycop.*, *Nux vom.*, *Pulsat.*, *Rhus tox.*, *Silic.*, *Sulphur*.

It is best antidoted by *Semen capi Lauroc.* (according to Helbig); *Gelsem.* (according to Ross Roberts), and *Nux vom.*

It antidotes: *Arsen.; Rhodod.; Lauroc.;* mercurial inhalations; lead colic.

Similar to: *Stramon.*, *Opium* (mind); *Pulsat.* (internal organs); *Nux |vom.*, *Ant. tart.*, (sensations); *Opium*, *Arsen.*, *Spigel.* (fever); *Lycop.* (skin); *Silic.* (modalities); *Nux vom.*, *Rhus tox.* (motions); *Coccul.*, *Ignat.*, *Nux vom.*, *Sepia* (sides of body).

NUX VOMICA.

Foison-nut.　　　　HAHNEMANN.　　　　*Loganiaceæ.*

¹ Mind.　Defective memory; manner shy and awkward.

Can't read or calculate, for she loses the connection of ideas; thinks she will lose her reason.

Time passes too slowly.

Delirium tremens, with oversensitiveness, nervous excitability and malicious vehemence.

Desire to talk about one's condition, with anxious reflections about it.

Inclined to find fault and scold; morose; stubborn; an insane desire when alone with her husband, whom she adores, to kill him.

Disinclination to work and great lassitude or weakness in the morning.

Cannot bear reading or conversation; irritable and wishes to be alone.

Anxiety, with irritability and inclination to commit suicide, but is afraid to die.

Despondent and buoyant alternately.

Hypochondriac mood of persons of sedentary habits, and of those who dissipate at night, with abdominal suffering and constipation; also when worse after eating, with sensitiveness.

Loss of energy.

Careful, zealous persons, inclined to get excited and angry, or of a spiteful, malicious disposition.

Irritable, morose, sullen; apt to become quarrelsome if disturbed.

Anger with habitual malicious, spiteful disposition.

Fiery, excited temperament.

Oversensitiveness to external impressions; noise; smells; light and music, or the most trifling ailments are unbearable and affect him much.

Oversensitiveness, every harmless word offends, every little noise frightens, anxious and beside themselves, cannot bear the least, even suitable, medicine.

Ailments after continued mental labor.

Worse after mental exertion.

After anger, chilliness alternating with heat, vomiting of bile and thirst; great laziness and aversion to occupy oneself.

² **Sensorium.** Stupefaction, confusion as from nightly reveling.

Vertigo: with loss of consciousness; falls forward; when stooping; as if the bed was turning in a circle; reeling in morning and after dinner; with pains in forehead, heat and redness of face.

Intoxication from drunkenness of previous day, with vanishing of sight and hearing; worse after dinner and in the sun.

Apoplexy, with stertorous breathing; dropping of the jaw, paralysis; attack preceded by vertigo, buzzing in ears, nausea and urging to vomit.

³ **Inner Head.** Congestion to the head with burning in it, and with heat and redness of the bloated face.

Burning in the forehead on awaking and after eating.

Stunning headache in morning after eating and in sunshine.

Bruised sensation of the brain, generally one (right) sided; better when lying on the painless side.

Pressive, boring pains in head, beginning in morning, less by evening; with dim sight, sour vomiting and palpitation; worse from mental exertion, light, noise, coffee, after eating.

Periodical headache in the forehead, sore as from ulceration, with constipation.

Semilateral headache from excessive use of coffee.

Pressing on vertex, as from a nail; as if the skull were pressed asunder.

Pressing as if something heavy were sinking down into head.

Tension in the forehead, as if it were pressed in, at night and in the morning, worse on exposing the head to the cold air.

Intense occipital headache; dizziness; pains in the eyes; stomach deranged.

Sensation as from a bruise in the back part of the head.

The brain seems to shake when walking or running in open air; better when wrapping head up, in warm room, and when at rest.

Head symptoms are worse from mental exertion, exercising in open air and after eating; better after rising in morning (except sick headache), in warm room; lying down or sitting quietly.

⁴ **Outer Head.** Scalp sensitive to touch, or to the wind; better from being warmly covered.

Liable to take cold on the head, mostly from dry wind, or from a draught.

Fetid sweat of one-half of the head and face which is cold, with anxiety, and dread of uncovering head; sweat relieves pain.

⁵ **Eyes.** Sight blurred by overheating.

Vision impaired by dissipation.

Photophobia, worse in the morning.

Atrophy of the optic nerve.

Hyperæsthesia of the retina; pains to the top of the head sleepless; awakens irritable in the morning.

Exudation of blood from the eyes. Ecchymoses.

Burning and smarting as from salt; canthi reddened.

Eyeballs (lower part) yellow.

Lids burn and itch, especially their margins; worse mornings.

Blepharospasmus.

Paresis of ocular muscles, worse from stimulants or tobacco.

⁶ **Ears.** Strong reverberation of sounds in the ear.

Tearing, stitching pains in the ears, extending to forehead and temples: worse mornings, evening in bed, and on entering a warm room.

External meatus dry and sensitive.

On swallowing, pushing out pain in the ear.

⁷ **Nose.** Oversensitive to strong odor—even fainting.

Smell before the nose like old cheese or brimstone.

Snuffles, especially of the newborn.

Nosebleed during sleep, when preceded by headache and red cheeks, or in the morning; from suppressed hemorrhoidal flow.

Coryza, dry at night, fluent by day; worse in warm room, better in cold air; sneezing early in bed; scraping in nose and throat.

Acrid discharge from the obstructed nose. Internal nose inflamed.

⁸ **Face.** Face: yellow; florid, with a yellow ground; pale distressed; yellow around mouth, eyes or nose.

Tearing in the infraorbital branch of the trigeminus; clear water from the eye and nostril of affected side; face numb; after abuse of coffee, liquors or quinine.

ı Intermittent neuralgia, worse in the infraorbital branch of trifacial, always markedly exacerbated in the morning; better sometimes when lying in bed.

Swelling of one cheek, with faceache and pain in cheekbone.

Pimples on the face, from dissipation.

Twitching of the muscles in the evening on lying down.

⁹ **Lower Face.** Painful peeling off of the lips, after excesses; crusts on the lips, or ulcers that burn and stick.

Lower jaw hangs down.

Submaxillary glands swollen, with stinging on swallowing.

¹⁰ **Teeth.** Toothache, with swollen face; worse from reading or thinking; tearing is worse from cold or cold things; better from warm drinks; worse from coffee or wine.

Stinging in decayed teeth; burning-stinging in a row of teeth.

Gum-boils, which seem about to burst.

Gums white, putrid, bleeding.

¹¹ **Tongue, etc.** Taste: bitter; sour; putrid in the morning, must rinse the mouth.

Tongue: heavily coated white or yellow; black and dark red, cracked on the edges; heavy, with difficult speech.

First half of tongue clean, sometimes red and shining; posterior, covered with deep fur.

¹² **Mouth.** Roof of mouth, throat and gums inflamed and swollen.

ı Small aphthous ulcers in the mouth and throat with putrid smell; bloody saliva runs out at night; gums scorbutic; coagulated blood is spit out; voice altered, as if speaking with a full mouth.

Mouth dry, parched, without much thirst.

¹³ **Throat.** Raw, sore, rough, as if scraped, causing hawking.

Pain as if the pharynx was constricted, or as if a plug was sticking in the throat, during empty swallowing.

❙Swelling of the uvula, stinging pains, with sensation of
a plug when swallowing saliva only.

❙Stitches into the ear, when swallowing; small fetid ulcers
in the throat; even in cases of a "nervous" character.

Throat worse while eating and still more afterward.

Allays irritation caused by topical applications; especially
if rawness and scraping are present.

¹⁴ **Desires.   Aversions.** Ravenous hunger, after drinking
beer.

Canine hunger, with aversion to bread, water, coffee and
tobacco.

Longing for brandy, beer, fat food or chalk.

Very hungry twenty-four hours or so before a spell of
dyspepsia.

¹⁵ **Eating and Drinking.** Milk sours on the stomach.

Bad effects of coffee; alcoholic drinks; debauchery.

After eating: sour taste; pressure in stomach an hour or
two after a meal, with hypochondriacal mood; pyrosis;
tightness about the waist, must loosen the clothing;
confused, cannot use the mind.

Two or three hours after a meal, epigastrium bloated,
with pressure as from a stone in the stomach.

After eating: 2, 3, 16, 17, 19, 26, 27, 29.   Warm food or
drinks: 10, 17, 27.   Cold food or drinks: 10, 16.

¹⁶ **Nausea and Vomiting.** Eructations: sour or bitter; putrid
in the morning.

Hiccough from overeating, or from cold drinks.

Heart-burn; water-brash; worse before breakfast; also
with drunkards.

Nausea: early in the morning; with fainting; after eating; from tobacco.

Vomiting: food, drink; bile; black substances; slime;
sour mucus; blood, after suppressed hemorrhoidal flow.

Vomiting of food that was taken a day or two before;
contraction of the pylorus.

¹⁷ **Stomach.** Region of stomach sensitive to pressure.

Indigestion after abuse of drugs; business anxiety; sedentary habits; long watching or debauchery, after too
high living.

Burning in the stomach; at the pylorus.

Clawing, cramping pains in stomach, with pressure and
tension between the scapulæ; pains extend to the chest
or down the back to the anus, with urging to stool.
θ Gastralgia.

Gastralgia worse from food, better from hot drinks; worse
in the morning before breakfast.

Pressure in epigastrium, as from a stone; worse mornings
and after meals.

[18] **Hypochondria.** Stitches in region of liver, worse from contact or motion.

Throbbing as from hepatic abscess.

Liver swollen, indurated, sensitive, with pressure and stinging; cannot bear the clothing tight; caused by high living, abdominal plethora, debauchery.

❙Jaundice, aversion to food, fainting turns; gall-stones; constipation nearly always present.

[19] **Abdomen.** Pressure under the short ribs, as from incarcerated flatulence; worse mornings and after meals.

Colic from indigestion, with water-brash; worse after coffee, brandy or overeating.

Flatulent colic, with pressure upward, causing dyspnœa, and downward, causing urging to stool and urination.

Periodical colic before breakfast or after meals.

Colic from suppressed hemorrhoidal flow.

❙Hernia; sensitive, bitter vomit; labored breathing.

Tension and fulness in loins, abdominal and renal region; hæmaturia, abdominal plethora.

[20] **Stool, etc.** Stools: small, slimy, bloody, with urging, ceasing after stool; mucous or watery, from indigestion or cold; like pitch, with blood.

Alternate constipation and diarrhœa.

Constipation, with rush of blood to the head; obstructed portal circulation; frequent, ineffectual urging; stools may be in hard masses.

Hemorrhoids, blind or flowing; abdominal plethora; congestion to the head; worse from high living or sedentary habits; with burning and sticking in rectum; anus burning, smarting and feels as if cut, some hours after stool.

Tearing in anus; constriction after mental exertion, after eating.

[21] **Urine.** Renal colic, especially in the right kidney, extending to genitals and right leg; worse lying on that side, better on the back.

Painful ineffectual urging to urinate; urine passes in drops, with burning and tearing; spasmodic strangury.

Before urinating, pressure on the bladder.

Urine: pale, later thick, whitish, purulent; reddish, with brick-dust sediment.

Hæmaturia, from suppressed hemorrhoidal flow or menses.

Spasmodic urethral stricture; paralysis of the bladder; urine dribbles.

[22] **Male Sexual Organs.** Easily excited desire, painful erections, especially in the morning; often excitable but power is weak.

During an embrace, the penis becomes relaxed.

Emissions during sleep; especially after onanism or from
too high living. Bad effects of sexual excesses.

Chancroid often relieved.

Orchitis, with stinging and spasmodic contraction, extending into the cords; the testicles being hard and retracted.

Increase of smegma.

Gonorrhœa: after abuse of copaiva and cubebs; thin discharge, with burning on urinating and frequent urging
to stool.

[23] **Female Sexual Organs.** Crampy, stitching pains in pelvis;
soreness across pubes.

Congestion of blood to the uterus.

Contractive, uterine spasms, colic, with discharge of coagula.

Pressure toward the genitals in the morning; prolapsus
uteri, from straining or lifting; bearing down toward the
sacrum, with ineffectual urging to stool, or pressing on
the bladder with urging to urinate.

Burning, heaviness, sticking in the uterus.

Metrorrhagia, especially at the climaxis, or from high living.

Hardness and swelling of the os tineæ.

Menses too early and profuse; flow dark, oversensitiveness
to nervous impressions; faints easily.

Leucorrhœa fetid, staining yellow.

Tingling and itching of the vulva, causing onanism.

[24] **Pregnancy.** During pregnancy: morning sickness; jaundice; colic; difficult breathing from upward pressure.

Abortion (especially for precursory symptoms).

Labor-pains: spasmodic, cause urging to stool or to urination; cause fainting; are worse in back; are too violent.

After-pains violent and protracted.

Lochia scanty and offensive.

[25] **Larynx.** Hoarseness, with roughness and scraping in throat.

Spasmodic constriction of the larynx after midnight, suffocating spells.

[26] **Breathing.** Spasms of chest from vapor of copper or arsenic.

Asthma, with fulness in the stomach; better after belching; oppression mornings or after eating; spasmodic
constriction of the lower part of the chest, worse from
cold air or exercise.

Short, slow, stridulous breathing.

[27] **Cough.** Dry, fatiguing, from titillation in the larynx;
worse after midnight and in the morning; causing pain
in the stomach and soreness in the abdominal walls;
worse after eating.

Cough worse from mental effort; ascending; cold; exertion; on awakening; from tobacco; drinking, eating;
from beer; better from warm drinks.

Whooping-cough worse in the morning; with vomituritio; splitting headache, the child hold its head; face blue; bleeding form eyes, nose and mouth.

Sputa yellow, grey, cold mucus, sour or sweetish, or bright red blood.

28 **Lungs.**   Roughness and rawness in the chest.

Pressing in the chest, as from a heavy load.

Sensation as if something was torn loose in the chest.

❘ Intercostal neuralgia, better when lying on the well side.

Congestion to the chest, with heat and burning.

Hæmoptysis; from anger; suppressed hemorrhoidal flow; debauchery; especially in drunkards.

29 **Heart.   Pulse.**   Heart feels tired; palpitation on lying down; frequent belching.

Palpitation: with orgasm of blood; from mental emotions; from protracted study; after eating, especially after spices or coffee.

Pulse: hard, full, accelerated; small, rapid; intermits every four or five beats.

31 **Neck.   Back.**   Neck stiff, with heaviness; from cold.

Tension, burning, pressing as from a stone between scapulæ.

❘ Cervico-bracial neuralgia, neck stiff, worse in the morning or after eating and from touch.

Burning or tearing in back.

Sudden stitches in back when turning, with dull pain while sitting.

Backache, must sit up to turn over in bed.

Pains in small of back, as if bruised or broken; worse 3 or 4 A.M.

Spine affected by sexual excesses.

32 **Upper Limbs.**   Shoulders pain, as if bruised.

Drawing pain, from shoulder to fingers.

Paralytic heaviness in shoulders, with weak arms.

Paresis of the arms, with shocks as if the blood would start from vessels; worse at night, or early in morning.

Arms go to sleep, numb, stiff feeling.

Veins in the hands enlarged.

Hands cold and sweaty, with cold nose.

33 **Lower Limbs.**   Darting pains from toes to hip, or from trochanter to hollow of knee; worse at stool, from motion or lifting, and at night.

Numbness and deadness of the legs.

Paralysis of the lower limbs: from overexertion, getting wet, sexual excesses, or after apoplexy; limbs cold, bluish, emaciated; jerks, tension of muscles, formication.

Sensation of paralysis, feeling as of a painful stripe down the inside of the thigh.

Knee-joints feels dry, with cracking when moved.

Arthritic inflammation of the knees, also with nodosities.

Bright red swelling of the legs, with black, painful spots.

Cramps in calves at night, also in soles, must stretch foot.

When walking, legs tremble; unsteady gait; drags feet.

[34] **Limbs in General.**   Sick feeling through all the limbs.

Bruised pains in limbs; in joints; worse during motion
   and at night.

Rheumatism, attacking mostly the muscles of the trunk,
   and the large joints; pale, tensive swellings; numbness
   or twitching, worse from the least jar or from cold.

Fingers and toes red with burning and itching, as if frozen.

[35] **Position, etc.**   Motion or exertion: 18, 26, 27, 33, 34, 40.
   Walking: 3, 33.   Running: 3.   Ascending: 27.   Must
   stretch the foot: 33.   Turning: 31.   Must sit up to turn
   over: 31.   Sitting: 3, 31, 36.   Stooping: 2.   Lying: 3,
   8, 21, 29, 36.

Worse in a horizontal position; better with the head high.
   Rest: 3, 6.

[36] **Nerves.**   Stitches through the body in jerks, feels sore all
   over, worse mornings.

Sudden failing of strength.

Trembling all over; mostly of the hands; in drunkards.

Great debility with oversensitiveness of all the senses.

Wants to sit or lie down.

Tendency to faint: from odors; in the morning; or after
   eating.

Paralysis: parts cold, numb, emaciated; caused by apoplexy or cerebral softening, with vertigo and weak
   memory; from sexual excesses; from the abuse of alcohol; after spasms; after poisoning with arsenic; after
   diphtheria.

Great reflex excitability.   See 1, etc.

Convulsions: from emotions, as anger; from indigestion;
   preceded by constipation, jaundice, etc.; begin with an
   aura from the epigastrium; opisthotonos with consciousness; limbs, rigid and go to sleep; choreic, with numbness; renewed by bright light, sudden jar, noise, or the
   least touch; deep sleep follows.

[37] **Sleep.**   Yawning, stretching; chilliness.

Sleepy in the early evening, but sleepless at night.

Drowsy all day, worse after meals.

Stupor, lower jaw dropped; deep sleep.

Night seems long; dreams full of bustle and hurry; springs
   up delirious, has frightful visions; awakens in fright
   from the least noise.

During sleep, blowing, snoring expiration.

Goes to sleep late from crowding of thoughts.

Awakens at 3 A.M. (with many complaints).

Awakens 3 A.M.; falls into a dreamy sleep at daybreak, from which he is hard to arouse, and feels then tired and weak.

Better after a short sleep, unless aroused.

[38] **Time.** Morning: 2, 3, 5, 6, 7, 11, 16, 17, 19, 22, 23, 24, 26, 27, 32, 36, 40. Evening: 3, 6, 8, 37, 40, 46.

Remission evening until midnight.

Night: 3, 7, 12, 32, 33, 34, 37, 40. After midnight: 25, 27, 31, 37, 40. Day: 7, 37.

[39] **Temperature and Weather.** Warmth of sun: 2, 3. Warm room: 3, 7. Warmth: 3, 4, 5, 6, 10. Cold, or cold air: 3, 4, 7, 10, 26, 27, 34, 40.

Worse in dry, generally better in wet weather.

Bad effects from sitting on cold stones.

Dry wind: 4. Getting wet: 33.

[40] **Chill. Fever. Sweat.** Chill: evening and night in bed till morning; worse when moving and from drinking; with hot face; alternating with heat; mornings, with constipation (in nursing children); not relieved by heat.

Sleep after chill.

Anticipating morning fever: chill with aching in the limbs, gaping; blue nails; no thirst; then thirst, long-lasting fever, with stitches in the temples; light sweat. Apyrexia marked by gastric and bilious symptoms; legs feel weak, paralytic.

Heat: at night without thirst; increase during least exertion or in the open air; averse to uncovering; or desire, but becomes chilled from uncovering, or is seized with colic; before the chill.

Congestive chills, with vertigo, anguish, delirium, vivid visions, distended abdomen; stitches in the sides and abdomen.

Sweat: after midnight and in morning; sour, offensive odor of musty straw; one-sided, or only on upper part of body; cold, clammy on face; relieves pains in limbs; chill and again sweat.

[41] **Attacks.** Periodical and intermittent affections.

[42] **Sides.** Right: 3, 18. Above downward: 17, 33. Below upward: 33.

[44] **Tissues.** Atrophy of infants, no appetite, or ravenous hunger; desire to eat, with frequent vomiting; constipation; sallow skin; face bloated.

Rheumatism especially of back or large joints; muscles palpitate and are cramped; parts feel torpid, paralytic.

[45] **Contact, Injuries, etc.** Touch: 4, 18, 36. Pressure: 17. Jar: 34. Straining or lifting: 23, 33. Must loosen clothing: 15, 18.

⁴⁶ **Skin.** Burning-itching all over; worse in the evening; itch-
ing with icterus.
Urticaria, with gastric derangements.
Ecchymoses, blue.
Boils, especially if several small ones unite.
Abscesses; often disperses them.

⁴⁷ **Stages and States.** Suits thin, irritable, choleric persons,
with dark hair, who make great mental exertion, or lead
sedentary life.
Debauchers who are irritable and thin.

⁴⁸ **Relationship.** Follows well after: *Arsen., Ipec., Phosphor.,
Sulphur;* is followed by *Bryon., Pulsat., Sulphur.*
Zincum does not agree well with *Nux vom.*
Complementary to *Sulphur.*
Antidotes to *Nux vom.:* wine, coffee (large doses); *Chamom.,
Coccul., Pulsat.*
Nux vom. is an antidote to : abuse of aromatics, drastics,
"hot medicines," narcotics, bad effects of coffee and al-
coholic drinks, tremors caused by mercury.
Compare with: *Graphit.* (gastralgia); *Laches.* (congestion
of liver); *Carb. veg., Caustic.* (catarrhal hoarseness).

OLEANDER.

Nerium oleander.   HAHNEMANN.   *Apocynaceæ.*

¹ **Mind.** Weak memory.
Absence of mind, want of attention.
Slowness of perception.
Difficult comprehension of what he reads.
Indolence, aversion to do anything.
Cannot bear contradiction, becomes enraged.
After mental exertion, flushes of heat.

² **Sensorium.** Vertigo: for a long time before the paralysis;
when rising from bed; when looking fixedly, or looking
down while standing.
Heaviness of the head; better when lying down.
Faintness, as from weakness; relieved by sweat.

³ **Inner Head.** Headache improved by looking cross-eyed.
Pressive pain from within outward, in the forehead.
Pain in the forehead, as if it would split.

⁴ **Outer Head.** Biting-itching on scalp, as from vermin, worse
back part of head and behind ears; better when first
scratching it; followed by burning and soreness, which
gives place to biting-itching; worse in evening when
undressing.

Humid, scaly, biting-itching eruption, especially on back part of head.

⁵ **Eyes.** When reading, burning and tension in the eyelids; lachrymation.

Double vision.

Eyes sunken.

⁶ **Ears.** Herpes and ulcers on and around the ears.

Cramp-like drawing on the auricle.

⁸ **Face.** Pale, sunken face in the morning, with blue rings around the eyes.

Alternate paleness and dark redness of the face.

⁹ **Lower Face.** Numbness of the upper lip.

Foaming at the mouth.

¹⁰ **Teeth.** Toothache only when masticating.

Drawing in the molar teeth at night when lying down, with anxiety, nausea and frequent micturition.

Bluish-white gums.

¹¹ **Tongue, etc.** Loss of speech.

Tongue: rough, dirty white, with elevated papillæ; coated white, with dryness of the mouth.

Food has a weak, insipid taste.

¹⁴ **Desires. Aversions.** Ravenous hunger, with trembling of hands and hasty eating, without appetite.

Much thirst, especially for cold water.

Wants brandy: 17.

¹⁵ **Eating and Drinking.** Violent empty eructations while eating.

After coffee: 21.

¹⁶ **Nausea and Vomiting.** Vomiting of food and bitter greenish water.

After vomiting, ravenous hunger and thirst.

¹⁷ **Stomach.** Pulsation in the pit of the stomach, as if the beats of the heart were felt through the whole thorax.

Emptiness in pit of stomach, even after eating; from nursing.

Sinking in pit of stomach, suddenly, with nausea or vomiting; wants brandy, which relieves.

¹⁹ **Abdomen.** Stitches and gnawing about the navel.

Rolling and rumbling in the intestines, with emission of a great quantity of fetid flatus.

²⁰ **Stool, etc.** Ineffectual urging to stool.

Rolling and rumbling, with emission of flatus, smelling like rotten eggs.

Stools thin, yellow, undigested, involuntary when emitting flatus.

Passes food undigested in the morning which he ate the day before.

First, diarrhœa, then hard, difficult stool; during pregnancy.

Stool and urine involuntary.

Diarrhœa, with intestinal ulcers. *θ* Tuberculosis.

Burning at the anus before and after stool.

²¹ **Urine.** Frequent profuse urination, especially after drinking coffee.

Urine brown, burning, with whitish sediment.

²⁵ **Larynx.** Viscid mucus in the trachea.

²⁶ **Breathing.** Oppressed breathing when lying; also as if the chest were too narrow, with long, deep breathing.

Stertorus breathing.

²⁷ **Cough.** Violent shaking cough, from tickling in the larynx.

²⁸ **Lungs.** Dull stitches in left chest, continuing during inhalation and exhalation.

Sensation of emptiness and coldness in the chest.

²⁹ **Heart. Pulse.** Dull, drawing pain over the heart, worse when stooping.

Palpitation, with weakness and empty feeling of chest, and at the same time fullness in pit of stomach.

Anxious palpitation; chest feels expanded.

Pulse: quick, skin hot; changeable, irregular; weak and slow mornings, full and rapid evenings.

³⁰ **Outer Chest.** Dull, lasting stitch in the sternum.

³² **Upper Limbs.** Hands tremble when writing.

Fingers stiff and swollen, with burning pains.

Veins on hands swollen.

Itch-like eruption on inside of wrist and between fingers.

³³ **Lower Limbs.** Itch-like eruption between nates.

Weakness of the lower limbs, with sensation in the soles as if "asleep," when walking.

Trembling knees, when standing.

Feet constantly cold.

³⁵ **Position, etc.** Motion: causes spasms.

Walking: 33.   Exertion: 40.   Writing: 32.   Rising: 2.
Standing: 2, 33.   Lying: 2, 10.

³⁶ **Nerves.** Painless paralysis.

Stiffness and coldness of limbs.

Loss of muscular power; trembling.

Violent spasmodic contractions of the muscles; more those of upper part of body and of left side.

³⁷ **Sleep.** Yawning: with trembling of lower jaw; with chilliness and trembling of muscles.

Restless sleep, frequent waking.

Voluptuous dreams, with seminal emissions.

³⁸ **Time.** Morning: 8, 29.   Evening: 4, 29.   Night: 10.

³⁹ **Temperature and Weather.** Undressing: 4.

⁴⁰ **Chill. Fever. Sweat.** Chilliness, want of animal heat, of external chill, internal heat; no thirst.

Chill all over, periodically; face hot, hands cold.

Periodical flushes of heat; worse after bodily or mental exertion.

⁴¹ **Attacks.** Periodical: 40.

⁴² **Sides.** Right: 36. Left: 28, 36.

⁴⁵ **Contact, Injuries, etc.** Scratching: 4.

⁴⁶ **Skin.** Violently itching eruption, bleeding, oozing out a fluid, forming scabs.

⁴⁸ **Relationship.** Antidote to *Oleand.: Camphor.*

OPIUM.

Poppy.   HAHNEMANN.   *Papaveraceæ.*

¹ **Mind.** Unconscious, eyes, glassy, half closed; face pale deep coma.

Drunkenness, with stupor, eyes burning and dry.

Vivid imaginations, exaltation of mind.

Imagines parts of body very large.

Thinks she is not at home.

Delirious talking, eyes wide open, face red, puffed up.

Mania-a-potu; with dulness of the senses, and at intervals sopor, with snoring; in old, emaciated persons; sees animals; affrighted expression of face.

Imbecility of will, as though annihilated.

Nervous and irritable.

Ailment from: excessive joy; fright; anger or shame.

After fright, the fear of the fright still remaining.

² **Sensorium.** Great sensibility to sound, light, and the faintest odors.

Apoplexy, with vertigo, buzzing in the ears, loss of consciousness, red, bloated, hot face; tetanic rigidity.

Congestion of blood to the head, with pulsations in it.

Great heaviness of the head.

On rising, fainting.

Vertigo, a sort of anxiety when rising; after typhus; also, from injuries of head.

Dull, stupid, as if drunk.

³ **Inner Head.** Headache aggravated on moving the eyes.

Chronic hydrocephalus.

⁵ **Eyes.** Obscuration of sight.

Amblyopia.

The pupils are dilated and insensible to light.

Contracted pupils. θ Cholera infantum.

Sensation as if the eyes were too large for the orbits.

Eyes glassy, protruded, immovable.

Staring look.

Red, half-closed eyes, dilated, immovable pupils; eyes burning, hot and dry.

Swelling of the lower lids.

The lids hang down, as if paralyzed.

⁶ **Ears.** Acuteness of hearing; clocks striking and cocks crowing at a great distance keep her awake.

Congestion to ears; hematorrhœa.

⁷ **Nose.** Loss of smell.

Stitches in the right nostril on taking a long inspiration.

Stoppage of nose; dry coryza.

⁸ **Face.** Bloated, dark, red and hot; red; pale, clay-colored, sunken countenance and eyes, with red spots on the cheeks; bluish (purple), swollen face.

Muscles of face relaxed, lower lip hangs down.

Trembling, twitching and spasmodic movements of facial muscles.

Corners of the mouth twitch; distortion of the mouth.

The veins of the face are distended.

❙ The face of a suckling, three to four weeks old, was like that of an old man.

⁹ **Lower Face.** The lower lip and jaw hang down.

Foam at mouth.

¹¹ **Tongue, etc.** Paralysis of tongue and difficult articulation.

Tongue quivering, coated dirty yellow, unctuous.

Black tongue.

Ulcers in the mouth and on the tongue.

¹² **Mouth.** Dry.

Ptyalism: spitting of blood.

Saliva lessened.

¹³ **Throat.** Dryness of the throat.

Inability to swallow; daily attacks of distention and strangulation.

¹⁴ **Desires. Aversions.** No thirst.

Violent thirst: aversion to food, or canine hunger without appetite.

Desire for spirituous liquors; costive.

¹⁵ **Eating and Drinking.** After wine: 1, 26. When drinking: 27.

¹⁶ **Nausea and Vomiting.** Unsuccessful vomituritio in drunkards.

Vomiting, first of food, then of a fecal-smelling substance; hiccough; great thirst, cold limbs; distorted face; ileus; incarcerated hernia.

Vomit: green, bloody or bitter, with violent colic and convulsions; of feces.

¹⁷ **Stomach.** Heaviness and pressure in the stomach.

Inactivity of the digestive organs.

46

[18] **Hypochondria.** Swelling of the spleen.

[19] **Abdomen.** Distended, with flatus; anti-peristalic motion, belching and vomiting; bowels seem absolutely closed, but with constant urging to stool and urine; anxiety, flying heat internally, stupefaction.

Squeezing pains, as if something were forced through a narrow space; shooting pains into testes and bladder; restless, anxious, changing position; face hot; pulse slow; nephralgia.

Crampy intestinal motions; rolling up, as of a hard body in right hypochondrium. θ Ileus.

Colic from lead.

Hard, bloated, tympanitic abdomen.

Laxness of abdominal organs.

∎Incarcerated umbilical and inguinal hernia; fecal vomit.

[20] **Stool, etc.** Stools: watery; black, fetid; frothy, with burning in anus and tenesmus; involuntary, offensive, thin; involuntary, after fright.

∎Cholera infantum, with stupor, snoring convulsions.

∎Asiatic cholera, typhoid symptoms or after too much camphor.

∎Constipation of corpulent, good-natured women and children.

Stool in hard, round, black balls; costive from inactive bowels; from spasmodic retention in small intestines, with feeling of pressing asunder.

∎Retention of stool, from ileus or paresis of intestines.

[21] **Urine.** Involuntary urination.

Urine: suppressed; drowsy, stupid; retained, bladder full, from nursing after passion of nurse; from contraction of sphincter or paralysis of fundus of bladder; passes with difficulty, as from atony; seldom and scanty, dark brown, brick-dust sediment.

Stream interrupted from spasm of neck of bladder; cutting in urethra.

Hematorrhœa.

[22] **Male Sexual Organs.** Excitement of the sexual organs and violent erections; or impotence.

[23] **Female Sexual Organs.** Menses profuse, violent colic, forcing her to bend over; urging to stool.

Amenorrhœa from fright; irresistible drowsiness; eclampsia.

Prolapsus uteri from fright.

Fetid discharge from uterus. θ After metritis.

Softness of uterus.

[24] **Pregnancy.** Violent movement of the fœtus.

Abortion threatening after great fright, especially if in the latter part of pregnancy.

During parturition: cessation of labor-pains; coma; retention of stool and urine; often from fright.

During and after labor, spasm, with loss of consciousness and drowsiness, open mouth; coma between paroxysms.

Suppression of lochia from fright, with sopor.

Newborn children, pale, breathless, cord pulsates.

ı Suckling of a few weeks, had not grown, but was like an old man. See 8. Limbs lax, skin wrinkled; the bones of the skull had lapped over during birth, the parietals over each other, and over the occiput.

²⁵ **Larynx.** Hoarseness, with dry mouth and throat, and white tongue.

Feeble voice, and requires a strong effort to talk loud.

ı Laryngismus stridulus.

²⁶ **Breathing.** Short inspiration, long, slow expiration, epigastrium drawn in; fine rales, constant cough, sopor, face bluish; great anguish and dread of suffocation; looks as if dying; slightly better from cold air and bending forward; worse from smoking or wine.

Difficult intermittent breathing, as from paralysis of lungs.

Rattling breathing; or deep snoring breathing, with wide open mouth; stertorous breathing.

Suffocative attacks during sleep, like nightmare. θ Diphtheria.

²⁷ **Cough.** Dry, tickling, paroxysmal, worse at night; with gaping, drowsiness, yet cannot sleep; or, with spasm of lungs and blue face; when drinking; with difficult sputa followed by gaping; sputa are frothy, containing blood and mucus.

ı Cough with dyspnœa and blue face. θ Diphtheria.

ı Cough, with profuse sweat on whole body. θ Diphtheria.

²⁸ **Lungs.** Tension and constriction of the chest.

Heat in the chest.

Blood thick, frothy, mixed with mucus; great oppression; burning about heart, tremor, feeble voice; anxious sleep, with starts; legs cold, chest hot; especially for drunkards.

²⁹ **Heart. Pulse.** Burning about the heart.

Pulsating arteries and swollen veins on the neck.

Pulse: varies; full and slow, with snoring; quick, hard, with anxious breathing; irregular and unequal; imperceptible; face purple; in cyanosis neonatorum.

³¹ **Neck. Back.** Back bent backward, spasmodically.

³² **Upper Limbs.** Twitching and spasmodic movement of the arms and hands, as in drunkards.

Paralysis of arms.

Veins of hand distended.

³³ **Lower Limbs.** Twitching and spasmodic movement of legs.

Weakness, numbness and paralysis of the legs.

Heaviness and swelling of the feet.

Feels as if her lower limbs were severed from her body and belonged to some one else.

³⁴ **Limbs in General.** Trembling of the limbs after fright.

Spasmodic jerkings and numbness of limbs.

Convulsive movements of the limbs.

Coldness of the extremities.

³⁵ **Position, etc.** Must lie down: 1. Rising up: 2. Moving eyes: 3. Changing position: 19. Bending forward: 26. Motion: 36. Lying on back: 37.

³⁶ **Nerves.** Spasms: from emotion, fright, anger, etc.; from approach of strangers (children); from crying. Throws limbs or stretches arms at right angles to body; or, tetanic rigidity, opisthotonos with rolling laterally. Spasm begins with loud screams; then foam at mouth; trembling of limbs; suffocation; eyes half open and upturned, pupils large and insensible to light. After attack deep sleep, face remains deep red and hot; stupor between spasms.

Twitching, trembling of head, arms, hands; now and then jerks of flexors; body cold; stupor; motion of body and uncovering head relieves.

Faints every fifteen minutes; shuts eyes; head hangs; unconscious; jerks; sighing.

Want of susceptibility to drugs; want of vital reaction.

Numbness and insensibility.

Paralysis, insensibility after apoplexy; also in drunkards; old people; retained stool and urine.

³⁷ **Sleep.** Heavy, stupid sleep, with red face.

Drowsiness or sopor; stertorous breathing; hot sweat.

Sleepy, but cannot go to sleep; face bloated.

Coma vigil.

Stupefying sleep, with the eyes half open and snoring.

During sleep, picking of bedclothes; groaning; voluptuous dreams.

Stupid sleeplessness, with frightful visions, before midnight.

ıSleeplessness, with acuteness of hearing; clocks striking and cocks crowing at a great distance, keep her awake.

³⁸ **Time.** Remission during the day and evening.

Aggravation night and morning.

Night: 27, 40. Before midnight: 37.

³⁹ **Temperature and Weather.** ıBed feels so hot she can hardly lie on it; better from cold; worse from heat.

Very susceptible to cold air.

Cold air: 26. Uncovering head: 36. Wants to uncover: 40.

⁴⁰ **Chill. Fever. Sweat.** Stiff and cold; chill and diminished heat, stupor; weak, scarcely perceptible pulse.

Coldness only of the limbs.

Chill after part of night, thirst, pains in limbs, head hot, sleepy; afterward heat, with sleep, headache, pale face, bilious vomit; then sweat, mostly on legs, with burning hot feeling.

Fever, whole body burning even when bathed in sweat, face red; stupor; snoring, mouth open; limbs twitch; wants to uncover.

During lucid intervals complains head is too hot. θ Typhus.

Flushed face, cold legs, sleepy, but cannot sleep.

Sweat over whole body, which is burning hot; sleep and snoring. Hot, profuse, morning-sweat, wants to be uncovered.

Sweat on upper part of body; lower part hot and dry.

Cold sweat on the forehead.

Typhoid type of fever, stupor, can scarcely be aroused; speechless; eyes half open; mild delirium or loud talking, fury, singing, desire to escape; the darker red the face the more it is indicated; impending cerebral paralysis from profound congestion.

[41] **Attacks.** Nightly epileptic attacks; combined with mental derangement.

[42] **Sides.** Right: 19, 42. Left: 18.

[44] **Tissues.** Plethora.

Morbus cœruleus.

Suppurations painless, also ulcers.

Burning or sensation of coldness in the veins.

Jerks, only the flexors active.

Increased excitability and action in voluntary muscles, with diminution of it in involuntary muscles.

Dropsical swelling of the whole body.

[45] **Contact, Injuries, etc.** Touch: 46.

[46] **Skin.** Dryness of the skin, without fever.

Very troublesome itching all over, fine pricking, rarely sensitive to touch.

Redness and itching of the skin.

Blue spots on the skin.

Paleness of the skin.

[47] **Stages and States.** Especially suitable for children and old persons.

Frequently suited to persons addicted to spirituous drink.

[48] **Relationship.** *Opium* is often indicated in ailments from charcoal vapors.

Opium antidotes: *Bellad., Digit., Laches., Mercur., Nux vom., Strychnia, Plumbum, Stramon., Tart. emet.*

Antidotes to *Opium:* strong coffee, *Bellad., Ipec., Nux vom., Vinum., Vanil. arom.*

OXALICUM ACIDUM.

Sorrel-acid.   NEIDHARD, 1844.   REIL, 1851. $C_2 O_3$.

[1] **Mind.** Diminished power to concentrate ideas.

Very much exhilarated; quicker thought and action.

As soon as he thinks about the pains they return.

[2] **Sensorium.** Vertigo: weakness and thirst; anxiety, headache and sweat; when looking out of the window; when rising from a seat; a swimming sensation on lying down.

Sensation of emptiness in the head, faint feeling, as if all the blood had left the brain.

Upper part of body, particularly the head, feels as if blood were coursing upward and outward.

[3] **Inner Head.** Dull headache of the vertex and forehead; heaviness.

Compression in head, sensation as from a screw behind each ear.

Pain between the vertex and occiput, at a spot pressing inwardly.

Headache, worse after wine; lying down; after sleep and on rising; better after stool.

[5] **Eyes.** Type blurs when reading.

Vanishing of sight, with giddiness and sweat; with nosebleed.

Linear objects appear larger and more distant.

Pain in both orbits, worse in left.

[7] **Nose.** Sneezing, with chilliness; with watery coryza.

Red, shining swelling of right side of nose, beginning at the tip and spreading thence.

[8] **Face.** Feeling of heat in the face.

Feeling of fulness in the face; face redder.

Face covered with cold sweat.

[9] **Lower Face.** Drawing pain, with rigidity near the angle of lower jaw, first and longest in left, then in right side.

[10] **Teeth.** Pain in decayed molar.

Gums bleed, are painful in spots.

Small ulcers on gums.

[11] **Tongue, etc.** Tongue swollen, sensitive, red, dry, burning.

Tongue: swollen, with a thick, white coating; coated white, with nausea, thirst and loss of taste.

Sour taste.

[12] **Mouth.** Watery saliva, or mucus in the mouth.

[13] **Throat.** Dryness in throat (morning), after diarrhœa.

Deglutition: especially painful mornings; difficult, with sour eructations.

Scraping in the throat, thick mucus accumulates.

¹⁴ **Desires.   Aversions.**   Appetite: increased; wanting, with loss of taste.

Thirst, with vertigo, loss of appetite, nausea, colic.

¹⁵ **Eating and Drinking.**   Sugar aggravates pain in the stomach; and wine the headache.

Drinking coffee: 20.

¹⁶ **Nausea and Vomiting.**   Heart-burn, worse evening.

Eructations empty or sour; also, sudden hiccough, with eructations.

Nausea, thirst, colic, after the diarrhœa.

¹⁷ **Stomach.**   Empty feeling, compelling one to eat.

Burning pain in stomach and throat.

Awakens at night with violent pressive pain, like a heavy weight, coming and going at intervals; flatulent discharge relieves.

Stomach sensitive; slightest touch causes excruciating pain.

¹⁸ **Hypochondria.**   Stitches in liver relieved by a deep breath.

Continuous pain in left hypochondrium, as if bruised; stitches.

¹⁹ **Abdomen.**   Colic about the navel, as if bruised, with stitches and difficult emission of flatulence; worse on moving, better when at rest.

Colic from eating sugar.

Burning in small spots in the abdomen.

²⁰ **Stool, etc.**   Constant involuntary stools.

Suddenly seized with distressing feeling in whole abdomen, twisting around navel, bearing down; dark, muddy, copious evacuation, 6 A.M.

Stool of mucus and blood.

Diarrhœa as soon as one drinks coffee.

Lying down causes return of diarrhœa.

Before stool; headache.

During stool: as if caused by the pain, headache; micturition (fainting, vomiting),

After stool: nausea and cramp in the calves; dryness in throat; relief of pain in small of back.

Pressing and straining in the rectum; tenesmus.

²¹ **Urine.**   Pain in region of kidneys.

Frequent and copious urination, which is clear, straw-colored.

Burning in urethra, as from acrid drops.

When urinating, pain in glans penis.

Thinking of urinating causes necessity to urinate.

²² **Male Sexual Organs.**   Great increase of sexual desire.

On lying down, erections without any cause, and afterward testicles and cords pain.

Testicles feel contused.

During a walk, pain and heaviness in the testicles, shooting along the cords.

²⁵ **Larynx.** Hoarseness and sensation· of mucus in larynx during talking.

▌Hoarseness and aphonia without soreness.

²⁶ **Breathing.** Difficulty of breathing, with constrictive pain in the larynx and wheezing; oppression more toward right side. *θ* Angina pectoris.

Jerking inspiration and sudden, forced expiration, as though he made a sudden effort to relieve intense pain by expelling the air from the lungs. *θ* Angina pectoris.

Paroxysms of short, hurried breathing, with intervals of ease.

²⁷ **Cough.** From tickling in larynx while walking in open air; larynx feels swollen.

Dry cough on taking violent exercise.

Mucus hawked up, thick, yellow-white, with a central black lump of the size of a pea.

²⁸ **Lungs.** ▌Sudden lancinating in left lung, depriving him of breath.

▌Congestion, inflammation localized at base of left lung.

Rheumatic pains in the left lung; better lying down.

When breathing, stitches in the chest and above the hip.

Dull, heavy, sore pain in the chest.

Pain in the middle of chest, through to the back.

²⁹ **Heart. Pulse.** Pain in the heart; soreness, stitches, from behind forward, or from above downward.

Sharp darting in heart and left lung, extending down to epigastrium. *θ* Angina pectoris.

Immediately after lying down in bed at night, palpitation for half an hour; three nights consecutively.

Heart-burn intermits when thinking of it.

Pulse increased in frequency, almost imperceptible, with deadly coldness, clammy sweats, livid nails.

³¹ **Neck. Back.** Pain under point of scapula, between shoulders, extending to loins.

Stitches from chest into scapula.

Back numb, weak. *θ* Angina pectoris.

Acute pain in back, gradually extending down the thighs, with great torture; seeks relief in change of posture.

Numbness, pricking, causing a cold sensation; back feels too weak to support the body.

Paralysis from inflammation of spinal cord, limbs stiff; paroxysms of dyspnœa.

³² **Upper Limbs.** Twitch first in left, later in right deltoid, with inclination to move.

Sharp, lancinating pains in the arms. *θ* Angina pectoris.

Arthritic pains in fingers, which are flexed.

Right wrist feels sprained, wants to stretch it; cannot
hold anything.

Hands feel heavy ; can move fingers but slowly.

Hands cold as if dead.

Fingers and nails livid.

Twitching of the fingers.

[33] **Lower Limbs.** Legs cold, powerless.   θ Angina pectoris.
Legs stiff, numb, weak.

Knees feel tired.

[35] **Position, etc.** Motion: 19, 32. Exertion: 27, 40. Walking:
22; in open air: 27.   Change of position: 31.   Rising:
2, 3.   Lying: 2, 3, 20, 22, 28, 29.   Rest: 19.

[36] **Neves.** Peculiar numbness, approaching to palsy.   θ Angina pectoris.

[37] **Sleep.** Yawning; sleepy during the day.
Awakens at night with palpitation.

[38] **Time.** Morning: 13, 20.   Afternoon: 40. Evening: 16, 40.
Night: 17, 29, 37.   Day: 37.

[40] **Chill.   Fever.   Sweat.** Chilliness: with sneezing (evening); after diarrhœa (afternoon).

Shaking chill, with red face (evening).

Creeping chill up the spine.

Heat from every exertion.

Flushes of heat, with sweat.

Sweat: clammy, with weakness; with giddiness.

[41] **Attacks.**   Symptoms recur in paroxysms; intermit for hours
or a day.

[42] **Sides.** Right: 7, 26 , 32. Left: 5, 9, 18, 28, 29. Left to right:
9, 32.   Above downward: 29, 31. Front backward: 31.
Behind forward: 29.

[43] **Sensations.**   Pain in small longitudinal spots.

Jerking pains, like short stitches, confined to small spots,
lasting only a few seconds.

[45] **Contact, Injuries, etc.**   Touch: 17. Shaving: 46.

[46] **Skin.**   Sensitive during shaving, as from chafing.

Skin mottled in circular patches.

[48] **Relationship.**   Antidotes to large doses: carbonates of lime
or magnesia.

Sugar, coffee and wine disagree.

PAREIRA BRAVA.

[21] **Uterine.**   Almost cartilaginous induration of mucous membrane of bladder.

I I Constant urging to urinate, violent pain in glans penis;

straining; pain extorts screams; must get down on all
fours to urinate; urine contains much viscid, thick,
white mucus or deposits a red sand.
ı Pains down the thighs during efforts at urination.
Urine has a strong ammoniacal odor.

[48] **Relationship.** Compare with *Chimaphial, Uva ursi* (spasm
and burning in bladder, ropy urine), *Hydrangea arb.,*
Berber. (latter has pains more in back and hips, and has
a yellow, loamy sediment).

PARIS QUADRIFOLIA.

Oneberry. STAPF. *Smilaceæ.*

[1] **Mind.** Loquacious mania.
Silly conduct.
Inclination to treat others with rudeness and contempt.
[3] **Inner Head.** Headache, aggravated by close thinking.
Dulness of the forehead, with headache.
Piercing and single stitches in the head.
Constrictive pressure in forehead and temples; the brain,
eyes and skin feel tense and the bones scraped; worse
from motion, excitement, or using the eyes.
[4] **Outer Head.** Scalp sensitive to touch; sore pain at small
spots on the forehead.
[5] **Eyes.** Feel too large, or swollen, and the orbits too small.
Eyes feel as if projecting, with a sensation as if a thread
was tightly drawn through the eyeball, and backward
into the middle of the brain; sight weak.
Feeling of contraction in internal canthi.
[6] **Ears.** Sudden pain in the ear, as if forced apart by a wedge.
[7] **Nose.** Discharge of red or greenish mucus on blowing the
nose.
Stuffed condition and fulness at the root of the nose; constant hawking of tenacious, white, tasteless mucus.
[9] **Lower Face.** Violent itching, biting and burning on the
edges of the lower jaw, frequently with red, small, easily
bleeding (miliary) eruption.
Tetters around the mouth.
Vesicles on the surface of the lower lip.
[11] **Tongue, etc.** Great dryness of tongue on awaking; tongue
feels too large.
Tongue white, with roughness; no thirst; bitter or lessened
taste.
[12] **Mouth.** Dryness of mouth in morning.

Tart saliva.

¹³ Throat.   Burning, stinging and scraping in throat.

Sore throat, as if a ball were lodged in it.

Tense, almost painless swelling on the roof of the mouth.
   θ Scarlatina.

¹⁵ Eating and Drinking.   Hunger very soon after a meal.

After eating, hiccough.

¹⁶ Nausea and Vomiting.   Belching, with pain.

¹⁷ Stomach.   Heaviness in stomach, as from a stone; relieved
   by eructation.

Weak, slow digestion.

¹⁹ Abdomen.   Rumbling and rolling in abdomen.

²⁰ Stool, etc.   Frequent soft stools.

Diarrhœic stools smell like putrid meat.

²¹ Urine.   Frequent micturition, with burning.

Dark red urine, with red sediment and a greasy-looking
   pellicle on the surface.

Acrid, excoriating urine.

Burning and stinging in the urethra.

²⁵ Larynx.   Periodical, painless hoarseness.

Hoarseness, voice feeble, continuous hawking of mucus,
   and burning in the larynx.

²⁶ Breathing.   Oppression of the chest, with desire to draw a
   long breath.

²⁷ Cough.   As from vapor of sulphur in the trachea or viscid
   phlegm in the larynx.

Expectoration of viscid, greenish mucus.

Constant hawking and gagging, on account of viscid,
   green mucus in the larynx and trachea.

²⁸ Lungs.   Stitches in the chest.

²⁹ Heart.   Pulse.   Palpitation of the heart during rest or
   motion.

Pulse full but slow.

³¹ Neck.   Back.   Nape of neck weary, as from a heavy load.

Neck feels stiff and swollen on turning it.

Dull pain in nape of neck, increasing at times in acuteness, with numbness, heat and weight; better from rest,
   and in the open air; worse from exertion.

Stitches between the scapulæ.

³³ Lower Limbs.   Laming pain in the feet.

Cold feet at night in bed.

³⁴ Limbs in General.   Stinging pains in limbs.

All the joints painful on motion.

³⁵ Position, etc.   Motion: 3, 29, 34. Turning head: 31.
   Exertion: 31. Rest: 29, 31.

³⁷ Sleep.   Restless, broken sleep, with many dreams.

³⁸ Time.   Morning: 12, 40. Evening: 40. Night: 33.

³⁹ Temperature and Weather.   Open air: 31. In bed: 33.

[40] **Chill. Fever. Sweat.** Chilliness mostly toward evening, with internal trembling.

Coldness of one (right) side, with warmth of other side.

During the chill, contractive sensation in the skin and in all parts of the body.

Chilliness, with goose-flesh.

Heat, descending the back, from the neck.

Heat, with sweat of the upper body.

Sweat in the morning, when waking, attended with frequent itching.

[42] **Sides.** Right: 40. Left: 40. Right to left: chest symptoms. Above downward: 40.

[43] **Sensations.** Stitches in all the limbs.

Contractive pressure in the joints.

Heaviness in all the limbs.

[45] **Contact, Injuries, etc.** Touch: 4.

[48] **Relationship.** Antidote to *Paris quad.*: *Coffea.*

Paris quad. is followed well by: *Ledum, Lycop., Rhus tox.*

PETROLEUM.

Rock-oil.   HAHNEMANN.   *Anthracite.*

[1] **Mind.** Did not know where she was in the street.

Delirium; thinks another person lies alongside of him, or that one limb is double.

Sadness and despondency, inclination to weep.

Excited, irritable, with inclination to be angry and to scold; anxious and irresolute.

Ailments from vexation, with fright.

[2] **Sensorium.** Vertigo on rising; often with bilious vomiting.

[3] **Inner Head.** Headache in forehead; every mental exertion causes him to become stupid.

Headache from anger.

Frontal headache, at times quite severe, but worse while the nausea remained.

Occipital headache, with general spasms and screaming; loss of appetite, constipation.

Pain from the occiput over the head to the forehead and eyes, with transitory blindness; he gets stiff; loses consciousness.

Pressing-stinging in the cerebellum.

Dull, pulsating pain in occiput.

Sensation as if everything in the head were alive.

Head feels numb, as if made of wood or as if bruised.

⁴ **Outer Head.** Sensation as of a cold breeze blowing on head.

Scalp very sore to the touch, followed by numbness; worse mornings; and on becoming heated.

Moist eczema, acute and chronic, worse on the occiput.

Falling off of the hair.

⁵ **Eyes.** Cannot open the eyes mornings; sight misty.

Aching in the eyes, worse in the evening and from light.

Ciliary blepharitis from conjunctivitis granulosa or from small-pox, with sticking and smarting in inner canthus.

Pannus in scrofulous patients; discharge from the eye white; cheeks rough.

Pains at the root of the nose, lids swollen, purulent discharge from eyes and nose.

Iritis, with dull pulsating in the occiput. θ Syphilis.

Fistula lachrymalis (of recent origin).

⁶ **Ears.** Sounds as of bells ringing.

Hardness of hearing; in old people.

Dryness and disagreeable sensation of dryness in the ear.

Eustachian tubes affected, causing whizzing, roaring, cracking, with hardness of hearing.

Polypus; wax increased, thick or thin.

Discharge of blood and pus from the ear.

Humid soreness behind the ear.

⁷ **Nose.** Slight epistaxis, relieving the headache.

Dry feeling in nose, frequent sneezing; adherent phlegm, blown out in small lumps; thick phlegm in posterior nares, worse mornings.

Swelling of the nose, with pain at its root; purulent discharge.

Fluent coryza, with hoarseness.

⁸ **Face.** Yellow complexion.

⁹ **Lower Face.** Easily dislocated jaw, in morning in bed, with much pain.

External swelling on left lower jaw, painful to touch and on stooping

Swelling of submaxillary glands.

Scurfs around mouth.

¹⁰ **Teeth.** Sensation of coldness in teeth.

Toothache from contact with fresh, open air, at night, and with swelling of cheek.

Numbness of teeth, they pain when biting on them.

Swelling of the gums, with stinging, burning pain when touching them.

Fistula dentalis.

¹¹ **Tongue, etc.** Taste: slimy, pappy; bitter; putrid; sour.

The tongue coated white in centre, with a dark streak along the edges.

¹² **Mouth.** Fetid smell from mouth.

Saliva, offensive smelling.

Great dryness of mouth and throat in morning, with much thirst.

Ulcers on the inner cheek, painful when closing the teeth.

[13] **Throat.** When swallowing, food enters into posterior nares.

Throat feels swollen and raw.

Stinging from throat into ear, when swallowing.

Throat dry, sore, pain in nape of neck when swallowing.

Hawking of a tough, disagreeably tasting phlegm, in mornings.

[14] **Desires. Aversions.** Hunger immediately after stool.

Ravenous hunger.

Aversion to meat and fat, as well as all warm, cooked food.

Loss of appetite.

Drinks all the time; passes water often.

Violent thirst (for beer).

[15] **Eating and Drinking.** After eating: giddiness; heat in the face; cutting in the abdomen; gastralgia better.

[16] **Nausea and Vomiting.** Sour, or bitter eructations.

Nausea and vomiting of bitter, green substances; worse from riding in a carriage, during pregnancy, and in the morning.

[17] **Stomach.** Pain in pit of stomach, as if something were tearing off.

Sensation of fulness or swelling of pit of stomach, with soreness when touched.

Violent pain in stomach, extending up into chest, with sweat and nausea.

Gastralgia, with pressing, drawing pains, better from eating.

Sensation of emptiness and weakness in stomach.

Weakness of digestion.

[19] **Abdomen.** Awake toward morning, with pinching colic, better from bending double.

Cold feeling in the abdomen.

[20] **Stool, etc.** Awakened early morning by urgent desire for stool, which is gushing, watery; sharp, cutting, colicky pains below the navel; rumbling.

Stools: slimy, preceded by colic; chronic diarrhœa; worse during the day; of bloody mucus; often profuse; yellowish, watery; weak feeling in bowels and rectum.

Diarrhœa during the day.

Diarrhœa: from cabbage, sour-krout; after riding in a carriage.

Stool insufficient, difficult, hard, in lumps.

Piles and fissures of the anus; great itching; scurf on borders of anus.

Excrescences on and in the anus, moist, irregular.

[21] **Urine.** Constant dripping of urine.

Frequent micturition, with scanty, brown, fetid urine.

Involuntary micturition, at night in bed.

Itching in the meatus urinarius (female) during micturition, preceded by an urgent desire to urinate.

Chronic blenorrhœa.

Contraction of the urethra. Burning in the urethra.

Chronic inflammation of pars prostatia urethræ, with frequent emissions and imperfect erection, chronic urethritis accompanying stricture.

[22] **Male Sexual Organs.** Sexual desire decreased in morning.

Gonorrhœa; chronic cases, with urethral itching.

Itching and humid herpes: on the scrotum; between scrotum and thigh; on the perineum.

[23] **Female Sexual Organs.** Aversion to an embrace.

Menses: too late and scanty; early and profuse; menstrual blood causes itching. .

Before the menses, throbbing in head; during menses, singing and roaring in the ears; lassitude.

Prolapsus uteri in patients reduced by chronic diarrhœa, occurring during the day.

Leucorrhœa, like albumen, profuse every day, or with nightly lascivious dreams.

Soreness and moisture on genitals, with violent itching.

[24] **Pregnancy.** During pregnancy, diarrhœa and vomiting, worse riding.

After confinement imagines there is another baby in bed which requires attention.

Itching and mealy covering of the nipples.

[25] **Larynx.** Dryness and scraping sensation in larynx.

Bronchial catarrhs. Hoarseness.

[26] **Breathing.** Cold air causes an oppressed feeling on chest.

Oppression of the chest, at night.

[27] **Cough.** Dry at night, coming deep from the chest, caused by a scratching in the throat; with stitches under the sternum.

[29] **Heart. Pulse.** Cold feeling about the heart.

Fainting, with ebullitions, heat, pressing on the heart and palpitation.

Pulse accelerated by every motion; slow during rest.

[30] **Outer Chest.** Herpes on the chest.

[31] **Neck. Back.** Stiff neck; it cracks when moved.

Herpes on the neck. Furuncles.

Pain in spine and pain all over body, with sciatica.

Pain in back, which does not allow him to move.

Great uneasiness and stiffness in small of back and coccyx in the evening.

Pain in the coccyx while sitting.

³² **Upper Limbs.** Fetid sweat in the axillæ.

Salt rheum on arms and hands, red, raw, burning; moist, or covered with thick crusts.

Deep, bloody rhagades on hands, thick crusts; worse during winter.

Brown or yellow spots on the arms.

Wrist feels sprained.

Burning in palms of hands.

³³ **Lower Limbs.** Leg swollen from knee to ankle, purplish, oozing, or covered with scales or scabs, which are easily detached; itching and burning like fire.

Spreading, sloughing ulceration of the leg.

Herpes on knee and ankles.

Ulcers on toes, originating in blisters.

Hot swelling of the soles, with burning.

Heel painfully swollen and red; chilblains.

Feet swollen; cold.

Feet tender and bathed in a foul moisture.

³⁴ **Limbs in General.** The limbs go to sleep and become stiff.

Rheumatic stiffness of the joints, with cracking when moved.

Rheumatic stiffness of shoulders and ankles; syphilis.

³⁵ **Position, etc.** Motion: 29, 31, 34. Rising: 2. Stooping: 9. Bending double: 19. Sitting: 31. Rest: 29.

³⁶ **Nerves.** Twitching in the limbs; epileptic attacks.

Violent trembling of the limbs; weak unto faintness.

³⁷ **Sleep.** With distressing dreams, as if somebody were lying alongside of him in bed.

³⁸ **Time.** Morning: 4, 7, 9, 12, 13, 16, 19, 20, 22, 40. Evening: 31, 40. Night: 1, 21, 23, 26, 27, 40, 44. After midnight: 40. Toward morning: 19, 20. Day: 20, 23, 40, 44.

³⁹ **Temperature and Weather.** Many ailments are worse before or during a thunder-storm.

Aversion to the open air and from it chilliness.

Warmth: 4, 17; of bed: 40. Open air: 10, 40. Cold air: 26. Winter: 32.

⁴⁰ **Chill. Fever. Sweat.** Chilliness through the body, followed by violent itching of the skin.

Chilliness in the open air.

Chill, with headache and excessively cold face and hands.

Shaking chill, 7 P.M., then sweat in the face, and later all over except the legs, which are cold.

Chill, especially toward evening, often with heat at the same time.

Heat in the evening after chill, with cold feet.

Heat after 12 P.M., and in morning in bed.

Flushes of heat all over, in frequent attacks during day.

Profuse sweat every night, or immediately after chill.

⁴⁴ **Tissues.** Hemorrhages, blood light red.

Swelling and indurations of glands; also after contusions.

Increased secretion of the mucous membranes.

Emaciation, with diarrhœa by day, none at night; in children.

⁴⁵ **Contact, Injuries, etc.** Touch: 4, 9, 10. Pressure: 10, 12.

Riding in carriage: 16, 20, 24.

Sprains and bruises.

After burns or scalds (cosmoline dressing).

⁴⁶ **Skin.** Itching herpes followed by ulcers.

Herpes: 22, 30, 31, 32, 33.

Chronic eczema, parts seem excoriated.

Itching, sore, moist surfaces or deep cracks.

Brown or yellow spots on the skin.

Welts and blisters, with raw feeling.

Unhealthy skin; small wounds ulcerate and spread.

Ulcers, with stinging pain and proud flesh; often deep» ulcers with raised edges.

⁴⁷ **Stages and States.** Light hair.

⁴⁸ **Relationship.** *Petrol.* antidotes: lead poisoning.

Antidote to *Petrol.: Nux vom.*

PHOSPHORUS.

Phosphor.   .HAHNEMANN.   *The Element.*

¹ **Mind.** Stupor, delirium, grasping at flocks.

Hysterical alternation of laughing and weeping.

Great indifference; answers no questions, or replies wrongly.

Gloomy, taciturn. Dejection, thought he would die.

Fearfulness, as if something were creeping out of every corner.

Anxious, restless: at twilight; when alone; about the future; during a thunder-storm; with palpitation.

Melancholy, sheds tears; or, with attacks of involuntary laughter.

Amativeness.

Apathy; indifference, even toward his own children.

Excitable, easily angered and vehement, from which he afterwards suffers.

Mind is overactive.

Irritability of mind and body; prostrated from the least unpleasant impression.

47

While reflecting, headache and dyspnœa; feeling of apprehension at pit of stomach; weak feeling in head.

Any lively impression is followed by heat, as if immersed
in hot water.

² **Sensorium.** Nervous vertigo; or, vertigo from abuse of
narcotics, coffee; also, on rising from bed, or a seat, with
fainting; worse mornings and after meals.

Confusion as from watching; confusion and heaviness,
worse in vertex and sinciput; vertigo, tendency to fall
forward. Better in cold air and with head uncovered.

❙Apoplexy, grasps at the head; mouth drawn to the left.

³ **Inner Head.** Cold, crampy pain on whole left side of head.

Sensation of coldness in cerebellum, with sensation of stiffness in the brain.

Pulsation in left temple. Headache over left eye.

Headache every other day.

Weight and throbbing in forehead on waking, better by
cold washing, worse on stooping; sometimes lasts all
day.

❙Impending paralysis of brain and collapse; burning
pain in brain.

Congestion to head; burning, stinging pains and pulsations commencing in occiput.

Sick headache, with pulsations and burning, mostly in
forehead; with nausea and vomiting, from morning
until noon; worse from music, while masticating and in
warm room.

Hot vertex after grief.

Headache in forehead as if a weight pressed it down into
the eyes.

❙Softening of brain, with persistent headache, slow answering questions, vertigo, feet drag, formication, numbness in the limbs.

❙Acute atrophy of brain and medulla oblongata, with
uræmia.

⁴ **Outer Head.** Scaly, bald spots on the head.

Head affected: from taking cold; from remaining in hot
rooms; after having the hair cut.

Tension in face and skin of forehead, frequently only one
side; worse from change of temperature and while
eating; better after eating; with anxiety.

Dandruff copious, falls out in clouds; roots of hair get
grey and hair comes out in bunches; scratching makes
itching worse, or burning and itching relieved at time,
but worse after scratching.

⁵ **Eyes.** When reading, letters look red.

After reading, dull pain deep in eyes; black spots pass
before the eyes, worse from looking at bright objects
and in lamplight; better in twilight.

Contracted pupils.

❙Glaucoma.

Momentary blindness, as from fainting.

Amblyopia from loss of fluids; also in Morbus Brightii.

Has stopped rapidly increasing myopia.

Paroxysms of nyctalopia; or, of a sensation as if things
    were covered with a grey veil.

Green halo around the candle.

Subacute conjunctivitis, lachrymation; swelling and sup-
    puration of lids, and meibomian glands, with itching
    and burning pains.

Aching in eyes, forehead and orbits.

Small burning spots on the eyeballs.

❙Fungus oculi.

Eyelids tremble and quiver; eyes fill with tears.

⁶ **Ears.** Difficult hearing, especially of human voice; also
    after typhus; hardness of hearing, with cold extremities.

Sounds reverberate in the ears; especially music.

Shooting through ears, especially at night; ear discharges.

Congestion to ears, with throbbing.

Noises in ears, roaring, from rush of blood.

Polypi in the ears.

⁷ **Nose.** Coryza: fluent, dulness of head, sleepiness, especially
    during the day and after meals; blowing blood from
    nose; alternating fluent and dry, with frequent sneez-
    ing; dry, forming crusts, adhering firmly; profuse dis-
    charge, flowing down into fauces; neck swollen; eyes
    staring, consequent on the resulting stagnation of blood;
    scarlatina.

Profuse discharge of green (or yellow) mucus from the
    nose; without coryza; also after frequent flowing of
    blood; polypus.

❙Polypi nasi, when they bleed easily.

Severe hemorrhage from nose, in diphtheria, following de-
    tachment of the membrane from the nose.

Sneezing causes pain in the throat.

Sensation of fulness in nose, especially high up in left
    nostril, with loose mucus.

Chronic inflammation of the nasal membrane, with sup-
    pressed or oversensitive smell.

Nose swollen, red, shining, and inner nose very dry.

Necrosis; periosteum raised and forms a new stratum of
    bone.

Wing-like motion of the alæ nasi.

Freckles on the nose.

⁸ **Face.** Face: pale, ashy; sickly yellow; livid; bloated, lips
    blue; hippocratic.

Circumscribed red spots on the cheeks.

Puffiness under the eyes.

Eyes sunken, with blue rings around.

Burning, throbbing, in region of antium.

Twitching, tearing, darting and tension in cheek-bones and jaw, with threatening caries.

Pains from forehead into eyes (right), and from vertex and temples down upon the zygoma.

Tearing about lower margin of right orbit, extending under right ear, involving also bones of face, as if everything was torn out.

⁹ **Lower Face.** Lips dry, with sooty coating.

Necrosis of the lower jaw, rarely of the upper.

Tearing in jaw-bones, evening worse lying down, better moving the jaw.

Parotitis, when suppuration sets in.

Tough, viscous expectoration, hangs on lips and tongue, in typhoid conditions.

Nose, lips, mouth and throat dry; no relief from water.

¹⁰ **Teeth.** Toothache; from washing clothes; from having the hands in cold or warm water.

Pricking and stinging in decayed teeth.

Gums stand off from teeth and bleed easily.

¹¹ **Tongue, etc.** Taste: bitter; slimy; sour, after drinking milk.

Tongue: dry, immovable, covered with black crusts, cracked, parched, or glossy; dry, coated white, with stinging in the tip; coated yellowish; coated only in the middle.

¹² **Mouth.** Aphthous patches on roof of mouth and tongue.

Soreness of mouth, easily bleeding.

Saliva increased, tasting saltish or sweetish.

¹³ **Throat.** Swelling of right tonsil; mucus in throat, removed with difficulty; is quite cold as it comes into mouth; mucus white, nearly transparent, in lumps.

Tonsils and uvula much swollen; uvula elongated; with dry and burning sensation. Muscular angina, with fatty degeneration.

Rawness and scraping in pharynx, worse toward evening; hawking in morning.

Dryness of throat day and night; it fairly glistens.

Sensation as of cotton in throat.

Burning in the œsophagus; spasmodic stricture.

¹⁴ **Desires. Aversions.** Wants to eat, but as soon as food is offered, does not want it.

Hunger: must eat during the chill, before he can get up; at night, feels faint.

Wants cold food and drink, ice cream, etc.

Thirst, longs for something refreshing.

Aversion to sweets, or to meat.

Want of appetite, from fulness in the throat.

Loss of appetite, alternating with bulimia; burning, cutting, pressing in stomach, nausea and vomiting.

15 **Eating and Drinking.** Bad effects from excessive use of salt.

After eating: sleepy; belches much even after a little food.

After eating: 2, 4, 7, 17, 26. Eating or drinking: 16, 17, 27. Drinking: 19; cold water: 17.

16 **Nausea and Vomiting.** Eructations: frequent, empty; -spasmodic; sour.

Regurgitation of food without nausea; also in mouthfuls.

Sourish, offensive fluid ejected in large quantity, looking like water, ink and coffee-grounds; after food, or even a swallow of water.

As soon as water becomes warm in stomach, it is thrown up.

Food scarcely swallowed, comes up again; spasms of œsophagus at cardiac end.

Constant nausea.

Vomiting: of bile; of blood.

17 **Stomach.** Severe pressure in stomach, after eating, with vomiting of food.

Oppression and burning in stomach; loss of appetite, inextinguishable thirst, worse after eating or drinking.

Cardialgia, with gnawing; worse from motion.

Cramps in stomach radiating to the liver.

Fulness and painfulness in stomach; sometimes a gurgling and stitching in pit of stomach.

Hemorrhage from stomach, better from drinking cold water.

Goneness in region of stomach.

Gastritis, with heart-burn, ending in an unconquerable scratching in the throat.

18 **Hypochondria.** Jaundice: with pneumonia or brain disease; during pregnancy; from nervous excitement.

Acute yellow atrophy of the liver; malignant jaundice.

Diffuse hepatitis; liver hard, large with subsequent atrophy.

19 **Abdomen.** Very sensitive abdomen, painful to touch; rolling and rumbling in abdomen; during and after drinking.

Painful feeling of weakness across whole abdomen, worse in hypogastric region after a short walk; must lie down.

Shooting in the abdomen, with empty feeling.

Sensation of coldness in the abdomen.

Abdomen flaccid, with chronic loose bowels.

Tympanitis, mostly about the cœcum and transverse colon.

20 **Stool, etc.** Stools: profuse, watery, pouring away as if from a hydrant, better after sleeping; copious, light colored; greenish, bloody; bloody, with small white particles,

like opaque frog's spawn; painless, blood-streaked, like flesh-colored water.

Chronic painless diarrhœa of undigested food, with much thirst for water during the night.

Frequent diarrhœa, during cholera time.

Painless, debilitating diarrhœa, worse mornings.

ǀConstipation, feces slender, long, dry, tough and hard, like a dog's; voided with difficulty.

Bleeding hemorrhoids.

Ulceration of the rectum, with discharge of pus and blood; tenesmus.

Anus feels as if it was open.

²¹ **Urine.** Profuse, pale, watery; frequent and scanty; turbid, whitish, like curdled milk, with brick-dust sediment and variegated cuticle on surface; with red sediment.

Hæmaturia, from debility after sexual excesses; blood deficient in fibrin.

Glycosuria, with phthisis.

Albumen and exudation cells in urine; Morbus Brightii.

Twitching and burning in the urethra, with frequent desire to urinate.

²² **Male Sexual Organs.** Sexual excitement, frequent erections and emissions, or irresistible desire for coitus.

Lascivious, strips himself, sexual mania.

Impotence after excessive excitement and onanism.

Hydrocele after gonorrhœal orchitis, with sexual weakness; also, after seminal losses.

²³ **Female Sexual Organs.** Nymphomania.

Sterility from excessive voluptuousness, or with late and profuse menses.

Metritis after frequent pregnancies; pyæmia and phlebitis; fair, graceful women.

Frequent and profuse metrorrhagia, pouring out freely and then ceasing for a short time. θ Cancer uteri.

Pain in left ovarian region and down the inner side of thigh.

Menses early, profuse, long-lasting; or early, scanty and pale; weeps before the menses; during menses, pains in the small of the back; palpitation.

Amenorrhœa, with blood-spitting; bleeding from the anus; or hæmaturia; menses suppressed, with milk in breasts.

Stitches upward, from vagina into pelvis.

Dull tearing in labia, during or after walking in open air.

Leucorrhœa: with chlorosis; instead of the menses; watery, slimy or acrid, causing blisters.

²⁴ **Pregnancy.** Labor-pains distressing, but little use; cutting pains through the abdomen.

Ulceration of the mammæ, with hardness; red spots or streaks; fistulous openings, with burning, stinging and watery, offensive discharge; also so soon as pus forms.

ı Cancer mammæ, with sharp, lancinating pains; or bleeding easily.

²⁵ Larynx. Hoarseness, with cough and rawness in larynx and bronchiæ; worse in the evening.

Aphonia: from prolonged, loud talking; catarrhal and nervous; larynx sensitive to touch.

Cannot talk on account of pain in larynx.

Larynx feels as if lined with fur.

Laryngeal croup; aphonia; rapid sinking; cold sweat; dropped jaw; sunken face; rattling breathing; also, with tendency to frequent relapses.

²⁶ Breathing. Asthma, with fear of suffocation.

Oppression and anxiety in the chest, worse evening and morning.

Stridulous inspiration in evening on falling asleep; nightly suffocative spells, as if lungs were paralyzed.

Spasmodic contraction of chest.

Noisy, panting breathing.

Difficult inspiration, chest feels full and heavy, with tension.

Short breath: after each cough; oppression and palpitation from a short walk; worse after evening

Fulness in the chest, as after eating too much.

²⁷ Cough. Dry, tickling, with tightness across chest; hollow, spasmodic, from tickling in chest; with trembling of whole body; with sticking in epigastrium; must press it with the hand; nervous, when anyone enters the room; from strong odors; before a thunder-storm.

Cough, with stitches over one eye, splitting headache, burning dryness in throat; hoarseness, aphonia; soreness and roughness in larynx; worse evening and night.

Cough worse from change from warm to cold air; from laughing, loud talking; change of weather; eating or drinking; lying on the left side or back.

While coughing, involuntary stool.

Sputa: mostly in morning; frothy, bloody, rust-colored; purulent, white and tough; cold mucus, tasting sour, salt or sweet.

²⁸ Lungs. Stitches in left chest, better lying on right side.

Burning, piercing soreness and tension in chest.

Congestion to chest; anxiety; worse from any emotion; cramp between scapulæ.

ı Broncho-pulmonary catarrh, with dilatation, or fatty degeneration of heart.

ı Pneumonia: dryness of air-passages; excoriated feeling in upper chest; great weight on chest or tightness; chest sore, bruised; well-developed co-existing bronchitis; hepatization, especially of lower half of right lung. Latter part of the period of deposit and early part of that of absorption.

Capilliary bronchitis; pulmonary œdema.

Pleuritis; late stages; heart dilated; purulent infiltration.

Threatened paralysis of the lungs, prostration, viscid sweat; small pulse; face sunken; rattling in the windpipe.

❙Tuberculosis in the tall, slender or rapidly growing; repeated hæmoptysis; great debility; frequent attacks of bronchitis.

²⁹ **Heart. Pulse.** Disease of the right heart, with consequent venous stagnation.

Palpitation from every motion; with rush of blood to the chest, especially in the rapidly growing youth.

Great pressure on the middle of the sternum; orthopnœa; dyspnœa, with inability to exert himself; palpitation.

Dilatation of the heart, following endocarditis, or fatty degeneration.

Pulse: accelerated, full and hard; sometimes double; small, weak and frequent.

³⁰ **Outer Chest.** Yellow spots on the chest.

³¹ **Neck. Back.** Back pains as if broken, impeding all motion.

Pain in small of back when rising from stooping.

Burning in a small spot in small of the back, better from
. rubbing.

Softening of the spine.

Progressive locomotor ataxia.

Pain in coccyx as if ulcerated, hindering motion, followed by painful stiff neck. θ Rachitis.

Pains in the sacrum after confinement.

³² **Upper Limbs.** Swelling of axillary glands.

Tearing in left shoulder, worse at night.

Arms weak, can hardly move them, they tremble.

Emaciation of the hands.

Tremor of the hands.

Finger-tips feel numb and insensible.

Periodical contraction of the fingers like cramp.

Veins on hands are distended.

Burning palms; or clammy sweat on the head and palms.

³³ **Lower Limbs.** Rheumatic stiffness of the knees; pains from knees to feet.

Swelling of the tibia.

Pains in the soles of the feet, as if bruised.

Nightly tearing in the feet, during pregnancy.

Feet swollen in the evening.

Feet icy-cold.

Twitching of the feet.

³⁴ **Limbs in General.** Hands and feet numb, clumsy; ankles feel swollen and as if the skin was tense.

Limbs tremble from every exertion; also icy-coldness of limbs.

When walking he makes missteps, from weakness.

Swelling of hands and feet, with stinging pains.

³⁵ **Position, etc.** Motion: 17, 31, 32. Walking: 26, 34; in
open air: 23. Change of position: 46. Exertion: 34.
Cannot exert himself: 29. Rising: 2, 31. Stooping: 3.
Must lie down: 19. Lying on back; on left side:
27; on right side: 28.

³⁶ **Nerves.** Oversensitive to external impressions: light, odors,
noises, touch, etc.

ı Pains tearing, drawing, tensive, excited by slightest chill;
body feels bruised, with sensation of coldness; open air
intolerable.

Frequent fainting; pale, cold; sudden syncope, lying as
if lifeless.

ı Epilepsy, with consciousness.

ı Spasms on the paralyzed side.

ı Paralysis; formication and tearing in the limbs; anæsthesia; increased heat.

³⁷ **Sleep.** Sleepy, coma vigil.

ı Stupor, burning heat of head; muttering delirium.
θ Pneumonia. Sopor, dry lips, black tongue, open mouth.

Sleepy all day, all night restless.

Restless, especially before midnight.

Awakens often from heat and ebullitions, or from hunger.

Feels in morning as if he had not slept enough, or as if
paralyzed.

Somnambulism.

³⁸ **Time.** Morning: 2, 13, 20, 26, 27, 37. Morning till noon:
3. Afternoon: 40. Evening: 13, 25. 26, 27, 33, 40.
Evening till midnight: 40. Night: 6, 14, 20, 26, 27, 32,
33, 37, 40, 44. Before midnight: 37. Day: 3, 7, 32.
Day and night: 13.

³⁹ **Temperature and Weather.** Warm room; 3, 4. Warm
washing: 10. Cold, cold washing: 2, 3, 10, 36. Change
of temperature: 4, 27. Thunder-storm: 1, 27. Uncovering: 40. Hair cut: 4.

⁴⁰ **Chill. Fever. Sweat.** Chill: generally only in the even-
ing; no thirst; worse from uncovering; veins on the
hands swollen; from evening until midnight, with great
weakness and sleep; at night, alternating with heat;
with diarrhœa; chill descends, heat ascends, the back.

Flushes all over, beginning in the hands.

Heat, with anxiety and burning in face and hands, afternoon and evening.

Sweat mostly on head, hands and feet, with increased
urine, or only on forepart of body.

Profuse night.sweat, worse during sleep. Clammy sweat.

Intermittent fever, heat at night, beginning in stomach;
faint and hungry; then chilly followed by internal heat,
especially in the hands, external cold continuing.

❙Typhoid forms of fever.

⁴¹ Attacks. Every other day: 3.

⁴² Sides. Right: 13, 28, 29. Left: 2, 3, 7, 23, 28, 32. Above downward: 23, 33, 40. Below upward: 40.

⁴⁴ Tissues. Ebulitions and congestions.

Fatty degeneration of liver, heart, kidneys, etc.; anæmia.

Chlorosis, with too rapid growth.

Hemorrhages from internal organs.

Small wounds bleed much. Fungus hæmatodes.

Sprains; joints easily dislocated.

Glands enlarged, especially after contusions.

Dropsy of the face, hands and feet.

Swelling of the bones; necrosis (lower jaw).

❙Exostoses, especially of the skull; tearing, boring pains; worse at night, or from least touch.

Hip-joint diseased; oozing a watery pus.

⁴⁵ Contact, Injuries, etc. Touch: 19, 25. Pressure: 27. Rubbing: 31. Scratching: 4. Contusions: 44.

⁴⁶ Skin. Burning in skin; or burning and stinging; restless, change of position.

Blood-boils.

Polypi bleeding readily.

Open cancers bleeding easily.

Vesicles around joints.

Brownish spots here and there. Red spots; petechiæ.

Dry, scaly, or pustulous eruptions; psoriasis on knees and elbows.

Scarlatina, with suddenly repelled rash; chest affected; typhoid symptoms, restless, yet apathetic.

Variola, with blood in the pustules; hemorrhagic diathesis.

Fistulous ulcers: erysipelatous; pus thin, ichorous; hectic.

⁴⁷ Stages and States. Tall, slender (slim) women; disposed to stoop.

Nervous, weak; desires to be magnetized.

Grows too rapidly.

⁴⁸ Relationship. Ill effects of excessive use: of salt; of camphor; of iodine.

Phosphor. follows well after: *Calc. carb., Chinchon., Kali carb., Lycop., Nux vom., Rhus tox., Silic., Sulphur.*

Complementary to *Cepa* and *Arsen.*

Antidotes to *Phosphor.: Nux vom., Coffea, Therb.*

Phosphor. antidotes: *Tereb., Rhus ven.*

Inimical: *Caustic.*

Acalypha Indica is excellent in the hæmoptysis of pulmonary tuberculosis; severe fit of dry cough, followed by spitting of blood.

PHOSPHORICUM ACIDUM.

Glacial phosphoric acid.   HAHNEMANN.   *HPO₃.*

[1] **Mind.** Unconsciousness, no complaints, even pinching is not noticed.

Weak memory.

Incapacity for thought in the morning.

Delirium: quiet with great stupefaction and dulness of the head; unintelligible muttering delirium.

Indifference and unwillingness to speak.

Answers either reluctantly and slowly, or short and incorrectly.

Homesickness, with inclination to weep.

Hysteria, in women of dark complexion, during change of life.

Sadness, grief and disposition to weep.

Ailments from grief, sorrow, homesickness or disappointed love; particularly with drowsiness, night-sweats toward morning, emaciation.

[2] **Sensorium.** Vertigo: in typhus, so that they fall; when they sit up; lying in bed, as if the feet were going up, with head remaining still; after reflection.

Stupefying pain in the forehead, with somnolency without snoring, the eyes being closed.

Confusion and painful cloudiness of the head, especially on awaking.

Sensation as if intoxicated, in evening, in warm room, with humming in head, which feels as if it would burst, when coughing.

[3] **Inner Head.** Chronic congestions to the head, caused by fright or grief.

School-girl's headache; from overuse of eyes.

Great heaviness of the head.

Headache forces one to lie down and is insupportably aggravated from least shaking or noise, especially music.

Headaches usually go from behind forward and are relieved by lying down.

[4] **Outer Head.** Periosteal pains compel motion.

Bones ache, feel as if scraped; better in motion; when lying, the pain shifts to side on which he lies.

Hair: turns grey, early; or flaxen and very greasy; falls off, especially after grief and sorrow.

Itching of the scalp.

[5] **Eyes.** Aversion to sunlight.

Sees colors, as of the rainbow.

Blindness, with frequent desire to wink.

Torpid amaurosis, caused by debilitating losses.

Eyes look glassy, lustreless; also with staring.

Pressing in eyes, as if eyeballs were too large.

Burning of eyelids and corners of eyes, especially in evening by candle-light.

Yellow spots in white of eye.

Margins of lids swollen, red, rounded; lashes fall out; pus
particles on the lashes or on the canthi.

Coldness of inner surface of eyelids.

⁶ **Ears.** Intolerance of noise, especially of music.

Nervous deafness, after typhoid diseases.

Dull hearing: stupefaction; especially to distant sounds.

Every sound re-echoes loudly in the ears.

Shrill sound in ears on blowing nose.

Otalgia, stitches in ears and drawing pains in cheeks and
teeth; aggravated only from music.

⁷ **Nose.** Fetid smell from the nose.

Sense of smell too acute.

Discharge of bloody pus from the nose.

Nosebleed in typhus, giving no relief.

Swelling on dorsum of nose, with red spots; scurfs.

⁸ **Face.** Skin of face feels tense, as if white of an egg had
dried on it.

Hippocratic face, lips and tongue very pale.

Sensation as if lower jaw was going to break.

Eruption on the face, yellow-brown crusts.

Burning in skin of cheeks.

Pimples on forehead and body of onanists.

Hairs of the beard fall out, especially after grief and
sorrow.

Sensation of coldness on one side of the face.

¹⁰ **Teeth.** Bleeding, swollen gums; tearing pains in teeth,
worse when warm in bed, and from heat or cold; burning in front teeth during the night.

Teeth become yellow and feel dull.

Hollow teeth ache only when food gets into them.

¹¹ **Tongue, etc.** Red streak in middle of tongue.

Tongue and lips pale in typhus.

Tough, clammy mucus in mouth and on tongue.

Burning in tongue; tongue swollen.

Smarting in mouth when masticating.

Tongue smarts only at night.

Bites the side of tongue involuntarily; also at night.

¹² **Mouth.** Dryness of mouth and throat; grey-whitish coating of tongue.

Tenacious mucus in mouth and fauces.

Cancrum oris following measles in syphilitic children.

[13] **Throat.** Dryness of palate and whole mouth, without thirst.

Velum palati feels excoriated, with burning.

Sore throat, soreness, scraping, stinging, worse swallowing food.

Hawks up tough mucus.

Nasal voice.

[14] **Desires. Aversions.** Loss of appetite; the little food taken comes up with acid eructations; half an hour after eating, crampy pains in stomach, with distress from acid eructations.

Unquenchable thirst.

Inclination for warm food.

Longs for something refreshing and juicy; bread is too dry.

Desire for beer and milk.

Averse to coffee, wine, beer, or spirituous liquors.

Sour food causes bitter eructations or flatulency.

Canine hunger: 37.

[15] **Eating and Drinking.** After eating: 36.

[16] **Nausea and Vomiting.** Nausea, as if at the palate.

[17] **Stomach.** Sensation as if the stomach were being balanced up and down.

Pressing in stomach, as from a heavy load.

[18] **Hypochondria.** Heaviness, stitches, burning of one spot in region of liver in passage of gall-stones; jaundice in scrofulous children, or from grief.

[19] **Abdomen.** Rumbling in abdomen, and noise as from water.

Meteoristic distention of the abdomen; rumbling and gurgling; painless stool.

[20] **Stool, etc.** Diarrhœa: does not debilitate; from acids; in young persons who grow too rapidly.

Stools: involuntary, liquid, grey; yellow, mixed with mucus; undigested, greenish-white, painless; escape with the flatus; yellow, watery, with meal-like sediment.

Hemorrhoids: bleeding, with intolerable pain in sitting; with cramps of the upper arm, forearm and wrist.

Intestinal hemorrhage in typhoid.

[21] **Urine.** ❙ Looks like milk mixed with jelly-like, bloody pieces; decomposes rapidly; passed in large quantities at night, clear like water.

Constant urging to urinate.

Involuntary urination.

Few drops of white, gleety discharge, mornings, and discharge of prostatic fluid in the evening.

[22] **Male Sexual Organs.** Erections, without sexual desire; morning when standing.

During coition, sudden relaxation of penis, preventing emission.

Weakness after coition; also after pollutions.

Emissions: frequent and debilitating, causing hypochondriasis; from weakness of the parts, with onanism and very little sexual excitement; during stool.

Onanism, when patient is distressed by the culpability of his indulgence.

Feeling of heaviness in glans, especially during urination; also, with tingling, oozing vesicles around the frænum; in balanorrhœa.

Swelling of the testes, with swelling and tension in the spermatic cords; testes tender to touch; gnawing pain or excoriated feeling in testes.

Inflammatory swelling of scrotum.

Formication of scrotum.

Hair of sexual parts falls off.

∎ Herpes preputialis, with tingling.

∎ Sycotic excrescences, chronic, with heat, burning and soreness when sitting or walking.

∎ Fig warts, complicated with chancre.

²³ **Female Sexual Organs.** Ovaritis and metritis, from debilitating influences; amenorrhœa.

Uterus bloated, as if filled with wind.

Dysmenorrhœa, with pain in region of liver.

Menses too early and too long.

Leucorrhœa yellow, mostly after menses, with itching.

Uterine ulcer with copious, putrid, bloody discharge; itching or corroding pain, or no pain.

²⁴ **Pregnancy.** Itching, pricking like flea-bites between mammæ, obliging her to rise at night.

Sharp pressure in left mamma. Scanty milk, debility, great apathy.

Deterioration of health from nursing.

²⁵ **Larynx.** Tenacious mucus in mouth and fauces, causes hawking.

Contraction in suprasternal fossa, worse when bending neck.

Horseness and roughness in throat, hindering speech.

Burning in throat and chest.

²⁶ **Breathing.** Dyspnœa, as from weakness of chest; caused by odors, by talking, or by any effort.

Opression of chest; with contraction; with anxiety; when beginning to walk; at night.

²⁷ **Cough.** Spasmodic tickling cough; as from "down" in the larynx, suprasternal fossa, and whole chest as far as the epigastrium; evening without, morning with, expectoration of dark blood, or tenacious, whitish mucus of sourish, herby taste.

Restless but weak with hæmoptysis.

28 Lungs. Burning in whole chest, with pressure.

Weak feeling in chest, from talking, coughing, or sitting too long; relieved by walking.

Spasm in chest and diaphragm, sudden and unexpected, must sit bent.

Loud rattling and whistling in chest, with but little cough.

29 Heart. Pulse. Stitches through the heart.

Palpitation: in children and young persons who grow too fast; after grief; after self-abuse.

Pulse irregular, sometimes intermitting one or two beats, generally small, weak or frequent, at times full and strong.

31 Neck. Back. Formication in the back.

Gnawing on the scapulæ.

Heaviness in lumbar region, increases to pain in the legs. θ Tabes dorsalis.

Burning pain in a spot about small of back.

Burning in lower half of body, from small of back to pit of stomach downward; extremities are cold to touch.

32 Upper Limbs. Tearing in shoulder and left hand.

Burning as from a red-hot coal, in different parts of arm and on shoulder.

Hydroadenitis in the axillæ.

Stiffness and cramp in joints.

Shriveled, dry skin of hands and fingers.

❙Wens on the hand, between metacarpel bones.

Sharply marked deadness of one-half of the fingers.

Hands tremble when writing.

Burning of hands and heaviness; blood rushes into them when they hang down.

Boring, drawing, digging pains in nerves, awaken him from sleep.

33 Lower Limbs. Heaviness and paralytic sensation in hip-joint, worse commencing to walk after sitting; better after walking a little.

Burning: in posterior muscles of thigh when standing, better when walking; in soles at night.

Ulcers on lower leg.

Pains in tibia at night.

Blisters on balls of toes; feet swollen and sweaty.

Beating, swelling and burning in joint of big toe.

34 Limbs in General. Drawing and twitching-tearing in limbs.

Smarting at night in bones of limbs.

Limbs feel weak, from loss of fluids, with no other pain than burning.

Formication in limbs.

Feeling as if periosteum were being scraped with a knife, after injuries.

Interstial distention of the bones; mercurial, syphilitic or
scrofulous.

Arthritic pains brought on by least cold, with irritable
cough; swallowing excites the pains; fear of touching
the parts.

Cold hands and warm feet.

Boils in the axillæ, on the shoulders and nates.

³⁵ **Position, etc.** Walking: 22, 26, 28, 33. Motion: 4, 28.
Going backward: 4. Sitting: 2, 20, 22, 28, 33. Must
rise: 24. Bending neck: 25. Lying down: 2, 3, 4, 36.
Standing: 22, 33. Lifting: 4. Rest: 4.

³⁶ **Nerves.** Child weak, pale, cold; painless stools.

Weak from loss of fluids, grief, sorrow or unfortunate love;
from suppression of eruptions; from talking.

Trembling, legs weak, stumble easily, or make missteps.

Fainting: after a meal; from less of fluids; from emotions;
with desire to lie down.

Cramps: spasmodic, in chest and diaphragm, in onanists.

Spasm, painful, in hip-joint.

Spasmodic jerking of head.

Twitching or quivering in muscles of thigh.

Tosses the hands about, restless in the evening.

³⁷ **Sleep.** Great drowsiness and apathy.

Lies in a deep sleep, but when aroused, fully conscious.
θ Typhoid.

Awakened by: canine hunger; dry heat; sensation of falling; sad thoughts.

³⁸ **Time.** Morning: 1, 21, 22, 27, 40. Evening: 2, 5, 27, 36,
40. Night: 10, 11, 21, 23, 24, 26, 33, 34, 40, 44, 45.
Day: 40.

³⁹ **Temperature and Weather.** Generally worse from uncovering, better from wrapping up.

Worse in snowy air.

Warm room: 2. Heat: 10; of bed: 10. Cold: 10.
Averse to uncover: 40.

⁴⁰ **Chill. Fever. Sweat.** Chills, with shuddering and shaking, always in the evening.

Chill and heat alternate frequently.

During the chill peculiar cold sensation in tips of fingers
and in abdomen, with weakness of arms and tearing in
wrist-joints.

Heat, but averse to uncovering.

Internal heat, without being hot to the touch.

Sweat: mostly on occiput and neck, with sleepiness during
daytime; profuse during night and in morning, with
anxiety; clammy.

Intermittent fevers: shaking chills over whole body, fingers being as cold as ice, without thirst, followed by heat,

without thirst; ∎excessive heat, depriving one almost of consciousness.

Thirst only during sweat.

Typhoid fever: 1, 2, 5, 6, 8, 11, 19, 20, 28, 29, 36, etc.

⁴² **Sides.**   Right: 18, 23. Left: 18, 24, 32. Above downward: 31.

⁴⁴ **Tissues.**   Hemorrhages, blood dark.

Painless swelling of glands.

Interstitial inflammation of bones; scrofulous, syphilitic or mercurial.

Bone diseases.

Periosteal inflammation, with burning, gnawing, tearing pains.

Caries, with smarting pains, not with necrosis.

Emaciation; also, of single parts.

External parts become black.

⁴⁵ **Contact, Injuries, etc.**   Touch: 31, 34, 40.

When after contusions periosteum feels as if scraped by a knife, worse at night.

Smarting in all wounds.

⁴⁶ **Skin.**   ∎Herpes dry or humid, squamous. ·

Itching between fingers, or in folds of joints, or on hands.

Exanthemata, suppressed by cold, cause brain symptoms; hardness of hearing or dropsy.

∎Variola.   In typhoid state, eruptions do not fill with pus, but degenerate into large blisters, which, bursting, leave surface excoriated; watery diarrhœa; with subsultus tendinum; fear of death.

Warts, indented, pedunculated.

Condylomata; with bone pains; complicated with chancre.

Ulcers: like carbuncles on the skin, with a coppery circumference; with smarting pain; flat and itching.

Parts get black.

⁴⁷ **Stages and States.**   Bad effects from growing too rapidly; as if beaten in back and limbs.

⁴⁸ **Relationship.**   *Cinchon.* before or after in colliquative sweat, diarrhœa and debility.

If in syncope after a meal, *Nux Vom.* is insufficient, give *Phosph. ac.*

After *Phosph. ac.* are frequently suitable: *Cinchon., Ferrum, Rhus tox., Veratr.*

Antidotes to *Phosph ac.: Camphor., Coffea.*

Distinguished in typhoid from *Mur. ac.* by pallor, grey or colorless stools; *Nitr. spir. dulc.* causes a sensorial apathy, a sort of half paralysis of the mental organs; can be aroused, when he answers slowly but relevantly, and again goes into a stupor. (Relieved in typhoid after *Phosph. ac.* failed.)

48

PHYTOLACCA DECANDRA.

Poke Root.   ALLENTOWN COLLEGE.   *Phytolaccaceæ.*

[1] **Mind.** Delirious.

Indisposition to mental exertion.

Disgust for business of day, on waking early in morning.

Melancholy, gloom.

Great fear, is sure will die.

Indifference to life.

Complete shamelessness and indifference to exposure of her person.

Irritability.

Restlessness.

Oversensitiveness to pain.

[2] **Sensorium.** Vertigo: with danger of falling; with dim vision; when rising from bed, feels faint; staggering.

[3] **Inner Head.** Pain in back of head and neck.

One-sided headache.

Pain extending back from the frontal region.

Shooting pain from left eye to top of head.

Heavy aching feeling in the head, at 1.30 P.M.

Sensation of soreness deep in brain.

Painful pressure on forehead and upper part of both eyes.

Pain in top of head, and a feeling as if the brain were bruised, when stepping from a high step to the ground.

Sick headache, worse in forehead; with backache and bearing down; comes every week.

[4] **Outer Head.** Tinea capitis; worse washing it when he is warm.

[5] **Eyes.** Photophobia.

Pupils contracted; tetanus.

Dimness of vision.

Burning, smarting, tingling pain in eyes; itching aggravated by gaslight; abundant flow of tears. *θ* Catarrhal ophthalmia.

Feeling of sand in eyes, with soreness and burning.

Sharp pain goes through ball of eye on reading or writing.

Reddish-blue swelling of eyelids, worse on left side, and in morning; hard, unyielding cellulitis.

Motions of one eye independent of the other.

Circumorbital pains in syphilitic ophthalmia.

[6] **Ears.** Shooting pains through both ears when swallowing; right side worse.

Eustachian tubes feel obstructed.

[7] **Nose.** Thin, watery discharge from nostrils increasing till the nose become stuffed.

Flow of mucus from one nostril, while the other is stopped;
both stopped up while riding.

Acrid discharge, excoriating.   θ Scarlatina.

⁸ **Face.**   Very pale; hippocratic; looking blue and suffering;
yellowish.

Cold sweat on forehead.

Blotches in face; worse in P.M., after washing and eating.

Swelling around left ear and side of face like erysipelas;
thence over scalp; very painful.

⁹ **Lower Face.** ╷Chin drawn closely to sternum, by convulsive
action of muscles of face and neck.   θ Tetanus.

╶ ╷Lips everted and firm.   θ Tetanus.

Upper lip excoriated.

Ulcers on lips.

Parotid and submaxillary glands swollen.

¹⁰ **Teeth.**   Disposition to bite the teeth together.

Difficult dentition.

¹¹ **Tongue, etc.**   Metallic taste.

Burnt feeling on back part of tongue.

Tongue: fiery red at tip; coated yellow and dry; thickly
coated at back part.

Tongue: hot, rough, tender and smarting at tip; also small
ulcers, like those caused by mercury; thick; protruding.

¹² **Mouth.**   Profuse saliva, sometimes yellowish, often thick,
ropy, tenacious; mercurial ptyalism, with inflamed
gums and teeth.

Small ulcers on inside of right cheek, very painful; he
cannot chew on that side.

Sensation of dryness in the mouth, with cough.

¹³ **Throat.**   Sore, worse right side; fauces dark, bluish-red;
worse swallowing saliva; feels as if a red-hot ball was
lodged in fauces; cannot bear touch of clothing about
neck.

Uvula large, transparent.

Tonsils large, bluish, ulcerated; throat feels as after choke-
pears; dry, rough, burning, smarting fauces.

Like a plug in throat, worse left side.

Dirty, wash-leather pseudo-membrane; mucus hawked
with difficulty, from posterior nares; hangs down in
strings; severe pains in head, neck and back; great
prostration; faint on rising.   θ Diphtheria.

Cannot drink hot fluids; choking; ulcers on tonsils.
θ Syphilis.

Pharynx dry, rough, feels like a cavern.

¹⁴ **Desires. Aversions.**   Great thirst.

Hunger soon after eating.

Loss of appetite.

¹⁵ **Eating and Drinking.**   After eating: 8.   Hot drinks: 13.

After lemonade: 20.

¹⁶ **Nausea and Vomiting.** Nausea, eructations of flatus and sour fluid.

Violent vomiting every few minutes.

Violent vomiting of clotted blood and slime, with retching, intense pain, and desire for death to relieve; purging and vomiting.

Vomiting in diphtheria.

¹⁷ **Stomach.** Bruised and sore feeling at pit of stomach.

Heat in stomach.

Pain in pit of stomach, as from a heavy blow or concussion there, followed by cramps in abdomen, and coolness,

Pain in region of pylorus.

¹⁸ **Hypocondria.** In right hopochondrium a sore spot, not larger than a dollar, extremely sensitive to touch.

¹⁹ **Abdomen.** Griping and cramps in abdomen.

Burning, griping pains in umbilical region.

Rheumatism extending to abdominal muscles.

Bearing down pains.

²⁰ **Stool, etc.** Stools: thin, dark brown; of mucus and blood, like intestinal scrapings; tenesmus; of bile.

Diarrhœa early in morning; after lemonade.

Constipation of the aged, or of those with weak heart.

Bleeding piles. Fissured rectum.

²¹ **Urine.** Weakness, dull pain and soreness in region of kidneys; most on right side, and connected with heat; uneasiness down the ureters; chalk-like sediment in urine.

Urine: albuminous; excessive or scanty; dark red, stains the vessel.

Pain in region of bladder before and during urination.

Urgent desire to pass water.

²² **Male Sexual Organs.** Gonorrhœa and gleet.

Orchitis; secondary syphilis.

Syphilis, chancres, ulcerated throat; ulcers on genitals.

²³ **Female Sexual Organs.** Menses too frequent and too copious; mammæ painful.

Painful menstruation in barren women; costive.

Ovaritis.

²⁴ **Pregnancy.** Pain in sacrum down to knees and ankles, then up to the sacrum; jerks here and there; after confinement.

Inflammation, swelling and suppuration of breasts.

Nipples very sensitive.

Breast hard as a stone, after weaning.

Nipples sore and fissured, with intense suffering on putting child to breast; pains seems to start from nipple, and radiate over whole body.

Excessive flow of milk, causing great exhaustion.

"Gathered breasts," with large, fistulous, gaping and angry ulcers, discharging a watery, fetid pus.

Mammary gland full of hard, painful nodosities.

25 Larynx. Hoarseness and aphonia.

Dryness of larynx and trachea, worse toward evening.

Burning in larynx and trachea, with a sensation of contraction of the glottis; labored breathing.

Spasms of glottis, eyes distorted, one eye moves independently of the other, thumbs clenched, toes flexed.

26 Breathing. Respiration difficult, oppressed; loud mucous rales.

Constant moaning and gasping for air. θ Diphtheria.

Faint, with sighing, slow breathing.

27 Cough. Hacking, dry, with hawking; excited by tickling in larynx or dryness in pharynx; worse at night as soon as he lies down.

Sputa thick, tough.

28 Lungs. Pains and suffocating feeling in throat and lungs.

Aching pains in chest and side, with cough.

Pain through mid-sternum, with cough.

29 Heart. Pulse. Shocks of pain in cardiac region; angina pectoris; pain goes into right arm.

Heart's action weak, with constipation.

Awakens with lameness near heart; worse during expiration; cannot get to sleep again.

Pulse: small, irregular, with great excitement in chest, especially in cardiac region; full, but soft.

30 Outer Chest. Rheumatism of lower intercostal, from exposure to cold and dampness.

31 Neck. Back. Convulsive action of muscles of face and neck. θ Tetanus.

Glands of right side of neck, hard.

Stiff neck; tonsils swollen.

Rheumatism in lumbar muscles.

Aching pain in lumbar region, day and night, with sore throat.

Pain streaking up and down the spine.

Aching in sacrum.

32 Upper Limbs. Both scapulæ ache continually.

Shooting pain in right shoulder-joint, with stiffness and inability to raise the arm; aching and tenderness along top of right trapezius.

Pain in arms, especially about attachment of deltoid muscles.

Finger-joints swollen, hard, shining.

Lame feeling in the arms.

33 Lower Limbs. Pains shooting from sacrum down outside of both hips.

Sharp, cutting pains in hip, drawing; leg drawn up, cannot touch the floor; hip disease on right side after mercury; or, in syphilitic children.

Rheumatism of left knee, hamstrings feel shortened.

Pains down from hips to knee; heavy dragging; neuralgic pains; all worse on outer part of thighs.

Nightly pains in periosteum of tibiæ.

Chronic rheumatism of left hip.

Ulcers and nodes on legs.

Feet puffed, soles burn; severe pains through ankles and feet; also, on dorsa of feet.

³⁴ **Limbs in General.** Severe pains in arms and legs from elbows and knees to fingers and toes ; worse from motion and contact; syphilis.

³⁵ **Position, etc.** Motion: 1, 5. Stepping down: 3. Rising from bed: 2. Lying: 27.

³⁶ **Nerves.** Great exhaustion, prostration, muscular paresis.

Legs weak, heavy; he staggers.

Tetanus; alternate spasms and relaxation of muscles; general muscular rigidity.

³⁷ **Sleep.** Frequent gaping.

Drowsiness.

Restlessness at night; pains drive him out of bed.

On waking, feels wretched.

³⁸ **Time.** Morning: 1, 5, 20, 31, 36, 40. Afternoon: 3. Evening: 25. Fight: 25, 27, 31, 33, 37, 44. Day and night: 31.

³⁹ **Temperature and Weather.** Damp weather: 3, 30, 44. Washing when warm: 4, 8. Cold: 30.

⁴⁰ **Chill. Fever. Sweat.** Coldness, faintness, dyspnœa; chill every morning.

Limbs cold, head and face hot.

Sweat cold on forehead; toes sweat.

Night-sweat.

⁴¹ **Attacks.** Every week: 3. Every morning: 40.

⁴² **Sides.** Right: 3, 6, 12, 13, 18, 21, 31, 32, 33. Left: 5, 8, 13, 29, 33. Left to right: 29. Below upward: 2. Above downward: 33. Above downward, then below upward: 24. Before backward: 3.

⁴³ **Sensations.** Pains flying like electric shocks; jerking pains; shooting, lancinating.

⁴⁴ **Tissues.** Loss of fat (animals).

It hastens suppuration.

Pus watery, fetid, ichorous.

Rheumatism and gout; pains shift; joints swollen, red; periosteum affected, especially in mercurialization and in syphilis; pains in middle of long bones or attachment of muscles; worse in damp weather, at night.

Glands inflamed, swollen.

Bones iflamed, swollen.

⁴⁵ Contact, Injuries, etc. Riding: 7. Touch: 13, 18, 24.

⁴⁶ Skin. Cool, shriveled, dry, lead-colored.

Barber's itch, local application of tincture.

Ringworm.

Boils, especially near the ulcers.

Black-looking, tettery, suppurative eruption.

Ulcers, with an appearance as if punched out; lardaceous bottom; syphilitic ulcerations.

Cancerous ulcers (also, on breast).

Erythematous blotches, irregular, slightly raised, pale red, ending in dark red or purple spots.

Rash.

Red spots, with syphilitic persons.

Scarlatina, with angina; acrid coryza; delirium; non-appearing eruption.

⁴⁸ Relationship. Antidotes to *Phytol.:* milk and salt; *Ignat.;* also, *Sulphur* against eye symptoms.

Opium is said to be an antidote for large doses. Coffee sometimes relieves vomiting.

PLATINA.

The Metal.   Staff.   *An Element.*

¹ Mind. Everything seems strange and horrible to her.

She thinks all persons are demons.

Illusion: everything around her is very small and everybody inferior to her in mind and body.

Delirium with fear of men, often changing with overestimation of oneself.

Disturbed state of mind, also religious, with taciturnity, haughtiness, voluptiousness and cruelty.

Mania, with great pride; fault-finding; unchaste talk; trembling and clonic spasms; caused by fright or anger.

Mood changing; cheerful or depressed.

Low-spirited, inclined to shed tears, worse in the evening; weeps with the pains.

Past events trouble her.

Much anguish; she feels as if she would lose her senses and die soon.

Satiety of life, with (taciturnity and) fear of death.

Great indifference.

Pride and overestimation of oneself; looking down with haughtiness on others.

Physical symptoms disappear, and mental symptoms appear, and vice versa.

After anger, alternate laughing and weeping, with great anguish and fear of death.

Mental disturbance after fright, grief or vexation.

3 **Inner Head.** Sensation of numbness in head and externally on vertex, preceded by a sensation of contraction of the brain and scalp; worse in evening and while sitting; better from motion and in open air.

Neuralgic headaches in sensitive or hysterical persons; cramp-like pressing inwards, with hot and red face, and roaring in head; pains gradually increase and as gradually decrease.

Numb feeling in the brain.

Sensation of water in the forehead.

4 **Outer Head.** Formication in one temple, extending to lower jaw, with sensation of coldness on that spot; worse in evening and when at rest, better from rubbing.

5 **Eyes.** Scintillations before the eyes; headache.

Sensation of coldness in the eyes.

Spasmodic trembling and twitching of the eyelids.

Objects appear smaller than they really are.

6 **Ears.** Ringing, rolling or rumbling sound in the ears.

Thundering jerks like distant cannonade, in right ear.

Otalgia with cramp-pain, often with rumbling in the ears.

Sensation of coldness in ears, with sensation of numbness extending to cheeks and lips.

7 **Nose.** Numbness and cramp-pain in nose.

Violent crampy pain at root of nose, with heat and red face.

Corrosive sensation on nose, as from something acrid.

8 **Face.** Pale, sunken; red and burning hot, with violent thirst, worse toward evening.

Sensation of coldness, tingling and numbness in one (right) side of face.

Cramp-pain, steady compressing, numb feeling and boring in malar bones.

9 **Lower Face.** Purple, net-like appearance on chin.

10 **Teeth.** Pulsating, digging through whole right jaw, worse toward evening and at rest; followed by numbness; pains come and go gradually.

11 **Tongue, etc.** Sensation as if the tongue were scaled.

Sweet taste on the tip of the tongue.

12 **Mouth.** Rhagades in the gums.

Sensation of coldness, especially in the mouth.

13 **Throat.** Cramp-like drawing in the throat, as if it were constricted.

Hawking of mucus, with scraping in throat.

Sensation as if the palate was elongated.

14 Desires. Aversions. Loss of appetite on account of depressed mood.

Ravenous appetite and hasty eating, detests everything around him.

Thirstlessness; or, thirst during heat.

15 Eating and Drinking. Worse on an empty stomach. After meals: 17.

16 Nausea and Vomiting. Eructations empty, mornings.

Continuous nausea, with great weakness, anxiety and trembling sensation, through the whole body.

17 Stomach. Pressure in stomach, especially after meals.

Sensation of constriction in pit of the stomach and in abdomen.

Burning in pit of stomach, extending into abdomen.

Jactitation of muscles in region of stomach.

19 Abdomen. Painter's colic; pain in umbilical region, extending through into back; patient screams and tries to relieve the pain by turning into all possible positions.

Pressing and bearing down in abdomen, extending into pelvis.

20 Stools, etc. Constipation; after lead poisoning; or while traveling; frequent urging, with expulsion of only small portions of feces, with great straining.

After an evacuation sensation of great weakness in abdomen or chilliness.

Itching-tingling and tenesmus at anus, especially in the evening.

Stools adhere to rectum and anus like soft clay.

21 Urine. Frequent micturition, with slow flow of urine.

Urine: pale, watery; red, with white clouds; turbid, depositing a red sediment.

22 Male Sexual Organs. Sexual desire excessive, with violent erections, especially at night.

Embrace with but little pleasurable excitement.

Morbid excitement inducing onanism, especially if prebubic.

23 Female Sexual Organs. Nymphomania, worse in the lying-in; tingling or titillation from genitals up into abdomen.

Painful sensitiveness and continual pressure in region of mons veneris and genital organs; body, except the face, feels cold. θ Prolapsus uteri.

Induration of the uterus; ulceration, with coexisting ovarian irritation.

Ovaries inflamed, with burning pains in paroxysms, stitches in the forehead. Also chronic ovaritis.

Frequent sensation as if the menses would appear.

Menses too early, too profuse and too short-lasting; flow
dark, clotted; preceded by spasms, much bearing down,
desire for stool, or backache; during the flow, pinching
in abdomen, excruciating pains in uterus, twitchings,
with screams; melancholy.

Metrorrhagia, the body feels as if growing large; genitals
very sensitive; nymphomania.

| Hemorrhages in clots, with uterine cancer, fibroids, etc.;
even the fibroid may be cured.

Leucorrhœa like white of egg, only by day, after urination
and after rising from a seat.

Pruritis vulvæ; voluptuous tingling, with anxiety and
palpitation of the heart.

Vulva painfully sensitive during coitus.

²⁴ **Pregnancy.** Contractions interrupted by sensitiveness of
vagina and external parts; labor-pains spasmodic, painful, but ineffectual.

After labor, so sensitive, she cannot bear touch of napkin.

²⁵ **Larynx.** Loss of voice.

Spasm of the glottis.

²⁶ **Breathing.** Difficult, anxious respiration.

Shortness of breath, as if the chest was constricted.

Deep breathing from sensation as of a weight on the chest.

²⁷ **Cough.** Hysterical dry cough, from stifling beneath upper
fourth of sternum.

²⁸ **Lungs.** Cramp-pain in left chest, gradually increasing and
decreasing in intensity.

²⁹ **Heart. Pulse.** Great anxiety and palpitation; commencing
endo or pericarditis.

Pulse regular, but small and weak, sometimes tremulous.

³¹ **Neck. Back.** Nape of neck weak; head inclines forward.

Cramp in posterior muscles of neck; tensive, numb feeling close to occiput, as if tied together.

Pains in back and small of back, as if bruised or broken;
worse from pressure or bending forward.

Pressing from small of back upon the pelvic organs.

Pain in small of back, going to groins and down limbs.

Numbness in sacrum and coccyx.

³² **Upper Limbs.** Weak, relaxed feeling in both arms, as after
holding a heavy weight, better from motion of arms.

Sore burning at the elbow, as if scraped.

³³ **Lower Limbs.** Weakness of thighs and knees, as if beaten.

Pain like after a severe blow, in left knee.

Tremulous restlessness in legs, with numb and torpid feeling when sitting; worse evenings.

Numb and tired feeling in feet, only while sitting.

³⁴ **Limbs in General.** Tension in limbs, as if wrapped tightly.

Cramp-like pains; numbness in limbs and joints.

Spasmodic, jerking and drawing pains in limbs and joints.
Ulcers on fingers and toes.

35 Position, etc.   Motion: 3, 32. Assumes every position: 19.
Rising from a seat: 23.   Bending backward: 31.   Rest:
4, 10, 36.   Sitting: 3, 33.

36 Nerves.   Spasmodic affections of hysterical women and of
children; tetanic-like spasms, with wild shrieks, alternating with catalepsy; spasms alternating with dyspnœa to suffocation; twitches of single muscles, trembling, shivering; worse at dawn.

Spasms from sexual erethism.

Tonic spasms, without loss of consciousness; face pale,
sunken; child, after the spell, lies on its back, kicks off
the clothes, and draws up its knees and spreads them
apart.

Paralytic weakness, worse at rest; numbness, stiffness and
coldness.

37 Sleep.   Great inclination to violent, almost spasmodic yawning.

Awakes, at night and has difficulty in collecting his senses.

During sleep, lies on back, arms over head, thighs drawn
up, and with legs uncovered.

Intense nervous wakefulness.

38 Time.   Morning: 36.   Afternoon: 37.   Evening: 1, 3, 4, 8,
10, 20, 33, 40.   Night: 22, 37.   Day: 23.

39 Temperature and Weather.   Open air: 3, 40.   Uncovered:
37.   Warm air: 40.

40 Chill.   Fever.   Sweat.   Chill in evening, with trembling
and tremulous feeling through whole body.

Shaking chill when going from room into open, even
warm, air.

Chilliness predominates, with irritability, which ceases
during the heat.

Heat, with sensation of burning in face, without any visible change in color of face.

Flushes of heat, interrupted by chilliness.

Gradually increasing, and in like manner decreasing heat.

Sweat only during sleep, ceases on wakening.

41 Attacks.   Pains increase and decrease slowly and gradually.

42 Sides.   Right: 10.   Left: 28, 33.   Front to back: 19.   Above
downward: 31.

43 Sensations.   Trembling through whole body: 16.

Dull pushing pains, as from a plug.

45 Contact, Injuries, etc.   Rubbing: 4.   Touch: 23, 24.   Pressure: 31.   Scratching: 46.

46 Skin.   Sensation of soreness, tingling, smarting and itching,
or pricking, stinging, burning, with inclination to
scratch on different parts of the body.

[47] **Stages and States.** Dark hair; rigid fibre.

Especially suited to females.

[48] **Relationship.** *Platin.* antidotes: bad effects of lead.

Antidotes to *Platin.*: *Pulsat., Spir. nitr. dulc.*

The facial neuralgia of *Verbasc.* is like a crushing with tongs, and occurs often twice a day.

PLUMBUM.

Lead, the metal, the acetate and carbonate. HARTLAUB.

[1] **Mind.** Wild delirium, with distorted countenance.

Much depression of spirits, especially with the colic.

Quiet and melancholic mood.

Anxiety, with restlessness and yawning.

[2] **Sensorium.** Stupefaction of head, he falls down unconscious.

Vertigo, especially on stooping, or when looking upward.

[3] **Inner Head.** Heaviness of head, especially in cerebellum.

Congestion of blood to head, with heat and beating in it.

Headache as if a ball was rising from throat into brain.

Paralysis occurring early; cerebro-spinal meningitis.

Meningitis, chronic, when the paralyzed parts soon fall away in flesh, the limbs become painfully contracted; frequent spells of colic with retraction of the abdomen.

[4] **Outer Head.** Great dryness of hair, it falls off even in beard.

[5] **Eyes.** Cloudiness before the eyes, inducing one to rest them.

Ophthalmia, lachrymation, photophobia, redness of the whole ball.

Yellowness of whites of eyes.

Pupils contracted.

Hypopion after iritis; nightly tearing pains in eye and forehead.

Eyeball feels too large.

Lids spasmodically contracted.

Paralysis of the upper lids.

[6] **Ears.** Stitches and tearing in ears.

Hardness of hearing; often sudden deafness.

[7] **Nose.** Erysipelatous inflammation of nose; vesicles on alæ.

Fetid odor before nose.

Much tough mucus in nose, which can only be discharged through posterior nares.

Cold nose.

[8] **Face.** Face pale, yellowish, like a corpse.

Bloated face. Swelling of one side of face.

The skin of the face is greasy, shining.

Painless peeling off of the lips.

⁹ **Lower Face.**   Lock-jaw.

Tearing in jaws, relieved by rubbing them.

¹⁰ **Teeth.**   Grinding of the teeth.

The teeth become black.

Yellow mucus on teeth.

Teeth hollow, decayed, crumbling off, and smelling offen-
sively.

Gums: swollen; show a lead-colored line; painful, with
hard tubercles.

¹¹ **Tongue, etc.**   Taste sweetish.

Tongue: dry, brown, cracked; coated yellow or green; inflamed, swollen; heavy, paralyzed; hurts as if bitten.

¹² **Mouth.**   Accumulation of sweetish saliva in mouth.

Froth in mouth.

Dryness of mouth.

Aphthæ, dirty-looking ulcers, and purple blotches in
mouth and on tip of tongue.

¹³ **Throat.**   Constriction in throat when trying to swallow,
with great urging to do so.

Sensation of a plug in throat.   Globus hystericus.

Tonsils inflamed, covered with small, painful abscesses.

Diphtheria, with tendency to sloughing.

Tough mucus in fauces and posterior nares.

Angina granulosa, going from left to right.

Fluids can be swallowed, but solids come back into mouth;
burning in œsophagus and stomach some hours after
eating; stricture from spasm.

¹⁴ **Desires.   Aversions.**   Great hunger.

No appetite, but violent thirst.

¹⁵ **Eating and Drinking.**   After eating: 13.

¹⁶ **Nausea and Vomiting.**   Eructations: empty; sweetish.

Gulping up of sweetish water.

Vomiting: of food and of discolored substances, with violent colic; of food, in morning, with great weakness; of
greenish and blackish substances; or of a thick white
substance, like white of egg in chronic gastritis.

Vomit has a fecal odor.

¹⁷ **Stomach.**   Violent pressure in stomach, and pain in back;
at times better bending backward, at others bending
forward; better from hard pressure.

¹⁹ **Abdomen.**   Violent colic, abdomen drawn in, as if by a
string, to the spine.

Cutting, contractive pains, with restless tossing; better
from rubbing, or hard pressure.

Constriction of intestines, naval violently retracted.

Abdomen hard as a stone; knots in recti muscles; anxious,
with cold sweat and deathly faintness.

Large, hard swelling in ileo-cœcal region, painful to touch and motion. θ Typhlitis.

Inflammation and gangrene of bowels.

Incarcerated hernia.

Intussusception, with colic and fecal vomiting.

20 **Stool, etc.** Stool: fetid, yellow and fecal; watery, with vomiting and violent colic; bloody masses; watery, dark, offensive.

Constipation, stools hard, lumpy, like sheep's dung; with urging and terrible pain from constriction or spasm of anus.

Light colored stools. θ Jaundice.

Fissures of the anus.

Anus feels as if drawn upward.

21 **Urine.** Morbus Brightii, contracted kidney.

Diabetes.

Necrotic cystitis from decomposed urea.

Urine: passed in drops; strangury; will not pass, as from atony of the bladder; dribbles, is high-colored and fetid.

22 **Male Sexual Organs.** Increased desire and violent erections.

Impotence.

Testicles: drawn up; feel constricted.

Genitals swollen and inflamed.

23 **Female Sexual Organs.** Cessation of menses on invasion of colic, may re-appear after paroxysm, or not again till next period.

Menorrhagia, with sensation of a string pulling from abdomen to back.

Wants to stretch limbs during ovarian pains; ovarian dropsy.

Climacteric period; dark clots alternately with fluid blood or bloody serum, with a sensation of fulness in pelvis and slight bearing down pains in small of back.

24 **Pregnancy.** Feeling as if there was not room enough in abdomen, at night in bed, must stretch violently.

Abortion from lead poisoning; or the child lives but a year or two.

25 **Larynx.** Constriction of larynx.

Aphonia from paralysis of the vocal cords.

26 **Breathing.** Want of breath; oppression from motion; short-breathed on going up stairs.

Heavy, difficult breathing.

Spasmodic dyspnœa.

27 **Cough.** With expectoration of blood or of pus after hemorrhage from the lungs; dry, spasmodic; worse lying on back and after getting out of bed in morning.

28 **Lungs.** Stitches in chest and sides.

Copious muco-serous or purulent expectoration.

Suppuration of lungs.

Circumscribed pulmonary mortification; also cheesy pneumonia.

²⁹ **Heart. Pulse.** Rush of blood to heart, during a rapid walk; anguish, cold sweat; stitches during inspiration; hypertrophy.

Pulse: variable, generally small and slow; contracted; at times hard and slow; at others small and accelerated; sinks even to 40.

³¹ **Neck. Back.** Tension in neck, extending to ears, when moving head.

Pains in back, better sometimes by bending forward, at others by bending backward.

Stitches in back and small of back.

³² **Upper Limbs.** Convulsive motion of arms and hands, with pain in joints.

Weakness and painful lameness of arms.

Wens on the hands.

³³ **Lower Limbs.** Drawing, pressive pains in sciatic nerve down to knee, with difficult walking and great exhaustion afterward; tubercular diathesis, with dry, hacking cough.

ⅠSciatica, when there is marked consecutive muscular atrophy; or earlier, when walking causes great exhaustion.

Cramps in the calves.

Swelling of the feet.

Fetid foot-sweat.

³⁴ **Limbs in General.** The pains in limbs are worse at night and are relieved by rubbing.

Paralytic weakness in extremities, especially on right side; hands and feet cold; total want of sweat.

³⁵ **Position, etc.** Inclination to take the strangest attitudes and positions in bed.

Walking: 29, 33. Motion: 19, 26, 31, 40. Going up stairs: 26. Stooping: 2. Bending backward or forward: 17, 31. Must stretch: 24. Lying on the back: 27. Turning eyes upward: 2. Rising: 27.

³⁶ **Nerves.** Paralysis: preceded by mental derangement, trembling, spasms, or by shooting, darting, intense, tearing pains in tracks of larger nerves; the parts emaciate: wrist-drop; caused by apoplexy, sclerosis of the brain or progressive muscular atrophy; alternating with colic.

Epilepsy, chronic forms; before the spell, legs heavy and numb, tongue swollen; afterward, long-lasting, stupid feeling in the head.

³⁷ **Sleep.** Somnolency.

Great sleepiness during the day.

Sleeplessness at night from colic.

³⁸ Time. Morning: 27. Evening: 16, 40. Night: 5, 24, 34, 37, 40. Day: 37.

³⁹ Temperature and Weather. Open air: 40, 46. In bed: 40.

⁴⁰ Chill. Fever. Sweat. Chill predominates, increasing toward evening, with violent thirst and redness of face.

Coldness in open air and when exercising.

Internal chill with external heat, in evening.

Chilliness in all the limbs.

Heat with thirst, anxiety, redness of face, and sleepiness.

Internal heat in evening and at night, with yellowness of the buccal cavity.

Sweat, anxious, cold and clammy; or want of sweat.

Sweat comes and goes, as soon as he gets into bed.

⁴¹ Attacks. The ailments develop themselves slowly and intermit for a time; intermission every third day.

⁴² Sides. Right; 33. Left to right: 13.

⁴³ Sensations. Sensation of constriction with pain and spasms in internal organs.

Tearing, sharp pains, with cramps.

⁴⁴ Tissues. Emaciation.

Dropsical swellings.

⁴⁵ Contact, Injuries, etc. Rubbing: 5, 9, 19, 34. Pressure: 17, 19. Touch: 19.

⁴⁶ Skin. Sensitive to the open air; dry, yellow, or pale bluish.

Dark brown spots on skin.

Decubitus.

Burning in ulcers; small wounds become easily inflamed and suppurate.

Gangrene.

⁴⁸ Relationship. Lead poisoning is antidoted by: *Alumen, Alum., Opium, Petrol., Nux vom.*, *Platin., Ant. crud., Coccul., Zincum.*

Alcohol as a preventive.

PODOPHYLLUM PELTATUM.

May Apple; Mandrake.   JEANES.   *Berberideæ.*

¹ Mind. Conscious during chill, but cannot talk, forgets the words he wishes to use.

Delirium, loquacity during heat; afterwards forgetful of what has passed.

Depression; imagines he is going to die, or be very ill.

Depression of spirits; also, in gastric affections.

Disgust for life, headache.

² Sensorium. Vertigo: while standing in open air; with tendency to fall forward; with sensation of fulness over eyes.

³ Inner Head. Stunning headache through temples, better from pressure.

Pressing in temples in forenoon, with drawing in eyes as if strabismus would follow.

Mist before eyes; then fleeting pains, worse at occipital protuberances, down the neck and shoulders, better when lying down in a quiet and dark place, and from sleep.

Head hot, rolling the head from side to side, moaning. θ Dentition.

Momentary darts of pain in forehead, obliging one to shut eyes.

Headache, alternating with diarrhœa.

Morning headache, with flushed face.

⁴ Outer Head. Sweat of the head during sleep, flesh cold. θ Dentition.

⁵ Eyes. Ulceration of cornea; conjunctiva hyperæmic; smarting, aching, heaviness (from grinding root).

Scrofulous ophthalmia, worse in morning.

⁸ Face. Hot, cheeks flushed. θ Infantile diarrhœa.

¹⁰ Teeth. Great desire to press gums together; jaws clenched; grind teeth at night; difficult dentition.

¹¹ Tongue, etc. Total loss of taste, could not tell sweet from sour; sleepless, restless.

Everything tastes sour.

Tongue: furred white, with foul taste; white, moist, shows imprints of teeth; dry, yellow.

¹² Mouth. Offensive odor from mouth.

Copious salivation.

Mouth and tongue dry, on awaking.

¹³ Throat. Sore throat right to left; left side sore, worse when swallowing liquids and in morning. Soreness of throat extends to ears.

Rattling of mucus in throat.

Goitre.

Pharynx dry, deglutition painful.

¹⁴ Desires. Aversions. Appetite variable, at times voracious.

Great thirst for large quantities of cold water.

Satiety from small quantity of food, followed by nausea and vomiting.

Moderate thirst during fever.

¹⁵ Eating and Drinking. After eating: regurgitation of food, sour; hot, sour belching; diarrhœa. Vomits food one hour after eating, craving appetite afterward; depression of spirits.

49

After acid fruit and milk, diarrhœa.

While eating: 18.

¹⁶ **Nausea and Vomiting.** Eructations: smelling like rotten eggs; hot, sour.

Regurgitation of food.

Gagging. θ Infantile diarrhœa.

Nausea and vomiting, with fulness of head.

Vomiting: of milk in infants, with protrusion of anus; of food, with putrid taste and odor; of thick bile and blood; with congestion of the pelvic viscera, during pregnancy.

¹⁷ **Stomach.** Hollow sensation in epigastrium.

Stitches in epigastrium from coughing.

Stomach contracts violently during retching.

Dyspepsia after abuse of calomel; tongue shows teeth prints; conjunctiva yellow; aching behind eyes; clayey stools.

Gastric catarrh.

¹⁸ **Hypochondria.** Fulness in right hypochondrium, with flatulence, pain and soreness.

Stitches, worse while eating.

Excessive secretion of bile; great irritability of the liver.

Torpidity of liver; jaundice.

Twisting pain in right hypochondrium, with sensation of heat there.

Chronic hepatitis; costive; jaundice; constantly rubbing and stroking hypochondrium with hands.

Jaundice with gall-stones; pain from region of stomach toward region of gall-bladder, with excessive nausea.

Jaundice, with hyperæmia of liver; fulness, soreness and pain; alternate constipation and diarrhœa.

¹⁹ **Abdomen.** Pain in bowels at daybreak, better from external warmth and bending forward while lying on side; worse lying on back.

Cramp-like pain in bowels, with retraction of abdominal muscles, 10 P.M., and again at 5 A.M. until 9 A.M.; lead colic.

Frequent but transient abdominal pains, during the day, better from pressure.

Rumbling in ascending colon.

Pain in transverse colon 3 A.M., followed by diarrhœa.

Sharp pain in right groin, preventing motion, latter months of pregnancy.

²⁰ **Stool, etc.** Stool: frequent, painless, watery, fetid discharges, gushing out; yellow-colored, with meal-like sediment; green, sour, with flatulence; morning, during dentition; greenish-yellow, slimy, bloody, gelatinous, mixed with feces; tenesmus and prolapsus ani; with

severe straining, much flatulence emitted; mucus, with spots and streaks of blood; black, only in morning; chalk-like, fecal, undigested; muco-gelatinous stools preceded by griping and colic; stools coated with shreds of yellow mucus.

Diarrhœa while being washed; after eating; dirty water soaking napkin through.

Diarrhœa, with great sinking at epigastrium, sensation as if everything would drop through the pelvis.

Stools pale, hard, dry or clayey; voided with difficulty; flatulence, headache.

Stools natural, but too frequent during the day, and exhausting.

Constipation of bottle-fed babies, with dry, crumbling stools.

Emission of fetid flatus.

Prolapsus ani, with stool, even from least exertion, followed by stool or thick, transparent mucus, or mixed with blood.

Piles, with prolapsus ani and long-standing diarrhœa, worse mornings; or constipation.

[21] **Urine.** Frequent nocturnal urination during pregnancy.

Enuresis, with involuntary urination during sleep.

Diminished urine; yellow, containing sediment.

Suppression of urine.

[23] **Female Sexual Organs.** Numb aching in region of left ovary; heat down thigh; third month of pregnancy.

Pain in region of ovaries, especially the right; also when extending down the antecrural nerve; worse straightening the leg. Sometimes pains go up to shoulder.

Ovarian tumor.

Sensation as if genitals would come out during stool.

Prolapsus uteri: after overlifting or straining; after parturition; with pain in sacrum; rumbling in ascending colon; prolapsus ani; or constipation.

Suppressed menses in young females, with bearing down in hypogastric and sacral regions, with pain from motion; better lying down.

Leucorrhœa, bearing down in genitals; costive; of thick, transparent mucus.

Swelling of labia during pregnancy.

[24] **Pregnancy.** During pregnancy; can lie comfortably only on stomach, early months: 19, 21, 23.

After-pains, with heat and flatulency; also with strong bearing down.

[26] **Breathing.** Inclined to breathe deeply; sighing.

Shortness of breath.

Sensation of suffocation, at first when lying down at night.

[27] **Cough.** With remittent fever; dry; loose; whooping, with constipation and loss of appetite.

[28] **Lungs.** Catarrh of chest during dentition.

[29] **Heart. Pulse.** Palpitation, with a clucking sensation rising up to throat, obstructing respiration.

Palpitation from mental emotion or exertion, with rumbling in ascending colon, heavy sleep, fatigue on awaking in morning, drowsy all forenoon.

Sensation in chest as if heart was ascending to throat.

[31] **Neck. Back.** Nape of neck stiff, with soreness of muscles of neck and shoulders.

Pain between shoulders, in the morning.

Pain under right scapula.

Flashes up the back, with stool.

Pain in lumbar region, withered sensation; worse at night and from motion.

Pain in loins, worse when walking on uneven ground, or from a misstep.

Backache after washing, with prolapsus uteri.

[32] **Upper Limbs.** Rheumatism in left forearm and fingers.

Pain from head into neck and shoulders, fingers numb.

Weakness of wrists, soreness to touch.

[33] **Lower Limbs.** Sharply defined ache in sacro-ischiadic foramen, with tenderness on pressure.

Pain and weakness in left hip, like rheumatism from cold, worse going up stairs.

Cramps, in calves, thighs and feet, with painless, watery stools.

Knee-joints crack during motion.

Joints weak, especially knees.

Legs heavy and stiff, as after long walk.

Aching of limbs, worse at night.

Feet cold.

Feet sweat, evening.

[35] **Position, etc.** Lying down: 3, 19, 23, 24, 26, 40. Going up stairs: 33. Walking: 31. Misstep: 31. Motion: 19, 20, 23, 29, 31, 33, 40. Exertion, washing: 31. Standing: 2. Bending forward: 19.

[36] **Nerves.** Slight paralytic weakness of whole left side.

Sudden shocks of jerking pains.

[37] **Sleep.** Heavy sleep; fatigue on waking.

Drowsy, half-closed eyes, moaning, whining, especially children.

Sleepy, especially forenoon.

Restless sleep, whining.

[38] **Time.** Morning: 3, 5, 19, 20, 29, 31, 37. Evening: 19, 33, 40. Night: 20, 21, 26, 31, 33. At 3 A.M.: 19. At 7 A.M.: 40. Day: 19, 20.

[39] **Temperature and Weather.**   Warmth: 19.   Washing: 20, 31.   Worse hot weather; diarrhœa.   Open air: 2.

[40] **Chill. Fever. Sweat.**   Chilliness while moving about during fever and in act of lying down, with sweat immediately afterward.

Chilly at first on lying down in evening, followed by fever and sleep, with talking and imperfect waking.

Chill 7 A.M., pressing in both hypochondria, dull aching in knees and ankles, elbows and wrists.

Backache before chill.

During fever: pain in head, thirst, shaking and cold sensation continue for some time.

Sweat, with sleep.

[42] **Sides.**   Right: 18, 19, 23, 31.   Left: 13, 23, 32, 33, 36.   Right to left: 13.

[44] **Tissues.**   Fulness of superficial veins.

Softness of flesh, with debility; children.

Relaxes the sphincters.

[45] **Contact, Injuries, etc.·**   Pressure: 3, 19, 33.   Overlifting: 23, 31.   Touch: 32.   Rubbing or stroking: 18.

[46] **Skin.**   Sallow skin; jaundice; also in children.

Skin moist, with preternatural warmth.

Scabs on skin.   Rawness and itching about genitals; also pustules (from grinding the root).

[47] **Stages and States.**   Bilious temperaments, especially after mercurialization.

[48] **Relationship.**   *Podoph.*, after *Ipec.* and *Nux vom.* failed, in vomiting.   Salt increases its action.

Antidotes to *Podoph.: Lact. ac., Nux vom.*

PSORINUM.

The Salt from a product of Psora. HERING.   *A Nosode.*

[1] **Mind.**   Thoughts vanish, after overlifting.

Memory so weak, cannot remember, does not even know his room.

Thoughts which he cannot get rid of; they constantly reappear in his dreams.

As if stupid in left half of head, morning.

Dull, stupid, foggy, as after a debauch, on awaking in night; dizziness, he falls down.

Dull all forenoon, disinclined to work.

Sad, depressed; even suicidal thoughts.

ᛙDespairs of recovery; thinks he will die, hopeless; especially after typhus, better from nosebleed.

¦ Religious melancholy.

Anxiety, full of fears, of evil forebodings.

Sentimental.

Cheerful, takes pleasure in his work.

Irritable, peevish, passionate, noisy; nervous, easily startled; restless, hands tremble.

Mental labor causes: fulness in head; intense headache; throbbing in brain; pain in left temple.

Every moral emotion causes trembling.

Severe ailments from even slight emotions.

² **Sensorium.** Vertigo: mornings; objects seem to go around with him; with headache; eyes feel pressed outward.

Fulness in vertex, as if brain would burst out.

Congestion to head, heat; awakened at night stupefied; could not recollect; after sitting still awhile had to rise to collect his senses.

³ **Inner Head.** Morning headache, with pressing in forehead, stupefaction, staggering, eyes feel sore.

Sensation as from a heavy blow received on forehead, awakens him; 1 A.M.

Pain as if brain had not enough room in forehead when rising in morning, a forcing outward; better after washing and eating.

Pain in back of head, as if sprained; pressure in right side of occiput as if luxated.

Cramp like, contractive headache.

Like hammers striking the head from within outward.

Pressing headache on small spots in forehead and temples, worse left side; feels intoxicated, stupid.

Congestion to head, cheeks red and hot, eruption on face reddens; great anxiety every afternoon after dinner. θ Fifth month of pregnancy.

⁴ **Outer Head.** Hair: dry, lustreless; tangles easily.

Viscid sweat about the head.

Whole head burns.

Pustules, boils on head, mostly scalp, which looks dirty and emits an offensive odor.

Moist, suppurating, fetid eruption. Also dry eruption.

Averse to having head uncovered; wears a fur cap even in hottest weather.

⁵ **Eyes.** Fiery sparks before eyes.

Objects seem to tremble for a few moments, get dark.

Aversion to light.

Confusedness before eyes, after anxiety.

Eyes feel tired in evening.

Photophobia when walking in open air.

Eyes water, inflamed; hurt so she can scarcely open them; pains over eyebrows, down nose, also back of head; complained mostly of her head.

Right eye inflamed, pressure as from foreign body when lids closed.

Ciliary blepharitis right to left, worse morning and during day; chronic cases.

Blepharitis, photophobia, child cannot open its eyes, lies on its face.

⁶ **Ears.** Humming or buzzing in left ear; afterward stinging; hard of hearing.

Discharge of reddish ear-wax.

ıExternal ears, raw, red, oozing; scabs form; sore pain behind ears.

ıOtorrhœa very offensive, purulent (watery, stinking diarrhœa).

Severe pain in ear, confined him to bed for four days; ear swollen; thought pain would drive him crazy.

Pustules on and behind concha.

Scabby eczema behind right ear came out, curing the child's old, dry deafness.

Herpes from temples over ears to cheeks; at times throws off innumerable scales; at others shows painful rhagades, with yellow discharge, forming scurfs; fetid humor; itching intolerable.

⁷ **Nose.** Loss of smell.

Smell of blood.

Nose sensitive when inhaling air.

Boring, stinging in right nostril, followed by excessive sneezing.

Burning, followed by thin nasal discharge, which relieves.

Tough mucus in nose; feels like a plug there; it nauseates him; better when stooping.

Catarrh, with cough and expectoration of yellow-green mucus.

Septum inflamed, large pustules.

⁸ **Face.** Pale, yellow, sickly; broad blue rings around eyes.

Burning heat and redness of face.

Pimples on forehead.

Cheek-bones pain as if ulcerated.

Ulcers in face.

Scabby face; especially cheeks from ears; lips and eyelids swollen, sore about eyes.

Red, small pimples on face, especially on nose, chin and middle of cheeks.

⁹ **Lower Face.** Upper lip swollen.

Lips dry, brown, black; ulcers on lips.

Lips painful, swollen.

Soreness of jaw, right side, around the ear; could not open his mouth, even wide enough to admit his fingers.

Corners of mouth ulcerated; sycotic condylomata.

Submaxillary and lingual glands swollen, sore to touch; at same time suppurating pustules on same place.

¹⁰ **Teeth.** Stitching in teeth from one side to other, radiating to head, with burning in right cheek, which is swollen.

Teeth feel so loose, fears they may fall out; worse from touch.

Ulcers on gums.

¹¹ **Tongue, etc.** Loss of taste, with coryza.

Taste: bitter, goes off when eating or drinking; foul, much mucus in mouth; less in fresh air.

Tongue: dry; tip dry, feels scalded; coated white; yellow; thickly covered with whitish-yellow slime.

¹² **Mouth.** Mouth dry, burning.

Tickling, burning; mouth inflamed, sore, worse from warm food; not annoyed by cold food.

Blisters inside lower lips; burning, painful.

¹³ **Throat.** Tough mucus in throat, hawking.

Throat burns, feels scalded.

Like a lump or plug in throat, impeding hawking of mucus.

Pain when swallowing saliva.

Difficult swallowing, throat feels swollen.

Ulcers on right side, with deep-seated pains and burning in fauces.

Tonsillitis; submaxillary glands swollen; fetid otorrhœa.

¹⁴ **Desires. Aversions.** Great appetite after a walk.

Must eat bread in middle of night, so hungry.

No appetite after typhus.

No appetite, but great thirst.

Loathing of pork.

¹⁵ **Eating and Drinking.** After eating: 2, 3. While eating: 11. Warm food: 12. Cold food: 12. Drinking: 11.

¹⁶ **Nausea and Vomiting.** Eructations: tasting like rotten eggs; sour, rancid.

Nausea: morning, with pain in small of back; all day, with vomiting; vomituritio, followed by vomiting, first of blood, then of a sour, slimy fluid.

¹⁷ **Stomach.** Cramps in stomach.

Sharp stinging in pit of stomach.

Weakness of stomach.

¹⁸ **Hypochondria.** Chronic hepatitis.

Deep, heavy pain in region of liver, worse from pressure or lying on right side, walking, coughing, laughing, or taking a long breath.

Stinging, sharp pain in region of liver and spleen.

Stitches in spleen, better when standing; worse when moving, and continuing if again at rest.

¹⁹ **Abdomen.** Colicky pains, better passing fetid flatus.

Pain in abdomen while riding.

Abdomen distended.

Painful bearing down, with painful, burning micturition.

Stinging, sharp pains in inguinal glands.

Pain through right groin when walking.

Inguinal hernia.

²⁰ **Stool, etc.** Stools: fluid, fetid, smell like rotten eggs or carrion; worse at night; of green mucus, mixed with blood; frequent, liquid

Griping and desire for stool while riding.

Chronic diarrhœa.

Costive; pain in small of back; blood from rectum.

Large quantities of blood from rectum, with hard, difficult stool.

Burning, hemorrhoidal tumors.

Soreness in rectum and anus when riding.

²¹ **Urine.** Involuntary urine, cannot hold it. θ Typhus.

Frequent, scanty urine; burning and cutting in urethra.

Urine thick, whitish, turbid, red deposit, cuticle forms on surface.

²² **Male Sexual Organs.** Impotence, want of emissions during coitus.

Aversion to coition.

Drawing in testcles and cords.

Male parts flabby, torpid.

Inflamed ulcer on glans, with swelling and heaviness of testicles.

Prostatic fluid discharged before urinating.

Sycotic excrescences on edges of prepuce, with itching and burning.

Painless, chronic blenorrhœa, stains linen yellow.

²³ **Female Sexual Organs.** Pinching in pubic region, in women.

Cutting in left loin; cannot walk without assistance.

Left ovary indurated after a violent knock; followed by itching eruption on body and face.

Knotty lump above right groin; even a bandage hurts.

Amenorrhœa: in psoric subjects, when tetter is covered by thick scurfs; with phthisis.

Dysmenorrhœa near climaxis.

Leucorrhœa, large lumps. unbearable in odor; violent pains in sacrum and right loin.

²⁴ **Pregnancy.** During pregnancy: congestions; fœtus moves too violently, abdomen tympanitic; nausea, vomiting.

Mammæ swollen, painful; redness of nipples, burning around them.

Pimples, itching violently, about nipples; oozing a fluid.

θ Second month of pregnancy.

Mammary cancer.

²⁵ **Larynx.** Hoarse when talking, phlegm sticks in larynx.
Tickling, throat as if narrowing, must cough to relieve it,
Talking very fatiguing.
²⁶ **Breathing.** Short-breathed.
Chest expands with great difficulty.
Cannot get breath.
Anxious dyspnœa, with palpitation.
Dyspnœa, worse sitting up to write, better lying down;
worse the nearer the arms are brought to the body.
Asthmatic attacks, with hydrothorax.
Stitches from behind forward, in chest and back, when
breathing.
²⁷ **Cough.** Dry, hacking, from titillation in trachea; dry, with
weakness, heaviness, or soreness in chest; evenings,
pains in throat and chest, caused by speaking, better
from quiet; with green mucous sputa, worse mornings
when awaking and evenings on lying down; coughs a
long time before expectorating.
Chronic blenorrhœa of the lungs, threatening phthisis.
²⁸ **Lungs.** Phthisis pulmonalis.
Burning-pressing in chest.
Pain in chest, great anxiety, by spells.
Hydrothorax.
Feeling, especially under sternum, as of ulceration of the
chest.
Chest symptoms better when lying down.
Sharp pain, right side, opposite tenth rib.
Pains in right side, worse from motion, laughing, cough-
ing; with sweat.
²⁹ **Heart. Pulse.** Pericarditis, psoric origin; better lying
quietly.
Rheumatic carditis; effusion, cannot lie down.
Pulse weak, feeble.
³¹ **Neck. Back.** Painful stiffness of neck, soreness and tear-
ing on bending backward.
Glands of neck swollen, pains thence to head.
Tearing and stitches between scapulæ.
Severe backache, as if bruised, cannot straighten out.
Pain in small of back, like weakness.
Small of back pains, worse from motion.
³² **Upper Limbs.** Attacks of lameness and soreness in right
shoulder, extending to hand.
Arms as if paralyzed and lame, from shoulders to hands.
Eruption in bends of elbows and around wrists.
Tearing in arms.
Copper-colored, red blisters on backs of hands.
Pustules on hands, near finger-ends, suppurating.
Itching between fingers; vesicles.
Sweaty palms, especially at night.

Small warts, size of pin's head, on left hand.

33 Lower Limbs. Pain in hip-joints as if dislocated, worse when walking, with weak arms.

Pains in legs, especially on tibia and soles, as from over-exertion in walking; legs restless, better on rising.

Sciatic pains; tension down to knee while walking.

Oozing blisters on legs, from small pustules, increasing in size, with tearing pains.

Dry herpes in bend of knees.

Chronic gonitis.

Ulcers on lower legs, with intolerable itching over whole body.

Feet go to sleep.

Heat and itching of the soles.

Eruption on insteps, soon becoming thick, dirty, scaly; suppurating; painful and itching at times, keeping him awake.

34 Limbs in General. Arthritis; rheumatism, especially in chronic form.

Tearing in left knee and left axilla.

Hands and feet tremble.

35 Position, etc. Rest: 18, 27, 33. Lying down: 26, 27, 28, 29; on right side: 18. Lies on face: 5. Cannot lie down: 29. Sitting up: 26. Standing: 18. Motion: 18, 28, 31. Exertion: 36, 46. Walking: 5, 14, 18, 19, 23, 33. Stooping: 7. Rising: 3, 33. Must rise: 2. Bending backward: 31. Cannot straighten out: 31. Overlifting: 1.

36 Nerves. Weakness, especially without structural diseased changes.

Debility after acute diseases; after typhus, with despair of recovery; thinks he is very ill, when he is not; appetite will not return; sweats from least exertion.

Nervous, easily startled.

Subsultus tendinum.

37 Sleep. Sleepy by day; sleepless at night, from intolerable itching; dyspnœa; congestion to head.

Sick babies will not sleep day or night, but worry, fret, cry.

Dreams vivid, continue after awaking.

Dreams of robbers, danger, traveling, etc.

Sleepless after 12 P.M., from congestion to head.

On awaking, cannot get rid of the one persistent idea.

38 Time. Morning: 1, 2, 3, 5, 16, 27. Afternoon: 2. Evening: 5, 27, 40. Night: 1, 2, 3, 14, 20, 32, 37. After midnight: 37. At 1 A.M.: 3. Day: 5, 16, 37.

39 Temperature and Weather. Feels a restlessness in his blood days before and during a thunder-storm.

Cough returns every winter.

Hot weather: 4. Warmth: 46. In bed: 46. Air: 7, 11.
Uncovering: 4. Washing: 3.

⁴⁰ **Chill. Fever. Sweat.** Chilly, evening, upper arms, thighs, with thirst; drinking causes cough.

Evening heat, delirium, great thirst, followed by profuse sweat.

Heat when riding in a carriage.

Profuse sweats.

Sweats easily, weak.

Typhus: picks bedclothes, reaches for objects in air.

⁴¹ **Attacks.** Every day same hour.

Every other day: headache, thirst, cold.

⁴² **Sides.** Right: 3, 5, 6, 7, 9, 10, 13, 18, 19, 23, 28, 32. Left: 1, 2, 3, 6, 18, 23, 32, 34. Right to left: 5. Side to side: 10. Within outward: 3, 4. Behind forward: 26. Above downward: 32, 33.

⁴⁴ **Tissues.** Body always has a filthy smell, even after a bath.

Thinner than usual; pale, exhausted.

Deeply-penetrating ichorous ulcers.

Caries.

Dropsy.

⁴⁵ **Contact, Injuries, etc.** Touch: 9, 10, 33. Pressure: 18, 30; of bandage: 23. Violent knock: 23. Scratching: 46. Riding: 19, 20, 40.

⁴⁶ **Skin.** Body itches intolerably; worse in bed and from warmth; scratches until it bleeds.

Skin dirty, greasy-looking, with yellow blotches here and there.

Fine red eruption, forming small white scales.

Whole surface scaly, dirty-looking, tawny; at times itching; desires scratching, which gives temporary relief.

Copper-colored pustules, no itching.

Itch: boils after itch.

Crusty eruptions all over.

After suppressed itch: urticaria, in attacks, after every exertion; tuberculosis; single pustules often appear.

⁴⁷ **Stages and States.** Scrofulous; nervous, restless, easily startled.

Psoric constitutions; especially when other remedies fail to permanently improve; lack of reaction after severe diseases.

Pale, sickly, delicate children.

⁴⁸ **Relationship.** Burning remaining (about nipples), yielded to *Carb. veg.*: 24.

Vomiting in pregnancy only relieved by *Lac. ac.*, was cured by *Psorin.*

Arnic. for a blow on ovary, followed by *Psorin.*

Follow *Psorin.* with *Sulphur*, mammary cancer.

Antidote: coffee.

PTELEA TRIFOLIATA.

Wafer Ash.   .   *Rutaceæ*

[1] **Mind.** Nervous, irritable, starts from a voice.

Sad, irritable; hurried manner, but dazed and confused, with muddled feeling in the head.

Disinclined to mental work, with languor rather than with inability.

Dazed, confused, as in a bilious attack.

Memory weak; forgetful as if intellection was slow; yet by collecting thoughts could recall things read many years ago.

[2] **Sensorium.** Confusion; raises a bitter fluid.

Vertigo, worse turning head or from sudden motions; with dulness and languor, rumbling about the navel, nausea, griping, aching in stomach; worse when writing, rising, or in a warm room.

[3] **Inner Head.** Headache, bones.

Splitting headache, worse mental exertion, stooping, or moving eyes; with nausea.

Dull aching in the forehead with depression and sour stomach; racking pain, with hurried manner and red face.

Pain from forehead to root of nose; sensation of a nail driven into the brain; worse in the morning on rising.

Throbbing over one eye. Darting pains over left eye, deep into head.

Hot flushes and pain in top of head and eyes.

Pain in left temple running across to the right.

Headache in the occipital region passing to the frontal, over the eyes.

Pressive feeling at the base of the brain, compared to the bruised headache of *Ipec.*

Headaches are worse from mental exertion, moving eyes, walking, noise, warmth, and on awaking, mornings.

[6] **Ears.** Intolerance of loud talking.

Ringing in the ears; slight giddiness.

[7] **Nose.** Breath seems so hot that it burns the nostrils. Nasal passages sore. Sneezing.

[8] **Face.** Expression: sickly, pale, especially around the eyes.

Color: yellow, skin dry and hard.

[10] **Teeth.** Carious teeth sensitive; gums sore. Teeth feel as if elongated.

[11] **Tongue, etc.** Coating: white fur, swollen; yellow, feels rough, papillæ red and prominent; brown-yellow, dry.

Taste: sour, morning; bitter.

Food seems tasteless.

¹² **Mouth.** Dry, with bitter taste.

Saliva profuse; drooling at night.

¹³ **Throat.** Pricking pains in throat; fauces inflamed, worse right side.

Hawking of mucus from the pharynx; lips and tongue dry.

¹⁴ **Desires. Aversions.** ▮Appetite voracious. Craves acid food.

▮Dislike things formerly enjoyed.

Repugnance to butter and fats, appetite poor; ▮also to animal food and to rich puddings.

Appetite poor with muddled feeling or pains in liver.

Thirst.

No thirst, with bitter taste.

¹⁵ **Eating and Drinking.** Worse from cheese, meat, pudding, etc.

▮Hepatic and gastric symptoms worse after meals.

¹⁶ **Nausea and Vomiting.** Eructations: sour; bitter; tasting of rotten eggs.

Nausea, rising of a bitter fluid, confused head, dizzy; sweat on forehead; bilious.

¹⁷ **Stomach.** ▮Sense of weight and fulness after even a moderate meal.

Distress in epigastrium and right hypochondrium, with drawing pains in fingers and ankles. ▮Burning distress; oppression; vomiting; chronic gastric catarrh.

Empty feeling. Faint feeling in stomach; sour risings.

▮Pressure at pit as from a stone, worse from a light meal.

Griping, cutting pains in the epigastrium; pressure causes nausea.

¹⁸ **Hypochondria.** ▮Liver swollen, sore on pressure, causing dull and aching pain; griping in the bowels; clothes feel too tight.

▮Weight, aching, distress in the hepatic region; dull pain, heaviness, better lying on the right side; turning to the left causes a dragging sensation.

Sharp, cutting pain in liver, worse from a deep inspiration.

¹⁹ **Abdomen.** Bloated, with weight on the stomach.

Soreness of the abdomen, worse bending body, feels like supporting it with the hands. Feeling of warmth.

Aching distress in bowels, back and legs.

Pulsation in the umbilical region synchronous with the heart.

Griping, colicky pains; heavy aching; throbbing; about the navel. Colic, bitter taste; with rumbling and discharge of wind from the bowels.

20 Stool, etc. Continual urging, with pressure on the rectum; with scanty or absent stool; rectal torpidity.

Diarrhœa: bilious, thin, fecal, dark, offensive, even cadaverous in smell, sulphuric in odor; with tenesmus; preceded by griping pains and rumbling; smarting in the anus.

Constipation. Passes balls of hard feces.

Diarrhœa and constipation alternately.

21 Urine. Smarting in urethra during and after micturition.

Scalding urine, scanty and difficult of retention.

Urine: clear or deep reddish-yellow, scanty; deposit of epithelia, phosphates and urates.

22 Male Sexual Organs. Sexual desire increased; later, lost.

26 Breathing. Feeling of pressure on the lungs and of suffocation when lying on the back; on awaking, 1 A.M.

28 Lungs. Uneasiness, difficulty in breathing, dull pain in right infraclavicular region, hacking cough; dulness on percussion (following gastric and hepatic symptoms).

31 Neck. Back. Aching distress in back, bowels and legs; rumbling of wind.

Lumbar pains: severe aching, distress, soreness, on awaking, or awakes him at 4 A.M.

34 Limbs in General. Aching; bruised feeling in muscles and joints on awaking. Drawing pains. Worse with gastro-hepatic symptoms.

35 Position, etc. Motion: 2, 3. Turning: 2. Rising: 2, 3. Stooping: 3. Walking: 3.

❙Lying right side: 18. Lying on left: 18. Bending: 19.

36 Nerves. Restless, uneasy; malaise.

·Feeling of weakness, languid, irritable; sick, faint sensations; as in bilious patients.

37 Sleep. Heavy sleep.

Awoke: 2 A.M., restless; headache, etc. At 4 A.M. aroused by gastric and hepatic symptoms.

38 Time. Morning: 3, 11.

Night: 11. 1 A.M.: 26   4 A.M.: 31, 37.

39 Temperature and Weather. Generally better in open air (except lung); worse in warm room. See 2, 46, etc.

40 Chill. Fever. Sweat. Chilliness, shivering; with the stool. Wants to be near the fire.

Dry, general heat; worse face and hands. Irritable, intolerant of noise.

Hot flushes and slight headache; feverish, hot head, dull frontal aching.

Sweat: profuse on awaking; on forehead during stool, or with raising of a bitter fluid.

44 Tissues. Mucous membranes are congested and irritated, with sense of roughness, smarting or prickling.

Causes congestion of liver, stomach and bowels, and
secondarily of the lungs. Is indicated briefly, when
there are irritability, dull, confused, frontal headache;
bitter taste, eructations like rotten eggs or bitter; swollen liver, relief from lying on right side, bilious stools;
languor, muscular soreness.

⁴⁵ **Contact, Injuries, etc.** Pressure: 17, 18.

⁴⁶ **Skin.** Itching all over as from flea-bites.

White blisters on a red base on right ear, discharging a
watery fluid; later desquamation or pus and scabs form;
boils.

Spots on limbs red, later purple; worse when warm or
excited; annoying itching. On disappearing they leave
yellowish marks like bruises.

⁴⁸ **Relationship.** Related to other Rutaceæ, and by the
possession of Berberina, also to *Podoph.*, *Berber.*,
Hydrast., etc.

From *Nux vom.*, *Ptelea* is distinguished by repugnance to
fat, offensive flatus; from *Mercur.* by relief of hepatic
symptoms when lying on right side.

PULSATILLA.

Wiesen Küchenschelle. HAHNEMANN. *Ranunculaceæ.*

¹ **Mind.** Fancies a naked man is wrapped in her bedclothes;
dreams of men.

Mania from suppressed menses.

Religious mania; sees the devil coming to take her; the
world on fire during night; fear, rage in spells or weeping; forgetful during lucid moments.

Easily moved to tears or laughter.

Silent mood, disgusted at everything.

In early morn depressed, full of cares about domestic
affairs.

Dread of men.

Tremulous anguish, as if death was near.

Anguish about the heart, even to suicide.

Mild, gentle, tearful, yielding, timid.

Peevish, changeable; pale; chilly. *θ* Children.

Envy; covetousness.

Fatigued by mental labor; head affected.

After slight emotions, difficult breathing; bad effects from
fright, mortification or excessive joy.

² **Sensorium.** Confusion of head, with pains, as after intoxication or watching.

Giddy, as if drunk; inclination to vomit.

Faint all the morning; frequent calls for water.

Apoplexy, unconscious; face blue-red, bloated; violent beating of heart, pulse collapsed, rattling breathing.

³ **Inner Head.** Stupefying headache, running chills, with humming in the head; worse when lying or sitting quietly or in the cold.

Soreness, as from subcutaneous ulceration in one or both temples; worse evening, at rest, in warm room; better when walking in open air.

Twitching-tearing in temple lain on; goes to other side when turning on to it; worse evenings, and on raising eyes upward.

Headache, as if it would burst; worse from moving eyes.

Stinging-pulsating in brain; worse when stooping.

Pulsating in evening, and from mental exertion; throbbing, with amenia.

Semilateral headache, also sometimes with nausea and vomiting.

❙Violent pain behind, on one side, as if a nail was driven in.

Beating, jerking, lacerating pains, or as if in a vise.

Headache from overloaded stomach, from pastry, fats, ice cream.

Acute pains in temples, with giddiness.

Pain as if brain was lacerated, on or soon after awaking.

Headaches worse from abuse of mercury; in warm room; better walking slowly in open air and from compression.

⁴ **Outer Head.** Rheumatic headache, worse on one side, and from 5 to 10 P.M.; crazing pains into the face and teeth.

Tingling, biting, itching on scalp, mostly on temples and behind ears, followed by swelling and eruptions; sore pain; worse evenings and when undressing; also, from getting warm in bed.

Tumors on scalp, suppurating and affecting the skull, worse lying on well side.

Fetid, often cold, sweat, at times on one side of head and face, great anxiety and stupor; worse at night and toward morning; better after waking and rising.

Disposition to take cold on head, worse when it gets wet; head sweaty.

⁵ **Eyes.** Oversensitive to light.

Flashing of fire, as if slapped in face.

Like a veil before eyes, better rubbing or wiping them.

Amblyopia: from suppression of any bloody discharge; from metastasis of gout or rheumatism; from gastric derangements; with heart disease; with coexisting diminished hearing.

50

Dim sight, especially on getting warm from exercise.

Dryness of eyes and lids, with sensation as if darkened by mucus, which out to be wiped away.

Stitches, especially from light and in sunshine.

Child frequently rubs its eye.

Pustular conjunctivitis, lachrymation more in open air or wind; discharge thick, yellow, bland, profuse.

Ophthalmia, with amenorrhœa.

Lids swollen, itch, burn, not excoriated, better from rubbing; subject to styes, especially on upper lid.

Granular lids, dry, or with excessive bland secretion; better in open air, but not in wind; granulations very fine.

Stinging, tearing pains, worse in the evening; rheumatic ophthalmia.

Fistula lachrymalis, discharging pus when pressed.

Ophthalmia neonatorum; profuse yellow, purulent discharge, gluing the lids.

Gonorrhœal ophthalmia; discharge suddenly suppressed.

⁶ Ears. Deafness: as if ears were stopped up; after suppressed measles; with otorrhœa; from cold after cutting hair; with hard, black cerumen. Can hear better on the cars.

Severe pain in ear, continuing through night, with paroxysms of increasing severity, but causing little concern during day; bland, nearly inoffensive, discharge of mucus and pus.

Roaring in ears, better out-doors; also, humming or tingling.

Phlyctenulæ (to prevent ulceration).

Otalgia, with darting, tearing pains, and pulsating at night.

External ear and meatus red and swollen; scabs on tragus.

⁷ Nose. Loss of smell, with catarrh.

Smell as of old catarrh; objective stench from nose.

Nosebleed: with suppressed menses; with dry coryza; in anæmia; blood coagulated.

Coryza, fluid or dry, loss of taste and smell, nostrils sore; wings raw; later yellow-green discharge; worse in-doors; chilliness, face pale, head confused; frontal headache.

Green, fetid, nasal discharge, with diminished taste and smell; chronic, thick, yellow, bland discharge.

⁸ Face. Red every evening; alternately red and pale; pale or yellowish, with sunken eyes; puffed, blue, red; cheeks and nose puffed.

Flushes in the face.

Facial neuralgia, nervous excitation coming at irregular intervals; worse when chewing, talking, or from hot or cold things in mouth.

Facial erysipelas, with stinging, pricking pain, skin peels off.

Skin of face painfully sensitive.

⁹ Lower Face. Gnawing, smarting around the mouth.

Lower lip swelled and cracked in the middle.

¹⁰ Teeth. Looseness of painful teeth.

Drawing, jerking, as if a nerve was put on the stretch and then let loose; shooting in gums.

Left side of face sensitive; stinging in decayed teeth.

Throbbing, digging in hollow teeth, with drawing extending to the eye; also, with otalgia.

Toothache worse in Spring; at night; from picking teeth; in warm room; in warmth of bed; when eating, but not from chewing; when sitting; from cold water, or from anything warm in the mouth; also during pregnancy; better walking around in open air.

¹¹ Tongue, etc. Loss of taste, with catarrh; nothing tastes good.

Taste: foul, especially in early morning; clammy wants to rinse mouth often; of putrid meat, with inclination to vomit, in morning; bitter mostly after swallowing food or drink, also, evening and morning.

Tongue: white or yellow, and coated with tenacious mucus; parched, dry, no thirst; feels in middle as if burned, even when moist, night and morning; feels too broad, too large.

Edges of tongue feel sore and as if scalded.

¹² Mouth. Dry in morning, without thirst.

Putrid smell from mouth, especially in morning.

Flow of sweetish saliva.

Constant spitting of frothy, cotton-like mucus.

¹³ Throat. As if raw and sore; stinging, with pressure and tension on swallowing; cutting, burning, during swallowing; stitches between acts of swallowing; as if swollen, or a lump in it, when swallowing.

Veins distended, throat inflamed, bluish-red.

Throat dry, worse mornings, with tough mucus in throat, especially in night and morning; much tenacious mucus in throat, like potash-salts.

Sore throat, with sense of dysphagia; she feels as though she would be choked.

Worse swallowing saliva and after food.

¹⁴ Desires. Aversions. Hunger: but knows not for what; eats greedily, followed by vomiting.

Food tastes too salt.

Appetite for: strong alcoholic drinks, beer; sour, refreshing things; herring.

Aversion to: fat food, pork, meat, bread, milk.

Thirst rare; when thirsty drinks often, but little at a time, it provokes inclination to vomit.

Thirstlessness, with moist or dry tongue.

15 Eating and Drinking. While eating: 10. After eating: 13, 16, 19, 26, 29, 37. Hot or cold food: 8, 10. Cold fruit: 16. After drinking: 16.

16 Nausea and Vomiting. Hiccough: after cold fruit; after drinking.

Eructations: tasting and smelling of food; bitter, bilious; rancid, sour.

Nausea, with colic, ceasing after vomiting.

Nausea at throat as from a worm crawling.

Vomiting: of blood, from a cold on stomach, or suppressed menses; of bilious matter; sour, green; chronic, after eating; caused by fruits, fats, pastry, ices; with pale face and chilliness.

17 Stomach. Pain in pit of stomach, during an inspiration; also, on pressure.

Weight as from a stone, early morning on waking; also an hour after eating, better by eating again.

Pressure in pit of stomach after every meal, vomiting of food.

Stitching pains, worse when walking or making misstep.

Crampy pains before breakfact or after meals.

Gnawing distress when stomach is empty; pressure and pinching after eating.

Stomach bloated, hard; flatulency.

Perceptible pulsation in pit of stomach.

Gastric catarrh, from ice cream, fruit and pastry; pain, as from subcutaneous ulceration.

Tension from stomach to chest.

18 Hypocondria. Darting, tensive pains in hepatic region.

Sticking in region of liver, also, particulatly when walking.

Feeling of lassitude in hypochondria.

19 Abdomen. Flatulent colic, evening after supper, or at night; oppressive flatulence in upper abdomen and hypochondria; shifting of flatus.

Colic: from cold, with diarrhœa; from ices, fruits, pastry; from getting feet wet.

Pain in lower chest and abdomen, obliging her to bend forward.

Abdomen and stomach distended; she must unlace.

Pressure in abdomen and small of back, as from a stone; lower limbs go to sleep when sitting; ineffectual desire for stool.

Cutting and dragging in hypogastric region around to loins, making her feel faint.

Painful sensitiveness of abdomen to touch.

Lumps in both groins, hard and painful.

20 Stool, etc. Stools: watery, only, or usually at night, sometimes unconsciously evacuated; greenish-yellow, slimy, very changeable; like bile, following rumbling in abdomen; offensive, corrosive; of white and bloody mucus.

Dysenteric stools, of clear yellow, red or green slime; pain in back, straining; tenesmus, from anus up along sacrum.

Dysentery during cholera times.

Discharge of blood and mucus during stool; face pallid; fainting; dysuria; frequent stools of mucus only, after dysentery.

Obstinate constipation, nauseous, bad taste in morning, must wash out her mouth; costive stools hard and large, after suppressed intermittent fever by quinine.

Desire for stool, insufficient or no evacuation of feces, but instead yellowish, sometimes blood-mixed mucus.

Painful protruding piles, with smarting and soreness.

Piles (blind) with menses; though generally with this remedy, they bleed.

[21] **Urine.**   Tenesmus and stinging in neck of bladder.

Continued pressure on bladder, without desire to urinate.

Ischuria, with redness and heat in region of bladder.

Frequent, almost ineffectual, urging to urinate, with cutting pains.

Desire to urinate, with drawing in abdomen.

Cannot retain urine; it is passed in drops, sitting or walking; involuntary when coughing, passing wind, or during sleep, the latter especially in little girls.

Urine increased, watery, colorless; or, scanty, red-brown.

Sediment reddish, bloody or mucous, jelly-like, sticking to vessel.

Hæmaturia, with burning at orifice of urethra and constriction in region of navel.

Burning in urethra.

After urination, spasmodic pain in neck of bladder, extending into thighs.   At end of urination, dropping of blood.

[22] **Male Sexual Organs.**   Desire too strong, almost priapism.

Long-lasting morning erections; emissions after onanism.

Sexual excesses resulting in headache; backache; limbs heavy.

Burning of testicles, without swelling.

Orchitis, with swelling of scrotum; from cold, contusion or checked gonorrhœa.

Spermatic cord inflamed by a badly-fitting truss.

Drawing, tensive pains, from abdomen through cords into testicles.

Hydrocele.

Prostate enlarged; feces flat, small in size; also acute prostatis.

Gonorrhœa, with thick, yellow, or yellow-green discharge.

Itching. burning on inner and upper side of prepuce.

²³ **Female Sexual Organs.** Tensive, cutting pain in uterus, which is very sensitive to touch and during coitus.

Pains in uterus, with amenorrhœa.

Prolapsus uteri, with pressure in abdomen and small of back, as from a stone; limbs tend to go to sleep; ineffectual urging to stool.

Metrorrhagia, blood changeable, stops and flows; profuse at times, at others intermittent, mixed with clots; at climaxis; in chlorosis; after abuse of quinine and iron.

First menses delayed.

Menstruation, too late, scanty and of short duration; flow thick, black, clotted; or thin, watery; or changeable in appearance; flows more during day while walking.

Menses suppressed, or flow intermittently; after getting feet wet; in chlorosis; from nervous debility; with throbbing headache; pressure in stomach; pain in uterus; dysuria; ophthalmia; morning nausea; or bad taste in mouth.

Crampy constriction of vagina; indurations; fistula; polypus.

Leucorrhœa: milky, thick, with swollen vulva; acrid, burning, painless, or with cutting in abdomen.

²⁴ **Pregnancy.** Threatened abortion; flow ceases and then returns with double force, ceases again, and so on.

Promotes expulsion of moles.

Labor-pains: deficient, irregular or sluggish; spasmodic; excite suffocation and faint spells, must have doors and windows open.

Retained placenta, want of action or spasmodic contraction.

Post-partum secondary hemorrhages from retained placenta or coagula.

After-pains too long or too violent; worse toward evening.

Lochia scanty, becoming milky; feverish, but no thirst.

Convulsions following sluggish or irregular labor-pains; unconscious; cold, clammy, pale face; stertorous breathing and full pulse.

Milk leg.

Mammæ: lumps in breasts of girls before puberty; or, escape of thin, milk-like fluid.

Breasts swollen, rheumatic pains extend to muscles of chest, also to shoulders, neck, axillæ and down the arms, change from place to place; during nursing.

Milk suddenly suppressed; lochia becomes milky, white.

After weaning: breasts swell, feel stretched, tense, intensely sore; milk continues to be secreted.

²⁵ **Larynx.** Hoarseness and roughness of throat; cannot speak aloud; hoarseness coming and going.

Aphonia nervosa returns at every motion; last cervical
vertebra feels sore, burning.

Constriction in throat, feels something there preventing
speech; cannot eat, weeps.

26 **Breathing.** Asthma: especially of children after suppression of rash; in hysteria, or with suppressed menses; in
the evening, especially after a meal.

Dyspnœa and vertigo, with weakness in head, when lying·
on the back; at night, in bed, as if throat or chest were
constricted; or as if fumes of sulphur had been inhaled;
morning, low down in chest.

Oppression of chest on walking fast, ascending an eminence, or exercising.

27 **Cough.** From irritation in pit of stomach; shattering, spasmodic, often in paroxysms of two coughs each; excited
by itching, scratching, and dry feeling, as from vapor of
sulphur in trachea and chest; dry at night, going off
when sitting in bed; loose by day; dry after every
sleep; evening after lying down, when warm in bed;
loose, vomits mucus; diarrhœa; worse at night; with
yellow mucus sputa, bitter or greenish; with purulent
expectoration; with expectoration of pieces of dark,
coagulated blood; menses suppressed.

Spitting of dark, coagulated blood; pain in lower part of
chest; anguish, shuddering; qualmishness.

28 **Lungs.** Phthisis florida, suppurative stage; chlorotic girls.

Soreness in chest; under clavicles.

Pain in chest, as if ulcerated.

Stitches in side only when lying, particularly at night.

Sticking in chest, worse from deep breath, or coughing.

Paroxysms of burning in chest.

Obstinate bronchial catarrh.

Congestion to cheek and heart at night; with anxious
dreams.

29 **Heart. Pulse.** Beating through chest interrupts sleep;
old maids.

Catching pain in cardiac region, better for a time from
pressure of hand. Pains, with but little or no anxiety.

Burning in region of heart.

Heaviness, pressure or sensation of fulness every evening.

Palpitation: in violent paroxysms, often with anguish and
obscuration of sight; trembling of limbs; from chagrin,
fright, or joy; with amenia, chlorosis; strong, with suppressed pulse; after dinner.

Pulse: accelerated, small and weak; frequent evenings,
with distended blood-vessels, slower in morning; often
scarcely perceptible.

30 **Outer Chest.** Chest pains as if bruised.

31 Neck. Back. Swelling of cervical glands.

Interscapular pain, worse by inspiration.

Curvature of upper part of spine.

Like cold water poured down back.

Stitches in small of back.

Pain in back and small of back, as from stooping long, or as if weary.

32 Upper Limbs. Severe pains in both shoulder-joins.

Hard, painful, throbbing glandular swelling in the right axilla.

Heaviness in arms from shoulders to fingers, numb feeling.

Arms feel as if broken and dislocated; worse on pressure and from movement.

Elbow swollen after a contusion.

Veins in forearms and hands swollen.

33 Lower Limbs. Pain as from festering, in muscles of buttocks, legs and soles.

Jerking pain in hip-joint, extending to knee.

Drawing, heaviness, weariness, in legs.

Legs hot, swollen, with tensive, burning pains.

Knees inflamed, swollen, with shooting pains.

Soft, white, shining swelling of knees.

Jerking, lacerating through left leg and foot, which becomes numb and œdematous; sensitive to touch; better from changing position.

Aching in calves, which are swollen.

Varices on legs.

Feet red, inflamed, swollen; also the soles. Swelling of top of foot.

Chilblains inflamed, bluish, itching.

34 Limbs in General. Redness and swelling of joints, with stinging pains.

Jerking, tearing, drawing in muscles, shifting rapidly from place to place; worse at night, from warmth; better from uncovering; towards evening pains more fixed with swelling of parts, when pains abate some.

Rheumatism: caused by getting wet, especially the feet; from protracted wet weather.

35 Position, etc. Motion: 19, 32, 33, 40. Exercise: 5, 26. Walking: 3, 10, 18, 21, 23, 26, 46. Rising: 4. Ascending: 26. Stooping: 3. Must bend forward: 19. Lifting eyes: 2, 3. Moving eyes: 3. Rest: 3. Sitting: 3, 10, 19, 21, 27. Lying: 3, 27, 29; on back: 26. Parts lain on: 3, 4, 43.

Pains worse changing from a long-maintained position.

36 Nerves. Hysteria; symptoms ever changing.

Epileptic convulsions, violent tossing of limbs, followed by relaxation, disposition to vomit, eructations; from suppressed menses.

Fainting fits, great paleness of face; shivering, coldness. Violent trembling all over.

Tired, worn out feeling, as from fatigue, but not better resting.

Nervous debility, with amenorrhœa.

37 Sleep. Yawning; drowsy by day; feverish somnolence.

Sleepless: after late supper, or eating too much; from ideas crowding on the mind; first part of night, sleeps late in morning.

Starts, talks, weeps, cries out in sleep.

Dreams: confused, frightful; anxious.

Talking, whining and screaming during sleep.

38 Time. Eearly morning: 1, 11. Morning: 2, 11, 12, 13, 20, 22, 23, 26, 29, 37, 40. 4 P.M.: 40. 5–10 P.M.: 4. Evening: 3, 4, 5, 8, 11, 19, 24, 26, 27, 29, 40. Night: 4, 6, 10, 13, 19, 20, 26, 27, 28, 34, 40, 46.

39 Temperature and Weather. Warmth: 5, 34; of bed: 4, 10, 26, 27. Warm room: 3, 10, 40. In-doors: 7. Sunshine: 5. Spring: 10. Cold: 46. Wet weather: 34. Open air: 3, 5, 10. Undressing: 4. Uncovering: 34. Washing: 40. Getting head wet: 4. Wetting feet: 19, 23, 34.

Generally pains better cool air; abdominal pains better warmth.

40 Chill. Fever. Sweat. Cold chills all over; chilly all the time, even in a warm room; chilly with the pains.

Chilly at lower abdomen and small of back; sleepy but no sleep.

One-sided coldness, with numbness.

Flitting chilliness; chills in spots, now here, now there; worse evening.

Chill 4 P.M., no thirst; anxiety, dyspnœa; vomiting of mucus when the chill comes on.

Heat, with red face, or one cheek red and one pale.

Internal dry heat, evening or night, without external heat.

Heat of right side or on upper part of body; lessened by moving or washing.

Heat of face or of one hand, with coldness of the other; body hot, limbs cold.

Attacks of anxious heat, as if water was poured over him.

Sweat: one-sided; only on face and head; more at night and in morning; soon ceasing when waking; sour, musty, at times cold; sweetish acid odor to sweat; at night, with stupid slumber.

Pains during sweat.

During apyrexia: headache; mucous diarrhœa, nausea and loss of appetite; enlarged spleen.

41 Attacks. Paroxysms of increasing severity.

Pains appear suddenly, leave gradually.

Wandering pains shift rapidly from part to part.

Symptoms ever changing.

⁴² **Sides.** Right: 10, 32, 40. Left: 10, 29, 33. Above downward: 21.

⁴³ **Sensations.** Tension in inner parts, or in joints.

Sensation of subcutaneous ulceration.

Tingling in parts lain on.

Pulsations through the whole body.

⁴⁴ **Tissues.** Hemorrhages, blood dark, easily coagulating.

Varicose veins; inflamed.

Circulation weak, sluggish, with paleness and constant chilliness; anæmia.

Inflammations of internal parts, with disposition to suppurate.

Affections of mucous surfaces; discharges thence are usually bland, yellowish-green, thick.

Emaciation, especially of suffering parts.

Chlorosis, especially after large doses of iron.

Glands swollen, painful, hot.

Scraping or tingling in periosteum; jerking boring in bones; incipiency of inflammation. Anasarca.

⁴⁵ **Contact, Injuries, etc.** Part touched feels bruised, ulcerated; skin sensitive.

Child wants to be carried slowly.

Better from tying clothes tightly.

Concussions; bruises, especially with injury of bones, sore pain when touched.

Touch: 19, 23, 33. Rubbing or wiping: 5. Pressure: 5, 29, 32; of clothes: 19; of truss: 22. Contusion: 22, 32. Riding in cars: 6.

⁴⁶ **Skin.** Pale; burning-itching here and there.

Urticaria, with diarrhœa; also in the summer; itching worse at night; from pastry or pork; from delayed menses; worse undressing, cool bath, etc.

Moles or freckles on young girls.

Erysipelas bluish, spreads rapidly; especially about buttocks and thighs; smooth skin.

Intertrigo, chafing, after abuse of chamomile tea. Rhagades. Chaps.

Bleeding tumors; changeable blood, most while walking during the day.

Measles even with typhoid symptoms; catarrh prominent; eruption tardy; earache; ophthalmia; short, dry cough, with pain in chest; or, rattling loose cough, which is prone to remain as a sequel.

Ulcers: bleed easily, with burning, stinging or itching around them; with hard or red areolæ; better from cold.

Wounds suppurate; pus thick, bland, too profuse.

⁴⁷ **Stages and States.** Sandy hair, blue eyes, pale face, inclined to grief and submissiveness.

Often indicated with women and children.

⁴⁸ **Relationship.** Complementary to *Sulph. ac., Lycop., Pulsat.*

It antidotes: *Cinchon.,* iron, *Sulphur, Sulph. ac.,* vapor of mercury, or of copper, *Coffea, Chamom., Bellad., Colchic., Lycop., Platin., Stramon., Sabad., Ant. tart.*

Pulsat. is antidoted by *Chamom., Coffea, Ignat., Nux vom.*

RANUNCULUS BULBOSUS.

Bulbous Crowfoot.   Franz.   *Ranunculaceæ.*

¹ **Mind.** Vanishing of thought on reflection.

Obtuseness of the senses.

Angry mood; quarrelsome.

² **Sensorium.** Vertigo, with danger of falling, when going from room into open air.

³ **Inner Head.** Pressing headache in forehead and on vertex, as if pressed asunder, with pressure on eyeballs and sleepiness; worse in evening or when entering a room from cold air; or vice versa.

Congestion of blood to head, sensation of fulness and enlargement of head.

Headache, with nausea and sleepiness.

The headache is caused or aggravated by a change of temperature.

⁴ **Outer Head.** Head feels too large.

⁵ **Eyes.** Hemeralopia, with heat, biting and pressure in eyes; lids and conjunctiva slightly red, with lachrymation; pus in the canthi.

Pressure in eyeballs.

Smarting and sore feeling in eye or canthus.

⁶ **Ears.** Stitches in ears, principally in evening.

⁷ **Nose.** Redness and inflammatory swelling of nose, with tension.

Scabs in the nostrils.

⁸ **Face.** Dry heat in face, with redness of cheeks, evenings.

Tingling in face, especially on nose and chin.

⁹ **Lower Face.** Spasms of the lips.

¹² **Mouth.** White saliva in mouth, tasting like copper.

¹³ **Throat.** Much viscid phlegm in throat.

Inflammatory burning pains in throat and on palate.

¹⁵ **Eating and Drinking.** After eating: 36.

¹⁶ **Nausea and Vomiting.** Spasmodic hiccough.

Nausea in afternoon and evening, sometimes with headache.

¹⁷ **Stomach.** Sensation of soreness and burning in pit of stomach, worse from touch.

Pressure in pit of stomach.

¹⁸ **Hypochondria.** Sensation of soreness in hypochondria, especially to touch.

Stitches in region of liver, extending up into chest.

Pulsations in left hypochondrium.

¹⁹ **Abdomen.** Colic and cutting pains in abdomen, and when pressing on it sensation as if everything were sore and bruised.

Burning soreness in abdomen.

Great tenderness of abdomen to touch.

²¹ **Urine.** Ulcers in the bladder.

²³ **Female Sexual Organs.** Leucorrhœa, at first mild, then acrid, corroding.

²⁶ **Breathing.** Short and oppressed, with pains in chest, and inclination to draw a long breath.

²⁸ **Lungs.** Stitches in chest.

Small, sore spot, as from subcutaneous ulceration θ After pneumonia.

Adhesions of the lungs (after inflammation).

²⁹ **Heart. Pulse.** Pulse full, hard, rapid in evening, slower in morning.

³⁰ **Outer Chest.** Chest feels sore, bruised; worse from touch, motion, or turning body (many cases of pleurodynia).

³¹ **Neck. Back.** Pain along inner edge of left scapula, often extending below its inferior angle, or through lower half of left side of thorax.

³² **Upper Limbs.** Spasmodic, rheumatic pain in arms.

Stitches in arms and hands.

Blister-like eruption in palms of hands.

³³ **Lower Limbs.** Drawing pain in the thighs, extending downward.

Cracking in joints (knee).

Corns sensitive to touch, smart and burn.

³⁵ **Position, etc.** Motion: 30. Turning body: 30. Cannot lie on side: 37.

³⁶ **Nerves.** Twitching of muscles.

Epileptic attacks.

Sudden weakness, with fainting.

Trembling of limbs, with oppression of breathing after fright or anger; aggravated in evening, and sometimes after eating, from change of temperature, especially from heat to cold.

³⁷ **Sleep.** Sleeplessness often with dyspnœa, heat and ebullitions; cannot lie on the side.

³⁸ **Time.** Morning: 29, 40. Afternoon: 16, 40. Evening: 3, 6, 8, 16, 29, 36, 40.

[39] **Temperature and Weather.** Room to open air: 2, 3. Open air to room: 3. Change of temperatnre: 36. Open air: 40.

[40] **Chill. Fever. Sweat.** Chilly, with heat in face, worse afternoon and evening; the well-covered chest is chilly out of doors.

Heat in evening, worse on right side of face, with cold hands and general uncomfortableness.

Heat, with internal chill at same time.

Sweat scanty and only in morning on awaking.

[42] **Sides.** Right: 18, 40. Left: 18, 31. Behind forward: 31. Above downward: 33.

[45] **Contact, Injuries, etc.** Touch: 17, 18, 19, 30, 33. Pressure: 19.

[46] **Skin.** Horn-like excrescences.

Vesicular eruptions, as from burns.

Shingles and intercostal neuralgia.

Flat, burning, stinging ulcers, with ichorous discharge.

Pemphigus.

Chilblains (external application).

[48] **Relationship.** Antidotes to *Ran. bulb.*: *Bryon.*, *Camphor.*, *Pulsat.*, *Rhus.*

Inimicals: alcohol, *Spir. nitr. dulc.*, *Staphis*, *Sulphur*, vinegar, wine.

RANUNCULUS SCLERATUS.

Nefarious Crowfoot.   Y. WATZKE.   *Ranunculaceæ.*

[1] **Mind.** Indolence and aversion to mental occupation in morning; low-spirited, depressed in evening.

Dulness of the head.

[2] **Sensorium.** Vertigo, with loss of consciousness.

[3] **Inner Head.** Gnawing pain in small spot on vertex or either temple.

[4] **Outer Head.** Sensation as if head was enlarged and too full.

Biting-itching on the scalp.

Scalp feels tense.

[5] **Eyes.** Smarting in eyes and canthi.

Painful pressing in eyeballs.

Eyes very weak and water much.

[6] **Ears.** Otalgia, with pressing or gnawing pain in head, and drawing pain in teeth.

[7] **Nose.** Lachrymation, with watery nasal discharge.

⁸ **Face.** Sensation as if face was covered with spider web.
  Drawing in face, with sensation of coldness.
  Face cold, livid.

¹⁰ **Teeth.** Drawing-stinging in teeth.

¹¹ **Tongue, etc.** Tongue exfoliated in spots, which are raw;
  mouth inflamed.
  Both sides of the tongue denuded like islands, the remaining parts thickly coated. θ Diphtheria.

¹³ **Throat.** Scraping or burning in throat.
  Swelling of tonsils, with shooting stitches in them.

¹⁵ **Eating and Drinking.** After meals: 16, 40.

¹⁶ **Nausea and Vomiting.** Eructations after meals, with
  taste of what has been eaten.

¹⁷ **Stomach.** Pain in the stomach, with fainting fits.
  Sensation of fulness in pit of stomach, increased by ex-
  ternal pressure, worse mornings.
  Sensation of soreness and burning in pit of stomach.

¹⁸ **Hypochondria.** Spleen swollen after intermittent fever and
  abuse of quinine.
  Dull pressure about liver, worse from a long breath.
  Stitches in liver, spleen or kidneys.

²⁰ **Stool, etc.** Frequent soft, or watery, fetid stools.
  Frequent sensation as though diarrhœa would set in.

²¹ **Urine.** Burns; strangury.

²² **Male Sexual Organs.** Stitches at glans penis.

²⁹ **Heart. Pulse.** Pulse quick, full, but soft, with heat at
  night.

³⁰ **Outer Chest.** Chest feels as if bruised, with sensation of
  weakness therein.
  Stitches in chest and intercostal muscles.
  External chest and sternum are painfully sensitive to
  touch.

³² **Upper Limbs.** Stitching, boring and gnawing in arms,
  especially violent in fingers.
  Itching between fingers, evenings.
  Swelling of fingers, mornings.

³³ **Lower Limbs.** Stinging, boring and gnawing in toes,
  especially violent in big toe.

³⁴ **Limbs in General.** Gout in fingers and toes.

³⁶ **Nerves.** Fainting with the pains.

³⁷ **Sleep.** Sleeplessness after midnight; with anxiety, heat
  and thirst, or with restlessness and tossing about.

³⁸ **Time.** Pains worse toward evening, decrease after midnight, when sleeplessness, tossing about, anxiety, heat
  and thirst set in.
  Morning: 1, 17, 32. Evening: 1, 30, 32, 38, 40, 43.
  Night: 29, 40. After midnight: 37, 38, 40. Toward
  morning: 40.

[39] **Temperature and Weather.** In-doors: 40. Open air: 40.
[40] **Chill. Fever. Sweat.** Chill or chilliness during meals.
Heat, evening in-doors, after walking in open air.
Dry heat at night, with violent thirst, mostly after midnight.
Sweat after heat, toward morning, mostly on forehead.
[42] **Sides.** Right eye and ear more affected than left.
[43] **Sensations.** Feels sore all over.
Smarting, itching, gnawing or boring in various parts, now here, again there: especially toward evening.
[45] **Contact, Injuries, etc.** Touch: 30, 43. Pressure: 17.
[46] **Skin.** Vesicular eruptions, with acrid, thin, yellowish discharge.

RHEUM.

Rhubarb.   HAHNEMANN.   *Holygonaceæ.*

[1] **Mind.** Child asks for different things, impetuously and with crying; dislikes even its favorite things.
Screaming of children, with urging and sour stools.
Not inclined to talk much.
Indolent, taciturn.
Morose.
Restless, with weeping.
[2] **Sensorium.** Vertigo and heaviness, with beating in head; worse while standing.
[3] **Inner Head.** Dull, stupefying headache, with bloated eyes.
Heaviness of head; heat rising up to it.
Pulsation in head, ascending from abdomen.
Sensation as if brain moved. when stooping.
[4] **Outer Head.** Sweat on hairy scalp.
[5] **Eyes.** Weak and dull, especially when looking intensely at an object.
Pupils dilated, with pressing headache; later contracted, with inward restlessness.
Pulsation in the eyes.
Convulsive twitching of eyelids.
Granulated upper eyelids.
[7] **Nose.** Stupefying drawing in root of nose, extending to tip, where it tingles.
[8] **Face.** Pale; one cheek red, the other pale.
Muscles of forehead are drawn together and wrinkled.
Tension of skin of face.
Cool sweat in face, most around nose and mouth.

[10] **Teeth.** Difficult dentition of children.

Toothache, with a cold sensation in teeth.

[11] **Tongue, etc.** Taste: sour; insipid, or nauseous; bitter, only of food, even of sweet things.

Tongue numb, insensible.

[12] **Mouth.** Salivation with colic or diarrhœa.

[14] **Desires. Aversions.** Desire for various things, but cannot eat them.

[15] **Eating and Drinking.** After eating prunes, colic.

After a meal, loose stool; colic, which is worse standing.

[16] **Nausea and Vomiting.** Nausea, as from stomach, or abdomen, with colic.

[17] **Stomach.** Fulness in stomach, as after eating too much.

Throbbing in pit of stomach.

[19] **Abdomen.** The wind seems to rise up in chest.

Violent pain with cutting, must lie doubled up; worse when standing.

Cutting and rumbling, as from flatulence.

Abdomen bloated, tense.

Like a lump around the navel.

[20] **Stool, etc.** Stool: brown and slimy; loose, thin, curdled, sour, fermented, turning green, reddening the anus.

Worse evening and night; fever in morning; worse from any motion, standing; after eating; during teething; in the lying-in from change of weather; during summer.

Before stool: ineffectual urging to urinate, cutting colic.

During stool: chilliness, cutting and constricting pains in abdomen; pale face; salivation; screaming (teething infants) with drawing up of limbs or stiffening body.

After stool: colic, ineffectual straining, worse from any motion.

Diarrhœa during inflammatory rheumatism.

Chronic diarrhœa sour, frothy; with moist tongue, thirst, loss of appetite.

Dysentery, after bloody stools have ceased, tenesmus, with brown, mush-like, slimy, sour stools.

[21] **Urine..** Burning in kidneys and bladder, before and during urination.

Bladder weak, must press hard to urinate.

Urine; increased; red, or greenish-yellow.

[23] **Female Sexual Organs.** Bearing down in uterine region, while standing.

[24] **Pregnancy.** After abortus, urinary complaints.

Milk of nursing women, yellow and bitter; infant refuses breast.

Diarrhœa in first days after confinement, with colic, tenesmus, prostration, restlessness, fear of death; the stools are watery, offensive.

Dentition difficult, with diarrhœa.

[26] **Breathing.** Dyspnœa, as from a load on upper part of the chest

[29] **Heart. Pulse.** Pulse generally unchanged, only a little accelerated, especially in evening.

[31] **Neck. Back.** Stiffness in sacrum and hips, cannot walk straight.

Violent cutting, as if in lumbar vertebræ, increased from stool.

[32] **Upper Limbs.** Darting pains in arms.

Twitching in arms, hands and fingers.

Bubbling sensation in elbow-joints.

Veins of hand distended.

Cold sweat on palms of hands.

[33] **Lower Limbs.** Twitching of muscles on thighs.

Sensation of fatigue in thighs.

Stiffness in bend of knee, with pain on motion.

Bubbling sensation from bend of knee to heel.

[34] **Limbs in General.** Limbs fall asleep, from lying on them, particularly the lower, in putting one over the other.

[35] **Position, etc.** Takes the queerest positions, in order to rest awhile; restless nights.

Standing: 2, 15, 19, 20, 23. Lying on affected parts: 34. Motion: 20, 33. Cannot walk erect: 31. Flexes limbs: 20. Extends limbs: 20. Puts hands over head: 37. Must lie doubled up: 19.

[36] **Nerves.** Exhaustion; weakness; also of children with the diarrhœa.

Weakness and heaviness in whole body, as if one were waking from a heavy sleep.

Child is pale, quarrels, frets in sleep; with convulsive startings in fingers.

[37] **Sleep.** Puts hands over head when falling asleep, and in sleep.

During sleep, heat, jerking motion of muscles in face or eyelids, trembling, moving limbs, bending the head backward.

Children cry and toss about all night; delirious talking; full of fear.

Walking while asleep.

On awaking from sleep, headache; bad odor from mouth.

Requires very little sleep and not much food.

[38] **Time.** Evening: 29.

[39] **Temperature and Weather.** General aggravation from uncovering, from cold; amelioration from wrapping up; from warmth.

Summer: 20. Change of weather: 20.

[40] **Chill. Fever. Sweat.** Chilliness, alternating with heat; or, internal, with external heat.

I

Heat all over, mostly on hands and feet, with cold face; no thirst.

Sweats easily in diseases without fever.

Sweat on scalp and forehead.

Cold sweat about nose and mouth.

Sweat stains yellow.

⁴² **Sides.** Symptoms mostly left-sided; going (in the sick) downward, or from right to left.

Right to left: 44. Below upward: 3. Above downward: 44.

⁴⁴ **Tissues.** Acute rheumatism, going from joint to joint, right shoulder to hip; left hip to right.

Lameness in wrists and knees after sprains and dislocations.

Anasarca.

⁴⁵ **Contact, Injuries, etc.** Sprains, etc.: 44.

⁴⁶ **Skin.** Child smells sourish, even if washed or bathed every day.

⁴⁷ **Stages and States.** Often suitable for children, sucklings, or during dentition.

⁴⁸ **Relationship.** After abuse of *Canth.* or *Magn. carb.*

Complementary to *Magn. carb.*

Rheum follows *Ipec.* well.

Antidotes to *Rheum: Camphor., Chamom., Coloc., Mercur., Nux vom., Pulsat.*

RHODODENDRON.

Yellow Snowrose. SEIDEL. *Ericaceæ.*

¹ **Mind.** Leaves out whole words in writing.

Great indifference, with aversion to all occupation or labor.

² **Sensorium.** Sensation of stupefaction and drowsiness in head on rising in morning.

Intoxicated from a little wine.

³ **Inner Head.** Pain in forehead and temples when lying in bed in morning; worse from drinking wine and in wet, cold weather; better after rising and moving about.

⁴ **Outer Head.** The scalp feels sore and as if bruised.

Violent drawing and tearing in bones and periosteum of cranial bones; worse when at rest; in the morning; during a thunder-storm and during wet, cold, stormy weather; better from wrapping the head up warmly; from dry heat and from exercise.

Biting-itching on scalp, especially in evening.

⁵ **Eyes.** Dimness of vision when reading and writing.

Shooting pain outward, worse before a storm.

Periodical, dry burning in eyes, worse in bright daylight and from intent looking.

Spasmodic contraction of eyelids.

Insufficiency of internal recti muscles.

⁶ **Ears.**   Otalgia (right ear); violent twitching pain.

Sensation in ear as from a worm.

Buzzing in ear, aggravated when swallowing.

⁷ **Nose.**   Diminished sense of smell.

Bleeding of nose, left side.

Soreness of inner nose, with scurf either yellow or black.

Violent sneezing, when rising in morning, with heat in face.

Thin, fluid and profuse discharge, with rheumatic or gouty symptoms.

One or the other nostril obstructed, less in the open air.

⁸ **Face.**   Chilliness over the face.

Violent tearing, jerking faceache; worse in the wind and from changes of weather; better while eating and from warmth.

⁹ **Lower Face.**   Lips dry, burning.

Vesicles on inner side of lower lip, sore when eating.

¹⁰ **Teeth.**   Toothache better from warm, than from the cold; pains leave completely during and for an hour or two after eating.

Toothache with earache.

Neuralgia of inferior and superior dental nerves; teeth loose; snags come away; gums swollen; pains worse from change of weather; better from warmth.

¹¹ **Tongue, etc.**   Taste lost.

Smarting vesicles under tongue.

¹² **Mouth.**   Increase of saliva in mouth, with dryness of throat.

¹³ **Throat.**   Constriction and burning in throat.

Sore throat.

¹⁴ **Desires.   Aversions.**   Easily satisfied with a small quantity of food; feels uncomfortable afterwards.

Thirst is generally wanting.

¹⁵ **Eating and Drinking.**   While eating: 8, 9.   After eating: 10, 19, 20; fruit: 20.   Drinking wine: 2, 3.   After drinking (especially cold water): 16, 17.

¹⁶ **Nausea and Vomiting.**   Gulping of a rancid or bitter fluid.

Nausea, water-brash, pressure at the stomach, better by belching.

Vomits after fluids, especially cold water; green, bitter vomit.

¹⁷ **Stomach.**   Pressure in stomach at night, after cold drinks.

Constriction and pressure at pit of stomach, with dyspnœa.

¹⁸ **Hypochondria.**   Periodical crampy pains under short ribs.

Pressing and drawing, with feeling of repletion in stomach and oppression of breathing.

Pains as from flatulence, worse in left hypochondrium.

Stitches in the spleen from walking fast: tension when stooping.

19 **Abdomen.** Distention in upper part of abdomen, with dyspnœa; evening and morning.

Much rumbling in abdomen, with eructations and discharge of fetid flatus.

Colic at navel, or feeling of repletion after eating.

20 **Stool, etc.** Stool papescent, yet tardy, requiring much urging.

Diarrhœa: painless, undigested; after meals; after fruit; from wet, cold weather; in morning with much flatus; or, with pains in limbs.

Dysentery in summer, renewed before a thunder-storm.

Drawing, extending from rectum to genitals.

Pulsation in anus.

21 **Urine.** ▮ Frequent urging to urinate, with drawing in region of bladder.

▮ Pain in urethra, as from subcutaneous ulceration.

Increased secretion of very offensive urine.

Greenish urine.

22 **Male Sexual Organs.** Desire weak; aversion to an embrace.

Emissions at night, with amorous dreams, later long-continned erections.

Testicles: especially the epididymis, intensely painful to touch; soreness extending into abdomen and thighs; drawn up, swollen, painful.

Induration and swelling of (left) testicle; after gonorrhœa, or with blenorrhœa.

▮ Hydrocele.

Itching and sweat of scrotum.

Soreness or sore sensation between genitals and thighs.

23 **Female Sexual Organs.** Menstruation too profuse and too early; with fever and headache.

Suppressed menstruation.

Pain in ovaries; worse in change of weather.

▮ Serous cysts of the vagina.

24 **Pregnancy.** After parturition, burning in uterine region, alternating with pains in limbs, fingers spasmodically flexed.

26 **Breathing.** Dyspnœa from constriction of chest.

27 **Cough.** Dry, exhausting, morning and evening, with oppression of chest and rough throat; with escape of urine.

28 **Lungs.** Shooting through left chest to back, when bending back and to the right.

29 **Heart. Pulse.** Boring pain in region of heart.

Heart's beat stronger.

Pulse slow and weak; or unchanged.

[30] **Outer Chest.** Chest sensitive to touch.
[31] **Neck. Back.** Stiff neck, gums and teeth sore, pains fly
about everywhere.

Shooting from back to pit of stomach.

Pain from small of back into arms.

Small of back pains, worse when sitting; worse in wet
weather.

[32] **Upper Limbs.** Drawing pains in arms, worse in wet weather.

Sensation as if blood ceased to circulate in arms, hands
feel warm.

[33] **Lower Limbs.** White swelling of knee, with intolerable
tearing pains, worse during rest and at night.

Sensation of coldness, skin wrinkles on lower legs.

Dropsical swelling of lower legs and feet.

Sensation lower legs and feet as if "asleep."

[34] **Limbs in General.** Heavy, weak feeling and formication
in back and limbs; worse at rest and in rough weather.

Sensation in joints as if sprained, with swelling and redness; with arthritic nodosities.

Drawing, tearing in periosteum, worse at night; in wet,
stormy weather; and at rest; better in motion; mostly
in forearms and lower legs.

Erratic, tearing pains in limbs.

[35] **Position, etc.** Rest: 4, 33, 34, 36, 40. Lying in bed: 3, 40.
Sitting: 31. Motion: 3, 4, 34, 36. Walking fast: 18.
Rising: 2, 3, 7. Stooping: 18. Bending back: 28; to
right side: 28.

[36] **Nerves.** Paralytic weakness during rest.

Great weakness after slight exertion.

[37] **Sleep.** Great sleepiness during the day, with burning in eyes.

Deep, heavy sleep before midnight, with sleepiness early
in evening, but sleeplessness after midnight; morning
sleep disturbed by pain and restlessness in body.

Awakes as if called.

[38] **Time.** Morning: 2, 3, 4, 7, 19, 20, 27, 37, 40. Day: 5, 37,
40. Evening: 4, 19, 27, 37, 40. Night: 17, 22, 33, 34,
37. After midnight: 37.

[39] **Temperature and Weather.** Warmth: 4, 8, 10. Dry heat:
4. Summer: 20. In bed: 40. Cold: 10. Open air:
7, 40. Wind: 8. Change of weather: 8, 10, 23. Wet,
cold weather: 3, 4, 20, 31, 34. Thunder-storm: 4, 5,
20, 34.

[40] **Chill. Fever. Sweat.** Chilliness in morning in bed, and
during day, if cold air blows on him.

Chilliness alternating with heat.

Persistent ice-cold feet in evening, continued long after
lying down in bed.

Heat in evening, with cold feet; feverish, with burning in
face.

Sensation of heat, especially in hands, although they feel cold to the touch.

Profuse debilitating sweat, especially when moving about in open air.

Offensive-smelling sweat in axillæ; spicy odor.

Formication and itching of skin, with sweat.

[41] **Attacks.** Pains in bones or skin in small spots; radiating from place to place.

[42] **Sides.** Right: 6. Left: 7, 18, 22, 28, 29. Within outward: 5.

[45] **Contact, Injuries, etc.** Touch: 22, 30, 40.

[46] **Skin.** Burning and tearing, with erysipelas.

[48] **Relationship.** Antidotes to *Rhodod.: Bryon., Clemat., Rhus*

RHUS TOXICODENDRON.

Poison Sumac. HAHNEMANN. *Anacardiaceæ.*

[1] **Mind.** Stupefaction, with tingling in head and pains in limbs, better in motion.

Absence of mind; forgetful; difficult comprehension; cannot remember the most recent events.

Incoherent talking; answers hastily or reluctantly, thought seems difficult; answers correctly but slowly; cannot hold mind on one subject long enough to answer.

Low, mild delirium, thinks he is roaming over fields, or hard at work.

Low-spirited, with prostration; inclination to weep, especially in the evening, with desire for solitude.

Fears he will be poisoned.

Anxiety, timidity; worse at twilight; restless change of place; wants to go from bed to bed.

Satiety of life, with fear of death.

Thoughts of suicide; wants to drown himself.

[2] **Sensorium.** Giddy, as if intoxicated, when rising from bed; with chilliness and pressure behind eyes.

Vertigo in the aged, worse when rising from lying, and from turning or stooping.

[3] **Inner Head.** Burning in forehead when walking.

Feeling as of a strapped board across the forehead.

Stupefying headache, with buzzing; worse when sitting or lying; in the cold, in the morning, from beer; better from warmth and motion.

Headache, must lie down; returns from the least chagrin.

Rush of blood to head, with humming, formication and throbbing; face glistening and red; restless, moving about.

Brain feels loose, when stepping or shaking the head.

Stitches extending to ears, root of nose and malar bones, with toothache.

Aching in occipital protuberances. (See end of 48.)

Meningitis in exanthematous fevers, or after getting wet; tingling limbs; high fever; restlessness.

⁴ **Outer Head.** Erysipelas of scalp, left to right, forming vesicles.

Eruption suppurating, moist, forming thick crusts, offensive itching; worse at night; hair is eaten off; extends to shoulders.

Scalp sensitive, worse on side not lain on, when growing warm in bed, from touch and combing the hair back.

⁵ **Eyes.** Great photophobia, profuse acrid lachrymation in morning and in open air; the cheek under the eye is dotted with red pimples; lids spasmodically closed.

Iritis: in rheumatic or gouty subjects; suppurative or where the ciliary body and choroid are involved, especially if of traumatic origin.

Pustules and superficial ulcers on cornea, with great photophobia; conjunctiva quite red, even to chemosis.

Sac-like swelling of conjunctiva, with yellow, purulent discharge.

Eyes red and agglutinated in morning.

Lids much swollen and inflamed.

Eyelids œdematous or erysipelatous, with scattered, watery vesicles; meibomian glands enlarged, cilia fall out.

Ptosis, also, paralysis of any of the muscles of eyeball, from getting wet; in rheumatic patients.

⁶ **Ears.** Hardness of hearing, especially of the human voice.

Otalgia, with pulsation in ear at night.

Bloody pus from the ears.

Parotitis, left side; especially suppurating, during scarlatina.

⁷ **Nose.** Loss of smell.

Epistaxis of coagulated blood, worse at night and when stooping, at stool, or from exertion; also in typhus, with some relief.

Spasmodic sneezing.

Discharge from the nose: of thick, yellow mucus; of green, offensive pus; of yellow ichor, with swollen cervical glands.

Fever-blisters and crusts under nose.

Tip of nose red and sensitive; nose sore internally.

Puffiness of nose.

⁸ **Face.** Fiery red; pale, sunken, nose pointed, blue around the eyes.

Erysipelas from left to right; face dark red, covered with

yellow vesicles; burning, itching and tingling with the stinging.

Burning, drawing, tearing in face; teeth feel too long; restlessness.

Milk crust.

Acne rosacea.

Impetigo on face and forehead.

⁹ **Lower Face.** Stiffness of jaws, cracking in articulation of jaw when moving it; jaw easily dislocated.

Corners of mouth ulcerated, fever-blisters around mouth; exanthema on chin.

¹⁰ **Teeth.** Painful, with stinging at root of nose, extending to malar bones.

Teeth feel too long and too loose, feel as if asleep.

Jumping, shooting, as if teeth were being torn out; or slow pricking, throbbing or tearing, extending into jaws and temples; face sore; worse at night, from cold, from vexation, better from external heat; crusty caries.

¹¹ **Tongue, etc.** Taste: putrid mornings and after eating; metallic; food, especially bread, tastes bitter.

Tongue: dry, red, cracked; has a triangular red tip; white, often on one side; yellowish; covered with brown mucus; takes imprint of teeth.

¹² **Mouth.** Mouth dry, with much thirst.

Saliva bloody; runs out of mouth during sleep.

Putrid breath.

Much tough mucus in mouth and throat.

¹³ **Throat.** Sore, feels stiff, after straining the throat.

Tonsil (right) covered with yellow membrane.

Sticking or stinging pain in tonsils, worse when beginning to swallow.

Feeling of swelling, with bruised pain; erysipelatous inflammation; parotids swollen; cellulitis of the neck; drowsiness.

Difficult swallowing of solids, as from contraction.

Œsophagitis. especially after corrosive substances.

¹⁴ **Desires. Aversions.** Hunger, without appetite.

No appetite, or wants only dainties.

Desire for oysters; sweets; beer.

Aversion to spirituous liquors; to meat.

Unquenchable thirst, wants cold drinks; worse at night, from dryness of mouth.

¹⁵ **Eating and Drinking.** After eating: 11, 16, 17, 19, 26, 37. Drinking: 40; ice water: 16, 17; beer: 3, 29, 37; coffee: 29; alcohol: 29.

¹⁶ **Nausea and Vomiting.** Eructations: with nausea; with tingling in stomach, worse when rising from lying.

Nausea: after ice water, or after eating, with sudden vomiting; with inordinate appetite and inclination to vomit; worse at night and after eating.

[17] **Stomach.** Stinging or pulsation in pit of stomach.

Fulness or heaviness, as from a stone, in stomach; after eating.

Pain in stomach and nausea, after ice water.

Pressure in pit of stomach, as if swollen, or as if drawn together.

[19] **Abdomen.** Soreness, as if beaten, in hypochondria and still more in abdomen; worse on the side lain on, when turning and when beginning to move.

Abdomen bloated, especially after eating.

Enteritis or peritonitis, with typhoid symptoms.

Colic, he must walk bent; worse at night; also after getting wet.

Typhlitis.

Sensation as if something was torn off in abdomen.

Visible contractions of abdomen above navel.

[20] **Stool, etc.** Stools: watery, mucous and bloody, with nausea, tearing down the thighs, and much tenesmus; frothy; white; painless and undigested; like the washing of meat; yellowish-brown, bloody, cadaverous-smelling and involuntary at night (typhoid).

Nightly diarrhœa, with violent pain in abdomen, relieved after stool or while lying prone.

Hemorrhoids: sore, blind; protruding after stool, with pressing in rectum, as if everything would come out.

Fissure of anus, with periodical, profuse, bleeding piles.

[21] **Urine.** Tearing in region of kidneys, œdema; after exposure to wet.

Urine: hot, white, muddy; pale, with white sediment; dark, becoming turbid.

Tenesmus vesicæ, discharges a few drops of blood-red urine.

Retention of urine; backache, restless, cannot keep quiet.

Urine passed in a divided stream.

Frequent urging day and night, with increased secretion.

Urine diminished, though he drinks much.

Urine voided slowly, spine affected; from getting wet.

Urine involuntary at night and while at rest.

[22] **Male Sexual Organs.** Erections at night; or with desire to urinate.

Swelling of glands and prepuce, dark, red, erysipelatous.

Scrotum becomes thick and hard, with intolerable itching.

Œdema of scrotum.

Humid eruption on genitals and between scrotum and thigh.

[23] **Female Sexual Organs.** Menses too early, profuse and

protracted; flow light colored, acrid, causing biting pain in vulva.

Amenorrhœa: from getting wet; with milk in breasts.

Metrorrhagia, blood clotted, with labor-like pains.

Bearing down, when standing or walking, back aches, better lying on something hard; prolapsus from over-exertion or straining.

Soreness in vagina hindering an embrace.

External genitals inflamed, erysipelatous.

[24] **Pregnancy.** During pregnancy: discharges of blood; pelvic articulations stiff when beginning to move.

Abortion impending from straining or overexertion.

Lochia vitiated and offensive, lasting too long or often returning.

Milk leg; also metritis, after delivery; with typhoid symptoms.

Mammæ: swell from catching cold, streaks of inflammation; galactorrhœa; milk vanishes, with general heat; milk cakes; discharges clots of milk and pus.

[25] **Larynx.** Hoarse from overstraining the voice.

Hoarseness and roughness in larynx, with roughness and soreness in chest.

Hot air arises from trachea.

Cold sensation in larynx, when breathing.

[26] **Breathing.** Oppression: as if the breath was stopped at tip of stomach; worse after a meal; anxious, as if not able to draw a long breath.

[27] **Cough.** Influenza; air-passages seem stuffed up; dry, hard, tickling cough; worse each evening until 12 P.M.; stiffness in back and limbs.

Cough: dry, teasing; caused by tickling in bronchia; uncovering, even a hand; with tearing pain in the chest, stitches, profuse sweat and pain in stomach; worse evening and before 12 P.M.; or in morning, soon after awaking; from talking, lying, or sitting still.

Sputa: acrid pus; greyish-green cold mucus, of putrid smell; pale, clotted or brown blood.

[28] **Lungs.** Stitches in chest, worse when at rest, and while sneezing and breathing; also when sitting crooked.

Tingling in chest, with tension in intercostal muscles; worse at rest.

Pneumonia: with typhoid symptoms, often from reabsorption of pus; also with tearing cough and restlessness, because quiet makes pain and dyspnœa worse.

Hæmoptysis: from overexertion, blowing wind instruments; blood bright; pain in lower part of chest; renewed from least mental excitement.

[29] **Heart. Pulse.** Uncomplicated hypertrophy, from violent exercise.

Organic diseases of heart, with sticking pains and soreness; numbness and lameness of left arm.

Chest and heart feel weak after a walk; trembling sensation of the heart.

Palpitation violent when sitting still.

Pulse: accelerated, weak, faint and soft; trembling or imperceptible; sometimes quicker than the heart's beat; irregular; affected by beer, coffee or alcohol.

³¹ **Neck. Back.** Stiff neck, with painful tension when moving.

Pains in shoulders and back, with stiffness as from a sprain.

Curvature of the dorsal vertebræ.

Spinal membranes inflamed, even myelitis; from getting wet or sleeping on damp ground.

Pains in small of back, better lying upon something hard.

Lumbago.

³² **Upper Limbs.** Tearing and burning in shoulder, arm lame, worse in cold, wet weather, in bed and at rest.

Axillary glands suppurating.

Hot swelling of hands in evening.

Rhagades on back of hand.

Warts on hands.

Swelling of the fingers.

Hang-nails.

³³ **Lower Limbs.** Coxalgia; involuntary limping; pains felt mostly in knee and worse from overexertion; pain worse at night.

Spasmodic twitching in limbs when stepping out.

Sciatica, right side, dull, aching pain, worse at night, in cold or damp weather; relieved by rubbing, heat and when warmed by exercise; numbness and formication.

Paroxysmal pains in legs from getting wet, especially when warm and sweaty.

Cramps in legs and feet, must walk about.

Ulcers: on legs, discharging profusely; on dropsical legs, discharging serum.

Swollen about ankles after too long sitting; feet swell in evening.

Intolerable itching of legs and feet at night; old rash.

³⁴ **Limbs in General.** Swelling and stiffness of joints from sprains, overlifting, or overstretching.

Phlegmonous erysipelas of limbs.

Rheumatoid pains in limbs: also with numbness and tingling; joints weak or stiff, or red, shining swellings of joints, stitches when touched; worse on beginning to move; after 12 P.M., and in wet, damp weather or places; better from continued motion.

Tearing pains in limbs, during rest.

³⁵ **Position, etc.** Motion: 1, 3, 9, 19, 24, 31, 33, 34, 36, 40.

Must change place: 1, 3, 21, 36. Must turn over: 37.
Turning: 2, 19. Stooping: 2, 7. Rising: 2, 16. Walking: 3, 23, 29. Stepping: 33. Must walk: 33. Must
walk bent: 19. Exertion: 7, 33. Shaking head: 3.
Rest: 21, 28, 34, 36. Lying: 3, 20, 23, 27, 31. Must
lie down: 3. Sitting: 3, 27, 28, 29, 33. Standing: 23.

³⁶ **Nerves.** Paralysis: after unwonted exertion; after parturi-
tion; rheumatic, from getting wet or lying on damp
ground; from sexual excesses; after ague or typhoid;
parts painless; or painfully stiff and lame, with tearing,
tingling and numbness.

Hemiplegia, right-sided; sensation as if "gone to sleep."

Great debility, soreness and stiffness, worse on beginning
to move; better from continuing motion, but soon fatigued, requiring rest again.

Restlessness, must change position.

³⁷ **Sleep.** Spasmodic yawning, yet not sleepy, with stitching
and pain as from dislocation of jaw.

Great sleepiness and lassitude after eating.

Heavy sleep, as from stupor.

Sleeplessness: from pain, more before 12 P.M., must turn
often to find any ease.

When intoxicated by beer, sleeps with mouth open and
head thrown back.

Dreams of great exertion; as rowing, swimming, etc.

³⁸ **Time.** Morning: 3, 5, 11, 27. 10 A.M.: 40. Evening: 1,
27, 32, 33, 40. 7 P.M.: 40. Night: 4, 6, 7, 10, 14, 16, 19,
20, 21, 22, 32, 33, 34. Before 12 P.M.: 27, 37. Day: 21.

³⁹ **Temperature and Weather.** Warmth: 3; of bed: 4. Heat:
10, 33. Cold: 3, 10. Uncovering: 27. Cold, open air:
5, 46. Cold, wet weather: 32, 33, 34. Getting wet or
damp in cold places: 3, 5, 19, 21, 23, 31, 33, 36, 46.

⁴⁰ **Chill. Fever. Sweat.** Constant chilliness, as if cold wa-
ter was poured over him, or as if the blood was running
cold through the veins, 7 P.M., feels cold when he moves.

Before the chill: dry cough; yawning; stretching; maxillary joint feels sprained.

Chills over the back, worse evenings; chill increased by
drinking.

Chill, with pains in limbs, restlessness; pale face, or alternating pale and red face.

Heat after chill, with sweat which relieves.

General heat, as from hot water or hot blood running
through veins.

General warmth with slight chills during motion; face
livid.

During fever, nettle-rash; thirst, drinking little and often.

Drowsy, weary, with yawning, 10 A.M., excessive heat,
without thirst.

Evening fever, with diarrhœa.

Sweat with pains; often with violent trembling.

Sweat: even during heat; except on face; with violent itching of the eruption; sour; musty, putrid; with thirst or thirstlessness.

⁴² **Sides.**   Right: 5, 13, 33, 36, 40. Left: 6, 29. Left to right: 4, 8.

⁴⁴ **Tissues.**   Acts on fibrous tissue.   Cellulitis.   Diseases of joints, stiffness; or when there are stitches in surrounding tendons, with tingling and burning.

Dropsy, with turbid urine.

Glands: swollen and hot, painful; indurated; suppurating.

Pain as if the flesh was torn loose from the bones; or as if the bones were being scraped.

Inflammation and swelling of long bones.

⁴⁵ **Contact, Injuries, etc.**   Touch: 4, 34.   Rubbing: 33. Straining: 23, 24, 25, 28, 34, 36.

⁴⁶ **Skin.**   Intolerable itching of skin; red, measly rash all over.

Itching all over, worse on hairy parts; after scratching, burning.

Urticaria: from getting wet; during rheumatism; with chills and fever; worse in cold air.

Eruption: herpetic; with incessant itching, burning and tingling; alternates with pains in chest and dysenteric stools.

Eczema: surface raw, excoriated; thick crusts, oozing and offensive.   Vesicles upon a red patch or with a spreading, red, erysipelatous base; internal pruritus followed by pains in the thighs after scratching.

Pustulous eruption.

Pemphigus, each bulla with a red areola.

Erysipelas.   Erysipelatous inflammations.   Zona.

Hardness of the skin, with thickening.

Carbuncles, bluish, gangrenous.

Variola, eruption sinks and turns livid; typhoid symptoms.

Scarlatina miliaria; rash dark, fever high; drowsiness and restlessness.

Chilblains.

⁴⁸ **Relationship.**   Complementary to *Bryon.*

Antidotes to *Rhus tox.: Bellad., Bryon., Camphor., Coffea, Crot. tig., Sulphur.*

Rhus antidotes: *Bryon., Ranunc., Rhodod., Tart. emet.*

After *Rhus* are frequently indicated: *Arsen., Bryon., Calc. ostr., Conium, Nux vom., Phosph. ac., Pulsat., Sulphur.*

Rhus tox. is frequently indicated after: *Arnic., Bryon., Calc. ostr., Calc. phosph., Chamom., Laches., Phosph. ac. Sulphur.*

Incompatible with *Apis.*

Rhus venenata is preferable in erythema nodosum; and

Rhus radicans in occipital headache; muscles sore; better moving and from warmth; caused by draught, dampness or by internal causes, as in typhoid.

RUMEX CRISPUS.

Yellow Dock. JOSLIN. *Polygonaceæ.*

[1] **Mind.** Low-spirited: with serious expression of face; with suicidal mood.

Irritable. Disinclined to mental exertion.

[3] **Inner Head.** Headache after waking in morning, preceded by a disagreeable dream.

Dull pains: on right side; in occiput; in forehead.

Darting pain, or sharp piercing in left side of head.

[5] **Eyes.** Pain in eyes, as from dryness; lids inflamed, worse in the evening.

[6] **Ears.** Ringing in the ears.

Itching deep in ears.

[7] **Nose.** Epistaxis, violent sneezing and painful irritation of nostrils.

Nose obstructed; dry sensation, even in posterior nares.

Fluent coryza, with sneezing; worse evening and night.

Yellow mucus, discharged through posterior nares.

[8] **Face.** Heat of face, redness worse evenings; dull headache.

[11] **Tongue, etc.** Bitter taste (morning).

Dry tongue and mouth: tongue feels as if burned.

Tongue coated white, yellowish-brown or reddish-brown.

Sudden change of voice at different times, or at same time on each day; or with the cough.

[13] **Throat.** Excoriated feeling in throat, with secretion of mucus in upper part of throat. אTח

Sensation of a lump in throat, not relieved by hawking or swallowing, it decends on deglutition, but immediately returns.

Aching in pharynx, with collection of tough mucus in fauces.

[15] **Eating and Drinking.** After meals: flatulency; heaviness in stomach or epigastrium; aching in left breast; pressure and distention in stomach.

[16] **Nausea and Vomiting.** Nausea at night, before diarrhœa.

[17] **Stomach.** Shooting from pit of stomach to chest; sharp in left chest; slight nausea; dull aching in forehead.

Aching and shooting in pit of stomach, and above it, on each side of sternum.

Sensation of fulness and pressure in pit of stomach, up into throat.

Tight, suffocative, heavy ache in epigastrium, through to back; clothes seem too tight; weak feeling in epigastrium, all worse when talking; frequently takes long breath.

[18] **Hypochondria.** Pain in hypochondrium from coughing, rapid walking or deep inspiration.

[19] **Abdomen.** Griping near navel, partially relieved by discharge of offensive flatus; flatulent colic soon after a meal.

Pain occurring, or worse during deep inspiration.

Sensation of hardness and fulness in the abdomen, with rumbling.

[20] **Stool, etc.** Stools: painless, offensive, profuse; brown or black, thin or watery; preceded by pain in abdomen; before stool. sudden urging, driving him out of bed in morning.

Morning diarrhœa, with cough from tickling in throat-pit.

Feces hard, tough, brown; costive.

Itching at anus, with discharge of offensive flatus.

Sensation as from pressure of a stick in rectum.

[21] **Urine.** Sudden urging.

Involuntary micturition, with cough.

Copious, colorless urine, in afternoon.

[25] **Larynx.** Tenacious mucus in throat or larynx, constant desire to hawk.

Hoarseness, worse evenings; voice uncertain.

Raw sensation in larynx, when coughing.

[26] **Breathing.** Frequent feeling as if she could not get another breath.

Suffocating feeling even down to epigastrium, as if tough phlegm must work up, with the cough; despair, even to suicidal feeling; prostrate, tearful, after attack.

[27] **Cough.** Hoarse, barking cough; in attacks, every night at 11 P.M., and at 2 and 5 A.M. (children).

Cough, with pain behind mid-sternum.

Dry, incessant, fatiguing cough, caused by tickling in the throat-pit, extending to behind sternum and to stomach. Soreness in larynx and behind sternum; rawness under clavicles; pain in stomach; stitches in left lung. Cough worse from changing rooms, evening after lying down; touching and pressing trachea or throat-pit, from the slightest inhalation of cool air, he covers his head with bedclothes, to make the air warmer.

Hawking, with burning soreness in larynx; later in left bronchus, renewed by strong exhalation and scraping.

[28] **Lungs.** Aching over anterior portion of both lungs.

Burning-sticking or burning-stinging pain in left chest near heart; worse from deep breathing and lying down in bed at night. *θ* Rheumatism.

Burning, shooting pain in right chest.

Sharp pain near left axilla.

Soreness behind stomach when breathing.

²⁹ **Heart. Pulse.** Heart feels as if it suddenly stopped beating, followed by a heavy throbbing through the chest.

Burning in region of heart.

Dull pain in region of heart; stinging; worse when lying down and breathing deeply.

Aching in heart, with throbbing of carotids and through body, shaking the bed; dyspnœa; worse when lying, had to sit up; face red, puffed, worse about eyes, which were red, lustreless.

Pulse accelerated, mostly when going up stairs.

³¹ **Neck. Back.** Pressing-aching in back, at lower border of scapula.

Sore or burning pain near sacro-iliac symphysis.

³² **Upper Limbs.** Pains in shoulder down to elbow, arms feel strained.

Hands cold, when coughing.

³³ **Lower Limbs.** Stitching in back of right hip; limping walk.

Legs ache.

Stitch-like pain in knee-joint, when standing.

Legs covered with small, red pimples.

Feet cold.

Feet sensitive.

Stinging in corns.

³⁵ **Position, etc.** Walking: 18. Ascending stairs: 29. Lying down: 27, 28, 29. Standing: 33. Must sit up: 29.

³⁶ **Nerves.** Great debility; averse to work; indifferent about his surroundings.

³⁷ **Sleep.** Unquiet sleep, dreams of danger and trouble.

Wakes early; with headache.

³⁸ **Time.** Morning: 3, 11, 20. Afternoon: 21. Evening: 5, 7, 8, 25, 27. Night: 7, 16, 27, 28. 11 P.M.: 27. 2 and 5 A.M.: 27.

³⁹ **Temperature and Weather.** Generally worse: from cool change of weather; when riding in cold wind; in cold, damp, raw weather.

Covering head: 27. Uncovering: 46. Cool air: 27, 46. Changing rooms: 27.

⁴⁰ **Chill. Fever. Sweat.** Chilly, worse on back; colic, nausea, stitches near middle of chest.

Sensation of heat, followed by that of cold, without shivering.

Flushes of heat worse on cheeks.

Sweat on waking from a sound sleep.

[42] **Sides.** Right: 3, 28, 33. Left: 3, 15, 17, 27, 28, 29.

[45] **Contact, Injuries, etc.** Touch or pressure: 17, 27.

[46] **Skin.** Itching in various parts, worse on lower limbs, while undressing.

Stinging-itching, or prickling-itching of skin.

Vesicular eruption, itching when uncovered and exposed to cool air.

RUTA GRAVEOLENS.

Rue.   HAHNEMANN.   *Rutaceæ.*

[1] **Mind.** Inclination to quarrel and contradict.

Dissatisfied with himself and others.

Anxious and low-spirited, with mental dejection.

Melancholy disposition toward evening.

[2] **Sensorium.** Vertigo: in the morning when rising; when sitting; when walking in the open air.

[3] **Inner Head.** Headache: as if a nail were driven into head; like a stupefying pressure on whole brain; after excessive use of intoxicating drinks.

Pulsative, pressing pain in forehead.

Stitching, drawing pain from forehead to temples.

Heat in head, with much restlessness.

[4] **Outer Head.** Large, painful swelling on scalp, as if originating in periosteum, sore to touch and preceded by rending pain.

Head externally painful, as if bruised or beaten.

Erysipelas of scalp, arising from wounds.

Humid scabs on head.

Periosteum, from temples to occiput, pains as if bruised.

Corrosive itching on scalp.

[5] **Eyes.** Itching at inner canthus and on lower lid, smarting after rubbing, eye becomes full of water.

Eyes burn, ache, feel strained, sight blurred, from fine sewing; reading too much, or otherwise overtaxing them; worse using them in evening.

Green halo around light in evening.

Spots on the cornea.

Eyes water in open air, not in-doors.

Spasms of lower eyelids, afterward lachrymation.

[6] **Ears.** Scratching pressure in ear, like from a blunt piece of wood.

Pain, as if bruised, in cartilage of ear, and under mastoid process.

7 Nose. Sweat on dorsum of nose.

Bleeding of nose, with pressure at root of nose.

8 Face. Erysipelas and swelling on forehead.

Pain, as if bruised, in periosteum of facial bones.

9 Lower Face. Lips dry and sticky.

12 Mouth. Gums painful, and bleed readily.

13 Throat. Sensation as from a lump in the throat on empty deglutition.

14 Desires. Aversions. Thirst for cold water, in the afternoon.

15 Eating and Drinking. After eating: sudden nausea; pinching in stomach after bread and butter; eructations and itching of skin after meat; replete as soon as he eats.

Intoxicating drinks: 3.

16 Nausea and Vomiting. Hiccough, with depression.

Nausea, sudden, while eating, with vomiting of the food.

17 Stomach. Burning or gnawing in stomach.

Dyspepsia from lifting heavy weights, with eructations and headache; cannot eat meat, it causes eructations and pruritus.

18 Hypochondria. Gnawing, pressing pain in region of liver.

Painful swelling of spleen.

19 Abdomen. Gnawing pain about navel.

Colic in children, from worms.

Colic, with burning or gnawing pain.

20 Stool, etc. Stool: soft, discharged with difficulty, from inactivity of the rectum; ❙rectum protrudes immediately on attempting a passage; lumpy, slimy; or bloody, with much flatus, seemingly only flatus; empty eructations, distended abdomen; feces often escape when bending over.

Frequent, unsuccessful urging, with prolapsus ani.

Constipation, alternating with mucous, frothy stools.

Tearing stitches in rectum, when sitting.

21 Urine. Urging constantly, could hardly retain urine; it forcibly retained, it could not be voided; severe pains.

Urination involuntary at night, and during day when walking.

Pressure on bladder as if continually full; at every step after urination, she feels as if bladder were full and moving up and down.

Frequent pressure to urinate, with scanty, green urine.

Spasmodic stricture of neck of bladder.

23 Female Sexual Organs. Corrosive leucorrhœa after irregular or suppressed menses.

24 Pregnancy. Metrorrhagia as a forerunner of miscarriage.

Prolapsus ani after confinement.

[25] **Larynx.** Sensation in larynx as from a bruise.
[26] **Breathing.** Short breath, with tightness of chest.
[27] **Cough.** With copious expectoration of thick, yellow mucus, with weak feeling in chest after it.
[28] **Lungs.** Gnawing pain in chest.
Phthisis after mechanical injuries of chest.
[29] **Heart. Pulse.** Anxious palpitation.
Pulse unchanged; or, somewhat accelerated only during heat.
[30] **Outer Chest.** On sternum a painful spot; also painful to pressure.
[31] **Neck. Back.** Pain on a spot, the size of palm of hand, below right scapula; worse in evening, after exertion, deep inspiration, or moving right arm; better from pressure.
Pain in back or coccyx, as if bruised.
Weakness in lumbar region; prolapsus recti.
Stitches in small of back when sitting, stooping or walking; better by pressure and when lying down.
[32] **Upper Limbs.** Pain in left elbow-joint, as from a blow; arm weak.
Wrists feel as if sprained, stiff; worse in wet, cold weather.
Ganglion of the wrist.
Hands numb and tingle after exercise.
Flat, smooth warts on inside of hand.
Contraction of fingers.
[33] **Lower Limbs.** Hip-bones feel bruised.
Anterior aspect of thighs feel bruised; painful to touch.
Shooting from back, down outside of left thigh on first moving or rising; hamstrings feel shortened. θ Sciatica.
Hamstrings feel shortened and weak, knees give way going up or down stairs.
Ankles pain after a sprain, or dislocation.
Pain in bones of feet, cannot step heavily thereon.
[34] **Limbs in General.** Rheumatism of right wrist and both feet; instep puffy; sour sweat.
[35] **Position, etc.** Restless and weak, turns and changes place frequently, when lying.
Motion: 33. Exertion: 31, 32. Walking: 2, 21, 31, 36, 40, 46. Ascending and descending: 33. Stooping: 31. Bending over: 20. Rising: 2, 33. Lying down: 31. Sitting: 2, 31. Rest: 44.
[36] **Nerves.** Tottering, as if thighs were weak; limbs pain when walking.
[37] **Sleep.** Much sleepiness during the day, with stretching.
Frequent waking at night.
Confused dreams.

[38] **Time.** Morning: 2, 40. Afternoon: 14, 40.. Evening: 1, 5, 31, Night: 21, 37. Day: 21, 37.

[39] **Temperature and Weather.** Warmth of stove: 40. In bed: 40. In-doors: 5. Open air: 2, 5, 40. Wet, cold weather: 32, 44.

[40] **Chill. Fever. Sweat.** Chill mostly left-sided; worse up and down back; shakes even near warm stove.

Chill with heat of face and violent thirst.

External and internal heat of face, with red cheeks and .cold hands and feet.

Frequent attacks of quick flushes of heat.

Heat, mostly afternoons, with anxiety, restlessness and dyspnœa; but no thirst.

Sweat, cold on face; morning in bed.

General sweat, after walking in open air.

[42] **Sides.** Right: 18, 31, 34. Left: 18, 32, 33, 40. Above downward: 33.

[44] **Tissues.** Bruised feeling all over, as from a fall or blow, worse in limbs and joints.

Bruises and other mechanical injuries of bones and periosteum; sprains; periostitis; erysipelas. Bone-pains with burning and gnawing, worse during rest and damp weather.

Dropsy.

[45] **Contact, Injuries, etc.** Touch: 4, 33. Pressure: 30, 31. Rubbing: 5. Riding: 46. Wounds: 4. Straining: 5, 17, 33, 44. Mechanical injuries: 28, 44.

[46] **Skin.** Itching of skin after eating meat.

Jaundice from liver complaints.

Ulcers and scabs on scalp, with copious discharge.

Skin becomes easily chafed, from walking and riding; also, in children.

Fistulous ulcers in lower legs.

[48] **Relationship.** *Ruta* antidotes *Mercur.*

SABADILLA.

Cebadilla.   STAPF.   *Liliaceæ.*

[1] **Mind.** No response to questions, loss of consciousness, then he jumps up and runs recklessly through the room.

Imagines: himself sick; parts shrunken.

Delirium during intermittents.

Mania; rage, quieted only by washing head in cold water.

Melancholy, from deep-seated abdominal irritation.

Anxious sensation, with qualmishness.

Easily frightened.

Thinking produces headache.

Mental exertion aggravates headache and produces sleep.

After fright, hysteric paroxysms.

2 **Sensorium.** Vertigo: things turn black before eyes, sensation of fainting; as if things were turning, especially when rising from a seat; more sitting than walking; felt stupid.

Dulness in head in influenza.

Beclouded, as after intoxication, without vertigo or pains.

3 **Inner Head.** Pressure in head, worse in forehead and both temples. θ Hay fever.

Stitches in temples.

Headache after a walk; on returning to room, a twisting, screwing pain from right side of head to both temples, and after going to bed, spreading over the whole head; returning daily.

Hemicrania, with tænia.

Headache from much thinking, or too close attention.

4 **Outer Head.** Fine prickling stitches in skin of forehead and scalp, when becoming warm.

Burning, crawling, itching on hairy scalp, better from scratching.

5 **Eyes.** Lachrymation when walking in open air, on looking at light, sneezing, coughing, or yawning.

Pressure on balls when looking up.

Margins of eyelids red.

Blue rings around eyes.

6 **Ears.** Difficulty of hearing.

Severe stitches in left ear.

Jerking pains, with itching in ear.

Itching of ears, with worms.

7 **Nose.** ∎ Spasmodic sneezing; hay fever.

∎ Fluent coryza; influenza; hay fever.

∎ One or other nostril stuffed up, inspiration through nose labored, snoring.

Itching in nose; agreeable titillation in alæ.

8 **Face.** ∎ Face feels hot, as after wine; red face and eyes; hay fever.

Swelling of the face, with spotted eruption.

9 **Lower Face.** Can hardly open mouth from pain in joints and muscles, with sore throat.

Lips hot, burn as if scalded.

Dry lips.

10 **Teeth.** Dull, troublesome pain in carious teeth, with sore throat.

Toothache, pain often extends over side of face; hot things, cold food, drink or air, produce or increase the pain.

Gums swollen; bluish.

[11] **Tongue, etc.** Taste: bitter; sweet; lost.

Tongue: sore, coated thick yellow; white in centre; moist, during fever; feels sore, as if full of blisters.

Cannot protude tongue, with sore throat.

Pain in tongue and down throat, deglutition difficult.

[12] **Mouth.** Cannot bear anything hot in mouth.

Anything cold in mouth, pains, during sore throat.

Mouth dry; throat sore.

Saliva: seemingly hot during pyrosis; copious; nausea, vomiting and vomiturition; sweetish, collects in mouth; jelly-like.

[13] **Throat.** Sensation of a skin hanging loosely in throat, must swallow over it.

Much tough phlegm in throat; must hawk.

Hawks bright red blood from posterior nares.

Stitches in throat, only when swallowing; tonsils swollen and inflamed, nearly suppurating; left to right.

Tonsillitis after coryza; suppuration; right tonsil remains somewhat swollen and indurated.

Dryness of fauces.

Constricted feeling deep in throat, as is œsophagus would be closed, as after swallowing an acid drink.

Continual desire to swallow, deeply cutting pains, whole body writhes.

Cannot swallow saliva on account of pain, must spit it out.

While swallowing and when not swallowing, feeling in throat of a body which he must swallow down.

Can swallow warm food more easily, in sore throat.

ı In an epidemic of sore throat, all cases which commenced on the left and extended to the right side.

[14] **Desires. Aversions.** Disgust: for all food; for meat; for sour things; for coffee.

No relish for food until she takes the first morsel, when she makes a good meal. θ Pregnancy.

Canine appetite, especially for sweets, farinaceous food, alternating with disgust for meat, wine and sour things.

No thirst, with moist tongue.

Desire for hot drinks. θ Angina.

Great thirst. θ Angina.

[16] **Nausea and Vomiting.** Eructations: in intermittents; rancid; sour.

Pyrosis, heat up into throat; copious salivation, saliva seemingly as hot as the body, but it is not.

Nausea: with chilliness; regurgitation, vomiturition in intermittents; and regurgitation of bitter mucus, leaving fatty taste.

Vomiting: of bile; with whooping-cough; of lumbrici; or

frequent nausea and vomiturition, with feeling of foreign
body in œsophagus.

[17] **Stomach.** Coldness in stomach.

Empty feeling in stomach.

Spasm of stomach, with short breath and dry cough.

Troublesome pressing bloatedness of stomach, with loss of
appetite.

Beating in left side of gastric region toward the back.

Burning in œsophagus and stomach, vomiturition, cutting
in abdomen, loose stool; nervous debility, twitchings.

Corroding, burning pain in stomach, when walking.

[18] **Hypochondria.** Stitching pains in hypochondria.

[19] **Abdomen.** Turning and twisting through whole abdomen,
as from a lump.

Spasmodic contraction of abdominal muscles, left side,
with burning pains; he bends over to left side.

Sensation as if a ball of thread was moving and turning
rapidly through abdomen.

Cutting in bowels, as with knives.

Burning, boring, whirling in region of navel.

Bloated abdomen.

Sensation as if abdomen was sunken in.

Rumbling in abdomen, as if empty.

[20] **Stool, etc.** Violent urging to stool, with croaking as from
frogs; sits a long while, then passes immense quantity
of flatulence; this is followed by an enormous evacuation; after that burning in abdomen, stool mixed with
blood.

Diarrhœa: of brown, fermented stool, swimming on the
water; liquid, mixed with blood and slime.

Burning in rectum after stool.

Crawling, itching in anus; ascarides.

Lumbrici; tænia; worm fever.

[21] **Urine.** Urging to urinate, especially in evening.

Urine dark, muddy, like clay water.

Burning in urethra when urinating.

[22] **Male Sexual Organs.** Pollutions, followed by loss of power
in extremities.

Lascivious dreams and emissions, with relaxed penis; afterward painful erections and extraordinary lassitude.

[23] **Female Sexual Organs.** ❙Nymphomania from ascarides.

Cutting pains, as from knives, in ovary.

Menses: too late, with painful bearing down, a few days
previous; decrease, flow by fits and starts and irregularly, sometimes stronger, sometimes weaker.

[24] **Pregnancy.** Gastric ailments. See 17.

[25] **Larynx.** While pressing on larynx, throat feels sore.

Hoarseness.

[26] **Breathing.** Sensation of narrowness in throat.

Shortness of breath, cardialgia, dry cough.

Breathing: heavy; anxious, during heat.

Wheezing in chest.

[27] **Cough.** Dry, from scratching or roughness in throat; especially in children, with lachrymation; during chill; also during apyrexia.

Hoarse cough, with hæmoptoë.

Cough worse: from cold, becoming cold; as soon as he lies down; violent spells recur at same hours, or at new and full moon.

Expectoration of tenacious, yellow mucus, of a repulsive sweet taste; or else of bright red blood, especially when lying down; influenza.

[28] **Lungs.** Pain and oppression in chest during apyrexia.

Stitches in side of chest, especially when inspiring or coughing.

Pleuritis, great paralytic debility.

Complains of coldness, with hot flashes intervening.

θ Pleuritis.

[30] **Outer Chest.** Red spots on chest.

[31] **Neck. Back.** Spine affected; after pollutions, excessive weakness shows itself in legs.

Bruised feeling in small of back and spine; also in sacral region.

[32] **Upper Limbs.** Sweat in axillæ.

Convulsions of arms.

Trembling of arms and hands.

Stitches in muscles of arms.

Red spots and stripes on arms and hands.

When writing, trembling of hand; old people.

Thick, fissured nails.

[33] **Lower Limbs.** Rheumatic pains in hips; severe stitching; worse during rest. better from motion.

Loss of power in legs.

Boring, tearing in thighs.

Stitches in muscles of thighs.

Severe burning and inflammation of tibia.

Feet swell, are painful on walking, feels every pebble.

Heaviness of feet.

Thick, inflamed, crippled toe-nails.

Horizontal fissures between and under toes.

Cold feet.

[34] **Limbs in General.** Paralytic drawing through all limbs.

[35] **Position, etc.** Motion: 33. Writing: 32. Walking: 2, 3, 17, 33; in open air: 5. Rising: 2. Sitting: 2. Lying: 27. In bed: 3. Rest: 33.

[36] **Nerves.** Great debility in intermittents.

Great paralytic weakness, in pleuritis.

Hysteria, after a fright.

Twitchings, convulsive tremblings; or, catalepsy, from worms.

Nervous diseases from worms, and firmly-seated abdominal irritations.

[37] **Sleep.**   Sleepy, can hardly overcome the inclination.

Sleepy before chill.

Many ideas occupy mind, prevent sleep, or make it light; evenings.

Sleep restless, tosses about; interrupted by frightful dreams.

Sleeps during heat.

[38] **Time.**   Morning: 40. Afternoon: 40. Evening: 21, 37, 40.

[39] **Temperature and Weather.**   Warmth: 4.   In room: 3. Cold washing: 1.

[40] **Chill.   Fever.   Sweat.**   Chill afternoon or evening, returning at the same hour; often without subsequent heat.

I Chill predominates; particularly on extremities, with heat of face.

Chills always run from below upward.

I Evening fever, with cold hands and feet and burning face.

Whole body feels hot; during coryza.

I Heat mostly of head and face, often interrupted by shivering, always returning at same hour.

Feverish; he feels sick, anxious, starts easily, trembles, breathes short and hot.

Sweat often during the heat; in morning hours with sleep.

Hot sweat in face, rest of body cold.

[41] **Attacks.**   Complaints return at precisely the same hour.

Worse every fourth day; worms.

[42] **Sides.**   Right: 3, 13.   Left: 6, 17, 19.   Right to left: 3. Left to right: 13.   Below upward: 40.

Most symptoms with the prover go from right to left See 13.

[43] **Sensations.**   Flying stitches over body at different places.

Burning-crawling here and there.

Whirling sensations in various parts.

Like a tape or string around various parts.

[44] **Tissues.**   Boring, cutting in bones.

[45] **Contact, Injuries, etc.**   Scratching: 4.   Pressure: 25.

[46] **Skin.**   Dryness of the skin.

Red spots and stripes, more marked in the cold.

[47] **Stages and States.**   Light hair ; muscles lax.

Children.

Old people.

[48] **Relationship.**   After *Acon.* and *Bryon.* failed in pleuritis, *Sabad.* cured.

Antidote: *Pulsat.*

SABINA.

Savin. STAPF. *Coniferæ.*

[1] **Mind.** Music is intolerable to her.

Much irritability of temper, hysteria.

Hypochondriacal mood.

Great tiredness and laziness, with a feeling of deep-seated inward trouble, which makes him melancholy and sad.

[2] **Sensorium.** Vertigo: especially in morning, fears she will fall; everything turns black before her eyes; suppressed menses; with congestions to, and heat in the head.

[3] **Inner Head.** Headache, especially in temporal eminences, suddenly appearing and slowly disappearing.

Frontal headache, pressing down on to eyes as if they would be pushed out; worse in morning on rising; better in open air.

Transitory tensive pain in forehead, as if skin had grown fast, with tension in eyes.

[6] **Ears.** Buzzing in ears.

[7] **Nose.** Redness of skin around alæ nasi, painful to touch.

[8] **Face.** Flushes of heat in face, chilliness all over, and coldness of hands and feet.

Pale face; eyes lustreless, with blue rings around them.

Pimples on cheeks and forehead.

[10] **Teeth.** Drawing toothache, caused by masticating.

Throbbing toothache, at night, as if the tooth would burst; worse from the heat of bed.

Swelling of gums around broken tooth.

[11] **Tongue, etc.** Bitter taste of food, of milk and coffee.

[12] **Mouth.** Offensive breath.

White saliva, becoming frothy when talking.

Dryness of mouth and œsophagus, without thirst.

[13] **Throat.** Sensation of a lump in throat; when trying to swallow, cannot; can swallow food.

[14] **Desires. Aversions.** Constant desire for acids and roasted coffee.

[16] **Nausea and Vomiting.** Heart-burn and sour eructations, especially when sitting crooked, which position also aggravates the other symptoms.

Paroxysms of nausea and qualmishness when she is in a crowd.

Frequent empty retchings.

Vomiting of bile, of undigested food eaten the day previous.

[17] **Stomach.** Stitches in pit of stomach, extending to back.

Frequent burning in pit of stomach, with drawing, twisting

and gurgling in bowels, bearing down toward sexual
organs.

[19] **Abdomen.** Tympanitis; bloatedness of the abdomen; rumbling in the evening in a warm room.

Labor-like pains in abdomen down to groins.

Soreness of abdominal muscles.

Pressing down toward genitals.

Slight sensation of motion in abdomen, as if something
were alive.

[20] **Stool, etc.** Stools: of blood and mucus; diarrhœic, with
much flatulence; frequent urging, finally a liquid portion is discharged, followed by a hard portion.

Hemorrhoids, with discharge of bright red blood, causing
pain in back, from sacrum to pubis.

[21] **Urine.** Vesical irritability, depending on gouty diathesis.

Diminished discharge of red urine, with strangury.

Frequent violent urging to urinate, with profuse discharge.

Retention of urine; discharge by drops, with burning.

Urine bloody and albuminous.

[22] **Male Sexual Organs.** Sexual desire increased, with violent
continuous erections.

Inflammatory gonorrhœa, with discharge of pus.

Hard swelling on penis.

Sycotic excrescences, with burning soreness.

Painfulness of prepuce, with difficulty in drawing it back.

[23] **Female Sexual Organs.** Almost insatiable desire for an
embrace.

Menses: too profuse, too early; partly fluid, partly clotted
and offensive; flows in paroxysms; with colic and labor-
like pains; with pains from sacrum to pubis.

Metrorrhagia increased by least motion, but often better
from walking.

Metritis, with hemorrhages.

Leucorrhœa: from suppressed menses; recurs every two
weeks; thick, yellow, fetid; with itching of pudenda.

Stitches from below upward, deep in vagina.

Condylomata, with sore, burning pains.

Cysts at the vulva, sensitive, or with tearing pains during
rest.

Chest symptoms relieved by pressing on chest with hand.

[24] **Pregnancy.** Promotes the expulsion of moles.

Tendency to abortion, especially at third month; discharge
of bright red, partly clotted blood, worse from any
motion; pain from sacrum to pubis; pains in the legs.

After-pains, with sensitiveness of the abdomen.

Metritis after parturition.

[26] **Breathing.** Shortness of breath.

[28] **Lungs.** Pressing pains in chest.

²⁹ **Heart. Pulse.** Palpitation at every motion, especially
    when ascending.

Pulse unequal; generally quick, strong and hard.

Violent beating of blood-vessels in whole body.

³² **Upper Limbs.** Arthritic stiffness and swelling of wrist-
    joint, with tearing and stinging, made almost insup-
    portable when the hand hangs down.

³³ **Lower Limbs.** Heaviness of the legs, with painfulness of
    thighs when walking.

Stinging pains in the hip-joins, in morning and when
    breathing.

Sensation of coldness in whole (right) leg.

Ulcers on the tibia, with lardaceous base.

Swelling, redness and stitches in big toe.   θ Gout.

³⁴ **Limbs in General.** Drawing, tearing pains in extremities,
    especially at night.

³⁵ **Position, etc.** Motion: 23, 24, 29. Walking: 23, 33. As-
    cending: 29. Rising: 3. Sitting crooked: 16. Rest:
    23. Lies on left side: 37. Hanging down of hand: 32.

³⁶ **Nerves.** Great lassitude and heaviness.

³⁷ **Sleep.** Sleeplessness and restlessness after midnight, with
    heat and profuse perspiration.

Lies on left side during sleep.

³⁸ **Time.** Morning: 2, 3, 33. Evening; 19, 40. Night: 10,
    34; 40. After midnight: 37. Day: 40.

³⁹ **Temperature and Weather.** Fresh air: 3. Heat of bed:
    10. Warm room: 19, 44.

⁴⁰ **Chill. Fever. Sweat.** Chill in evening with attacks of
    shivering.

Great chilliness during day.

Shivering, with obscuration of sight, followed by sleepi-
    ness.

Burning heat of whole body, with great restlessness.

Flushes of heat in face, rest of body chilly, hands and
    feet cold.

Sweats easily. Sweats every night.

⁴¹ **Attacks.** Every two weeks: 23.

⁴² **Sides.** Right: 33. Below upward: 23. Behind forward:
    23, 24.

⁴⁴ **Tissues.** Drawing pains through long bones.

Red, shining swelling of affected parts.

Arthritic complaints; tearing, stinging in joints after they
    become swollen; worse in heated room; better in cool
    air or cool room. Arthritic nodes.

Chlorosis.

Throbbing in all blood-vessels.

⁴⁵ **Contact, Injuries, etc.** Touch: 7, 23, 24.

⁴⁶ **Skin.** Black pores in skin, especially of face.

Fig-warts, with intolerable itching and burning; exuberant granulations.

[47] **Stages and States.** Chronic ailments of women: arthritic pains, tendency to miscarriage.

[48] **Relationship.** *Sabin.* is useful after *Thuja*, in condylomata. Antidote to *Sabin.: Pulsat.*

SAMBUCUS NIGRA.

Black Elder.   HAHNEMANN.   *Caprifoliaceæ.*

[1] **Mind.** Sees images when shutting eyes.
Delirium without fever.
Anxiety: with vomiting; with sweat.
Very easily frightened; trembling anxiety and restlessness.
Fright followed by suffocative attacks, with bluish, bloated face.

[3] **Inner Head.** Dizziness, with tension in head when moving it, sensation as if it were filled with water.
Sudden jerks through head.
Pressive pain on temporal bones.

[4] **Outer Head.** The head is bent backward.
Erysipelas over whole left side of head, ear much swollen, confined to bed and could not move.
Scurfs on head, with intolerable itching.
Skull feels as if stretched.

[5] **Eyes.** Child could not open eyes, could not bear light, awaking from sleep, with screaming.
Eyes half open in sleep.

[6] **Ears.** Great swelling, heat, redness and lump just under right ear, in neck, accompanied by a very sharp pain.

[7] **Nose.** Breathing through nose impeded, with dry coryza, especially in infants.
Sniffles of children.
Nose seems perfectly dry and completely obstructed.

[8] **Face.** Pale, bluish, or red; pale, collapsed covered with cold sweat; appears much older and yellow; bloated, dark blue; red spotted.
Burning heat and redness of face.
Burning heat of face, with icy-cold feet.
On awaking, face breaks out in a profuse sweat, which gradually extends over body.
Tension and numbness, as from swelling of cheeks.

[10] **Teeth.** Tearing and stinging in teeth, with sensation of swelling in cheek.

[13] **Throat.** Dryness of throat and mouth, with thirstlessness.

[14] **Desires. Aversions.** Thirst, but drink is not palatable.

[15] **Eating and Drinking.** Worse after eating fruit.

[16] **Nausea and Vomiting.** Everything makes him feel sick. Vomiting, first of food, later of bile.

[19] **Abdomen.** Colic pain, with discharge of much flatulence, from taking cold.

Painful pressure in abdomen, with nausea, when leaning against a hard edge.

Great soreness in abdomen.

[20] **Stool, etc.** Stools: frequent, watery; thin, slimy, with much wind, followed by urging; pressure in stomach and navel; abdomen large.

[21] **Urine.** Frequent urging to urinate, with profuse discharge of urine.

[23] **Female Sexual Organs.** Menses too profuse, also menorrhagia.

[24] **Pregnancy.** Mammæ red and swollen.

Milk diminished.

Debilitating sweat after childbirth.

[25] **Larynx.** Voice: hollow; hoarse, with much tough mucus in the larynx.

Patient woke at night, with agonizing fits, spasms of epiglottis, with agony and fear of suffocation; springing up in bed and struggling for breath.

[26] **Breathing.** Anxious, loud; quick, wheezing, crowing.

Oppression of chest, with pressure in stomach, and nausea.

Nightly suffocative attacks, with great restlessness; shedding of tears and throwing about of arms.

Suffocating attacks after midnight.

Child suddenly awakens, nearly suffocated, sits up in bed, turns blue, gasps for breath, which it finally gets; spell passes off; it lies down again, aroused sooner or later in same manner.

[27] **Cough.** Hollow, dry, at night; deep and dry before chill; with regular inhalations, but sighing exhalations; suffocative, hollow, deep, whooping, caused by spasm of chest, expectoration of small quantities of tough mucus, only during day; suffocative, with crying, children; worse about midnight; during rest; lying in bed, or with head low; from dry, cold air.

Sputa: very yellow, as if colored by bile; taste saltish.

[29] **Heart. Pulse.** Orgasm in whole body.

Occasional omission of heart-beat.

Pulse generally very frequent and small; sometimes slow and full, sometimes intermitting.

[30] **Outer Chest.** Pressure under sternum, with a counter pressure from spine toward sternum.

Compression of chest violent, trembling from pain.
31 Neck. Back. Sweat on throat and neck, with children.
32 Upper Limbs. Paralytic heaviness in elbow-joint.
Trembling of hands when writing.
Stitches in wrist.
Dark blue bloatedness of forearms and hands.
Muscles between little finger and next very sore.
33 Lower Limbs. Sharp, deep stitches in tibia.
Œdemtious swelling of feet, extending to legs.
Icy-cold feet: with warmth of body; with hot face.
34 Limbs in General. Hands and feet bloated and blue.
35 Position, etc. Motion: 3, 40. Springing up: 25. Sitting
up: 26. Bending back: 4. Throws arms about: 26.
Rest: 27. Lying: 40; with head low: 27. Leaning:
19. Cannot move: 4.
36 Nerves. Great weakness.
General trembling, with anxiety and ebullitions of blood.
37 Sleep. Sleepiness, without sleep.
Frequent awakening, as in a fright, with anxiety, trembling, dyspnœa, as if he would suffocate.
Slumber, with eyes and mouth half open.
During sleep, dry heat; after awaking, profuse sweat.
38 Time. Morning: 40. Night: 6, 25, 27, 37, 40. About or
after midnight: 26, 27. Day: 27.
39 Temperature and Weather. Dry, cold air: 27. Uncovering: 40.
40 Chill. Fever. Sweat. Chill running over whole body,
with crawling sensation here and there.
Dry heat on falling asleep, after lying down.
Dry heat, without thirst, shuns uncovering.
Hot body, with cold hands and feet during sleep; on
awaking the face breaks out into a profuse sweat, which
extends over the body, and continues more or less during the waking hours; on going to sleep again, the dry
heat returns.
Hectic flush.
Profuse night-sweat.
Profuse weakening sweat, day and night, lasts through the
apyrexia: 24.
42 Sides. Right: 6, 33. Left: 4.
43 Sensations. Feeling of great soreness, as if beaten all over;
headache.
44 Tissues. Œdema, anasarca.
45 Contact, Injuries, etc. After contusions, tension in dark
red swelling.
Pressure: 19. Scratching: 46.
46 Skin. Bloated, dark red swelling.
47 Stages and States. Scrofulous children.

Formerly fat or robust people become emaciated.

After violent emotions, grief, anxiety, or excess in sexual indulgence.

⁴⁸ **Relationship.** Ailments from abuse of *Arsen.*

Sambuc. follows well after *Opium*, in consequences of fright.

Antidotes to *Sambuc.: Arsen., Camphor.*

SANGUINARIA CANADENSIS.

Bloodroot.   G. BUTE.   *Papaveraceæ.*

¹ **Mind.** Confused, relieved by eructations.

Anxiety and feeling of dread. Anxiety precedes vomiting and delirium.

Moroseness, with nausea; cannot bear a person to walk in room.

Angry irritability; moroseness.

² **Sensorium.** Sensation as if paralyzed and unable to move while lying on her back, with full consciousness of her surroundings.

It seems as if events that transpired in dreams were of weeks and months duration.

Vertigo in cold weather.

Sensation as if in railroad car, and every one about her talked rapidly, begs to be held.

Vertigo: with long-continuing nausea, debility and headache; on quickly turning head and looking upward; on lying down at night; on rising from stooping; in cold weather.

³ **Inner Head.** Periodical sick headache; begins in morning, increases during day, lasts until evening; head feels as if it must burst, or as if eyes would be pressed out; or, throbbing, lancinating pains through brain, worse on right side, and especially in forehead and vertex; followed by chills, nausea, vomiting of food or bile; must lie down and remain quiet; relieved by sleep.

Headache begins in occiput, spreads upward and settles over the right eye.

Severe headache, only relieved by pressing back up against something hard.

Headache, rheumatic, running up posterior auricular region.

⁴ **Outer Head.** Soreness in spots, especially temporal regions.

Distention of veins in temples; feel sore when touched.

⁵ **Eyes.** Diminished power of vision.

Dimness of eyes, with sensation as if hairs were in them.
Pupils dilated.

Neuralgia in and over right eye.

Yellowness of sclerotica, with icterus.

Catarrhal ophthalmia, granular lids.

Ophthalmia, followed by ulceration of cornea.

Copious lachrymation: following the burning and dryness; tears hot; with coryza.

⁶ **Ears.** Painful sensitiveness to sudden sounds; right ear worse.

Beating, humming, with congestion of blood.

Burning of the ears, cheeks red.

Earache, with headache, singing in ears, and vertigo.

Beating under ears, at irregular intervals, often only a couple of strokes.

⁷ **Nose.** Loss of smell.

Nasal polypi.

Fluent coryza, with frequent sneezing; worse right side.

Ulcerative ozæna, with epistaxis.

Rose cold and subsequent asthma; sick and faint from odor of flowers.

⁸ **Face.** Distention of veins of face, with excessive redness, a feeling of stiffness, and veins sore to touch.

Circumscribed redness of one or both cheeks.

Red cheek, with burning in ears.

Cheeks (and hands) livid.   θ Typhoid pneumonia.

Paleness of face, with disposition to vomit.

Neuralgia in upper jaw, extending to nose, eye, ear, neck and side of head; shooting, burning pains; must kneel down and hold head tightly to the floor.

⁹ **Lower Face.** Lips feel dry.

Swelling of lips toward evening.

Under lips burns, is swollen, hard and blistered; blisters dry up and form crusts, which drop off.

Stiffness in articulation of jaws.

¹⁰ **Teeth.** Toothache from picking the teeth, or in hollow teeth when touched by the food.

Spongy, bleeding and fungoid condition of gums.

¹¹ **Tongue, etc.** Loss of taste, with a burnt feeling on tongue.

Sweet articles taste bitter, followed by burning in fauces.

White coated tongue, with slimy, fatty taste.

Tip of tongue burns as if scalded.

Tongue sore; pain like a boil.

Red tongue, feels as if in contact with something hot.

¹² **Mouth.** Fetid breath, clammy mouth, sticky teeth.

Sores on gums and roof of mouth.

¹³ **Throat.** Burning, especially after eating sweet things.

Roof of mouth and uvula sore and burning.

53

Ulcerated sore throat.

Throat feels swollen, if to suffocation, with pain when swallowing, and aphonia. Tonsillitis, promotes suppuration.

Heat in throat, better inspiring cold air; throat so dry it seems as if it would crack.

Pearly coating on palate and fauces. θ Diphtheritis.

Burning in pharynx and œsophagus.

¹⁴ **Desires. Aversions.** Craving for he know not what, with loss of appetite; wants piquant articles.

Sugar tastes bitter, and causes burning.

Craves food: 16.

¹⁵ **Eating and Drinking.** Sweet things aggravate, produce burning.

Soon after eating: feels empty; difficult breathing, nausea, water-brash, lassitude almost to fainting, cold sweat until 12 P. M., after a little food.

While eating: 27.

¹⁶ **Nausea and Vomiting.** Eructations; disposition to vomit; pale face.

Nausea intense, in paroxysms: worse when stooping, with flow of saliva; followed by nettle-rash, heart-burn, eructations, with headache and chills, followed by vomiting, and sometimes diarrhœa.

Vomiting: craves food to quiet the nausea; of bitter water; of sour, acrid fluids; of ingesta; of worms; preceded by anxiety; with headache and burning in stomach; head better afterward.

¹⁷ **Stomach.** Soreness and pressure in epigastrium, aggravated by eating.

Burning in stomach, with headache.

Gastritis, with burning, vomiting, headache.

Jerking in stomach, as if from something alive.

Goneness, with sick headache.

Sudden attacks of constriction in pit of stomach, as if suffocating.

¹⁸ **Hypochondria.** Heat streaming from breast toward liver.

Liver torpid; skin yellow; colic.

Violent stitches in splenetic region.

Pains in left hypochondrium, worse when coughing, better from pressure and when lying on left side.

¹⁹ **Abdomen.** Flatulent distention of abdomen in evening, with escape of flatus from vagina (os uteri being dilated).

Indurations in abdomen.

Cutting bellyache from right to left iliac fossa, thence to rectum.

Soreness in abdomen, aggravated by eating.

Colic, with torpor of the liver.

Feeling as from hot water pouring from breast into abdomen, followed by diarrhœa.

[20] **Stool, etc.** Stools thin, fecal; bright yellow; undigested; watery.

Escape of much flatus upward and downward; also, with diarrhœa. It relieves the cough.

Diarrhœa following coryza, pains in chest and cough.

Urging, but no evacuation, with sensation of a mass in lower part of rectum, and discharge of offensive flatus only.

Alternate diarrhœa and constipation.

Hemorrhoids.

[21] **Urine.** Dark, yellow urine, with icterus.

Urine scanty, high-colored, reddish sediment on standing.

Copius and frequent nocturnal urination, clear as water.

[22] **Male Sexual Organs..** Seminal emissions.

Gleet; old cases.

[23] **Female Sexual Organs.** Climacteric disorders, especially flashes of heat and leucorrhœa.

Menses: at right time, offensive smelling, bright red flow; clots, like lumps of flesh; later, blood darker, and less offensive; scanty, headache, from occiput to frontal region, head as if bursting; face red and hot.

Os uteri ulcerated; fetid, corrosive leucorrhœa.

Uterine polypi.

Flatus from uterus: 19.

[24] **Pregnancy.** Threatened abortion, with nausea, pains in loins, extending through hypogastric and iliac regions, and down the thighs.

Mammæ: stitches in both; sore to touch under right nipple, and painful soreness of the nipples.

[25] **Larynx.** Chronic dryness in throat, sensation of swelling in larynx, and expectoration of thick mucus.

Aphonia, with swelling in throat.

Dryness in throat, with soreness, swelling and redness.

[26] **Breathing.** Short, accelerated, constrained breathing; extreme dyspnœa; cheeks and hands livid; compressible pulse. θTyphoid pnuemonia.

Asthma, especially after the "rose cold," worse from odors.

Painful, sighing respiration.

Inclination to take deep inspiration, which increases constriction of chest, and causes tearing pains in chest, worse right side.

[27] **Cough.** Wheezing, whistling cough; metallic sounding; stridulous breathing; croup.

Cough dry, caused by: tickling in throat-pit; ticking in stomach.

Dry cough, awakening him and not ceasing until he sits
up in bed and passes flatus, upward and downward.

Whooping-cough, constricted, spasmodic action across
throat beneath the jaws; cough worse at night, with
diarrhœa.

Hæmoptysis during phthisis pulmonalis.

Sputa: thick mucus; rust-colored; offensive, purulent.

²⁸ Lungs. Sharp piercing midway between sternum and right
nipple.

Pain in right chest to shoulder, can only with difficulty
place hand on top of head.

Stitches on lower part of left breast to shoulder.

Cramps in chest.

Burning in chest, also stitching; he lies on the back;
sputum is tough, rust-colored and difficult; pulse quick
and small; face and limbs cold, or hands and feet burning hot, and cheeks circumscribed red and burning,
worse in afternoon; extreme dyspnœa. θPneumonia.

Breath and sputa smell badly, even to the patient; belches
before and after cough; after cough heat, then gaping;
circumscribed red cheeks; diarrhœa; night-sweats; pains
in legs.

²⁹ Heart. Pulse. Painful stitches or pressing pain in region
of heart.

Palpitation before vomiting, with great weakness.

Irregularity of heart's action and pulse, with coldness,
insensibility, etc.

Weak feeling at the heart.

Pulse: hard, frequent; small and quick; irregular, with
great weakness.

³⁰ Outer Chest. Burning in sternum.

Severe soreness under right nipple, worse from touch.

³¹ Neck. Back. Pain in nape of neck.

Dull pain along inner edge of left scapula, worse from
breathing.

Rheumatic pains in neck, shoulders and arms, worse at
night.

Pain in sacrum, from lifting.

Lumbago, from lifting; or, myalgia of great muscles of
back

Soreness down muscles of back; pains shift about; feels
pain more when drawing long breath.

³² Upper Limbs. Itching in axilla before catamenia.

Rheumatic pain in right arm and shoulder; worse at night;
on turning in bed; cannot raise the arm.

Burning in palms, redness of hands, and severe burning.

Ulceration of the roots of all the nails on both hands.

Panaritium, first right, then left fingers.

33 Lower Limbs. Rheumatic pain in left hip; also, inside of right thigh.

Bruise-like pain in thigh, alternating with burning and pressure in breast.

Pain through hips, extending down right limb.

Wandering pains worse at night.

Knees are stiff.

Left leg and foot swelled in evening, with violent burning pain, did not know where to lay the limb; limb externally cold; worse until 12 P.M.

Sharp pain in right ankle and great toe-joint.

Burning of soles of feet, worse in bed.

Cold feet, afternoon.

34 Limbs in General. Burning of hands and feet, worse at night.

Rheumatic pains, worse in those places least covered with flesh, but not in joints; on touching the painful part, pain vanishes and appears on some other part.

Rheumatism in all joints, with swelling and spasmodic pains.

35 Position, etc. Motion: 40. Walking: 36. Rising: 2. Stooping: 16. Turning quickly: 2; in bed: 32. Indisposed to move: 36. Cannot find rest: 33. Restricted motion of right arm: 28, 32. Must sit up: 27. Must kneel down: 8. Lying down: 2, 27; on side: 17, 18; on back: 2, 17, 28. Must lie down: 3. Looking upward: 2.

36 Nerves. Lameness of right arm.

Paralysis of right side.

Lassitude, torpor, languor; not disposed to move or make any mental exertion, worse damp weather.

Limbs weak while walking in open air.

37 Sleep. Sleepless at night, wakes with fright, as if he would fall.

Dreams: of sailing on sea; of business matters; frightful.

Drowsiness, causing mental and bodily indolence.

38 Time. Morning: 3. Afternoon: 28, 33, 40. Evening: 3, 9, 19, 27, 33, 40. Until 12 P.M: 15. Midnight: 33. Night: 2, 27, 31, 32, 33, 34, 37. Day: 3.

39 Temperature and Weather. In bed: 33, 40. Cold weather: 2. Damp weather: 35. Atmospheric changes: 44. Cold, open air: 13, 36.

40 Chill. Fever. Sweat. Chill, with headache, nausea, pain under scapula on motion; shivering in back, worse evening in bed.

Slight flushes of heat, followed by chills, then face flushed, hands hot, qualmish feeling all over; lassitude.

Heat flying from head to stomach.

Burning heat, rapidly alternating with chill and shivering.

Afternoon fever, with circumscribed red cheeks. Fever
2 to 3 P.M. daily.

Flushes of heat.

Fever and delirium.

Slight chill, violent fever, headache and delirium.

Copious sweat; cold sweat.

Typhus, with the characteristic headache.

41 Attacks. Headache usually recurs every seven days; increases in severity from morning till evening.

42 Sides. Right: 3, 5, 6, 7, 18, 19, 24, 26, 28, 30, 32, 33, 36.
Left: 6, 18, 28, 29, 31, 33. Right to left: 19, 32.
Above downward: 19, 24, 33, 40. Below upward: 28.
Up and down: 20, 27.

43 Sensations. Heat flying from head to stomach.

Sensation as if hot water was poured from breast into
abdomen.

An uncomfortable prickling sensation of warmth spreading over whole body.

Slow, shooting pains, with long-continued thrills.

44 Tissues. Languid circulation, limbs cold, skin pallid, sensitive to atmospheric changes.

Veins distended, feel sore.

Surging of the blood.

Red or grey hepatization of lungs.

Polypi, nasal and uterine.

Carbuncles.

Warts.

Fungous excrescences.

45 Contact, Injuries, etc. Pressure: 3, 8, 18. Touch: 5, 6,
8, 10, 24, 30, 34. Lifting: 31.

46 Skin. Heat and dryness.

Itching and nettle-rash before the nausea.

Old, indolent ulcers, with callous borders and ichorous
discharge; dirty granulations, dry, sharp-cut edges.

Icterus, during prevalent intermittent fever.

Prickling sensation of warmth, spreading over body.

Eruption on face of young women, with menstrual troubles,
especially deficiency.

48 Relationship. After *Bellad.* fails in scarlatina.

As a dynamic remedy for the narcosis of opium.

Sanguin. antidotes: *Rhus rad.*

SARSAPARILLA.

A root from South America.   HAHNEMANN.   *Smilaceæ.*

¹ **Mind.**   Mental depression caused by the pains.

  ı Anxiety, with the pains; also after seminal emissions.

Morose, with inclination to work.

Gloomy, desponding, without known cause; debility.

Irritable, impatient or changeable.

Thinking about the food he has been eating makes him sick.

² **Sensorium.**   Dull, stupid feeling, cannot keep the mind on his study.

Staggers, falls forward, in the open air.

Vertigo while looking steadily, with nausea, mornings.

³ **Inner Head.**   Headache, with nausea and sour vomiting.

Pressure, or pressure with stitches, in left side of forehead.

Pains from occiput darting forward to eyes.

Shooting from right parietal region to temple or face.

Throbbing in top of head, worse from walking; aching in forehead, occiput or temples.

Pressing in vertex, increasing and decreasing slowly.

⁴ **Outer Head.**   Sensitiveness of scalp; falling off of the hair.

Mercurio-syphilitic affections of the head.

⁵ **Eyes.**   White paper looks red in evening.

  ı Obscuration before eyes as from a fog; mist when reading; worse after seminal emissions.

Eyes pain from light of day.

Stitches in eyes.

Internal canthi bluish and bloated; headache from behind forward; abuse of mercury.

Ophthalmia after checked tetter.

Itch-like eruption on eyelids.

⁶ **Ears.**   Words reverberate in ear.

Sound in head when talking as if a bell was striking.

Burning-itching scab on ear-lobe.

⁷ **Nose.**   Stoppage of nose for years.

Scabby eruption on and under the nose.

⁸ **Face.**   Eruption like milk-crust; child cries, is restless.

Itching eruption on forhead, with burning; becoming humid on scratching.

Pimples of various sizes on face.

Heat of face; sweat on forehead, in evening in bed.

⁹ **Lower Face.**   Stiffness and tension in muscles and articulation of jaw.

Herpes on upper lip.

[10] **Teeth.** Sensitiveness of upper front teeth.

Tearing in teeth, from cold air and cold drink.

[11] **Tongue, etc.** Taste of food bitter.

Taste: bitter in the morning; sweetish.

Tongue coated white.

Mercurial aphthæ on tongue and roof of mouth.

[13] **Throat.** Spasmodic contraction of throat, with dyspnœa, must loosen his cravat.

Dryness and roughness of throat in morning.

Ulcers on the soft palate.

[14] **Desires. Aversions.** Want of appetite, the thought of food disgusts him.

Want of thirst.

[15] **Eating and Drinking.** Burning in stomach, especially after eating bread.

After eating: bitter eructations (also during); feels as if he had eaten nothing; diarrhœa.

After eating: 1, 20. After eating bread: 15. Cold drinks: 10.

[16] **Nausea and Vomiting.** Nausea when thinking of food.

[17] **Abdomen.** Rumbling, with sensation of emptiness in the abdomen.

Burning, or cold feeling in abdomen.

External abdomen very sensitive to touch.

[20] **Stool, etc.** Constipation, violent urging to urinate, stool small, with much bearing down.

Stool with much wind, colic and backache; also after any food which disagrees.

Blood with the stool.

[21] **Urine.** Tenderness and distension over region of bladder.

Passes gravel or small calculi; blood with last of urine.

Tenesmus of bladder, with discharge of white acrid pus and mucus.

Urging ineffectual; urging with the constipation.

Painful retention of urine.

Urine: bright and clear, but irritating; often and copious, must rise at night; scanty, slimy, flaky, sandy; copious, passed without sensation.

Sand in urine or on diaper; child screams before and while passing it.

During urination air passes from bladder.

Urine passes in a thin, feeble stream, or in drops without pain.

Severe pain at conclusion of urination.

[22] **Male Sexual Organs.** Seminal emissions, lascivious dreams, with backache, prostration, vertigo.

The least excitement causes an emission, even without sexual feeling. Bloody pollutions.

Spermatic cords swollen, sexual excitement makes them ache and sensitive.

Offensive odor about the genitals.

Herpes on the prepuce.

Gonorrhœa checked by cold, wet weather, or by mercury, followed by rheumatism.

23 Female Sexual Organs.   Menses too late and scanty, preceded by urging to urinate; itching eruption on forehead; flow acrid; soreness inside of thighs.

During menses, griping in pit of stomach, in direction of small of back.

Leucorrhœa on walking; pain at meatus urinarius after urinating.

Nipples withered, small, retracted.

26 Breathing.   Shortness of breath, he must loosen the neckcloth and vest.

Stoppage of breath as if by a spasm, with constriction of throat.

27 Cough.   From a tickling in chest, or with rattling on chest.

28 Lungs.   Stitches from back through to chest with every motion.

29 Heart.   Pulse.   Palpitation of heart without fear; mostly during day.

Ebullition of blood and protruding veins.

Pulse accelerated (in the evening), slow in the morning.

30 Outer Chest.   Breast-bone feels as if bruised.

31 Neck.   Back.   Neck emaciated; marasmus of children.

Cervical glands indurated; abuse of mercury.

Stitches in back from the least motion.

❙Pains from small of back down spermatic cords; after emissions.

Pain down a part of spine, across hips, and down thighs; difficult urination.

32 Upper Limbs.   Stitches in joints of arms, hands and fingers, on motion.

Deep rhagades on fingers, with burning pains.

Finger-tips feel as if ulcerated.

33 Lower Limbs.   Stitches in legs, especially from motion.

Weakness in thighs and knees.

Red spots on calves.

Icy-coldness of feet before going to bed.

Burning in tips of toes, which are sensitive to pressure.

Rheumatic pains at night, in the feet.

34 Limbs in General.   Limbs immovable, as if paralyzed.

Trembling of hands and feet.

Hands and feet peculiarly weary.

Rheumatism, bone-pains, after mercury or checked gonorrhœa; pains worse at night, in damp weather or after taking cold in the water.

35 Position, etc.   Worse from moving the diseased part or from bodily exertion.

Motion: 28, 31, 32, 33. Walking: 3, 23. Must rise: 21
Lies on back: 37.

[36] **Nerves.** Fainting attacks, with difficult stool.
Paralysis, muscles atrophied.

[37] **Sleep.** Sleepiness at night; awakens frequently.
Dreams: lascivious, without erections; of fatal accidents.
Sleeps lying on the back.

[38] **Time.** Morning: 2, 11, 13, 29. Forenoon: 40. Evening:
5, 8, 29, 40. Day: 5, 29. Night: 21, 22, 33, 34, 37.
Day and night: 40.

[39] **Temperature and Weather.** Better in open air, as long
as one does not move about.
Worse in Spring and Summer; eruptions.
Warm room: 46. Heat: 47. In bed: 8. Open air: 2, 46.
Cold air: 10, 46. Cold, wet weather: 22, 34, Getting
wet: 34.

[40] **Chill. Fever. Sweat.** Chilliness predominating (day and
night).
Frequent shuddering, mostly in forenoon, running from
feet upward.
Worse during chilliness; better as he becomes warm.
Heat in evening, with ebullitions and palpitation of heart.
Sweat on forehead, during evening heat.

[41] **Attacks.** Increasing and decreasing slowly: 3.

[42] **Sides.** Right: 3. Behind forward: 3, 5. Above downward:
20, 31. Below upward: 40.

[44] **Tissues.** Scrofulous diseases.
Great emaciation, skin becomes shriveled, or lies in folds.

[45] **Contact, Injuries, etc.** Touch: 19. Pressure: 33; of clothing: 26.

[46] **Skin.** Rash as soon as he goes from warm room into cold air.
Dry, red pimples, only itching when exposed to heat.
Rhagades, deep, burning.
Base of eruption is much inflamed; child cries much, and
is very uneasy; crusts become detached in open air, and
the skin adjoining chapped.
Herpetic ulcers, extending in a circular form; forming no
crusts, red, granulated bases, white borders; skin ap-
pears as after the application of a warm compress; se-
rous, reddish secretions.
Ulcers after abuse of mercury.
Shriveled skin.

[47] **Stages and States.** Dark hair.
Sycosis.

[48] **Relationship.** *Sarsap.* is frequently used after abuse of
mercury.
Sarsap. and *Sepia* follow each other well.
Antidotes to *Sarsap.*: *Bellad.*, *Mercur.*
Vinegar appears, at first. to increase the effect of *Sarsap.*

SECALE CORNUTUM.

Ergot.   *A nosode from the rye, called a parasite.*

No Proving.*

[1] **Mind.** Stupid, half sleepy state.
  Impaired power of thinking.
  Delirium : quiet ; wandering.
  Mania : with inclination to bite ; with inclination to drown
    oneself ; room is a troubled sea into which she desires
    to plunge. She thinks two are sick, one recovers, the
    other dies.
  Uncomfortableness and depression.
  Fear of death.
  Anxiety, sadness, melancholy.
  Great anguish ; wild with anxiety.
  Apathy, indifference.

[2] **Sensorium.** Feeling of lightness of head, most in occiput.
  Giddiness ; unsteady gait.
  Heaviness of head and tingling in legs.
  Unconsciousness, with heavy sleep, preceded by tingling
    in head and limbs.

[3] **Inner Head.** Pulsations in head, with giddiness, so that
    she cannot walk.
  Pain and confusion, most in occiput.
  Congestion in the head and chest.

[4] **Outer Head.** Hair falls out.
  Twisting of head to and fro.

[5] **Eyes.** Photophobia.
  Obscuration of sight.
  Double or triple vision.
  Blue and fiery dots flying before the eyes.
  Pain in eyes, with feeling as if they were spasmodically
    rotated.
  Stitching pain in eyes.
  Cataracta senilis.
  Pupils generally dilated.
  Suppressed secretion of tears.
  Injection of the conjunctiva.
  Eyes sunken, surrounded by a blue margin.

---

* A collection of the monographs of epidemics, supposed to have been
caused in Germany and France, principally by the ergot and other mixtures
which spoil the bread, was made in 1825, by C. Hering, and left the next year,
on his departure for Surinam, with Trinks, who had it completed by some
of his assistants, and published. Later additions are mostly cases of poisoning.

Paralysis of upper eyelids, from coal gas.

Immovable state of eyelids after facial erysipelas.

Eyes looked fixed, wild, glazed.

⁶ **Ears.** Undue sensitiveness of hearing, so that even the slightest sound re-echoed in her head and made her shudder.

Confused hearing.

Singing in ears and difficult hearing.

Humming and roaring in ears, with occasional deafness.

❙Hard hearing, after cholera.

⁷ **Nose.** Sneezing.

Nosebleed: blood dark, runs continuously, with great prostration, small, thread-like pulse, in old people, or drunkards; of young women.

Nose stopped up, yet watery discharge running from it.

⁸ **Face.** Pale; pinched, pale, earthy looking; dark red and swollen; contracted and discolored, with sunken eyes, blue rings around eyes.

Wan, fearful countenance.

Tingling in face.

Muscular twitchings, usually commence in face and then spread all over body, sometimes increasing to dancing and jumping.

Spasmodic distortion of the mouth and lips.

Forehead hot.

⁹ **Lower Face.** Lockjaw.

Lips deathly pale.

¹⁰ **Teeth.** Looseness of the teeth.

Grinding of the teeth.

Bleeding from the gums.

¹¹ **Tongue, etc.** Tongue, thickly coated with yellowish-white; dry, tenacious substance; discolored, brown or blackish; deathly pale.

Slight, but unpleasant warmth on tongue, during day.

Spasm of tongue, projecting it from mouth, forcing it between teeth and rendering speech indistinct.

Feeble, stuttering, indistinct speech, as if the tonge was paralyzed.

¹² **Mouth.** Bloody or yellowish-green foam at the mouth.

Increased secretion of saliva.

Much acid fluid in mouth.

Spitting of blood.

¹³ **Throat.** Dryness of soft palate, throat and œsophagus, with thirst.

Burning in throat, with violent thirst.

Painful tingling in throat and on tongue.

¹⁴ **Desires, Aversions.** Hunger, as from long fasting.

Disgust for food, especially for meat and fatty things.

Thirst, during all stages of fever.

Unquenchable thirst.

Desire for: sour things; lemonade.

16 Nausea and Vomiting. Eructations: with disagreeable taste; sour; tasteless, but with subjective, disagreeable empyreumatic odor.

Nausea; inclination to vomit; painful retchings.

Vomiting of food; of a yellowish-green, frothy mass; first of contents of the stomach, then only mucus; of mucus mixed with lumbrici; of decomposed matter.

Vomiting of large quantities of dark brown slime, bile and shreds; typhoid.

Hæmatemesis, patient lies still; great weakness, but no pain; abdomen soft.

17 Stomach, Anxiety and pressure in pit of stomach, with great sensitiveness to touch.

Severe anxiety and burning at pit of stomach.

Pain in pit of stomach.

Violent pressure in stomach, as from a heavy weight.

Warmth and feeling of repletion.

Burning in stomach.

Painful constriction of epigastrium.

18 Hypochondria. Enlargement of liver.

Acute pain in hepatic region.

Inflammation and gangrene of liver.

Burning in the spleen.

19 Abdomen. Distention of the belly.

Flatulence, with rumbling.

Painful sensitiveness and rumbling, with continued nausea and confusion of head.

Inclination to colic, diarrhœa, and bloatedness of abdomen.

Pain in lower belly, preventing an upright posture, even forcing him to lie doubled up in bed.

Continual bearing down in lower abdomen.

Burning in abdomen.

Cold feeling in abdomen and back.

Strong pulsation in umbilical region.

Lumps and welts in abdomen; in affections of the uterus.

20 Stool, etc. Stools: watery, slimy; offensive, watery; watery, yellowish or greenish, discharged rapidly with great force, or even involuntary; painless, without effort, with great weakness.

Colliquative diarrhœa.

Cholerine, with more retching than vomiting.

ⅠCholera Asiatica, with collapse, face sunken, distorted, particularly the mouth; crawling sensation as from ants.

Paralysis of the rectum.

Bleeding from the bowels.

[21] **Urine.** Unsuccessful urging to urinate.

Retention of urine. Ischuria paralytica.

Urine: pale, watery.; bloody in old people. Enuresis in old age.

Urinary deposit looking like white cheese.

Discharge of thick, black blood from bladder. θ Kidney affections.

[22] **Male Sexual Organs.** After lightness in occiput, violent dragging in spermatic cord, causing sensation as if the testicle was being drawn up to the inguinal ring.

After sexual excess, palpitation of the heart.

[23] **Female Sexual Organs.** Menses: too profuse, and lasting too long; with tearing and cutting colic, cold extremities, cold sweat, great weakness and small pulse; or with violent spasms.

Menstrual blood: thin and black; black, lumpy, or brown fluid, and of disgusting smell.

Uterine hemorrhage, worse from the slightest motion.

Passive hemorrhage of very fetid, or dark blood.

Atonic hemorrhage, during the critical age.

Uterine ulcer, feels as if burnt, discharges putrid, bloody fluid.

Burning pains in greatly distended uterus, which felt hard and was painful to touch.

Leucorrhœa brownish and offensive; like cream; from weakness and venous congestion.

Ulcers on outer genitals discolored and rapidly spreading.

[24] **Pregnancy.** Arrested development of the fœtus.

Threatened abortus: more especially at the third month; with copious flow of black, liquid blood; false labor-pains, with bloody discharge.

After abortus: difficult contraction of uterus; thin, black, foul-smelling discharge.

During pregnancy: frequent and prolonged forcing pain, particularly in thin, ill-conditioned women; cramps in calves.

During labor: prolonged bearing down and forcing pains in the uterus; pains irregular; pains too weak; pains feeble, distant or ceasing; everything seems loose and open, no action; fainting fits; after labor; retained urine.

Strength of uterus weakened by too early or perverted efforts.

Labor ceases, and twitchings or convulsions begin.

Puerperal convulsions, with opisthotonos.

Retained placenta, with constant strong bearing down in abdomen; or with relaxed feeling of parts.

After-pains: too long and too painful.

Lochia: dark, very offensive; scanty or profuse; painless or accompanied by prolonged bearing down pain.

Suppression of lochia followed by uterine inflammation.

Lack of milk, with much stinging in mammæ.

[25] **Larynx.** Voice: hollow, with difficult breathing; feeble and inaudible.

Thickening of the mucous membrane of the air-passages.

[26] **Breathing.** Respiration: slow; labored and anxious: oppressed.

[27] **Cough.** Hard, hoarse cough, with little expectoration.

Concussive cough.

Spitting of blood, with or without cough.

[28] **Lungs.** Cramp in the chest.

Spasmodic shocks, from right half of chest into right arm and right leg.

Pains over nearly all the front of chest, worse from coughing and motion.

[29] **Heart. Pulse.** Palpitation, oftener at night, with congestion and frequently intermitting pulse.

Pulse: often unchanged even during violent attacks; generally slow and contracted, at times intermittent or suppressed; somewhat accelerated during the heat; small; empty, weak; thread-like in hemorrhages.

[31] **Neck. Back.** Tenderness of lower cervical and upper dorsal spinous processes, with stiffness of the neck.

Gentle creeping sensation in back, as if a soft air was blowing through it.

Tingling in back, extending to fingers and toes.

Pains at sacrum, with bearing down, as if parts would be forced out, worse when moving. •

"Kink" in the back.

Spine disease, with gressus vaccinus.

Pressure upon affected portion, causes pain there as well as through chest; exciting an irritation to cough; aggravation from every exertion, or strain upon the spine.

[32] **Upper Limbs.** Spasmodic jerks of the hand, with flexion of hand at wrist, or of forearm.

Numbness and insensibility of hands.

Burning in hands.

Hands deathly pale.

Coldness and numbness of right hand, with tingling of the ring and little fingers.

Loss of feeling in back of fingers.

Loss of muscular power and of feeling in hand.

Fingers convulsively drawn in toward palm, clasping thumb.

Rough rash all over the arm.

Fingers bent backward, or spasmodically abducted.

Painful swellings of fingers.

Violent pains in finger-tips.

Gangrene of fingers.

³³ **Lower Limbs.** Hammering, tearing pain in both thighs, increased by motion.

Legs heavy and tired.

Tingling in legs.

Creeping feeling in anterior femoral and posterior tibial regions.

Shuffling gait, as if the feet were dragged along.

Rheumatic pains of joints.

Cramp in calves.

Burning in feet.

Swelling of feet, with black spots.

Toes drawn up toward dorsum of foot.

Tingling in toes.

Gangrene of toes.

³⁴ **Limbs in General.** Lassitude, heaviness, trembling of limbs.

Limbs cold, covered with cold sweat.

Formication; prickling; tingling; numbness in limbs.

Cramps in hands and toes.

Painful jerkings in limbs at night.

Paraplegia.

³⁵ **Position, etc.** Motion: 28, 31, 33. Walking: 3. Exertion: 31. Stretching the limb out: 34. Lies still: 16. Lies doubled up: 19.

³⁶ **Nerves.** Spasmodic twitchings.

Irregular movements of whole body.

Spasms, with the fingers spread out.

Convulsive jerks and starts in the paralyzed limbs.

Painful contractions in the flexor muscles.

Tetanic spasms, with full consciousness, followed by great exhaustion.

Sudden and great exhaustion.

Loss of power of voluntary motion. Feels as if walking upon velvet; paralysis from disease or lower part of spine, sensory, then motor.

Sinking spells at 3 A. M.

³⁷ **Sleep.** Frequent yawning.

Inclination to sleep; drowsiness.

Sleep at night disturbed by frightful dreams.

Great sleepiness; deep, heavy sleep, stupor.

Restless and sleepless; from formication which worries.

³⁸ **Time.** During the day: 11. Night: 29, 34, 37. 3 A. M.: 36:

³⁹ **Temperature and Weather.** Aversion to heat or to being covered.

May feel cold, but does not wish to be covered.

Desire for fresh air.

Cold better: 44. Heat worse: 44.

⁴⁰ **Chill. Fever. Sweat.** Disagreeable sensation in back, abdomen and limbs.

Skin cold, with shivering.

Violent chill of but short duration; followed soon after by internal burning heat, with great thirst.

Burning fever, interrupted by shaking chills.

Cold limbs, cold sweats, great weakness.

Cold stage preceded by vomiting, succeeded by moderate sweating.

Severe and long-lasting dry heat, with great restlessness and violent thirst.

Sweat, especially on upper body.

Cold, clammy sweat over the whole body.

Profuse sweats. Colliquative sweats.

[42] **Sides.** Right: 28, 32, 33.

[43] **Sensations.** Formication under the skin.

Burning in all parts of body, as if sparks were falling on them.

[44] **Tissues.** Dissolution of blood corpuscles, blood thin; passive hemorrhages.

Neuralgia caused by pressure on branch of a nerve by a distended vein.

Thrombosis of abdominal vessels.

Tumefaction of glands. I Lymphatic tumors.

I Collapse from choleroid diseases.

Rapid emaciation of paralyzed parts.

Ulcers, worse from external warmth.

Gangrene: from anæmia; external injuries, application of leeches or mustard; better from cold, worse from heat; dry, of old people.

[45] **Contact, Injuries, etc.** Touch: 17, 23. Pressure: 31, 44.

The slightest wound causes bleeding for weeks.

Straining: 31.

[46] **Skin.** Cold and dry; dingy, wrinkled, dry and insensible; desquamation.

Petechia and miliary eruptions.

Variola, pustules of abnormal appearance, either fill with a bloody serum, or dry up too soon.

Varicose ulcers aud enlarged veins in old people.

[47] **Stages and States.** Irritable, plethoric subjects.

Nervous temperament.

Women of very lax muscular fibre.

Feeble, cachectic women; thin, scrawny.

Very old, decrepit persons.

[48] **Relationship.** Resembles in cholera morbus, *Colchic.*

Cinchon. follows well after *Secale.*

Similar to *Arsen.*, but cold and heat act opposite.

Cinnam. increases labor-pains, checks profuse hemorrhage, and is used instead of Ergot.

54

SELENIUM.

HERING. *The Element.*

[1] **Mind.** Great dulness, with complete insensibility and indifference to his surroundings.

Very forgetful, especially in business; during slumber, however, he remembers all that he had forgotten.

A kind of stammering; he uses the syllables of words in wrong connections; therefore pronounces some words incorrectly.

Difficult comprehension.

Total unfitness for any kind of work.

Great talkativeness when excited.

Mental labor fatigues him much.

[2] **Sensorium.** Vertigo: on lifting head or rising up; on moving about, with nausea, vomiting, faintness; worse after breakfast and dinner.

[3] **Inner Head.** Headache from lemonade, tea or wine; every afternoon.

Violent stinging over left eye, when walking in sun, or from strong odors; with increased secretion of urine, and melancholy.

[4] **Outer Head.** Hair falls off when combing; also of eyebrows, whiskers and genitals; tingling-itching on scalp in evening, oozing after scratching; tension and sensation of contraction of scalp.

[5] **Eyes.** Itching vesicles on edges of eyelids and on eyebrows.

Spasmodic twitching of left eyeball.

[6] **Ears.** Ear stopped.

More ear-wax, hardening in his deaf ear.

[7] **Nose.** Itching in nose and on borders of wings.

Inclination to bore fingers into nose.

Yellow, thick, jelly-like mucus in nose.

Discharge of dark blood from nose.

Phlegm in choanæ.

Coryza, ending in diarrhœa.

Complete obstruction of the nose, chronic.

[8] **Face.** Greasy, shining skin of face.

Twitching of muscles of face.

‖ Comedones.

Great emaciation of face and hands.

[10] **Teeth.** Picks teeth until they bleed; toothache.

Teeth covered with mucus.

[14] **Desires. Aversions.** Want of appetite in morning, with white-coated tongue.

Aversion to food much salted.

Great longing for ardent spirits.

Hungry during the night.

[15] **Eating and Drinking.** After eating; violent beating all over body, worse in abdomen; must lie down.

Salt food agravates.

After eating: 2. From lemonade, tea, wine: 3.

[18] **Hypochondria,** Searching pain in region of liver, worse in taking a long breath, with sensitiveness to external pressure; followed by a red, itching rash in region of liver.

Stitches in spleen when walking.

[20] **Stool, etc.** Stool: hard and so impacted that it requires mechanical aid; mucus or blood passes with last portion; contains threads of fecal matter like hair.

Papescent stool, with tenesmus and feeling in anus as after a hard stool.

[21] **Urine.** Dark, scanty; red in the evening.

Sediment coarse, red, sandy.

Involuntary urination when walking; drips after stool or micturition.

[22] **Male Sexual Organs.** Erections slow, insufficient; semen emitted too rapidly and with long-continued thrill; weak, ill-humored after an embrace, weakness in loins.

Semen thin, without normal odor.

Lewd thoughts, but physically impotent.

Prostatic juice oozes while sitting, during sleep, when walking, and at stool.

Itching on the Scrotum.

[23] **Female Sexual Organs.** Catamenia copious and dark.

[24] **Pregnancy.** During pregnancy throbbing in abdomen.

[25] **Larynx,** Voice husky when beginning to sing, or from talking long; hawks transparent lumps every morning, sometimes bloody.

[26] **Breathing.** Frequent deep breathing with moaning.

[27] **Cough.** In morning, straining chest, with expectoration of mucus and blood.

[31] **Neck. Back.** Neck stiff on turning head.

Pain as from lameness in small of back, in morning.

[32] **Upper Limbs.** Tearing in hands at night, with cracking in wrists.

Emaciation of hands.

Itching in palms; vesicles on and between fingers.

Dry, scaly eruptions, itching palms; syphilitic eruptions.

[33] **Lower Limbs.** Cracking of the knee-joint on bending it.

Flat ulcers on the lower legs.

Emaciation of the legs.

Itching around the ankle, in the evening; blisters on toes.

Cramps in calves and soles.

Legs feel weak, with fear of paralysis after typhus.

[35] **Position, etc.** Motion: 2. Walking: 3, 18, 21, 22. Least exertion: 40. Bending: 33. Rising: 2. Lifting head: 2. Turning head: 31. Must lie down: 36.

[36] **Nerves.** Irresistible desire to lie down and sleep; strength suddenly leaves him.

[37] **Sleep.** Sleepless before 12 P.M.: light sleep, least noise awakens him. Starts on falling asleep.

Dreams of quarrels and cruelties.

Hungry in the night.

Awakens early and always at same hour.

Worse after a siesta on hot days. Pains worse after sleep.

[38] **Time.** Morning: 14, 25, 27, 31. Afternoon: 3. Evening: 4, 21, 33, 37. Night: 14, 32, 33, 37.

[39] **Temperature and Weather.** Every draft (even if warm) causes pain in limbs, head, etc.

Sun: 3. Hot weather: 37.

[40] **Chill. Fever. Sweat.** Chill alternating with heat.

External heat, burning in skin and only in single spots.

Sweat: profuse on chest, arm-pits and genitals; from least exertion; as soon as he sleeps; stains yellow, or white and stiffens the linen.

[41] **Attacks.** Same hour: 37.

[42] **Sides.** Right: 18, 42. Left: 3, 18.

[44] **Tissues.** Great emaciation, especially of face, thighs and hands.

[45] **Contact, Injuries, etc.** Pressure: 18. Scratching: 4, 46.

[46] **Skin.** Red rash in region of liver.

Frequent tingling on small spots of the skin, with great irritation to scratch; spots remain humid.

Itch checked by mercury or sulphur.

Flat ulcers.

[47] **Stages and States.** Blondes

[48] **Relationship.** Antidotes to *Selen.: Ignat., Pulsat.*

Incompatible: *Cinchon.,* wine.

SENEGA.

Seneca Snake-root. *Polygallaceæ.*

[1] **Mind.** Cheerful, but irritable, easily becomes vehement when excited. Phlegmatic.

Anxiety with accelerated breathing.

[2] **Sensorium.** Confused feeling in the head.

Dulness, with pressure and weakness of the eyes.

Slight vertigo before the eyes.

³ Inner Head. Head feels heavy.

Sort of aching in forehead, sinciput and occiput; comes
every day, is felt when sitting in a warm room and is
accompanied by pressure in eyes, that does not bear
touch, though headache is not worse from pressure; bet-
. ter from exercise in open air.

Pressing pain in forehead and orbits after dinner, especially
in left side of head; relieved in the open air.

⁵ Eyes. Aching over the orbits, eyes tremble and water when
he looks at an object intently or steadily; eyes weak and
watery when reading.

Weakness of sight and flickering, must wipe the eyes
when reading, but they are aggravated thereby.

Evenings, on walking towards setting sun, seems to see
another sun beneath the first; on turning eyes outward
it appeared like a compressed oval, and disappeared
when head was bent backwards and when eyes were
closed.

Promotes absorption of lens fragments after operation for
cataract.

Paresis of the left oculo-motor nerve, with paralysis of the
superior rectus muscle; patient could see clearly only
by bending head backwards, which relieved double
vision.

Drawing and pressure in the eyeballs, with diminution of
visual power.

Eyes pain as if pressed out, or as if balls were being expanded, especially in the evening and in candle-light.

Hypopion in scrofulous patients.

Cilia hang full of hard mucus; smarting of the conjunctiva,
as if soap was in the eyes; mornings; blepharitis; sometimes lids stick so after sleep, they must be soaked before they can be separated.

⁷ Nose. Troublesome dryness of the Schneiderian membrane.

Smell before the nose as of a malignant ulcer.

Sneezes so often and so violently head grows dizzy and
heavy; followed by thin coryza.

¹¹ Tongue, etc. Coated white, yellowish-white, or slimy in
the morning, with slimy, unpleasant taste.

Taste: bad, with rumbling in stomach; metallic; like
urine.

¹³ Throat. Mouth and throat dry; tenacious mucus difficult
to hawk up; scraping and roughness; constriction in the
fauces; hawking.

¹⁶ Nausea and Vomiting. Eructations, which relieve the
mucus and hawking.

Nausea with vomiturition; burning in the stomach.

[17] **Stomach.** Pressure below the pit of the stomach; sense of gnawing hunger.

Digging pain in the epigastrium, disposition to flatulence and to outbursts of ill-humor.

[20] **Stool, etc.** Purging, vomiting and anxiety; watery stools, spurting from the anus.

Stools scanty, hard, or dry and large, insufficient.

[21] **Urine.** Urine diminished, dark colored, foams when shaken.

Urine acrid, increased in amount.

Urging and scalding before and after micturition; mucous shreds in the urine; on cooling becomes thick and cloudy, or deposits a thick sediment, yellowish-red, with upper stratum yellow and flocculent.

[25] **Larynx.** ❙Tenacious mucus causing hawking or coughing; often an irritating, shaking cough, as in old cases of bronchitis.

Sudden hoarseness when reading aloud.

❙Hoarse; throat so dry it hurts when he talks.

[26] **Breathing.** Short breathing and oppression of the chest on going up stairs.

Dyspnœa as from stagnation in the lungs; also on awaking and during chill. See 37, 40, etc.

[27] **Cough.** Dry, with oppression of chest and roughness in throat; short, hacking, from mucus or from irritation in larynx, worse in the open air ❙❙and from walking fast.

❙Cough often ends in a sneeze (often in common colds).

Shaking cough like whooping-cough from burning and tickling in the larynx in the morning, with copious, tough, white, mucous sputum (like white of egg).

❙Soreness of the chest, dry cough, throat dry, hoarseness; later much mucus in bronchi and trachea.

Cough worse evenings, at night, during rest, sitting, lying on (left) side, and in a warm room.

[28] **Lungs.** Orgasm of blood; oppression with flushes of heat; oppression especially during rest; tightness.

Certain movements cause pain, as if chest was too tight; disposed to expand the chest, this leaves soreness.

Shooting stitches in the chest, worse during inspiration, during rest.

Dull stitches and burning pain in left chest when lying on the right side.

❙Walls of chest sensitive or painful when touched, or when he sneezes (often as a remnant of colds on the chest).

Burning sore pain under the sternum, especially during motion and on deep inspiration.

Stepping hard, walking fast or running, causes pulling sore pain, as if through mediastinum.

Accumulation of much mucus in larynx, trachea and chest.

Is said to be useful for hydrothorax after inflammations in chest.

²⁹ **Heart. Pulse.** Violent boring pain in region of heart.

Heart's beat shakes the whole body; violent palpitation while walking.

³¹ **Neck. Back.** Pressing pain between the scapulæ especially when stepping hard, or on other movements which concuss the chest.

Pulse rather hard and accelerated.

³⁵ **Position, etc.** Many symptoms worse during rest. But see 27, 28.

Exercise: 3. Motion: 28. Bending head back: 5. Going up stairs: 26. Walking, walking fast: 5, 27, 28, 30. Sitting: 3, 27. Lying on side: 27, 28.

³⁶ **Nerves.** Debility, with stretching of the limbs, confusion, heaviness and beating in the head.

Legs feel weak; joints feel lame.

Weakness seems to originate in the chest.

Lassitude and slight trembling of upper limbs.

Faintness, walking in open air.

³⁷ **Sleep.** As soon as he lies down evenings, heavy sleep.

Restless sleep, full of dreams; awakens often from dull stitches and tightness in chest.

³⁸ **Time.** Day: 3. Evening: 5, 27. Night: 27. Morning: 5, 11, 27.

³⁹ **Temperature and Weather.** Warm room: 3, 27. Open air: 3, 27, 36, 40.

⁴⁰ **Chill. Fever. Sweat.** Chilliness, weakness of feet; chill in open air; dyspnœa.

Shuddering over back, heat in face, weak, burning eyes, beating headache, difficult breathing, body feels bruised.

Flushes of heat: see 28. Skin hot. Skin becomes warmer and moister.

⁴⁴ **Tissues,** ❙ Diseases of mucous membranes; especially of the lining of larynx, trachea and bronchi.

❙ ❙ Catarrhs that tend to leave sore and tender places in the walls of the chest, as though there were left circumscribed spots of inflammation.

⁴⁵ **Contact, Injuries, etc.** Touch: 3, 28, 46. Stepping hard: 28, 31. Wiping eyes: 5.

⁴⁶ **Skin.** Burning veisicles, itching when touched.

Bites of poisonous, enraged animals.

⁴⁷ **Stages and States.** Best suited for the phlegmatic, also for fat children predisposed to catarrh; or to the sluggish, who react from colds imperfectly.

⁴⁸ **Relationship.** Compare: *Sapon., Calc. carb., Caustic., Baryt.*

(in fat children); *Aspar*, (bronchial and cystic catarrh, both drugs have difficult detachment of mucus, turbid urine with burning, etc. *Senega*, more a shaking cough; *Aspar.*, one that causes gagging; latter has, too, more weakness of heart, and more tendency to gravel and gout in old people); *Bryon.*, *Scilla*, *Hepar*, *Cubebs*, *Co-paiba* (last two in frothy urine with mucous shreds).

SEPIA.

Ink of Cuttlefish.   HAHNEMANN.   *Mollusks.*

¹ **Mind.** Weak memory.
Heavy flow of ideas.   Inability for mental activity.
Fits of involuntary weeping and laughter.
Aversion to one's occupation.
Sadness about one's health and her domestic affairs.
Dread of being alone.
Anxiety: with fear, flushes of heat over the face; about real or imaginary evils.
Antagonistic states; imagines what he does not want to; uses wrong words knowing them to be so, etc.
Great indifference even to one's family, to those one loves best.
Is easily offended and inclined to be vehement.
Great irritability alternating with indifference.
Greedy, miserly.
Great excitability in company.   Restless, fidgety.
After overexertion of the mind, as with bookkeepers, etc.
² **Sensorium.** Stupefaction of the head.
Momentary attacks of giddiness when walking in open air or while writing.
Congestion of blood to the head.   Heaviness of the head.
³ **Inner Head.** Paroxysms of hemicrania; stinging pain from within outward, in one (mostly left) side of head or forehead with nausea, vomiting and contraction of pupils; worse in-doors and when walking fast; better in open air, and when lying on painful side.
Boring headache from within outward, forenoon till evening, feels as if he would die; worse from motion and stooping; relieved by rest, when closing eyes, from external pressure, and sleep when enough has been had.
Shooting pains in-out, especially over left eye, extorting cries, with vomiturition.
Pressing or bursting headache as if eyes would fall out, or

head burst, worse from stooping, motion, coughing or
shaking the head; continued hard motion relieves
headache.

Pulsating headache in cerebellum, beginning in morning,
lasting till noon, or sometimes till evening; aggravated
from least motion, when turning eyes, when lying on
back; better when lying on side, when closing eyes,
when at rest and in dark room.

Beating: in head; in occiput.

Headache, with aversion to all food.

⁴ **Outer Head.** Involuntary jerking of head backward and
forward, especially forenoons and when sitting.

Fontanelles remain open, with jerking of head, pale,
bloated face, stomacace, green, diarrhœic stools.

Sensation of coldness on vertex, worse when moving head
and stooping; better when at rest and in open air.

Disposition to take cold from dry, cold wind, or getting
head wet.

Sweat on head smelling sour, with faintish weakness in
evening before sleep or in morning.

Violent itching, like from insects, on occiput or behind ears.

Eruption on vertex and back part of head, dry, offensive
stinging, itching and tingling, with cracks; feeling sore
when scratching.

Sensitiveness of roots of hair, worse in evening, to contact,
to cold North wind, when lying on painless side, burning after scratching.

Falling off of the hair.

⁵ **Eyes.** Dulness of sight; also when writing; sees only one-
half of the object clearly, the other half is obscured.

Many black spots before eyes. Green halo around candle-
light.

Great sensitiveness of eyes to light of day.

Prickling in eyes, evenings from candle-light.

Yellow color of whites of eyes.

Lachrymation, morning and evening.

Burning in eyes in morning.

Inflammation of eyes, with redness of white, stitching and
pressure in eyes.

Follicular conjunctivitis, worse in summer; eyelids will
close.

Redness of eyelids, with styes on them.

Nightly agglutination of eyes, or dry scurf on the eyelids
on waking.   •

Pustules on cornea, also fungus hæmatodes.

Acne-like pustules on edges of lids; the latter feel tight.

Painful heaviness of upper lids on awaking.

⁶ **Ears.** Oversensitiveness to noise, particularly music.

Humming in ears, followed by loss of hearing.
Stitching in ears.
Discharge of thin matter from ear.
Much itching in affected ear.
Tetters on lobe of ear, behind ears and in nape of neck.
Stitches in parotid glands which swell, with tensive pain
on turning the head.

⁷ **Nose.** Great sensitiveness to odors.
Loss of smell, or fetid smell before the nose.
Epistaxis, also during pregnancy and with hemorrhoids.
Fluent coryza, sneezing, early morning. Dry, worse left
nostril.
Swollen, inflamed nose; nostrils sore, ulcerated and scabby.
Blowing of large lumps of yellow-green mucus or yellow-
green crusts with blood, from the nose.
Painful eruption on tip of nose.

⁸ **Face.** Small red pimples on forehead; rough forehead.
Face: pale; yellow.
Yellow saddle across nose; yellow spots on face; yellow
around mouth.
Tetters around mouth, with itching of face.
Swelling of under lip, soreness, burning pain and a pricking as of a splinter in lip; or, ulcers covered with large
thick scurfs; corrosive ichor oozes from under the scabs;
epithelioma.
Inflammation and swelling of one side of face, from the
root of a decayed tooth.
Intermittent prosopalgia, with congestion of eyes and head,
jerking pains, like electric shocks upwards.

⁹ **Lower Face.** Swelling of submaxillary glands.

¹⁰ **Teeth.** Toothache: drawing in upper molars; in a hollow
tooth, extending to ear; throbbing; stitching.
Early decay of the teeth. Teeth feel dull.
Swelling of gums, dark red, painful, bleeding from slightest
touch. Gums painful, as if burned.

¹¹ **Tongue, etc.** Taste: bitter; saltish; putrid or offensive.
Food tastes too salt.
Tongue painful, as if sore or scalded; vesicles; white-
coated.

¹² **Mouth.** Offensive smell from the mouth.
Profuse flow of salt saliva; yet throat is very dry.

¹³ **Throat.** Pain in throat, as if raw, when swallowing; also
stitching and scraping from empty deglutition.
Inflammation of throat, worse on left side. Sensation of
a plug.
Much mucus in throat. Hawking of mucus in morning.

¹⁴ **Desires. Aversions.** Canine hunger; or, no appetite, nothing tastes good.

Aversion to food, particularly meat.

Desire for vinegar; also, for wine.

Thirstlessness; or, much thirst in the morning.

¹⁵ **Eating and Drinking,** During and immediately after eating the pains are renewed or aggravated.

After eating: eructations; empty or bitter tasting; hiccough.

After drinking milk: 20. From acids: 28.

¹⁶ **Nausea and Vomiting.** Eructations: frequent with efforts to vomit; bitter; sour; taste like rotten eggs.

Heart-burn, extending from stomach to throat.

Nausea: after eating, also in morning fasting; from smell of food; when riding in a carriage.

Vomiting: of bile and food in morning of milky fluid; during pregnancy.

¹⁷ **Stomach.** Sensitiveness of pit of stomach to touch.

Painful sensation of emptiness in stomach and abdomen.

Pressure in stomach, as from a stone; after eating.

Pain in stomach after the simplest kind of food.

Cramp in stomach.

Stitches, or, burning in stomach. Beating in pit of the stomach.

Twisting in stomach and rising in throat, tongue becomes stiff, speechless, afterward the body may become rigid.

Hardness in pyloric region.

¹⁸ **Hypochondria.** Stitches: in region of liver; also, when riding; in left hypochondrium; better lying on painful side.

¹⁹ **Abdomen.** Colic: with great distention and sensitiveness of abdomen; recurring toward evening.

Rumbling in abdomen, especially after eating.

Abdomen puffed up. Pot-belliedness of mothers.

Brown spots on abdomen.

²⁰ **Stool, etc.** Diarrhœa: jelly-like stools, with colic and tenesmus; of green mucus; sour-smelling; debilitating; worse after drinking milk, especially if boiled.

Unsuccessful urging to stool, only wind and mucus passed; sensation of lump in rectum.

Stool insufficient, retarded, like sheep-dung.

Pain in rectum during and long after stool; hard, knotty, insufficient stool, mixed or covered with mucus; involuntary straining.

Sense of weight in anus, not relieved by evacuation.

Discharge of blood with stool.

Pain in rectum extending to genitals.

Heat, burning, and swelling of anus.

Almost constant oozing of moisture from rectum.

Soreness between the buttocks.

[21] **Urine.** Urging to urinate from pressure on bladder.

Frequent micturition, even at night.

Involuntary discharge of urine at night, especially during first sleep.

Mucous discharge, periodical, not at each micturition; sometimes pieces of coagulated mucus clog up urethra.

Urine: turbid, with sediment of red sand; blood-red, with white sediment and a cuticle on the surface; very offensive, with much white sediment; with dark brown admixture.

Smarting in urethra, when urinating.

Difficulty of urinating, especially in morning; a feeling as if drops came out of the bladder, which is not the case.

Gleet, no pain, discharge only during the night, a drop or so staining the linen yellowish.

[22] **Male Sexual Organs.** Increased sexual desire, with weakness of the genitals; profuse sweat, especially on the scrotum; itching around the genitals.

Emissions, also after onanism. Semen watery.

After emission, burning in forepart of urethra, languid and drowsy, sensitive to damp air.

During coition, insufficient erection and but little thrill.

After coition, great weakness in the knees.

[23] **Female Sexual Organs.** Pain in Uterus, bearing down comes from back to abdomen, causes oppression of breathing, crosses limbs to prevent protusion of parts.

Stitches, or shooting, lancinating pains mostly in neck of uterus, go up to umbilicus and pit of stomach.

Prolapsus: of the uterus; of the vagina; with constipation.

Induration of neck of uterus.

Dropsy of uterus.

Tenderness of female parts to touch. Coition painful to women.

Menses: too early and too profuse; even with mania; too late and too scanty; suppressed.

Metrorrhagia during climateric age; or, during pregnancy, especially fifth and seventh months.

Amenorrhœa at age of puberty or later.

Redness, swelling, and itching eruption on inner labia.

Leucorrhœa: yellow or greenish water; like pus; of badsmelling fluids, accompanied by much itching in genital organs.

[24] **Pregnancy.** Soreness of abdomen of pregnant women; feel the motions of child too sensitively.

Abortion after the fifth month.

Offensive, excoriating lochia.

Bleeding and soreness of nipples, preceded by itching.

Nipples crack very much across the crown.

[25] **Larynx.** Hoarseness: with tickling in larynx and bronchi; with coryza and dry cough from titillation in throat.

Sensation of dryness in larynx.

Roughness and soreness of larynx and throat.

[26] **Breathing.** Oppression of chest and shortness of breath when walking. Severe oppression toward evening.

After emotions of mind, loses breath and gets palpitation.

[27] **Cough.** Dry cough: especially evening in bed, till midnight, frequently with nausea and bitter vomiting; during sleep, without waking; from tickling in larynx, or, in bronchi, toward morning.

Cough every evening, not ceasing until he coughs loose a little phlegm.

Paroxysms of spasmodic cough resembling whooping-cough, excited by tickling in chest, from larynx to the stomach; daytime without, morning with expectoration of yellow, green or grey pus, or, of a milk-white, tenacious mucus, generally of saltish taste.

Cough and coryza, with sneezing, commences every morning before getting out of bed, and lasts until 9 A. M.

Irritation to cough so sudden and violent can scarcely inhale at all.

Cough worse: when at rest; when lying on left side; from acids.

Coughs phlegm loose, but cannot get it up.

Expectoration profuse, purulent, offensive, green, tasting salty only in morning; ❙of blood while lying down.

[28] **Lungs.** Sensation of emptiness in chest.

Great pressure on chest, more left side.

Stitch in left side of chest and scapula, when breathing or coughing.

Sensation of soreness in middle of chest.

Chest symptoms relieved by pressing on chest with hand.

[29] **Heart. Pulse.** Palpitation of heart after emotions of mind.

Interruption of the beating of the heart most after dinner; alarmed; quivering motion.

Wakes up with violent beating of the heart.

Palpitation, with anxiety about things which happened years ago.

Congestion of blood to chest, with violent palpitation of heart.

An occasional hard "thump" of the heart.

[30] **Outer Chest.** Brown spots on chest.

[31] **Neck. Back.** Pain in back and small of back, particularly with stiffness, improved by walking.

When stooping, sudden pain in back as if struck by a hammer, relieved by pressing back against something hard.

Weakness in small of back when walking, generally from disease of the uterus.

Belching relieves pain in back.

32 Upper Limbs. Humid tetter in arm-pit.

Pain, as from dislocation, in shoulder-joint, after exertion.

Lameness and falling asleep of arms and fingers.

Drawing in arms down to fingers.

Bruised pain in arms.

Herpes on elbow (scaling off).

Stiffness in wrist-joint.

Heat in hands during day, with nervous excitement.

Cold hands even in warm room, and from hands chill through whole body.

Skin on palms peels off.

Itch and scabs on hands, soldier's itch.

. Panaritium with violent beating and stitching pains.

Painless ulcers on tip of finger; or, on the joints.

33 Lower Limbs. Coxagra, with lancinating stitches, must get out of bed for relief; pains worse from rising, but better from slow walking.

Sciatica, better during pregnacy; pains 3 to 5 A. M., veins swollen.

Lower limbs go to sleep, when walking.

Icy-coldness of lower limbs.

Swelling of limbs and feet, worse when sitting or standing, better when walking.

Swelling of knee, soft, painless.

Cracking in knee-joint.

Sensation of running as from a mouse, in lower limbs.

Coldness in legs and feet, especially in evening in bed, when the feet get warm, the hands get cold.

Burning, or, heat of the feet at night.

Feet swollen, with sensation as if fallen asleep.

Profuse sweat of feet; or, sweat of unbearable odor causing soreness of toes.

Tension in tendo-achillis, also swelling of the tendon.

Sciatica becomes chronic, localizing in the heel.

Ulcer on the heel.

34 Limbs in General. Stiffness of joints.

Arthritic pains in joints.

Jerking and twitching of head and limbs, during the day.

Limbs go to sleep easily, after manual labor.

Weakness of joints, especially the knees.

Patient fears the joints cannot bear the exertion of lifting.

35 Position, etc. Rest: 3, 4, 27. Lying on painful side: 3; on painless side: 4; on left side: 27; on back: 3. Sitting: 4, 33. Standing: 33. Rising: 33. Stooping: 3, 4, 31. Motion: 3, 40. Exertion: 32, 40. Walking: 2,

3, 26, 31, 33, 36, 40.   Stretching: 36.   Kneeling: 36.
Legs crossed: 23.   Writing: 2.   Shaking head: 3.   Moving head: 4.   Turning head: 6.   Closing eyes: 3.
Turning eyes.

³⁶ **Nerves.**   Restless, fidgety.

Hysterical spasms.   Sensation of ball in inner parts.

Jerking and twitching of head and limbs.

Spasms in buttocks in bed, at night, when stretching out the limb.

Twitching of limbs during sleep.

A short walk fatigues much.

Paralysis, with atrophy.

Fainting: after getting wet; from riding in a carriage; while kneeling in church.

³⁷ **Sleep.**   Great sleepiness in daytime or too early in evening.

Frequent awaking from sleep without cause or because he thinks he has been called.

Talks aloud during sleep.

Awakens in morning at three o'clock and cannot go to sleep again.

Wakeful, sleeplessness from rush of thoughts.

Restless sleep.

³⁸ **Time.**   Morning: 4, 5, 7, 13, 14, 16, 21, 27.   Forenoon till evening: 3.   Morning and evening: 5.   Evening: 4, 5, 19, 26, 27, 33, 38, 40.   Evening till midnight: 27, Night: 21, 27, 33, 36.   3 A.M.: 37.   Day: 27, 32, 34, 37, 40.

³⁹ **Temperature and Weather.**   Warm room: 3, 32.   In bed: 27, 33, 46.   Open air: 2, 3, 4, 40.   Cold winds: 4. Damp air: 22.   Getting wet: 4, 36.

⁴⁰ **Chill.   Fever.   Sweat.**   Want of natural bodily warmth.

Shuddering during the day, without chill.

Chilliness evening, in open air, and from every motion.

More thirst with the chill than with the heat.

Heat with attacks of chilliness, with thirst.

Intermittent fever, with thirst during the chill.

Flushes of heat from least motion ; or, as if hot water was poured over him, then sweat, weakness, faintness.

Heat ascends.

Morning-sweat after awaking, profuse.

Sweat, more when walking and from the least exertion. Sweat more after a nervous shock and when sitting quietly after exertion.

Night-sweat: on chest, back and thighs; from above downward to the calves, every third night; smelling sour; offensive; or, like elder blossoms.

⁴² **Sides.**   Right: 18.   Left: 3, 7, 13, 18, 27, 28.   Within outward: 3.   Below upward: 23, 40.   Above downward: 32, 40.

Pains extend from other parts to the back.

⁴³ **Sensations.** Sensation of a ball in inner parts.
Tingling in outer parts.
Excessive sensitiveness to pain.

⁴⁴ **Tissues.** Bad effects from loss of fluids.
Painless swelling of the lymphatic glands.
Erysipelas, generally pustulous.
Arthritic affections of the joints.
Crippled nails.

⁴⁵ **Contact, Injuries, etc.** Touch: 4, 10, 17, 23. Pressure: 3, 28, 31. Scratching: 4. Riding: 18, 36.

⁴⁶ **Skin.** Itching in face, on arms, hands, back, hips, feet, abdomen and genitals.
Itching often changes to burning, when scratching.
Soreness of the skin; humid places in bends of knees.
Brown, or, claret-colored, tetter-like spots.
Humid tetter, with itching and burning.
Vesicles, itching, followed by abundant desquamation.
Ringworms; boils; pustules; pemphigus.
Ulcers: painless, on joints or tips of fingers or toes; itching, stinging and burning.

⁴⁷ **Stages and States.** Especially suited to persons with dark hair; for women, and particularly during pregnancy, in childbed, and while nursing.

⁴⁸ **Relationship.** *Sepia* is frequently indicated after : *Pulsat., Silic., Sulphur.*
Antidotes to *Sepia*; Its action is reduced by vegetable acids; the most powerful antidote, is inhalation of *Spir. nitr. dulc.;* less powerful *Ant. crud.* or *Ant. tart.;* when the circulation is much excited, *Acon.*
Sepia antidotes: *Calc. ostr., Cinchon., Mercur. Phosphor., Sarsap., Sulphur,* Rhus-poisoning (with desquamation).
Incompatible: *Laches.*

SILICEA.

HAHNEMANN.

¹ **Mind.** Confusion of mind. Difficulty in fixing attention.
Wishes to drown herself.
Screaming violently.
Over-anxious about himself; low-spirited; weeps every evening.
Gloomy, feels as if she would die.
Desponding, melancholy, tired of life. Also melancholic

with weak arms, aching sacrum, burning of feet, with sweat; all better after a seminal emission.

Compunctions of conscience about trifles.

Indifferent, apathetic.

Yielding, faint-hearted, anxious mood.

When crossed has to restrain himself, to keep from doing violence.

Child obstinate, headstrong; cries when kindly spoken to.

Restless, fidgety, starts at least noise.

Reading and writing fatigue, cannot bear to think.

² **Sensorium.** Vertigo: as if one would fall forward; ascending from dorsal region, through nape of neck into head; worse from motion, or, looking upward; accompanied by nausea; with rachitis; from excessive use of the eyes; when riding; with sleepiness.

Fainting, when taking cold from suppressed foot-sweat.

³ **Inner Head.** Cold feeling from nape of neck to vertex, extreme heaviness of head.

Congestion of head; cheeks hot; slight burning in soles of feet.

Burning in head, with pulsation and sweat of head: worse at night, from mental exertion, talking; better by wrapping the head up warmly.

Shooting from nape to vertex.

Violent periodic headache, vertex, occiput or forehead; one-sided as if beaten; throbbing in forehead; coming in night, with nausea, vomiting.

Violent headache, with loss of reason.

Loud cries, nausea to fainting; subsequent obscuration of sight; megrim.

Obstinate morning headaches, with chilliness and nausea.

Headaches, with, or followed by, severe pain in small of back; heaviness and uncomfortable feeling in all the limbs.

Tearing, frequently one-sided, with stitches through eyes and in cheek-bones.

Pulsating, beating, most violent in forehead and vertex, with chilliness.

Headache from occiput through to right supraorbital region.

Headache worse: from mental exertion; excessive study; noise; motion, even jarring of room by footstep; light; stopping; talking; cold air; touch. Better: from wrapping head up warmly; hot compresses; in warm room; lying down in dark.

Headache every seventh day.

Vibratory shaking sensation in head when stepping hard, with tension in forehead and eyes.

55

[4] **Outer Head.** Open fontanelles; head too large and rest of body emaciated, with pale face; abdomen swollen, hot.

Cephalæmatoma neonatorum.

Tearing in scalp, worse from pressure and at night.

Lumps rise on the head, hair falls out, scalp sensitive to touch, even to the hat; tearing pains.

Profuse head-sweat; body dry; likes wrapping up; sweat sour; face pale; emaciated; large abdomen; weak ankles.

Patches of eruption on scalp, exfoliating thin, dry furfuraceous scales.

Eruption on back of head, moist or dry, offensive, scabby, burning, itching, discharging pus.

Itching pustules on scalp and neck very sensitive; better wrapping up warmly.

Phagedenic ulcer on forehead painful and discharging offensive pus.

[5] **Eyes.** Long-lasting photophobia; daylight dazzles eyes.

Letters run together, appear pale; dim vision after suppressed foot-sweat.

Occasional lightning-like flashes in eyes and a feeling as if something obscured the vision; nervous sensation in head.

Black spots before eyes; a persistent speck before right eye.

Momentary loss of sight, with uterine affections; pregnancy, etc.

Cataract; also after suppressed foot-sweat, or preceding ringworms.

Day blindness, with sudden appearance of furuncles.

Amblyopia from abuse of stimulents; nervous, sensitive persons.

Tearing, shooting, or, at times, throbbing, stinging pains in eyes, in paroxysms; pains worse in draught or before a storm.

Ulceration of cornea; sloughing ulcer; non-vascular, with photophobia.

Pustular keratitis after psoriasis.

Opaque cornea after small-pox.

Spots and cicatrices on cornea.

▮ Corneal fistula,

Eye inflammed from traumatic causes; abscesses.

Hypopion.

Lachrymation in the open air.

Fistula lachrymalis; bone affected.

Swelling of right lachrymal sac, skin over it inflammed; glistening; throbbing pain; tears hot; worse evening.

▮ Big styes; also to prevent their recurrence.

Blepharitis, with agglutination in morning.

[6] **Ears.** Oversensitiveness to noises.

Ringing or roaring in the ears.

Hissing in the perforated ear.

Stoppage of ears, which open at times with a loud report.

Difficult hearing, especially of human voice and during full moon; also with chronic suppuration.

Otalgia, with stitches from in out.

Otitis interna.

Itching in the eustachian tube; chronic coryza.

Itching in both ears.

Increased secretion of thin cerumen.

Otorrhœa: scabs cover the purulent secretion in the ear; discharge offensive, watery, curdy; with soreness of inner nose and crusts on upper lip; after abuse of mercury; with caries.

Caries of mastoid process.

Scabs behind ears.

Hard swelling of parotid; suppuration, especially if slow, painless.

⁷ **Nose.** Loss of smell.

Much sneezing, with acrid coryza.

Dryness and stoppage after checked foot-sweat.

Nosebleed.

Coryza long-lasting, oft-returning.

Nose stuffed up: or, alternately dry and fluent; obstructed mornings, fluent during day.

With every fresh cold, stoppage and acrid discharge; makes inner nose sore and bloody.

Gnawing and ulcers high up in nose, with great sensitiveness of place to contact.

Nose inwardly dry, excoriated, covered with crusts.

Swelling of nasal mucous membrane; chronic coryza.

Intolerable itching of tip of nose.

Cold nose.

⁸ **Face.** Face: pale, cachectic; body cool and sweaty; earthy; yellow; distorted.

Pains, worse after being a short time in bed.

Skin of face cracks.

Acne on forehead and backs of hands.

Induration of cellular tissue of face; also following parulis.

Lupus; serrated ulcers with greyish, purulent surfaces; corroding, threatening to perforate the cheek.

Blood-boils on cheeks.

Sycosis menti.

⁹ **Lower Face.** Articulation of jaw spasmodically closed.

Pains more in jaw-bones than teeth; jaw swollen; toothache.

Caries of lower jaw; necrosis.

Dry and parched feeling of lips.

Scabby eruption on lips, which smarts.

Ulcers on vermilion border of lower lip.

Cancer of lower lip; ulcer greyish, superficial, excruciatingly painful.

Painful or painless swelling of submaxillary glands.

10 **Teeth.** Difficult dentition; gums sensitive, blistered; frequently grasping at gums.

All her teeth feel long and loose.

Carious teeth, pains worse at night and on inhaling cold air.

Throbbing toothache, swelling of periosteum.

Stinging toothache, preventing sleep.

Gums very sore; inflamed; gum-boils.

Discharge of offensive matter from openings near root of teeth or from gums.

Erysipelatous swelling on gums and roof of mouth after teeth were extracted.

11 **Tongue, etc.** Taste: of blood, morning; of soap-suds; bitter, morning, with thick mucus in throat ; of rotten eggs.

Loss of taste and appetite.

Sensation of a hair on forepart of tongue.

Tongue coated with brownish mucus.

One-sided swelling of tongue.

Ulcer on right border of tongue, eating into it, and discharging much pus. θ Carcinoma.

12 **Mouth.** Saliva runs out.

Suppuration of salivary glands.

Stomacace; mouth gangrenous, with perforating ulcer of palate.

13 **Throat.** Tough slime in the fauces.

Tonsils swollen, each effort to swallow distorts face.

Tonsillitis when the suppurating gland will not heal.

Pricking in throat, as from a pin, causing cough.

Throat feels as if filled up, as if he could not swallow; frequent cough bringing up white, frothy, saltish mucus; worse toward evening.

❙ Paralysis of the velum palati; food is ejected through the nose.

Painful swallowing, no inflammation; hysteria.

Swallowing difficult, as from paralysis.

Foods gets easily into the choanæ.

14 **Desires. Aversions.** Canine hunger, with nervous, irritable persons.

Want of appetite; excessive thirst.

Wants only small quantity of preserves.

Averse to warm, cooked food; desires only cold things, disgust for meat.

15 **Eating and Drinking,** Small quantities of wine cause ebulitions and thirst.

16 **Nausea and Vomiting.** Eructations: sour; tasting of food; loud, uncontrollable.

Nausea; with violent palpitation of the heart; after every exercise, which raises bodily temperature; after eating a little; vomiting of tenacious mucus, hiccough.

Vomits: whenever he drinks; ingesta, at night.

Morning vomiting, with nanseau, much exhaustion.

Intense heart-burn, sensation of a load in epigastrium.

Water-brash, with chilliness.

17 Stomach. Burning or throbbing in pit of stomach.

Sensitiveness of pit of stomach to pressure.

Pressure as after eating too much.

Induration of pylorus.

Anguish in pit of stomach, attack of melancholy.

Cutting feeling; or, at other times weight, crampy sensation, tightness at pit of stomach.

18 Hypochondria. Beating soreness in liver; worse on motion, when walking, when lying on right side.

Throbbing, ulcerative pain in region of liver, worse from touch or walking.

Hardness, distention of liver; abscess of liver.

19 Abdomen. Pressure, clothing across abdomen feels too tight, after eating.

Colicky pains in lower abdomen, with straining and increased pain during stool.

Colic; from worms; with constipation or difficult stool; with yellow hands, blue nails; with reddish, bloody stools.

Abdominal pains relieved by warmth.

Flatulence, much rumbling.

Distended, hard, hot abdomen, especially in children.

Inguinal glands inflamed.

Inguinal hernia.

20 Stool, etc. Sharp stitches in rectum when walking.

Stools; pap-like, offensive; contain undigested food, with great exhaustion, but painless; child has sweaty hands and feet; watery, weakening; liquid, slimy, frothy, mucous or bloody.

Constipation, stool large or composed of hard lumps, light colored; expulsion difficult, as from inactivity of rectum; when partly expelled it slips back again.

Hemorrhoids intensely painful, boring-cramping from anus to rectum or testicles; protrude during stool, become incarcerated; suppuration.

Fistula in ano; also with chest symptoms; I fissura ani; costive, or sticking pains at coccyx.

21 Urine. Suppuration of the kidneys; abscesses.

Continuous urging, with scanty discharge; also at night.

I Frequent micturition with distress from irritable sphincter.

Weakness in urinary organs; constant desire to urinate.

Profuse urination relieves headache.

Involuntary micturition at night; also in children, with
worms and in chorea.

Urine: light colored; suppressed; turbid, sediment of red
or yellow sand.

²² **Male Sexual Organs.** Sexual desire increased or decreased,
weak power but increased desire, ejaculation premature.

Painful erections, before rising in morning; frequent violent erections.

After coition, sensation on right side of head as if paralyzed; soreness of limbs. (But see 1.)

Thick, fetid pus from urethra. θ Gonorrhœa.

Red spots and itching on corona glandis.

Slight swelling of penis and testicles.

Squeezing pain in testicles.

Itching humid spots on genitals, mostly on scrotum; sweat
on scrotum.

Hydrocele; scrofulous children.

²³ **Female Sexual Organs.** Increased desire, with spinal
affection.

Nymphomania, with plethora.

Nausea during an embrace.

Menses: too early and scanty; too late and too profuse;
irregular, every two or three months.

Menstrual flow strong-smelling, acrid.

Amenorrhœa, with suppressed foot-sweat; pain in abdomen.

Metrorrhagia, offensive foot-sweat; icy-cold body; painful
hemorrhoids.

Bloody discharge between periods.

Leucorrhœa: profuse, acrid, corroding; milky, preceded
by cutting around the navel.

Prolapsus uteri from myelitis.

Pressing-down feeling in vagina; parts tender to touch.

Serous cysts of the vagina.

Itching at the pudendum; of the genitals.

²⁴ **Pregnancy.** Threatened abortion; hemorrhage after the
abortion.

Promotes expulsion of moles; shooting pains.

While nursing: sharp pains in breast or uterus, pain in
back, increase of lochia; pure blood flows every time
child nurses; complains every time she puts child to
breast.

Aversion of child to mother's milk; refuses to nurse, or,
if it does nurse, it vomits.

Milk suppressed.

Mammæ swollen, dark red, sensitive, burning pains prevent rest at night; also, suppuration of mammæ. Induration, burning pains; limbs go to sleep.

Hard lumps in mammæ.

Great itching of swollen mammæ; scirrhus.

Darting, burning in left nipple.

Nipple is drawn in like a funnel.

Scirrhus near right nipple, hard as gristle, uneven surface.

Nipple ulcerates; is very tender.

25 Larynx. Hoarseness, roughness of larynx.

Husky voice; worse morning; chronic coryza.

Fibrous, painless swelling on larynx, connected with thyroid cartilage.

26 Breathing. Shortness of breath and panting from walking fast, or from manual labor.

Arrest of breathing when lying on back; when stooping; when running, also after running; when coughing.

Oppression of chest, she cannot take a long breath.

Asthma, worse when lying down; spasmodic cough; spasm of larynx; pulsations in the chest; often with profuse, purulent sputa.

27 Cough. Dry with hoarseness; with soreness in chest; excited by tickling in throat-pit; hollow, spasmodic; loose, day and night; with profuse expectoration; vomiting of tenacious mucus in the morning; with purulent sputa; awakens him at night; worse from motion; scanty mucous expectoration.

Expectoration: profuse, fetid, purulent, green; only during day; of 'viscid, milky, acrid mucus; at times pale, frothy blood; often tastes greasy.

Colds fail to yield; sputum persistently muco-purulent and profuse.

28 Lungs. Lungs feel sore.

Stitches in chest and sides through to back.

Excruciating, deep-seated pains in chest.

Pain under sternum.

Inflammation of lungs resulting in suppuration.

Dropsy of chest; also in stone-cutters.

Empyema after pleurisy.

Congestion to chest; chilly body.

29 Heart. Pulse. Palpitation of heart while sitting, so that he had to hold on to something.

Violent hammering palpitation, after every quick or violent motion.

Pulse: small, hard, rapid; frequently, irregular and then slow.

30 Outer Chest. Painless throbbing in sternum.

Tightness across chest; after suppressed foot-sweat.

Eruption like varicella, covering the breast; itching violently.

31 Neck. Back. Cervical glands and parotids swollen, indurated.

Stiff back after sitting.

Rheumatism of lower cervical vertebræ.

Violent tearing between scapulæ.

Constant aching in centre of spine.

Spinal irritation, paralytic symptoms; cold feet; constipation.

Aching in loins, shooting down the legs.

Spinal curvature to right, painful to touch and motion.

Spina bifida.

Psoas abscess.

Spasmodic pain in small of back; does not allow him to rise.

Lame feeling in region of sacrum.

Pain across small of back on getting out of bed in the morning.

Aching, beating, throbbing in lumbo-sacral region.

Coccyx hurts after riding; coccygodynia.

32 Upper Limbs. Offensive axillary sweat.

Bones of arms feel bruised.

Shaking of left arm; before epilepsy.

Right arm and wrist weak; cannot raise anything.

Arms go to sleep when resting on them.

Limbs tremble; forearm jerks so, could not feel the pulse; after bleeding.

Wen on tendons of extensors of fingers.

Paralysis of hands; also in leprosy.

Enchondroma, right hand.

Moist tetter on hands.

Profuse sweat on hands.

Bone felons; deep-seated pains; worse from warm bed; burning, stinging, aching in superficial parts.

Run-arounds; ulceration about nails; hang-nails.

Contraction of flexor tendons; very painful when moving fingers.

Finger-tips burn.

Nails: yellow, crippled, brittle or crumpled; blue in fever.

33 Lower Limbs. Suppuration and caries of hip-joint.

Trembling of legs, with extreme nervousness.

Sensation of loss of power in legs.

Gonocace, pains stinging, lancinating; swelling, doughy; fistulous openings, with hard edges, discharging greenish-yellow pus.

Cramps: in the calves; in soles.

Cold legs and feet, after suppressed foot-sweat.

Feet give way under her, when walking.

Offensive foot-sweat, with rawness between toes.

Ingrowing toe-nails, offensive discharge.

Itching on soles, driving to despair.

³⁴ **Limbs in General.** Twitching of limbs, day and night.
Limbs: go to sleep easily; sore and lame; evenings.
Stinging in limbs at night.
Limbs cold; transient, local sweats of feet and arm-pits.
Sweat on hands and feet after fever.

³⁵ **Position, etc.** Rest: 32. Wants to lie down: 36, 37. Can't
stand: 36. Lying down: 3, 26; on back: 26; on right
side: 18. Sitting: 29, 31. Can't rise: 31. Motion: 2,
3, 18, 27, 29, 31, 32. Exertion: 16, 40. Walking: 18,
20, 26, 33, 36. Running: 26. Jarring: 3. Stooping: 3.
Descending: 3. Rising: 31, 36. Stepping: 3. Writing:
2. Looking up: 2. Closing eyes: 1. Moving eyes: 3, 5.

³⁶ **Nerves.** Restless: fidgety; starts at least noise.
Trembling in all the limbs, hands in particular; at times
she was quite unable to lift a cup of tea.
Hysteria, paralysis, and obstinate neuralgia, caused by
dissipation, or hard work with close confinement.
Spasms spread from solar plexus to brain; come at night
or during new moon; attacks preceded by coldness of
left side, shaking and twisting of left arm. θ Epilepsy.
Convulsions after vaccination.
Child slow in learning to walk.
Sense of great debility, wants to lie down.
ı Paralysis from tabes dorsalis.
ı Progressive locomotor ataxia.

³⁷ **Sleep.** Sleepy but cannot sleep.
Sleepless; from ebulitions.
During sleep starts, jerkings of the limbs, snoring.
Somnambulism.
Dreams: lascivious, pleasant; anxious, of murders, horrid
things.
Night-sweats; obstinate morning headache; chilly, nau-
seated.
Erections and urging to urinate awake him.
Feels unrefreshed, wishes to remain in bed.

³⁸ **Time.** Morning; 3, 7, 11, 22, 25, 27, 37. 6 A.M.: 40. After-
noon: 40. 3–5 P.M.: 40. Evening: 1, 5, 13, 15, 34, 40.
11 P.M.: 40. Night: 3, 4, 10, 21, 22, 24, 27, 34, 36, 40,
46. Day: 27, 40, 46. Day and night: 27, 34.

³⁹ **Temperature and Weather.** Warmth: 10, 19. Warmth
of bed: 4, 8, 32, 40. Warm room: 3. Warm wraps: 3,
4, 40. Hot compresses: 3. Cold: 10. Cold or open
air: 3, 5, 10. Debility during thunder-storm. Draft:
3. Undressing: 4.

⁴⁰ **Chill. Fever. Sweat.** Want of animal heat; always
chilly, even when exercising.
Suffering parts feel cold.
Left side suddenly cold, before epilepsy.

Chill in bed in evening.

Frequent chilliness, with occasional feverishness.

Fever during dentition.

Frequently during day, short flushes of heat, principally in face.

Violent general heat, violent thirst in afternoon, evening and all night.

Fever worse at night.

Periodically returning heat during day, no previous chill; followed by slight sweat.

Sweat only on head and face; sweat from least exertion.

Warm sweat from epilepsy.

Profuse sweat. θ Typhus.

Sweats periodically: 11 P.M., 6 A.M., or 3 to 5 P.M.

Night-sweats; sour or offensive; debilitating; mostly after midnight.

Typhoid forms of fever, great debility, profuse sweat; desire to be magnetized.

Spotted fever; also in slow convalesence.

[41] **Attacks.** New moon; 36. Increase of moon: 1. Full moon: 6. Every seventh day: 3.

[42] **Sides.** Right: 3, 5, 6, 7, 11, 18, 22, 24, 31, 32. Left: 6, 24, 29, 32, 36, 40, 43. Below upward: 2, 3, 31. Above downward: 31. Front to back: 19, 28. Within outward: 3, 6.

[43] **Sensations.** Feels as if she was divided into halves and that the left side did not belong to her.

Susceptible to nervous stimuli, to magnetism; exhaustion from suppuration.

Wandering pains; sudden pains passing quickly over body.

Prickling-tingling in various parts.

[44] **Tissues.** Fungi easily bleeding.

Discharges and excretions offensive; pus, stools, sweat of feet, etc.

Hemorrhages: from nose, stomach, bowels, or lungs.

Swelling, inflammation, also, suppuration of glands.

Inflammation, swelling, ulceration and necrosis of bones.

❙ Dropsy. Emaciation. Rachitis.

Fibrous parts of joints, especially of the knee, inflamed.

Children, while growing, suffer with violent pains, swelling of limbs and congestion.

Cellular inflammation; boils, abscesses, etc., stage of suppuration; tardy recovery; subsequent induration.

Malignant and gangrenous inflammations.

❙ Cancer.

❙ Fistulous openings, discharge offensive, parts around hard, swollen, bluish-red: 48.

[45] **Contact, Injuries, etc.** Touch: 3, 4, 5, 7, 18, 23, 27, 31. Pressure: 4, 17, 19, 31. Scratching: 30. Riding: 2, 31.

After a fall, periostitis; spine disease; ulcers near spine.

Erysipelas of scalp after injury to bones.

Ailments from vaccination.

Small foreign bodies under skin; promotes expulsion.

⁴⁶ Skin.   Skin wax-like.   θ Tuberculosis.   θ Caries.

Yellow, earthy skin; sometimes covered with pityriasis.

Itching exanthema; small pustules filled with lymph, dying quickly.

Eruption burns only by day.   θ Acne.

Small wounds suppurate profusely.

Eczematous, impetiginous, or herpetic eruptions.

Rhagades around eyelids, lips, etc.

Rose-colored blotches.

Small blisters.

Pemphigus.

Zona.

Erysipelas, with suppuration; deep-seated, phlegmonous erysipelas.

Boils come in crops; tendency to boils; leave indurations.

Abscesses speedily "point," but secretion of pus is too scanty.

Malignant pustule.

Ulcers: from suppuration of membranous parts; phagedenic; extend in depth; after abuse of mercury; offensive, with ichor, proud flesh, stinging, burning, itching; edges hard, high or spongy.

Carbuncles: 29, 31, 46.

Large, fleshy warts, suppurating.

Variola; suppuration exhausts the patients, and dessication delays; bone diseases as sequelæ.

⁴⁷ Stages and States.   Especially suitable for children, large heads, open sutures; much sweat about head; large bellies.

Nervous, irritable persons, with dry skin, profuse saliva, diarrhœa, night-sweats.

Weakly persons, fine skin, pale face; light complexion; lax muscles.

Hereditary rheumatism.

Scrofulous diathesis. Rachitic, anæmic conditions: caries.

Oversensitive, imperfectly nourished, not from want of food, but from imperfect asimilation.

Stone-cutters; chest affections and total loss of strength.

⁴⁸ Relationship.   *Silic.* is frequently indicated after: *Bellad., Bryon., Calc. ostr., Cina, Graphit., Hepar, Ignat., Nitr. ac., Phosphor.*

After *Silic.: Fluor. ac.*, which also antidotes its abuse; *Hepar*, if pimples appear around the ulcer.

Laches., Lycop., Sepia, also follow well.

Silic. antidotes; the abuse of mercury, but does not follow the potentized *Mercur.* well ; *Sulphur.*

Antidotes to *Silic.: Fluor. ac., Hepar.*

Complementary to *Thuja.*

Compare Gettysburg water (soreness between vertebræ, worse on motion, pus from joints, as in caries of vertebræ, hip-joint disease, etc.).

SPIGELIA.

Pinkroot.   HAHNEMANN.   *Loganiaceæ.*

[1] **Mind.** Weak memory.

Disinclined to mental work.

Restless and anxious; solicitude about the future.

Gloomy, suicidal mood.

Afraid of pointed things, as pins; easily irritated or offended.

[2] **Sensorium.** Vertigo: as if he would fall, worse in morning on rising, with headache, depriving him of his senses; when looking down or turning the eyes ; with nausea.

[3] **Inner Head.** Nervous headache, worse from thinking, from noise or anything jarring; face pale; anxious palpitation; nausea and vomiting.

Tearing in forehead, paroxysmal, with fixed eyes.

Boring from within outward, in the forehead, vertex or cerebellum.

Pulsating stitches in frontal protuberances.

Stitches in left side of head and out of left eye.

Pressing headache, mostly in right temple; worse from least motion or noise; better at rest, and lying with head high.

Headache beginning at cerebellum (in morning), spreading over left side of head, causing violent and pulsating pain in left temple and over left eye; periodical.

Dull stitches from within outward, on top of head ; worse from touch and after washing, but better while washing it.

Feels as if the head would burst.

Painfulness of cerebellum, with stiff neck.

Headache when stooping, as from a band around the head.

[4] **Outer Head.** Shaking in brain, worse when moving head or stepping hard.

Tension on the scalp.

Scalp feel sore to touch.

Head feels as if too large.

⁵ Eyes. Feels as if feathers were on the lashes; worse wiping them.

Farsighted.

Photophobia; oversensitive retina.

Asthenopia (accommodative), slight retinitis; neuralgia; or with anæmia of the optic nerve from excessive tea drinking.

Dilated pupils.

Sharp, stabbing, sticking pains through ball back into head, or radiating: worse from moving eyes and at night.

Eyeballs feel too large.

Boring pains, supraorbital and temporal.

Superciliary ridge pains; worse from any change in the weather.

Bluish ring around the cornea; iris discolored.

Rheumatic ophthalmia, profuse lachrymation, with or without pain; ptosis.

Strabismus, with worms.

Upper lids feel hard and immovable; stabbing pain in eyes.

Lids inflamed and ulcerated.

Chronic twitching of eyelids.

Great inclination to wink.

⁶ Ears. Hearing oversensitive, in neuralgia and headache.

Periodical deafness; ears feel as if stuffed.

Otalgia, with pressing pain as from a plug.

⁷ Nose. Violent nosebleed; also with endocarditis.

Coryza fluent; with dry heat, no thirst; eyes water; headaches, with hoarseness, and anxiety about the heart.

Copius offensive mucus, flows through posterior nares, causing choking at night.

Tickling and itching in nose.

Herpetic eruption on nose.

⁸ Face. Bloated, distorted; worse morning on awaking; pale, sickly; yellow around the eyes; red; sweaty.

Prosopalgia, mostly left-sided, with tearing, shooting, burning into eye, malar bone and teeth; periodical; from morning until sunset, worse at noon; worse from motion or noise; with lachrymation, ciliary neuralgia, palpitation; cheek dark red.

⁹ Lower Face. Lips dry, pale, cracked.

Neuralgia radiating to nose, face, temples and neck.

¹⁰ Teeth. Toothache: throbbing in decayed teeth; pressing outward, teeth feel cold; better while eating; worse after eating; from cold water; and at night, driving out of bed.

¹¹ Tongue, etc, Taste like putrid water.

Stammering; with abdominal ailments.

Tongue: coated yellow; burning, with blisters; cracked.

¹² **Mouth.** Breath fetid.

Mouth dry on awaking mornings, with stinging.

Mouth feels dry and pricks as from pins, yet filled with tenacious and nauseous saliva.

White or yellow mucus in mouth and throat.

¹³ **Throat.** Sensation as of a worm rising in throat.

Tingling in œsophagus.

¹⁴ **Desires. Aversions.** Ravenous hunger, with nausea and thirst.

Loss of appetite, with violent thirst.

Desire for alcoholic drinks.

¹⁵ **Eating and Drinking.** Worse before breakfast: 16.

Better during and generally after eating.

¹⁶ **Nausea and Vomiting.** Nausea before breakfast, with sensation of a worm rising in throat; better after eating; sickly, pale face. *θ* Worms.

Vomits food, with sour rising like vinegar.

¹⁷ **Stomach.** Pit of stomach sensitive to touch.

Pressure in stomach as from a hard lump.

¹⁸ **Hypochondria.** Stitches in region of diaphragm, left side, arresting the breathing.

Heavy pressure in precordial region, causing constriction and anxiety; with cutting and griping in bowels, as from wind.

¹⁹ **Abdomen.** Cutting colic at navel.

Pressure in umbilical region as from a hard lump.

²⁰ **Stool, etc.** Emission of fetid flatus.

Stools: of mucus with tenemus; large lumps of mucus without feces; of feces with masses of worms; hard like sheep's dung and enveloped in mucus.

Itching and tickling in anus and rectum. *θ* Ascarides.

²¹ **Urine.** Copious; with frequent urging, mostly at night; drips involuntarily, with burning in orifice of urethra; with whitish sediment.

²² **Male Sexual Organs.** Erections with voluptuous fancies, but without sexual desire.

Swelling of one-half of corona glandis.

Tingling around corona glandis.

²⁴ **Pregnancy.** Stitches under either nipple.

²⁶ **Breathing.** Short-breathed, worse when talking, with red cheeks and lips.

Dyspnœa and suffocating attacks when moving in bed, or raising arms; must lie on right side, or with head high. *θ* Heart disease.

²⁷ **Cough.** At night with catarrh; dry, hard; with worm-affections; with dyspnœa, which is worse when bending forward.

[23] **Lungs.** Constriction in chest, with anxiety and difficult breathing.

Stitches in chest, worse from least movement, or when breathing.

Sensation of tearing in chest.

Trembling feeling, worse from any movement.

Can lie only on right side, with head high. *θ* Hydrothorax.

[29] **Heart. Pulse.** Stitches about heart: sometimes synchronous with pulse; with anxiety and oppression; open with commencing valvular disease, endocarditis, etc.

Purring feeling over heart; wave-like motion, but synchronous with the pulse.

Palpitation: violent, worse bending forward; high fever; stitch pains; when he sits down, after rising in the morning; from deep inspiration or holding the breath; from worms; from least motion.

Systolic blowing at the apex.

❙ Nervous palpitation, with intermittent pulse.

Pulse: irregular; strong, but slow; trembling.

[30] **Outer Chest.** Painful contraction of muscles.

Shootings under left clavicle, or on a line with the heart.

[31] **Neck. Back.** Rheumatism of nape of neck, with painful numbness; worse lying on back.

Stitches in back, also when breathing.

[32] **Upper Limbs.** Trembling of arms.

Stitches in bends of elbows and joints of hands and fingers.

Contraction of flexors of fingers.

[33] **Lower Limbs.** Sprain of the foot.

Lancinating pain on sole of foot, when standing.

[34] **Limbs in General.** Stinging or stitching in joints.

Hard nodosities on hands and toes.

[35] **Position, etc.** Rest: 3. Standing: 33. Sitting: 29. Lying on back: 31; with head high: 3, 26, 28; on right side: 26, 28. Rising: 2, 29, 36. Motion: 3, 4, 5, 8, 26, 28, 29, 40. Must move: 36. Stooping: 4. Bending forward: 27, 29. Stepping hard: 4. Raising arms: 26. Jarring: 3. Looking down: 2. Turning eyes: 2.

[36] **Nerves.** Restless; cannot keep limbs still at night.

Body painfully sensitive to touch; part touched feels chilly; or, tingling through body.

Body feels heavy and sore, when rising from a seat.

[37] **Sleep.** Sleepy by day, even mornings; goes to sleep late.

Sleep restless, unrefreshing.

[38] **Time.** Morning: 2, 3, 8, 12. 40. Morning till sunset: 8. Noon: 8. Night: 5, 7, 10, 21, 27, 36, 40. Day: 37.

[39] **Temperature and Weather.** Washing: 3. Change of weather: 5. Cold: 10. Desire to uncover: 40.

[40] **Chill. Fever. Sweat.** Chill: often recurs at the same

hour each morning; alternates with heat or sweat; on some parts, others being hot; from least movement; spreads from chest.

Heat especially in back; in flushes, at night, with thirst for beer; on face and hands, with chill in back; with desire to uncover.

Offensive-smelling night-sweat, with heat at same time.

Clammy sweat on hands.

Cold sweat.

⁴¹ **Attacks.** Periodical: 3, 8.   Same hour every day: 40.

⁴² **Sides.**   Right: 3.   Left: 3, 8, 18, 29, 30. Before backward: 5.   Within outward: 3.

⁴⁴ **Tissues.**   Dropsy of internal parts.

Painful glandular swellings.

Rheumatism attacking the heart.

⁴⁵ **Contact, Injuries, etc.**   Touch: 3, 4, 17, 36.   Wiping: 5.

⁴⁶ **Skin**.   Pale, wrinkled, yellow, earthy.

⁴⁸ **Relationship.**   *Spigel.* follows: *Acon.* (endocarditis), and is followed well by *Arsen., Digit., Kali carb.* (heart symptoms), *Act. rac., Zincum.*

Spigel. is antidoted by: *Aurum* (restlessness in limbs), *Coccul., Pulsat.*

SPONGIA TOSTA.

Common Sponge, roasted.   HAHNEMANN.   *Spongida.*

¹ **Mind.**   Mental dulness.   Difficult comprehension.

Irresistible desire to sing, with excessive mirth.

Disposition to weep.

Paroxysms of anxiety.

Fear of the future; tired of life.

Obstinancy.

Aggravation from excitement.

² **Sensorium.**   Vertigo: with danger of falling; at night when awaking, with nausea.

Congestion of blood to head, with throbbing and pressure in forehead.

³ **Inner Head.**   Stitches in temples, worse left.

While lying, feels a strong pulsation, worse about the ear on which she is lying.

Dull headache in right side of brain, on coming into warm room, from the open air.

Headache in back part of head.

Headache as if skull would burst, in vertex and forehead.

⁴ **Outer Head.** Sensation as if hair were standing on end on vertex.

Violent itching on scalp.

Head bent backward; neck stiff.

Yellow, scabby eruption. ❙ Favus.

⁵ **Eyes.** Double vision; better lying down.

Pressing and stinging in eyes,

Coldness of eyes.

Lachrymation and headache, when looking fixedly at one spot.

Redness of eyes, with lachrymation and burning.

Pressing heaviness of eyelids.

Eyes protruding, staring.

⁶ **Ears.** Hardness of hearing.

Congestion of blood to ears; burning.

Suppuration of external ear.

⁷ **Nose.** Bleeding of nose, especially when blowing it.

Nose stuffed up. θ Whooping-cough.

Fluent coryza; hoarseness; croupy cough; after dry, cold winds.

Nasal mucus viscous, grows thick. θ Membranous croup.

Nose pinched, cold.

⁸ **Face.** Pale, with sunken eyes; red, with anxious expression.

Heat on one side of face, renewed when thinking of it.

Swelling of cheeks.

Itching and stinging on cheeks.

Cold sweat on face.

Cramp-like pain from left articulation of jaw to cheek; evenings, while eating, or when walking in open air.

⁹ **Lower Face.** Eruptions on the lips.

Swelling of the submaxillary glands, with tension.

¹⁰ **Teeth.** Feel dull and loose when masticating.

Itching and stinging in the teeth.

¹¹ **Tongue, etc.** Taste: bitter, only in the throat; sweetish in the mouth.

Difficulty of speech.

Tongue brown, dry.

Mouth and tongue full of vesicles, with burning and stinging pains.

¹² **Mouth.** Raw.

Mouth burning, dry. θ Croup.

Saliva diminished; or, with whooping-cough, increased.

¹³ **Throat.** Burning and stinging in throat; rawness and scratching.

Penetrating tickling in throat, toward ear.

Sore throat, worse after eating sweet things.

❙ Thyroid gland swollen even with the chin; at night suffocating spells, barking, with stinging in throat and soreness in abdomen.

6

 ❙ Throat externally swollen ; suffocating attacks.

Relief of throat symptoms, when lying on back.

¹⁴ **Desires. Aversions.** Insatiable appetite and thirst.

¹⁵ **Eating and Drinking.** While eating: 8. Sweet things: 13, 27. Cold drinks: 27. Warm food or drink: 27.

¹⁷ **Stomach.** Ulcerative feeling in pit of stomach, must lie on back.

Drawing, as if growing together, in pit of stomach, as far as throat, when it seems to press the windpipe so she can hardly breathe.

Cannot tolerate tight clothing about stomach.

Stitches in region of stomach.

Stomach feels flaccid, and as if standing open.

¹⁸ **Hypochondria.** Pressure in hypochondria.

¹⁹ **Abdomen.** Rumbling in abdomen, worse evenings and mornings.

Violent action of abdominal muscles during inspiration.

Viscera drawn up against diaphragm.

Swelling and inflammation of (left) inguinal gland.

²⁰ **Stool, etc.** Costive; stool hard, insufficient, with tenesmus.

Itching, biting and soreness at anus; discharge of ascarides.

²¹ **Urine.** Frequent urging to urinate. with small discharges.

Urine frothy; sediment thick, greyish-white or yellow.

Involuntary discharge of urine.

²¹ **Male Sexual Organs.** Testicles swollen, head; screwing, squeezing, with stitches up into cord; any motion of bed or clothing brings on a throbbing. θ Maltreated orchitis. θ After checked gonorrhœa.

Heat in male genitals.

²³ **Female Sexnal Organs.** Menses too soon, too profuse; preceded by colic, backache, soreness in sacrum and craving in tomach, palpitation; during menses, drawing in all limbs; awakes with suffocating spells.

²⁵ **Larynx.** Hoarseness, cough, coryza.

Hoarse, voice cracked or faint, choking sensation ; whistling inspiration.

Voice gives out when singing or talking.

Feeling of a plug in larynx.

❙ Laryngismus stridulus.

Larynx sensitive to touch, and when turning neck.

Talking hurts the larynx.

❙ Inflammation of larynx, trachea and bronchi.

Attacks of mucous rattling in windpipe; strangling at times.

Feeling of stoppage in windpipe.

Starts from sleep suddenly, with contraction of larynx.

²⁶ **Breathing.** Wheezing, anxious, worse during inhalation, with violent laboring of abdominal muscles; whistling, sawing, between coughs. θ Whooping-cough. θ Croup.

Dyspnœa: severe, on lying down; exhaustion worse in chest after every exertion; sudden weakness, tottering while walking, blood seems to rush into chest as if it would burst; with frothy, white sputa and much retching; an hour after, slight coughing brings up grey, lumpy mucus; relieved by bending body forward.

❙Sensation as if he had to breathe through a dry sponge.

Asthma: from taking cold, cannot lie down; sibilant ronchi; after menses.

Awakens with suffocating sensation.

²⁷ **Cough.** Dry, barking, hollow, croupy; wheezing, asthmatic; caused by burning, tickling in larynx, like a plug or valve; or, by feeling of accumulation of mucus and weight in chest.

Cough worse from: sweets; cold drinks; smoking tobacco; lying with head low, room too warm; dry, cold winds; every excitement. Better from: eating or drinking warm things.

❙Chronic cough, violent attacks, brought up small, hard tubercle.

Sputa scanty, tenacious, yellow, indurated, slightly sour tasting; loosened mornings, but must be swallowed again.

❙Profuse sputa of mucus, cannot lie down. θ Pneumonia in stage of resolution.

²⁸ **Lungs.** Congestion in chest from least movement or exertion; dyspnœa, nausea, faintish weakness.

Burning, soreness, rawness, with heaviness, in chest.

❙Tuberculosis beginning in apex of (left) lung.

Constrictive spasmodic pain through chest and larynx.

Stitches in both sides of chest.

²⁹ **Heart. Pulse.** ❙Angina pectoris; contracting pain in chest, heat, suffocation, faintness and anxious sweat.

❙Aneurism of aorta; dry, paroxysmal cough, worse lying down.

❙Palpitation: violent, with pain, grasping respiration; suddenly awakened after midnight, with suffocation, great alarm, anxiety. θ Valvular insufficiency.

Attacks of oppression and cardiac pain; worse lying with head low.

❙Rheumatic endocarditis, loud blowing with each heartbeat.

Stinging, pressing pains, in precordial region.

Pulse frequent, hard, full or feeble.

³¹ **Neck. Back.** Painful stiffness of muscles of neck and throat.

Cold neck, evenings.

Pressing pain in small of back.

[32] **Upper Limbs.** Twitching of muscles of left shoulder.

Heaviness and trembling of forearms and hands.

Large vesicles on forearm.

Swelling of hands and stiffness of fingers.

Numbness of ends of fingers.

Redness and swelling of finger-joints, with tension on bending them.

Cramp-like pain in ball of right thumb, lasting all day; on motion of hand it spreads to thumb.

[33] **Lower Limbs.** Thigh spasmodically drawn forward or backward.

Thighs numb, cold, with fever.

Feeling of lameness from right knee to right hip.

Stiffness of legs.

Heat in feet; veins distended.

[34] **Limbs in General.** Stiffness in limbs.

Trembling in all the limbs.

[35] **Position, etc.** Motion: 28, 32. Walking: 3, 8, 26. Exertion: 26, 28. Turning neck: 25. Bent forward: 26. Bent backward: 4, 27. Sitting: 3. Must sit up: 25. Cannot lie down: 26, 27. Lying: 3, 5, 26, 29; on back: 3, 13, 17; on affected side: 3; with head low: 27, 29.

[36] **Nerves.** Feeling of numbness of lower half of body.

Great debility and prostration.

[37] **Sleep.** Stupid slumber with the fever.

Sleepy, gaping, no activity, afternoons.

Lies asleep with head low.

Sleepless, with violent ebullitions.

Lies awake, eyes closed and sees animated images.

Awakens in a fright; suffocating; starts out of sleep.

After siesta, legs numb.

[38] **Time.** Morning: 25, 27, 40. Afternoon: 37. Evening: 8, 40. Morning and evening: 19. Night: 2. Before midnight: 27. After midnight: 29.

[39] **Temperature and Weather.** Warm room: 3, 27. Warm stove: 40. Open air: 3, 8. Dry cold winds: 7, 27.

[40] **Chill. Fever. Sweat.** Chill, with shaking even near warm stove; mostly across the back.

Violent heat after chill, dry, burning all over except thighs, which remain numb and chilly.

Flushes of heat, returning when thinking thereof.

Anxious heat, red face, weeping, inconsolable.

Heat, sweat, itching of skin.

ꛁ Typhoid fever.

Sweat: general in morning; cool on face, evenings.

[42] **Sides.** Right: 3, 32, 33. Left: 3, 8, 19, 28, 32. Both sides: 28, Below upward: 33. Within outward: 3.

[43] **Sensations.** The whole body feels heavy.

44 Tissues.   Ebullitions, distended veins.

Swelling and induration of glands.

Dropsy in cavities of body.

45 Contact, Injuries, etc.   Touch: 25, 46,   Pressure: 17.

Scratching: 46.   Worse from motion of bed.

46 Skin.   Sensitive to touch.

Red, itching blotches on skin.

❙ Herpes.

47 Stages and States.   Light hair.   Skin and muscles lax.

Often indicated with children and women.

48 Relationship.   *Spongia* follows well after: *Acon., Hepar.*

After *Spongia* are often indicated : *Bromium, Hepar.*

SQUILLA.

Squills.   HAHNEMANN.   *Liliaceæ.*

1 Mind.   Great anxiety of mind, with fear of death.

Angry about trifles.

Aversion to mental or bodily labor.

2 Sensorium.   Vertigo in morning, with nausea.

Beclouded and dizzy in head.

3 Inner Head.   Drawing, lancinating headache.

Pulsation in head when raising it.

Headache in morning on waking, with pressing pains.

Contractive pain in both temples.

Quickly passing pain in occiput, from left to right.

Stitching pain in right side of forehead.

4 Outer Head.   Painful sensitiveness of vertex, mornings.

5 Eyes.   Left eye looks much smaller than right; upper eye-lid swollen.

Contraction of pupils.

6 Ears.   Tearing pain back of left ear.

7 Nose.   Child sneezes during cough; eyes water; rubs eyes and nose.   θ Measles.

Acrid, corrosive, fluent coryza in morning..

Humid eruptions under nose, with stinging-itching.

8 Face.   Changeable expression and color of face.

During the heat, redness of face, followed by paleness, without coldness.

9 Lower Face.   Lips: twitch, and are covered with yellow crusts; black and cracked.

11 Tongue, etc.   Food tastes bitter, especially bread ; or sweetish, especially soup and meat.

12 Mouth.   Much viscid mucus in mouth.

[13] **Throat.** Burning in palate and throat; dryness in throat.

[14] **Desires. Aversions.** Insatiable appetite.
> Desire for acids. Thirst for cold water, but the dyspnœa
> allows her to take but a sip at a time.

[15] **Eating and Drinking.** After eating: 27. Cold drinks: 27.

[16] **Nausea and Vomiting.** Empty eructations.
> Nausea; during morning cough; continuous, in pit of
> stomach, alternating with a pain in abdomen, as with
> diarrhœa.

[17] **Stomach.** Pressure in stomach, as from a stone.

[19] **Abdomen.** Cutting pain in abdomen, as from flatulence.
> Painful sensitiveness of abdomen and region of bladder.

[20] **Stool, etc.** Painless constipation.
> Frequent discharge of very fetid flatulence.
> Diarrhœa, stools very offensive, watery, during measles, or
> looking black ; slimy fluid, in frothy bubbles.

[21] **Urine.** Continuous, painful pressure on bladder.
> Urine : increased, pale, with frequent urging ; involuntary ;
> scanty, dark red. θ Hydrothorax.
> When urinating, feces escape.

[23] **Female Sexual Organs.** Atony of cervix uteri.

[26] **Breathing.** Moaning, with open mouth ; wheezing ; rattling,
> with pleurisy, must sit up ; short, from least exertion.
> So out of breath cannot drink ; child seizes the cup eagerly
> but can drink only in sips.

[27] **Cough.** Dry, night and morning ; short, rattling, disturbing
> sleep ; spasmodic from mucus in the trachea, or creep-
> ing sensation in chest ; with headache ; dyspnœa ; spirt-
> ing of urine ; stitches in chest or pain in abdomen ;
> caused by cold drinks ; during measles ; after eating :
> from every exertion.
> Sputa white or reddish mucus ; sweetish, or empyreumatic
> or offensive in odor.
> The loose morning cough is more fatiguing than the dry
> evening cough.

[28] **Lungs.** Stitches : in chest, especially when inhaling and
> coughing ; in sides of chest. θ Pleurisy.
> Pains in chest are worse in morning.
> Especially suitable in pneumonia and pleurisy, after blood-
> letting.
> Heaviness on chest; congestion of blood to chest.

[29] **Heart. Pulse.** Pulse small and slow, slightly hard.

[31] **Neck. Back.** Stiffness of neck.

[32] **Upper Limbs.** Sweat in arm-pit.
> Convulsive twitching of arms ; cold hands.

[33] **Lower Limbs.** Convulsive twitching of legs.
> Cold foot-sweat.   Sweat only on toes.
> Soles red and sore when walking.

34 Limbs in General. Tearing and restlessness in upper and lower extremities.

Convulsive twitchings and motions of limbs, worse in morning and evening, and during motion.

Soreness in bends of joints.

35 Position, etc. Motion: 34, Walking: 33, 40. Exertion: 26, 27. Sitting: 40. Must sit up: 26. Raising head: 3.

37 Sleep. Frequent yawning, without sleepiness.

Restless sleep, with much tossing about.

38 Time. Morning: 2, 3, 4, 7, 16, 27, 28, 34. Afternoon and evening: 40. Evening: 27, 34, 40. Night: 40. Night and morning: 27.

39 Temperature and Weather. Uncovering: 40.

40 Chill. Fever. Sweat. Chill internally at night, with external heat.

Chilliness toward evening when walking, not while sitting.

Heat dry, burning, mostly internally.

Heat of whole body, with cold hands and feet, with aversion to being uncovered ; face pale after the heat.

Sensation of great heat in the body, in afternoon and evening, generally with cold feet.

Whenever he uncovers himself during heat, he suffers from chilliness and pain.

Sweat wanting.

42 Sides. Right: 3, 5. Left: 5, 6. Left to right: 3.

46 Skin. Eruptions like itch, with burning, itching.

Excoriation in bends of limbs.

48 Relationship. Useful after *Bryon.*

STANNUM.

Tin.   HAHNEMANN.   *Element.*

1 Mind. Forgetful and absent-minded.

She cannot get rid of an idea once fixed in her head.

Visions by day of fancied things.

Feels like crying all the time, but crying makes her worse.

Sadness, with aversion to men and disinclination to talk.

Continued restlessness and anxiety.

Cannot muster sufficient courage to do anything.

Sullen, answers unwillingly and shortly.

Thinking makes her feel wretched.

From giving directions in her domestic affairs, great palpitation of the heart, and anxiety.

2 Sensorium. Vertigo: when reading, with loss of thought; worse walking in open air or raising head.

³ **Inner Head.** Headache every morning, over one or the other eye, mostly left, gradually extending over whole forehead, increasing and decreasing gradually; often with vomiting.

Migraine, cerebral in origin, rather than gastric; atrocious pains with congestion, severe, painful constriction in forehead and temples; coldness of trunk and limbs; vomiting followed by marked relief.

Painful jerks through left temple, forehead and cerebellum, leaving a dull pressure, worse during rest, better from motion.

Throbbing headache in temples.

Heaviness in head, during rest and motion, evenings.

⁴ **Outer Head.** Burning in forehead, with nausea, better in the open air.

⁵ **Eyes.** Weak, lustreless eyes.

Pupils contracted.

Pustular swelling at inner canthus of left eye, like a lachrymal fistula.

Pressive pain in inner canthus, as from a stye.

Biting in eyes, as from rubbing with a woolen cloth.

Agglutination of lids at night.

⁶ **Ears.** Ringing in left ear.

Shrieking noise in ear when blowing the nose.

Ulceration of ear-ring hole.

⁷ **Nose.** Oversensitive smell.

Stuffed feeling and heaviness, high up in nostrils.

Dry coryza on one side, with soreness, swelling and redness of the nostril.

⁸ **Face.** Flushes of heat in face from any movement, better in open air; one cheek hot and red.

Face pale, sunken eyes, mind dull.

Prosopalgia: pains increase and decrease gradually; after suppressed chills by quinine.

¹⁰ **Teeth.** Feel loose, elongated, with painful jerking shortly after eating.

¹¹ **Tongue, etc.** Taste: sour; sweet; offensive; everything bitter but water.

Difficult, weak speech, occasioned by weakness.

Tongue: red; with yellow mucous coating.

¹² **Mouth.** Fetid smell from mouth.

¹³ **Throat.** Cutting in throat as from knives, when swallowing.

Hawks mucus, with soreness in throat; voice then becomes higher for singing.

¹⁴ **Desires. Aversions.** Hunger, except in evening; cannot eat enough.

Appetite irregular, with hypochondriasis.

Aversion to beer; it tastes flat or bitter.

¹⁵ **Eating and Drinking.** After eating: 10, 16, 19. Warm
drinks: 27.

¹⁶ **Nausea and Vomiting.** Eructations bitter, after eating.
Nausea after eating, followed by vomiting of bile; or undigested food.
Vomiting: of blood; of bile and mucus on awaking in
morning; of water when smelling cooking.

¹⁷ **Stomach.** Hæmatemesis, worse when lying, better from
pressure on stomach: slight touch causes a feeling of
subcutaneous ulceration.
Cardialgia, pains gradually come and go, extend to navel,
and are better from hard pressure; sickly expression.
Uneasy, knows not what to do with himself; pains relieved
by walking, yet so weak he must soon rest.
Sinking, "gone" feeling in epigastrium.

¹⁸ **Hypochondria.** Occasionally through day, great epigastric
weakness and hunger, but cannot eat.
Burning in hepatic region; stinging.
Boring stitches in left hypochondrium.
Hysteric spasms in region of diaphragm.

¹⁹ **Abdomen.** Empty feeling after eating.
Cutting about navel, with bitter eructations, hunger and
diarrhœa; better from hard pressure.
Hernia, better from pressure on abdomen.
Abdomen sore, as from subcutaneous ulceration.

²⁰ **Stool, etc.** Stools; green, curdy, with much colic; with
bitter eructations: hard, dry, knotty or insufficient, with
renewed desire afterwards.
Rectum inactive; much urging even with soft stool.
Passes worms; colic; sickly face.

²¹ **Urine.** Profuse and pale, then scanty, brown and sometimes
white, like milk.
After urination, continued urging.
Deficient urging, as from insensibility of bladder, which
feels dull, yet the secretion is scanty.

²² **Male Sexual Organs.** Voluptuous feeling in genitals, end-
ing in an emission.
Emissions without dreams.

²³ **Female Sexual Organs.** Menses too early and too profuse;
preceded by melancholy; pain in malar bones, which
continues during menses.
Bearing down in uterine region; prolapsus uteri.
Displacement of vagina; worse during stool; feels so
weak she must drop down suddenly, but can get up
quite readily.
Leucorrhœa: with great debility; of yellow, white or
transparent mucus.

²⁴ **Pregnancy.** Spasmodic labor-pains; they exhaust her, she
is out of breath.

Child refuses the mother's milk.

25 Larynx. Voice deep, hoarse, hollow; higher, after hawking up mucus.

Roughness and hoarseness, the latter momentarily better by coughing.

Laryngeal phthisis, with constant, short, irritating, hacking cough and aphonia; empty feeling in chest.

26 Breathing. Attacks of asthma, preceded by symptoms of ordinary cold, 4 to 5 A.M.; attacks increase and decrease gradually.

Disposition to take a deep breath; causing a feeling of lightness.

Evening dyspnœa; must loosen the clothing.

Crowing, snorting respiration.

Oppressed breathing, from every movement, when lying down and in the evening.

27 Cough. Dry, evening in bed; concussive, in paroxysms of three coughs; caused by mucus in chest, and by stitches and dryness in trachea; sputa like the white of an egg or yellow-green pus, sweetish, putrid, sour or saltish; during the day, with copious, green, salty sputa; most profuse in morning.

Accumulation of much mucus in trachea, easily thrown off by coughing; afterward soreness or stiches in chest.

Cough caused by talking, singing, laughing, lying on (right) side and from drinking anything warm.

28 Lungs. Tension across upper part of chest, with emptiness in lower.

Chest so weak he cannot talk; empty feeling in chest.

Hæmoptysis, with tendency to copious expectoration.

Phthisis mucosa, with the characteristic cough, weakness and sputa; profuse sweats.

Stitches in left side of chest, when breathing or lying on that side; knife-like below left axilla.

Great sore feeling in chest.

29 Heart. Pulse. Pulse frequent and small.

31 Neck. Back. Weakness of nape of neck.

Stitches in back; in small of back and into limbs.

32 Upper Limbs. Jerking in muscles of arm when resting it; fingers jerk when holding the pen.

Weakness and heaviness of arms, especially the right; worse from motion.

Swelling of the hands, evening.

Painful hang-nails.

33 Lower Limbs. Weakness and heaviness, especially of thigh and knee-joint, must sit down.

Swelling of ankles, evenings.

34 Limbs in General. Paralytic heaviness of limbs; worse using the arm or walking, particularly descending.

Insupportable restlessness of all the limbs.
³⁵ **Position, etc.**   Motion: 3, 8, 26, 32, 34, 40.   Exercise: 36.
  Holding pen: 32.   Exertion of dressing: 37.   Walking:
  2, 17, 34.   Descending: 34, 36.   Raising head: 2.   Must
  drop down suddenly: 23.   Must sit down: 33.   Rest:
  3, 32.   Must rest: 17.   Lying down: 26; on right side:
  37; on left side: 28.
  Always lies on her back with one leg stretched out and the
  other drawn up. θ Pregnancy.
  Must lie on right side, with pleuritic effusion.
³⁶ **Nerves.**   Feels as if she would faint.
  Paralysis mostly left-sided; feeling of a load in affected
  arm and corresponding side of chest; from emotions,
  spasms, or onanism.
  Faint sensation after going down stairs, can go up well
  enough.
  Trembling, worse from slow exercise.
  Hysterical spasms, with pain in abdomen and in diaphragm.
  Epilepsy : with tossing of limbs, clenching thumbs, opisthotonos; unconsciousness; with sexual complications;
  during dentition, with symptoms of worms.
³⁷ **Sleep.**   Sleepy during day ; goes to sleep late at night.
  Restless, the child moans during sleep, or supplicates in a
  timid manner.
  So weak on awaking, it puts her out of breath to dress.
³⁸ **Time.**   Morning: 3, 16, 27.   4 to 5 A. M.: 26.   10 A. M.: 40.
  4 to 5 P. M.: 40.   Evening: 14, 26, 27, 32, 33, 40.   Night:
  5, 37.   Night and morning: 40.   Day: 1, 18, 27, 37.
³⁹ **Temperature and Weather.**   Open air: 2, 4, 8.
⁴⁰ **Chill.   Fever.   Sweat.**   Chill: 10 A. M., finger-tips numb, or
  in the evening over the back; only on head, with thirst;
  slight, but with chattering teeth, as from convulsion of
  masseter muscles.
  Heat from 4 to 5 P. M., with sweat.
  Burning head in limbs, mostly in hands, every evening.
  Anxious heat, as if sweat would break out.
  Thirst after the heat.
  Sweat: smells mouldy, musty; debilitating, night and
  morning, most profuse on neck; debilitating, from least
  movement.
  Hectic fever.
⁴¹ **Attacks.**   Every morning: 3.   Every evening: 40.   Grad-
  ual increase and decrease : 3, 8, 17, 26.
⁴² **Sides.**   Right: 18, 32.   Left: 3, 6, 18, 28, 36.   Above down-
  ward: 31.
⁴⁵ **Contact, Injuries, etc.**   Touch: 17.   Pressure: 17, 19.
⁴⁸ **Relationship.**   *Stannum* follows well after *Caustic.*
  Similar to: *Silphium,* (latter has profuse, thin, stringy,

sputa), *Myosotis* (in phthisis mucosa, sweat, emaciation, etc.), *Silic.*, *Phosphor.*, etc.

Complementary to *Pulsat.*

Antidoted by *Pulsat.*

STAPHISAGRIA.

Stavisacre.　　　　HAHNEMANN.　　　　*Ranunculaceæ.*

[1] **Mind.**　Want of memory and heavy weight between eyes.

Child throws or pushes things away indignantly.

Indifference, low-spirited, dulness of mind; after onanism.

Hypochondriacal, apathetic, with weak memory; caused by unmerited insults; sexual excesses, or by persistently dwelling on sexual subjects.

Very sensitive to least impression; the least word that seems wrong, hurts her.

Fretful peevishnsss, with excessive ill-humor.

Great indignation about things done by others or by himself; grieves about the consequences.

Ailments from indignation with vexation, or reserved displeasure.

[3] **Inner Head.**　Dull feeling of head, with inability to perform any mental labor.

Sensation of a round ball in forehead, sitting firmly there even when shaking the head.

Pressive, stupefying headache, especially in forehead.

Headache, as if brain was compressed, worse in forehead.

Brain aches, as if torn to pieces, morning on rising from bed, worse from motion, better from rest and warmth; headache passes off with much yawning.

Sharp, burning, needle-like stitches in left temple.

Dull stitches in right temple, worse from touch.

Feeling in occiput as if hollow, or as if the brain was not large enough for the space.

[4] **Outer Head.**　Painful drawing at various spots, worse from touch.

Humid, itching, fetid eruption on occiput, sides of head and behind ears, scratching changes place of itching, but increases the oozing.

Painful sensitiveness of scalp, skin peels off, with itching and smarting, worse in evening, and from getting warm.

Hair falls off, mostly from occiput and around the ears, with humid, fetid eruption, or dandruff on the scalp.

Pressing, stinging and tearing pains in bones and in periosteum of cranium; swelling and suppuration of bones (caries), with putrid-smelling sweat, day and night; worse from motion and contact.

Burning-stinging on head, mostly on left-temple; worse from heat of bed, at 3 P.M., and when lying on it.

⁵ **Eyes.** On looking at sun, hot water runs out of left eye, scalding cheek and making eye smart.

ı Syphilitic iritis, with bursting pain in eyeball, temple and side of face.

ı Arthritic opthalmia, pains extending to teeth; eyes burn on least exertion, as if very dry, yet lachrymation is constant.

ı Blepharitis, margins of lids dry, with hardened styes, or tarsal tumors.

Left upper tarsal edge itches, relieved by rubbing.

Styes, nodosites, chalazæ on eyelids, one after the other, sometimes ulcerating.

ı Anchylops, leaving a small, hard tumor.

ı Steatoma on conjunctiva palpebrarum.

ı Polypi of conjunctiva.

⁶ **Ears.** Hardness of hearing, with swelling of tonsils, especially after abuse of mercury.

Stitches in the ears.

⁷ **Nose.** Scratching in choanæ.

Ulceration of nostrils, with scabs deep in nose.

Violent coryza, one nostril is stuffed up, with much sueezing and lachrymation; with nasal voice.

⁸ **Face.** Countenance sunken, nose peaked, eyes sunken, with blue margins around them.

Inflammation of bones of face; boring pains.

Brown and blue color of face when getting angry.

Eruption dry, itching, painful, skin rough.

⁹ **Lower Face.** Lips full of ulcers and scurfs, with burning pains.

Easy dislocation of jaw.

Painfulness of the submaxillary glands, with or without swelling.

¹⁰ **Teeth.** Black, crumbling, carious; show dark streaks.

Toothache during menses.

Gnawing, tearing in decayed teeth; shooting into ear, throbbing in temples; worse from cold drinks and touch, but not from biting on them.

Fistula dentals.

Gums white, swollen, ulcerating, spongy, bleed when touched.

¹¹ **Tongue, etc.** Taste: flat; of food, bitter.

¹² **Mouth.** Painful excrescence on inside of cheek.

Stomacace; mouth and tongue full of blisters.

Constant accumulation of water in mouth.

[13] **Throat.** Dry and rough, with soreness when talking and swallowing.

While talking she swallows continually.

Swelling of tonsils, also after abuse of mercury.

[14] **Desires. Aversions.** Extreme hunger, even when stomach is full of food.

Appetite for bread or milk.

Longing only for thin, fluid food (soup).

Great desire for wine, brandy or tobacco.

Want of thirst.

[15] **Eating and Drinking.** After eating: 14, 19, 20; meat: 27. After drinks: 19, 29. Cold drinks: 10.

[16] **Nausea and Vomiting.** Belching makes a scratching in throat, irritable larynx, and then is followed by cough.

Bitter eructations after sour food.

Water-brash.

[17] **Stomach.** Sensation as if stomach were hanging down, relaxed.

[19] **Abdomen.** A feeling of weakness in abdomen, as if it would drop, wants to hold it up.

Spasmodic cutting in abdomen after eating and drinking.

|Swollen abdomen (in children), with much colic.

|Colic: after lithotomy; with urging to stool, or with urging to urinate and squeamishness, worse after food or drink.

Painful swelling of inguinal glands.

[20] **Stool, etc.** Flatus; hot; smells like rotten eggs.

Stool: retarded, but soft; escapes with the flatus; costive, with much urging.

After the least food or drink, griping and dysenteric stool.

Hemhorrhoids. with enlarged prostate; intense pain in back and through the whole pelvis.

[21] **Urine.** Frequent urging to urinate, with scanty discharge in a thin stream, or discharge of dark urine by drops.

Profuse discharge of watery, pale urine, with much urging.

Urine involuntary, acrid, with burning; neither straining nor external pressure causes a discharge, especially after difficult confinement.

During and after micturition, burning in urethra; after micturition, urging as if the bladder was not emptied.

[22] **Male Sexual Organs.** Sexual desire excited.

Effects of onanism: face sunken; abashed look: nocturnal emissions; backache; weak legs; organs relaxed.

Seminal emissions followed by great prostration; dyspnœa.

Atrophy of the testicles.

Testicles inflamed, with burning-stinging, and pressing-drawing

Shooting-drawing in the cord. Right testicle feels as if
compressed

Aching in outer side of left testicle when walking, worse
from touch.

Voluptuous itching of scrotum.

Soft, humid excrescences on and behind corona glandis.

²³ **Female Sexual Organs.** Very sharp, shooting pains in
ovary, which is exquisitely sensitive to pressure.

Menses: irregular, late and profuse; sometimes wanting;
first of pale blood, then dark and clotted; occasionally
spasmodic uterine contractions.

Granular vegetations of vagina.

Painful sensitiveness of sexual organs, especially when
sitting.

Spasmodic pains in the vulva and vagina.

Stinging-itching of the vulva.

²⁵ **Larynx.** Sensation of constriction and pressure in throat-
pit after anger, aggravated when swallowing.

Rawness in larynx from talking.

Feeble voice from weakness of vocal organs, after anger.

Hoarseness, with much tenacious mucus in larynx and
chest.

²⁶ **Breathing.** Dyspnœa, with constriction; also, after seminal
emissions.

²⁷ **Cough.** Spasmodic, hollow, with expectoration of yellow,
tough, purulent mucus at night; only during the day;
after vexation or indignation; worse after eating meat.

Sputa loosened at night and generally swallowed.

²⁸ **Lungs.** Soreness and rawness in chest, especially when
coughing.

²⁹ **Heart. Pulse.** Palpitation: from the least motion; from
mental exertion; from music; after siesta.

Trembling beating of the heart.

Pulse frequent and small; often trembling.

³¹ **Neck. Back.** Painful swelling of the glands of the throat,
neck and axillæ.

Pain in small of back, as after overlifting; worse at rest,
at night and in morning, and when rising from a seat.

Violent stitches upward in the back.

Suppurating swelling in psoas muscles.

Rheumatic drawing, pressure and tension in neck, with
stiffness.

³² **Upper Limbs.** Herpes: with scabs on elbows; on hands.

❙Osteitis of the phalanges of fingers.

Numbness in tips of fingers.

❙Arthritic nodosities on the fingers.

³³ **Lower Limbs.** Nates ache while sitting; pain extends to
small of back, sacrum and hip-joint.

Pulsating in hip-joint, as from beginning suppuration.

Legs painfully weak, especially the knees.

Stitches in knee and knee-joint.

Crural neuralgia, stinging, stitching pains during movement.

On putting foot to the ground, pricking in balls of feet, as
if toes would be drawn down.

³⁵ **Position, etc.**   Motion: 3, 4, 23, 29, 33, 44.   Exertion: 5,
40.   Walking: 22. Stepping: 33. Stretching: 37. Ris-
ing from a seat: 31.   Rest: 3, 23, 31.   Sitting: 23, 33.
Lying on affected part: 4.   Leaning against something: 3.

³⁶ **Nerves.**   Nervous weakness.   Paralysis on one side, from
anger.

Twitches at night.

Convulsions, with loss of consciousness, retraction of the
thumbs and foaming at mouth.

³⁷ **Sleep.**   Violent yawning and stretching, bringing tears to
eyes.

Sleepy all day, awake all night, body aches all over.

•Goes to sleep late: from crowding of ideas; because the
herpes or ulcers burn and itch.

³⁸ **Time.**   Morning: 3, 31. 3 P. M.: 4 40. Evening: 40. Night:
5, 27, 31, 36, 37, 40, 4g. After midnight: 40. Toward
morning: 40. Day: 27, 37.

³⁹ **Temperature and Weather.**   Warm room: 40.   Heat of
bed: 4.   Sun: 5.   Wants to uncover: 40. Open air: 40.

⁴⁰ **Chill.   Fever.   Sweat.**   Chill and coldness predominate.

Chill: 3 P. M., better exercising in open air; in evening,
with heat in face; ascending from neck over head, or
running down back; more in a warm room.

Heat: wants to uncover; thirst; external after 12 P. M.,
followed by chill toward morning; burning at night,
mostly on hands and feet.

Sweat: profuse; cold on forehead and feet; at night smelling like rotten eggs; with desire to uncover.

Teritan fever, with symptoms of scurvy; constipation.

Before and after argue, ravenous hunger.

⁴² **Sides.**   Right: 22, 23.   Left: 4, 5, 22.   Above downward:
23, 40.   Below upward: 31, 40.

⁴⁴ **Tissues.**   Stiffness and sensation of fatigue in all the joints,
on motion.

Painful swelling of glands.

Bones, especially those of the fingers, imperfectly developed.

Swelling and suppuration of bones and of periosteum;
shooting, tearing, or boring pains.

Arthritic nodosities on joints.

⁴⁵ **Contact, Injuries, etc.**   Mechanical injuries from sharp,
cutting instruments.

Touch: 10, 22, 23. Contact: 4. Pressure: 23. Rubbing: 5. Scratching: 4, 46. Combing: 4.

[46] **Skin.** Herpes: dry, with scabs on joints; chronic, with nightly twitching; burn after scratching.

Ulcers, in scurvy.

Fig-warts: dry, pediculated; after abuse of mercury.

[48] **Relationship.** Abuse of mercury or *Thuja.*

Coloc. and *Staphis.* act well after each other.

Antidote to *Staphis.: Camphor.*

Incompatible: *Ran bulb.*

STICTA PULMONARIA.

Lungwort Lichen.   BURDICK.   *Lichens.*

[1] **Mind.** General confusion of ideas, inability to concentrate them.

Feels as if she must talk, whether listened to or not.

[3] **Inner Head.** Dull sensation in head, with sharp pains in vertex, side of face and lower jaw.

Darting in temporal region.

Dull, heavy pressure in forehead and root of nose.

Catarrhal headache before discharge sets in.

[5] Sick headache; must lie down, worse from light and noise; nausea and vomiting, nearly to faintness.

[5] **Eyes.** Burning in eyelids, with soreness of ball in closing lids or turning eyes.

Profuse mild discharge; catarrhal conjunctivitis.

[7] **Nose.** ǀ Constant need to blow nose, but no discharge results.

Feeling of fulness and heavy pressure at root of nose; tingling in right side of nose; loss of smell; dry coryza.

Excessive and painful dryness of mucous membrane; secretions dry rapidly, forming scabs difficult to dislodge. θ Influenza.

[8] **Face.** Darting pains in side of face.

[9] **Lower Face.** Darting pains in lower jaw.

[13] **Throat.** Soft palate feels like dry leather, causing painful deglutition.

[18] **Hypochondria.** Dull pain in right hypochondrium. θ Catarrh.

Full feeling in left hypochondrium.

[19] **Abdomen.** Rumbling as if full of yeast, with severe pain from sternum to spine.

[27] **Cough.** Dry, worse evening and night, can neither sleep nor lie down; dry, noisy; spasmodic stage of whooping-

57

cough; severe, dry, racking, caused by tickling right
side of trachea, below larynx; splitting frontal headache; loose morning, less free during day; pain left
side, below scapula; tickling in larynx and bronchi; incessant, wearing or racking, in consumptives; croupy.

²⁸ **Lungs.** Oppression of chest and feeling of a hard mass
there; hard, racking cough, excited by inspiration.

²⁹ **Heart. Pulse.** Dull, oppressive pain in cardiac region.

³⁰ **Outer Chest.** Pulsation along right side of sternum to
abdomen.

³² **Upper Limbs.** Hands sweat profusely.

³³ **Lower Limbs.** Bursitis, especially about knee.

³⁴ **Limbs in General.** Darting pains in arms, fingers, joints,
thighs, toes.

Swelling and stiffness of hands and feet.

Heat and circumscribed redness of joints; inflammatory
rheumatism.

³⁵ **Position, etc.** Cannot lie down : 27. Must lie down : 3.

³⁶ **Nerves.** As soon as night came, her feet and legs would
dance and jump around in spite of her; had to hold
them; hysteria, after loss of blood.

Legs, as if floating in air; she felt light and airy, without
any sensation of resting on the bed.

General feeling of dulness and malaise, and when a catarrh
is coming on.

³⁷ **Sleep.** Sleepless: from nervousness, or from cough; after
surgical operations.

·⁸ **Time.** Morning: 27. Evening and night: 27.

⁴² **Sides.** Right: 7, 18, 27, 30. Left: 18, 27. From before
backward: 18.

STRAMONIUM.

Jamestown-weed.   HAHNEMANN.   *Solanaceæ.*

¹ **Mind** Dulness of senses; also before a rash.

Coma, spasms; later, snoring, unconscious, jaw hangs,
hands and feet twitch, eyes roll; pupils dilated; automatic grasping of hands towards nose, ears, etc.; difficult to swallow liquids.

Unconscious, stupid.

Awakens terrified, knows no one, screams with fright,
clings to those near (child).

Feels stupid, with indifference to everybody and everything.

Memory weak; loses thoughts before she can give them
   utterance; weeps about her weak mind; also after sunstroke.

Hallucinations, which terrify the patient; sees ghosts,
   hears voices back of his ears; sees strangers or imagines
   animals are jumping sideways out of ground, or running
   at him.

Strange, absurd ideas; thinks herself tall, double, or lying
   crosswise; one-half of body cut off, etc.

Says he converses with spirits; prays fervently; sermonizes.
Ecstatic.

Delirium with grand ideas; general paralysis.

Delirium: shy, hides himself; tries to escape; conscious
   of her condition; full of fear; talks incessantly, absurdly,
   laughs, claps her hands over head, wide-open eyes; great
   sexual excitement, during night.

❙Lies on the back, knees and thighs flexed, hands joined;
   delirium alternating with tetanic convulsions.

Mania: for light and company; cannot bear to be alone;
   runs about; rage; proud, haughty; merry, exaltation.

❙Hydrophobia; water, a mirror or anything bright excites
   convulsions; screams; bites; mouth dry; pupils large;
   unconscious. (Best drug, change dose till cure certain.)

❙Talks in a foreign tongue. θ Typhus.

Loquacious, talks all the time, sings, makes verses.

Melancholic, fears death, weeps all the time.

Pangs of conscience; thinks he is not honest.

Alternate exaltation and melancholy.

Alternation of delirium and somnolence.

On being reprimanded, pupils dilate immediately (child).

❙After fright: St. Vitus dance; epilepsy; mania; melancholia.

² **Sensorium.**   Vertigo: cannot walk in dark, or with eyas
   closed; staggering, obscuration of vision, red face; reeling as if drunk.

³ **Inner Head.**   Tormenting sensation of heat in whole head,
   mostly vertex, with great dulness; after sunstroke.

Pressure on forehead when rising, could only half open
   eyes, could not look up.

Headache congestive, morning; worse toward noon, gradually decreasing toward evening; pains terrible, fears
   going mad, would run or press head against a wall.

Pulsating in vertex; fainting.

Heat, pulsating about vertex, attacks of fainting, loss of
   sight and hearing, face bloated, turgid; convulsive motions of head, frequently raising head from pillow, or
   bending it backward; better lying still.

Sensation of lightness of head.

ı Pain in head; nausea, delirium, eyes wild, staring,
inflamed; frenzy, convulsive spasms and twitchings of
nerves, hands and feet become cold, pulse sinking.
θ Meningitis.

Headache, with loss of sight and hearing.

Rheumatic headache, with dulness; difficult thinking;
worse on vertex or forehead; worse evening and night.

Tearing in neck and over head, shunning light; better
from warmth; worse from cold; worse on getting up in
morning.

⁴ **Outer Head.**   Jerks head up from pillow.

Boring head into pillow.

Head bent backward.

Moves head, thrusts it in all directions: in spasms, mostly
to the right.

Supports head with hands while bending or rising; after
sunstroke.

⁵ **Eyes.**   Light dazzles; shuns light; convulsions from bright
light or brilliant objects.

Hemeralopia.

Illusions in colors, often dark, less often blue and red.

Double vision, obliquely.

Vision cloudy, as through a veil.

Total blindness.   θ Typhus.

Pupils dilated; sometimes immovable and insensible to
light.

Eyes: wide open, staring; brilliant; wild and red; protrude; vacillate; vessels injected; contorted; rolling;
squinting; half open, in sleep; inflamed.

⁶ **Ears.**   Very sensitive to noises; least noise startles him.

Hardness of hearing.

Sensation as of wind rushing out of ear.

Otalgia, left side, violent pains remitting somewhat at
night, better when covering head warmly.

⁷ **Nose.**   Nose feels stopped, yet he breathes freely.

Nasal discharge yellow, bad smelling.

Nosebleed: dark, in lumps; with whooping cough.

⁸ **Face.**   Red, bloated, hot; red, eyes wild; hot and red, with
cold hands and feet; circumscribed redness of cheeks;
pale.

Forehead wrinkled; frowning (often in brain diseases).

ı Thinks face elongated.   θ Hysteria.

ı One-sided erysipelas, with meningitis; spasmodic symptoms alternately with paralytic.

ı Prosopalgia nervosa pains maddening, spasmodic starts
and shocks through body, throws arms upward; skin of
forehead wrinkled.

Pain in cheek near left ear, as if sawing the bone; muscles in oscillating motion.

⁹ **Lower Face.** Moves lips back and forward.

Lips: red; with yellow streak on vermilion border, as in malignant fevers; dry; or sore and cracked.

Lock-jaw after convulsions.

Mouth spasmodically closed.

Lower jaw hangs.

¹⁰ **Teeth.** Grinding the teeth.

Sordes on teeth.

¹¹ **Tongue, etc.** Taste: bitter; all food tastes like straw to her.

Stammering: distorts face; makes great effort to speak; mouth drawn now to right, again to left.

Speechless; sometime with spasmodic laughter at night, weeping during day.

Tongue: whitish, with fine red dots; point redder than usual; dry, red; dry and parched; pale red, in constant motion; swollen, coated dry; yellow in centre, dry; swollen, hangs out of the mouth.

¹² **Mouth.** Mouth and throat so dry, they glisten; thirst.

Salive increased; drivelling. ❙ More saliva with chills and fever.

Viscid slime in mouth.

Whole inner mouth as if raw.

¹³ **Throat.** Difficult swallowing, with stinging, pressing pain in submaxillary glands.

Averse to fluids; shrinks from the proffered cup.

Averse to water, even sight of it causes spasm; constriction of throat, froth, spitting; hydrophobia: 36.

Feeling as of boiling water rising in throat.

Spasm of œsophagus, worse trying to swallow.

¹⁴ **Desires. Aversions.** Appetite either increased or decreasd.

Violent thirst.

Troublesome thirst, even with much saliva.

Thirstless, sometimes with cold or hot stage and sweat; averse to water during fever.

Aversion to water: 13.

¹⁶ **Nausea and Vomiting.** Hiccough; restless at night, screaming in sleep.

Nausea: flow of very salt saliva; but cannot vomit.

Vomiting: dark green, mixed with food; in evening; vomits bile.

❙ Diaphragmitis, delirium; burning along diaphragm; short-breathed; spasms; struggles against water offered.

¹⁷ **Stomach.** Drawing in back part of stomach.

Inflammation, burning; anxiety.

Intense pain, vomits nearly all food.

Cardialgia, eructations, vomiting all food; emaciation.

Epigastrium tense, hard, painful.

¹⁹ **Abdomen.** Heat, anxiety in abdomen.

Wind in abdomen awakens her; screams, thinking herself full of creeping things.

Abdomen hard, tense; tympanitic; distended, but not hard.

Colic: with rumbling; violent, coming on suddenly, in evening, with faint sensation and cold shivers.

20 Stool, etc. Stools: black, preceded by writhing in bowels, and delirium; smelling like carrion, blackish; painless, diarrhœic.

▮Cholera infantum; foul-smelling stools; strabismus; awakes with fright; pale face.

Constipation: with convulsions; cardialgia; alternating with diarrhœa.

Hemorrhoids: painful; bleeding.

Coagulated blood passes from the anus.

21 Urine. Kidneys secret less or none, in acute diseases, especially of children.

Urine: clear, profuse, passed suddenly, at night; also after delirium; copious, with spasms; passed involuntarily; suppressed, especially in cerebral diseases; dribbles slowly, feebly; despite urging no stream forms, no pain.

During urination: rigors, rumbling in belly.

22 Male Sexual Organs. Exalted sexual passion.

Child constantly has hand on the genitals, with spasms.

▮Onanism causing epilepsy.

23 Female Sexual Organs. Nymphomania; lewd talking; sings obscene songs; has smell of semen.

Excessive menstrual flow; drawing in thighs, abdomen and upper limbs.

Menstrual flow very watery.

During menses; loquacity; strong smell as of semen.

After menses: sobbing, whining.

Dysmenorrhœa.

▮Metrorrhagia, loquacity, singing, praying; sometimes passing large coagula.

24 Pregnancy. During pregnancy: mania; faceache; full of strange ideas.

Threatened abortion; unceasing talking, singing, imploring.

Puerperal convulsions, with copious sweating.

Scanty lochia; puerperal mania, milk still copious; many hallucinations; talks foolishly.

25 Larynx. Voice: higher and finer; screeching; indistinct.

Constriction of larynx and thoracic muscles.

26 Breathing. Rattling breathing: toward 12 P.M.; in whooping-cough; in chill or sweat.

Frequent inspiration and expiration, breath oppressed.

Breathing: short, difficult; anxious, during heat or sweat.

Spasms of muscles of chest; single parts twitch; spasmodic
motions of arms; sometimes chest fixed, breathes only
with diaphragm and abdominal muscles.

Inspiration slow, expiration quick.

27 Cough. ı Of drunkards.

Periodical, painless, spasmodic cough, shrill, screeching
tone; worse morning; from touching throat; from walking in wind; in vaulted rooms; after debauch; after
fright; from looking at bright objects; from drinking
water.

ı Whooping-cough, barking, croup-like, with suffocating
contraction of chest, violent beating of heart, rattling,
anxiety, congestion, blood-spitting; convulsions.

28 Lungs. Pain in breast, cough and other peri-pneumonic
symptoms during recovery from meningitis.

29 Heart. Pulse. Palpitation.

Beating of heart, so increased by motions he cannot speak
for hours; trembling, twitching as in chorea; murmurs
instead of regular sounds; consequent on fright.

Pulse: full, strong; frequent, hard; irregular; small and
spasmodic; slow, in typhus; sometimes trembling or imperceptible; sometimes double and very quick, with
quiet respiration.

30 Outer Chest. ı Red rash on chest. θ Typhus.

31 Neck. Back. Constant pain in cervical and upper dorsal
vertebræ.

Bending backward.

Drawing pain in spine.

Spot in back pains when touched.

Put right arm often to small of back and draws mouth, as
if he had severe pain.

32 Upper Limbs. Raises arm above head, claps hands, makes
graceful, gyratory motions.

Grasping about with hands, as if reaching for things;
searching for things; picking.

Grasps the throat; sighing, groaning.

Hands and arms tremble.

Clapping hands over head.

Hands clenched (not thumbs) but they can be opened.

Difficult to bring hand to tumbler or carry latter to mouth.

ı Panaritium, pain intolerable, drives to despair; relieves
pain of suppuration.

33 Lower Limbs. Coxalgia, left side; also for violent pains
when abscesses form.

ı Inside right thigh red, swollen. θ Typhus.

Spasmodic rigidity of lower limbs.

Paralysis of lower limbs; loss of speech; staring.

Constant trembling of feet.

[34] **Limbs in General.** Arms agitated, lower limbs quiet.

Drawing, laming, somewhat spasmodic pains in muscles.

Fingers and heels numb, latter sometimes painful, rheumatic headaches.

Limbs feel as if "gone to sleep."

Cold hands and feet.

[35] **Position, etc.** Lying: 3. Inclined to lie down: 36. Rising: 2, 4. Raises head: 3, 4. Bends backward: 3, 4. Bending: 4, 31. Motion: 4. 29. Walking: 36.

[36] **Nerves.** Great inclination to lie down.

Totters as if giddy, cannot make even a few steps without help.

Frequent twitching; sudden jerks through the body.

Trembling of limbs.

‖Convulsions, especially opisthotonic, from bright, dazzling objects, water or touch. Child rigid as a board.

‖Chorea from fright; creeping in limbs, then violent movements generally crosswise; rotate arms over head; jump up, climb over tables, etc.

‖Hysteria preceded by great sensitiveness, weeping and laughing alternately; sexual excitement.

‖Spasms; abdomen puffed; alternation of clonic and tonic; body very hot; continually changes character.

Said to be very effective for hydrophobia (vary the dose even to the production of symptoms).

‖Epilepsy from fright; attacks sudden, with screams, afterwards drowsy; aching in stomach; periodical. Gives warning of approach by premonitory symptoms.

‖Catalepsy, limbs can be moved by others. Tonic spasms.

Muscles will not obey the will.

Paralysis of one, convulsions of other side.

Left side paralyzed, stammering, unconnected words, sheds tears.

‖Paralyzed limbs after apoplexy.

[37] **Sleep.** Drowsy by day; staggering and drowsy.

Sleepy, but cannot sleep; after the convulsions.

Snoring, deep sleep.

Coma, rattling respiration, bloody froth at mouth. θ Scarlatina.

Falls into a deep sleep; deep breathing, snoring.

Sleepless, tosses about.

During sleep: laughs; screams; starts; sexual excitement; emissions; spasms; sits up, looks about, talks incoherently.

Awakens: with a solemn air of importance; all things seem new: screaming, seems frightened, knows no one, shrinks away, or jumps out of bed.

[38] **Time.** Morning: 3, 7, 27. Afternoon: 40. Evening: 3,

16, 19. Night: 1, 3, 6, 11, 16, 21, 26, 28. Toward midnight: 26. After midnight: 20. Toward morning: 7. Day: 11, 37.

[39] **Temperature and Weather.** Warmth: 3. Warm covering: 6. Cold: 3. Vaulted rooms: 27. Sunstroke: 1, 3, 4.

[40] **Chill. Fever. Sweat.** Chilly, as from cold water down her back.

Chills: run down back; and general coldness, with red face and twitchings; with great sensitiveness to uncovering; with heat in head.

❘ Fever in children; cry out in sleep; start, jerk; eyes half open, pupils large; suppressed urine.

Anxious heat with vomiting.

Afternoon, first heat of head and face, then general coldness, then general heat.

Heat; anxious, with vomiting; delirium, thirst and sweat; of whole body, face vivid red; at same time sweat.

Covers up during heat.

Sweat: cold all over; with delirium; with impaired vision, or shunning light; oily of putrid odor.

[41] **Attacks.** Worse during equinoxes: 36.

Worse in summer: spasms, ecstasy.

Attacks of epilepsy come periodically: 36. Gradually decreasing: 3. Suddenly appearing: 19, 21.

[42] **Sides.** Right: 4, 33. Left: 6, 8, 33, 36. Right to left: 11.

[43] **Sensations.** Painful sensations as if joints were loose, with anguish therefrom.

Arms and legs feel as if separated from body.

[44] **Tissues.** Mitigates the terrible pains of tumors, abscesses.

❘ Plethoric, especially young persons.

❘ Emaciated, cries day and night; cough.

❘ Anasarca, after scarlatina.

[45] **Contact, Injuries, etc.** Touch: 31, 36. Pressure: 3.

[46] **Skin.** Whole skin and conjunctivæ red, like crimson.

Skin hot and dry.

Worse when eruptions are suppressed, or do not come out well.

❘ Burns.

❘ Entire face swollen, muttering delirium, small-pox before vesicles form.

Restless, skin itching; rash coppery-red, skin, dry, hot.

Measles, before eruption, with convulsions, frightful visions of rats and mice, seem frightened, try to hide; spasm of œsophagus; body hot, face red, puffed.

[47] **Stages and States.** Children especially; chorea, mania, fever.

Young, plethoric persons.

⁴⁸ **Relationship.** In metrorrhagia from retained placenta, with
clapping hands, delirium, loquacity, etc., *Secale* acts
better than *Stramon.*
Ailments from: vapor of *Mercur.*, *Plumbum.*
Antidotes to *Stramon.*: *Bellad.*, *Hyosc.*, *Nux vom.*; against
large doses: lemon. juice; senna (cerebral symptoms);
tobacco injections; vinegar.
Stramon.: useful in whooping-cough after *Bellad.* had
acted too powerfully.

SULPHUR.

Brimstone.   HAHNEMANN.   *Flowers of Sulphur.*

¹ **Mind.** Weak memory, particularly for names. .
Dulness; difficult thinking; misplaces or cannot find
proper words when talking or writing.
Foolish happiness and pride, thinks herself in possession
of beautiful things; even rags seem beautiful (also when
recovering from spasms).
Indisposed to everything (work, pleasure, talking or
motion), in the evening.
Disgust, up to nausea, about any effluvia arising from his
own body.
Melancholy mood; dwelling on religious or philosophical
speculations; anxiety about his soul's salvation; indifferent about the lot of others.
Hypochondriac mood through the day; merry in evening.
Peevish; irritable; quick-tempered.
Excitable mood, easily irritated, but quickly penitent.
Great obstinacy, dislike to have any one near him.
² **Sensorium.** Vertigo: while sitting or standing, with nosebleed, in the morning; when stooping; when rising
from bed; when walking in open air; when crossing a
river; with nausea; with vanishing of sight; with inclination to fall to the left side; worse after meals, particularly after dinner.
Rush of blood to head, with roaring in ears and heat of
face, worse when stooping, talking, in open air; better
sitting in warm room.
Heaviness and fulness in forehead, worse when raising the
head to a sitting posture; worse after sleep; after talking; better when sitting, or when lying with the head
high.
³ **Inner Head.** Tearing or stitches in forehead or temples,

from within outward; worse from eating or stooping; better when pressing head together, and when moving about.

Shooting in forehead from in-outward; worse from stooping or eating; better from pressing teeth together, and when moving head.

Pressure in temples and tight feeling in brain when thinking or doing mental work.

Painful tingling on vertex and in temples.

Sensation of emptiness in occiput; worse in open air and from talking; better in-doors.

Drawing and tearing through head.

Headache every day, as though head would burst.

Throbbing headache at night.

Sick headache, very weakening, once a week, or every two weeks; pains generally lacerating and stupefying, numbing.

Every step is felt painfully in head.

⁴ **Outer Head.** Sensitiveness of vertex, pressing pain when touched; worse in evening; from heat of bed; in morning when awaking; smarting and burning after scratching.

Roots of hair painful, especially to touch.

Severe itching on forehead, also on scalp.

Dry, offensive, scabby, easily bleeding, burning eruption begins on back of head and behind ears, with sore pain and cracks; better from scratching.

Humid, offensive eruption, with thick pus, yellow crusts, itching, bleeding and burning.

Contractive pain as from a band around cranium, with sensation as if flesh was loose, followed by inflammation, swelling and caries of bones; worse in wet, cold weather, and when at rest; better from motion.

Hair dry, falling off, scalp sore to touch, itching violently, in the evening, when getting warm in bed.

▮ Fontanelles close too late.

Drandruff.

⁵ **Eyes.** Photophobia, with stitches; worse in sultry weather.

Shunning light, during the sweat.

▮ Retinitis, caused by over-use of eyes, congestion of optic nerve.

▮ Obscuration of sight; like a gauze before eyes. Cataract.

Halo around gas or lamplight.

Shortsightedness.

Pustular inflammation of cornea, or conjunctive, with marked lachrymation.

Superficial and deep ulcers on cornea, intense redness of eye, great photophobia.

Inflammation of eyes, or lids, itching, smarting, burning, feeling like from sand.

┃ Painful inflammation of eye, from presence of foreign body (after *Acon.*).

Ulceration of margins of lids.

Lids swollen, burn and smart, with itching; aggravation from bathing eyes.

Dryness of eyes in room, lachrymation in open air.

Agglutination of lids at night.

Lids drawn together spasmodically, in morning.

⁶ **Ears.** ┃ Hardness of hearing, preceded by oversensitiveness of hearing.

Humming or hissing in ears.

Wabbling as if water was in ears.

Stinging in left ear.

┃ Purulent, offensive otorrhœa, worse left ear.

┃ Catarrhal discharge, every eighth day.

┃ Ears very red; with children.

⁷ **Nose.** Smell before the nose as from an old catarrh.

Nosebleed at 3 P.M., with vertigo, afterwards nose sore to touch.

Bloody discharge when blowing the nose.

Profuse catarrhal discharge of burning water.

Fluent, burning coryza, out-doors, nose stopped up in-doors.

Chronic stoppage; also of one nostril.

Dry ulcers, or scabs in nose.

Swelling and inflammation of nose; red nose.

┃ Freckles and black pores on nose.

⁸ **Face.** Face: pale, sickly looking; pale, eyes sunken, and with blue margins; spotted red; circumscribed redness of the cheeks; freckled.

Erysipelas, beginning at right ear and spreading over face.

Swelling of the cheek, with pricking pain.

⁹ **Lower Face.** Painful eruptions around the chin.

Herpes at the corners of mouth.

Bright redness of lips, particularly with children.

Swelling of lips, especially upper lip.

Lips dry, rough, and cracked.

Burning, twitching, or trembling of lips.

¹⁰ **Teeth.** Great sensitiveness of teeth.

Teeth feel too long.

Tearing toothache on left side.

Pulsating and boring in teeth, worse from heat.

Toothache coming on in open air, or from least draught, or at night in bed, or from washing with cold water; ' with congestion to head, or with stitches in ears.

Painful feeling of looseness of teeth.

Swelling of gums, with beating pain in them.

Bleeding of gums.

¹¹ **Tongue, etc.**   Taste; sour; bitter; sweetish; foul, when
 awaking in morning.

 Talking: 2, 28, 36.

 Tongue; white with red tip and borders, mostly in acute
  diseases; white or yellow; brown and dry; furred in
  morning, but wears off during day (chronic cases).

¹² **Mouth,**   Ptyalism from abuse of mercury, or during a fever.

 Saliva profuse, with nauseous taste, "all her trouble seems
  to be caused by this nauseous saliva."

 Bad smell from mouth, mostly after eating.

 Blisters in mouth ; thrush.

¹³ **Throat.**   Sensation of a lump in throat; dryness of throat.

 Stitches in throat when swallowing.

 Painful contraction of throat when swallowing.

 Burning up into throat, with sour eructations.

 Sensation as of a hair in throat.

 Sore throat, great burning and dryness, first right then
  left side.

 Elongation of palate; swelling of palate and tonsils.

 Pharyngeal wall looks dry.

 Whole back part posterior to palatine arches appears in a
  state of ulceration or sloughing.

¹⁴ **Desires.   Aversions,**   Great craving for food, especially
 with little children.

 Drinks much, eats little.

 Violent thirst for beer; longing for brandy.

 Desire for sweets, and diseases from eating sweet things ;
  also in pale, lean children with large abdomens.

 Milk disagrees, causing sour taste and sour eructations.

 Aversion to meat.

¹⁵ **Eating and Drinking.**   After eating but little, feels fulness
 in stomach.

 After eating: 2, 3, 16, 17 ; and drinking: 19. After eating
  sweet things: 14, 19.

¹⁶ **Nausea and Vomiting.**   Hiccough.

 Eructations: generally empty, or tasting of the food; sour;
  after eating; as soon as he presses on stomach.

 Regurgitations; sour; of food and drink.

 Vomiting: of food, especially early in morning, and in
  evening; first watery, then of food; sour ; of blood.

 Nausea: in morning; after each meal.

¹⁷ **Stomach.**   Sensitiveness to touch in region of stomach.

 Marked weakness about 11 A.M., empty, gone, or faint
  feeling.

 Pressure at stomach, also after eating.

¹⁸ **Hypochondria.**   Stitches, or pressing pain in region of liver.

 Swelling and hardness of liver.

Stitches in spleen, worse when taking a deep inspiration, and when walking.

Stitches in left side of abdomen, when coughing.

[19] **Abdomen.** Intestines feel as if strung in knots, worse from bending forward.

Rolling and rumbling in bowels, as if empty.

Incarcerated flatulence in left side of abdomen, with heaviness, fulness and constipation.

Colic after eating or drinking, obliging one to bend double, worse from sweet things.

Painful sensitiveness of abdomen, to touch, as if internally raw and sore.

Painful swelling of inguinal glands.

Big belly and emaciated limbs, with children.

[20] **Stool, etc.** Stools: brown, watery, fecal; green mucus; bloody mucus; undigested; frothy; sour; changeable; fetid.

Diarrhœa: at night, with colic, tenesmus, watery-white, mucous stools of sour smell; driving out of bed in morning, painless; fetid, watery or involuntary; of scrofulous children; as if bowels were too weak to retain their contents.

The odor of stool follows him as if he had soiled himself.

Dysenteric stools at night, with colic and violent tenesmus; blood in mucus in thready streaks.

Frequent unsuccessful desire for stool.

Alternation of constipation and diarrhœa.

Constipation; stools hard, knotty, insufficient.

Hemorrhoids, blind, or flowing dark blood, with violent bearing down pains from small of back toward anus.

Suppressed hemorrhoids, with colic, palpitation, congestion to lungs; back feels stiff as if bruised.

Lancinating pain from anus upward, especially after stool.

Pulsating pain in anus, all day. Itching, burning and stinging at anus.

Anus swollen, with sore, stitching pains. Stools excoriate.

[21] **Urine.** Retention of urine.

Frequent micturition, especially at night; large quantities of colorless urine after hysteric spasms. Nocturnal enuresis.

Urine fetid, with greasy-looking pellicle on it.

Burning in orifice of urethra, during micturition.

Redness and inflammation of orifice of urethra.

Painful desire, with discharge of bloody urine, requiring great effort.

Mucous discharge from urethra.

[22] **Male Sexual Organs.** Involuntary discharge of semen, with burning in urethra.

Coldness of penis; weak sexual powers; impotence.

Inflammation and swelling, with deep rhagades, burning and redness of prepuce, with phimosis.

Deep suppurating ulcer on glans and prepuce, with puffed edges.

Phimosis, with discharge of fetid pus.

Testicles relaxed, hanging down.

Offensive sweat around genitals.

Soreness and moisture of scrotum.

²³ **Female Sexual Organs.** Menses: too late; of short duration; or, suppressed; blood thick, dark, acrid, sour-smelling, makes the thighs sore.

Before the menses: headache; cough in evening; nosebleed.

During menses: nosebleed; rush of blood to head; weak, faint spells.

Bearing down in pelvis, toward genitals.

Sterility, with too early and too profuse menstruation.

Leucorrhœa of yellow mucus, corroding, preceded by pains in abdomen.

Burning in vagina, is scarcely able to keep still.

Sore feeling in vagina, during coition.

Troublesome itching of vulva, with pimples all around.

Labor-like pain over the symphysis.

Weak feeling in genitals.

²⁴ **Pregnancy.** Promotes expulsion of moles.

After nursing, nipples smart, burn and bleed; chapped nipples.

Suppuration of mammæ, with chilliness in forenoon, heat in afternoon.

Hemorrhoids in childbed.

²⁵ **Larxnx.** Voice rough, hoarse, with much mucus on chest; aphonia.

Talking fatigues and excites the pains; shooting pains through left chest to back.

Catarrh, with fluent coryza, chilliness, rawness of chest and cough.

²⁶ **Breathing.** Shortness of breath and oppression, on bending arms backward.

Nightly suffocative fits; wants doors and windows open.

Difficult breathing, with visible beating of heart.

Rattling in chest, worse after expectoration.

²⁷ **Cough.** Dry, choking; short, dry, with stitches in chest, or under left scapula; dry, with hoarseness, dryness in throat and watery coryza; with much rattling of mucus in chest; loose, with soreness and pressure in chest; expectoration of thick mucus; rattling in trachea, hoarseness; expectorating greenish lumps of sweetish taste.

Expectoration of bloody pus.

When coughing: headache, as if bruised or torn; sometimes vomiting; pain in abdomen.

Spasmodic whooping-cough, two paroxysms in quick succession.

In the paroxysm the successions follow each other rapidly.

Cough excited by tickling in the larynx, as if caused by
"down," evening and night without, morning and day
with, expectoration of dark blood, or of yellow, greenish, purulent, or milk-white, watery mucus; usually of
sourish, sometimes putrid, flat, or saltish taste, or like
.the offensive discharge of an old catarrh.

²⁸ **Lungs** Congestion of blood to chest.

Feeling as if a lump of ice was in right chest.

Stitches through chest, extending into left scapula; worse
lying on back and during least motion.

Pain in chest from overlifting, or after inflammation of
lungs.

Burning in chest rising to face.

Pain as if chest would fly to pieces, when coughing or
drawing a deep breath.

Weakness in chest; in evening while lying down; when
talking.

❙Exudation, after pneumonia.

²⁹ **Heart. Pulse.** Palpitation of heart, worse when going up
stairs or when climbing a hill.

Sensation as if heart was enlarged.

Pulse full, hard and accelerated, at times intermittent.

³⁰ **Outer Chest.** Shooting in sternum.

³¹ **Neck. Back.** Sensation as if vertebræ were gliding one
over the other, when turning in bed.

Cracking in cervical vertebræ, especially on bending backward.

Stiffness in neck or back.

Pain in small of back, on rising from a seat.

Gnawing pain in small of back.

Stitches in scapulæ.

Pain in small of back, after heavy lifting and taking cold
at the same time.

❙Curvature of spine, vertebræ softened.

³² **Upper Limbs.** Pain as if sprained, or as if bruised in left
shoulder.

Rheumatic pains in shoulders, especially the left.

Lacerating pains in shoulders and shoulder-joints, especially at night.

Drawing and tearing in arms and hands.

Sweat in arm-pit, smelling like garlic.

Rhagades on hands, especially between fingers, on finger-
joints and in palms.

Thick red chilblains on fingers.
Numbness of fingers, in morning.
Hang-nails.
Cold hands and feet.

33 Lower Limbs. Heaviness of limbs when walking.
Swelling of knees, white or red.
Dropsy of the knee-joints.
Stiffness of knee and ankle-joints.
Cramp: in calves at night, also with diarrhœa; in soles at
every step.
Burning soles, wants them uncovered.
Soles cold and sweating.

34 Limbs in General. Chillblains thick and red, with cracks
on joints.
Corns, with aching and stinging pains.
Limbs "go to sleep."
Tearing in limbs, muscles and joints, from above down-
ward.
Weakness, cracking, swelling of joints.
Gouty or rheumatic complaints, with or without swelling.
Pain in limbs, worse when covered with feather covering.

35 Position, etc. Rest: 4. Lying: 28; with head high: 2.
Motion: 1, 4, 28, 31. Turning in bed: 31. Moving
head: 3. Stooping: 2, 3. Bending forward: 19. Bending backward: 31. Rising: 2, 31. Walking: 2, 3, 18,
33, 36. Crossing a bridge: 2. Ascending: 29. Standing: 2. Sitting: 2. Must bend double: 19. Bending
arms backward: 26. Every step: 33.

36 Nerves. ❙Child jumps, starts and screams fearfully.
Frequent spasmodic jerking in whole body.
Great debility and trembling; talking fatigues.
Weak, faint spells, frequently during day, after nursing
or night-watching, with great sleepiness.
❙Epilepsy, with stiffness; sensation like from a mouse
running up arms to back, before the fit.
Unsteady gait, tremor of hands.
Cannot walk erect, stooped shoulders.

37 Sleep. Heavy, unrefreshing sleep.
Child falls asleep as soon as tenesmus ceases.
Drowsy in afternoon and after sunset; wakeful at night.
Easily awakened, takes short naps.
Sleep, with half-open eyes.
Talks loudly while asleep.
Jerks and twitches during sleep.
Awakens with a start or scream.
Dreams: vivid; anxious.

38 Time. Morning: 2, 4, 5, 11, 16, 20, 27, 32, 40. Forenoon:
24. 11 A.M.: 17. Afternoon: 24, 37, 40. 3 P.M.: 7.

Evening: 1, 4, 16, 20, 23, 27, 28, 37, 40. Night: 3, 5, 10, 20, 21, 26, 27, 32, 33, 37, 40. Day: 1, 3, 11, 20, 27, 36, 40.

³⁹ Temperature and Weather. Warm room: 2, 5. In-doors: 3, 7. Warmth of bed: 4, 10, 46. Covering: 34. Wants to be uncovered: 33, 40. Sultry weather: 5. Heat: 10. Open air: 2, 3, 5, 7, 10, 26. Draught: 10. Wet and cold weather: 4. Washing in cold water: 10.

Children dislike being bathed.

⁴⁰ Chill. Fever. Sweat. Chill: mostly internal and without thirst, generally in evening, but also at other times; external, with simultaneous internal heat and red face; with thirst, preceded by heat; spreading from the toes; running up the back.

Heat: afternoon or evening, skin dry, much thirst; in soles; or cold feet, with burning soles, seeks a cool place for them, or puts them out of bed.

Frequent flushes of heat, sometimes ending with a little moisture and faintness.

Sweat: at night and in the morning hours; profuse, sour-smelling, the whole night; in the evening, most on the hands; at night, only on the nape and occiput.

⁴¹ Attacks. Every eighth day: 6. Every one or two weeks: 3.

⁴² Sides. Right: 8, 18, 28. Left: 2, 6, 10, 18, 19, 25, 27, 28, 32. Right to left: 13. Front to back: 25. Within outward: 3. Below upward: 20, 40. Above downward: 34.

⁴³ Sensations. Sensation as of a hoop or band around parts.

⁴⁴ Tissues. Scrofulous and rickety complaints.

Emaciation of children, face has a very old look.

Dry, flabby skin.

❙Glandular swellings indurated or suppurating.

Borders of mucous membranes are very red.

⁴⁵ Contact, Injuries, etc. Touch: 4, 7, 17, 19. Pressure: 3, 16. Stepping (jar): 3, 33. Scratching; 4, 46. Over-lifting: 28, 31.

⁴⁶ Skin. Voluptuous itching and tingling, with burning or soreness after scratching.

Itching, worse in warm bed.

Bright redness of whole body in scarlatina.

Freckles. Yellow, brown, flat spots.

Skin rough, scaly, scabby.

Herpes, scabby and scurfy.

Sore feeling of the skin, with disposition to exertion.

Soreness in folds of skin.

Ecchymosis from a slight bruise.

Rhagades after washing.

Furuncles, particulary on the nates.

Eruptions: 4, 5, 7, 8, 9, 12, 22, 23, 24, 33, 34.

Erysipelas, with throbbing and stinging.

Dropsical swelling of external parts.

Ulcers: with raised, swollen edges, bleeding easily, surrounded with pimples; with tearing, stinging pains and
discharging fetid pus.

⁴⁷ **Stages and States.** Especially suitable for lean, stoop-
shouldered persons.

❙ Body offensive despite washing.

⁴⁸ **Relationship.** *Sulphur* frequently serves to rouse the reactive power of the system, when carefully selected remedies have failed to produce a favorable effect, especially
in acute disease.

Sulphur, Calc. ostr. and *Lycop.;* or, *Sulphur, Sarsap.* and
Sepia, frequently follow in the order given.

Complementary: *Aloe soc.*

Sulphur antidotes: *Cinchon., Jodium, Mercur., Nitr. ac.,
Rhus tox., Sepia;* ailments from the abuse of the metals
generally; tremors caused by *Arsen.*

Antidotes to *Sulphur: Acon., Camphor., Chamom., Cinchon.,
Mercur., Pulsat., Rhus tox., Sepia.*

Compare: *Myrt. comm.* in stitches through upper left chest.

SULPHURICUM ACIDUM.

Sulphuric Acid.   HAHNEMANN. SO_3.

¹ **Mind.** Must do everything in a great hurry.

Unwilling to answer; says yes or no with difficulty, pulse
very small and frequent.

Disheartened.

Inclined to weep.

Irritable, restless.

Mental excitability.

² **Sensorium.** Sensation in forehead as if brain was loose
and falling from side to side; worse when walking in
the open air; better when sitting quiet in room.

Rush of blood to head in headache.

³ **Inner Herd.** Painful shocks in forehead and temples,
worse in forenoon and evening.

Headache as if a plug were thrust quickly, by increas-
ingly severe blows, in head.

Gradually increasing and suddenly ceasing headache.

⁴ **Outer Head.** Hair turns grey, falls out; eruption on scalp,
very sore; worse in open air.

⁵ **Eyes.** Fill with tears, when reading.

Tension in eyelids in morning; difficult to open them.

Deep blue circle under right eye.

Feeling as of a lump in right outer canthus; on closing
eye seems to move to inner canthus, and to return on
opening.

In chronic inflammation of eyes more frequent useful in
beginning, later *Sulphur.*

⁶ **Ears.** Hardness of hearing; feeling as of leaf lying before
ear.

Buzzing in right ear.   θ Neuralgia.

⁷ **Nose.** Nosebleed: oozing of dark, thin blood; evenings;
worse from smelling coffee; of old people.

Coryza, alternately dry and fluent; with loss of smell and
taste, hunger, sore eyes and tension in forehead.

⁸ **Face.** Crusta lactea, with stringy, yellow stools.

Face: deadly pale; feels as if white of an egg had dried on
it.

Dry, shriveled spots in face (with hemorrhoids).

Pain commencing at 9 P. M. in ramus of lower jaw and temple of right side, better from warmth, and from lying on
affected side.   Comes gradually, leaves suddenly.

⁹ **Lower Face.** Shooting, stinging pain in red scar on lower
jaw.

Lips peel off.

¹⁰ **Teeth.** Toothache; worse in evening in bed, aggravated by
cold; better from heat.

Dull toothache concentrating in right eye-tooth; hurts
when eating and on pressure.   Pain increases slowly,
ceases suddenly.

Destruction of teeth.   θ Diabetes mellitus.

¹¹ **Tongue, etc.** Loss of taste.

Talking difficult, as from want of elasticity of the parts.

Tongue dry, ⸗

¹² **Mouth.** Sensation of dryness.

Much saliva.

Aphthous mouth and gums; yellowish and painful.

¹³ **Throat.** Thick yellow membrance on fauces, tonsils, teeth,
lips; sticks like glue; impeded deglutition; voice thick;
parotids swollen, hard; sopor; stench from mouth.

ı Stringy, lemon-yellow mucus hangs from posterior nares
in diphtheria.

Roughness in throat.

Lancinating pain in throat.

Stinging in throat and chest at same time.

Constricted feeling in throat.

¹⁴ **Desires. Aversions.** Desire: for fresh fruit; for brandy.

Loss of appetite and great debility.

¹⁵ **Eating and Drinking.** Water causes a cold of the stomach
if not mixed with alcoholic liquor.

Ailments: from drinking brandy (symptoms are palliated by drinking wine); from eating oysters.

After eating, pain in stomach, and rising of food by the mouthful.

After warm food: 40.   Coffee (odor of): 7. 27.   Cold water: 27.   Alcoholic drinks: 29.   Wine: 40.

[16] **Nausea and Vomiting.**   Belching after cough.

Chronic heart-burn, sour eructations.

Nausea with chilliness.

Sour vomit, first water, then food.

Vomiting, of drunkards.

Raising of mucus so sour that it sets teeth on edge.

[17] **Stomach.**   Coldness and relaxed feeling in the stomach.

Dyspepsia.

[18] **Hypochondria.**   Spleen enlarged, hard and painful; hurts when coughing.

[19] **Abdomen.**   Labor-like pains in abdomen, extending to hips and back.

Colic, with sensation as if a hernia would protrude.

Violent protrusion of an inguinal hernia.

[20] **Stool, etc.**   Diarrhœa, with great debility.

Stools: diarrhœic, with passage of much flatus; watery and very offensive, like rotten eggs; bright yellow, mucous, looking stringy or chopped, cholera infantum ; of hard, small, black lumps, mixed with blood, with violent pinching in anus.

Hemhorroids feel damp, painful to touch, itch violently; stools cause violent burning, stinging, tearing pains, or the tumors prevent passage.

[21] **Urine.**   Diminished secretion of brown urine, becoming turbid, like loam-water, on standing.

Sediment like blood and a cuticle on the urine.

Pain in bladder if the call to urinate is postponrd.

[22] **Male Sexual Organs.**   Erections.

Orchitis, right side.

[23] **Female Sexual Organs.**   Menses too early and too profuse.

Distressing nightmare before the menses.

In climaxis, spitting of blood ; costive.

Leucorrhœa ; acrid or burning; milky or transparent; of sanguineous mucus, with a sensation as if the menses would appear.

Prolapsus of vagina; parts look greenish and smell badly.

[24] **Pregnancy.**   Nausea and vomiting during pregnancy.

Sterility, with menses too early and too profuse.

[25] **Larynx.**   Hoarseness, with dryness and roughness in throat and larynx.

Larynx painful ; feels inelastic, causing difficulty in talking.

[26] **Breathing.** Shortness of breath

[27] **Cough.** Dry, two short hacks ; soreness between scapulæ ; tiredness ; from irritation in chest, with expectoration, in the morning, of dark blood, or of a thin, yellow, blood-streaked mucus, tasting sour ; after cough, belching ; in the open air, worse from walking, riding, cold water, and odor of coffee.

Cough and hæmoptysis after typhus.

[28] **Lungs.** Stitches in chest ; about heart.

Sensation of great weakness in chest.

Burning in left side of chest up to throat.

Shooting, stinging, now in scapula, again in arm-pit, or in chest.

Profuse hemorrhage from the lungs : tuberculosis.

Ulcerations in different parts of lungs.

[29] **Heart. Pulse.** Palpitation of heart, with or without fear or anxiety,

Shooting through the heart.

Pulse : small, feeble, accelerated ; affected by alcoholic drinks.

[30] **Outer Chest.** Sternum sore, as if beaten.

[31] **Neck. Back.** Stiffness in back on rising in morning.

Blood-boils on the back.

Large suppurating swellings on right side of neck.

[32] **Upper Limbs.** Stitches : in shoulder-joints on lifting the arms ; in finger-joints.

Tension in elbow-joint.

Chilblains on hands.

Red swelling on back of hand, not painful.

Blue spots on the arms.

After erysipelas, inflamed swelling of little finger.

[33] **Lower Limbs.** Knees painfully weak.

Ankles weak, can't walk.

Feet cold, swollen.

Distention of veins of feet.

Stitching in corns.

Red itching spots on tibia.

Blood-red, very painful scar on tibia.

[35] **Position, etc,** Lying : 8. Sitting : 2. Rising : 31. Motion : 40. Exercise : 40. Walking : 2, 27, 33. Lifting arms : 32.

[36] **Nerves.** Sensation of tremor all over, without trembling.

Debility, great exhaustion.

[37] **Sleep.** Goes to sleep too late, wakens too early.

During sleep twitches, especially of fingers.

[38] **Time.** Morning : 5, 27, 31, 40. Forenoon : 3. Evening : 3, 7, 10, 40. 9 P. M.: 8. Day : 40.

[39] **Temperature and Weather.** Warmth : 8, 10. In bed : 10, 40. In-doors : 2, 40. Open air : 2, 4, 27, 40.

⁴⁰ **Chill. Fever. Sweat.** Frequently chilly during day; worse in-doors, better out-doors when exercising.

Frequent chills, running down the body.

Heat in evening and in bed.

Flushes of heat, with sweat. *θ* Climaxis.

Sweat: excessive, mostly on upper body; from motion, continued after sitting down; sour; cold, immediately after eating warm food; mornings; at night, profuse; lessened by drinking wine.

⁴¹ **Attacks.** Itching of skin every Spring; formation of single pustules.

Gradually coming, suddenly ceasing: 3, 8, 10.

⁴² **Sides.** Pressing, stinging pains inward.

Right: 5, 6, 8, 10, 22, 31. Left: 18, 28, 29. Above downward: 40.

⁴⁴ **Tissues.** Scars become blood-red or blue, and painful.

Painful sensitiveness of glands.

Veins (of feet) distended.

Weak and exhausted from some deep-seated dyscrasia.

Hemorrhages of black blood from all the outlets of body.

⁴⁵ **Contact, Injuries, etc.** Bad effects from mechanical injuries, when there are bruises, chafing, lividity of skin.

Scratching seldom relieves itching, but changes its locality.

Pressure: 10.   Touch: 20.   Riding: 27.

⁴⁶ **Skin.** Scars turn blood-red and hurt.   Blue spots like ecchymoses.

Red itching blotches on skin.   Yellow skin, livid spots.

Gangrenous tendency after a bruise.

⁴⁷ **Stages and States.** Frequently indicated for old people, particularly women.

Child sour despite careful washing.

Light-haired people.

In climacteric years, flushes of heat.

⁴⁸ **Relationship.** Follows well after *Arnic.*

Pulsat. is complimentary and antidotal.

Sulph. ac. antidotes bad effects of lead water.

TABACUM.

Tobacco.   HARTLAUB.   *Solanaceæ.*

¹ **Mind.** Forgetful; slow perception.

Idiotic; epileptic idiocy.

Cheerful, merry, loquacious.

Melancholy; anxiety, better from weeping.

Sudden anxiety, with angina pectoris; also, with oppression of the chest, driving him from place to place.

Diseases originating in cerebral irritation, followed by marked gastric symptoms.

² **Sensorium.** Vertigo: excessive heaviness in the head; with qualmishness in stomach; better out of doors.

³ **Inner Head.** Sick headache, coming on early in morning, intolerable by noon; deathly nausea, violent vomiting greatly aggravated by noise and light.

Headache better in open air.

⁵ **Eyes.** Dimsightedness, as through a veil, evenings; also with double vision.

Heat and burning in eyes; eyeballs injected, cornea covered with mucus, must wipe it off.

Pupils dilated.

Contraction of lids.

⁶ **Ears.** Nervous deafness.

Sensation as if ears were closed.

Ears burning hot and red.

⁷ **Nose.** Smell feeble. Nasal catarrh with sensation of crawling in nostrils.

⁸ **Face.** Emaciation and death-like pallor of the face; cold, covered with sweat.

Face blue, pinched.

Face is drawn, distorted; eyes sunken; blue around them.

Lips cracked, swollen, covered with a brown crust: 48.

Glowing heat in face, with redness frequently only on one side.

Violent tearing in bones of face and teeth.

¹⁰ **Teeth.** Drawing, rending toothache.

¹¹ **Tongue, etc.** Cannot speak. θ Angina pectoris. Difficult speech.

¹³ **Throat.** Dry and choky, can hardly swallow; burning in throat and mouth.

Violent constriction of throat. θ Angina pectoris.

Much viscid phlegm in throat, difficult to raise.

Uvula œdematous.

Pharynx feels as if burning, raw and scraped.

¹⁴ **Desires. Aversions.** Great thirst. θ Cholera infantum.

Constant hunger; nausea if stomach is not satisfied; or disgust for food.

¹⁵ **Eating and Drinking.** Sensitive to smell of wine; fumes all but intoxicate her.

¹⁶ **Nausea and Vomiting.** Nausea and vomiting on least motion. θ Cholera infantum.

Nausea and cold sweat remaining after *Veratr.* and *Secale* checked stools. θ Cholera.

Eructations: sour, hot; also of small amounts of food; or, loud, noisy.

Vomiting: nausea, as soon as he begins to move; during
pregnancy, deathly nausea; of water; of sour fluid,
with mucus.
Seasickness, deathly nausea; pallor; coldness; worse
from least bodily movement; better on deck in fresh,
cold air.

[17] **Stomach.**   Spasmodic pressure in pyloric region.
Writhing in pit of stomach. θ Cardialgia.
Sticking in pit of stomach through to back.
Sinking, weakness, relaxed sensation.
Various distressing sensations, as burning, cramps, sudden
shocks on falling asleep, etc.

[18] **Hypochondria.**   Pressure, heaviness or stitches in liver.
Liver enlarged, pressure on it sends pain to pit of stomach.

[19] **Abdomen.**   Gurgling in bowels.
Shifting of flatulence.
Abdomen tympanitic, costive; also with severe pains in
spells, worse eating, yet so hungry, cannot refrain.
Violent burning, must shriek, horrible pains.
Spasms of bowels.
Violent contractions in abdominal muscles; naval retracted.
Strangulated hernia; nausea, deathly faintness, cold; cold
sweat; vomiting; sudden cerebral hyperæmia.

[20] **Stool, etc.**   Sudden papescent, yellow-green or greenish,
slimy stools; tenesmus; shifting flatus.
Costive; stools like the sheep's, evacuated with difficulty.
Body cold, abdomen hot; not satisfied until clothing is all
off of abdomen. θ Cholera infantum.
Stools yellow, sometimes greenish slime; vomiting, de-
bility; cold sweat. θ Cholera infantum.
Cholera, body cold, face distorted, spasms; vomiting, or,
no stool or vomit; collapse.
Soft stool, tenesmus; burning backache.

[21] **Urine.**   Renal colic; violent pains along ureters (worse
right); cold sweat, pale face, fainting, deathly nausea,
great exhaustion.

[22] **Male Sexual Organs.**   Nocturnal emissions.

[23] **Female Sexual Organs.**   Stitching pains in abdomen, genitals, urethra, etc.
Climacteric troubles; much mental confusion; giddy;
weak and faint.

[24] **Pregnancy.**   Morning sickness: 16.

[25] **Larynx.**   Voice weak and hoarse.

[26] **Breathing.**   Paroxysms of suffocation.   Hurried, anxious,
irregular respirations.
Dyspnœa; costiveness.
Asphyxia.
Sticking under sternum, with inability to take deep breath.

[27] **Cough.** Dry cough.

Whooping-cough, violent straining and vomiting, stitches in pit of stomach, inability to breathe deeply; hiccough, as if he would suffocate, after the cough.

[28] **Lungs.** Tightness across upper part of chest, with angina pectoris.

[29] **Heart. Pulse.** Palpitation in attacks at night, tight across chest, with angina pectoris.

Oppression at heart; pulse feeble, irregular. θ Cholera.

Violent beating of heart and carotids.

Sudden precordial anguish.

Violent palpitation lying on left side; goes off when turning to right.

Pulse: quick, full, large; imperceptible, small, intermittent; excessively slow; soft, feeble.

[31] **Neck. Back.** Neuralgic pains up into neck, with angina pectoris; also with tightness in the throat.

Pains between shoulders. θ Angina pectoris.

Violent pain in small of back and loins; usually better walking.

Throbbing in sacral region, evening.

[32] **Upper Limbs.** Left arm exhausted, painful.

Cramps in arms and hands; in single fingers, especially while washing; early morning.

Spasmodic contraction in arms and hands.

Hands feel lame, cold; then burning, with bloated finger-tips.

Hands icy-cold; body warm.

Trembling of the hands.

[33] **Lower Limbs.** Legs from knees down icy-cold.

Cannot walk, with angina pectoris.

Formication in left leg, from knee to toes.

Tremor and disabling weakness of the feet.

[34] **Limbs in General.** Coldness, trembling of limbs; cold sweat.

Cramp, tearing in limbs.

[35] **Position, etc.** Lying on left side: 29. Lying on right side: 29. Motion: 16, 31.

[36] **Nerves.** Weary, languid; tremor.

Horrid pains, with involuntary muscular contractions of muscles.

Spasmodic contraction of muscles, spasms, general insensibility, relaxation.

[37] **Sleep.** Drowsiness, going off in open air. ❙ Stupefying sleep at night.

Sleepless; jerking and twitching in sleep.

[38] **Time.** Morning: 3, 24, 32. Noon: 3. Evening: 31, 40. Night: 22, 29, 37.

[39] Temperature and Weather. Cold air: 16. Open air: 3, 37. Washing: 32. Clothing must be removed: 20.

[40] Chill. Fever. Sweat. Coldness and shuddering in whole body, evenings. Icy-coldness of legs, from knees to toes. Body, warm, hands icy-cold; or, body cold. θ In cholera. Sweat: cold, hands, forehead, face; viscid, cold; profuse.

[41] Attacks. Symptoms come in paroxysms.

[42] Sides. Right: 18, 29, 46. Left: 29, 32, 33.

[44] Tissues. Emaciation, especially of back and cheeks.

[45] Contact, Injuries, etc. Motion of vessel: 16. Touch: 46.

[46] Skin. Cold; in cholera; livid, with angina pectoris. Red spots in face and on right shoulder, burning when touched. Itching, with red or yellow spots on chest and shoulders; vesicles.

[48] Relationship. *Tabac.* antidotes: *Cicut., Stramom.* Antidotes to *Tabac.: Ipec.,* vomiting; *Arsen.,* chewing tobacco; *Nux vom.,* gastric symptoms next morning after smoking; *Phosphor.,* palpitation; *Ignat., Pulsat.,* hiccough; *Clemat.,* toothache; *Sepia,* neuralgia right side of face, dyspepsia, chronic nervousness; *Lycop.,* impotence; wine, spasms, cold sweat from excessive smoking. *Plant. maj.* has several times caused an aversion to tobacco.

TARAXACUM.

Dandelion.   HAHNEMANN.   *Compositæ.*

[1] Mind. Constant muttering to himself. θ Typhus. Inclined to talk, laugh and be merry. Undecided, shunning labor, but after beginning, works well.

[2] Sensorium. Vertigo when walking about; apyrexia of ague.

[3] Inner Head. Drawing pain in left temple while sitting, ceasing when walking and standing. Needle-like stitches in left temple while sitting, ceasing when standing. Violent tearing in occiput. θ Typhus. Pressure, with heaviness, in lower part of occiput.

[4] Outer Head. Head falls now to left, now to right side.

[5] Eyes. Aversion to light; stinging-burning in eyes.

[6] Ears. Drawing pain in external ear.

[7] Nose. Nosebleed; left side.

[8] Face. Hot and red. Pimples on cheeks, alæ nasi and corners of mouth.

⁹ **Lower Face.** Upper lip cracked.

¹⁰ **Teeth.** Feel dull; set on edge, as from acids, when chewing food.

¹¹ **Tongue. etc.** Taste: bitter, before eating; sour, saltish, especially of butter and meat.

White spots on the tongue amongst the red.

Tongue: coated white, cleans off in patches, leaving dark red, tender, very sensitive spots; mapped tongue.

¹² **Mouth.** Sour water accumulates in the mouth.

Accumulation of saliva in mouth, with sensation as if larynx was pressed shut.

¹³ **Throat.** During and after swallowing food, aching across clavicles, up left side of neck into her ear; gullet feels too small for the food.

¹⁵ **Eating and Drinking.** After eating: 11, 13, 40. While eating: 13. After drinking: 40.

¹⁶ **Nausea and Vomiting.** Eructations bitter; hiccough.

❙Eructations for several days, returning after drinking.

Belching, gagging, nausea at night. *θ* Ague.

Nausea: with headache, anxiety; and vomiting, after fat food.

¹⁸ **Hypochondria.** Liver enlarged, indurated.

Pain in region of the spleen. *θ* Ague.

¹⁹ **Abdomen.** ❙Motions in abdomen, as if bubbles were forming and bursting.

❙Hysterical tympany; eructations after drinking; bubbles of wind burst in abdomen, etc.

Abdomen puffed. *θ* Jaundice.

Stitching pains, especially in the sides.

²⁰ **Stool, etc.** Ineffectual urging, with much pressing; scanty, hard stool. *θ* Ague.

Stool difficult, even if not hard. *θ* Ague.

Voluptuous itching in perineum, compelling scratching.

²¹ **Urine.** Frequent, profuse and pale urine.

²² **Male Sexual Organs.** Shooting upward and spreading over pubic region each time after urinating; epididymitis.

²³ **Female Sexual Organs.** Suppressed menses.

²⁸ **Lungs.** Stitches in chest.

Boring, digging in chest.

Twitching in right intercostal muscles.

³¹ **Neck. Back.** Tearing from ear down to neck.

Rolling and gurgling in right scapula.

Pressing stitches along spine, mostly in sacrum, with dyspnœa.

³² **Upper Limbs.** Twitching in muscles of arms.

Numbness in left arm, side of head and ear.

Pressive pain in right middle, ring and little finger.

Hands hot.

Finger-tips icy-cold.

³³ Lower Limbs. Stitching pain in left thigh.

Pressive pain in left calf.

Jerking pain in right calf, ceases quickly when touched.

Tearing pains only in lower limbs, worse during rest. *θ* Typhus.

Burning in knees, legs, toes.

Drawing pain on dorsum of right foot, when standing; ceases when sitting.

Severe, or fine stitching pains in right sole.

³⁴ Limbs in General. Can move limbs, but they feel as if bound or powerless.

Limbs painful to touch and to improper position.

³⁵ Position, etc. Rest: 33. Wants to lie down : 36. Standing : 3, 33. Sitting : 3, 33, 37. Improper position : 34. Walking : 2, 3.

³⁶ Nerves. Exhausted, inclined to sit or lie down; semi-conscious.

Debility, loss of appetite, profuse sweat every night; thirst; restless sleep.

³⁷ Sleep. Yawning, sleepy when sitting.

At night on waking, heat, mostly of face and hands.

Sleep disturbed by : dreams ; sweat.

³⁸ Time. 8 P.M. : 40. Night : 16, 36, 37, 40.

⁴⁰ Chill. Fever. Sweat. Chilliness all over; at night, with sweat and gastric ailments.

Chill, after food or drink.

Chill in open air.

Nose and hands cold at 8 P.M. ; when he falls asleep, sweat breaks out, mostly on head.

Long-lasting chill; copious sweat; pain in spleen.

Copious, debilitating night-sweats, causing biting on skin.

Sweat, mostly with thirst.

⁴² Sides. Right : 4, 26, 28, 31, 32, 33. Left : 3, 4, 7, 13, 18, 32, 33, 40.

⁴⁴ Tissues. Neuralgia and rheumatism after typhus.

⁴⁵ Contact, Injuries, etc. Touch : 33, 34. Scratching : 20.

⁴⁶ Skin. Pimply, sycotic skin.

Stinging in skin.

TELLURIUM.

Precipitated Metal.   HERING.   *The Element.*

¹ Mind. Forgetful.

Quiet disposition.

Rough, angular disposition.

² **Sensorium.** Vertigo : morning after rising from bed ; worse when walking, sitting up, or turning head ; pulse accelerated, nausea, vomiting of food ; better lying perfectly quiet ; when going to sleep.

³ **Inner Head.** Brain feels as if beaten, on slightest movement. Heaviness and fulness in head in morning.

Violent (linear) pain in a small spot over left eye ; pain short, sharp and defined.

⁵ **Eyes.** Deposit of a chalky-looking white mass on anterior surface of lens.

Pterygium.

Purulent discharge ; eczema impetiginoides on lids.

Left upper lid worse ; lachrymation, itching and pressure ; scrofulous ophthalmia.

Herpes conjunctiva bulbi ; veins enlarged, running horizontally towards the cornea, ending in little blisters near edge of cornea ; worse from crying.

⁶ **Ears.** Dull, throbbing pain day and night, thin, watery, excoriating discharge.

Vesicular eruption on membrana, then suppuration and perforation.

Membrana tympani permanently injured and hearing greatly diminished.

Itching and swelling, with painful throbbing in external meatus ; in three or four days, discharge of a watery fluid, smelling like fish-pickle, which causes vesicles wherever it touches ; ear is bluish-red, as if œdamatous ; hearing impaired.

Sensation : as if something suddenly closed up in the ear ; as if air whistled through left eustachian tube, when snuffing or belching, air passes through it.

⁷ **Nose.** Fluent coryza, lachrymation and hoarseness when walking in open air.

⁸ **Face.** Sudden flashes of redness over the face.

Twitching and distortion of facial muscles, worse when talking.

Ringworm.

¹⁰ **Teeth.** Salivation ; gums bleed easily and profusely.

¹² **Mouth.** Breath has a garlic-like odor.

¹³ **Throat.** Sore throat, dry sensation in fauces, better when eating and drinking.

¹⁵ **Eating and Drinking.** See 13.

¹⁷ **Stomach.** Weak feeling, like faintness in the stomach, after congestion of blood in head and nape.

¹⁹ **Abdomen.** Pinching in abdomen.

²⁰ **Stool, etc.** Flatus peculiar and stinking.

²¹ **Urine.** Increased urination.

High-colored, acid urine.

Drop sticking at mouth of urethra.

²² **Male Sexual Organs.**   Increased sexual desire.

Herpes on scrotum and perineum.

²⁹ **Heart.   Pulse.**   Dull pain in region of heart, when lying on left side; better when lying on back.

Palpitation of heart, with throbbing through whole body and full pulse, followed by sweat.

³¹ **Neck.   Back.**   Painful sensitiveness of spine, from last cervical to fifth dorsal vertebra; sensitive to pressure and touch.

Pain in sacrum.   See sciatica.

³³ **Lower Limbs.**   Pain in sacrum, passing into right thigh down sciatic nerve, worse when pressing at stool, coughing, laughing, also when lying on the affected side. θ Sciatica.

³⁵ **Position, etc.**   Lying quietly: 2; on left side: 29; on back: 29; on affected side: 33.   Sitting: 2.   Rising: 2.   Walking: 2, 7.   Motion: 3.   Turning head: 2.

³⁸ **Time.**   Morning: 2, 3.   Day and night: 6.

³⁹ **Temperature and Weather.**   Open air: 7.

⁴⁰ **Chill.   Fever.   Sweat.**   Chilly, with the pains.

Sweat on face.

Sweat on spots, with increased itchings of these places.

⁴² **Sides.**   Right: 33.   Left: 3, 5, 6, 29.   Above downward: 33.

⁴⁵ **Contact, Injuries, etc.**   Touch: 31.   Pressure: 31.

⁴⁶ **Skin.**   Ringworms: cover the whole body, more distinct on lower limbs; on single parts.

TEREBINTHINA.

Oil of Turpentine.   HARTLAUB.   *A volatile oil.*

¹ **Mind.**   Stupefaction; deep sleep; uræmia; fainting.

Mind clear, then unconscious, followed by inability to concentrate his mind.

Dull, languid; relieved by free micturition.

² **Sensorium.**   Sudden vertigo, with obscuration of sight.

³ **Inner Head.**   Dull headache, with colic.

Intense pressure and great fulness of head.

⁵ **Eyes.**   Iritis; urinary symptoms present.

Pains in and over eye, worse at night or 1 to 3 A. M.

Eye dark red, face red on affected side.

⁶ **Ears.**   Sensation in ears as of the striking of a clock.

⁷ **Nose.**   Violent nosebleed.

⁸ **Face.** Earthy color of the face, sunken features.

¹⁰ **Teeth.** Scorbutic affections, with hæmaturia.

¹¹ **Tongue, etc..** ❙ Tongue smooth, glossy, as if deprived of papillæ. θ Typhoid.

¹⁵ **Eating and Drinking.** After eating: 16.

¹⁶ **Nausea and Vomiting.** Sickness at stomach after eating.

¹⁷ **Stomach.** Dull pain in epigastrium.

Pressure as if he had swallowed a bullet, which had lodged in pit of stomach.

¹⁸ **Hypochondria.** Burning in right hypochondrium.

¹⁹ **Abdomen.** ❙ Distended abdomen: tympany in typhoid, puerperal fever, etc., tongue agreeing; frequent colic; constipation.

Worms: with foul breath, choking sensation, dry, hacking cough; burning and tingling at the anus, with sensation as if ascarides were crawling about; sometimes with spasms.

²⁰ **Stool, etc.** Intestinal catarrh and diarrhœa, with nephritis.

Hemorrhages from bowels, with ulceration; epithelial degeneration.

Stools watery, greenish, mucous and watery; worse in morning.

Violent burning in rectum and at anus after stool.

²¹ **Urine.** Affections of kidneys, worse from living in damp dwellings.

Burning and drawing from right kidney to hip.

Pressure in kidneys when sitting, better from motion.

Frequent urination at night, with intense burning.

Urine: black, with coffee-grounds sediment; great emaciation and weakness; clear, watery, profuse; incontinence at night; scanty, turbid, dark, epithelial sediment; albuminous; bloody, the blood thoroughly mixed with the urine; containing sugar.

Sensitiveness of hypogastrium, tenesmus of bladder, strangury; burning in region of kidneys; urine deposits a slimy, thick, muddy sediment; urine smells of violets.

²² **Male Sexual Organs.** Gonorrhœa, with strangury, tenesmus of bladder, smarting in urethra, chordee.

²⁴ **Pregnancy.** Burning and bearing down in uterus; burning urination. θ Puerperal metritis.

²⁶ **Breathing.** Difficult respiration, as if from congestion of lungs.

Asthma, worse from motion.

²⁷ **Cough.** Bronchial catarrh, with spitting of much phlegm.

Dry cough, no expectoration, or blood-streaked sputa.

²⁸ **Lungs.** Hemorrhage from lungs.

Unbearable burning and tightness across chest, with great dryness of mucous membranes, or profuse expectoration.

[29] **Heart. Pulse.** Pulse: increased in force and frequency; feeble, rapid.

[34] **Limbs in General.** Intense pains along larger nerves.

Sciatica in rheumatic patients; the urinary symptoms agreeing.

[35] **Position, etc.** Motion: lessens pains; increases asthma.

Sitting: 31. Motion: 21, 26. Climbing: 36.

[36] **Nerves.** Weakness, languor.

[38] **Time.** Morning: 20. Night: 21.

[39] **Temperature and Weather.** Damp dwelling: 21.

[40] **Chill. Fever. Sweat.** Rigors, followed by feverish heat through whole body; headache, red face. θ Bright's disease.

Fever, with violent thirst.

Profuse sweat.

[42] **Sides.** Right: 18, 21.

[44] **Tissues.** Dryness, burning of mucous membrane of air-passages.

Dropsy, with kidney affections.

Emaciation.

[48] **Relationship.** *Tereb.* in antidoted by *Phosphor.*

Compare: *Canthar., Copaiva.*

THERIDION CURRASSAVICUM.

Orange Spider.   HERING.   *Araneideæ.*

[1] **Mind.** Time passes too quickly.

Talkative, inclined to mental exertion; hilarity.

Want of self-confidence; hysteria: 36.

Great aversion to work; especially to his usual avvocation.

[2] **Sensorium.** Vertigo: with nausea, even to vomiting; worse from stooping, from least movement; on closing eyes; on board a vessel; with cold sweat.

[3] **Inner Head.** Violent frontal headache, with throbbing, extending to occiput.

Headache, on beginning to move.

Headache which she cannot describe nor even make clear to herself.

Throbbing over left eye and across forehead; sick stomach, worse on rising from lying; worse from persons walking over the floor; from least noise.

Head feels thick, thinks it belongs to another; that she can lift it off.

Sunstroke.

59

⁴ **Outer Head.** Itching on scalp.

⁵ **Eyes.** Flickering before eyes in frequent paroxysms, even when closing the eyes; like a veil before eyes; she must lie down; also in hysteria.

Sensitive to light; things look double; fluttering, nausea and cold hands.

Hard, heavy, dull pressure behind eyes.

⁶ **Ears.** Worse from least noise, every sound penetrates her whole body, especially the teeth, makes vertigo worse.

Rushing in both ears like a water-fall.

Itching behind ears, she would like to scratch them off.

⁷ **Nose.** Sneezing; watery discharge, worse evening.

❙ Chronic catarrh, discharge offensive-smelling, thick, yellow, or yellowish-green.

⁸ **Face.** Pale.

⁹ **Lower Face.** Feels immovable mornings when awaking.

¹¹ **Tongue, etc.** Salty taste; or, mouth feels furred, benumbed.

¹² **Mouth.** Feels numb; or, slimy.

¹⁴ **Desires. Aversions.** Desire for wine, brandy or tobacco.

Appetite for acidulous drinks.

Constant desire for food or drink, but he knows not for what.

Much thirst.

¹⁶ **Nausea and Vomiting,** Nausea: on rising in morning; from sounds; with vertigo; on closing eyes; like sea-sickness; from sparkling before eyes; on motion; from talking; from fast riding in a carriage.

¹⁸ **Hypochondria.** Violent burning pain in hepatic region, worse from touch; retching, bilious vomit.

❙ Abscess of liver; relieves vertigo and nausea.

¹⁹ **Abdomen.** Pain in groins; after coitus; in groin on motion.

²⁰ **Stool, etc.** Small soft stool, daily, with much straining.

²¹ **Urine.** Increased urination.

Seminal emission during siesta.

²² **Male Sexual Organs.** Desire lessened.

²³ **Female Sexual Organs.** Hysteria: during puberty; at climaxis.

²⁶ **Breathing.** Increased inclination to take deep breaths, to sigh.

²⁸ **Lungs.** Violent stitches up high in chest beneath left shoulder through into throat.

❙ Phthisis florida, in beginning.

²⁹ **Heart. Pulse.** Anxiety about heart; sharp pains radiate to arm and left shoulder. θ Climaxis.

Pulse slow, with vertigo.

³³ **Lower Limbs.** Itching and nodes on nates.

Feet swell.

³⁵ **Position, etc,** Motion: 2, 3, 16, 19. Exertion: 36. Walk-

ing: 40. Must lie down: 5. Stooping: 2. Rising: 3, 16.

³⁶ **Nerves.** Weak, limbs tremble, sweating.

Faints after every exertion.

³⁷ **Sleep.** Sleepy all morning.

Deep night sleep

During sleep, bites point of tongue.

³⁸ **Time.** Morning: 9, 16, 37. Evening: 7. Night: 39.

³⁹ **Temperature and Weather.** Sun: 3. Cannot get warm: 40.

⁴⁰ **Chill. Fever. Sweat.** Shaking chill: with foam at mouth; during headache, with vomiting.

Bones pain, as if they would fall asunder: coldness, cannot get warm.

Sweats easily, after walking.

⁴² **Sides.** Right: 18. Left: 3, 28, 29.

⁴⁴ **Tissues.** ‖Scrofula when other remedies fail: rachitis, caries, necrosis, "to reach the root of the evil and destroy cause."

⁴⁵ **Contact, Injuries, etc.** Touch: 18. Jar of persons walking on floor: 3. Motion of vessel: 2. Riding in a carriage: 16.

⁴⁶ **Skin.** Skin: 4, 6, 33.

⁴⁸ **Relationship.** *Therid.* follows well after *Calcar.* and *Lycop.*

Antidotes to *Therid.*: *Acon.* against sensitiveness to noises and violent paroxysms; *Moschus*, nausea; *Graphit.*

THUJA.

Arbor vitæ.　　　　　HAHNEMANN.　　　　　*Coniferæ.*

¹ **Mind.** Cannot think, talks slowly, as if hunting for words; uses wrong words.

Fixed ideas: as if a strange person was at his side; as if soul and body were separated; as if made of glass; as if a living animal were in abdomen.

Insane women will not be touched or approached.

Hurried, with ill-humor; talks hastily.

Disinclined to talk, worse on awaking mornings.

Feels as if she cannot exist any longer; quiet, shunning everybody.

Extremely scrupulous about least thing.

Dissatisfied, quarrelsome; overexcited, angry at trifles.

Music causes weeping, and trembling of feet.

² **Sensorium.** Vertigo: with eyes shut, ceases on opening

them; when rising from sitting; on stooping; looking upward or sideways.

³ Inner Head. Tearing in forehead, temples and occiput; worse at night.

❙ Pain in left frontal eminence as from a nail.

Pressing in vertex, as from a nail; worse afternoon and from 3 to 4 A.M.; better in motion and after sweat.

Boring through temples.

Headaches worse from sexual excesses; overheating; better from exercise in open air, looking upward and turn-in the head backward.

Headache worse from tea.

⁴ Outer Head. Scalp sensitive to touch or pressure of pillow; better if rubbed; violent burning, tearing, stitching pains, worse in warm bed.

Eruption moist, corroding on occiput and temples; worse from touch, better from rubbing.

White, scaly dandruff; hair dry and falling out.

Sweat smelling like honey, mostly on uncovered parts.

Wants head and face warmly wrapped.

⁵ Eyes. Flames of light, mostly yellow; looking into light of day, sees spots like bottles of water moving.

Amblyopia; blurred sight better from rubbing; aching back into the head.

Acts prominently on the sclerotica; useful in episcleritis, sclero-choroiditis anterior, and commencing scleral staphyloma.

❙ Iritis, with condylomata on the iris; sharp sticking in the eye with much heat above and around the eye.

Better when eyes are warmly covered; if uncovered, feels as if a cold stream of air was blowing out through them; but sometimes a dull aching in the eye is relieved in the open air.

Granular lids, when granules are large, wart-like.

❙ Chronic conjunctivitis, worse whenever his night's rest is disturbed.

❙ Dry, bran-like tinea ciliaris; lashes imperfect and irregular.

Inflammatory softening of inner surface of lids.

❙ Excellent for tarsal tumors.

⁶ Ears. Inner ear feels swollen, with increased hardness of hearing.

Noise in ear as from boiling water.

Stitches from neck into ear.

❙ Watery, purulent otorrhœa, smelling like putrid meat.

⁷ Nose. Smell in nose as of fish-brine.

Coryza fluent out-doors, dry in the room.

Blows out much thick, green mucus, mixed with blood

and pus; later brown scabs form; nose sore; red crup-
tion on the alæ, often moist; the latter worse from excesses.

Painful scabs in nostrils.

⁸ **Face.**   Red and hot, netted with veins; circumscribed burning, red cheeks; bloated, dropsical, erysipelatous.

Skin hot and red, peels off when washed.

Eruption leaves livid spots.

Faceache, from left malar to ear, teeth, nose and head;
painful spots burn like fire, and are sensitive to the
sun; also, after checked eruption.

❚ Boring in left malar bone, relieved by touch.

Skin of the face greasy.

⁹ **Lower Face.**   Lips pale, swollen, peeling off.

White, flat ulcers on inside of lips and in corners of mouth.

¹⁰ **Teeth.**   Decay at roots (as in sycosis), the crown remaining
sound; crumble, turn yellow.

Toothache from tea; also when better from cold water and
worse in warm room.

Gums swollen, inflammed, dark red in streaks; with white
suppurating margins.

¹¹ **Tongue, etc.**   Taste: sweet; of putrid eggs, morning; food
seems not salt enough; of bread, as if dry and bitter.

Tongue swollen, worse right side.

Bites the tongue frequently.

❚ Ranula bluish, surrounded by varicose veins; jelly-like
or grey.

¹² **Mouth.**   ❚ Aphthæ; ulcers in the mouth.

¹³ **Throat.**   Feels raw, dry, as if from a plug, or as if constricted when swallowing.

Much mucus in throat, hawked up with difficulty.

Swallowing painful, especially of saliva.

Mucous tubercles in the fauces.

¹⁴ **Desires.   Aversions.**   Craving alternates with want of
appetite.

Thirst, especially at night; longs for cold food and drink.

¹⁵ **Eating and Drinking.**   While eating: 16. After breakfast:
20.   Drinking: 17; cold water: 28   Eating or drinking cold things: 27.   Tea: 10, 48,   Coffee: 20.   Fat
food: 20.   Onions: 20.

¹⁶ **Nausea and Vomiting.**   Eructations: rancid, or acrid; of
air, while eating.

Vomiting of mucus, or of greasy substances.

¹⁷ **Stomach.**   The fluid he drinks falls audibly into stomach.

Pit of stomach swollen; sensitive.

❚ Indurations in the stomach.

¹⁸ **Hypochondria.**   Stitches in hypochondria, now right, then
left.

[19] **Abdomen.** While sitting, stitching in abdomen, as from needles.

Upper part of abdomen drawn in.

Flatulence, as if an animal were crying in abdomen.

Abdomen big, puffed; protrudes here and there, as from the arm of a fœtus; motions therein, as if it contained something alive (in old maids).

Ileus; spasmodic stricture, as if something alive was pushing out.

Soreness of the navel.

Painful swelling of inguinal glands.

[20] **Stool, etc.** Stool: pale; yellow, watery, expelled forcibly, with much noisy flatus, with blood; oily or greasy; gurgling, like water from a bung-hole.

Diarrhœa: daily after breakfast; after vaccination; fat food; onions; or coffee.

Ineffectual urging, with erections.

Stool in hard balls; obstinate constipation, from inactivity or intussusception.

Hemorrhoids: during stool pains are so great she has to desist; burning violently while walking; anus fissured; sensitive to touch; often with warts.

Abrasions of the anus; oozing of fluid from the anus.

[21] **Urine.** Kidneys inflamed; feet swollen.

Stitches from rectum to bladder.

Bladder feels paralyzed; has no power to expel urine.

Frequent urging, with profuse flow, more toward and in the evening; with stitches in urethra.

Involuntary urination at night, or when coughing.

After urinating, feels as if a drop were running down urethra.

Continued urging; passes a few drops of blood.

Wants to pass water, but feels as if a tape prevented.

Urine: too frequent and too copious; contains sugar, foams; dark red in the morning; deposits a brown mucus; with dark, cloudy sediment, in rheumatism.

Burning, smarting in urethra.

[22] **Male Sexual Organs.** Nightly painful erections, causing sleeplessness.

Round, unclean, elevated ulcers, surrounded with redness; moist, painful.

❙Chancres, with pains, as from a splinter sticking.

❙Gonorrhœa: scalding, when urinating, urethra swollen; urinal stream forked; discharge yellow, green, watery; often with warts; with red erosions on the glans.

❙Checked gonorrhœa, causing: articular rheumatism; prostatitis; sycosis; impotence.

Swelling of the prepuce.

❙Sycotic, moist excrescences on prepuce and glans.

Left testicle drawn up.

Aching in testes, as if contused, worse when walking.

Sweetish-smelling sweat on the scrotum.

²³ **Female Sexual Organs.** Embrace prevented by extreme sensitiveness of vagina.

Menses too short and too early ; preceded by profuse sweat.

Erosions at the os uteri, like aphthæ. Mucous leucorrhœa.

❙Cauliflower excrescences, bleeding easily, and offensive.

❙Left ovary inflamed, worse at each menstrual nisus ; distressing pain, burning when walking or riding ; must lie down.

Pains in vulva and perineum ; cramp when rising from a seat ; erysipelas vulvæ.

❙Condylomata, moist, suppurating, stinging and bleeding.

❙Erectile tumors, with burning.

²⁴ **Pregnancy.** Child moves so violently it awakens her, and causes cutting in bladder, with urging to urinate ; pains in left sacro-iliac articulation, running into groin.

❙Abortion, at the third month.

Labor-pains weak and ceasing.

²⁵ **Larynx.** Sensation as of a skin in larynx.

²⁶ **Breathing.** Short-breathed : from mucus in the trachea ; from fulness and constriction in hypochondria and upper abdomen.

Asthma worse at night, with red face ; coughing spells or sensation of adhesion of the lungs.

²⁷ **Cough.** Evenings, after lying down, sputum is loose and easier when he turns from the left to the right side ; only during the day, or in the morning after rising ; as soon as he eats or drinks anything cold.

Sputa : green, taste like old cheese.

²⁸ **Lungs.** Spasm of lungs from drinking cold water.

Stitches in chest from drinking anything cold.

²⁹ **Heart. Pulse.** Palpitation : periodical, in rest or motion ; from ascending ; anxious, when awaking, mornings ; audible, with violent congestion to the chest.

Violent pulsations in evening.

Pulse full, accelerated, evening ; slow and weak, morning.

³⁰ **Outer Chest.** Skin on clavicles blue.

³¹ **Neck. Back.** Cervical glands swollen.

Skin on neck brown, greasy.

Burning from small of back to between scapulæ.

Pulsating in the back.

❙Spine curved, stands bent forward ; pot-bellied.

Cramp-like pain in lumbar region after long standing ; when attempting to walk, feels as if he would fall.

³² **Upper Limbs.** Herpes on the elbow.

Finger-tips: erysipelatous, with tingling; numb and cold, as if dead.

³³ **Lower Limbs.** Hip-joint feels relaxed, when walking, leg feels as if made of wood.

Hip aches, leg becomes elongated.

Tips of toes red and swollen.

Fetid sweat on toes.

Suppressed foot-sweat.

Nets of veins, as if marbled, on soles of feet.

³⁴ **Limbs in General.** Stitches in limbs and joints.

Joints crack when limb is stretched.

❙ Nails crippled, brittle, or soft.

Rheumatism, with numb feeling; worse in warmth, from moving at night, after 12 P.M.; better from cold and after sweating.

³⁵ **Position, etc.** ˎMotion: 3, 29, 34. Exercise: 3. Walking: 20, 22, 23, 31, 35, 40. Ascending: 29. Rising: 23, 27. Stands bent forward: 31. Stooping: 2. Long standing: 31. Looking upward or sideways: 2, 3. Turning head backward: 3. Limb stretched; 34. Lying: 27; on left side: 37. Turning from left to right side: 17. Must lie down: 23. Parts lain on: 37. Sitting: 19. Rest: 5, 29.

³⁶ **Nerves.** Limbs go to sleep.

Sensation of lightness of body when walking.

Paralysis of one side.

❙ Jerks of the upper part of the body. *θ* Chorea.

Debility worse mornings.

Nervous symptoms accompany or depend upon affections of skin or mucous membranes; hence, neuralgia from checked eruptions; from suppressed gonorrhœa, etc. See 48.

³⁷ **Sleep.** Heavy, cannot get awake mornings.

Sleeplessness: sees apparitions on closing the eyes; parts lain on painful; from heat and restlessness; from mental depression.

Dreams anxious when sleeping on left side.

³⁸ **Time.** Morning: 1, 11, 20, 27, 28, 36, 37, 40. Afternoon.: 3, 40. Evening: 21, 27, 29, 40. Night: 3, 5, 14, 21, 22, 26, 33. After midnight: 34, 40. 3 to 4 A.M.: 3. Day: 5, 27.

³⁹ **Temperature and Weather.** Sun: 8. Warmth: 34, 37. Warm wraps: 4, 5. Warm bed: 4. Room: 7. Covered parts: 40, 46. Uncovered parts: 4, 5, 40. Out-doors: 7. Open air: 3, 5. Cold: 34. Washing: 8.

⁴⁰ **Chill. Fever. Sweat.** Chill: in attacks, mostly evenings; on left side, which feels cold to the touch; after 12 P.M. and in the morning, without thirst; internal, with external heat and violent thirst; then sweat.

Heat: mornings, chills afternoons; evenings, mostly in face; dry, of covered parts; burning, in the face, without redness.

Sweat: only on covered parts; general, except the head; when walking in the morning, mostly on the head; during sleep, stops when he awakens; oily, fetid, smelling sweat.

⁴¹ Attacks. Periodically: 29. Third month: 24.

⁴² Sides. Left: 3, 8, 22, 23, 24, 29, 40. Right: 11. Right to left: 18.

⁴⁴ Tissues. Emaciation and deadness of affected parts.
Sycosis.
❙ Affects prominently epithelia, first causing hardening, hypertrophy; then softening.
Indurations; later, softening.
Œdema about the joints.
Flesh feels as if beaten off the bones.

⁴⁵ Contact, Injuries, etc. Touch: 1, 4, 8, 20, 40. Pressure: 4. Rubbing: 4, 5. Scratching: 46. Riding: 23.

⁴⁶ Skin. Looks dirty; brown here and there; brown-white spots.
Pemphigus, painful.
Hair thin, grows slowly, splits.
Zona.
Epithelioma.
Eruptions, only on covered parts, burn violently after scratching.
Bleeding fungous growths.
White, scaly, dry, mealy herpes.
Nævus.
❙ Condylomata; warts, seedy, pediculated; moist, mucous tubercles.
Ulcers flat, with a bluish-white bottom.
Blood-boils on the back.
Small-pox, stage of maturation.
Bad effects of vaccination: emaciation; sleeplessness; diarrhœa; restlessness; trembling; neuralgia; paresis, etc.

⁴⁸ Relationship. *Thuja* follows well after: *Mercur.*, *Nitr. ac.*
Complementary to *Silic.*
Thuja antidotes: abuse of tea; *Mercur.*, *Sulphur*, *Iodium*, *Nux vom.*
Antidotes to *Thuja*: *Chamom.*, for nightly toothache; *Coccul.*, for the fever; also, *Camphor.*, *Mercur.*, *Pulsat.*, *Sulphur.*
Cinnab. is preferable for warts on prepuce.
Compare with *Spigel.*, *Coccinella* (both in tic douleureux).
Asaf. (nervous ailments from checked skin symptoms).
Ant. tart. develops the variola-pustule; *Thuja* dries it up.

TRILLIUM PENDULUM.

Wake Robin. No Proving. *Smilaceæ.*

⁷ **Nose.** Profuse epistaxis, passive.

¹⁰ **Teeth.** Bleeding from cavity after extraction of a tooth.

¹⁷ **Stomach.** Heat and burning in stomach, rising up into œsophagus.

Sinking in stomach, with hemorrhages.

²⁰ **Stool, etc.** Dysentery when discharges are mostly of blood.

²³ **Female Sexual Organs.** Displaced uterus, with consequent menorrhagia; flow profuse.

Gushing of bright red blood from uterus, at the least movement; later, blood pale from anæmia.

Menses often come on after overexertion, too long a ride, etc.; profuse flow.

Leucorrhœa: bloody, with great prostration; yellow, creamy, profuse, between menses.

Climaxis, with weak sight, anxious look; pale; faint; flow returns every two weeks.

²⁴ **Pregnancy.** Threatened abortion; profuse hemorrhage.

Lochia too profuse.

²⁷ **Cough.** Troublesome, copious, purulent sputa; hectic; hæmoptysis.

³¹ **Neck. Back.** Pain in back, with uterine hemorrhages.

³³ **Lower Limbs.** Legs cold, with hemorrhages.

³⁵ **Position, etc.** Motion: 23. Overexertion: 23. Long ride: 23.

⁴¹ **Attacks.** Every two weeks: 23.

⁴⁴ **Tissues.** Hemorrhages usually bright red, profuse; also when sacro-iliac synchondroses feel as if falling apart, wants to be bound tightly.

Feels as if bones were broken; with hemorrhages.

Crowding sensation in the veins like a tightening up of the parts, worse in those of legs and ankles.

URTICA URENS.

Nettle. No Proving. *Urticaceæ.*

¹⁴ **Desires. Aversions.** Loss of appetite; itching of anus; itching of nose; nocturnal restlessness.

²⁰ **Stool, etc.** Dysentery.

Intense itching of anus from worms.

[21] **Urine.** Suppressed; upper body œdematous.

[22] **Male Sexual Organs.** Itching and stinging of scrotum.

[23] **Female Sexual Organs.** Pruritus vulvæ.

[24] **Pregnancy.** Insufficiency, or entire want of secretion of milk after parturition.

Arrests the flow of milk after weaning.

[28] **Lungs.** Hæmoptysis, from violent exertion of lungs.

[32] **Upper Limbs.** Continuous pain in right deltoid.

[35] **Position, etc.** Exertion: 28.

[38] **Time.** Night: 14.

[41] **Attacks.** Symptoms recur annually.

[42] **Sides.** Right: 32.

[43] **Sensations.** Stinging, burning sensations, in any part.

[45] **Contact, Injuries, etc.** Rubbing: 46.

[46] **Skin.** Nettle-rash: itching and burning of the skin as if scorched; raised, red blotches; fine, stinging points; pale and requires constant rubbing.

Burns involving only the skin; intense burning, itching.

Consequences of suppressed urticaria.

USTILAGO.

Corn Smut.   BURT.   *Maidis Fungi.*

[1] **Mind.** Great depression of spirits; irritable.

[2] **Sensorium.** Frequent attacks of vertigo; things whirl before the eyes, are double; or, white specks come into view and blot all else.

[3] **Inner Head.** Feeling of fulness of head, with dull, pressive frontal headache.

Pain on top and side of head; climaxis.

[5] **Eyes.** Twitching of eyes, they seem to revolve in circles and dart from object to object.

[6] **Ears.** Constant dull pain in left ear, caused by extension from inflamed tonsil.

Eyes feel hot on closing lids.

Eyes smart, balls ache; profuse lachrymation.

[8] **Face.** Sudden pallor; evening, while sitting.

[11] **Tongue, etc.** Slimy, coppery taste.

Pricking sensation in tongue, with a feeling as if something was under its root pressing it upward.

[12] **Mouth.** Saliva profuse; bitter.

[13] **Throat.** Dryness of fauces, with difficult degluition; with burning distress in stomach.

Tonsils congested, inflamed; left one very large, dark colored, with dull pain, worse from swallowing.

Feeling as of a lump behind larynx, producing constant desire to swallow.

Sharp, lacinating pain in right tonsil.

Burning in œsophagus at cardiac orifice.

¹⁴ **Desires. Aversions.** Loss of appetite, followed by canine hunger.

¹⁶ **Nausea and Vomiting.** Eructations of food, strongly acid.

¹⁷ **Stomach.** Goneness in epigastrium; climaxis.

Faint feeling, a number of times in epigastrium, with pain in region of liver and bowels.

Burning distress in sternum and stomach, with fine neuralgic pains.

Repeated fine, sharp, cutting pains in epigastrium.

¹⁸ **Hypochondria.** Pain in region of right lobe of liver.

¹⁹ **Abdomen.** Fine, cutting, colicky pains every few minutes; relieved by hard stool, followed by dull pains in bowels.

Pain in left inguinal region while walking.

²⁰ **Stool, etc.** Black, lumpy stools; costive.

²¹ **Urine.** First increased and light, with great desire; later, scanty and dark; hæmatemesis.

²² **Male Sexual Organs.** Erotic fancies; emissions; prostrated, dull, lumbar pains, despondent, irritable.

Seminal emissions, irresistible tendency to masturbation.

²³ **Female Sexual Organs.** Constant aching, referred to the mouth of the womb.

Displaced uterus, with menorrhagia; cervix tumefied; bleeds when touched.

For days oozing of dark blood, with small coagula; uterus enlarged, cervix tumefied or dilated.

Menses scanty, with ovarian irritation.

Bearing down as if everything would come through.

Burning distress in ovaries.

Acute pain worse in left ovary, with swelling; pains intermittent; shoot rapidly down legs.

Menses profuse, frequent coagula.

Between menses constant suffering under left breast, at margin of ribs.

Climaxis: vertigo, metrorrhagia.

²¹ **Pregnancy.** Produces abortion.

Labor pains deficient; os soft, pliable, dilatable.

²⁸ **Lungs.** Sharp tearing in left side from top of chest down to sixth or seventh rib, aggravated by breathing.

²⁹ **Heart. Pulse.** Burning pain in cardiac region.

³⁵ **Position, etc.** Sitting: 8. Walking: 19.

³⁷ **Sleep.** Troubled, tosses about, dreams are troublesome; heat over body.

³⁸ **Time.** Evening: 8. Night: 40.

³⁹ **Temperature and Weather.** In a warm room felt oppressed, faint.

⁴⁰ **Chill· Fever. Sweat.** Internal heat through body, but worse in eyes, which are sensitive to light and sore to touch; pulse normal.

General heat during night after sleep.

⁴¹ **Attacks.** Every few minutes: 19.

⁴² **Sides.** Right: 13, 17, 18. Left: 6, 13, 19, 23, 28, 29. Above downward: 28.

⁴⁵ **Contact, Injuries, etc.** Touch: 23, 40.

VALERIANA.

Valerian.　　　　　　　　Franz.　　　　　　　*Valerianeæ.*

¹ **Mind.** Easy comprehension. Intellect predominates over mind.

Passes quickly from one subject to another.

Intellect confused; replies incoherently.

Erroneous ideas; thinks she is some one else, moves to edge of bed to make room; imagines animals lying near her which she fears she may hurt. *θ* Typhoid fever.

Ecstasy. Thinks himself distinguished.

Mild delirium, with great excitement and trembling. *θ* Typhoid.

Fear, especially evening in dark, palpitation, trembling.

Changeable; hypochondrical anxiety or trembling excitability.

Hysteria, overexcitable, changeable disposition and ideas.

² **Sensorium.** Feels light, as if flying in the air.

Vertigo, when stooping.

Oversensitive.

³ **Inner Head.** Headache appearing suddenly, or in jerks.

Pressing, as from a stupefying constriction in forehead, drawing into orbits; face pale; worse evening, at |rest and in open air; better from movement, in room and when changing position.

One-sided drawing headache from a draft of air.

Headache in sunshine.

Stinging or pressing in forehead, extending to orbits.

⁴ **Outer Head.** Icy-cold sensation in vertex from continuous pressure of the hat.

⁵ **Eyes.** Vivid light like lightning, accompanied by dark spot to the side of the line of vision.

Luminous appearances before eyes in evening in dark. Clearsighted.

Better from light; worse in dark.

Expression of eyes peculiary wild; hysterical neuralgia.

Edges of lids inflamed, with biting, stinging.

[8] **Face.** Cheeks red and hot, especially in open air.

White blisters, with elevated red base, on cheek and upper lip, painful to touch.

Fierce pains through left side of face, darting into teeth and ear; muscles twitch; hysterical neuralgia.

Facial pains, appearing suddenly and in jerks.

Spasmodic twitching and drawing in the cheek-bones.

[9] **Lower Face.** Lips incrusted.

[10] **Teeth.** Stinging pain in teeth.

[11] **Tongue, etc.** Taste as of rancid tallow; greasy.

Tongue thickly coated, foul.

[14] **Desire. Aversions.** Voracious hunger, with nausea.

[15] **Eating and Drinking.** Worse on an empty stomach; better after breakfast.

After dinner: 10. When eating: 40.

[16] **Nause and Vomiting.** Eructations like putrid eggs, morning on waking.

Heart-burn, gulping of a rancid fluid which does not rise into the mouth.

Nausea, with sensation as from a string hanging down throat; profuse ptyalism.

Nauseated, faint; lips white, body icy-cold.

[17] **Stomach.** Pressing, aching in pit of stomach, as from something forcing a passage through it; neuralgia of limbs.

[18] **Hypochondria.** Sudden warm rising from epigastrium, with difficult breathing. θ Hysteria.

[19] **Abdomen.** Distended, hard.

Colic: hysterical, especially evenings in bed; after dinner; from hemorrhoids: from worms.

[20] **Stool, etc.** Discharge of ascarides.

Thin, watery diarrhœa, with lumps of coagulated milk; diarrhœa of children.

Greenish, papescent stool, passing with blood; constant pressing and violent screaming; diarrhœa of children.

[21] **Urine.** Increased and more frequent.

During urination, much straining and prolapsus recti.

Sediment of urine red or white.

[23] **Female Sexual Organs.** Menses too late and scanty.

[24] **Pregnancy.** The child vomits as soon as it nurses; after the mother has been angry.

[26] **Breathing.** Choking in throat-pit on point of falling asleep, she awakens as if suffocating.

Inspirations grow less deep and more rapid until they

cease; then she catches her breath by a sobbing effort; so on in spells. θ Asthma.

²⁸ **Lungs.** Frequent jerks and stitches in chest, with a sensation as if something pressed out; worse in lower part of chest.

²⁹ **Heart. Pulse.** Stitches in region of heart.

Pulse rapid, somewhat tense, or small and weak.

³¹ **Neck. Back.** Spine irritated, in beginning of typhoid fever.

Pain in the loins, as from cold or overlifting.

Bubbling pressure above anus in coccygeal region.

³² **Upper Limbs.** Rheumatic pains in scapulæ.

Darting along the arms, shoulders and face; hysterical neuralgia.

³³ **Lower Limbs.** Pain in hip and thigh, intolerable when standing, as if thigh would break; ischias.

Acute, crampy, tearing pain in posterior muscles, especially those of calf, better in morning and when rubbing affected part; worse toward evening and when quiet.

³⁴ **Limbs in General.** Rheumatic pains in limbs, rarely in joints; worse during rest after previous exertion; better from movement.

Arms and legs move normally, but when at rest, jerk and twitch. θ Hysteria.

³⁵ **Position, etc.** Motion: 3, 34. Exertion: 34, 40. Changing position: 3. Stooping: 2. Rest: 3, 34. Standing: 33.

³⁶ **Nerves.** Agitation of all nerves, jerks, twitches, trembling.

³⁷ **Sleep.** Sleepless, restless tossing; nightly itching, muscular spasms.

Cannot sleep before 12 P.M.

Worse on awaking.

³⁸ **Time.** Morning: 16. Evening: 1, 2, 3, 5, 19, 40. Night: 37, 40. Before midnight: 37.

³⁹ **Temperature and Weather.** Room: 3. In bed: 19. Sun: 3. Open air: 3, 8. Draught: 3.

⁴⁰ **Chill. Fever. Sweat.** Chill: of short duration; followed by long-lasting heat, with dulness of head and thirst; begins in neck and runs down the back. Fainting during cold stage.

Long-lasting heat, often with sweat on the face. Heat predominates.

Increased heat evenings, and when eating.

In evening, spells of fugitive heat, with thirst; no shivering; with the neuralgia of limbs.

Sweat profuse, worse at night or from exertion, with violent heat.

Frequent and suddenly ceasing attacks of sweat, mostly on forehead.

Better after sweat.
[41] **Attacks.** Sudden: 3, 40. Frequent: 40.
[42] **Sides.** Right to left: neuralgia of legs. Left: 8, 29. Above downward: 40.
[44] **Tissues.** Red parts become white.
[45] **Contact, Injuries, etc.** Better from rubbing; neuralgia of limbs.
  Decubitus soon. θ Typhoid.
  Slight wounds cause spasms.
  Touch: 8. Pressure: 4.
[46] **Skin.** Painful eruptions.
  White miliaria on chest and back. θ Typhoid.
  Skin too dry and warm; hysterical neuralgia.
[47] **Stages and States.** Nervous, irritable, hysterical.
[48] **Relationship.** *Valer.* useful after abuse of chamomile tea.
  Antidotes to *Valer.*: *Camphor., Coffea, Pulsat.*

VERATRUM ALBUM.

White Hellebore.   HAHNEMANN.   *Melanthaceæ.*

[1] **Mind.** Stupid from excess in alcoholic drinks.
  Never speaks the truth; does not know herself what she is saying.
  Thinks himself distinguished; squanders his money.
  Delirium, heavy, soporous sleep; restless, thirsty, cramps in legs, cold sweat, tingling; irregular pulse. θ Cerebro-spinal meningitis.
  Mania: with desire to cut and tear, especially clothes; with lewdness and lascivious talk.
  Loquacity, he talks rapidly.
  Talks much about religious things; praying.
  Disposed to talk about faults of others, or silent; but if irritated, scolding, calling names.
  Kissing everybody; before menses.
  Impudent behavior in childbed.
  Curses all night and complains of stupid feeling, with headache and ptyalism.
  Dislikes to talk, except in delirium.
  Cannot bear to be left alone.
  Fearfulness; starts; with running about and shouting.
  Anxious, restless, easily frightened, whining, weeping, apathetic delirium, blue face. θ Typhoid.
  Anxiety, as after committing an evil deed, worse evening and after dinner.

Despair about his position in society; feels very unlucky.

Despair of her salvation; with suppressed catamenia.

After fright: fear, anxiety; coldness; fainting; involuntary diarrhœa.

Consequences of injured pride or honor.

² **Sensorium.** Vertigo; with cold sweat on forehead; with loss of vision, sudden fainting; from opium eating; from abuse of tobacco or alcohol.

Heaviness of the head, things seem to whirl in a circle. θ Typhoid.

Faints from least exertion; from slight wounds; from violent pains; after loss of fluids; anxiety, nausea, convulsive twitchings.

³ **Inner Head.** Paroxysms in various parts of brain, partly as if bruised, partly pressure.

Burning in brain.

Neuralgia of head with indigestion; features sunken.

Head hot and covered with sweat; headache; children rub the head, cannot bear to be left alone; put hands to head. θ Typhoid.

Headache: nausea, vomiting, pale face; stiff neck, profuse micturition; as if brain was torn to pieces; chronic, coming on in afternoon, lasting through night; drawing in both arms; better towards morning; frequent micturition.

Violent pains drive to despair; or, great prostration with headache; fainting, with cold sweat and great thirst; nausea, vomiting and diarrhœa; or, obstinate constipatiou.

⁴ **Outer Head.** Head burning hot; limbs alternately hot and cold.

Scalp very sensitive, with headache.

Like a piece of ice on head; or, sensation of warmth and coldness at the same time on scalp, the hair being sensitive.

Plica polonica.

Cold sweat on forehead, with many complaints.

Compelled to rub forehead, with a kind of insensibility. θ Typhoid.

⁵ **Eyes.** Black motes or specks before eyes, with diplopia; photophobia; worse on rising from bed or chair.

Hemeralopia.

Eyes: turned upward, showing only whites; distorted, protruding; fixed, watery, sunken, lustreless; full of tears; lids livid, blue edges.

Pupils: contracted; dilated, with weak sight; fails to recognize those near, or does so but slowly.

Tearing pains in eyes, depriving one of sleep; worse in cold, damp weather. θ Rheumatic ophthalmia.

Excessive dryness of lids.

Lids: heavy, can scarcely lift them; trembling.

Profuse lachrymations and cutting pains, with feeling of dryness and heat.

⁶ **Ears.** Deaf, as if ears were stopped, one or both.

⁷ **Nose.** Smell before the nose as from manure, or from smoke.

Nose: grows more pointed, seems longer; face cold; icy-cold; mouth cold.

Epistaxis: right sided, only at night in sleep; face deathly pale, body cold; pulse slow, intermittent.

Boring in the nose.

Nose inside feels too dry.

⁸ **Face.** Restless, wild look; pale, distorted face.

Blue or green circles around eyes.

Face: collapsed, pale, bluish; nose more pointed; of leaden hue; red in bed, becomes pale on rising; alternately pale and red.

Neuralgia; drawing, tearing pains, with bluish, pale face, sunken eyes; prostration.

Tearing in cheeks, temples and eyes, with heat and redness, driving to madness; worse in damp weather; right side; especially in anæmic persons.

Spasms of muscles when masticating.

Lock-jaw.

Risus sardonicus.

⁹ **Lower Face.** Lips: bluish or hanging down; rubbing the mouth and nose; dry, black, parched.

Black around mouth and nostrils. *θ* Typhoid.

¹⁰ **Teeth.** Violent toothache, throbbing; face swollen, cold sweat on forehead.

Toothache drives to madness, nervous, excitable persons.

Teeth heavy, as if filled with lead.

Grinding teeth.

¹¹ **Tongue, etc.** Taste: bitter; as from peppermint; flat or sweetish; putrid.

Tongue: cold, withered; swollen, dry, cracked and too red; white, with red tip and edges; coated yellowish-brown; back part black.

Speech lisping, stammering; or as if tongue was too heavy. *θ* Typhoid.

¹² **Mouth.** Froth at the mouth; spasms.

Mouth dry; saliva lessened.

Burning in mouth and throat.

Constant flow of saliva, like water-brash.

¹³ **Throat.** Dryness in throat, which cannot be removed by drinking.

Scraping or roughness in throat.

Sensation of dust in throat.

Sensation of constriction of throat.

Chronic catarrh of œsophagus.

Feeling of distention in pharynx.

[14] **Desires. Aversions.** Craves fruit, juicy food; or saltish things.

Appetite voracious; after typhoid : 40.

Hunger and appetite between paroxymsms of vomiting.

Much thirst, drinks frequently, but only a little at a time.

Thirst for the coldest drinks; wants everything cold; often during pregnancy.

Aversion to warm things.

Appetite diminished, mouth as if lined with mucus; flat or sweetish taste.

[15] **Eating and Drinking.** After dinner: 1. Eating: 19. Warm food: 18. Fruit: 20. Eating and drinking cold things: 27. Drinking: 13, 14, 16, 40. Alcoholic drinks: 1, 2. Opium eating: 2. Tobacco: 2.

[16] **Nausea and Vomiting.** Bitter eructations.

Hiccough, after hot drinks.

Nausea : with sensation of fainting, generally with violent thirst.

Vomiting: violent, with continuous nausea and great prostration; of thin, blackish or yellowish substances; of bile and blood, black; of food and drink, or drink only ; of food, or of acid, bitter, foamy; white or yellow-ish-green mucus; whenever he moves, or drinks; with vertigo, pale face, clean tongue, good appetite, hiccough, fainting.

Painful retraction of obdomen during vomiting.

[17] **Stomach.** Anguish in pit of stomach.

Pains coming gradually, first in epigastrium, then radiating upward and to both sides, reaching to back between lowest point of scapula: becomes agonizing, then gradually subsides; shakes with cold. θ Gastrodynia.

Gastric catarrh, great weakness, cold, sudden sinking.

Hæmatemesis, with slow pulse, coldness, fainting fits, cold sweat; nausea when moving or rising.

Chronic weakness of stomach: from dampness of climate and want of fresh air; from abuse of quinine.

[18] **Hypochondria.** Hyperæmia of liver, with gastric catarrh, putrid taste, disgust for warm food, great pressure in hepatic region, alternating with vomiting and diarrhœa.

Spleen swollen. θ Intermittents.

Spasm of diaphragm during prevailing south winds, in persons with cold hands, great oppression and anxiety in chest.

Diaphragmitis, with peritonitis, vomiting, coldness.

[19] **Abdomen.** Burning in abdomen as from hot coals.

Colic: after a cold; after abuse of quinine; from fruits
and vegetables; abdomen swollen, sensitive; no flatus
either way; cold sweat; with burning pain, twisting,
cutting, with nausea and vomiting, worse from food;
better after wind passes.

Peritonitis, with vomiting and diarrhœa, skin cold;
features sunken; pulse small, weak; restless, anxious.

Great sinking and empty feeling.

Intussusception of bowels; great anguish; rushes about
bent double, pressing the abdomen.

Cold feeling in abdomen.

Abdomen distended, very sensitive; colic.

Incarcerated hernia, not inflamed; anti-peristaltic action.

Cold sweat.

Protrusion of inguinal hernia during cough.

Cured a case of abdominal complaint going from left to
right.

²⁰ Stool, etc. Intestinal catarrh, coming on suddenly at night,
in Summer; vomiting and purging.

Stools: watery, greenish, mixed with flakes; gushing,
profuse, rice-water discharges, with tonic cramps, commencing in hands and feet, spreading all over; sunken,
even hippocratic face; Cholera Asiatica; watery, inodorous; watery, gushing, flaky; thin, papescent, mucous;
green, gushing, exhausting, after fright; involuntary.

Unconscious discharge of thin feces when passing flatus.

Cholera morbus, worse at night; cold sweat on forehead;
vomiting and purging at same time; after fruits.

Constipation: chronic stools, large and hard; or, first part
large, latter part smaller; stools in round, black balls;
chronic, with children; as from inactivity of rectum.

Hemorrhoids, with disease of lungs, or pleura.

Painless discharge of masses of blood in clots, with sinking
feeling.

²¹ Urine. Continuous urging to urinate.

Frequent micturition with violent thirst and hunger.

Urine: scanty, red-brown, or suppressed; greenish.

Involuntary urination; during cough, also during typhoid.

²³ Female Sexual Organs. Nymphomania of lying-in women;
also before menses.

Metritis, with fits of vomiting, delirium, anxiety; vomiting
and diarrhœa; body hot, limbs cold.

Menses: too early, too profuse; suppressed, with despair of
salvation, or with blood-spitting.

Amenorrhœa, with nervous headache, leaden face, nausea,
vomiting and diarrhœa.

Dysmenorrhœa, with prolapsus; vomiting, diarrhœa, exhaustion.

Strangulated prolapsed vagina, with cold sweat, exhausting vomiting and diarrhœa.

[24] **Pregnancy.** Abortion threatened; pains, with cold sweat, nausea, vomiting.

During pregnancy: wants to wander about house; taciturn; haughty; thirst; vomiting.

Labor-pains exhaust her; fainting on least motion.

Lochia suppressed, with nymphomania.

Eclampsia parturientium; pallor, collapse, anæmia, or violent cerebral congestion, with bluish, bloated face, wild shrieks, tearing the clothing.

Puerperal mania, wants to kiss every one.

[25] **Larynx.** Spasmus glottidis.

Paroxysms of constriction of larynx, suffocative fits, with protruded eyes.

Debility great, catarhal symptoms slight; influenza during cholera seasons.

Hollow, hoarse voice.

[26] **Breathing.** Dyspnœa. Oppression.

Contractive spasm of chest.

Asthma in damp, cold weather; in early morning; better throwing head back; inclination for motion; cold sweat of upper part of body; worse from cold drinks.

[27] **Cough.** Dry, tickling, after walking in sharp, cold air; dry, spasmodic, rattling, but nothing loosens; deep, hollow, ringing, whooping, excited by tickling in lowest branches of bronchi, expectoration of yellow, tough, tenacious mucus of bitter, saltish, sour, or putrid taste; spasmodic; cyanosis, cold sweat; blood-spitting; after great exertion; loud barking, in hysteria; worse morning and late evening until 12 P.M.; going into warm room; getting warm in bed; change of weather; eating and drinking cold things, especially water; crying (children); vexation.

Convulsive stage of whooping-cough.

Epidemic whoop-cough, worse Spring or Autumn.

[28] **Lungs.** Constant rattling of mucus, but cannot expectorate; sticky sweat about head; weak; frequent irregular pulse; bronchitis of the aged.

Capillary bronchitis.

Acute bronchial catarrh, in the emphysematous.

Rattling in lungs, fear of suffocation; frothy, serous sputa; blue face; œdema of lungs.

Stitches in sides of chest.

[29] **Heart. Pulse.** Strong palpitation of heart, with chorea.

Violent, visible, anxious palpitation, with fainting.

Tumultuous, irregular contractions of heart, forerunners of paralysis.

Intermittent action of heart in feeble persons, with some obstruction to hepatic circulation.

Palpitation in the anæmic; agony of death, legs cold; difficult breathing, better at rest or lying down.

Pulse: frequent, small, hard; slow, soft, intermittent; sometimes slower than heart-beat.

[31] **Neck. Back.** Neck so weak, child can scarcely keep it erect, especially in whooping-cough.

Tingling in fingers, causing anxiety and painful jerks of limbs.

During exercise, rheumatic pain between scapulæ from nape to small of back; worse going to stool.

Bruised feeling in sacral region.

[32] **Upper Limbs.** Neuralgia in brachial plexus, as if beaten or bruised.

Arms: feel cold when raising them; feel as if too full and swollen.

Paralytic and bruising pain in arms.

Arm trembles, when anything is grasped.

Tingling in hands and fingers, causing anxiety.

Hands icy-cold, blue.

[33] **Lower Limbs.** Difficult walking; first right, then left hip-joint feels paralytic.

Shocks in right hip.

Electric jerks in limbs; worse in bed, must sit up and let legs hang out of bed; must walk about. *θ* Rheumatism.

Pains in feet, especially the knees, as if heavy stones were tied to the parts; must move about for relief.

Limbs: stiff in forenoon and while standing; rheumatism; alternately hot and cold, head hot; cold.

Cramps in the calves.

Sudden swelling of the feet.

Feet icy-cold.

[34] **Limbs in General.** Painful paralytic weakness in upper and lower limbs.

Limbs go to sleep, also when lying down.

❙ Pains in limbs resembling a bruise, worse during wet, cold weather; worse in warmth of bed; better when walking up and down.

[35] **Position, etc.** Children are easier when carried about quickly.

Must walk about during pains: 33, 34. Walking: 27, 33, 34. Rushes about bent double: 19. Wanders about house: 24. Motion: 16, 17, 24, 26. Exertion: 2, 27. Grasping anything: 32. Raising arms: 32. Standing: 33. Must sit up: 33. Sitting: 37. Rising: 5, 8, 17, 36. At rest: 29. Lying down: 29, 34. Must lie down: 36. Arms stretched above head: 37.

[36] **Nerves.** Trembling, jerking.

Puerperal convulsions: 24.

Convulsions caused by religious excitement; also of children; anxiety, pale face, cold sweat on forehead; cough before or after spasm; sometimes syncope after spasm.

Tonic spasms, with contraction of spasms of hands and soles of feet.

Cramps, with profuse alvine discharges; 48.

Excessive weakness; also after abuse of *Cinchon.*

Child feeble, with a sort of hectic; whooping-cough.

Paralysis: after cholera; from debilitating losses.

Must lie down; anguish, cold sweat on forehead when he rises.

Sudden sinking of strength.

[37] **Sleep.** Sleepiness.

Uninterrupted sleep for three days. θ Typhoid.

Drowsy, starts as if frightened, preventing sleep; fever follows.

Arms stretched above head, moaning, during sleep.

Nightly anxiety and sleeplessness.

Dreams: of being drowned; of being bitten by a dog and cannot escape; of being hunted; of robbers, with frightened awakening and a fixed idea that the dream is true.

[38] **Time.**   Morning: 3, 26, 27, 40.   Forenoon: 33.   Afternoon: 3.   4–5 P.M.: 19.   Evening: 1, 27, 40.   Night: 1, 3, 5, 7, 20, 40.   Before midnight: 27.

[39] **Temperature and Weather.** Hot summer weather: 20, 46. South winds: 18.   Warmth of bed: 27, 33, 34.   Warm room: 27.   Spring and Autumn: 27.   Fresh air: 17. Every draught of air aggravates.   Change of weather: 27.   Cold, sharp air: 27.   Cold, damp weather: 5, 8, 17, 26, 34.   Aversion to being covered.

[40] **Chill. Fever. Sweat.** Chill and coldness: mostly external, with internal heat, and cold, clammy sweat; running downward; shaking chill with sweat, which soon passes off into general coldness.

Chill increased by drinking; lessened after getting out of bed.

Whole body icy-cold.

Chill of nursing children.

Chill and heat alternating, now here, again there, on single parts.   •

Heat: mostly internal, with thirst but no desire to drink; in the evening, with sweat; ascends.

Profuse sweat, morning, evening, or all night; also with every stool.

Sweat cold, clammy; offensive; bitter-smelling; or staining yellow; but always with deathly pale face.

General cold sweat, worse on forehead.

Intermittent types often pernicious during cholera; also after abuse of quinine.

Rheumatic fever, with profuse sweat, great weakness and diarrhœa.

Typhoid forms of fever, especially in cholera seasons; also when vital forces suddenly sink.

⁴¹ **Attacks.** Coming and increasing gradually: 17. Suddenly in Summer: 20. Spring and Autumn: 2. Last three days: 37.

⁴² **Sides.** Right: 7, 8, 18, 33. Left: 18, 19, 29. ▌Right to left: 33. Left to right: 8. Above downward: 40. Below upward: 40.

⁴⁴ **Tissues.** Skin and muscles lax.

Anæmia of the skin.

Pyæmia.

Anasarca: vomiting, purging, great prostration.

⁴⁵ **Contact, Injuries, etc.** Rubbing: 3, 4, 9. Pressure: 19, 46. Slight wounds: 2.

⁴⁶ **Skin.** Wrinkled skin; skin remains in folds after pressure.

Skin blue, purple, cold.

Rash over body, or on face and hands.

Dry eruptions like itch.

Desquamation of indurated or thickened portion of skin.

Erysipelas.

Measles tardy and pale; skin often livid; hemorrhages, but no relief; drowsy; weak; cold; thready pulse; also for spasmodic cough and vomiturition.

Scarlatina in hot, summer weather; eruption bluish; pulse • feeble; burning heat of limbs alternating with coldness.

⁴⁷ **Stages and States.** Children.

Anæmia.

Lean, choleric or melancholy persons.

⁴⁸ **Relationship.** *Veratr.* is frequently indicated after *Arsen.*, *Cinchon.*, *Cuprum*, *Ipec.*, *Phosph. ac.*

After *Veratr.* are frequently indicated: *Arsen, Arnic.*, *Cinchon, Cuprum, Ipec.*

Similar to: *Cuprum* (but latter has cough, better drinking, cramps, with scanty discharges); *Bryon.* (constipation); *Jatr. curc.* (vomit of albuminous matter; spurting, watery diarrhœa; abdomen and calves flattened by cramp); *Ric. comm.* (cholera-collapse, vomiting and purging still continuing).

Veratr. may be indicated: in stupefaction from alcohol; after abuse of *Cinchon.;* in colic from copper; bad effects from opium eating; or, from tobacco.

Veratr. antidotes: *Arsen.*, *Cinchon.*, *Ferrum.*

Antidotes to *Veratr.: Acon.*, *Camphor.*, *Cinchon.*, *Coffea.*

VERATRUM VIRIDE.

Green Hellebore.   BURT.   *Melanthaceæ.*

[1] **Mind.** Stupefaction; congestion.

Mental confusion, loss of memory; vertigo; cerebral hyperæmia.

Insanity from cerebral congestion.

Puerperal mania; silent, suspicious; will not see her physician, he seems to terrify her; fears being poisoned; sleepless, can hardly be kept in her bedroom.

Depression of spirits.

[3] **Inner Head.** Headache from nape of neck, with vertigo, dim vision, dilated pupils.

Congestion to head: from high living, abuse of stimulants; during dentition.

Fulness in head, throbbing arteries; increased sensitiveness to sounds; buzzing in the ears; double or partial vision. θ Sunstroke.

Meningitis, high fever, intense congestion, later rolling of head; vomiting; or, face haggard, cold, and pulse slow; breathing labored.

[4] **Outer Head.** Severe frontal headache, with vomiting.

[5] **Eyes.** Dimness of vision, with dilated pupils.

Green circles around the candle, which turn to red.

Traumatic erysipelas of eyelids.

Twitching, contortion of eyes, rolling of eyeballs; paralysis of lids.

[6] **Ears.** Deafness from moving quickly, with faintness.

Roaring in ears; congestion; nausea, vomiting.

Ears cold and pale.

[7] **Nose.** Profuse secretion of mucus from the nose.

[8] **Face.** Cold, bluish, covered with cold sweat; nose pinched, cold, blue; paleness of the lips and around alæ nasi.

Convulsive twitchings of facial muscles.

Face flushed; cerebral congestion.

[9] **Lower Face.** Mouth drawn down at one corner.

Lips dry; mouth dry, or thick mucus in mouth.

[10] **Teeth.** Dentition; cerebral congestion, excited pulse; convulsions.

[11] **Tongue, etc.** Tongue: yellow, with red streak down the middle; feels scalded.

[12] **Mouth.** Copious secretion of saliva.

[13] **Throat.** Dryness and heat in throat, with severe hiccough.

Burning in fauces and œsophagus, with constant inclination to swallow.

Spasm of œsophagus, with or without rising of frothy, bloody mucus.

Sensation as of a ball rising into œsophagus.

[16] **Nausea and Vomiting.** Heart-burn, with bitter, sour rising.

Vomiting: long-continuing; of glairy mucus after food; of blood; of bile.

Vomiting, with inflammatory or cerebral disease.

Smallest quantity of food or drink is immediately rejected.

[17] **Stomach.** Sharp, flying pains in epigastrium and umbilical region passing to pubes.

Excruciating pain, covering a space the size of hand, in lower part of stomach.

Intense drawing, twisting pains in stomach, as if it was drawn tightly against spine, causing pain in dorsal region.

Pains culminate every five minutes in severe vomiting.

[19] **Abdomen.** As if drawn in, following cramp in stomach.

Pains at right of umbilicus, passing down to groin.

Enteritis, with high fever, great vascular excitement; vomiting; dark, bloody stools.

[20] **Stool, etc.** Stools: bloody; black, in typhoid; copious, light, mornings; mushy, preceded and followed by cutting in bowels.

Hemorrhoids red and dark blue; neuralgic pains in the rectum.

[21] **Urine.** Increased, pale; deposits a reddish sentiment.

Specific gravity of urine diminished.

[23] **Female Sexual Organs.** Menstrual colic, preceded by great congestion and troublesome strangury; plethoric women.

Suppressed menses, with cerebral congestion; plethora.

[24] **Pregnancy.** Vomiting during pregnancy.

Puerperal convulsions, during labor, after blood-letting; furious delirium; arterial excitement; cold, clammy sweat.

[26] **Breathing.** Labored, must sit up, cold sweat on the face; decreased from 40 to 16, pneumonia.

Oppression of the chest.

[27] **Cough.** Short, dry, hacking; loose, rattling; worse going from warm to cold.

[28] **Lungs.** Congestion of chest, with rapid respiration, nausea, vomiting; dull burning in region of heart.

Pneumonia, pulse hard, strong, quick; or, engorgement of lungs, with faint feeling in stomach, nausea, slow or intermittent pulse.

[29] **Heart. Pulse.** In cardiac region: burning; prickling; or, dull aching.

Heart's beat: loud, strong, with arterial excitement; low and feeble; fluttering.

Faintness and blindness; when rising from lying; from sudden motions; better lying quietly.

Pulse: suddenly increases and gradually decreases below normal; slow, soft, weak; irregular, intermittent.

³¹ Neck. Back. Aching in back of neck and shoulders.

Muscles of back contracted, drawing head backward.

Opisthotonos; arterial excitement; hands and feet cold; shocks in limbs; congestion of brain and spine, loss of consciousness.

Heat and redness down spine; back of head hot. *θ* Spotted fever.

³³ Lower Limbs. Pain in either great trochanter when lying on it.

Lancinating pain in right hip.

Right ankle feels as if dislocated, can scarcely walk; later left.

³⁴ Limbs in General. Rheumatism, especially in left shoulder, hip and knee; high fever; scanty red urine.

Flying pains; pains in joints; shuddering; rheumatism.

Cramps in legs, fingers, toes.

Pain, especially about the condyles.

³⁵ Position, etc. Moving: 6, 29. Walking: 33. Rising: 29. Must sit up: 26. Lying, quietly: 3; on affected side: 33.

³⁶ Nerves. Twitchings and contortions of body, unaffected by sleep; froth about lips; champing of teeth; difficult swallowing; head jerking or continually nodding; sexual excitement; chorea.

Violent spasms, like galvanic shocks.

Convulsions after scarlet fever, great dilatation of pupils; inability to sleep.

❚Opisthotonic convulsions in anæmic subjects from exhausting diarrhœa.

Trembling, as if child was frightened and on verge of a spasm.

Convulsions, with opisthotonos; anæmia from diarrhœa.

Paralysis; tingling in limbs; cerebral hyperæmia.

³⁷ Sleep. Sleeplessness; cross, quarrelsome; also in acute fever.

Coma; blue face; spasms.

Restless sleep; dreams of drowning; of being on water.

³⁸ Time. Morning: 20.

³⁹ Temperature and Weather. Sunstroke: 3. Going from warm to cold: 27.

⁴⁰ Chill. Fever. Sweat. Coldness of whole body, cold sweat on face, hands, feet.

Chilliness, with nausea.

Coldness, with pale skin, flabby muscles; quick, but weak pulse.

Typhoid fevers when pulse is full, hard, frequent; pain violent in back of head; delirium; black stools.

Irritative fever, with cerebral congestions, causing convulsions; children.

⁴⁴ **Tissues.** Congestions, especially of base of brain, chest, spine, stomach.

Dropsy, with fever. θ After scarlatina.

⁴⁵ **Contact, Injuries, etc.** Rubbing relieves pains and itching.

⁴⁶ **Skin.** Itching of different parts, better from rubbing.

Tingling and pricking in skin.

Skin cold, clammy, bluish, insensible, shriveled.

Eruptions, with intense fever.

Measles, during febrile stage, especially if pulmonary congestion is impending; convulsions before eruption.

Scarlatina, with intense arterial excitement. Rheumatism, carditis, dropsy, as sequelæ.

Small-pox, intense fever, restlessness, excessive pain.

⁴⁷ **Stages and States.** Full-blooded, plethoric.

⁴⁸ **Relationship.** *Ver. vir.* cured spasms from strychnine.

VIBURNUM OPULUS.

Cranberry Tree. *Caprifoliaceæ.*

¹ **Mind.** Depressed.

Unable to concentrate mind on usual mental labor.

² **Sensorium.** Vertigo: inclines to turn to left; on rising, as if would fall forward; on closing eyes.

³ **Inner Head.** Dull frontal headache; and throbbing, extending to eyeballs, worse mental exertion, better moving about.

Frontal headache, occasional vertigo, incapacitates for study; with profuse and frequent urination.

Dull, heavy headache, mostly over eyes, worse on left side, at times extending to vertex and occiput, principally when delayed menses should appear; worse sudden jar, bending over. false step, movement.

Severe pain in left parietal region, sharp, penetrating brain, worse every cough, moving head, when bowels move.

⁵ **Eyes.** Heaviness over eyes and in balls, must, at times, look twice to be sure of seeing an object.

Eyes burn; profuse flow of tears.

Sore feeling in eyeballs.

⁶ **Ears.** Sharp, jerking pains as from knife.

Wakens at night with pain in ears, deep in bone.

External ear sore as if bruised; cannot lie on it; must rub ear, it feels as if pinned to head.

[8] **Face.** Flushed and hot.

[11] **Tongue, etc.** Dry; broad and white, centre brown, takes print of teeth.

Taste: coppery; disagreeable.

[12] **Mouth.** Lips and mouth dry.

[16] **Nausea and Vomiting.** Constant nausea; also relieved while eating; followed by vomiting.

Deathly sick at stomach as if could not live, every night; worse least motion.

[17] **Stomach.** Food lies heavily.

Stomach felt faint and nauseated, must lie down (for ten days after menses cease).

Goneness as if empty.

Aching, better stretching body and throwing stomach forward.

[18] **Hypochondria.** Spleen: darting pain, deep-seated; feels as if hot fluid was running through splenic vessels, better walking about room.

Intense pain in splenic region, faintness, better by sweat.

Severe throbbing pain under left floating ribs, better from hard pressure and walking; cannot lie on left side.

[19] **Abdomen.** Tender and sensitive, worse about umbilicus.

Cramping colic pains in lower abdomen, almost insupportable, coming suddenly and with terrible severity.

[20] **Stool, etc.** Constipation: stools of large, dry, hard balls, voided with such difficulty as to need mechanical aid; much tenesmus, or inactive rectum.

Dark blood after stool.

Diarrhœa profuse, watery, with chills, and at same time, cold sweat that rolls off of forehead.

[21] **Urine.** Urine: clear, profuse, frequent; sensation after micturition as if urine was still flowing; during menses and also with headache.

[22] **Male Sexual Organs.** Seminal emissions without dreams.

[23] **Female Sexual Organs.** Before menses: severe bearing down, drawing in anterior muscles of thighs; heavy aching in sacral region and over pubes; occasional sharp, shooting pains over ovaries; pains make her so nervous she cannot sit still; excruciating, cramping, colicky pains in lower abdomen, and through womb; pains begin in the back and go around, ending in cramps in uterus.

During menses: nausea; cramping pain and great nervous restlessness; flow ceases for several hours, then returns in clots. Flow scanty, thin, light colored, with sensation of lightness of head, faint when trying to sit up. Spasmodic or membranous dysmenorrhœa.

Leucorrhœa thin, yellow-white, or colorless, except with the stool, when it is thick, white, blood-streaked.

²⁴ **Pregnancy.** ‖Threatened abortion; intense cramp in uterus and bearing down; or, pain around from back, ending in excruciating cramp in lower abdomen (many cases).

³¹ **Neck. Back.** Neck stiff, with pain in occiput.

Tired, bruised pain in muscles of back, from point of scapula to wing of ilium on each side, better from firm pressure.

³⁴ **Limbs in General.** Buzzing feeling in hands, as if they would burst.

³⁵ **Position, etc.** Walking: 18. Moving: 3. Rising: 1. Lying: 17. Stretching: 17. Sitting up: 23.

³⁷ **Sleep.** Restless, unrefreshing.

³⁸ **Time.** Worse evening and night: 6, 16.

³⁹ **Temperature and Weather.** Worse in a warm room. Better in open air.

⁴⁰ **Chill. Fever. Sweat.** Chill from 8 to 1 A.M., or 12 M. followed by severe headache.

⁴² **Sides.** Left side most affected.

⁴⁵ **Contact, Injuries, etc.** Pressure: 6, 18, 31. Sudden jar: 3.

⁴⁸ **Relationship.** Compare: *Cauloph., Act. rac., Gelsem., Sepia, Chamom., Secale., Xanthox., Coccul., Pulsat., Symphoricarpus* (uterine nausea).

Viburnum, in a threatened abortion, relieved; but renewed symptoms differing only in the appearing of an irritable, peevish state of mind, required *Chamom.*, which cured.

VIOLA ODORATA.

Sweet Violet.   Wm. Gross.   *Violaceæ.*

¹ **Mind.** Weakness of memory; or, increased mental activity, easy comprehension. The intellect predominates over the emotions.

Very restless, talking much. θ Measles.

Hysterical; inclined to weep, without knowing why.

² **Sensorium.** Vertigo while sitting.

³ **Inner Head.** Congestion of blood to head, with pricking in forehead.

⁴ **Outer Head.** Head feels heavy and sinks forward.

Tension in scalp, extending to upper part of face.

⁵ **Eyes.** Eyelids drawn down, as from sleepiness.

⁶ **Ears.** Aversion to music, especially to violin; worse from music.

Stitches in and around the ears.

[7] **Nose.** Numbness of the tip of the nose.

[8] **Face.** Hot forehed.

Tension below eyes and above nose to temples.

[12] **Mouth.** Aphthæ of infants.

[19] **Abdomen.** Distention of abdomen.

[20] **Stool, etc.** Helminthiasis.

Stool natural or constipated; dyspnœa.

Itching of anus, every afternoon.

[24] **Pregnancy.** During pregnancy, dyspnœa.

[25] **Larynx.** Hoarseness followed by coryza.

[26] **Breathing.** Difficulty of breathing, with painful exhalation, anxiety, palpitation of the heart. θ Hysteria.

Dyspnœa, with occasional cough; worse in day time than at night. θ Pregnancy.

Shortness of breathing and violent dyspnœa, as if a stone were lying on chest.

Soft, noiseless breathing.

[27] **Cough.** By day chiefly, in long-lasting spells, dry, short, violent, with much dyspnœa.

Whooping-cough in nervous, thin, little girls.

Sputum profuse, clear, ropy, jelly-like.

[28] **Lungs.** Oppression of chest, as from a weight, awakening her at night. θ Hysteria.

[32] **Upper Limbs.** Slight trembling of arms; dyspnœa.

Rheumatic affection of upper limbs.

Aching in right wrist.

ı Rheumatism of the (right) wrist; especially in females.

Drawing in elbow-joint and dorsum of hand.

[33] **Lower Limbs.** Œdematous swelling of lower limbs, with stitching pains.

[35] **Position, etc.** Sitting: 2.

[36] **Nerves.** Trembling of limbs.

Relaxation of all muscles.

Great nervous debility.

Hypochondriasis.

[38] **Time.** Afternoon: 20. Night: 26, 28, 40. Day: 26.

[39] **Temperature and Weather.** After having stayed up in a cold room during the fall season: hoarseness.

[40] **Chill. Fever. Sweat.** Chilly disposition.

[41] **Attacks.** Fvery afternoon: 20.

[42] **Sides.** Right: 32.

[43] **Sensations.** Tension in outer parts.

Transient burning on various places.

[46] **Skin.** Dry, warm skin, want of sweat; only palms moist; measles running an irregular course.

[47] **Stages and States.** Hysteria.

Tall, thin, nervous girls; mild, impressive; of fair complexion; tuberculous.

Females 32.
[48] **Relationship.** Is followed well by *Corall.* (whooping-cough; *Cina* (worms).

XANTHOXYLUM.

Prickly Ash. *Rutaceæ*

[1] **Mind.** Nervous, frightened feeling.
Depression and weakness.
[3] **Inner Head.** Dulness. Bewilderment; pain in back of head,
Throbbing headache; over right eye, with nausea.
Pain over the eyes with throbbing above root of nose.
Aching and flashes of throb-like pain as if top of head was about being taken off.
Tightness of the scalp: 23.
[7] **Nose.** Right nostril seems filled up. Discharge of mucus, of dry and bloody scales.
[12] **Mouth,** Peppery taste in mouth, fauces and throat.
[13] **Throat.** Peppery sensation; soreness, with expectoration of tough mucus.
Feeling of a bunch in left side of throat when swallowing, shifting to right.
[14] **Desires. Aversions.** No appetite.
[16] **Nausea and Vomiting.** Sense of oppression at stomach; frequent chills: 40.
[17] **Stomach.** Feeling of fulness or pressure. Fluttering.
[20] **Stool, etc.** Griping pains 7 A.M., with thin, brown stools, mixed with mucus.
[21] **Urine.** Profuse, light colored urine: nervous women.
[23] **Female Sexual Organs.** ▮Ovarian pains extending down the genito-crural nerves: 33.
▮Dreadful distress and pain; headache; menstrual flow too early and profuse; pains down the anterior of thighs; neuralgic dysmenorrhœa.
[24] **Pregnancy.** ▮After-pains, when of the above character and with profuse lochia.
[25] **Larynx.** Hoarse, husky feeling in the throat.
[28] **Lungs.** Desire to take a long breath. Tight feeling about the chest, inclined to gape.
[33] **Lower Limbs.** ▮Severe neuralgic pains in the course of the genito- crural nerves: 23.
Excessive weakness of lower limbs; chlorosis.
[34] **Limbs in General.** Pains in the limbs, neuralgic, shooting; Numbness and weakness.

[36] **Nerves.** Pricking sensation; shocks as from electricity.
Numbness, worse on left side.

[40] **Chill. Fever. Sweat.** Chills, pains in limbs; nausea: 16.
Flashes of heat.   Sense of heat in veins.

[44] **Tissues.** Acts upon the nervous system, mostly upon the
sensory nerves, but causes a marked depression of vitality, a non-reactive state; hence its use in chlorosis,
measles, neuralgia, etc., when there is sensorial and
bodily depression.
Mucous membrane smarts as from pepper.   Catarrh.

[46] **Skin.** Measles, dulness, bewilderment, drowsiness, want of
sufficient development of the eruption (see catarrhal
symptoms.   Clinical, but trustworthy).

[48] **Relationship.** Compare with: *Act. rac., Gelsem., Bellad.*

ZINCUM.

Zinc.   Franz.   *Eement.*

[1] **Mind.** Unconscious; signs of effusion into the brain; feet
constantly moving; often from undeveloped eruptions.
Weak memory, with stinging pains in the head.
Repeats all questions before answering them.
Stares as if frightened on waking, and rolls from side to
side.
Sensitive to others talking.
Low-spirited at noon; lively in the evening or vice versa.
Thinks of death calmly; or hypochondriacal, with gastric
symptoms; pressure in spine and fear of death.
Child cross toward evening; brain affected.

[2] **Sensorium.** Vertigo in occiput, with falling to left when
walking; stupefaction and dulness of intellect, especially
afternoon and evening.

[3] **Inner Head.** Pressure on root of nose, as if it would be
pressed into head.
Sharp pressure on a small spot in forehead, evenings.
Hemicrania, worse after dinner; tearing and stinging.
Cramp-like, tearing pain in right and left temple.
Pressure on top of head, worse after dinner; frequent dizzi-
ness, then nausea and vomiting of bile; face pale;
costive; cerebral depression.
Sore pain in head.
Internal headaches, mostly semilateral, or in sinciput or
occiput; worse from wine, in warm room, and after eat-
ing.

61

Headache from drinking even small quantities of wine.

⁴ **Outer Head.** Sensation of soreness of vertex, as from soreness or ulceration; worse in evening in bed and after
eating; better after scratching.

Hair falls out on vertex, causing complete baldness, with
sensation of soreness of scalp.

⁵ **Eyes.** Sensitive to light; brain affected.

Amaurosis; during severe headache; passing away with
the headache; with contracted pupils.

Eyes dim, watery.   θ Brain affections.

Sees luminous bodies.   θ After operations.

Iritis (syphilitic), worse at night, with hot, scalding tears.

Conjunctivitis, pains worse at night; inflammation more in
inner canthus.

Pterygium.

Upper lids heavy, as if paralyzed.

Granular lids, after ophthalmia neonatorum.

⁶ **Ears.** Cracking and detonation in ear.

Frequent acute stitches in right ear near tympanum.

Earache of children, especially boys.

Otorrhœa of fetid pus.

⁷ **Nose.** Dry; brain affected.

Coryza, with hoarseness and burning in chest.

Nose feels sore internally.

Swelling of one side of nose, with loss of smell.

⁸ **Face.** Pale, alternately with redness; brain affections;
earthy, with wandering expression; waxy, white or yellow, in typhus.

Burning, jerking, stitching in infraorbital nerve, with
bluish eyelids; worse from least touch and in evening.

Scirrhus on right cheek, size of a walnut.

Cold sweat on forehead.

⁹ **Lower Face.** Lips and corners of mouth cracked, with
yellowish ulceration.

Thick, viscid humor on the lips.

¹⁰ **Teeth.** Herpes (yellowish in mouth from sea-bathing).

Drawing, or smarting and stinging in roots of (upper)
front teeth and in hard palate.

Gums painful while eating, ulcerated, white, bleed easily.

Teeth feel long and loose, with swelling of submaxillary
glands.

Grits the teeth.

¹¹ **Tongue, etc.** Taste: sweetish; metallic; like spoiled cheese;
bloody; bitter, in fauces.

Tongue: dry, don't want to talk; coated at root and dry
(brain diseases); swollen on left side; hindering talking; covered with vesicles.

¹² **Mouth.** Increased flow of saliva, with crawling in inner
surface of cheek.

[13] **Throat.** Herpetic-like eruption on tonsils, soft palate and
root of tongue; whitish, somewhat elevated, ulcerated
spots in mouth. θ Sequelæ to gonorrhœa.

Pain in posterior part of hard palate and in velum palati,
especially when yawning.

Dryness of throat, evening; mucus collects from posterior nares; soreness in throat; tearing in posterior
fauces, more between acts of empty deglutition or after
eating.

Cramp-like, strangling pain externally in muscles, when
swallowing.

[14] **Desires. Aversions.** Aversion to: meat, fish, and sweet
things; to cooked or warm things.

Thirst, with heat in palms.

Insatiable hunger, but no appetite for breakfast, with hurried deglutition.

[15] **Eating and Drinking.** After eating: 3, 4, 16, 19, 26, 31,
40.

Worse from: sugar (heart-burn); wine (nearly all symptoms); milk (sour eructations).

[16] **Nausea and Vomiting.** Sweetish rising into throat, with
sweet taste in mouth, or taste of blood.

Eructations, with pressure in middle of spine.

Heart-burn; swollen feet and varicose veins during pregnancy.

Subdued nausea, with universal, tremulous feeling.

Nausea in stomach, with retching and vomiting of bitter
mucus; renewed by least motion.

As soon as first spoonful reaches stomach, up it comes.

Vomiting of blood or of sanguineous mucus, with effort.

[17] **Stomach.** Spasm of stomach and hypochondria, and a constriction in œsophagus, with dyspnœa and increased
heat of the body; worse during inspiration.

Burning in pit of stomach when pressing thereon; in
evening.

Burning in pit of stomach, before breakfast, extending
into œsophagus.

Hæmatemesis.

Sensation like a worm creeping up from pit of stomach
into throat, causing coughing.

[18] **Hypochondria.** Cramp-pains in region of liver, with
dyspnœa and hypochondriasis after eating.

Liver enlarged, hard and sore to touch; feet swollen;
vomits bloody phlegm.

Stitches in spleen, worse from pressure.

[19] **Abdomen.** Pressure and tension in abdomen.

Flatulent colic, worse from wine, toward evening or during
the night, and at rest; loud rumbling and rolling; re-

traction of abdomen; hot, moist, fetid, flatus passing off without relief; lead colic.

Violent bearing down in abdomen after a difficulty, scanty stool; relieved by passing flatus.

Inguinal hernia.

20 Stool, etc. Stool: frequent, small, sometimes involuntary; pitch-like; or dry, brittle and granulous; soft, papescent, or thin, with pale blood; difficult; hard, dry, insufficient, expelled with much pressure.

Diarrhœa involuntary, with stupor.   θ Typhus.

21 Urine. Violent pressure of urine on bladder; sits with legs crossed, and though bladder feels as if full, none passes.

Can only pass water while sitting bent backward; much sand in urine.

Urine turbid, loam-colored, in morning.

Frequent micturition of pale, yellow urine, which, on standing, deposits a white, flaky sediment.

Involuntary urination while walking, coughing and sneezing.

22 Male Sexual Organs. Easily excited; the emission, during an embrace, is too rapid; or, difficult and almost impossible.

Long-lasting and violent erections.

Copious discharge of prostatic juice, without any cause.

Orchitis: from a bruise, with drawing and retraction of one or the other testicle, goes from right to left; after checked otorrhœa.

Atrophy of testicles.

Spermatorrhœa; emissions without dreams, face pale, sunken, blue rings around eyes.

Hair falls off from genitals.

Removes buboes, syphilitic or otherwise, in left inguinal region.

23 Female Sexual Organs. Irresistible sexual desire at night; desire for onanism.

Boring pain in left ovarian region, better from pressure, but entirely relieved only during menstrual flow.

Amenorrhœa, with alternately red and pale face.

Dysmenorrhœa when, during menses, limbs feel heavy, with violent drawing about knees, as if they would be twisted off; sudden oppression of stomach, she has to loosen her dress; chilliness.

Menses: too early and too profuse, lumps of coagulated blood pass away, mostly when walking; flow most profuse at night.

Ulceration of uterus, discharge bloody, acrid, but ulcers are rather destitute of feeling.

Leucorrhœa: of bloody mucus after menses, causing itch-

ing of vulva; of thick mucus, three days before and
after menses.

Cutting colic, succeeded by leucorrhœa.

Pruritus vulvæ causes masturbation.

Varicose veins of external genitals, with fidgety feet.

²⁴ **Pregnancy.** Tendency to miscarry. •

Puerperal convulsions if an eruption (especially a long-
standing one) has recently disappeared.

Mammæ swollen and sore to touch; catamenia suppressed.

Soreness of nipples.

²⁶ **Breathing.** Asthma, evening after eating, from flatus, with
increase of dyspnœa, when expectoration stops, decreasing when it recommences.

²⁷ **Cough.** All night, with dull pains in chest; spasmodic,
child puts hands to genitals; with varicose veins on
legs; with shooting in scrobiculum, leaving when sputum is raised; worse after eating sweets; wine; also
during menses.

Sputa: yellow, purulent; blood-streaked; tenacious;
sweetish, putrid, or metallic-tasting; pure blood, morning and during day.

²⁸ **Lungs.** Pain in chest, as if cut to pieces, with constrictive
sensation.

Burning in chest.

Coldness in chest.

Stitches in left chest and in heart, at every beat.

Sensation of emptiness behind sternum.

²⁹ **Heart. Pulse.** Severe pain in cardiac region, some swelling and great tenderness.

Feels as if a cap were over the heart; spine affected.

Irregular, spasmodic action of heart; occasionally one
violent thump.

Violent pulsations in blood-vessels, during heat.

Pulse: irregular, or small and frequent, evenings, slow
mornings; increased by wine; scarcely perceptible.

³¹ **Neck. Back.** Nape of neck feels weary and tired, from
writing or any exertion. Stiffness and tension of neck.
Tearing pains.

Burning in shoulder-blades; tension between shoulder-
blades.

Burning along whole spine, worse sitting.

Pain in small of back on turning over in bed at night.

Pain in small of back, when sitting, or when in act of
sitting down; diminished by continuous walking.

Pain at last dorsal vertebræ.

³² **Upper Limbs.** Lameness and deadness of hands; they look
bluish. •

Weakness, numbness and tremor of hands, when writing.

61*

Cracked and dry skin of hands, even in mild weather.
Chilblains itch and swell.

³³ **Lower Limbs.** Varices in legs, with fidgety feet.
Formication in calves.
Sensation of stagnation in blood of legs.
Inflammation of tendo-achilles, erysipelatous; worse from
touching heel to ground and from wine.
Feet are sweaty and sore about toes; fetid.
Paralysis of feet, from suppressed foot-sweat, by getting
wet; worse from wine.
Chilblains, worse from scratching and friction.
Coldness of feet at night.

³⁴ **Limbs in General.** Rheumatism, tearing, lameness and
trembling; or crampy pains; or twisting in affected
limbs and frequent jerking of whole body during sleep;
worse from being overheated and from exertion.
Great weakness: of limbs; especially of lumbar region
and bends of knees, when walking in open air.
Sudden sensation of weakness in limbs, with canine hunger.

³⁵ **Position, etc.** While writing: 31, 32. Walking: 2, 21,
23, 31, 34. From overexertion: 31, 34. Motion: 16.
Sitting: 31. At rest: 19. Must sit bent: 21.

³⁶ **Nerves.** Twitching in various muscles. The whole body
jerks during sleep.
Hands tremble; grasps at flocks; or slides down in bed.
Chorea, depressed spirits, health suffers; caused by fright;
suppressed eruptions; worse after wine.
❘ Beginning of locomotor ataxia, when lightning-like pains
are marked and intense.
Spasms: child cross before attack, body hot, restless at
night, fidgety feet, right side twitcheg; pale children,
during teething.
Neuralgia after zoster; better from touch.

³⁷ **Sleep.** Drowsiness: with frequent gaping; and yet cannot
sleep, head feels so light.
During sleep: cries out, awakens with fear; limbs and
body jerk.

³⁸ **Time.** Acts better when given in evening.
Morning: 21, 27, 29. Forenoon: 40. Noon: 1. Afternoon: 2. Evening: 1, 2, 4, 8, 13, 17, 19, 26, 29. Night:
5, 19, 23, 27, 36, 40, 46. During the day: 27, 40.

³⁹ **Temperature and Weather.** Complaints from overheat-
ing: 34. Warm room: 3. Open air: 34, 40. Getting
wet: 33. Sea-bathing: 10.

⁴⁰ **Chill. Fever. Sweat.** Chills: begin after eating dinner;
in open air; on approach of a storm; run down back;
alternate with heat; external, with increased internal
warmth; from touching anything cold.

Heat: internal, with cold sensation in abdomen and on
feet; anxious sensation of heat, without any external
heat, during the night; of face, with cool body in forenoon; in flushes, with violent trembling and short, hot
breath.

Sweat: profuse all night, wants to uncover; easy during
day, from exercise; offensive.

⁴² **Sides.** Right: 6, 8, 18, 36. Left: 2, 11, 18, 22, 23, 28.
Right to left: 22.   Above downward: 40.

⁴⁴ **Tissues.**   Especially in the anæmic; brain exhausted; not
able to develop exanthemata.

Dropsy, with uneasiness in renal region.

⁴⁵ **Contact, Injuries, etc.** Scratching: 4, 33. Touch or pressure: 8, 17, 18, 23, 24, 33, 36, 46.

⁴⁶ **Skin.**   Itching in bends of joints.

Pains, seemingly between skin and flesh.

Rhagades, mostly between fingers, bad even in mild
weather.

Sudden itching here and there, especially in evening in
bed, goes off by contact.

Dry herpes over whole body.

Neuralgia, following herpes zoster.

⁴⁸ **Relationship.**   *Zincum* is followed well by *Ignat.*, but not
by *Nux vom.*, which disagrees.

Antidotes to *Zincum: Hepar., Ignat.*

Incompatible *Chamom., Nux vom.*

Zincum picricum (preferable with dull, heavy, periodic,
occipital headache; pains in small of back as if struck).
Zincum sulph. is useful in persistent dysenteric discharges; cutting pains in side of abdomen; also good
when cannot sleep because of jerking of legs.

ZINGIBER.

Ginger.   FRANZ.   *Zingibereæ.*

¹ **Mind.** Forgetful.

Not in least anxious in midst of physical suffering from
threatened suffocation.

Good-humored.

Irritable and chilly; also during menses.

² **Sensorium.**   Vertigo, limbs heavy.

Head feels too large.

³ **Inner Head.**   Rush of blood, worse about temples.

Pressure into forehead and root of nose when stooping.

Frontal headache over eyes and at root of nose; also when he exerts himself.

Headache, worse over left eye; aching over eyebrows, followed by nausea; later over right eye and pressing in left occiput, worse in warm room, but continued in cold, damp air, in motion or sitting.

Heavy pressure in head from without inward, when walking in cold, damp air.

⁵ **Eyes.** Weakness of sight; dimness of cornea.

Eyes sensitive to light, with stinging pain in eyeballs.

Feeling as from sand in eyes.

Smarting, burning in eyes.

⁷ **Nose.** Sneezing, and ineffectual attempts.

Watery coryza, right side, then left, more in open air.

Dryness and obstruction in posterior nares, with discharge of thick mucus.

Ozæna.

⁸ **Face.** Face red and hot.

Exhausted look, blue under eyes, before menses.

¹⁰ **Teeth.** Pressure and drawing in roots of teeth.

¹¹ **Tongue, etc.** Taste of food remains; especially that of bread.

Slimy, bad taste in morning.

¹² **Mouth.** Mouth and posterior nares dry, the latter stopped up.

Breath smells foul to herself, as from disordered stomach.

¹³ **Throat.** Increased mucous secretion, no fever.

¹⁴ **Desires. Aversions.** Much thirst, mouth·dry, also with heat in head.

No desire to smoke.

¹⁵ **Eating and Drinking.** After bread: headache, pressure in stomach.

Complaints from eating melons.

¹⁶ **Nausea and Vomiting.** Belching and diarrhœa.

Nausea: on rising; much rumbling; after morning stool.

Vomits slime; old drunkards.

¹⁷ **Stomach.** Weak digestion; stomach heavy like a stone; fidgety; cramps in soles, hoarseness.

¹⁸ **Hypochondria.** Heavy pain in right hypochondrium, toward the back, worse from deep breathing.

Stitches in spleen; stinging.

¹⁹ **Abdomen.** Contracting colic passes through abdomen while standing; soon after, desire for stool.

Sore pain on a small place right side of abdomen.

Flatulency; costive; gout.

Sharp pain in left iliac region.

²⁰ **Stool, etc.** Diarrhœa: from impure water; from water containing coal oil; of brown mucus, worse morning; worse from deranged stomach; from cold, damp weather.

Hemorrhoids, hot and painful.

Burning redness, itching at anus and higher up the back.

21 Urine. Dull aching: and hot sensation in left kidney; in both kidneys, with frequent desire to urinate.

Complete retention of urine after typhus.

Urine: thick, turbid; dark brown; of strong smell.

While urinating, pain in orifice of urethra.

22 Male Sexual Organs. Yellow, nightly discharge from, urethra.

23 Female Sexual Organs. Menses too early and profuse, dark, clotted; irritable; exhausted look before; drawing pain in sacrum.

25 Larynx. Hoarseness.

Smarting below larynx followed by cough, with mucous rattling.

26 Breathing. Asthma humidum; loosens the phlegm.

Painful respiration; more difficult at night, must sit up in bed; worse two or three hours every A.M. *θ* Asthma.

27 Cough. Dry, hacking; from tickling in larynx on left side of throat; from smarting or scratching; with pain in lungs, difficult breathing; morning sputum, which is copious.

28 Lungs. Stitches through chest, pains in chest, pleuritic.

Stinging pains after motion, also stinging-pressing in region of heart.

31 Neck. Back. Backache as from weakess; worse sitting and leaning against something.

Lower part of back; as if beaten; or, lame from walking or standing; feels stiff.

32 Upper limbs. Heavy, lame feeling in upper arms; numbness worse forearm.

Rheumatic, drawing pains in back of hands.

Heat of palms of hands.

33 Lower Limbs. Pains in hip-joints; joints stiff, lame.

Burning, stinging, tingling in feet.

Painful swelling of feet.

Heels ache after long standing.

Cramps in soles.

34 Limbs in General. Dull, heavy feeling; also with dizziness.

Joints weak; back lame.

35 Position, etc. Stooping: 3. Standing: 19, 31, 33. Motion: 3, 28. Must sit up: 26. Sitting: 3, 31. Lying down: 31. Wants to lie down: 36. Exertion: 3. Walking: 3, 31. Rising: 16. Leaning against something: 31.

36 Nerves. Foaming at mouth, free urination, spasms.

Wants to lie down.

Faintish weakness.

37 Sleep. Sleepy, worse afternoons.

Coma.

Sleepless in night, awakens 3 A.M.; falls asleep again late in morning.

[38] **Time.** Morning: 11, 16, 20, 26, 27, 37. Afternoon: 37. Evening: 31. Night: 22, 26, 37. 3 A.M.: 37. Day: 6.

[39] **Temperature and Weather.** Warm room: 3. Open air: 7, 40. Cold, damp air; 3, 20°

[40] **Chill. Fever. Sweat.** Chilly in open air; in evening; chill goes upward.

Hot and chilly at the same time.

[41] **Attacks.** Every morning: 26.

[42] **Sides.** Right: 3, 7, 18, 19. Left: 3' 7, 18, 19, 21, 28. Left to right: 3. Right to left: 7. Without inward: 3 Below upward: 40.

[46] **Skin.** Skin feels relaxed, pliable.

Itching on scalp, beard, genitals.

[48] **Relationship.** Antidote to *Zingib.*: *Nux vom.*

ZIZIA.

Meadow Parsnips. *Umbelliferæ.*

[36] **Nerves.** Spasmodic movements of the muscles of the face and extremities. Spasmodic twitching during sleep (confirmed in chorea).